ARCHIVES OF

SURGERY

VOLUME 87

JULY THROUGH DECEMBER, 1963

AMERICAN MEDICAL ASSOCIATION Publication

STATEMENT OF OWNERSHIP, MANAGEMENT AND CIRCULATION
(Act of October 23, 1962: Section 4369, Title 39, United States Code)

Publisher: File two copies of this form with your postmaster.

1. DATE OF FILING: September 30, 1963

2. TITLE OF PUBLICATION: Archives of Surgery

3. FREQUENCY OF ISSUE: Monthly

4. LOCATION OF KNOWN OFFICE OF PUBLICATION *(Street, city, county, state, zip code)*
535 North Dearborn Street, Chicago, Cook, Illinois 60610

5. LOCATION OF THE HEADQUARTERS OR GENERAL BUSINESS OFFICES OF THE PUBLISHERS *(Not printers)*
535 North Dearborn Street, Chicago, Cook, Illinois 60610

6. NAMES AND ADDRESSES OF PUBLISHER, EDITOR, AND MANAGING EDITOR

PUBLISHER *(Name and address)*
American Medical Association, 535 North Dearborn Street, Chicago, Illinois 60610

EDITOR *(Name and address)*
J. Garrott Allen, M. D., 535 North Dearborn Street, Chicago, Illinois 60610

MANAGING EDITOR *(Name and address)*
Gilbert S. Cooper, 535 North Dearborn Street, Chicago, Illinois 60610

7. OWNER *(If owned by a corporation, its name and address must be stated and also immediately thereunder the names and addresses of stockholders owning or holding 1 percent or more of total amount of stock. If not owned by a corporation, the names and addresses of the individual owners must be given. If owned by a partnership or other unincorporated firm, its name and address, as well as that of each individual must be given.)*

NAME	ADDRESS
None	

8. KNOWN BONDHOLDERS, MORTGAGEES, AND OTHER SECURITY HOLDERS OWNING OR HOLDING 1 PERCENT OR MORE OF TOTAL AMOUNT OF BONDS, MORTGAGES OR OTHER SECURITIES *(If there are none, so state)*

NAME	ADDRESS
None	

9. Paragraphs 7 and 8 include, in cases where the stockholder or security holder appears upon the books of the company as trustee or in any other fiduciary relation, the name of the person or corporation for whom such trustee is acting, also the statements in the two paragraphs show the affiant's full knowledge and belief as to the circumstances and conditions under which stockholders and security holders who do not appear upon the books of the company as trustees, hold stock and securities in a capacity other than that of a bona fide owner. Names and addresses of individuals who are stockholders of a corporation which itself is a stockholder or holder of bonds, mortgages or other securities of the publishing corporation have been included in paragraphs 7 and 8 when the interests of such individuals are equivalent to 1 percent or more of the total amount of the stock or securities of the publishing corporation.

10. THIS ITEM MUST BE COMPLETED FOR ALL PUBLICATIONS EXCEPT THOSE WHICH DO NOT CARRY ADVERTISING OTHER THAN THE PUBLISHER'S OWN AND WHICH ARE NAMED IN SECTIONS 132.231, 132.232, AND 132.233, POSTAL MANUAL *(Sections 4355a, 4355b, and 4356 of Title 39, United States Code)*

October 1962 thru September 1963	AVERAGE NO. COPIES EACH ISSUE DURING PRECEDING 12 MONTHS	SINGLE ISSUE NEAREST TO FILING DATE
A. TOTAL NO. COPIES PRINTED *(Net Press Run)*	47,117	48,042
B. PAID CIRCULATION 1. TO TERM SUBSCRIBERS BY MAIL, CARRIER DELIVERY OR BY OTHER MEANS.	46,045	46,984
2. SALES THROUGH AGENTS, NEWS DEALERS, OR OTHERWISE.	none	none
C. FREE DISTRIBUTION *(including samples)* BY MAIL, CARRIER DELIVERY, OR BY OTHER MEANS.	1,072	1,058
D. TOTAL NO. OF COPIES DISTRIBUTED. *(Sum of lines B1, B2 and C)*	47,117	48,042

I certify that the statements made by me above are correct and complete.

(Signature of editor, publisher, business manager, or owner)
Russell H. Clark, Business Director

POD Form **3526** Aug. 1963

Surgical Training in Canada

ANGUS D. McLACHLIN, MD, LONDON, ONT, CANADA

Surgical training in Canada is a product of its needs and resources, its ethnic background, and its association with a large and very friendly neighbor to the south.

There are centers in Canada where density of population and research and treatment facilities warrant the highest degree of surgical specialization. In contrast, sparsely settled areas isolated by great distances and vagaries of the weather need general surgeons who can deal with everyday problems and emergencies in the small local hospitals.

Stemming as it did from France and the British Isles, Canada has kept bonds that show clearly in the training and qualification of its surgeons. The Royal Colleges of Surgeons with their great tradition and demanding admission examinations have long been a challenge to young Canadians seeking academic recognition. The primary examinations of the English College were held in Canada in 1929, 1930, and 1931. The senior Canadian surgeons responsible for the organization of the Canadian Royal College in 1929, many of them Fellows of one of the older Royal Colleges, naturally sought a Royal charter for formation of the new College, and molded it and its examination system after the pattern that had so influenced their own formative years. Surgeons from French Canada were similarly attracted to France and particularly to Paris with its system of graduated hospital appointments and competitive examinations. The senior surgeons at Laval and the University of Montreal usually held higher diplomas from Paris. Many French-speaking and a much smaller proportion of English-speaking Canadian surgeons are bilingual. An awareness of continental surgery and a delightful Gallic flavor are very evident in our national surgical societies.

Surgeons in the United States and Canada have a long history of common effort. Canadians were active in the inauguration of the American College of Surgeons, and indeed part of the inscription reads: "Founded by Surgeons of the United States and Canada, 1913." Canadians have been made welcome in national and regional surgical societies in the United States and have held senior offices in these organizations. They have known at first hand the training requirements of the American College of Surgeons and later of the American Board of Surgery. Problems in grading of medical schools and in approval of hospitals for graduate training in surgery have been shared. It is small wonder that the requirements are very much alike and that training approved for the examination of the American Board or of the Canadian Royal College is likely to be acceptable on either side of the border. In the British Isles the final Fellowship examinations are taken early in a young surgeon's career, and indeed the degree is a prerequisite to the final years of training. In both the United States and Canada qualifying examinations in surgery are written at the end of the training period. The training system in Canadian surgery is like the American. The style of examination is closer to that of the British Isles especially in the written papers. The four questions to be answered in three hours are often of an essay type that may prove a real hurdle to the student who has difficulty in marshalling his knowledge and presenting it well. I would like to think that Canadian surgery has adopted what suited it best from its elders and friends but at the same time has established an identity of its own.

Presidential Address. Presented at the 20th Annual Meeting of the Central Surgical Association, Chicago, Feb 22, 1963.

Surgical training as we now understand it dates in Canada only from the beginning of this century. The Canadian Association of Clinical Surgeons founded by university teaching surgeons in 1909 sought to improve teaching methods but had not yet developed the residency system. At that time the internship after graduation was a rotating type and seldom lasted more than one year. Practical training in surgery, if taken at all, was by preceptorship. The Royal Colleges of Surgeons in the British Isles were held in great esteem. Young Canadians began the pilgrimage to the British Isles and the hard grind entailed in passing the primary and final Fellowship examinations. If successful, a few visited surgical centers in the British Isles and on the continent. The majority, their funds exhausted, returned to Canada with little addition to their practical skill in surgery but with proof that they had mastered anatomy and the physiology of that period and had good knowledge of what had been written about surgery. With or without a teaching appointment their final training was usually in the bitter school of unsupervised trial and error. That many of them became very competent is a compliment to their individual ability and effort and not to the training system. E. W. Archibald and W. E. Gallie began their careers at the turn of the century and had a great influence in the training of Canadian surgeons.

Edward William Archibald graduated from McGill in Medicine in 1896 and studied at Montpellier in France. He had a supreme command of the English and French languages and in addition could lecture in German. His basic research in the biliary system and pancreas and particularly in the production of pancreatitis has stood the test of time. A pioneer in chest surgery he became president of the American Association for Thoracic Surgery. Well known and respected in American as well as in Canadian surgery, he held the presidency of the American Surgical Association. His presidential address to that Society in 1935 entitled: "Higher Degrees in the Profession of Surgery" added impetus to the formation of the American Board of Surgery in 1937. An honorary Fellow of the Royal College of Surgeons of England, he was familiar with teaching methods in Canada and the United States, in the British Isles, and on the Continent. The modern training of surgeons at McGill took origin from E. W. Archibald and continued under the guidance of his pupils Fraser B. Gurd (who founded the McGill Diploma Course in Surgery), G. Gavin Miller, R. R. Fitzgerald, P. G. Rowe, D. R. Webster, and H. Rocke Robertson. The Diploma Course has now been succeeded by a plan of training fitted to the requirements of the Royal College of Surgeons of Canada.

William Edward Gallie graduated in Medicine from the University of Toronto in 1903. After initial training in Toronto he worked in the Hospital for Ruptured and Crippled in New York and later became a Fellow of the Royal College of Surgeons of England by examination. Returning to the staff of the Hospital For Sick Children in Toronto he became chief surgeon to that hospital in 1921 and then in 1929 chief surgeon to the Toronto General Hospital and Professor and Head of the Department of Surgery in the University of Toronto. He did fundamental work in tendon fixation, the repair of bone and the fate of bone grafts, and in the transplantation of fibrous tissue, especially fascia, in the form of living sutures. He held the presidency of the American Surgical Association, the American Orthopaedic Association, and the American College of Surgeons, the last for an unprecedented six years during World War II. Having served the Royal College of Surgeons of England as Hunterian Professor he was in 1947 awarded the Honorary Gold Medal of the College. This had been granted only 21 times since its inception in 1822. In spite of his original contributions and his many honors Dr. Gallie may be remembered best for the plan of surgical training he established in Toronto and his influence on surgical training in all Canada. He had an abiding interest in the training of young men and an infectious enthusiasm toward surgery and life that stimulated all who came under his influence. He was held in affectionate reverence by the group he had trained, the happily named "Gallie Slaves." R. M. Janes and F. G. Kergin have carried on the direction of the Toronto school of surgery. Dr. Gallie's interest in surgical training extended beyond his own university. With his aid the R. S. McLaughlin Foundation has provided Fellowships for young surgeons from any Canadian medical school who had completed their ordinary training and had been assured teaching posts. The additional training in Canada or abroad provided to these future teaching surgeons has strengthened all Canadian medical schools. Since Dr. Gallie's death the endowment of the McLaughlin-Gallie visiting professorships permits outstanding teachers to spend a considerable time at one or more Canadian medical schools each year.

Many others contributed, but W. E. Gallie and E. W. Archibald were responsible for the first centers in Canada. They were the first Lecturers in Surgery when the Royal College of Canada began to hold annual meetings.

The first organized training of surgeons on this continent was by William S. Halstead in Baltimore in the early years of this century. Full-time clinical appointments in surgery began in Baltimore and Boston in 1913 and spread across the continent, with variants in the strict or geographical full-time principles. Under this clinical and research guidance the modern residency systems with their essential of graduated transference of responsibility gradually evolved. C. L. Starr of Toronto became the first full-time professor of surgery in Canada in 1921, and W. E. Gallie succeeded him. Duncan Graham had become Professor of Medicine in Toronto in 1919, the first full-time appointment in the British Commonwealth. The success of the Toronto School in graduate training, both medical and surgical, may have been in part due to this early adoption of the full-time principle. The majority of the twelve Canadian university departments of surgery now have a small full-time core, though much of the teaching is done by part-time staff.

The Royal College of Physicians and Surgeons of Canada was incorporated in 1929 by an Act of the Parliament of Canada on petition from the Canadian Medical Association. The intent was to provide for physicians and surgeons in Canada a higher medical qualification signifying training and competence in a special branch of medicine or surgery. The College is divided into medical and surgical divisions, and a Fellow in Surgery is designated "Fellow of the Royal College of Surgeons of Canada." The College is bilingual, and in the French language the name of the College is "Le Collège royal des Médicins et Chirurgiens du Canada," and a Fellow in Surgery is designated "Associé du Collège royal des Chirurgiens du Canada." The charter members were Professors of Medicine and Surgery and Obstetrics and Gynaecology, and subsequently other distinguished Canadian physicians and surgeons were included. Admission to Fellowship by examination began in 1932.

Initially Fellowship of the Royal College of Surgeons of Canada was only in General Surgery. Since 1947, Fellowship may be held in General Surgery, Cardiovascular and Thoracic Surgery, Neurosurgery, Obstetrics and Gynaecology, Ophthalmology, Orthopaedic Surgery, Otolaryngology, Plastic Surgery, and Urology.

Canadian hospitals have organized their training programs to comply with the requirements of the Royal College, and the universities of Canada have given close cooperation in providing instruction in the basic sciences and opportunity for basic and clinical research. About two thirds of all hospitals approved by the Royal College are affiliated with medical schools.

The prescribing and maintenance of standards of training and examination have been and continue to be the predominant interest and concern of the College. A searching examination, both written and practical, has limited Fellowship to those who have attained excellence in a specialty. In consequence the Fellowship has high prestige in Canada and is a requirement for admission to the staff of most teaching hospitals. As of September, 1961, there were 1,443 Fellows of the Royal College of Surgeons of Canada.

On request from the Canadian Medical Association, the Royal College began a program of certification of specialists in Canada in 1942. Certificates were first granted without examination to a selected group of Canadian physicians and surgeons who were considered to have adequate training and ability. Certification in general surgery and the surgical specialties by examination began in 1946, and certification without examination came to an end in 1947. The specialist certificate is intended to ensure a high standard of clinical competence in the specialty concerned but has a less searching examination in the broad fields of surgery and the basic sciences. Certificants are encouraged to attend the meetings of the College but are not members. The double standard of surgical qualification was not ideal but did identify to Canadians seeking surgical care those who had competence in the field and undoubtedly filled a real need. The initial difference in training requirements between Certification and Fellowship was that in Certification one of the four years of training past the rotating internship could be spent in supervised practice. As need became less acute and training programs expanded, the long-desired single standard of training in certification and fellowship has become possible in most specialties. In further effort to reach a single standard, qualification is already only by means of the Fellowship examination in some of the specialties and others are to follow the same pattern.

The training requirements are as elastic as possible within the limitation of providing adequate clinical experience. After graduation from medical school the average training taken would be a rotation year, three years of resident training in clinical surgery, and a year in clinical research or in one of the basic sciences. Since the examination cannot be taken before the end of the training period the candidate would then prepare for the written examination in October to be followed by the oral examination in November. A minimum of 5½ years will have been necessary between graduation from medical school and the completion of the training and the qualifying examinations. Some, and particularly the group who have teaching appointments, will go on to further training. A few having taken Fellowship in General Surgery will sit the Fellowship again in one of the other surgical specialties when they have satisfied the training requirements.

In Canada in 1961, with a total population of 18,049,000 there were 7,215 doctors who held a specialist certificate from the Royal College and who were engaged in the active practice of their specialty in Canada. This represented 34.9% of the total number of doctors in Canada. Half the specialists' certificates are held by surgeons. In comparison, in 1954 in the United States 65,000 doctors representing 41.9% of the total physicians in that country were practicing a specialty. The ideal number of specialists would be hard to determine, but Canada does seem reasonably well supplied. The most frequent certification in the small towns in Canada is that in General Surgery.

From its beginning the Fellowship had envisaged an examination which would be "a severe test of the knowledge, ability and judgment of the candidate." The pass rate has always been low and had stabilized at about 40% until recently when it has fallen as low as 30%. With Certification by examination in 1946 the number of candidates gradually increased. Between 1950 and 1954 the pass rate in Certification had been about 80%. This fell off gradually until it is now about 60% of candidates. The fall-off in pass rate coincided with a sudden increase in the number of candidates. Several factors may be significant. A rapid increase in the number seeking training led to training in hospitals that were not experienced in teaching or had inadequate facilities. Some of these hospitals had approval for only one or two years of training. The College has made statements advising against fragmentation of training but has not yet enforced them. An increase in severity of the examination has perhaps been true in Certification in an effort to bring its level closer to that of Fellowship, but is less likely in Fellowship where the level has been long established. There is in Canada real concern over the high failure rate in the Fellowship examinations and the hardship this imposes on young men who have in good faith taken a long period of training. This was very evident at the last annual meeting of the College in Edmonton in January, 1963. The majority of the Fellows at large and of the Council of the College are now qualified by examination, and there is naturally a strong feeling that the standard should be maintained. Some of the training centers have been able to show a very acceptable pass rate over a period of many years and have come to believe that candidates with upper third of class standing and good records as rotating interns will be likely to pass the Fellowship in Surgery at the first attempt if they have been subjected to good training. Training programs in Canada are this year being subjected to an on-the-scene review by experienced teachers capable of assessing their real value. A report is due before the annual meeting of the College in 1964. It would be most unfortunate if the standard of the Royal College of Surgeons of Canada, which has done so much to improve Canadian surgery, was lowered to meet controllable inadequacies in the trainees or their training. Preserving Certification perhaps only in General Surgery for the occasional candidate who has warranted training but proves unable to reach the Fellowship level would be preferable to lowering the standard of Fellowship. The Canadian Fellowship had in its beginning a primary examination in the basic sciences. This had proven unsatisfactory and was abandoned in 1944 in favor of the present single examination at the end of the training period. In 1953 a revised form of the primary examination, that would be taken in the earlier years of training and would screen out candidates with little apparent chance of success in the final examinations, was considered very carefully. There were many arguments for and against the plan, but it was finally believed unwise. A primary examination in addition would permit closer association with the other Royal Colleges in the British Isles and the Commonwealth. In these colleges success in the primary examination of one College will be accepted for admission to the final examination of the others. This does not seem feasible in Canada in the near future.

The final problem of the disappearing service patient and the associated difficulty in delegating surgical responsibility in the training of surgeons is now upon Canada. Some of the provinces are already under forms of universal medical care, and all political parties are committed to it. The Royal College of Physicians and Surgeons of Canada in its brief to the Royal Commission on Health Services has given sound advice. Included in the brief are recommendations that approved hospitals be provided the means to establish attractive clinical teaching units for the care of all classes of patients who wish to be treated in such units; that Faculties of Medicine whose budgets are intended primarily to meet the cost of undergraduate medical education be given financial assistance in meeting the cost of graduate training programs, including the engaging of additional teaching staff in both clinical and preclinical departments; that the resident staff in teaching hospitals be that recommended by the heads of the clinical departments and that the resident staff have adequate remuneration; and that basic and clinical research be supported in the belief that the health care of the people of a country will not in the long run be better than the provision which that country makes for medical research. The recommendations of the Farquharson Report concerning increased support for medical research in the Faculties of Medicine and in the teaching hospitals were supported.

Canada has developed a system of surgical training and qualification that will identify to the patient seeking surgical care those with special training and skill. At the upper level of Fellowship in the Royal College of Surgeons of Canada a broad knowledge of surgery and the basic sciences must be combined with a high level of clinical competence. In the future every effort should be made to bring all Canadian surgery to this higher standard. Careful assessment of the present training programs and strengthening of universities and teaching hospitals at both basic and clinical levels will do much to help. This must probably all be accomplished within some plan of universal medical care.

Angus D. McLachlin, MD, Faculty of Medicine, University of Western Ontario, London, Ontario.

Massive Gastroduodenal Hemorrhage

Changing Concepts of Management

HENRY G. KELLEY, MD; GEORGE N. GRANT, MD; AND DAN W. ELLIOTT, MD, COLUMBUS, OHIO

The high mortality and wide variation in treatment of massive upper gastrointestinal hemorrhage indicate that its management is far from satisfactory. Therefore, Wangensteen's introduction of gastric hypothermia for control of acute hemorrhage has seemed a welcome innovation.[9] Two other clinics have published experience with this procedure, citing nine[7] and ten[4] cases, respectively, and expressing encouragement although eight of these patients died. This new procedure has been employed only in the most seriously ill, so that a high mortality at first may be expected. The value of gastric hypothermia probably can be assessed only if its impact is measured on an entire institution's experience with serious gastrointestinal hemorrhage. These considerations, plus dissatisfaction with all present types of emergency operation for the control of hemorrhage, have led to a review of the entire experience with this problem at the University Hospital from 1950 through 1962.

This interval provides experience adequate to evaluate the results of three different operative procedures: two-thirds gastric resection, vagotomy with hemigastrectomy, and vagotomy with pyloroplasty. Each of these has had a period of predominant use during this study, while the influence of gastric hypothermia is limited to the last two years.

Presented at the 20th Annual Meeting of the Central Surgical Association, Chicago, Feb 21-23, 1963.

From the Department of Surgery, The Ohio State University College of Medicine, University Hospital.

Aided by a grant from the Central Ohio Heart Association of Columbus, Ohio.

Methods and Materials

The hospital records were reviewed of all patients admitted to University Hospital from 1950 to 1962 with a diagnosis of gastrointestinal hemorrhage. Although 1,092 patients had gastroduodenal hemorrhage, only 417 cases were included in the study which met the following criteria for massive hemorrhage: (1) active bleeding and (2) one or more of these: (*a*) shock, (*b*) hemoglobin below 7 gm% or hematocrit below 25, or (*c*) six pints (3,000 cc) of blood required within 24 hours to maintain a stable blood pressure. Mild and chronic hemorrhage present no real problem in emergency surgical management and were excluded. Esophageal varices and known blood dyscrasias were excluded because each of these presents intricate and difficult entities in surgical management peculiar to itself. The lesions included in the study are gastric, duodenal, and marginal ulcer; benign and malignant tumors of the stomach; hiatus hernia; diffuse gastritis; and those cases in which no definitive diagnosis could be made.

Each record was reviewed in a standard manner and the data placed on IBM cards for accurate tabulation. No case that met the above criteria was excluded, whether or not other severe disease or trauma was present. In many cases, the hemorrhage suggested stress ulceration. The management of these patients was in no way controlled, and, therefore, this is a retrospective study.

The initial management of the 417 patients with massive gastroduodenal hemorrhage was fairly uniform. Estimation of initial blood loss was made, six pints of blood were cross-matched for each patient, and prompt replacement was begun. As each pint was administered, another was added to the reserve, so that there were always six pints available for operation, if necessary. A Levin tube was placed in the stomach to follow the rate of hemorrhage. Laboratory studies included a complete blood cell count, urinalysis, blood urea nitrogen, prothrombin time, bleeding and clotting time, and sulfobromophthalein (SBP) retention if cirrhosis was suspected. Hemoglobin and hematocrit determinations were repeated every four hours. The results were promptly placed on the "hemorrhage sheet" described by Elliott et al.[2] On this sheet there is recorded graphically in one place the data most useful in following the course of the patient: blood pressure, pulse rate, each pint of blood replacement, and the resulting change in hemoglobin level. Thus, this graph will disclose whether or not the patient is responding satisfactorily to nonoperative treatment.

Emergency upper gastrointestinal x-rays were taken when the site of bleeding was unknown and after the patient's blood pressure was stable. These were obtained in 26% of the patients coming to operation. No restriction was placed on the fluoroscopist, so that a complete examination could be carried out.

The need for operative intervention was based on: (1) continued hemorrhage after five pints (2,500 cc) of blood or more had been administered in any 24-hour period, and (2) continued hemorrhage after 48 hours of treatment. The same criteria were used for operative intervention in the 21 patients treated initially with gastric hypothermia. The operative procedure carried out to control the hemorrhage in each patient was the choice of the operating surgeon. No effort was made to separate the mortality and morbidity of the residents' cases from those of the senior surgeons.

Gastric hypothermia was accomplished as recommended by Wangensteen.[6] The gastric hypothermia machine consists of a refrigeration unit with a pump which passes a solution of 50% ethanol through a coaxial nasogastric tube into an intragastric balloon. The unit is a closed system in which a constant volume of coolant at a constant temperature is circulated between the reservoir of the refrigeration unit and the intragastric balloon. The temperature of the coolant going into the stomach was maintained between 0 to 10 C.

Prior to insertion of the cooling balloon, the stomach was lavaged through an Ewald or a No. 18F Levin tube with 1,000 cc of iced isotonic saline solution to remove all clots. A Levin tube was left in the stomach to monitor the control of hemorrhage. The volume in the intragastric balloon varied between 500 and 1,000 cc. The patient's body temperature was effectively maintained above 95 F (35 C) with heating blankets. All patients were sedated prior to and throughout the cooling procedure. Gastric hypothermia was continued for 24 hours after all evidence of hemorrhage had ceased.

Results

Sixty per cent (249 of the 417 patients) responded to the initial regimen of nonoperative therapy, a proportion which substantially agrees with previous experience.[2] There were 16 deaths in the hospital after bleeding had stopped, due largely to other diseases exacerbated by the bleeding episode, yielding a mortality rate for nonoperative treatment of 8%.

Altogether, 250 patients were operated upon, and the cause or site of hemorrhage

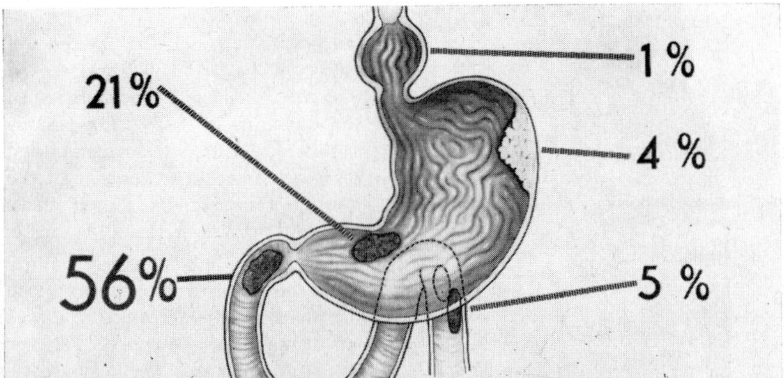

Fig 1.—Sites of hemorrhage in 250 operative cases: the variety of lesions proven at operation.

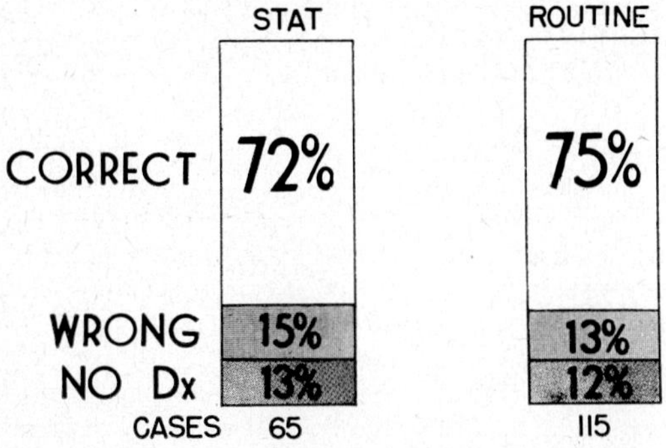

Fig 2.—Preoperative x-ray diagnosis. Emergency gastroduodenal x-rays gave results as good as elective examinations.

was determined in 94% (Fig 1). Duodenal ulcer accounted for the bleeding in well over one half of the cases and gastric ulcer in an additional one fifth. No cause or site of bleeding could be found in 6% of the cases, despite diagnostic gastrotomy and thorough exploration.

Preoperative x-rays could be compared with the operative findings in 180 of these patients. The x-ray diagnosis was correct in three out of four, whether the examination was done as an emergency or later in the routine daily schedule (Fig 2). X-rays were indeed misleading in one patient out of seven, by indicating a lesion which was not present at subsequent laparotomy.

Definitive surgery was carried out electively in 99 of these patients after the bleeding had been controlled, with an operative mortality of 3%. In contrast, 151 patients required operation as an emergency to stop the hemorrhage and 29 died, for a mortality of 19% (Fig 3).

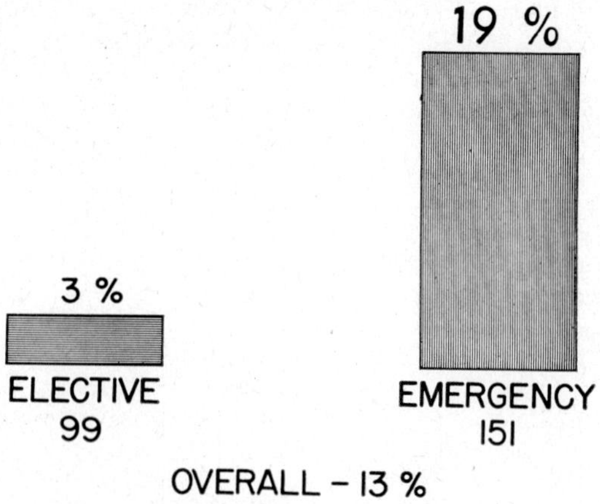

Fig 3.—Operative mortality in 250 cases. Mortality is significantly higher in emergency surgery.

Clearly, these cases concern the surgeon most, since they are responsible for the high mortality in the entire series. While there is general agreement on the need for prompt operation if any, there is no such agreement on the details of the procedure to be employed. In this hospital there have been three successive waves of enthusiasm for three different kinds of operation during the past 13 years. In Fig 4, the type of procedure actually used in the 151 uncontrolled bleeders is shown by its per cent of the total for each year. The two-thirds gastric resection was performed in the greatest number of cases during the first three years of this study but declined in use after that. Vagotomy with hemigastrectomy became the predominant operation from 1955 to 1959 and was the most frequently employed procedure in this 13-year period. During the latest four years, after the enthusiastic re-

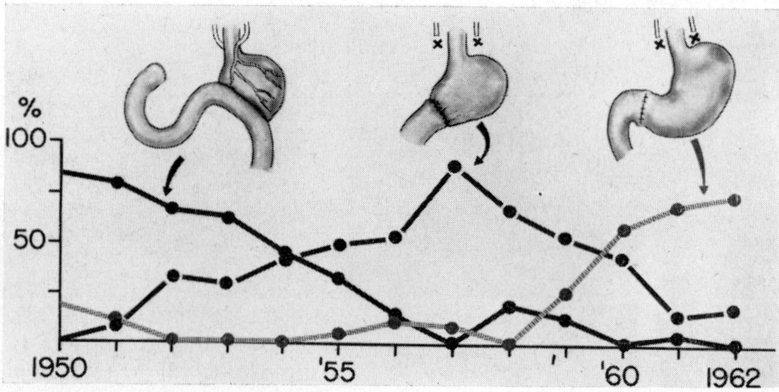

Fig 4.—Type of operation in 151 uncontrolled bleeders. Three waves of enthusiasm have been seen for three different operations to stop bleeding since 1950.

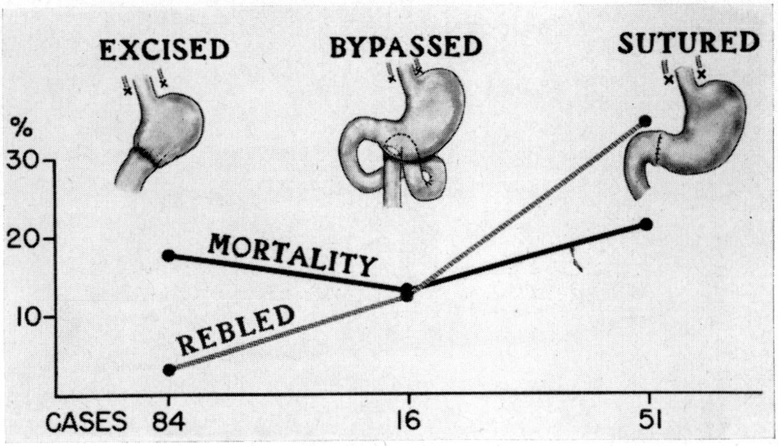

Fig 5.—Management of bleeding point. Rebleeding is less with excision of the original bleeding point, but the mortality is high for all three methods of management.

port of Weinberg,[10] vagotomy and pyloroplasty with oversewing of the bleeding point gained sharply in popularity.

Among all of these operations there were fundamentally three methods for handling the bleeding point: It could be totally excised as in the two-thirds resection or the hemigastrectomy with vagotomy. It was bypassed in a relatively few cases, as when gastroenterostomy with vagotomy was performed for duodenal ulcer. The bleeding point was left in the gastrointestinal stream in the pyloroplasties with vagotomy, although carefully ligated. Regardless of the method for managing the bleeding point or the nature of the operation performed, the mortality rate remained high, as shown in Fig 5.

Significant postoperative rebleeding within the gastrointestinal tract, requiring three pints or more of blood, rarely occurred when the original bleeding point was totally excised (Fig 5). In contrast, such rebleeding occurred in one third of the patients when the original lesion was left in continuity, as in the pyloroplasty group. Rebleeding may have accounted for a portion of the mortality in this group. Among all the patients who rebled, 45% subsequently died.

Emergency intervention to control hemorrhage had actually been required in about 40% of the cases seen each year until the advent of gastric cooling in 1960. As the use of hypothermia has rapidly increased, emergency operation has declined to one-half its former incidence, or 20% in 1962 (Fig 6). Gastric cooling has actually been employed in 21 cases, and 4 of these subsequently required operation, accounting for the overlap in the graph in Fig 6.

Each of the 21 patients treated initially by gastric hypothermia was considered a

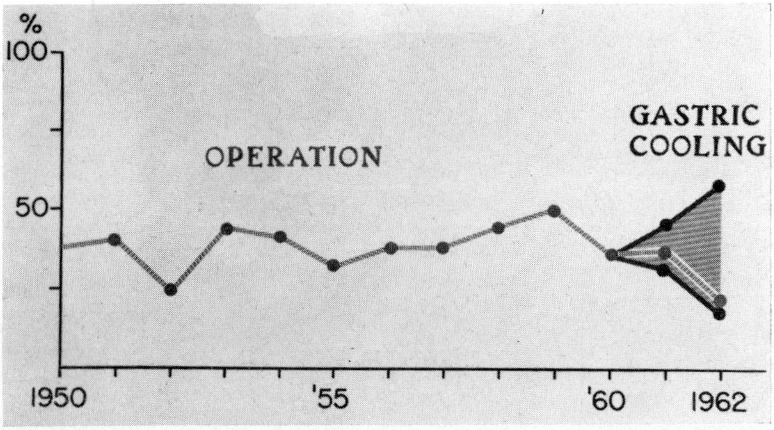

Fig 6.—Per cent requiring intervention (417 cases). Gastric cooling has reduced the incidence of emergency operations to one half.

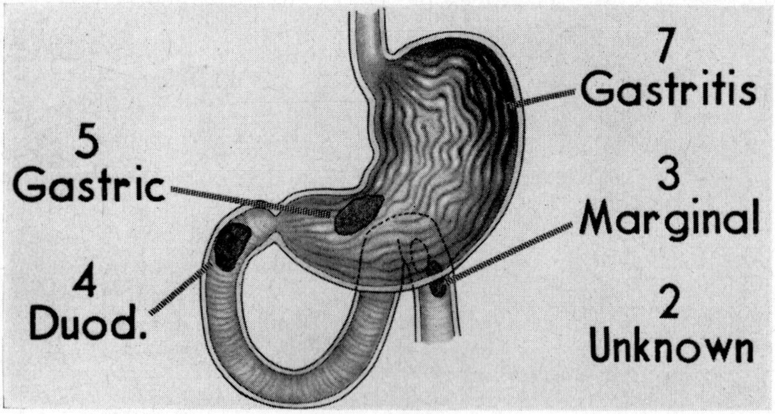

Fig 7.—The variety of lesions in 21 poor-risk patients treated by gastric cooling.

Control of Hemorrhage by Gastric Hypothermia

Lesion	Cases	Hemorrhage Controlled
Diffuse gastritis	7	6
Gastric ulcer	5	4
Duodenal ulcer	4	3
Marginal ulcer	3	1
Unknown site (stress)	2	2
Totals	21	16

poor candidate for an operation of any type, usually because of severe concomitant disease. Fig 7 shows the variety of lesions treated for massive hemorrhage by gastric cooling. In the seven cases with gastritis and the two with an undiagnosed bleeding site the hemorrhage was a manifestation of secondary or stress ulceration. The results with respect to the control of bleeding in each of these lesions are listed in the Table. There were no important complications directly related to the cooling procedure. Fig 8 summarizes the over-all results in this small group. In 16 out of 21 (76%), the bleeding was controlled. Four of these patients died later of severe concomitant disease. In five, the bleeding continued, and one of these five died. Operation was performed in the other four with one additional death. Among the four patients operated upon, the prior effort at hypothermia did not seem to affect adversely their subsequent postoperative course, in keeping with the experience of others.[4] Out of the 21 patients subjected to gastric refrigeration 6 died, for a mortality rate of 29%. This did not seem high for this severely afflicted small group.

Altogether, there were 167 uncontrolled bleeders (151 were operated upon and an additional 17 had gastric cooling). Some inquiry was made as to why these patients should have had such a high mortality. It was found that 44% of this group had a serious life-threatening disease outside the gastrointestinal tract before the onset of hemorrhage. Such a disease was present in 72% of the patients that died as against 37% of those who lived (Fig 9). Especially such acute lesions as cerebral trauma,

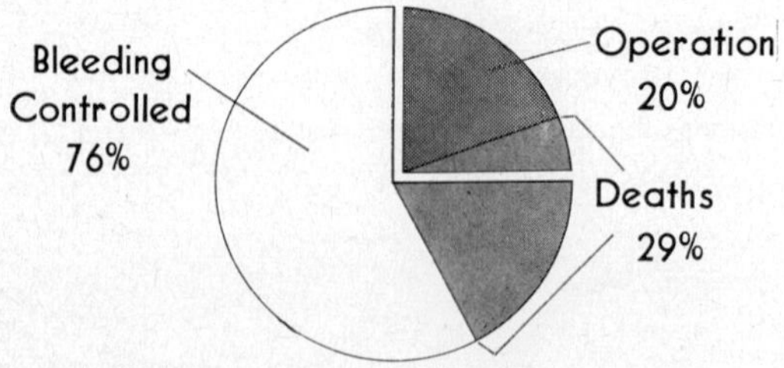

Fig 8.—Results of gastric cooling in 21 poor-risks patients. The bleeding was controlled in three fourths of those cooled, and in the remainder an operation was performed.

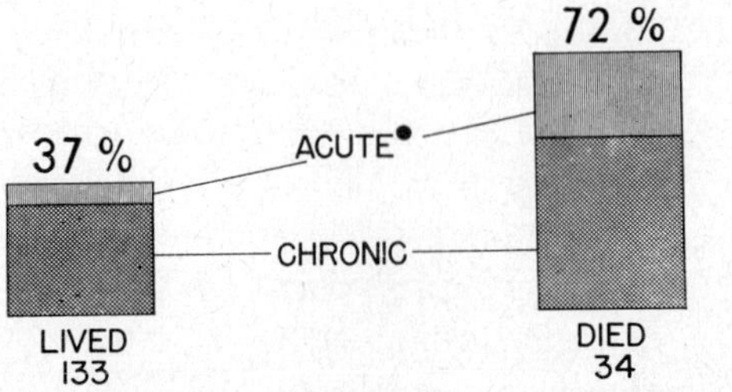

Fig 9.—Almost half (44% in 167) of the uncontrolled bleeders had another severe disease as well.

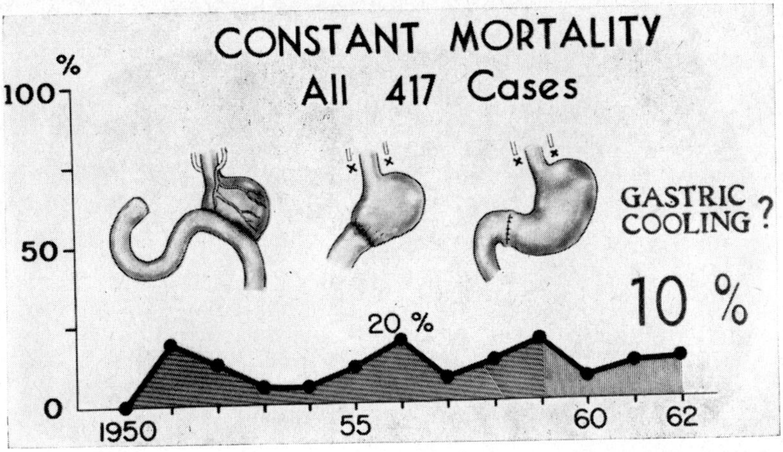

Fig 10.—Despite changes in operative procedures from time to time, the mortality remains high and has been only slightly influenced by gastric cooling.

extensive burns, serious pancreatitis, ruptured intracranial and abdominal aneurysms contributed significantly to the deaths in this series.

The newer procedures, such as vagotomy with pyloroplasty or gastric cooling, are usually tried first in only the most critically ill patients. Therefore, their true value can be appreciated only from an examination of an entire institution's experience following their introduction. For this reason, the annual mortality for all 417 patients included in the study has been plotted in Fig 10. It shows a widely fluctuating mortality rate, rising to peaks of 20% in the bad years regardless of the type of operation in predominant use. Since the introduction of gastric cooling, the over-all mortality has ranged about 10%. It is too early to be sure that this figure will be improved, but experience to date with gastric hypothermia appears to warrant further investigation and trials.

Comment

Mixter and co-workers, in 1956, reviewed the trends in management of massive gastroduodenal hemorrhage over a 28-year period, in an effort to shed light on the problem of a persistently high mortality. They summed up their findings by condemning exclusively nonsurgical treatment and advocating early gastric resection.[5] Stewart [8] and others [1,3] have reached these same conclusions.

While one or another operative procedure has been advocated from time to time, this study indicates no distinct advantage for one operation over another with regard to final outcome. Weinberg's [10] ulcer ligation with vagotomy and pyloroplasty is technically safer and tolerated better by critically ill patients. However, it was disappointing indeed to find in this small series (51 cases) that the incidence of postoperative rebleeding (36%) mitigated the early good results. Consequently, the mortality for this lesser procedure has been no better than that after two-thirds gastric resection or vagotomy and hemigastrectomy.

Probably the selection of the proper operation to control hemorrhage in a massively bleeding patient is a highly individual matter. Vagotomy with pyloroplasty and ligation of the bleeding point may well be the best operation for an elderly and critically ill patient bleeding acutely. On the other hand, it would probably not be best for a younger and more vigorous patient with recurrent bouts of hemorrhage.

A significant factor in the high mortality of massive gastroduodenal hemorrhage is the high proportion of patients (44%) with other serious lesions. These are the problem patients, for whom no operation has proved satisfactory. They are surely logical candidates for gastric hypothermia, once simpler nonoperative measures fail and operation seems imminent. The small experience reported here with 21 such critically ill people encourages further use of this modality.

If, out of an institution's entire experience, only the most severely ill are selected for gastric cooling, this procedure will encounter a seemingly high mortality. On the other hand, those not selected for cooling may well exhibit improved results. Thus, the true value of gastric hypothermia, or any other new therapy for massive gastroduodenal bleeding, will be measured in a declining annual mortality rate for the institution as a whole.

Summary

The records have been reviewed for 417 patients with truly massive gastroduodenal hemorrhage treated from 1950 through 1962. In 40%, the bleeding would not stop. Emergency operation was performed in 151 patients with an operative mortality of 19%, contrasted with 3% in those having elective surgery. There was no difference in the results of three different operations: two-thirds gastric resection, vagotomy with hemigastrectomy, and vagotomy with pyloroplasty and oversewing of the bleeding point.

During the past two years, gastric hypothermia has been employed in an additional 21 poor-risk patients. Bleeding was controlled in 16, and 15 survived. Gastric hypothermia has significantly reduced the need for emergency operation and promises to help improve the management of this difficult lesion.

Henry G. Kelley, MD, Department of Surgery, The Ohio State University College of Medicine, University Hospital, Columbus 10, Ohio.

REFERENCES

1. Darin, J. C.; Polacek, M. A.; and Ellison, E. H.: Surgical Mortality of Massive Hemorrhage From Peptic Ulcer, Arch Surg 83:71 (July) 1961.

2. Elliott, D. W.; Hartle, R.; Marshall, F.; and Zollinger, R. M.: Response to Transfusion as Guide in Management of Upper Gastrointestinal Hemorrhage, AMA Arch Surg 77:386 (Sept) 1958.

3. Karlson, K. E.; Enquist, I. F.; Dennis, C.; and Fierst, S.: Results of Three Methods of Therapy for Massive Gastroduodenal Hemorrhage, Ann Surgery 148:594 (Oct) 1958.

4. Miller, R. E.; Moscarella, A. A.; and Fitzpatrick, H. F.: Local Gastric Hypothermia, Arch Surg 86:272 (Feb) 1963.

5. Mixter, G., Jr.; Imparato, A. N.; and Hinton, J. W.: Massive Hemorrhage From Peptic Ulcer: The Changing Therapy Over a 28 Year Period, Ann Surg 145:783 (May) 1957.

6. Nicoloff, D. M.; Griffen, W. O., Jr.; Salmon, P. A.; Peter, E. T.; and Wangensteen, O. H.: Local Gastric Hypothermia in the Management of Massive Gastrointestinal Hemorrhage, Surg Gynec Obstet 114:495 (April) 1962.

7. Richman, A., and Anthony, D.: Experiences With Localized Gastric Hypothermia in Massive Upper Gastrointestinal Bleeding, Amer J Dig Dis 8:113 (Feb) 1963.

8. Stewart, J. D.; Cosgriff, J. H.; and Gray, J. G.: Experiences With the Treatment of Acutely Massively Bleeding Peptic Ulcer by Blood Replacement and Gastric Resection, Surg Gynec Obstet 103:409 (Oct) 1956.

9. Wangensteen, O. H.; Root, H. D.; Jenson, C. B.; Imamoglu, K.; and Salmon, P. A.: Depression of Gastric Secretion and Digestion by Gastric Hypothermia: Its Clinical Use in Massive Hematemesis, Surgery 44:265 (Aug) 1958.

10. Weinberg, J. A.: Treatment of the Massively Bleeding Duodenal Ulcer by Ligation, Pyloroplasty and Vagotomy, Amer J Surg 102:158 (Aug) 1961.

Treatment of Postgastrectomy Stomal Ulcer by Gastric Freezing

EUGENE F. BERNSTEIN, MD; ARTHUR S. McFEE, MD; ROBERT L. GOODALE, JR., MD; ARTHUR J. MADSEN, MD; AND OWEN H. WANGENSTEEN, MD, MINNEAPOLIS

Introduction

The development of stomal ulcer following gastric resection for duodenal ulcer, whether manifested by recurrent ulcer symptoms or by upper gastrointestinal tract bleeding, represents a difficult and challenging problem. Almost invariably surgery has been necessary to correct the situation, with vagotomy and/or further resection as the conventional surgical approach. Vagotomy is the simpler and lesser procedure and has been widely employed in the management of stomal ulcer in recent years.

Gastric freezing for the definitive control of the peptic ulcer diathesis is a direct outgrowth of successes with milder forms of gastric hypothermia for the control of massive upper gastrointestinal hemorrhage.[1] Gastric cooling for this latter purpose followed studies in frogs and dogs in which it was observed that gastric digestion was completely suspended at temperatures of 10 to 15 C. In fact, subsequent studies have shown virtual suspension of gastric digestion at temperatures below 10 C, as a result of the decreased secretion of HCl at temperatures of 10 to 15 C and inhibition of peptic activity at temperatures below 30 C.[2]

How Gastric Freezing Thwarts the Peptic Ulcer Diathesis.—The beneficial effects of gastric freezing are a result of selective injury to the secretory apparatus of the stomach. Extensive animal experimentation has demonstrated: (1) depression of gastric secretion from intact canine stomachs and suppression of secretion in isolated canine gastric pouches, and (2) significant protection against development of ulcer attending known ulcer-provoking situations in the experimental animal.[3-5]

Extensive trials with gastric freezing were made in dogs to determine the limitations of safety factors, before the method was applied to man.[6] In October, 1961, clinical application of gastric freezing for duodenal ulcer was initiated in this clinic. At first, only patients with chronic duodenal ulcer, referred for elective surgery, were offered gastric freezing in lieu of operation. As experience with the safety and efficacy of the method increased, indications for its use were extended to other manifestations of peptic ulcer, including patients with stomal ulcer who had undergone one or more surgical procedures and who still suffered from ulcer symptoms.

Our experience in cases with chronic unobstructed duodenal ulcer with classical indications for elective surgery suggests that relief of symptoms, marked secretory depression, and healing of ulcer craters may be expected in approximately 50% of instances with a single freeze.[7] Unresponsive cases, or those in whom symptoms recur, are treated with subsequent additional episodes of freezing, at intervals of two to twelve months, as appears necessary.

Experimental studies in the animal laboratory indicate that multiple episodes of gastric freezing produce extensive gastric mucosal atrophy, in distinction to relatively mild and transient histologic changes seen following a single freeze. Such changes may

Presented at the 20th Annual Meeting of the Central Surgical Association, Chicago, Feb 21-23, 1963.

Advanced Research Fellow, American Heart Association (Dr. Bernstein).

Department of Surgery, University of Minnesota Medical School.

This work was supported by grants from the United States Public Health Service and the Donald J. Cowling Funds for Surgical Research.

still be seen, but in lesser degree, as late as six months after the final freeze, and in some instances prolonged secretory depression also may be observed in dogs whose stomachs have been subjected to multiple episodes of freezing.

The striking initial secretory depression following a single freeze appears transient in man, too, with return to control secretory levels by six months. However, during this period, the patient's ulcer crater has healed, and dietary strictures and medication have been dispensed with. Many patients then remain asymptomatic, despite return of secretory values to prefreeze control levels.

These lessons, learned from an experience with gastric freezing in over 200 patients with chronic duodenal ulcer, have been applied to other manifestations of the peptic ulcer problem. This presentation will summarize our experience with gastric freezing for stomal ulcer.

Indications

Patients with stomal ulcer subjected to gastric freezing have been divided into two groups. Approximately half of our patients had one or more episodes of upper gastrointestinal hemorrhage after primary surgery for duodenal ulcer. In this group, a stomal ulcer often was not demonstrable by x-ray studies at the time gastric freezing was instituted. The extent of the bleeding, however, very definitely suggested the presence of an erosive or ulcerative process at the neostoma.

The other group of patients had recurrence of ulcer symptoms after gastric surgery, and a stomal ulcer crater was almost invariably demonstrable. In fact, some of these craters were very large.

Prefreeze Studies.—Before undertaking gastric freezing in any group of patients, a prefreezing gastrointestinal x-ray series is mandatory. In patients with a likely neostomal ulcer, it is important to ascertain whether a crater is present and to note the degree of impairment, if any, in emptying of the residual gastric pouch. In patients with intact stomachs, any grade of gastric retention is regarded as a contraindication to gastric freezing. An intact stomach should not retain more than 40% of a 12 oz barium meal after one hour and should be essentially empty by two hours. Secretory studies are performed routinely before and after freezing to observe its effect upon the gastric secretory response. These studies include (1) an eight-hour unstimulated overnight aspiration, (2) a Hollander test, using insulin to evoke vagal-stimulated gastric secretion, and (3) a peptone gastric analysis, which primarily concerns the antral gastrin secretory mechanism in patients with intact stomachs.

While the unreliability of these tests following partial gastrectomy is recognized, careful placement of a nasogastric tube, under fluoroscopy, has resulted in obtaining evidence of significant acid concentration in a number of such patients who appeared achlorhydric when first studied. These tests constitute an important item in evaluating the effects of gastric freezing, especially upon intact stomachs.

In the presence of a demonstrable stomal ulcer crater, accompanied by symptoms including hemorrhage or recurrent ulcer following prior surgery, achlorhydric secretory studies would not be a contraindication to gastric freezing. However, persistence of active gastric secretion in the presence of recurrent symptoms and a demonstrable neostomal ulcer crater constitutes incontrovertible evidence of ulcer recurrence.

Technique

Only slight modifications have been made in adapting the technique originally described for freezing the intact stomach[6] to the postgastrectomy stomal ulcer patient. The patient is fasted for at least 12 hours while secretory studies are performed. Thirty minutes prior to freezing, premedication is administered. This includes 50 mg of meperidine hydrochloride (Demerol), 25 mg of chlorpromazine (Thorazine), 60 mg of phenobarbital, and 0.4 mg of atropine. The

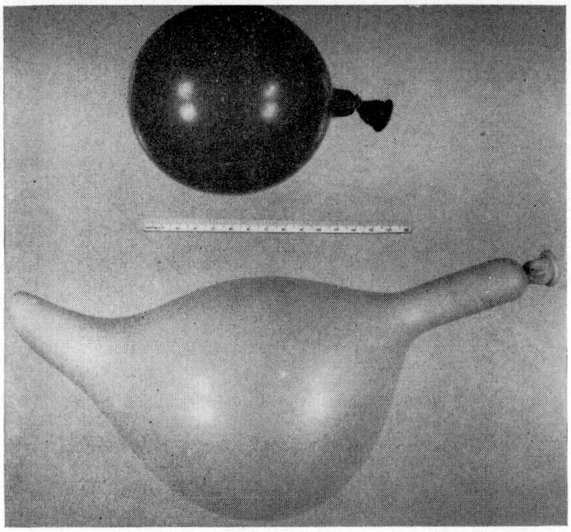

Fig 1.—Small round balloon used in patients with post-Billroth II gastric pouch, and stomach-shaped balloon employed when the stomach is intact, or after gastroenterostomy or Billroth I resection.

patient is placed on an Aqua-K-Thermia warming blanket and is covered with an electric blanket.

The systemic temperature is monitored throughout the procedure, and a downward drift in the body temperature of more than 2 C (3.5 F) during gastric freezing is distinctly unusual. The throat is anesthetized by spraying with 5% hexylcaine hydrochloride (Cyclaine), after which the patient is urged to gargle employing the same solution. An appropriate balloon is selected, based on the x-ray appearance of the size of the stomach. In general, after the Billroth II type of gastrectomy, a small round balloon which readily distends to a volume of 400 to 500 cc is employed (Fig 1). This is tied to the end of the double lumen tubing of the Swenko Gastric Hypothermia unit (Fig 2), much in the same manner as the stomach-shaped balloon is attached for freezing the intact stomach. In some patients, after a Billroth I gastric resection, or after gastrojejunostomy, the stomach-shaped balloon has been employed.

In the earlier patients with neostomal ulcer subjected to gastric freezing, the balloon was simply passed into the gastric pouch, after roughly measuring the length of tubing on the patient's chest. The balloon was then inflated gradually to the point of discomfort from distention but without provoking pain.

Fig 2.—The gastric freezing apparatus which is employed in both primary and postresection peptic ulcer disease.

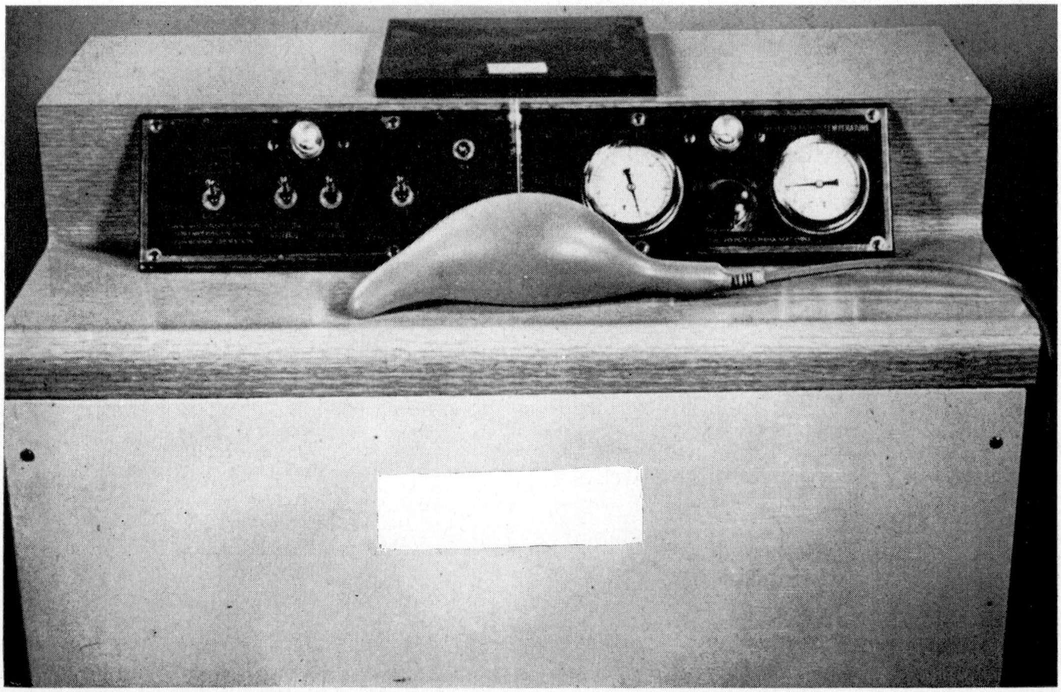

In general, this degree of distention averaged 400 cc. More recently, the balloon has been passed regularly under fluoroscopic control to position it accurately in the residual gastric pouch (Fig 3 and 4). Gastric freezing was performed over a period of 60 minutes, with inflow temperatures varying between −15 to −17 C and outflow temperatures of −10 C in 14 of the 33 patients. In 12 additional patients with stomal ulcer, the freezing time was 45 minutes, and in 7 the duration of the gastric freeze was 50 minutes.

Fig 3.—*A*, x-rays demonstrate discrete jejunal ulcer crater directly opposite the stoma of a Billroth II anastomosis, just prior to gastric freezing. *B*, round freezing balloon, filled with methylglucamine diatrizoate (Gastrografin), has been positioned and filled under fluoroscopic guidance. Double lumen tube is then fixed in place, methylglucamine diatrizoate washed out, and perfusion with alcohol carried out.

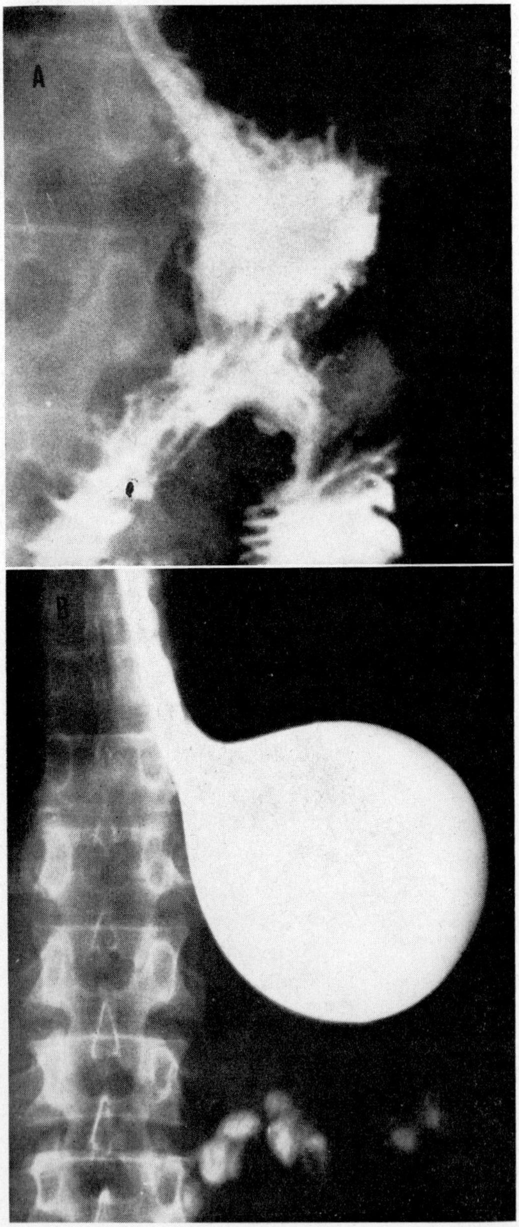

We began by freezing the intact stomach for 60 minutes. After the observation of several instances of melena and the occurrence of gastric ulcer in 6 patients, the duration of freezing was reduced to 45 minutes. At this time, inflow and outflow temperatures were established at −17 C and −10 C instead of the earlier levels of −20 C (inflow) and −12 C (outflow). Meanwhile the end hole of the inflow tube was sealed, and provision for outflow was made through a number of side vents (32 holes made in the distal 2 cm of the tube with a heated 22 gauge needle). The direct thrust of the cold alcohol through the inflow tube upon the same area of the balloon and stomach is thus eliminated. No complications were noted in this group of patients and so the time was advanced again to an hour's freeze. The subsequent development of one gastric ulcer has again persuaded us to reduce the time of freezing to 50 minutes, which we are currently employing. The technical details of the freezing procedure have been defined clearly and must be very carefully observed, particularly with regard to:

1. Duration of freezing
2. Balloon volume and fit of stomach
3. Perfusion rate
4. Temperatures—inflow and outflow
5. Balloon thickness
6. Systemic temperature

Any modification or alteration in any of these items could affect the situation very materially and would necessitate reassessment of new guide lines in the experimental laboratory prior to clinical application. Moreover, anyone taking up gastric freezing would be well advised to test the performance of his machine and the accuracy of the temperature depression recorded over the range of temperature herein desired, employing a mercury thermometer for the purpose.

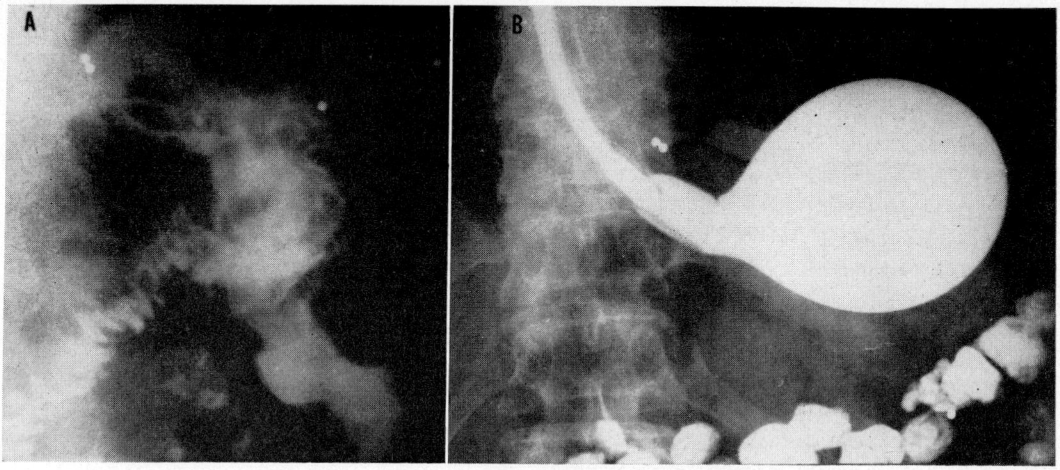

Fig 4.—*A*, a large jejunal ulcer crater is demonstrated opposite and just distal to the gastric pouch. *B*, the freezing balloon is in place, and is filled adequately and completely to distend the residual acid secreting tissue.

On completion of the freeze, a 15-minute thawing period is permitted with the balloon distended but not perfused. Then, the balloon is emptied and gently removed. Within two hours the patient is permitted to eat and drink. Follow-up gastric secretory studies and x-rays are performed at intervals of six weeks and at three, six, and twelve months. In fact, our present plan is to follow this group of patients indefinitely.

Results

To date, 33 patients with postgastrectomy neostomal ulceration have been treated by gastric freezing. All but 2 were males. Of these, 23 had recurrent bleeding or ulceration after a Billroth II gastrectomy, 3 after a Billroth I gastrectomy, 1 after a segmental gastrectomy, and 6 after gastrojejunostomy. Four of the patients with Billroth II resections and 1 with a gastrojejunostomy had complemental truncal vagotomies. In 15 of these patients there was x-ray evidence of an active stomal ulcer crater, although the evidence was not altogether unequivocal in 2. Eighteen patients had demonstrable free acid in their eight-hour unstimulated overnight analysis prior to freezing, a figure that ranged as high as 60 and 63 mEq of free acid in 2 patients with prior Billroth II gastrectomies. After their initial freeze, 9 of these 18 patients became achlorhydric, and 6 others

TABLE 1.—*Stomal Ulcer Treated by Gastric Freezing*

Number of patients treated: 33		
Number with x-ray evidence of crater: 15 (debatable in 2)		
Previous operation:		
1. (a) Billroth II	19	
(b) Billroth II and complemental vagotomy	4	
2. Billroth I	3	
3. Segmental resection	1	
4. Gastrojejunostomy	6	
Demonstrable free acid on unstimulated overnight aspiration:		
Prefreeze	18	
Postfreeze (immediate)	9 (6 had marked reduction)	
6 weeks postfreeze	4 of 12 studied (3 of these subsequently refrozen)	
Duration of freeze:		
45 min	12	
60 min	14	
50 min	7	
Refreeze: 9 patients		
Indications:		
Recurrent melena	2	
Persistent pain and crater	7	
Interval of refreeze:		
2-3 wk	2	
6 wk	3	
3 mo	3	
5 mo	1	
	Frozen Once (24)	Refrozen (9)
Present Status:		
Excellent (asymptomatic)	9	0
Good results, but few persistent symptoms	5	8
Death from other causes, but good symptomatic relief until death	2	0
Death from other causes, without good relief	1	0
Failure, operated upon	0	1
Frozen too recently for evaluation	7	0

TABLE 2.—*Current Status of Patients With Marginal Ulcer Treated by Gastric*

Duration of Follow-Up	Clinical Status: Excellent (Asymp.)	Clinical Status: Good (Few symptoms, crater healed)	Clinical Status: Failure	Too Early for Evaluation	Secretory Status, Immediate: Achlorhydric	Secretory Status, Immediate: Marked Depression	Secretory Status, Immediate: No Dep.	Secretory Status, Immediate: Not Done
Single Freeze								
6 mo or more (4)	3 *	1	0	0	3	0	0	1
3-6 mo (4)	4	0	0	0	2	1	1	0
6 wk-3 mo (7)	4 *	3	0	0	4	2	1	0
Less than 6 wk (9)	0	1	1 *	7	8	0	0	0
Multiple Freeze								
3-6 mo (2)	0	2	0	0	2	0	0	0
Less than 3 mo (7)	0	6	1	0	6	1	0	0

* Includes one patient who has died of unrelated causes.

had marked reductions (greater than 50%) in the amount of free acid obtained in the overnight secretion. In the 3 other patients, the postfreeze acidity was essentially that of the prefreeze control values, although in 1 of these the postfreezing values actually were higher than the observed prefreeze control values.

Postfreezing follow-up data are available on all 26 patients whose stomachs were frozen initially more than six weeks ago. Of these, 9 are asymptomatic and achlorhydric, with healed ulcer craters at intervals up to eight months after freeze. Five others had good results but have a few persistent symptoms.

Three patients have died from causes unrelated to the freezing but were successfully controlled up to the time of death. One died of myocardial infarction seven months after gastric freezing with an excellent clinical result from the gastric freeze over this period of life; the second died one month after gastric freezing, after surgery for pancreatic abscess, secondary to a long-standing history of chronic pancreatitis; the third suffered a myocardial infarct six weeks after freezing but was free of ulcer pain for this brief interval. Thus, 16 of the 26 patients followed had control of their stomal ulcer process with a single freeze. Of the remaining 10, one

TABLE 3.—*Current Status of Patients With Marginal Ulcer Treated by Gastric Freezing Analyzed*

Operative Procedure	Clinical Status: Excellent (Asym.)	Clinical Status: Good	Clinical Status: Failure	Too Early for Evaluation	Secretory, Immediate: Achlorhydric	Secretory, Immediate: Marked Depression	Secretory, Immediate: No Dep.	Secretory, Immediate: Not Done
Single Freeze								
Billroth II (15)	9 *	1	0	5	10	3	1	1
Billroth II and vagotomy (2)	1 *	0	0	1	2	0	0	0
Pyloroplasty and segment resection (1)	0	1	0	0	1	0	0	0
Gastrojejunostomy (6)	1	3	1 *	1	4	1	1	0
Multiple Freeze								
Billroth II (4)	0	3	1	0	3	1	0	0
Billroth II and vagotomy (2)	0	2	0	0	2	0	0	0
Billroth I (3)	0	3	0	0	3	0	0	0

* Includes one patient who has died.

Freezing

After Freezing			
Late (Three Mo or More)			
Achlor-hydric	Marked Dep.	No Dep.	Not Done
3	1	0	0
2	0	0	2
5	2	0	0
0	0	0	8
0	0	0	2
0	0	0	7

failure is described above; the others have been subjected to refreezing.

The residual gastric pouches of nine patients have been refrozen for recurrent melena (two patients) or for persistent pain and persistent x-ray evidence of an ulcer crater (seven patients). The gastric pouches of two of these patients were refrozen within three weeks of their initial freeze, while in three the refreeze was done six weeks after the first freeze, and in four patients an interval of three months or more intervened after the initial attempt at controlling the peptic ulcer diathesis by freezing. Of these nine, eight are now known to be essentially asymptomatic; one is considered a failure

According to Operative Procedure

Status			
Late			
Achlor-hydric	Marked Dep.	No Dep.	Not Done
8	0	0	7
1	0	0	1
0	1	0	0
2	0	0	4
0	0	0	4
0	0	0	2
0	0	0	3

and has been operated upon. One patient's stomach has been frozen a third time after an episode of melena one year after the first two freezes which were two weeks apart. In each instance refreezing has been performed with the aid of fluoroscopic placement of the gastric balloon and controlled fluoroscopic distention of the balloon to fill the gastric pouch adequately.

The three patients treated for ulcer recurrence after a Billroth I procedure were not affected significantly by their first freeze and have been subjected to a second freeze; all are included in the group discussed above. This recital will serve to emphasize the importance of technical factors in gastric freezing. Complete filling of the entire residual gastric pouch appears to be considerably easier after a Billroth II resection than is the case in the intact stomach.

Of six patients followed for six months or longer after the initial freeze, only one has had a recurrent x-ray crater with evidence of continued free HCl. He has been treated by a second gastric freeze. The three remaining patients have been followed for eight months without evidence of ulcer recurrence, pain, bleeding, or x-ray demonstration of an ulcer crater after a single session of gastric freezing.

Report of Cases

Case 1.—A 39-year-old white male had x-ray confirmation of duodenal ulcer for 20 years. Six years prior to admission he underwent total colectomy and ileostomy for ulcerative colitis. A Billroth II gastric resection for the duodenal ulcer was performed 18 months prior to admission. After resection the patient had an episode of melena approximately every 30 days. X-rays taken on admission demonstrated a definite marginal jejunal ulcer (Fig 5*A*). Gastric freezing was performed on Sept 27, 1962, for 45 minutes with an outflow temperature of the perfusate of —11 C. Secretory studies were achlorhydric both before and after the freeze.

For three weeks following the freeze, he continued to have typical ulcer pain, but the pain then disappeared. When re-examined on Nov 27, 1962, two months after freezing, he was no longer taking ulcer medication or on an ulcer diet and had gained three pounds. There has been no bleeding since freezing the residual gastric pouch. X-ray studies revealed complete healing of the jejunal ulcer (Fig

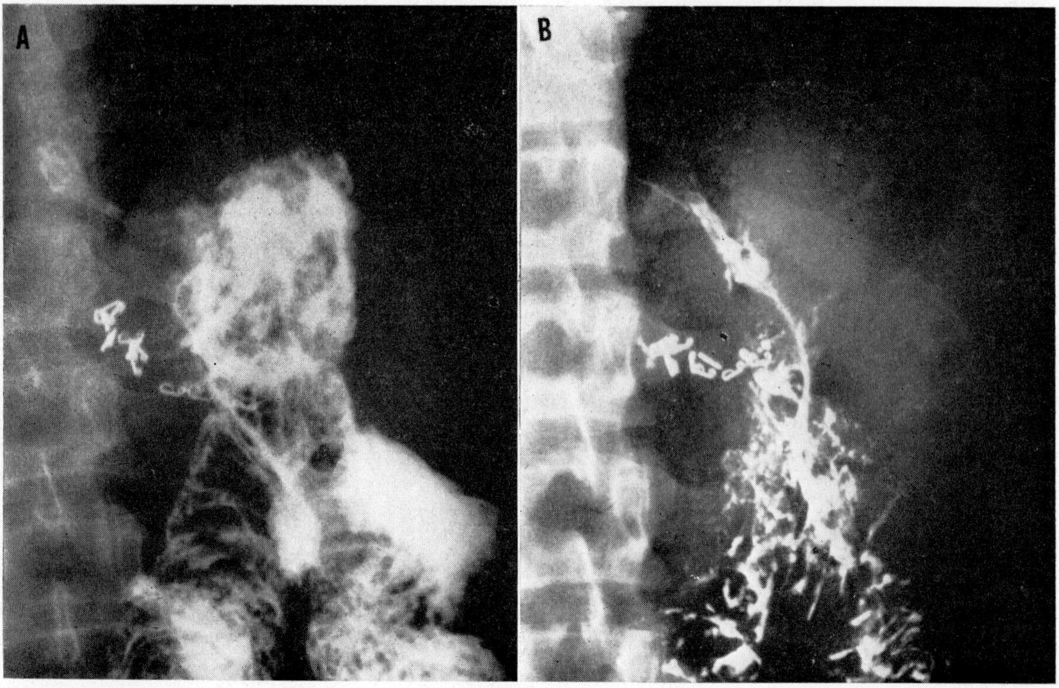

Fig 5 (case 1).—*A*, a large, rounded jejunal ulcer crater is demonstrated directly opposite the gastric stoma, one day prior to freezing. This patient also had a previous total colectomy and ileostomy for ulcerative colitis. During the 18 months between his gastric resection and the freeze, he had an episode of melena almost every month. *B*, two months after freezing, x-rays reveal complete healing of the stomal ulcer. Patient has remained asymptomatic and is no longer taking ulcer medications or observing an ulcer diet.

5*B*). Current secretory studies indicate continued achlorhydria.

Case 2.—A 46-year-old female had a peptic ulcer history dating from 1947, when she had several episodes of hematemesis, and was treated by a Billroth II gastric resection. In January, 1948, she had a gastrointestinal perforation due to a stomal ulcer, treated by closure and vagotomy. Since 1960, this patient was transfused on four occasions for anemia, associated with hematemesis in one instance. The presence of dull, gnawing, right upper quadrant pain radiating into the left lower chest demanded the ingestion of Gelusil.* On admission, a serum calcium of 11.5 mg% and phosphorus of 2.3 mg% were considered highly suggestive of parathyroid disease. Gastrointestinal x-rays revealed a definite jejunal stomal ulcer (Fig 6). Triple histamine stimulated gastric analysis prior to freezing contained 48 degrees of free acid and 68 degrees of total acid.

Gastric freezing was performed on Aug 14, 1962, for 60 minutes, with outflow temperatures averaging —12 C and a volume of 175 cc.

Laparotomy performed on Aug 20, 1962, confirmed the diagnosis of carcinoma of the pancreas, with direct invasion of the gastrojejunostomy and multiple hepatic metastases. Biopsy established the diagnosis of adenocarcinoma, metastatic to the liver, confirming the preoperative diagnosis of the Zollinger-Ellison syndrome. Repeat gastrointestinal series on Oct 10, 1962, indicated persistence of the same large chronic ulcer crater at the level of the anastomosis, probably in the wall of pancreatic tumor. There was, in addition, a new shallow ulcer crater in the proximal portion of the afferent jejunal loop, and also a shallow posterior wall ulcer in the lower portion of the lesser curve aspect of stomach. Unstimulated eight-hour overnight gastric analysis repeated on Oct 10, 1962, contained 1,275 cc, at pH 3.0 with 10 degrees of free acid. Peptone and Hollander tests were achlorhydric.

On follow-up examination, on Jan 20, 1963, the crater was unchanged and a gastric analysis revealed 350 cc at pH 1.9 with 20 degrees of free acid. In addition the patient noted the return of a few mild ulcer symptoms. Refreezing was therefore performed, with fluoroscopic control, on Jan 22, 1963. The patient noted marked improvement in symptoms following this second freeze, and gastric aspiration following the freeze contained 500 cc at pH 3.2, with 5 degrees of free acid.

* An antacid absorbent containing magnesium trisilicate and low reactive aluminum hydroxide gel.

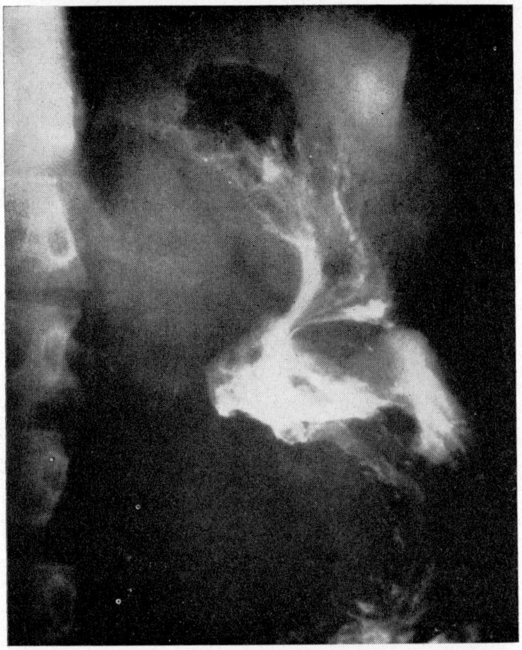

Fig 6 (case 2).—Prefreeze x-ray in a patient with a proven Zollinger-Ellison syndrome due to a malignant pancreatic tumor with direct invasion of the gastrojejunostomy stoma. The patient suffered severe ulcer pain accompanied by melena. A constant deformity of the jejunal loop, consistent with a larger crater, is seen. After freezing, this patient has been free of ulcer pain and bleeding for five months, although the crater (considered to be due to direct invasion by the malignancy at laparotomy) has not healed.

Comment

Stomal ulcer, after performance of an adequate gastric resection or partial gastrectomy and truncal vagotomy, has been attributed to the initial severity of the peptic ulcer diathesis, drug-induced hypersecretion, pancreatic tumors, and a syndrome of polyglandular disease. Such surgical inadequacies as incomplete vagotomy, poor gastric drainage, antral exclusion, insufficient resection, and a long afferent jejunal loop in the Billroth II operation directly prejudice a favorable long-term result of the operation. A number of drugs, including steroids, reserpine, caffeine, alcohol, and salicylates, also have been associated with increased gastric secretion and have been implicated as etiologic factors in recurrent ulceration.

Since 1955, the medical world has been alerted to another (Zollinger-Ellison) syndrome, characterized by marked gastric hypersecretion, hypertrophic gastric rugae, duodenal nodularity, failure to respond satisfactorily to a well-augmented medical regimen, rapid recurrence of ulceration after adequate or radical surgery, and persistent diarrhea.[8] The presence of a primary jejunal ulcer or unusually low-lying duodenal ulcer also suggests the possibility of a Zollinger-Ellison pancreatic tumor.[9,10] In addition, an abnormally high incidence of peptic ulceration has been described in association with multiglandular endocrine disease involving the pituitary, adrenal, and parathyroid glands, as well as the pancreas.[11-21] Unless an isolated pancreatic tumor can be demonstrated at operation, Zollinger has come to recommend total gastrectomy for this severe manifestation of the peptic ulcer diathesis.[22]

One patient in the presently reported stomal ulcer group has been treated satisfactorily for recurrent gastric hemorrhage from the Zollinger-Ellison syndrome by gastric freezing (case 2).

Gastric freezing appears to offer a safe and simple form of treatment for the patient with a recurrent episode of peptic ulceration, without the associated hazards of reoperation and postsurgical difficulties. To date, there has been no mortality in the entire group of 298 patients treated by gastric freezing either directly or indirectly attributable to the freezing procedure. In the stomal ulcer group, there has been one serious complication, a gastric perforation, which closed and healed spontaneously on conservative treatment.

In general, relief of pain, healing of ulcer craters, and the absence of further upper gastrointestinal tract bleeding has been observed regularly. Evidence of return of gastric secretion, recurrent bleeding, or reulceration has been treated by additional episodes of freezing. To date, more than one episode of freezing has been employed in nine patients. Only one of the stomal ulcer patients treated so far by gastric freezing has required surgery, although laparotomy was performed in one additional patient to confirm the presence of a pancreatic malignancy with multiple metastases. In this group of patients with stomal ulcer, as in the other 36 patients in the over-all freeze group treated with multiple episodes of gastric freezing to date, there has been no evidence of harm from refreezing.

Summary and Conclusions

Gastric freezing has been employed in the treatment of 33 patients with postgastrectomy stomal ulcer. Control of ulcer symptomatology, depression of gastric secretion, and x-ray evidence of healing has been observed in all but 9, following a single freeze. Eight other patients were satisfactorily controlled by refreezing. Only 1 has required surgery for control of his stomal ulcer. While follow-up in these patients is still relatively short, these results are encouraging and warrant further clinical studies and observations. Refreezing has been performed with impunity in 9 instances of recurrent or persistent stomal ulcer disease.

There has been no mortality either directly or indirectly attributable to gastric freezing among 298 * patients subjected to the freezing procedure. One major complication was observed among the group of 33 patients with stomal ulcer—perforation with a small dissection tract which healed completely on conservative treatment.

Gastric freezing appears to be a useful adjunct in the treatment of the postgastrectomy stomal ulcer patient and may come to replace surgery in many instances in the management of this condition.

Eugene F. Bernstein, MD, Department of Surgery, University of Minnesota Medical School, Minneapolis, 14, Minn.

* This group now (5-10-63) numbers 387 patients with 490 episodes of gastric freezing. There has been no mortality. The stromal ulcer freeze group now totals 39 patients.

REFERENCES

1. Wangensteen, O. H.; Root, H. D.; Jenson, C. B.; Imamoglu, K.; and Salmon, P. A.: Depression of Gastric Secretion and Digestion by Gastric Hypothermia: Its Clinical Use in Massive Hematemesis, Surgery 44:265, 1958.

2. Peter, E. T.; Bernstein, E. F.; Sosin, H.; Madsen, A. J.; Walder, A. I.; and Wangensteen, O. H.: The Role of Temperature in Controlling Gastric Digestion, JAMA 182:894, 1962.

3. Wangensteen, O. H.; Peter, E. T.; Nicoloff, D. M.; Walder, A. I.; Sosin, H.; and Bernstein, E. F.: Achieving "Physiological Gastrectomy" by Gastric Freezing: A Preliminary Report of an Experimental and Clinical Study, JAMA 180:439, 1962.

4. Wangensteen, O. H.; Peter, E. T.; Bernstein, E. F.; Walder, A. I.; Sosin, H.; and Madsen, A. J.: Can Physiological Gastrectomy Be Achieved by Gastric Freezing? Ann Surg 156:579, 1962.

5. Peter, E. T.; Bernstein, E. F.; Walder, A. I.; Madsen, A. J.; Sosin, H.; and Wangensteen, O. H.: The Effect of Profound Gastric Hypothermia (Gastric Freezing) Upon Various Phases of Gastric Secretion, Surg Forum 13:269, 1962.

6. Peter, E. T.; Bernstein, E. F.; Sosin, H.; Madsen, A. J.; Walder, A. I.; and Wangensteen, O. H.: Technique of Gastric Freezing in the Treatment of Duodenal Ulcer, JAMA 181:760, 1962.

7. Bernstein, E. F.; Sosin, H.; Madsen, A. J.; McFee, A. S.; Goodale, R. L., Jr.; Allcock, E. A.; and Wangensteen, O. H.: Results of Gastric Freezing for Peptic Ulcer, Univ Minn Med Bull 34:108, 1962.

8. Zollinger, R. M., and Ellison, E. H.: Primary Peptic Ulcerations of the Jejunum Associated With Islet Cell Tumors of the Pancreas, Ann Surg 142:709, 1955.

9. Forty, F., and Barrett, G. M.: Peptic Ulceration of the Third Part of Duodenum Associated With Islet-Cell Tumours of Pancreas, Brit J Surg 40:60, 1952.

10. Oberhelman, H. A., Jr.; Nelson, T. S.; Johnson, A. N., Jr.; and Dragstedt, L. R., II: Ulcerogenic Tumors of the Duodenum, Ann Surg 153:214, 1961.

11. Cope, O.: Hyperparathyroidism: Diagnosis and Management, Amer J Surg 99:394, 1960.

12. Jackson, C. E.: The Association of Peptic Ulcer With Hereditary Hyperparathyroidism, Gastroenterology 37:35, 1959.

13. Mieher, W. C., Jr.; Hartsock, R. J.; Geokas, M. C.; Ballard, H. S.; and Frame, B.: Peptic Ulcer as a Manifestation of Familial Polyendocrine Disease, JAMA 179:854, 1962.

14. Moses, A. M.: Gastrointestinal Manifestations of Primary Hyperparathyroidism: Experience at Mount Sinai Hospital and Review of Literature, J Mount Sinai Hosp NY 25:339, 1958.

15. Ostrow, J. D.; Blanshard, G.; and Grey, S. J.: Peptic Ulcer in Primary Hyperparathyroidism, Amer J Med 29:769, 1960.

16. Riddick, F. A., Jr., and Reiss, E.: Hyperparathyroidism: Analysis of Recent Experiences, Clinical Spectrum, and Diagnostic Tests, Ann Intern Med 56:183, 1962.

17. Rogers, H. M.; Keating, F. R., Jr.; Morlock, C. G.; and Barker, N. W.: Primary Hyper-

trophy and Hyperplasia of Parathyroid Glands Associated With Duodenal Ulcer: Report of Additional Case With Special Reference to Metabolic Gastrointestinal and Vascular Manifestations, Arch Intern Med 79:307, 1947.

18. Schiffrin, M. J.: Relationship Between the Parathyroid and the Gastric Glands in the Dog, Amer J Physiol 135:660, 1942.

19. Spiro, H. M.: Hyperparathyroidism, Parathyroid "Adenomas" and Peptic Ulcer, Gastroenterology 39:554, 1960.

20. Wilder, W. T.; Frame, B.; and Haubrich, W. S.: Peptic Ulcer in Primary Hyperparathyroidism: An Analysis of 52 Cases, Ann Intern Med 55:885, 1961.

21. Block, M. A.; Smith, R. F.; Haubrich, W. S.; and Horn, R. C.: Surgical Problems in Management of Islet-Cell Tumors With Gastric Hypersecretion, Arch Surg 85:270, 1962.

22. Zollinger, R. M.; Elliott, D. W.; Endahl, G. L.; Grant, G. N.; Goswitz, John T.; and Taft, D. A.: Origin of the Ulcerogenic Hormone in Endocrine Induced Ulcer, Ann Surg 156:570, 1962.

A Critical Evaluation of Total Gastrectomy

KENT W. BARBER, JR., MD; WILLIAM H. ReMINE, MD; JAMES T. PRIESTLEY, MD; AND ROBERT P. GAGE, MS, ROCHESTER, MINN

Since Schlatter performed the first successful total gastrectomy in 1897, many reports on this subject have appeared, especially in the last two decades. Prior to the report of Finney and Rienhoff in 1929, the literature consisted largely of occasional reports of one or two successful cases. These authors collected 67 cases in which total gastrectomy had been performed with a mortality rate of 53.8%. Since 1929, a number of series of total gastrectomies have been reported.

Pack and McNeer, in 1943, completed an excellent collective review of the literature on total gastrectomy for cancer, and they included an original report of 20 cases of their own. The collective operative mortality rate was 37.6%. Lahey and Marshall,[5] in 1944, reported on 73 cases in which total gastrectomy had been performed with a mortality of 33%. Waugh and Fahlund, in 1945, reported 77 cases of total gastrectomy performed at the Mayo Clinic from 1917 through 1943 with an over-all mortality rate of 44.2%.

Read at the meeting of the Central Surgical Association, Chicago, Feb 21-23, 1963.

Fellow in Surgery, Mayo Foundation (Dr. Barber); Section of Surgery (Drs. ReMine and Priestley); Section of Biometry and Medical Statistics (Mr. Gage).

Beginning in the late 1940's, reports appeared in the literature, which illustrated that modern improvements in surgery were associated with a reduction in the previously high mortality rate to a reasonable level. Longmire, in 1947, presented 20 cases with a mortality rate of 10%; Wangensteen, in 1949, presented 28 cases with a mortality rate of 3.5%; and Lahey and Marshall,[6] in 1950, reported 64 cases with a mortality rate of 9.4%. In 1952, ReMine and Priestley reported 108 cases in which total gastrectomy had been performed during the years 1945 to 1949, inclusive, with a mortality rate of 12.9%. Marshall and Uram reported 127 cases, in 1954, with a mortality rate of 8.7%, and, in 1956, Ransom reported 50 cases with a mortality rate of 18.0%. Fly and coworkers, in 1958, reported a mortality rate of 16.4% in 134 cases in which total gastrectomy had been performed during the years 1950 to 1954 at the Mayo Clinic. More recent series reported by Welch and Wilkins, in 1958, Cornell and co-workers, in 1960, and Rush and co-workers, in 1960, showed hospital mortality rates to be 8.3%, 5.6%, and 16.4%, respectively.

McNeer and Pack, in 1954, stimulated interest by first reporting a mortality rate of

TABLE 1.—*Total Gastrectomy for Carcinoma of Stomach, 1917 Through 1961: Hospital Mortality*

	Total			1960 to 1961			1950 to 1959		
		Died in Hospital			Died in Hospital			Died in Hospital	
Associated procedure	Patients	No.	%	Patients	No.	%	Patients	No.	%
Partial pancreatectomy, splenectomy, omentectomy	52	15	28.8	4	1	25.0	30	8	26.7
Splenectomy, omentectomy	239	40	16.7	21	3	14.3	147	26	17.7
Omentectomy	51	6	11.8	0	0		28	2	7.1
None	72	29	40.3	0	0		1	0	0.0
Total	414	90	21.7	25	4	16.0	206	36	17.5

26.3% for cases in which "extended" total gastrectomy, which included en bloc resection of omenta, spleen, and tail of the pancreas, had been carried out. McNeer and associates,[10] in 1956, reported a mortality rate of 23.3% for similar cases, and, in 1960, Lawrence and McNeer reported a rate of 19.2%. Welch and Wilkins, in 1958, reported a mortality rate of 15.4% where extended total gastrectomy had been performed for cure. In their extended gastrectomy, portions of contiguous structures such as the transverse colon, pancreas, and liver were excised together with the primary tumor—sometimes the spleen was included in the specimen.

One of the earliest reports of late results after total gastrectomy was by Lahey, in 1950, who reported a three-year survival rate of 21%. ReMine and Priestley reported an 18% five-year survival rate in 1952, while Marshall and Uram reported a 14.7% five-year survival rate in 1954. Fly and coworkers in 1958 presented a series of 188 cases in which total gastrectomy had been performed for cancer with survival rates of 17.6% for three years, 12% for five years, and 8.8% for ten years. Rush, Brown, and Ravitch, in 1960, reported a 9% five-year survival rate. In 1960, Lawrence and McNeer presented the first long-term results following extended, radical, total gastrectomy; they reported a 21.4% five-year survival rate.

Material and Methods

The present study was based on a group of 479 patients on whom total gastrectomies were performed during the years 1917 through 1961, inclusive. The majority of these operations were carried out for gastric neoplasm (439 patients including 25 with sarcoma), but a few were done for benign gastric lesions which, for the most part, could not be accurately diagnosed at the time of operation, and two were done for esophageal squamous cell epithelioma. Total gastrectomy was employed for malignant lesions only when all involved tissue could not be removed by subtotal gastrectomy. Over a period of many years, this procedure has been used in approximately 15% to 20% of all patients who have had gastric resections performed for cancer at the Mayo Clinic.

TABLE 2.—*Total Gastrectomy: Hospital Mortality According to Type*

				Type o					
	Total			Esophagojejunostomy With Enteroanastomosis			Esophagojejunostomy Without Enteroanastomosis		
		Died in Hospital			Died in Hospital			Died in Hospital	
Period, Years	Patients	No.	%	Patients	No.	%	Patients	No.	%
Before 1940	36	22	61.1	25	16	64.0	9	4	44.4
1940-1949	180	40	22.2	116	25	21.6	48	12	25.0
1950-1959	234	41	17.5	143	22	15.4	33	7	21.2
1960-1961	29	4	13.8	20	2	10.0	0	0	—
Total	479	107	22.3	304	65	21.4	90	23	25.6

According to Operative Procedure

1940 to 1949			Before 1940		
	Died in Hospital			Died in Hospital	
Patients	No.	%	Patients	No.	%
18	6	33.3	0	0	
70	10	14.3	1	1	100.0
22	3	13.6	1	1	100.0
42	11	26.2	29	18	62.1
152	30	19.7	31	20	64.5

Associated Surgery

We have usually performed a "conservative" total gastrectomy for malignant lesions of the stomach, that is, we have removed adjacent structures only when there has been evidence of involvement in these areas (Table 1). Of 414 patients operated on for carcinoma of the stomach, only 52 or 12.6% had what could be termed an "extended radical operation" with removal of part of the pancreas, in addition to the spleen and portions of the esophagus, duodenum, and omentum. This procedure was performed, in most cases, only when involvement of the pancreas was apparent or suspected. From 239 patients or 57.8%, the spleen and omentum were removed; from 51 or 12.3%, only the omentum was removed. No associated structures were removed from 72 patients or 17.4%; all but one of these patients were operated on before 1950. In a few cases, removal of additional structures, such as portions of the diaphragm, liver, or colon, was carried out.

of Anastomosis

Anastomosis					
Esophagoduodenostomy			Roux-Y and Miscellaneous		
	Died in Hospital			Died in Hospital	
Patients	No.	%	Patients	No.	%
1	1	100.0	1	1	100.0
14	3	21.4	2	0	0.0
42	8	19.0	16	4	25.0
4	0	0.0	5	2	40.0
61	12	19.7	24	7	29.2

It is of interest and of some practical significance that operative mortality is definitely higher when a more extensive operation is performed. Thus for the years 1950 to 1961, the mortality for total gastrectomy, partial pancreatectomy, splenectomy, and omentectomy was 26.5%; for total gastrectomy, splenectomy, and omentectomy, 17.3%; and for total gastrectomy and omentectomy, 7.1%. These figures cannot be accepted as showing differences in operative mortality strictly depending on the extent of the operative procedure, as, in general, it is true that more extensive lesions were present when more extensive operations were performed. Nevertheless, they may be of some significance, as one might reasonably expect an increase in operative mortality as the scope of operation is extended.

Restoration of Gastrointestinal Continuity

Several methods were used to restore gastrointestinal continuity in the present series of patients (Table 2). In most cases (63.4%), continuity was reestablished after total removal of the stomach by an end-to-side esophagojejunal anastomosis, with an enteroanastomosis between the jejunal limbs. In a small group (18.8%), end-to-side esophagojejunal anastomosis was used without an additional anastomosis between the jejunal limbs. In 12.7% of the patients, end-to-end esophagoduodenal anastomosis was employed, and the Roux-Y type, or some other type, of anastomosis was used in the remaining 5%.

Table 2 shows that during the years 1940 to 1959, the operative mortality rate was lower when an enteroanastomosis between the jejunal limbs was employed in association with end-to-side esophagojejunal anastomosis than when it was not used. Attention is drawn to our experience in this regard, as some surgeons have reported differently and have suggested that the jejunojejunal anastomosis should be omitted. In our practice, this anastomosis is omitted only under unusual circumstances. It serves to assure decompression of the proximal jejunal loop

TABLE 3.—*Total Gastrectomy: Survival Rates*

Diagnosis	Three Years or More After Operation * Patients at Risk	Survived No.	Survived %	Five Years or More After Operation * Patients at Risk	Survived No.	Survived %	Ten Years or More After Operation * Patients at Risk	Survived No.	Survived %
Carcinoma	275	42	15.3	242	24	9.9	152	12	7.9
Sarcoma	14	8	57.2	14	7	50.0	9	4	44.4
Benign	26	23	88.5	25	21	84.0	18	11	61.2

* Inquiry as of Jan 1, 1961: 3-year group includes patients operated on 3 or more years before inquiry, that is, in 1957 or earlier; 5-year group, those operated on in 1955, or earlier; 10-year group, those operated on in 1950, or earlier. Hospital mortality is excluded in calculation of survival rates.

as well as to prevent reflux esophagitis. It is apparent from the data in Table 2 that we do not employ replacement operations in association with total gastrectomy. It is also apparent that there has been a gradual reduction in operative mortality over the years, although in our experience the risk of total gastrectomy remains definitely higher than for partial or subtotal gastrectomy.

Pathologic Characteristics

The pathologic diagnosis was adenocarcinoma of the stomach in 414 of the 479 patients; sarcoma, either leiomyosarcoma or lymphosarcoma, in 25; and a benign lesion in 38. In two cases, the diagnosis was squamous cell epithelioma of the esophagus. Thus, total gastrectomy was performed on some patients who did not have a malignant lesion; this was done because of a large indurated gastric ulcer which was thought to be malignant, because of an ulcerating lesion adjacent to the esophagogastric junction which likewise was considered to be malignant, or, in the exceptional case, because of recurrent peptic ulceration. Total gastrectomy is not recommended for benign lesions, except under most exceptional conditions of which the Zollinger-Ellison syndrome might be an example.

Survival Rates

Survival rates, based on follow-up data on patients who survived operation, are grouped according to pathologic diagnosis (Table 3). The three-year survival rate for patients who had total gastrectomy performed for carcinoma was 15.3%; the five-year rate, 9.9%; and the ten-year rate, 7.9%. These rates are somewhat lower than those reported by ReMine and Priestley, in 1952, and by Fly and co-workers, in 1958. It may be that in recent years total gastrectomy has been employed in a higher percentage of patients with less favorable lesions than in former years. This possibility is supported by the fact that in our experience the operability and resectability rates of patients with cancer of the stomach have gradually increased. As a corollary, it might be mentioned that, unfortunately, the percentage of patients undergoing resection for gastric cancer with lymph-node involvement has not decreased.

Our five-year survival rates are compatible with those of other series recently reported in the literature: Welch and Wilkins, in 1958, reported 380 cases with a 12.9% five-year survival rate. Stensrud, in 1959, reported 160 personal cases with a 10.5% five-year survival rate. Rush and co-workers, in 1960, reported 70 cases with a five-year survival rate of 9.0%. These comparative results demonstrate that total gastrectomy is a worthwhile procedure for a limited number of patients with extensive carcinoma of the stomach.

Our experience with patients who have had total gastrectomy for sarcoma is limited. For 14 patients, the three-year survival rate was 57.2%, the five-year rate, 50.0%, and the ten-year rate, 44.4%. These rates are definitely better than those for the larger group of patients with carcinoma.

TABLE 4.—*Total Gastrectomy for Carcinoma of Stomach: 5-Year Survival Rates According to Grade of Malignancy*

Grade of Malignancy (Broders')	Five Years or More After Operation * Patients at Risk	Survived No.	Survived %
1 and 2	19	8	42.1
3	40	7	17.5
4	183	9	4.9
Total	242	24	9.9

* Inquiry as of Jan 1, 1961. Included here are data on only those patients operated on in 1955, or earlier. Hospital mortality is excluded in the calculation of survival rates.

Of the 25 patients surviving total gastrectomy for benign disease, 21 or 84% survived five years; of 18 patients, 61.2% survived ten years. It is of interest that 17 of those who lived five years were still living at the time of the present study.

Two factors which influence survival rates most significantly are the histologic grade of the lesion (Broders') and the presence or absence of lymph-node metastasis. Table 4 shows that, although the majority of lesions were of a high grade, 42.1% of the patients with grade 1 and grade 2 lesions survived five years, while only 17.5% and 4.9%, respectively, of the patients with grade 3 and grade 4 lesions did so. Nineteen per cent of the patients without lymph-node metastasis lived five years, but this figure was reduced to 5.9% when patients had lymph-node metastasis (Table 5).

Whether extension of total gastrectomy to include routine partial pancreatectomy significantly increases survival rates, we believe remains to be determined. Partial pancreatectomy was performed in only 52 of our 414 cases with cancer and was usually employed in these cases for actual or suspected pancreatic involvement by the carcinoma. Our data, therefore, supply no information as to whether routine inclusion of the tail of the pancreas, in all cases in which total gastrectomy is performed, would or would not increase survival rates. According to our experience, however, the hospital mortality rate for these 52 patients was

TABLE 5.—*Total Gastrectomy for Carcinoma of Stomach With and Without Metastasis to Lymph Nodes: 5-Year Survival Rates*

Lymph-Node Metastasis	Five Years or More After Operation * Patients at Risk	Survived No.	Survived %
Present	170	10	5.9
Absent	72	14	19.4
Total	242	24	9.9

* Inquiry as of Jan 1, 1961. Included here are only those patients operated on in 1955, or earlier. Hospital mortality is excluded in the calculation of survival rates.

28.8%, which is significantly higher than for patients from whom a portion of the pancreas was not removed. This has been found also in the series reported by McNeer and Pack in 1954, in which the mortality rate for extended radical total gastrectomy (including a portion of the pancreas) was 26.3%, while that for "simple" total gastrectomy was 11.4%; Welch and Wilkins, in 1958, reported mortality rates of 27.7% and 15.4%, respectively, for these procedures; and more recently Lawrence and McNeer reported 19.2% and 22.2%, respectively.

In calculating five-year survival rates according to associated procedures (Table 6), it is evident that increasing the extent of the operation to include partial pancreatectomy did not improve the prognosis. As just mentioned, however, in most of our cases partial

TABLE 6.—*Total Gastrectomy for Carcinoma of Stomach: 5-Year Survival Rates According to Associated Procedures*

Associated Procedure	Five or More Years After Operation * Patients at Risk	Survived No.	Survived %
Partial pancreatectomy, splenectomy, omentectomy	24	2	8.3
Splenectomy, omentectomy	139	15	10.8
Omentectomy	37	3	8.1
None	42	4	9.5
Total	242	24	9.9

* Inquiry as of January 1, 1961. Included here are data on those patients operated on in 1955, or earlier. Hospital deaths are excluded in calculation of survival rates.

pancreatectomy was performed for apparent involvement, not as a routine procedure.

General Health of Survivors

Follow-up studies are available regarding the well-being of 46 patients who have survived total gastrectomy for periods ranging from less than 5 years (10 patients) to more than 15 years (nine patients). In spite of total removal of the stomach, 76% of the group of 46 patients considered their health to be good. All patients lost weight prior to operation, but 35 (76%) of the group gained weight after operation. Of these, 11 regained their normal weight, one was within 5 pounds of his normal preoperative weight; eight were within 10 pounds, five were within 15 pounds, and 10 were within 25 pounds.

Only 12 patients or 26.2% of the 46 stated that they ate as much as they had prior to operation; 13 patients ate three fourths as much; 18 patients, one half as much; and three patients, one fourth as much. As could be expected, only 16 patients ate only three meals a day, while the remainder made a habit of eating at several times a day in addition to their regular mealtimes. Approximately one half of the group experienced some fullness after eating; seven other patients had mild to moderate symptoms of dumping. Approximately 40% of the patients had loose stools or diarrhea postoperatively. Anemia was known to develop postoperatively in approximately three fourths of the group, but it responded satisfactorily to medication.

What is important concerning rehabilitation of patients after total gastrectomy is that 76% of the survivors or 35 patients were able to return to their former jobs, usually within six to eight months after surgery.

Comment

The results of the surgical treatment of carcinoma of the stomach are far from satisfactory; yet, in our series patients surviving total gastrectomy, 42 of 275 or 15.3% survived three years or more, 24 of 242 or 9.9% survived five years or more, and 12 of 152 or 7.9% survived ten years or more after operation. Although these numbers are small, they demonstrate that some people with carcinoma of the stomach can survive for appreciable periods after total gastrectomy for cancer. The results of total gastrectomy for sarcoma, on the other hand, have been more encouraging, as 50% of these patients have survived five years. Most of the patients with sarcoma received postoperative irradiation.

One of the unresolved questions pertaining to performance of total gastrectomy for cancer relates to the extent of the operation which should be routinely performed. Welch and Wilkins (1958) stated that the "extended" total gastrectomy constituted the procedure of choice for patients who had a cancer of the body or fundus of the stomach and were in reasonably good condition. Lawrence and McNeer (1960) advocated this procedure for lesions situated proximally in the stomach when evidence of metastasis to adjacent lymph nodes is present.

To us, it would seem unwise for all surgeons who might perform total gastrectomy to remove a portion of the pancreas routinely until the evidence regarding the value of this practice is more complete and convincing. In this evaluation, survival rates must of course be balanced against operative mortality rates. Although a theoretical "case" can be made for increasing the extent of operation for many different types of cancer, actual experience must provide the final answer. It appears that, at some stage in this process, the law of diminishing returns would make itself evident. We believe that total gastrectomy should not be employed if it is apparent that all areas of malignant involvement cannot be removed. In other words, total gastrectomy is not an appropriate palliative procedure.

Summary

Experience with 479 patients who underwent total gastrectomy at the Mayo Clinic during the years 1917 through 1961, inclusive, was reviewed. Most of these patients (414) were operated on for adenocarcinoma.

The over-all hospital mortality rate from 1917 through 1961 was 22.3%, with the rate being 13.8% in 1960 to 1961, inclusive. Extended radical total gastrectomy, including an *en bloc* resection of the greater and lesser omenta, the spleen, and the distal portion of the pancreas, was carried out in 52 patients in whom actual involvement of the pancreas was noted. End-to-side esophagojejunal anastomosis with enteroanastomosis between the limbs of the jejunal loop was the type of restoration of gastrointestinal continuity used most often (63.4% of cases). It was found that 9.9% of patients who had total gastrectomy for carcinoma survived five years, and 7.9% survived ten years. Total gastrectomy was employed only in instances where the malignancy could not be extirpated by a less extensive resection.

Mayo Clinic, Rochester, Minn.

REFERENCES

1. Cornell, G. N.; Gilder, H.; Moody, F.; McSherry, C. K.; and Beal, J. M.: The Use of Jejunal Interposition With Total Gastrectomy, Ann Surg 152:430-444 (Sept) 1960.

2. Finney, J. M. T., and Rienhoff, W. F., Jr.: Gastrectomy, Arch Surg 18:140-162 (Jan) 1929.

3. Fly, O. A., Jr.; Priestley, J. T.; Comfort, M. W.; and Gage, R. P.: Total Gastrectomy: Mortality and Survival, Ann Surg 147:760-768 (May) 1958.

4. Lahey, F. H.: Total Gastrectomy for All Patients With Operable Cancer of the Stomach (Editorial), Surg Gynec Obstet 90:241-248 (Feb) 1950.

5. Lahey, F. H., and Marshall, S. F.: Indications For, and Experiences With, Total Gastrectomy: Based Upon 73 Cases of Total Gastrectomy, Ann Surg 119:300-320 (March) 1944.

6. Lahey, F. H., and Marshall, S. F.: Should Total Gastrectomy Be Employed in Early Carcinoma of the Stomach? Experience With 139 Total Gastrectomies, Ann Surg 132:540-560 (Sept) 1950.

7. Lawrence, W. J., Jr., and McNeer, Gordon: An Analysis of the Role of Radical Surgery for Gastric Cancer, Surg Gynec Obstet 111:691-696 (Dec) 1960.

8. Longmire, W. P., Jr.: Total Gastrectomy for Carcinoma of the Stomach, Surg Gynec Obstet 84:21-30 (Jan) 1947.

9. Marshall, S. F., and Uram, H.: Total Gastrectomy for Gastric Cancer: Effect Upon Mortality, Morbidity, and Curability, Surg Gynec Obstet 99:657-675 (Dec) 1954.

10. McNeer, G.; Lawrence, W., Jr.; Ortega, L. G.; and Sunderland, D. A.: Early Results of Extended Total Gastrectomy for Cancer, Cancer 9:1153-1159 (Nov Dec) 1956.

11. McNeer, G., and Pack, G. T.: Postoperative Mortality Following Total Gastrectomy, Cancer 7:1010-1015 (Sept) 1954.

12. Pack, G. T., and McNeer, G.: Total Gastrectomy for Cancer: A Collective Review of the Literature and an Original Report of 20 Cases, Surg Gynec Obstet 77:265-299 (Oct) 1943.

13. Ransom, H. K.: Cancer of the Stomach: A Report on Cases Treated by Total Gastrectomy, Gastroenterology 30:191-205 (Feb) 1956.

14. ReMine, W. H., and Priestley, J. T.: Late Results After Total Gastrectomy, Surg Gynec Obstet 94:519-525 (May) 1952.

15. Rush, B. F., Jr.; Brown, M. W.; and Ravitch, M. M.: Total Gastrectomy: An Evaluation of Its Use in the Treatment of Gastric Cancer, Cancer 13:643-648 (May-June) 1960.

16. Schlatter, C.: A Unique Case of Complete Removal of the Stomach—Successful Esophago-Enterostomy—Recovery, Med Rec 52:909-914 (Dec 25) 1897.

17. Stensrud, N.: Late Results After Total Gastrectomy for High Gastric Carcinoma, Ann Surg 150:63-66 (July) 1959.

18. Wangensteen, O. H.: Technical Suggestions in the Performance of Total Gastrectomy: The Posterior Esophagojejunal Buttress; Use of Air-Vent Suction Drain; Accompanying Coincidental Superior Mesenteric Ganglionectomy to Improve Reservoir Capacity, Surgery 25:766-775 (May) 1949.

19. Waugh, J. M., and Fahlund, G. T. R.: Total Gastrectomy, Surg Clin N Amer 25:903-917 (Aug) 1945.

20. Welch, C. E., and Wilkins, E. W., Jr.: Carcinoma of the Stomach, Ann Surg 148:666-681 (Oct) 1958.

DISCUSSION

On papers by Drs. Grant et al, Bernstein et al, and Barber et al.

Dr. Louis T. Palumbo, Des Moines, Iowa: Dr. Grant and associates have presented a subject which continues to be one of our major surgical problems. Their results reflect the favorable downward trend in mortality associated with this most fearsome complication of duodenal or gastric ulcers.

Recently we completed a study of 702 of our cases treated for bleeding during the past 16 years. Average age of the patients was 55 years; 17% were 60 years or older. A total of 331 (47%) were massive bleeders, and in 157, or 47% of the cases, emergency surgery was necessary. From 1946 to 1957, a partial gastrectomy, of the three-fourth type, Billroth II anastomosis, with removal of the ulcer was performed in all patients.

Eighty-one patients were in this group; there were ten deaths, a mortality rate of 12.8%.

From 1957 to 1963, sixty patients were operated upon as an emergency measure for massive bleeding. In this group we employed our distal antrectomy, removing 25% or less of the stomach, with a bilateral vagectomy, using a Billroth II anastomosis. There were three deaths, or a 5% mortality. During the past 1½ years, we have performed a pyloroplasty with vagotomy in only the poor-risk and the elderly patients and in those cases where resection of the ulcer would be difficult. This procedure was performed upon 16 patients; there were two deaths, a mortality rate of 12.5%.

In the group of patients with moderate or massive hemorrhage who had stopped bleeding upon admission to the hospital and for whom the surgical-medical team recommended delayed surgical intervention, the mortality was much lower, being 5.9%. It was 9.7% for patients over 50 years of age as compared to 3.3% for patients under 50.

In recent years our mortality rate continues to show a progressive decline. This is based upon many factors, among which are earlier surgical intervention and that younger patients are being referred for surgical treatment earlier and during an episode of bleeding.

The mortality rate is greatly influenced by the degree and duration of hemorrhage, the age of the patients, the degree of liaison between physician and surgeon, the effectiveness of organized positive treatment and ancillary supportive measures, surgical judgment and experience, and, *finally,* the surgical procedure performed.

Dr. Walter Gerwig, Jr., Clarksburg, W Va: After such a tremendous number of cases as have been reported by Dr. ReMine and his co-workers, I feel reluctant to state the small number of our patients.

In 1956, we began to employ interposition of a piece of transverse colon between the esophagus and the duodenum in an attempt to improve the nutritional balance in the postgastrectomy patient.

This slide merely depicts the nature of the preparation using the transverse colon. You will note it is in an antiperistaltic position. By the use of this preparation it was our hope that we could restore continuity, that we would be able to stimulate both bile and pancreatic secretion by enabling the food to go over the duodenum, and finally we thought it would provide a reservoir that might have some triturary action.

We have recently reported a five-year follow-up of the nine patients we had. Five of them were operated on for malignant disease and did not survive.

The four patients who have survived were operated on for benign lesions. It will be noted that all of them still suffer from anorexia, and that anemia and weakness play a rather important part, with the exception of the first patient shown. There is a considerable amount of weight loss, as evidenced from their best weight to their current weight. Copious regurgitation occurred in three of the four patients. This is interesting because the propulsive action of the colon in the reverse peristaltic position would fill up with secretions, and lying down at night would result in the patient almost drowning in his own intestinal juices. Fetid eructations unfortunately have persisted for over five years in one of the individuals.

There was a great deal of discussion in the symposium this morning concerning bile esophagitis. We had that to a very distressing degree in one patient, who required a transection of the common duct and ultimately Roux en Y reconstruction. Pain was a factor in one patient. They all agreed their bowel habits were quite normal, but I think they had so many problems higher up that they paid very little attention to their lower intestinal tract.

Dr. Stanley Hoerr, Cleveland: I should like to emphasize the importance of terminology and semantics when we try to communicate with each other in a disease as subjective as duodenal ulcer. We have learned, for example, to distinguish massive bleeding occurring rapidly from massive bleeding occurring slowly. The problems they present are quite different.

The first paper pointed out the distinction between patients requiring a transfusion of six units of blood and those merely having a low hemoglobin. I think it is equally important for us to distinguish between patients requiring an emergency operation and those who do not. It has been helpful to us to distinguish between "emergency," "urgent," and "elective" operations for hemorrhage. We use the term "emergency" to apply to patients who have to be taken to the operating room unscheduled and "urgent" to apply to those who cannot wait indefinitely but perhaps who can wait a few hours until they can be done as part of a regular schedule.

I think this concept will be useful in evaluating the place of gastric cooling. Like Drs. Grant, Kelley, and Elliott, we too feel that gastric cooling is going to have a place, particularly in the poor-risk patient, in converting someone who might otherwise require an emergency operation into someone who can be tided over into an urgent, but scheduled, operation.

Finally, I think it is going to be extremely important to distinguish between gastric cooling and gastric freezing. Cooling we believe has proved its place. Freezing we believe has yet to be proved. I think perhaps it might be well to let more time elapse before we pass judgment on gastric freezing.

I noticed on one slide shown by Dr. Bernstein that he said it was "too early to evaluate" certain of the patients who had had a gastric freezing. I suggest that it is "too early to evaluate" any of the patients whom he reported; perhaps we should set a minimum five-year limit for follow-up as a standard, just as we do in cancer.

I know Dr. Wagensteen and his associates were well aware of the need for a long-term follow-up, and they will get it for us. I do believe the rest of us should wait for them to find out just what these late results will be, before we all go out and buy freezing machines and start treating ulcers in this fashion.

Dr. Howard E. Dorton, Lexington, Ky: The gravity of the bleeding ulcer problem is clearly emphasized in this excellent presentation by Drs. Grant, Kelley, and Elliott. Their mortality rates are essentially the same as those reported from other good medical centers. I doubt seriously if much improvement can be made on those figures as long as resection is routinely employed.

In 1947, in an effort to improve on these mortality figures (which were much higher then), we began using a simpler procedure, that of ligation of the bleeding point, followed by vagotomy and pyloroplasty. Since that time we have employed it on 141 consecutive bleeders of all degrees of severity—53 of these were massive bleeders—and this without mortality, with not a single instance of recurrent bleeding in the immediate postoperative period, and with only three late recurrences of ulcer bleeding.

Since we have had scattered reports of an occasional failure with the method, we thought it might be appropriate to re-emphasize some of the technical points that we consider responsible for our success with the method.

Adequate exposure can be made easier by wide Kocherization of the duodenum and intraluminal elevation and exposure of the ulcer with ordinary Sawyer proctologic retractors, as illustrated in this mock bleeding ulcer preparation from the dog laboratory. Secure transfixion of the ulcer base is easy to accomplish with this exposure. The ulcer is oversewn with heavy chromic catgut. We do not use silk because we fear it might cause granuloma formation and recurrent bleeding.

Of course, a complete vagotomy and a wide-open pyloroplasty is a must. We prefer the Finney operation. Equally important is the postoperative management.

We think it is vitally necessary to suppress, insofar as possible, the remaining gastric phase of gastric secretion to prevent the recently placed sutures from being digested away by acid of antral hormonal origin. This we accomplish by means of constant suction on our feeding-suction gastrostomy tube. We look with disfavor upon overflow drainage from a gastrostomy tube because this would not neutralize the antral phase; in fact, it would stimulate gastrin formation. We use constant suction for five days, and then, when the patient is placed on oral feedings, he is instructed in postural drainage of the atonic vagotomized stomach after every intake to keep the stomach as dry as possible between feedings. I apologize for reciting these technical points in detail, but I feel sure they are responsible for our continuing success with the method.

Above all, we adhere to the doctrine that there is no substitute for survival and that this predominant factor should far outweigh any argument regarding the long-term efficacy of any other procedure of greater magnitude.

Dr. Robert M. Zollinger, Columbus, Ohio: Dr. Bernstein and associates have now extended the principle of gastric freezing to a most challenging group of ulcer patients. I am sure their patients readily welcomed this new form of treatment since they have already been disappointed with the results of surgery. If surgeons adhered more to establish physiologic principles and performed the operation properly there should be fewer and fewer recurrent ulcers unless a potent gastric secretogogue is being produced outside the stomach.

A review of 105 recurrent ulcers seen on our surgical service implicated the surgeon in three out of five cases. Blind devotion to a particular technique combined with either incomplete or nonphysiologic procedures were the usual causes. In one fourth of our patients the recurrent ulceration was associated with drugs, in our opinion, rather than the fault of the operation. One or all of the following were consumed by these patients each day: more than ten cups of coffee, two packages of cigarettes, three cocktails, or twelve tablets containing acetylsalicylic acid. Drugs given for the control of arthritis or hypertension were responsible in some instances. In one half of Dr. Bernstein's cases, there was gastrointestinal bleeding without a proven ulcer by x-ray. Certainly, we would all agree that withdrawal of such potent gastric secretogogues or irritants should control the ulcer diathesis and make either surgery or gastric freezing unnecessary except for the control of persistent massive hemorrhage.

Recurrent ulcer associated with the endocrine glands is a more serious problem and occurred in one in ten of our patients. Removal of a parathyroid adenoma or the solitary nonbeta-cell adenoma of the pancreas should suffice. Unfortunately the ulcerogenic tumors of the pancreas are often malignant as well as multiple, making total gastrectomy mandatory to control the fulminating ulcer diathesis. Since irradiation has not controlled the output of acid in these patients, we have advised total gastrectomy even in the presence of liver metastasis. The method of Dr. Bernstein offers a much better solution to the problem, and I would support gastric freezing in these unfortunate patients although I suspect the beneficial effect would be very short. I would like to suggest to these workers that they study the return of gastric acidity in dogs which have had gastric hypersecretion induced by complete pancreatic duct ligation.

I would like to ask Dr. Bernstein how he is going to approach the recurrent ulcer problem in patients having the mechanism for the continuous overproduction of gastrin from either a distended antrum or a retained antral stump. To this group should be added the patient who has had an enteroenterostomy as a part of a Billroth II resection. Finally, I would like to ask him about the nutritional status of these patients after freezing, and, lastly, how many times does he advise refreezing before correcting the cause by another surgical procedure?

Dr. John A. Gius, Iowa City: I am prompted by Dr. Hoerr's reference to semantics and peptic ulcer. The term "diathesis" has been used to connote a generalized predisposition which underlies ulcer development. I would suggest that our current preoccupation with local lesions of the stomach and duodenum and disturbances in the gastric secretory mechanism per se promises to perpetuate an unrewarding search for new therapeutic modalities, new operations, and new answers for a problem we do not understand.

May I suggest that there are other aspects of the ulcer problem which need to be studied in the human? One aspect was suggested by the discussion regarding a patient treated by gastric freezing who died of coronary occlusion, and another who died from cerebral hemorrhage.

I would like to suggest that the ulcers and these vascular accidents were all part of the same problem. And further, that the concept of a vascular basis for ulcerogenesis, propounded by Rudolf Virchow and others over a hundred years ago, needs to be restudied.

Some observations we have made at the University of Iowa may be pertinent. In microscopic observations of blood vessels in patients, we found formations of the small vessels of the lower lip which appear to correlate with the tendency to gastroduodenal ulceration. I think these vascular changes are part of an underlying diathesis. Perhaps all the vessels are so affected but those of the upper gastrointestinal tract are especially vulnerable to acid-peptic digestion when a variety of internal or external environmental conditions exist.

Dr. Charles B. Puestow, Chicago: It may sound a little discouraging that only 9.8% of resected patients are alive at the end of five years and 7.9% are alive at the end of ten years, but that does not mean that all the rest died of cancer. In the large series of gastric resections that we have performed, we have found as many patients who have died in less than five years and who at autopsy showed no evidence of cancer as we have had survive the operation for a five-year period. Of course, by resecting the stomach we do not cure coronary sclerosis and other diseases.

The second point I wish to make concerns the results Dr. ReMine has reported from a symptomatic point of view—the return of the patient to work, the loss of symptoms, the apparent restoration to good health of this large group of patients with total gastrectomy in whom he did not make a substitute stomach.

You learned this morning to make a substitute stomach adds about two hours more to the operation. It adds a good deal more bleeding. If a surgeon can get as good results by doing an end-to-side anastomosis and an enteroanastomosis as he would by making a substitute stomach, is it not better to do the less extensive procedure?

I would like to ask Dr. ReMine if he feels that his postoperative morbidity, both immediate and long range, is no greater than in patients in whom substitute stomachs have been made.

Dr. Charles L. Eckert, Albany, NY: Suspecting that most of you read the *New England Journal of Medicine* but that probably many of you do not get back to the section on correspondence, I thought it might be pertinent to read a short piece of a letter replying to a letter Dr. Stephen Wagensteen and Dr. Robert Smith addressed to Dr. Claude Welch concerning his annual review on abdominal surgery.

They were commenting about his failure to separate gastric hypothermia from gastric freezing. In reply, Claude Welch had this to say:

"Gastric freezing used experimentally for the control of duodenal ulcer is followed regularly by destruction of the gastric mucosa. Furthermore, inadvertent palpation may rupture the frozen stomach and lead to a fracture extending from cardia to pylorus. Also, hemorrhages occur a week to ten days after freezing in a number of instances. Finally, damage to the gastric wall may be serious. Thus, in one case in the Massachusetts General Hospital severe hemorrhage five days after gastric freezing required operation. Death followed resection since the stomach was so necrotic that it failed to hold the sutures."

I think this simply serves to emphasize that gastric freezing is a form of selective destruction of gastric mucosa, and, providing all factors concerned with this selective destruction are carefully controlled, it may be done with a safety that has been demonstrated by the group from Minneapolis. But I am most fearful, as Dr. Hoerr was, that if the rest of us try to adapt our machines willy-nilly to freezing the stomach, a great many tragedies are going to happen that should be avoided.

Dr. Daniel W. Elliott, Columbus, Ohio: Whenever a new procedure is introduced for the treatment of desperately ill people, such as those with serious gastroduodenal hemorrhage, there is a tendency at first to use the new procedure only in those patients who are very ill and who obviously are going to die if the standard resections are carried out. This has happened at our hospital in the selection of patients for pyloroplasty and vagotomy, and, as you saw, the same tendency is apparent in the selection of patients for gastric cooling to control hemorrhage. As a result, only a relatively few patients have had each of these procedures, and their mortality rate appears high. However, if the more seriously ill patients are selected out for the new procedures, then the record ought to be much improved for the remaining patients. Such considerations make it quite clear that the only way to measure the impact of a new procedure is to examine the entire record of a hospital or a similar institution as a whole. This has been done in the present study, and we are encouraged. Although there has been only a slight improvement in our mortality rate, this improvement may be significant since it extends over the entire hospital's experience with gastroduodenal hemorrhage.

Dr. E. F. Bernstein, Minneapolis: I would like to support the paper by Dr. Elliott and has group. At the University of Minnesota, using essentially the same strict criteria, approximately 75% of a group of over 90 massive upper gastrointestinal bleeders have been controlled over the past five years.

We agree with Dr. Hoerr that gastric freezing is still to be considered essentially an experimental venture. At the same time we would like to believe that other university centers, willing to take this up with an eye to open objective observation and comparison of results, will be encouraged to do so. We are currently engaged in long-term follow-up studies.

Regarding Dr. Zollinger's comments, there are, to be sure, a number of patients in the stomal ulcer group with no demonstrable hydrochloric acid prior to freezing. However, with upper gastrointestinal hemorrhage, recurrence of ulcer symptoms, or x-ray evidence of a crater, we feel the diagnosis of a stomal ulcer is justified.

Repeated gastric freezing will produce gastric atrophy, but this appears to be temporary in the experimental animal. Seven or eight gastric freezes of the intact canine stomach over a period of four weeks are followed by return to fairly normal secretory valves in many dogs within a few months. However, in the isolated canine Heidenhain or Pavlov pouch, a single freeze may produce complete achlorhydria, even to augmented histamine, for as long as 18 months (the length of our observations).

We have created two experimental ulcer-provoking situations in the dog, although not the one Dr. Zollinger suggested, described by Dr. Elliott. We have observed that gastric freezing reduces considerably the incidence of ulcer provoked by intramuscular implantation of histamine in beeswax, as well after transplantation of the antrum as a diverticulum to the colon (*Ann Surg* 156:579, 1962).

In answer to Dr. Eckert's question, we are troubled by the circumstance that some investigators have been unable to duplicate our experimental findings, in which gastric freezing has been demonstrated to be quite safe in the experimental animal. Certainly our experience in man, which currently includes somewhat more than 300 patients treated without mortality either directly or indirectly related to the freezing, indicates the procedure is safe. Moreover, it is effective in depressing gastric secretion long enough in most instances to permit ulcer craters to heal.

The experience of Dr. Welch (*New Eng J Med* 268:331 [Feb 7] 1963) cited by Dr. Eckert in his discussion will serve to emphasize the importance of technique. There is real hazard in gastric freezing, I am certain, if the guide lines defined by us previously are not closely followed. We do not observe destruction of the gastric mucosa in the experimental animal following freezing in which these guide lines are carefully followed. These critical items of technique involve the actual temperature of the perfusing alcohol, the systemic temperature of the perfused animal, the thickness and distention of the gastric balloon, and the duration of the freezing period. Among 143 patients whose stomachs were frozen for either 45 or 50 minutes not a single instance of postfreezing melena or gastric ulceration has been observed.

It would appear that a relatively narrow zone divides safe freezing, attended by secretory depression, and gastric necrosis accompanied by irrevocable complications. We are continuing to explore this border area to define more exactly safe and effective means of attaining our desired ends. If morbidity as well as mortality can be completely deleted, gastric freezing should come to play an important role in the control of some aspects of the peptic ulcer diathesis.

Dr. William H. ReMine, Rochester, Minn: Interposition procedures are fascinating and perhaps useful. They seem to satisfy some basic urge that we have to restore patients to as near physiologic state as possible. However, their effectiveness in this respect is not borne out in the experimental animal. There is nothing physiologic about some of the procedures that have been used except to restore continuity. Some of these procedures were used at our institution in 1962. Our series extended only through 1961 so that we might have an adequate follow-up period to report upon. Five Roux en Y procedures were performed during 1962 also.

In answer to Dr. Puestow's question, considerably more morbidity is associated with interposition procedures than with the one we have been accustomed to using, namely esophagojejunostomy with enteroenterostomy below it. If one desires to create a pouch or a repository for food, a simple procedure that has worked very well in our experience and that we are using more and more frequently is that of extending the enteroenterostomy up as far as necessary to create a pouch. It is the old pantaloon type of procedure described many years ago. In most instances this provides a satisfactory pouch for food to repose in, so that it can mix adequately with material coming from the proximal jejunum, the pancreas, and the biliary tree.

It is particularly important to have some way of bypassing the esophagojejunal anastomosis to prevent reflux esophagitis, but we do not have any procedure that will prevent it completely. With many of the old procedures in which an enteroenterostomy was not done below, the occurrence of stricture and stenosis of the esophagojejunal anastomosis was not necessarily the fault of the original anastomosis but was really the fault of the reflux esophagitis that occurred later.

Experimental Attempt to Delay Alimentary Transit After Small Bowel Exclusion

WALTER H. GERWIG, JR., MD, AND ALFRED GHAPHERY, MD, CLARKSBURG, W VA

Extensive resections of the small bowel can now be performed with minimal immediate mortality. Surgeons no longer need to harbor great concern for the procedure itself but must recognize that the maintenance of adequate nutrition continues to be a serious problem. In cases of superior mesenteric artery occlusion, often a major portion of the small bowel and, frequently, the right half of the colon must be resected. Such patients, even if they survive surgery, usually die of starvation within months. It is a frustrating and helpless experience to watch an individual deteriorate because the bowel is unable to provide adequate utilization of ingested food.

The response to extensive resection of the small intestine in man is followed by a variable and unpredictable outcome. This depends upon the magnitude of the resection, the length and viability of the remaining bowel, the presence or absence of the ileocecal valve, and possibly a number of additional factors which are not as yet clearly understood. The resection of all of the small bowel and the right half of the colon, which is frequently mandatory in cases of superior mesenteric artery occlusion, is in most instances followed by diarrhea, weight loss, steatorrhea, hypoproteinemia, hypocalcemia, anemia, and death. There are, however, occasional reports now appearing with increasing frequency of long-term survivals following such resections.[1,2] It is also noteworthy that successful massive resections in infants have been accomplished.[3,4] These, of course, represent the exception and serve as a vexatious stimulus in dramatically demonstrating the unquestionable feasibility of success while adeptly concealing the nebulous physiologic factors which lead to this success.

Massive resections of the small intestine, and particularly massive and total resections of the stomach, have resulted in an enormous amount of surgical research aimed at correcting the resultant gastrointestinal tract imbalance. Total gastric resection has led to numerous studies aimed at creating pouches to replace the resected stomach. Ileocolic

Presented at the 20th Annual Meeting of the Central Surgical Association, Chicago, Feb 21-23, 1963.

Chief of Surgery, Veterans Administration Hospital, Clarksburg, W Va, and Professor of Surgery, West Virginia University Medical Center (Dr. Gerwig); Surgical Resident, West Virginia University Medical Center, Currently assigned to Veterans Administration Hospital, Clarksburg (Dr. Ghaphery).

segments have been utilized,[5,6] with specific interest in the ileocecal valve, but such pouches appear to be of minimal benefit. Additional studies,[7] including a five-year re-evaluation,[8] have demonstrated that a transverse colon substitute pouch following total gastrectomy left a great deal to be desired. One of us (W. H. G.) has recently demonstrated in the dog that the stomach, even though denervated and excluded from the alimentary tract, is able to exert a beneficial influence in maintaining body weight.[9] Empirically, it is suspected that the mechanism of influence is most likely transmitted through the blood stream. These observations again reflect the many perplexing problems of the gastrointestinal tract which must yet be solved before the success of the surgeon's technical skill can be complemented by an equally successful sound patient in good nutritional and physiological balance.

The queries of researchers have probed with equal vigor the more difficult problem of maintaining nutrition and life in the patient with massive small bowel resection. It has also been shown in dogs that resection of 75% or more of the small intestine will result in early death.[10] Both in man and in the experimental animal, such resections are associated with a markedly reduced transit time for the passage of food through the gastrointestinal tract. Frequent, bulky stools ultimately lead to malnutrition, cachexia, and death. Many forms of therapy have been instituted to correct this deficit in maintaining nutrition. Since the greatest impairment seems to be in the absorption of fat and in protein assimilation, low-fat, high-carbohydrate diets have been utilized but found to be of questionable value.

The effect of vagotomy on the intestinal transit time has also been the subject of extensive investigation. It has been reported that prolongation of the transit time occurs in the small bowel of man after vagotomy.[11] Other workers indicate that vagotomy does not produce a marked effect on intestinal activity, although they did demonstrate a difference in the number, duration, and frequency of peristaltic waves between the normal and vagotomized dog.[12]

Renewed enthusiasm has recently developed for the reversal of a portion of the small bowel, which is interposed so as to produce an antiperistaltic segment. This appears to prolong the transit time of food through the bowel and decrease somewhat the loss of water, fat, and nitrogen. As previously mentioned, the resection of 75% of the small bowel of dogs invariably resulted in death. However, it has now been shown that the interposition of an antiperistaltic segment of bowel in this same type of resection will enhance the possibility of survival.[13] Further investigation of this approach indicates that if the interposed segment is 15 cm or longer, it usually causes obstruction; but if the segment is approximately 5 cm, the delay in transit time without obstruction is achieved.[14]

A case report which dramatically demonstrates the clinical application of this research was recently published.[15] The patient was an 84-year-old female in whom a short, reversed segment of jejunum was inserted after massive intestinal resection of over 90% of the small bowel and over half of the colon. This was performed for a superior mesenteric artery occlusion with gangrene. The patient is still living and demonstrates the feasibility of using a reversed small bowel segment to help control the malabsorption problem.

It would appear that if a segment of small bowel were available in cases of massive resection so that one could produce an antiperistaltic segment, the patient would benefit to some degree, possibly a degree sufficient to maintain life.

Unfortunately, the desired segment of bowel is frequently not available to the patient with superior mesenteric artery thrombosis, so that death by malnutrition or other related causes can readily be predicted. One might, therefore, explore possibilities for utilizing other tissues to delay transit time through the bowel, with the hope of improving nutrition. The effects of vagotomy in delaying transit time also merit further consideration.

In this investigation, a cylinder of gastric tissue is created and interposed in an antiperistaltic fashion between the duodenum and colon. We felt that such a substitute may serve to delay transit time of food through the gastrointestinal tract, with the hope that increased absorption of water, fat, and nitrogen will be achieved. The hazards of gastric tissue lying adjacent to the large bowel and the ulcerations that frequently result in the latter are recognized. This particular arrangement of gastric and colonic tissue differs, however, in one important respect, viz, the gastric and colonic tissues are immediately adjacent to and bathed by the alkaline juices of the pancreas and hepatic bile. This should serve to neutralize the acid that might result from the interposed gastric segment. The possibility exists also that the addition of vagotomy to the procedure may serve to diminish the volume of acid produced. The effect, if any, of vagotomy on transit time is also being studied.

Ludwig Thiry, an Austrian physiologist (1817-1897), created one of the oldest types of intestinal fistulas which consisted of a segment of intestine isolated with intact blood and nerve supply. The continuity of the intestine was restored by an end-to-end anastomosis. One end of the isolated segment of intestine is closed and the other end brought out of the abdomen. Luigi Vella, an Italian physiologist (1825-1886), brought both open ends of the intestine to the outside, thus the Thiry-Vella fistula.

It is recognized that exclusion of the entire small bowel as a Thiry-Vella fistula does not physiologically duplicate in detail actual resection of the bowel. Further studies with actual resection are to be undertaken in the future when this preliminary study is completed.

Method

Mongrel dogs were used as the experimental animal, and the subjects were divided into three groups. In each of the three groups, the large

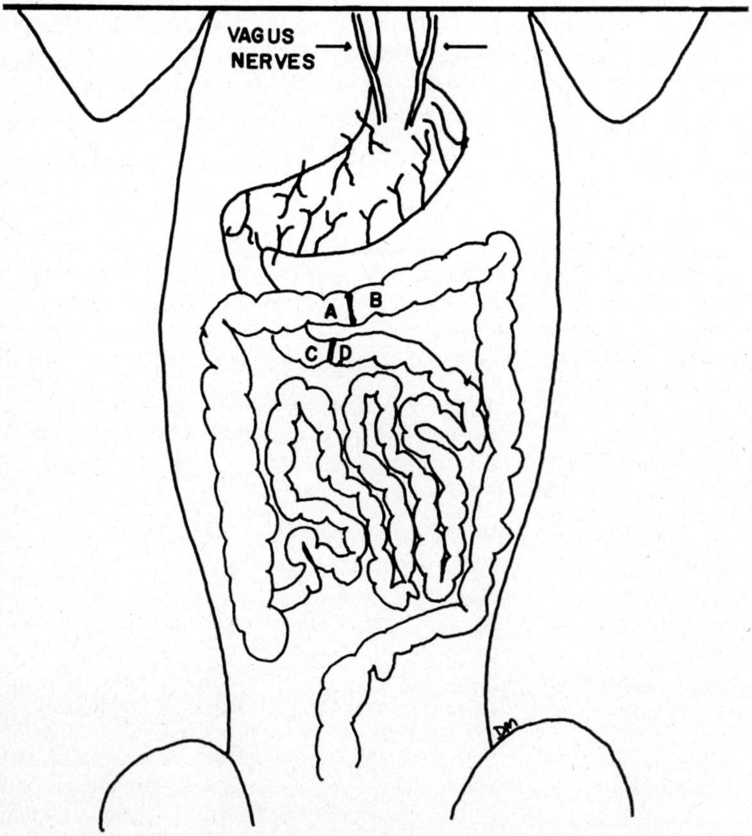

Fig 1.—Showing sites of transection for creation of an extensive Thiry-Vella fistula.

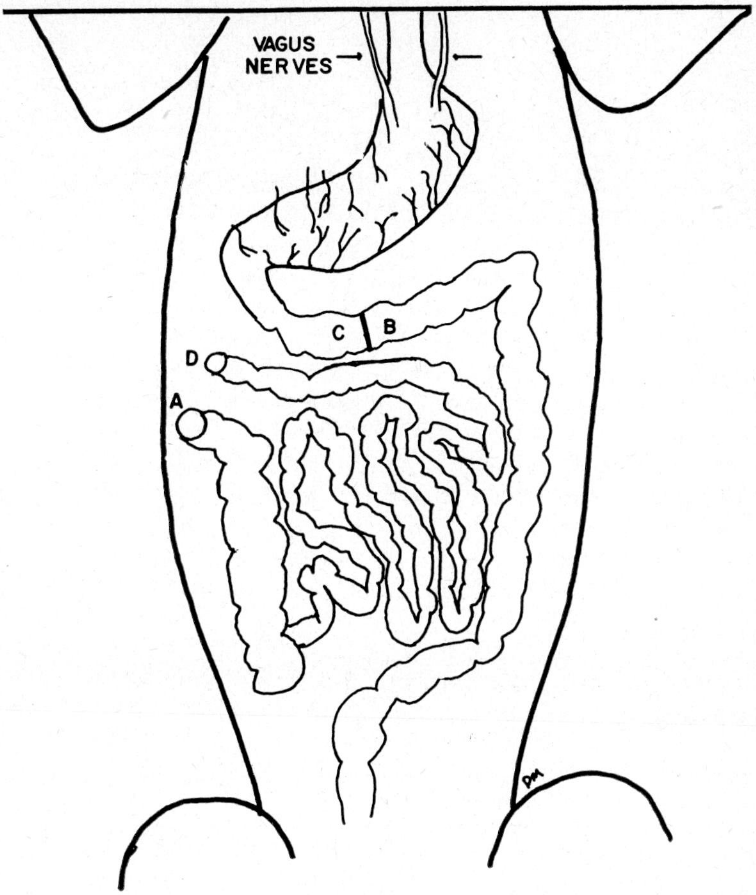

Fig 2.—Control Thiry-Vella fistula preparations.

bowel was transected as near to its midportion as possible, the proximal end being "point A" and the distal end, "point B." Next, the small bowel was transected at the duodenum. Since there is no ligament of Treitz, the site of transection was arbitrarily chosen as the point just distal to the level at which the pancreas is in direct contact with the duodenum. The proximal segment of transected duodenum was designated "point C" and the distal end, "point D" (Fig 1).

Rather than subject the animals to the trauma of massive resection, points A and D were brought out of the abdomen through individual openings, thus defunctionalizing the entire small bowel and a portion of the large bowel as a Thiry-Vella fistula. In extensive superior mesenteric artery occlusion, this is the portion that would require removal.

The animals were studied in three groups:

Group I. A Thiry-Vella fistula was created and a duodenocolic anastomosis performed, points C and B being the sites of anastomosis with points A and D the fistula stomas (Fig 2).

Group II. The same procedure was performed as in Group I, in addition to which a bilateral vagotomy was added.

Group III. Defunctionalization of the bowel with the Thiry-Vella fistula was again undertaken. A cylinder 6 to 7.5 cm in length and 2 cm in diameter was prepared from the greater curvature of the stomach. This cylinder of gastric tissue, with its omentum and blood supply intact, was rotated 180 degrees on its own axis and interposed between the duodenum, point C, and the colon, point B (Fig 3). It is hoped that by placing the tube in an antiperistaltic position, the transit time of food to the large bowel might be delayed and thereby contribute to an increase in the absorption of water, fat, and nitrogen.

The decrease in stomach size resulting from this preparation is not expected to contribute to weight loss since, as mentioned above,[9] the stomach, even though denervated and excluded from the alimentary tract, is able to exert a beneficial influence in maintaining body weight.

Postoperative care consisted of nothing by mouth for two days. Liquids were then allowed during the next 24 hours. Solids in the form of canned dog food were begun on the fourth postoperative day. Fluids were given subcutaneously on the basis of 10 cc per pound for an indefinite length of time,

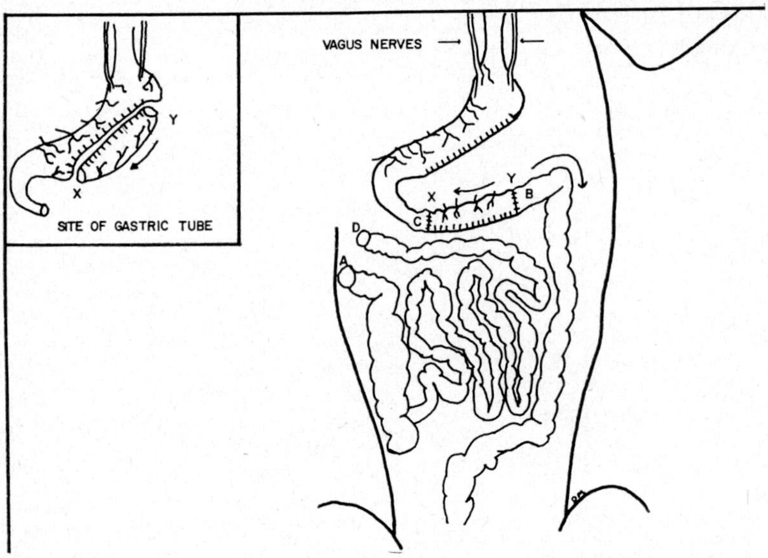

Fig 3.—Thiry-Vella fistula with interposition of an antiperistaltic tubular segment obtained from the greater curvature of the stomach.

depending on the hydration status of the animal. Atropine 1.5 mg, b.i.d., plus Kaopectate (kaolin and pectin) 60 cc, q.d., were given when alimentation was begun. Supplementary vitamins included 1 cc of B complex and 1 cc of ascorbic acid daily. Calcium gluconate was given in increments of 3 cc every four days. Daily weight determinations were recorded on all animals.

Results

Any animal that did not survive for a period of six days was considered to have succumbed as a result of the surgical procedure and has not been included in our tabulations. The five dogs in Group I with the Thiry-Vella fistula and duodenocolic anastomosis all died in a relatively short time. None of the animals lived longer than 36 days. The average postoperative survival period was 22 days. Weight loss in this group was gradual but progressive and measured 50% of the total body weight.

The second group, consisting of six dogs with the Thiry-Vella fistula and duodenocolic anastomosis, plus the vagotomy, had a postoperative average survival time of 36 days. All dogs of this group are dead with a single exception, now 68 days postoperative. Weight loss was less than that of Group I and consisted of 34% of the total body weight.

Group III was comprised of six dogs with the Thiry-Vella fistula and the created, interposed cylinder of greater gastric curvature. The postoperative mortality rate associated with creation of the gastric cylinder was initially quite high, being approximately 60%.

Creation of the gastric cylinder was in itself not technically difficult. The most frequent complication was a leak along the anastomotic line of the gastric cylinder and colon, specifically at the junction of the gastric cylinder suture line with the anastomotic suture line of the cylinder and colon.

In this group with the Thiry-Vella fistula and the interposition, three of the six animals are still living, the average postoperative survival time being 43 days. The body weight loss is estimated at 29%.

All animals of each of the three groups had diarrhea as expected. All required daily parenteral fluids to maintain hydration, even though alimentation was satisfactory for both liquids and solids.

The results are depicted graphically in Fig 4.

Conclusion

It would appear from this study that vagotomy may exert some influence on increasing survival time following massive resection of the small bowel. The effect of interposing a cylinder of greater gastric curvature in an antiperistaltic direction between the duode-

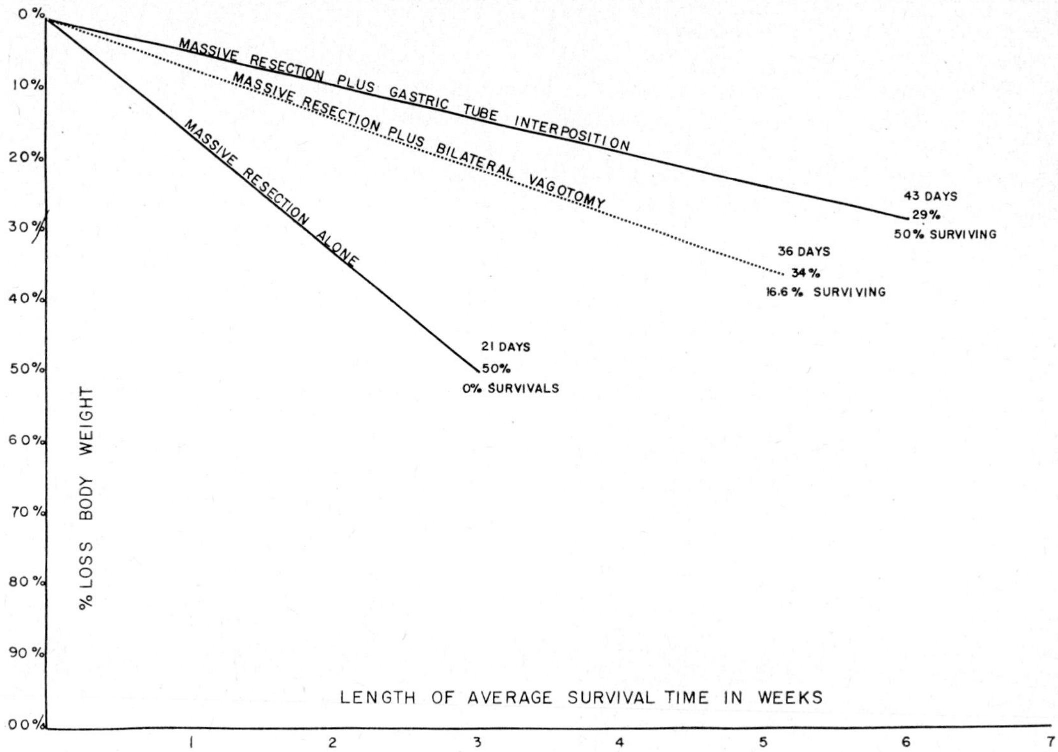

Fig 4.—Results in the three groups depicted graphically.

num and colon also appears to possess some beneficial effects.

Walter H. Gerwig, Jr., MD, Chief of Surgery, Veterans Administration Hospital, Clarksburg, W Va.

REFERENCES

1. Cogswell, H. D.: Massive Resection of the Small Intestine, Ann Surg 127:377, 1948.

2. Meyer, H. W.: Sixteen-Year Survival Following Extensive Resection of Small and Large Intestine for Thrombosis of the Superior Mesenteric Artery, Surgery 51:755, 1962.

3. Lawler, W. H., and Bernard, H. R.: Survival of an Infant Following Massive Resection of the Small Intestine, Ann Surg 155:204, 1962.

4. Gallant, V. J.: Successful Massive Resection of Small Intestine in a Newborn Infant: Case Report, Harper Hosp Bull 19:185, 1961.

5. Hunnicutt, A. J.: Replacing Stomach After Total Gastrectomy With Right Ileocolon, AMA Arch Surg 65:1, 1952.

6. Johnson, A.; Goldman, P.; Davis, C.; Harper, H.; McCorkle, H. J.; and Gardner, R.: An Experimental Study of the Nutrition of Animals Following Gastrectomy, Surg Forum 3:40, 1952.

7. Keshishian, J. M.; Harrison, I.; McClelland, J. R.; Miller, H. D.; and Gerwig, W. H., Jr.: Substitute Pouch Following Total Gastrectomy, Amer Surg 21:811, 1955.

8. Gerwig, W. H., Jr.: Transverse Colon Substitute Pouch Following Total Gastrectomy: A Five-Year Re-Evaluation Study, Amer J Surg 103:15, 1962.

9. Gerwig, W. H., Jr.: The Denervated, Excluded Gastric Pouch: Influence on Total Body Weight, Surgery 52:451, 1962.

10. Hammer, J. M.; Seay, P. H.; Hill, E. J.; Prust, F. W.; and Campbell, R. B.: Intestinal Segments as Internal Pedicle Grafts, AMA Arch Surg 71:625, 1955.

11. Dennis, C.; Eddy, F. D.; Frykman, H. M.; McCarthy, A. M.; and Westover, D.: Response to Vagotomy in Idiopathic Ulcerative Colitis and Regional Enteritis, Ann Surg 128:477, 1948.

12. Faik, S.; Grindlay, J. H.; and Mann, F. C.: Effect of Vagotomy on Intestinal Activity, Surgery 28:546, 1950.

13. Hammer, J. M.; Seay, P. H.; Johnston, R. L.; Hill, E. J.; Prust, F. H.; and Campbell, R. B.: The Effect of Antiperistaltic Bowel Segments on Intestinal Emptying Time, AMA Arch Surg 79:537, 1959.

14. Stahlgren, L. H.; Umana, G.; Roy, R.; and Donnelly, J.: A Study of Intestinal Absorption in Dogs Following Massive Small Intestinal Resection

and Insertion of an Antiperistaltic Segment, Ann Surg 156:483, 1962.

15. Gibson, L. D.; Carter, R.; and Hinshaw, D. B.: Segmental Reversal of Small Intestine After Massive Bowel Resection, JAMA 182:952, 1962.

16. Markowitz, J.; Archibald, J.; and Downie, H. G.: Experimental Surgery, ed 4, Baltimore: The Williams & Wilkins Company, 1959, chap 9, p 221.

DISCUSSION

Dr. Louis T. Palumbo, Des Moines, Iowa: This is an interesting study and may prove to benefit patients who have extensive small and large bowel resections for regional enteritis or because of superior mesenteric artery thrombosis or infarction.

In 1947, we combined bilateral vagus resection with a 75% partial gastrectomy for treatment of chronic duodenal ulcer. One of our reasons for this was to bring about a delayed gastric emptying and delayed small bowel transit time, both of which might reduce the incidence and severity of the dumping syndrome and might have a favorable effect upon bowel activity.

In collaboration with our x-ray department, repeated follow-up gastrointestinal x-ray examinations and motor meal studies were carried out in patients who had a partial gastrectomy with or without vagus resection and in our group with a distal antrectomy (25% or less of the stomach resected) with bilateral vagectomy.

The average emptying time of the gastric remnant in the partial gastrectomy group was 45 minutes, whereas in the partial gastrectomy-vagectomy series it was 180 minutes, and in the antrectomy-vagectomy series it was 80 minutes, during the first year after surgery. However, later follow-up studies in both series revealed an emptying time of 30 to 40 minutes, the same as in the partial gastrectomy series.

Repeated barium motor meal x-ray studies of the small bowel were considered normal in 87% in the partial gastrectomy group as compared to 60% in the partial gastrectomy-vagectomy and antrectomy-vagectomy groups. In the remaining 40% the small bowel pattern revealed clumping, segmentation, puddling, and hypomotility with a delayed transit time. By the end of the first year after surgery, in 90% of the antrectomy-vagectomy group the motor meal studies were within normal range without any further evidence of disturbed motility or pattern. This was not so in the partial gastrectomy-vagectomy series.

Vagal denervation of the gastrointestinal tract results in atonicity and dilatation of the stomach and delayed small bowel transit time with x-ray changes in the motor meal patterns. Within a year, usually, tonicity is regained and motor function returns to near normal in most instances. This may be accounted for by the local control assumed by the intrinsic autonomic nervous system nerve supply of Auerbach's and Meissner's plexuses.

Dr. John M. Hammer, Kalamazoo, Mich: In 1949-1950 I was interested in producing a chronic ulcer. I wanted to get away from the Mann-Williamson preparation because of the starvation factor, and Dragstedt's antral transplant ulcers were too acute, so I reversed the duodenum in dogs and was able to produce ulcers more chronic than either of the other two. These ulcers occurred in about six months.

These preparations were interesting in that not only did they produce ulcers but there was a marked dilatation of the reversed loop and the bowel above. Following these animals along by means of x-rays, and so on, we found marked delay in emptying time which lasted up to eight hours. After four hours, a good deal of the barium was still in the dilated duodenum and stomach. After 24 hours, there was still some barium present.

Because of this marked delay in emptying time, we thought that probably by resecting segments of bowel and reversing the distal loop we could delay the emptying time in some of these small bowel problems. We took a series of dogs and took out approximately 90% of the bowel in some of the animals. By reversing a segment about two inches in length, we were able to delay the emptying time.

We found again marked dilatation above the segment. There was marked delay in emptying time. These animals in this series survived much longer than the controls. Our control dogs died usually within a matter of several months, whereas these dogs went on and apparently maintained their weight.

I personally have not reversed a segment in a human, although I have had some patients who have had rather massive resections. I employed it in one patient with a gunshot wound of the abdomen, in whom I took out all but 30 inches of jejunum and anastomosed that to the transverse colon. At the time he was injured by the gunshot blast he had an abdomen full of pig hocks and spaghetti, so there was quite a bit of chemical peritonitis. He has gotten along very well. Probably he has enough adhesions to delay his emptying time.

Dr. Gerwig has apparently created a Thiry-Vella fistula and has taken most of the small bowel and colon out of the food line. He has also made a Heidenhain pouch which he has put in between the duodenum and the colon. From his results he has delayed the emptying time both with this method and with vagotomy, but his animals have not survived long enough so that I believe we can draw any conclusions.

This is an interesting procedure, and it would be interesting to see how the animals would react if he removed the Thiry-Vella fistula, because even though it is defunctionalized he is probably losing fluids and electrolytes through this preparation.

As far as his animals not developing ulcers is concerned, with the reversion segment, they have not lived long enough to develop an ulcer of the type I produced by reversing the duodenum. I think his work is very interesting and probably should be continued to see what his long-term results will be.

Dr. Arnold J. Kremen, Minneapolis: By raising a lake of gastric mucosa Dr. Gerwig has gained an additional eight to ten inches. How much this will contribute in the way of absorptive surface is a little hard to understand, but the experiment has not gone too long and it is well worth following.

I have been interested for some years in this problem. Some years ago I presented some experimental data relating to various segments of the intestinal tract which can best be taken out of the stream and sacrificed. In the dog, apparently, the proximal small bowel can be taken out of the stream or sacrificed with very little nutritional defect, whereas the terminal ileum would seem to be a most important area; and indeed one of the very important areas for preservation of some state of nutritional normalcy is the ileocecal valve.

Some abdominal catastrophes are such that it is impossible to save the ileocecal valve. In some instances of mesenteric thrombosis the right colon is involved in the process. To my knowledge—and I have searched over the years for a number of people who have had long-term survivals of very massive intestinal sacrifice—aside from Dr. Mayer's case that was mentioned previously, and a few others, the vast majority of them are people who have had a few inches of terminal ileum and ileocecal valve that have been preserved. It is in this group that I believe most of our spectacular survivals of massive intestinal resections have come about.

Another point I would like to make very briefly is that there have been around the country a number of patients (not a large number) who have been characterized as having the Pickwinian syndrome of extreme obesity, upon whom an attempt at treatment has been carried out by short-circuiting a segment of small intestine. I have done a few. Howard Payne in California has done a few, and he recently reported his experience to the Pacific Coast Surgical Society. Some have been done in the East.

There has been some correspondence between people relating to this. Whether this is a purposeful procedure or not remains to be evaluated. I would approach this procedure with extreme caution, and I think it should not be done except when all other means of controlling obesity have been exhausted. I do not mean the obese patient of 250 lb (113.4 kg), but patients of 450 lb (204.1 kg). I have had a few of these patients with a few very gratifying successes, and in a few it has been amazing that one can bypass 75% of the small intestine, mostly proximal small intestine, and see the patient lose from 280 lb (127.0 kg) to 250 lb (113.4 kg) and stabilize there for the next few years at 250 lb (113.4 kg), with no more than 25% of the intestinal tract functioning on stream.

Dr. Alfred Ghaphery, Clarksburg, W Va: As stated in the presentation, the small bowel and right colon were excluded from the alimentary tract as a Thiry-Vella fistula rather than subjecting animals to the trauma of massive resection. Realizing the physiological differences that exist between simple exclusion and massive resection, the exclusion was undertaken in this preliminary study so that the merits of each preparation could be better evaluated. It is well to point out that even though the exclusion was the procedure performed, the extensive weight loss and the very short survival time appear to be almost identical to and comparable with the outcome had actual resection been undertaken.

Standardization of the interposed segment of gastric tissue was achieved by creating the tube over a piece of rubber tubing that was preliminarily used as a stent so that we might be assured that each interposed segment would be of identical measurement. In this manner, all interposed segments were relatively equal.

Effect of Serotonin Loading on Histamine Release and Blood Flow of Isolated Perfused Liver and Lung

THOMAS C. MOORE, MD; LARS NORMELL, MD; AND BEN EISEMAN, MD, LEXINGTON, KY

Considerable experimental and clinical evidence has been accumulated in recent years to indicate that a significant increase in the discharge of serotonin (5-hydroxytryptamine) into the vascular system occurs in both the postgastrectomy dumping and the metastatic carcinoid syndromes. The precise roles of the release of serotonin in the production of the physiologic changes and symptoms which occur in these syndromes is not entirely clear. The cardiac lesions which are found in the carcinoid syndrome are limited to the right side of the heart, and there is experimental evidence that serotonin is inactivated by the lung. Although experimental "dumping" is associated with a significant increase in serotonin in portal venous blood, a corresponding increase in systemic venous and arterial blood has not been demonstrated. In addition, there is evidence that serotonin is inactivated by the liver as well as the lung.

The purpose of this study is to evaluate, by means of serotonin loading of isolated perfused liver and lung, the possible role of serotonin-induced histamine release in the dumping and carcinoid syndromes.

Experimental Method

Freshly excised canine liver and lung were perfused in sterile isolated chambers with fresh and aseptically drawn, heparinized canine blood. Principles of aseptic surgical technique were observed throughout removal and perfusion of the isolated liver or lung from heparinized animals and were monitored by blood cultures obtained at intervals during the perfusion. Intravenous pentobarbital sodium was used for anesthesia. Heparinization of donor animals was carried out with intravenous heparin injections ranging from 2.5 to 10 mg per kilogram. A pump-oxygenator system was employed in the liver perfusions. The details of the liver perfusion set up have been described previously.[4] The temperature, pH, oxygen saturation, bile production, and perfusion pressures in hepatic artery and portal vein were monitored and kept within physiologic limits. Constant perfusion pressures were maintained.

Both methyl methacrylate (Lucite) and stainless steel chambers were used for lung perfusions (Fig 1). Ethylene oxide pressure sterilization was employed for the Lucite chambers. The steel chambers were autoclaved. The majority of the perfusions were carried out in steel chambers. The pulmonary artery perfusion cannula was inserted into the main pulmonary artery through an incision in the right ventricle and secured by a right ventricular purse-string ligature and an umbilical tape ligature around the pulmonary artery. The left atrium was vented for free flow of pulmonary venous return into the funnel-shaped bottom of the perfusion chamber. Redundant portions of the heart were excised. Oxygenated pulmonary venous blood drained by gravity into a graduated reservoir which was used to measure pulmonary blood flow. Blood from this reservoir was propelled by a Sigma motor pump through coils immersed in a constant temperature bath into an elevated second reservoir with a runoff circuit (Fig 2). This reservoir was used to maintain a constant pressure of pulmonary arterial inflow. The trachea was secured to a metal cannula in the removable top of reservoir was used to maintain a constant pressure of pulmonary arterial inflow. The trachea was secured to a metal cannula in the removable top of the perfusion chamber which was connected to a Harvard respirator. A constant respiratory volume and rate were used in each perfusion. Pressures in the respiratory circuit and the pulmonary arterial line were measured continuously during the perfusion by means of transducers and recorded on a Gilson multichannel recorder. The pH, lung temperature, and oxygen saturation also were monitored.

Presented at the 20th Annual Meeting of the Central Surgical Association, Chicago, Feb 21-23, 1963.

From the Department of Surgery, University of Kentucky Medical Center.

Supported by USPHS grants No. AM-05621-02 and No. HE-06738-02, the Kentucky Division of the American Cancer Society, and the Fred Rankin Surgical Fund.

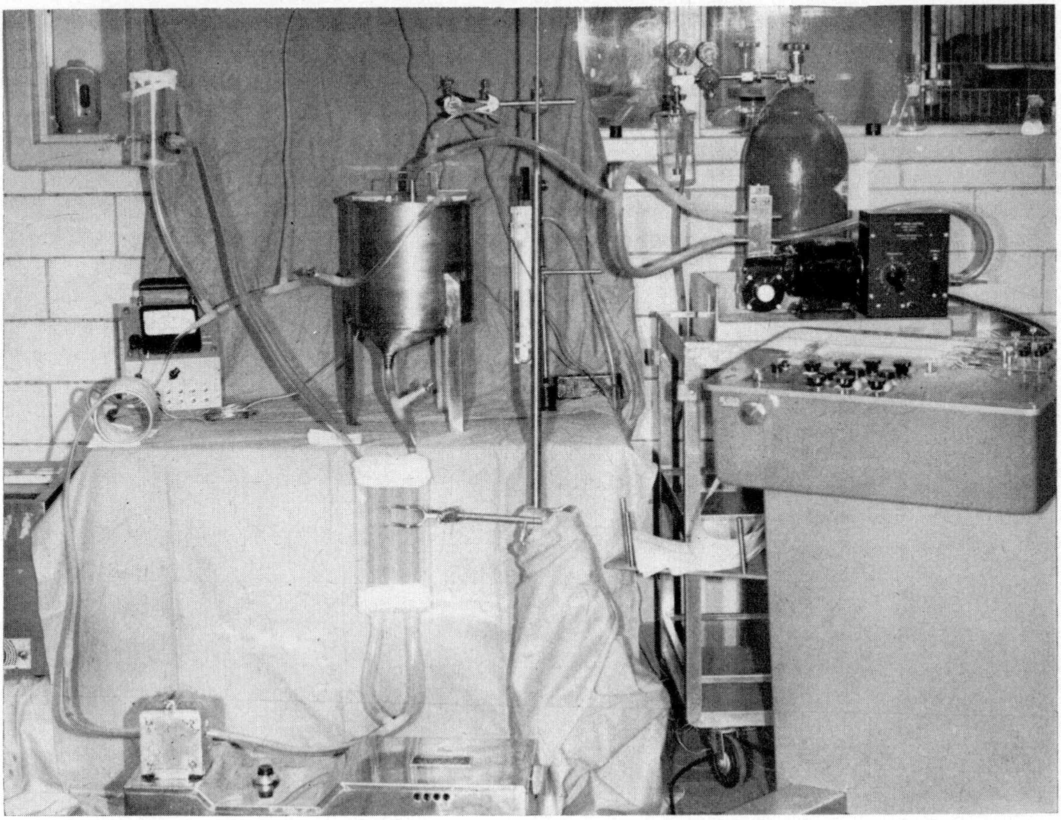

Fig 1.—Sterile isolated lung perfusion setup employing the stainless steel lung perfusion chamber.

After baseline blood samples were obtained, serotonin loads of from 0.5 to 15 mg were given to the 3-liter liver perfusion system via the portal venous reservoir and to the 1.3-liter lung perfusion system via the pulmonary arterial line. The majority of the loads were of 0.5 mg, and all but 8 of the 57 serotonin loads were in the 0.5 to 2.0 mg range. Blood samples for histamine determination were obtained at 3, 5, 10, 30, and 60 minutes after loading. Whole blood histamine concentrations were measured by the fluorometric assay method of Shore, Burkhalter, and Cohn.[20] The quantitative measurement was carried out in a Turner fluorometer with an excitation at 360 mμ and the fluorescence at 450 mμ. A blank and standards were carried throughout the entire procedure to make the proper adjustments.

Whole blood histamine was measured rather than plasma histamine in order to determine the liberated histamine. Plasma histamine determinations give an inaccurate picture of the total amount of histamine liberated, since nearly one half of injected histamine passes from the plasma into the cell fraction of blood during the first hour after injection. Histamine loading of the perfusion system with the organ removed has revealed a fall of plasma histamine concentrations during a one-hour run. This does not occur when whole blood determinations are made. Lindell and Viske[11] found no inactivation of C^{14} isotope labeled histamine by blood cells or plasma. They also found that about 5% of added labeled histamine had entered the cell fraction after five minutes and that after one hour 35% to 47% of the tagged histamine was in the cell fraction.

The capacity of the method of histamine determination employed in this study to differentiate between histamine and one of its major breakdown products, methyl histamine, was confirmed by demonstrating that no elevation in histamine levels occurred when significant amounts of methyl histamine were added to whole blood. Whole blood histamine determinations were made at the standard intervals before and after control serotonin loading of the perfusion system with the organ absent.

Results

Control Loadings.—Five control runs were made with no organ in the perfusion system. A load of 0.5 mg of serotonin was given in all, and whole blood histamine concentrations were made at the standard intervals. In none of the runs was the whole

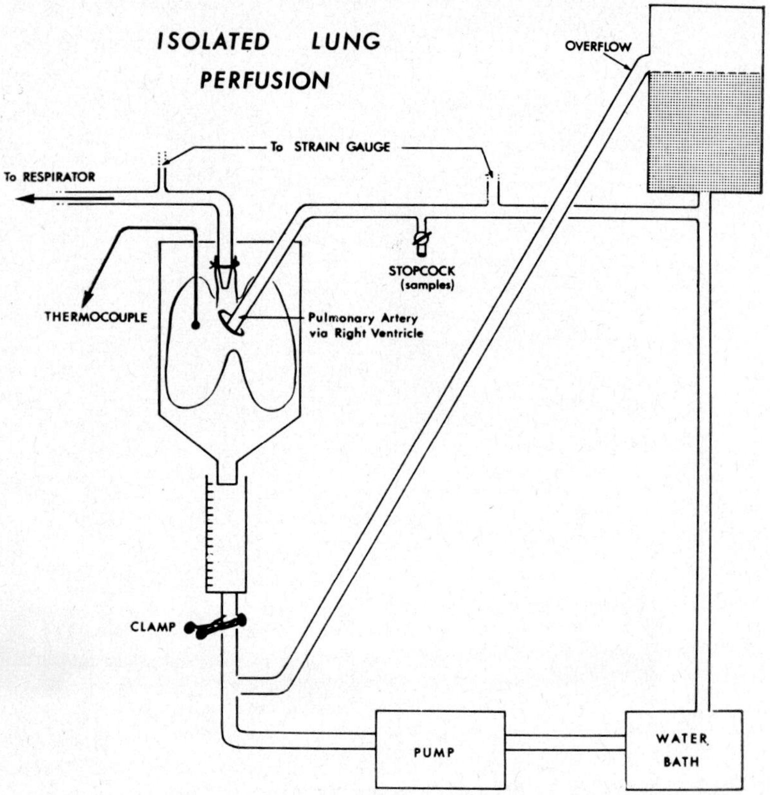

Fig 2.—Diagram of the lung perfusion system.

blood histamine elevated above the two preloading baseline concentrations.

Liver Perfusions.—Seventeen serotonin loadings were given in 13 liver perfusions. The loadings ranged from 0.5 to 5.0 mg. A significant release of histamine was observed in eight loadings in seven perfusions (Table 1). The per cent of peak histamine rise above the mean baseline concentration in this group of perfusions ranged from 249 to 1,250 and averaged 609.

Histamine release did not occur during nine loadings in six perfusions. Failure of histamine release occurred during eight consecutive serotonin loadings in perfusions two through six. During this period, heparin, an inhibitor of histamine release, was given in comparatively high concentrations (approximately 10 mg/kg) to the dogs being used as donors of blood for the perfusion system. A reduction in the amounts of heparin used (to the 2.5 to 3.0 mg/kg range) resulted in

TABLE 1.—*Summary of Experimental Data From Isolated Liver Perfusions in Which Serotonin Loading Was Associated With Histamine Release*

Perfusion No.	Serotonin Load (Mg)	Whole Blood Histamine (μg/Ml) Baseline	Baseline	3 Min	5 Min	10 Min	30 Min	60 Min	Per Cent Peak Histamine Rise Above Mean Baseline
1 a	0.5	0.074	0.088	0.250	0.147	0.407	0.147	0.147	502
b	2.0	0.103		0.157	0.162	0.260	0.598	0.038	581
7 a	5.0	0.090	0.090	0.103	0.259	0.233	0.207	0.155	288
8 a	5.0	0.062		0.120	0.034	0.224	0.172	0.068	361
9 a	5.0	0.041	0.041	0.083	0.291	0.083	0.041	0.041	710
11 a	5.0	0.010	0.014	0.040	0.029	0.121	0.047	0.150	1250
12 a	5.0	0.041	0.044	0.106	0.046	0.041	0.050	0.023	249
13 a	5.0	0.021	0.016	0.016	0.168	0.157	0.103	0.065	933

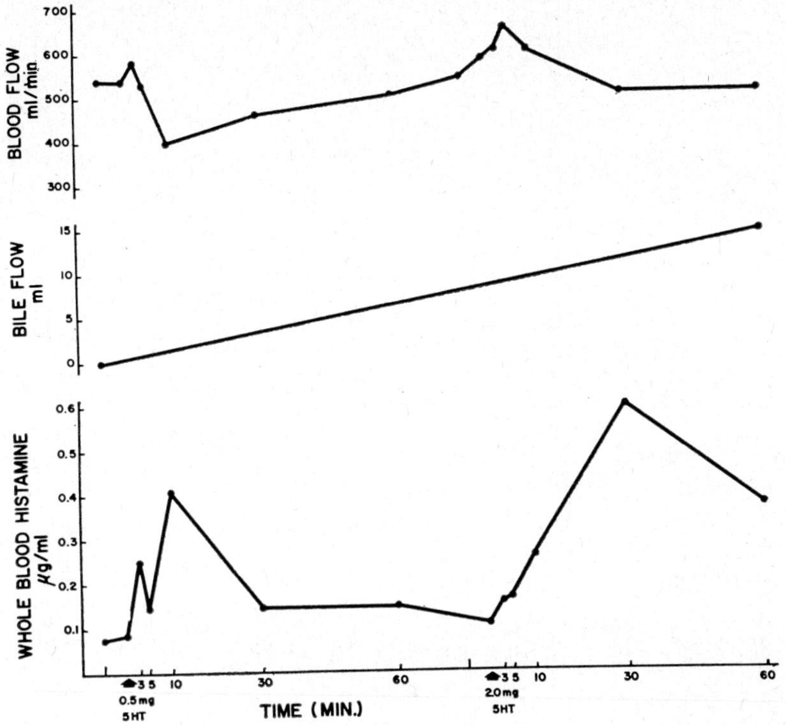

Fig 3.—Graph illustrating blood flow and histamine release responses of the isolated canine liver (perfusion No. 1) to acute serotonin loadings of 0.5 and 2.0 mg. In both loadings blood flow is increased and histamine is released.

a return of more consistent histamine release in response to serotonin loading.

Compound 48/80, a known and potent histamine releaser, was first used to evaluate the adequacy of the histamine release mechanism of the perfused organ in liver perfusion No. 6. Neither serotonin nor compound 48/80 released histamine. Compound 48/80 monitoring of the histamine release mechanism was used in seven subsequent liver perfusions. In all perfusions in which compound 48/80 released histamine, serotonin also was found to release histamine (Fig 3). Neither serotonin nor compound 48/80 released histamin in perfusion No. 10. Thus in eight monitored liver perfusions, there was 100% correlation between serotonin and compound 48/80 release of histamine. In perfusions in which histamine release was comparatively large, compound 48/80 appeared to be a more potent releaser of histamine than serotonin. In perfusion No. 11, the peak histamine after compound 48/80 loading was 2,600% of the baseline concentration, and in perfusion No. 13 it was 1,322% of the baseline.

In 13 of the 14 serotonin or compound 48/80 loadings in which histamine release occurred, the endogenous histamine was cleared effectively from the perfusate by the isolated liver.

The 17 serotonin loadings produced an increase in hepatic blood flow in 11, no change in three, and a decrease in flow in three (Fig 4). The increase in flow ranged from 50 to 200 cc in perfusions with preloading flows ranging from 500 to 900 cc per minute. Two of the three decreases in flow occurred in perfusions with flows of 400 cc per minute or less. Compound 48/80 reduced hepatic blood flow in all of eight loadings. In the six perfusions with preloading flows over 500 cc per minute, compound 48/80 produced marked reduction in flow—to 20% and less of the preloading flow. Terminal histamine loading resulted in marked reduction of flow in all of seven perfusions.

Lung Perfusions.—Forty-one serotonin loadings were given in 25 isolated lung perfusions. Thirty-seven of the loadings were in the 0.5 to 2.0 mg range, 26 being at the 0.5 mg level. A release of histamine was

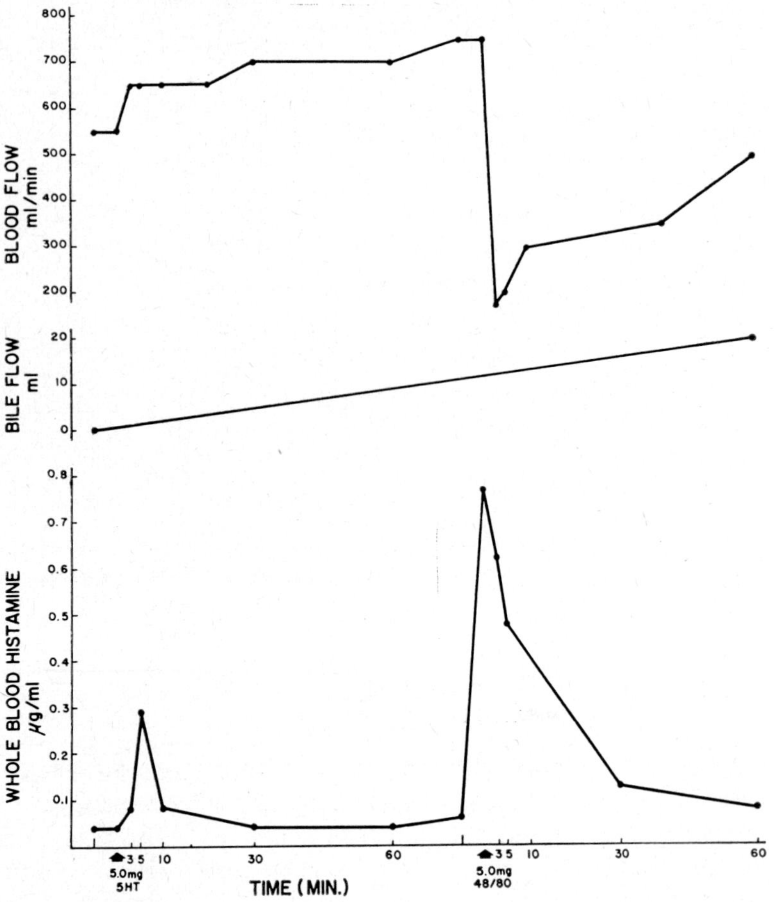

Fig 4.—Blood flow changes and histamine release in response to serotonin and compound 48/80 loading of liver perfusion No. 9.

observed in the initial 16 loadings and in 27 of the 41 (Table 2). The peak postloading histamine concentration ranged from 142% to 2,620% of the mean baseline level and was more than 200% in 22 of the 27 (Fig 5).

Three loadings were known anoxic runs which were made after initial loadings had shown histamine release. In all three runs there was a failure of histamine release (Fig 6).

The reasons for the failure of histamine release in 11 loadings were not clear. Some of these loadings occurred during the period of excessive heparinization of donor blood. Some improvement in the incidence of histamine release occurred when heparinization was reduced and glucose was added to the perfusion system. The addition of glucose to the system also appeared to increase the rate of clearance of the endogenous, liberated histamine from the perfusate (Fig 7).

Compound 48/80 monitoring of the histamine release mechanism was carried out after 14 serotonin loadings. Five serotonin loadings which led to histamine release were followed by histamine release with compound 48/80 (Fig 8). In seven monitored serotonin loadings, neither serotonin nor compound 48/80 released histamine. In one run serotonin but not compound 48/80 released histamine. In one run the reverse occurred. Thus, the histamine release response to serotonin and compound 48/80 was similar in 12 of the 14 monitored serotonin loadings.

Histamine release in one perfusion was evaluated by lung biopsy demonstration of reduction in histamine content after serotonin loading. Histamine content was 2.68μg per gram of wet weight prior to 1.0 mg serotonin loading. The content fell to 1.31μg after the first loading and to 0.614μg and 0.811μg after the second 1.0 mg serotonin loading.

Table 2.—*Summary of Experimental Data From Isolated Lung Perfusions in Which Serotonin Loading Was Associated With Histamine Release*

Perfusion No.	Serotonin Load (Mg)	Whole Blood Histamine (μg/Ml) Baseline	Baseline	3 Min	5 Min	10 Min	30 Min	60 Min	Per Cent Peak Histamine Rise Above Mean Baseline
35 a	0.5	0.26		0.48	0.64	0.48	0.54	0.50	246
36 a	0.5	0.20		0.38	0.40	0.46	0.42	0.46	230
37 a	0.5	0.19	0.18	0.70	0.74	0.98	0.90	0.86	530
b	0.5	0.50	0.49	1.16	1.00	1.21	1.15	1.15	244
38 a	0.5	0.22	0.22	0.68	0.50	0.55	0.62	0.60	309
b	0.5	0.34	0.35	0.60	0.47	0.50	0.63	0.50	183
39 a	0.5	0.44	0.44	0.94	0.98	1.00	1.00	1.00	227
b	0.5	0.50	0.50	1.16	1.20	1.22	1.20	1.20	240
40 a	0.5	0.20	0.22	0.70	0.73	0.75	0.82	0.79	390
b	0.5	0.26	0.27	0.98	0.99	0.99	1.25	1.00	472
41 a	0.5	0.080	0.092	0.312	0.227	0.395	0.177	0.249	465
b	0.5	0.129		0.207	0.375	0.189	0.270	0.189	291
42 a	0.5	0.06	0.05	0.60	0.40	0.75	0.65	0.55	1364
b	0.5	0.55		0.50	0.91	0.95			173
43 a	0.5	0.06	0.06	1.34	1.21	1.44	1.31	1.23	2400
b	0.5	0.98		1.03		1.40	1.63	1.35	166
48 a	2.0	0.053		0.048	0.037	0.118	0.075	0.010	223
50 a	2.0	0.042	0.042	0.090	0.042	0.069	0.090	0.053	214
b	15.0	0.063		0.092	0.069	0.069	0.069	0.069	142
51 a	0.5	0.059		0.023	0.140	0.119	0.023	0.047	237
54 a	0.5	0.01	0.01	0.058	0.038	0.262	0.67	0.029.	2620
b	0.5	0.047		0.074	0.047	0.121	0.074		257
56 a	0.5	0.027	0.054	0.102	0.025	0.044	0.035	0.040	255
59 a	1.0	0.024	0.021	0.029	0.020	0.048	0.020		213
b	1.0	0.038		0.058	0.058	0.020	0.067		176
60 a	2.0	0.005	0.105	0.005	0.005	0.020	0.045		450
62 a	5.0	0.064	0.064	0.069	0.139	0.495	0.366	0.238	773

This was followed by a no-loading, biopsy perfusion as a control. The histamine content per gram of wet weight did not fall below the baseline preloading level in numerous biopsies taken throughout the perfusion.

The serotonin loadings consistently produced a rather marked fall in pulmonary blood flow (Fig 9). The fall in flow was of comparatively short duration, generally lasting from 10 to 15 minutes. The fall in flow

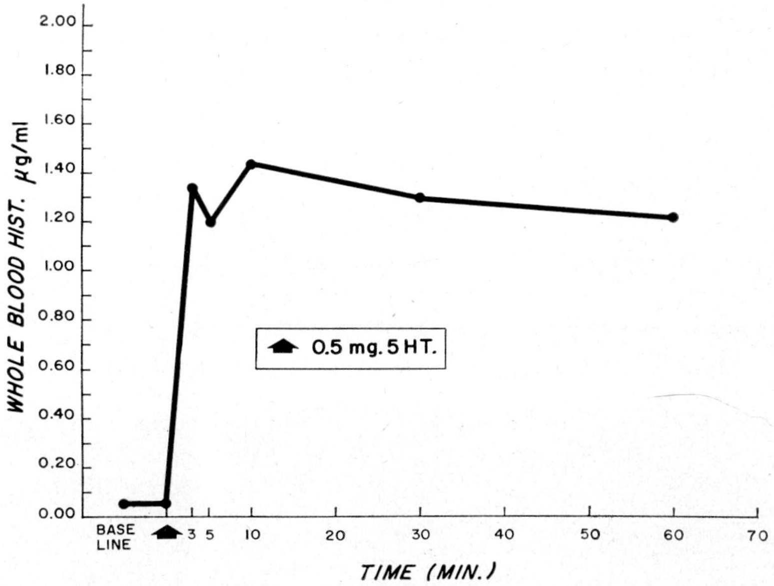

Fig 5.—Histamine release from the isolated perfused lung in response to serotonin loading.

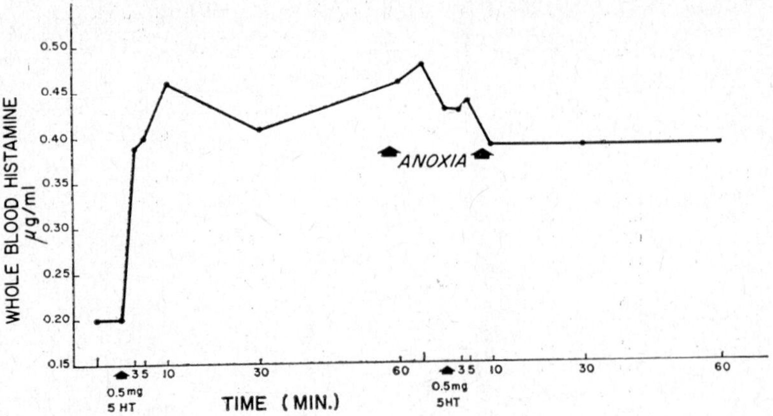

Fig 6.—Graph showing anoxia inhibition of histamine release by serotonin loading after prior loading of the same perfusion prior to anoxia had led to histamine release.

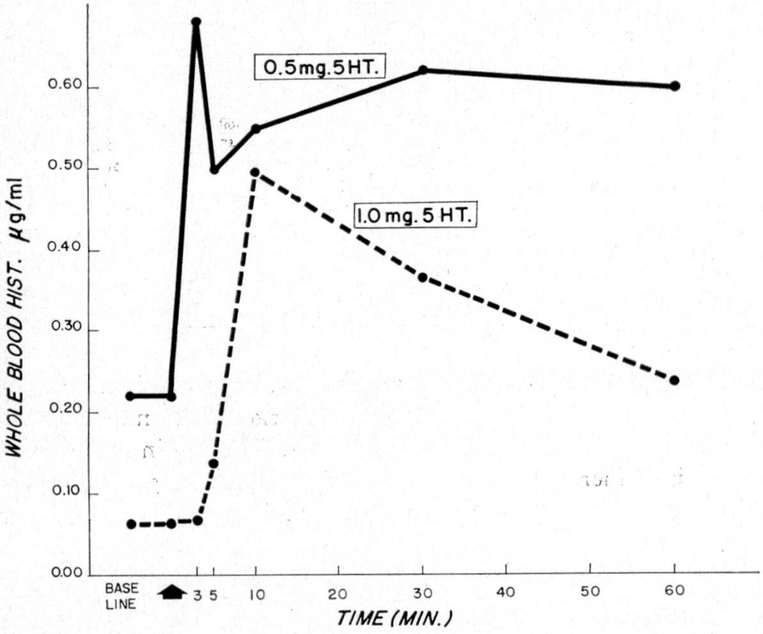

Fig 7.—Graph illustrating the role of added glucose in the fate of endogenous, released histamine after serotonin loading of the isolated perfused lung. Endogenous histamine is cleared from the perfusate more rapidly when additional glucose is added (perfusion loading 62a—broken line) than when the perfusion is carried out without the addition of glucose (36a—unbroken line).

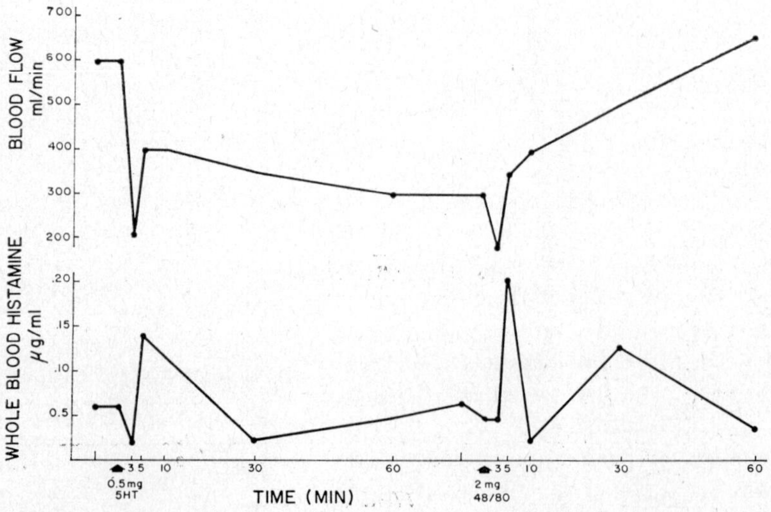

Fig 8.—Histamine release and reduction in blood flow responses to serotonin and compound 48/80 loading of lung perfusion No. 51.

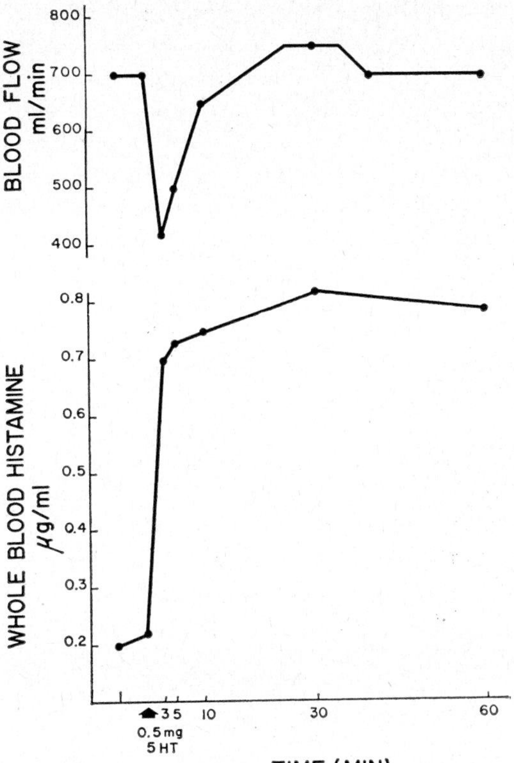

Fig 9.—Histamine release and blood flow changes in response to serotonin loading of the isolated perfused lung system (No. 40).

with compound 48/80 in equal weight loadings was consistent but less severe than observed with either serotonin or histamine loading.

Comment

The findings in these experiments indicate that serotonin loading of both the isolated perfused liver and lung systems results in a release of histamine. Although histamine release was not observed in all experiments, compound 48/80 monitoring of the histamine release mechanism indicated that the failure of serotonin to release histamine was accompanied by a like failure of 48/80 to release histamine. This observation suggests that the release failure was due to some blockade of the histamine release mechanism. Studies of histamine release have been notoriously treacherous due to the large number of agents and circumstances which can block histamine release. The use of excessive amounts of heparin, an inhibitor of histamine release, doubtless caused difficulty in some of the perfusions. In other experiments, there was no clear explanation for the blockade of the histamine-release mechanism.

The release of histamine is an important part of the anaphylactic and allergic reactions. A number of toxins, venoms, and proteolytic enzymes also may act as histamine releasers. Other types of histamine releasers are discussed in detail by Paton.[15] They include large molecular weight materials such as dextran and polyvinyl pyrolidine (PVP), certain surface active materials such as lysolecithin and the detergent Tween 20,* and a group of relatively simple monobasic compounds. Another group of histamine liberators includes compound 48/80 and propamidine. These substances act the first time they are administered and cause no tissue damage. Much remains to be learned concerning the production, storage, release, function, and metabolism of histamine and the relationship of the mast cell to these processes. Some interesting new ideas relative to the role of histamine in metabolic processes have been reviewed in a recent article by Kahlson.[10]

Blockade of histamine release may occur in anoxia and in the presence of metabolic inhibitors. Histamine release appears to depend on metabolically active mast cells.[25] It is of interest that histamine release is not inhibited by blockade of aerobic metabolism if glucose is present.[1,18,19] The energy for histamine release in these circumstances is derived independently of the Krebs cycle, presumably from the Embden-Meyerhof cycle. Other factors of importance in histamine release have been reviewed recently by Uvnäs.[23] These factors include a peak release temperature of 40 C, the presence of some calcium ions, and a pH in a relatively limited range around 7 C. Heating of tissues briefly to 45 C blocks histamine release. Thiopental also is a blocker of histamine release. The role of heparin in the blockade of histamine

* Polyoxyethylene sorbitan monolaurate.

has been emphasized by Higginbotham and Dougherty.[8]

Feldberg and Smith [6] in 1953 reported the release of histamine from living tissue by serotonin. The serotonin was given as an acute loading of 2.5 mg into the arterial line of a perfused skin flap or gastrocnemius muscle of the cat. The arterial infusion of the gastrocnemius muscle was with Tyrode's solution and that of the skin flap with Locke's solution. An infusion pressure of 60 to 200 cm of water provided a venous outflow of 2 to 4 ml per minute. The serotonin loading produced a marked temporary reduction in flow. The venous outflow was collected and assayed on the atropinized guinea pig's ileum for histamine concentration. Both serotonin and tryptamine released a significant amount of histamine and were more active in this respect than propamidine and the other amines and amidines examined by MacIntosh and Paton [12] in 1949 and more active than the opium alkaloids and morphine derivatives examined by Feldberg and Paton [5] in 1951.

Indirect evidence of histamine release by serotonin was reported in 1956 by Page and McCubbin.[14] They found that the antihistamine drugs promethazine (Phenergan) and diphenhydramine (Benadryl) inhibited or prevented the arterial depressor response to intravenous serotonin infusion in cats and dogs. When the blockade by the antihistamine drugs was complete, as judged by the lack of response to injected histamine or compound 48/80, infusion of serotonin did not alter arterial pressure in six experiments. Additional indirect evidence is to be found in the clinical observation of Pernow and Waldenström [16] that histamine excretion was greater than normal in seven of nine cases of carcinoid tumor.

The finding of an increase in circulating histamine in some serotonin-secreting carcinoid tumors, the right-sided location of cardiac lesions and the higher concentration of serotonin in portal and hepatic venous and right heart blood than in systemic arterial blood in this syndrome suggest that the metastasizing carcinoid syndrome may involve more than a mere physiologic response to elevated serotonin levels. It also is of interest that, although the physiologic role of serotonin is to decrease rather than increase gastric acid secretion, an increased incidence of peptic ulceration has been reported in patients with the carcinoid syndrome. The peripheral hypertension and flush responses are difficult to attribute solely to a vasoconstrictor such as serotonin. Furthermore, the available experimental evidence, although limited, suggests that the lung inactivates serotonin. Starling and his associates [21,24] in the early 1920's were able to remove a vasoconstrictor substance from defibrinated blood by perfusion through the lungs. It now is generally accepted that the vasoconstrictor substance was serotonin. Gaddum and his associates,[7] in 1953, reported the destruction of serotonin in the isolated perfused cat lung. If serotonin is a releaser of histamine from the lung and is destroyed by the lung, it may be that some portion of the carcinoid syndrome is due to serotonin-induced release of histamine. It also may follow that antihistamine drugs, especially those which also have an antiserotonin effect such as cyproheptadine, may be of value in controlling some of the unpleasant symptoms associated with the malignant carcinoid syndrome.

The discharge of serotonin into the portal venous system in response to an experimental dumping challenge of 50% dextrose injected into the proximal small intestine appears to be well established. Toh [22] in 1954 described the release of serotonin in the portal venous system from the dog's gastrointestinal tract. The release of serotonin in response to intestinal intraluminal sucrose solutions of varying tonicity was reported in 1949 by O'Hara, Fox, and Cole.[13] Drapanas and associates [2] and Peskin and associates [17] in 1962 demonstrated that the symptomatology of the experimental dumping syndrome, produced by the rapid instillation of hypertonic glucose solution into the proximal small intestine of dogs, was associated with a rise in the portal venous concentration of serotonin. Peskin also reported that the associated reduction in plasma volume was minimal. Drapanas, however, experienced difficulty in demonstrating convincing concomitant elevations in systemic arterial serotonin concentrations and in correlating these levels with the time of onset of the symptoms of "dumping." Drapanas [8] has recently found that approximately 80% of instilled serotonin is inactivated in a single passage through the liver. Johnson and his associates [9] have reported the successful use of serotonin antagonists, including cyproheptadine, in blocking the vasomotor symptoms of experimental and clinical "dumping." It is of interest that the three drugs used by them share an additional pharmacologic property—they are antihistaminics. These findings by other investigators and the observations in the experiments recorded here suggest that serotonin-induced release of histamine from the liver as well as the lung may be responsible for some of the vasomotor and related symptoms of the dumping syndrome.

Summary and Conclusions

1. Serotonin loading of the isolated perfused liver and isolated perfused lung systems results in the release of histamine.

2. Histamine is not released in all serotonin loading of the two systems. Compound 48/80 monitoring of the histamine-release mechanism has indicated that a failure of serotonin to release histamine has been associated with a like failure of compound 48/80 to release histamine in the same perfusion setup and that the failure of serotonin to release histamine in the occasional liver and lung perfusion is due presumably to some unexplained blockade of the histamine-release mechanism.

3. The literature pertaining to histamine-releasing substances and to the mechanism and blockade of histamine release is reviewed briefly.

4. It is suggested that serotonin-induced release of histamine may be involved in the production of the vasomotor and related symptoms encountered in the malignant carcinoid and dumping syndromes.

5. Blood flow of the isolated perfused liver generally is increased slightly to moderately by serotonin loading, while both compound 48/80 and histamine loading result in a marked reduction in flow. Loading with all three drugs produces a significant reduction in pulmonary blood flow.

Thomas C. Moore, MD, Department of Surgery, University of Kentucky Medical Center, Lexington, Ky.

REFERENCES

1. Diamant, B., and Uvnäs, B.: Evidence for Energy-Requiring Processes in Histamine Release and Mast Cell Degranulation in Rat Tissues Induced by Compound 48/80, Acta Physiol Scand 53:315, 1961.

2. Drapanas, T.; McDonald, J. C.; and Stewart, J. D.: Serotonin Release Following Instillation of Hypertonic Glucose Into the Proximal Intestine, Ann Surg 156:528, 1962.

3. Drapanas, T.: Personal communication to the author.

4. Eiseman, B.; Knipe, P.; McColl, H. A.; and Orloff, M. J.: Isolated Liver Perfusion for Reducing Blood Ammonia, AMA Arch Surg 83:356, 1961.

5. Feldberg, W., and Paton, W. D. M.: Release of Histamine From Skin and Muscle in the Cat by Opium Alkaloids and Other Histamine Liberators, J Physiol 114:490, 1951.

6. Feldberg, W., and Smith, A. N.: Release of Histamine by Tryptamine and 5-Hydroxytryptamine, Brit J Pharmacol 8:406, 1953.

7. Gaddum, J. H.; Hebb, C. O.; Silver, A.; and Swan, A. A. B.: 5-Hydroxytryptamine: Pharmacologic Action and Destruction in Perfused Lungs, Quart J Exp Physiol 38:255, 1953.

8. Higginbotham, R. D., and Dougherty, T. F.: Mechanism of Heparin Protection Against a Histamine Releaser (48/80), Proc Soc Exp Biol Med 92:493, 1956.

9. Johnson, L. P.; Sloop, R. D.; Jesseph, J. E.; and Harkins, H. N.: Serotonin Antagonists in Experimental and Clinical "Dumping," Ann Surg 156:537, 1962.

10. Kahlson, G.: New Approaches to the Physiology of Histamine, Perspect Biol Med 5:179, 1962.

11. Lindell, S. E., and Viske, K.: A Note on the Distribution of C^{14} Histamine Added to Blood, Brit J Pharmacol 17:131, 1961.

12. MacIntosh, F. C., and Paton, W. D. M.: The Liberation of Histamine by Certain Inorganic Bases, J Physiol 109:190, 1949.

13. O'Hara, R. S.; Fox, R. D.; and Cole, J. W.: Serotonin Release Mediated by Intraluminal Sucrose Solutions, Surg Forum 10:215, 1959.

14. Page, I. H., and McCubbin, J. W.: Arterial Pressure Response to Infused Serotonin in Normotensive Dogs, Cats, Hypertensive Dogs and Man, Amer J Physiol 184:265, 1956.

15. Paton, W. D. M.: The Release of Histamine, Progr Allerg 5:79, 1958.

16. Pernow, B., and Waldenström, J.: Determination of 5-Hydroxytryptamine, 5-Hydroxyindole Acetic Acid and Histamine in 33 Cases of Carcinoid Tumor (Argentaffinoma), Amer J Med 23:16, 1957.

17. Peskin, G. W., and Miller, L. D.: The Role of Serotonin in the "Dumping Syndrome," AMA Arch Surg 85:701, 1962.

18. Rothschild, A. M.: Effect of Metabolic Inhibitors on the Release of Histamine by Anaphylatoxin and by Antigen in Vitro, Experientia 17:555, 1961.

19. Rothschild, A. M.; Vugman, I.; and Rocha e Silva, M.: Metabolic Studies on the Release of Histamine by Compound 48/80 in the Rat Diaphragm, Biochem Pharmacol 7:248, 1961.

20. Shore, P. A.; Burkhalter, A.; and Cohn, V. H., Jr.: A Method for the Fluorometric Assay of Histamine in Tissues, J Pharmacol Exp Ther 127:182, 1959.

21. Starling, E. H., and Verney, E. B.: The Secretion of Urine as Studied on the Isolated Kidney, Proc Royal Soc [Biol] 97:321, 1925.

22. Toh, C. C.: Release of 5-Hydroxytryptamine From the Dog's Gastrointestinal Tract, J Physiol 126:248, 1954.

23. Uvnäs, B.: Mechanism of Histamine Release From Mast Cells, Chemotherapia (Basel) 3:137, 1961.

24. Verney, E. B., and Starling, E. H.: Secretion by the Isolated Kidney, J Physiol 56:353, 1922.

25. Westerholm, B.: The Influence of Anoxia on 48/80-Induced Histamine Release From Rat Skin, Acta Physiol Scand 50:300, 1960.

DISCUSSION

Dr. Theodore Drapanas, Buffalo: There is not much doubt now that a humoral mechanism does in fact exist, and that serotonin is intimately involved in this mechanism, as evidenced in animals by a prompt increase of serotonin in portal blood simultaneously with an increase in peripheral blood flow, thoracic duct lymph flow, and diminution of pancreatic juice flow during a dumping challenge. In addition, if you give serotonin to patients intravenously, symptoms of flushing, palpitation, and weakness are produced which are identical to the early vasomotor responses seen in dumping.

Our concern has been how this mechanism is mediated. Are both serotonin and histamine involved? There are many difficulties involved in the study of these fluorescent amines. Thiopental and heparin both inhibit serotonin and histamine release, as Dr. Moore has pointed out, and consequently the use of these agents in experiments produces inconsistent results. The washing of syringes used to collect blood samples and of glassware by common laboratory detergents results in a marked quenching of fluorescence. To confuse the problem further, most of the serotonin antagonists now on the market are not only potent antihistaminics but also very good tranquilizers.

Despite the strong evidence that serotonin is released by the intestinal mucosa with resulting elevation in portal blood levels, we have had difficulty in obtaining convincing parallel elevations in systemic blood serotonin levels.

Using an experiment outlined here, we determined clearance across the liver bed by infusing serotonin into the portal system and getting levels of serotonin in the portal vein and in the hepatic vein branch.

I think Dr. Moore has shown very nicely or has commented on the fact that although we have a marked rise in portal vein serotonin, the hepatic vein rises are not convincing. This does not, however, exclude the possibility that some of the intermediate aldehyde breakdown products of serotonin are also biologically active. Unfortunately these substances are chemically evanescent, very unstable, and impossible to assay at the present time.

Dr. Moore has presented convincing experimental evidence that histamine may be liberated by serotonin in both liver and lung, and he has pointed out the similarity in biological action of these pressor amines. Histamine liberation would also explain the gastric hypersecretion and the increased incidence of peptic ulceration noted in patients with the carcinoid syndrome. I would suspect that histamine might be similarly released anywhere in the body where mast cells might be found. Perhaps the final answer will rest on further studies of the relationship of the mast cell to these processes.

I would like to ask the authors if they have performed studies on systemic histamine levels in animals or patients following a dumping challenge. Second, is histamine released when lung, liver, and perhaps other tissues are perfused in situ with a serotonin load in the blood stream?

Dr. Thomas C. Moore, Lexington, Ky: As Dr. Drapanas has indicated, studies related to histamine release are very pesky indeed. The abstract in your program states that histamine is not released from the liver. This was the result of our overheparinization, and the statement in the program is actually incorrect. In the first two liver loadings we carried out, histamine was released, and in the next eight loadings we were not able to obtain a release of histamine. We started monitoring at this point with Compound 48/80. We also wished to check this finding with the lung, and found we were unable to get a release of histamine from the lung as we had done in the previous 16 loadings. This prompted us to probe more deeply into the entire problem of histamine release.

We find there are many substances used in a perfusion setup, as employed here, which do inhibit the release of histamine. The barbiturates do this: heparin inhibits the release. The optimum pH for histamine release is around 7 and the optimum temperature around 40 C. A certain amount of calcium ion is necessary in a system for the release of histamine. Many other factors are involved.

In regard to Dr. Drapanas' questions concerning the increase of histamine in the systemic circulation following a dumping challenge, we have not carried this out, nor have we carried out in situ loadings with serotonin. We felt that in our isolated system, we were able at least to collect as much as possible (more so in the lung than in the liver) of the liberated histamine and perhaps get some of the results without having the added problem of the blood perfused throughout the entire body. It appears that when histamine release does occur it is a fairly rapid and comparatively sizeable release.

Effects of Various Drugs on Exotoxin (Cl Perfringens) Toxicity

Pretreatment With Chlorpromazine, Phenoxybenzamine, Heparin, and Cortisone

PAUL NORA, MD, AND HAROLD LAUFMAN, MD, CHICAGO

The cell-free filtrates of various bacteria are known to exert toxic effects upon the mammalian organism, leading to irreversible shock and death. Gram-negative bacteria of the colonially smooth variety characteristically yield a cell-wall lipopolysaccharide complex identified as an endotoxin. Certain anaerobic bacteria such as the clostridia produce a protein substance designated as an exotoxin which also causes lethal effects and has been implicated in a variety of afflictions ranging from intestinal strangulation obstruction to gas gangrene infections. Both endotoxin and exotoxin may cause irreversible shock and death. The terminal pathologic findings after lethal injections of these substances are identical.[3] In fact, hemorrhagic necrosis of the intestinal mucosa appears to be a finding common to irreversible shock due to many causes, including hemorrhage,[1] epinephrine injections,[2] etc.

In contrast to this uniformity in autopsy findings, we have found that the physiologic course of animals following exotoxin injection is strikingly different from that observed in endotoxin-injected animals.[3] For example, endotoxin produces a hemoconcentration (elevated erythrocyte count and elevated hematocrit) within four hours, whereas exotoxin produces a depressed erythrocyte count and depressed hematocrit within this period; endotoxin causes a rather rapid leukopenia, whereas exotoxin injection leads to a steadily increasing leukocytosis lasting about 12 hours; endotoxin, in lethal doses, causes a steady decline in blood pressure following a brief rebound from hypotensive levels, whereas exotoxin, after the initial reaction, does not result in severe hypotension until just before death (Fig 1).

In the light of these findings, the present study was undertaken to determine the effects of pretreatment with certain drugs on exotoxin shock and to compare these results with those of pretreatment on endotoxin shock. The four drugs chosen were those found to exert a salutary effect on endotoxin shock when used as pretreatment: chlorpromazine, phenoxybenzamine, heparin, and cortisone. None of these drugs has yielded significant results when used as postshock treatment in the experimental animal.

Presented at the 20th Annual Meeting of the Central Surgical Association, Chicago, Feb 21-23, 1963.

With the technical assistance of Clem McDonald and Gregory Louviaux.

From the Department of Surgery, Northwestern University Medical School.

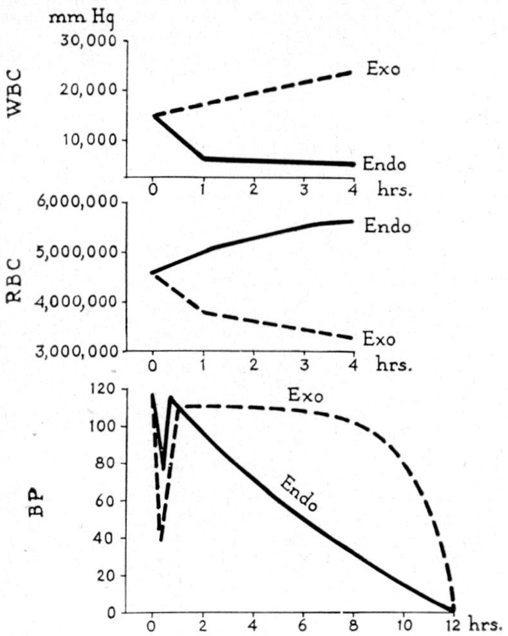

Fig 1.—Comparison between average responses of erythrocyte count, leukocyte count, and blood pressure to lethal doses of exotoxin (lecithinase) and endotoxin (lipopolysaccharides).

Materials and Methods

Ninety-six dogs were used in the study. The first 22 animals were employed for pilot experiments from which the choice of anesthesia and the dosage of exotoxin were determined. The remaining 74 dogs were subjected to studies in pairs, one treated and one untreated.

The exotoxin which we employed was lecithinase, the α-exotoxin of *Clostridium perfringens.* One of the problems in the use of this enzyme is its variable toxicity. It is available only as a liquid whose toxicity varies with shelf-life, as well as from batch to batch. Hence, the toxicity of each injection had to be confirmed by injecting paired dogs of equal weight, one as an untreated control, the other as a pretreated animal. The dose of lecithinase which led to death in about 12 hours was found to vary from 35 minimum lethal dose (MLD) to 44 MLD per kilogram.

The anesthetic employed was morphine sulfate, 2 mg/kg. We learned that the synergistic effects of pentobarbital and central nervous system depressants such as chlorpromazine often led to excessive suppression of vital functions or even death. Lillehei[4] had found the same phenomenon in his endotoxin experiments and advised us to use the morphine for basal anesthesia and to avoid the use of barbiturates.[5]

Hourly determinations of blood pressure, erythrocyte count, hematocrit, leukocyte count, and platelet count were made on all animals. Blood pressure was determined by femoral artery cannulation. Autopsies were performed on all animals. In pilot experiments we learned that a 72-hour survival was tantamount to permanent survival, and therefore we used the 72-hour survival as our end point.

The four drugs which were employed for pretreatment of exotoxin-injected dogs had previously been tested for pretreatment of endotoxin-injected[6] dogs. The doses of each of these drugs and the length of pretreatment were as follows:

Group I. Seven pairs of dogs, one of each pair pretreated with chlorpromazine 25 mg/kg, 30 minutes prior to a lethal injection of lecithinase. The alternate dog of each pair received a lethal injection of lecithinase alone and acted as a control.

Group II. Seven pairs of dogs, one of each pair pretreated with phenoxybenzamine hydrochloride 0.5 mg/kg in 1,000 cc of saline intravenously one hour prior to the injection of a lethal dose of lecithinase. The alternate dog of each pair received a lethal injection of lecithinase alone and acted as a control.

Group III. Six pairs of dogs, one of each pair pretreated with heparin sodium 12 mg/kg in 1:1,000 solution ten minutes prior to the injection of a lethal dose of lecithinase. The alternate dog of each pair received a lethal injection of lecithinase alone and acted as a control.

Group IV. Six pairs of dogs, one of each pair pretreated with hydrocortisone acetate 15 mg/kg intramuscularly daily for five days prior to and including the day of injection of a lethal dose of lecithinase. The alternate dog of each pair received a lethal injection of lecithinase alone and acted as a control.

Results

Every one of the 26 untreated dogs which had received an injection of exotoxin died in 10 to 18 hours (Table 1). Survival data of the pretreated groups were as follows.

Group I. Chlorpromazine.—Four of seven pretreated dogs survived. The three pretreated nonsurvivors had a mean longevity

TABLE 1.—*Exotoxin*

Pretreatment	Animals	Survivors	Remarks
None	26	0	Average survival 13 hr ± 8
Chlorpromazine, 30 min, 25 mg/kg	7	4	3 dogs survived 36 hr ± 10.1
Phenoxybenzamine, 1 hr, 0.5 mg/kg	7	4	3 dogs survived 10 hr ± 4.2
Heparin, 10 min, 12 mg/kg	6	0	Average survival 4 hr ± 3.6
Hydrocortisone, 5 days, 15 mg/kg	6	3	3 dogs survived 10 hr ± 5.8

of 36 hours ± 10.1. Until shortly before death these animals appeared quite healthy but, at autopsy, demonstrated the typical hemorrhagic infiltration of intestinal mucosa found in untreated exotoxin-injected animals. Average survival time of untreated dogs in this group was 12 hours.

Group II. Phenoxybenzamine.—Four of seven pretreated dogs survived, but the three nonsurvivors had a mean longevity of 10 hours ± 4.2, not significantly different from that of untreated exotoxin-injected dogs. Average survival time of untreated dogs in this group was 14 hours.

Group III. Heparin.—All pretreated dogs died, with a mean survival time of 4 hours ± 3.6. The mean survival time of untreated dogs in this group was 16 hours.

Group IV. Hydrocortisone.—Three of six pretreated dogs survived. The average longevity of the nonsurvivors was 10 hours ± 5.8, whereas that of the untreated dogs in this group was 12 hours.

Comment

Although endotoxin and exotoxin are chemically unrelated and apparently produce different physiologic responses early in the toxic state after injection, both toxins ultimately lead to hypovolemia, irreversible shock, and death. Acute hemorrhagic necrosis of the intestinal mucosa is the most striking autopsy finding in both instances, as it is also in death following irreversible shock from hemorrhage, epinephrine, or superior mesenteric artery occlusion.[6] In exotoxin shock homeostatic mechanisms apparently support the blood pressure until shortly before death, while in endotoxin shock the blood pressure falls steadily as effective plasma volume is depleted.

Longerbeam and co-workers[7] studied the effects of pretreatment with a variety of drugs in dogs subjected to lethal endotoxin shock (Table 2). He found that chlorpromazine, phenoxybenzamine, and cortisone when used as pretreatment each reduced the mortality rate due to endotoxin shock, prevented most of the changes in plasma volume, hematocrit, and plasma hemoglobin, and also prevented the characteristic intestinal changes of irreversible shock from occurring. Although this group of investigators found no beneficial effect from heparin, Hardaway[8] reported a 50% survival rate in endotoxin shock dogs pretreated with heparin.

TABLE 2.—*Endotoxin* *

Pretreatment	Animals	Survivors	Remarks
None	90	6	Average survival 10.3 hr ± 5.5
Chlorpromazine, 30 min, 25 mg/kg	10	6	
Phenoxybenzamine, 1 hr, 0.5 mg/kg	10	9	
Heparin, 10 min, 30 mg/kg	10	1	1 dog survived 12.1 hr
Hydrocortisone, 5 days, 15 mg/kg	10	9	

* Adapted from R. C. Lillehei (reference 6).

In our experiments with lethal exotoxin shock, chlorpromazine, phenoxybenzamine, and cortisone appeared to offer about the same salvage rate when used as pretreatment in dogs subjected to lethal endotoxin shock. Heparin was of no value. Our results, then, closely resemble those reported by Lillehei in endotoxin-injected dogs, and it would appear from casual observation that both endotoxin and exotoxin toxicity respond equally well to the same drugs.

However, in our group of exotoxin-injected dogs pretreated with chlorpromazine, there was a remarkable difference in clinical appearance between pretreated and unpretreated dogs, even among the animals which did not survive (Fig 2). All seven of the chlorpromazine pretreated dogs lived a minimum average of 36 hours during which time they appeared quite healthy. A rather rapid deterioration and death then occurred in three dogs, while four remained well. This observation was in marked contrast to that of dogs in any other group. In the groups pretreated with phenoxybenzamine and with cortisone, the ultimate survival rates were about the same as that of dogs pretreated with chlorpromazine, but the nonsurvivors lived no longer than unpretreated dogs and never showed a beneficial response to pre-

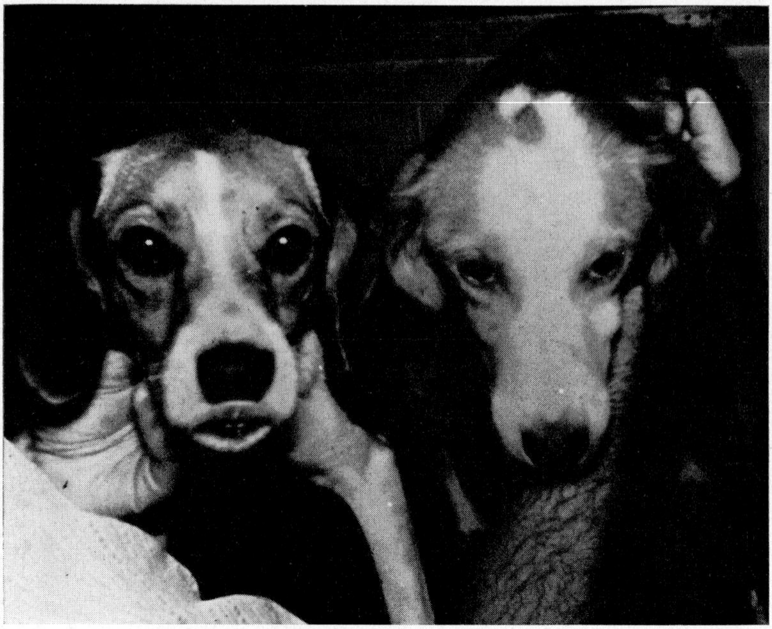

Fig 2.—Appearance of exotoxin-injected dogs six hours after injections. Neither of these dogs were permanent survivors, but note the state of well-being of the dog on the left side which had been pretreated with chlorpromazine.

treatment. Heparin pretreatment actually appeared to shorten the lives of exotoxin-injected dogs.

It has been surmised that the protective action of chlorpromazine and phenoxybenzamine is their ability to moderate the severe vasospastic phenomena induced by endotoxin shock.[9] Cortisone appears to suppress vasoconstrictive actions of endogenous catecholamines.[10]

In our exotoxin-injected dogs, the early physiologic responses (erythrocyte, leukocyte, platelet counts, hematocrit, etc) were unaltered by pretreatment regardless of whether the dogs eventually survived or not. The difference between survival or death appeared to depend upon events leading to a terminal drop in blood pressure. None of the surviving dogs showed evidence of hemorrhagic necrosis of the intestinal mucosa, a finding common to all dogs which died (Fig 3 and 4).

Much more is known about the mechanism causing death in endotoxin shock than in exotoxin shock. It may well be that their ultimate mechanisms are the same, although the rate at which they occur and the intermediate physiologic responses are different. Among other things, it is necessary to study catecholamine concentrations in the blood at various stages of exotoxin shock. The intensity and persistence of the vasoconstriction in exotoxin shock appears to be considerably greater than in endotoxin shock, as evidenced by the prolonged maintenance of blood pressure after lethal injections of

Fig 3.—*Left,* gross appearance of intestinal mucosa of exotoxin-injected dog pretreated with chlorpromazine and surviving until sacrifice. *Right* hemorrhagic appearance of unpretreated exotoxin-injected dog.

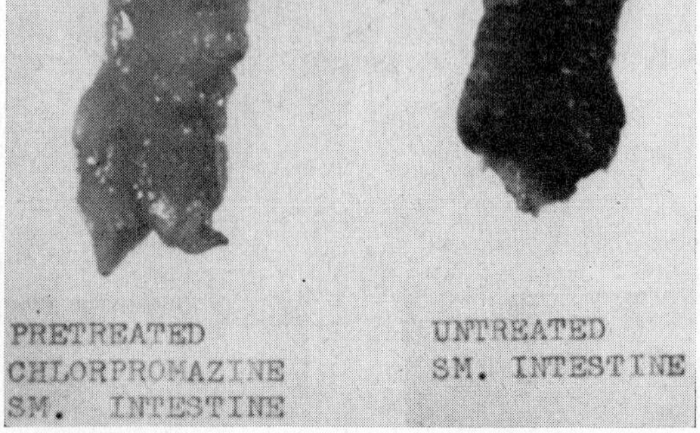

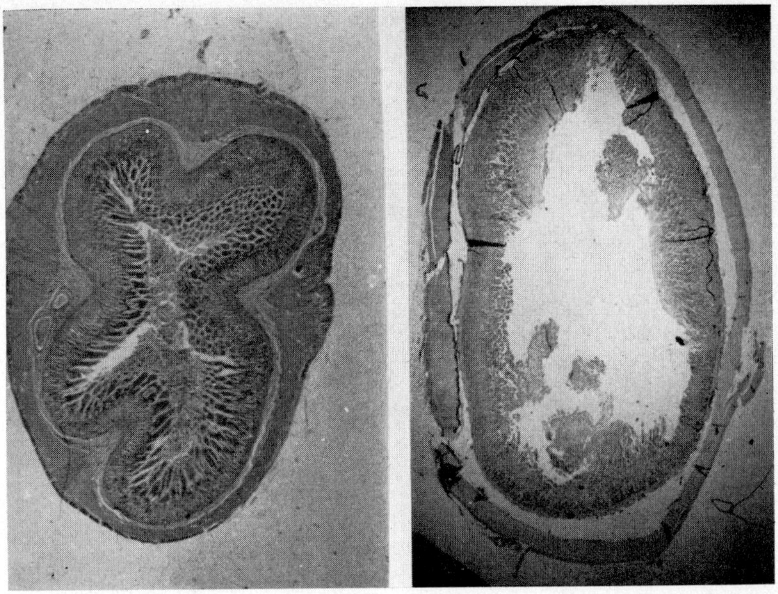

Fig 4.—*Left,* histological appearance of intestinal mucosa of exotoxin-injected dog pretreated with chlorpromazine and surviving until sacrifice. *Right,* hemorrhagic appearance of unpretreated exotoxin-injected dog.

exotoxin. Depression of erythrocyte count in exotoxin shock may well be a function of the hemolytic activity of the enzyme lecithinase rather than one of hemodilution.[11] Blood volume determinations in exotoxin shock are undependable because of severe hemolysis caused by the lecithinase. Whereas hydrocortisone and phenoxybenzamine appear to be the best drugs for pretreatment of endotoxin shock in the dog,[9] our results indicate that chlorpromazine is the best drug thus far tested for pretreatment of exotoxin shock.

Although the dog already in shock responds adversely to the drugs which are beneficial as pretreatment,[10] the human being may respond more satisfactorily. For example, Collins [12] has reported beneficial effects of chlorpromazine in posthemorrhagic shock in man when the drug was given in addition to blood transfusions. Thus far, no reports have been made on the results of post-treatment with these drugs in exotoxin shock in man.

Summary

Irreversible shock due to lecithinase, the α-exotoxin of *Clostridium perfringens,* caused hemorrhagic necrosis of the small intestinal mucosa and death, similar to that seen after irreversible shock due to hemorrhage, endotoxin, and epinephrine. Physiologic responses of erythrocyte count, leukocyte count, and blood pressure are significantly different in the first four hours after exotoxin injection from those found after endotoxin injection. Depressed hematocrit and leukocytosis are characteristic of exotoxin shock, whereas hemoconcentration and leukopenia occur in endotoxin shock. Blood pressure is maintained in exotoxin shock until shortly before death, whereas it drops steadily until death from endotoxin shock. Pretreatment of groups of exotoxin-injected animals with four drugs, chlorpromazine, phenoxybenzamine, heparin, and cortisone, revealed that all but heparin yielded at 50% to 60% salvage rate after lethal exotoxin injections. However, chlorpromazine caused a significant prolongation in survival time and support of state of well-being in nonsurvivors, while the other drugs did not.

Paul Nora, MD, Department of Surgery, Northwestern University Medical School, Chicago 11, Ill.

REFERENCES

1. Lillehei, R. C.: Intestinal Factor in Irreversible Hemorrhagic Shock, Surgery 42:1043-1054 (Dec) 1957.

2. Poole, T. R., and Watts, D. T.: Peripheral Blood Epinephrine Levels in Dogs During Intravenous Infusion, Amer J Physiol 196:145-148, 1959.

3. Nora, P. F.; Lobbes, K. E.; and Laufman, H.: Comparison of Toxicity of Endotoxin, Exotoxin, Bacterial Cells, and Strangulation Obstruction, Surg Forum 13:356, 1962.

4. Lillehei, R. C., and MacLean, L. D.: Physiological Approach to Successful Treatment of Endotoxin Shock in Experimental Animal, Arch Surg 78:464-471 (March) 1959.

5. Lillehei, R.: Personal communication to the authors.

6. Lillehei, R. C.; Longerbeam, J. K.; and Rosenberg, J. C.: The Nature of Irreversible Shock: Its Relationship to Intestinal Changes, reprint from Bock, K. D., ed.: Shock: Pathogenesis and Therapy; An International Symposium, Berlin, Springer-Verlag, 1962.

7. Longerbeam, J. K.; Lillehei, R. C.; Scott, W. R.; and Rosenberg, J. C.: Visceral Factors in Shock, JAMA 181:878-883 (Sept 8) 1962.

8. Hardaway, R. M.; Husni, E. A.; Geever, E. F.; Noyes, H. E.; and Burns, J. W.: Endotoxin Shock: A Manifestation of Intravascular Coagulation, Ann Surg 154:791 (Nov) 1961.

9. Lillehei, R. C., and MacLean, L. D.: The Intestinal Factor in Irreversible Endotoxin Shock, Ann Surg 148:513 (Oct) 1958.

10. Spink, W. W.: Endotoxin Shock, Ann Intern Med 57:538 (Oct) 1962.

11. Furr, W. E., Jr.; Bourdeau, R. V.; Roach, H. D.; and Laufman, H.: In Vivo Effects of Clostridium Welchii Lecithinase, Surg Gynec Obstet 95:465, 1952.

12. Collins, V. J.; Jaffee, R.; and Zahony, I.: Shock: A Different Approach to Therapy, Ill Med J 122:350-353 (Oct) 1962.

Staphylococcus Enterocolitis

ROBERT J. GARDNER, MD; GEORGE C. HENEGAR, MD; AND FREDERICK W. PRESTON, MD, CHICAGO

The diagnosis of staphylococcus enterocolitis was not made on the surgical service of the Veterans Administration Research Hospital from the opening of the hospital in 1953 until 1959. Ten patients, seven of whom died, seen during 1959 and 1960, have been previously reported.[8] Since then there have been eight cases, the last six of which were managed without a fatality. The entire series of eighteen patients is analyzed in this report.

Staphylococcus enterocolitis is an inflammatory condition of the small and large intestine characterized by profuse exudation into the bowel lumen, enterotoxic shock, and the presence of coagulase-positive hemolytic *Staphylococcus aureus* often in pure culture in the stool. Other names for the disease which are given in the literature are pseudomembranous enterocolitis, membranous enterocolitis, diphtheritic enteritis, staphylococcal enteritis, micrococcic enteritis, and antibiotic enteritis.

Some authors state that pseudomembranous enterocolitis is an uncommon entity with multiple etiologic factors often unrelated to the administration of antibiotics and is a disease which occurred approximately as frequently in the era before antibiotics as it does today.[4,5,9] These authors make a distinction between pseudomembranous enterocolitis and staphylococcus enterocolitis, a milder more common illness, which is separate as to both etiology and prognosis but has similar symptomatology. Dearing's studies show that patients with pseudomembranous enterocolitis may have *Micrococcus pyogenes* (*S aureus*) in pure culture in the intestine or that the pseudomembrane may exist without culturable *M pyogenes*. Furthermore, patients with symptoms of staph-

Presented at the 20th Annual Meeting of the Central Surgical Association, Chicago, Feb 21-23, 1963.

From the departments of surgery, Veterans Administration Research Hospital and Northwestern University Medical School.

This work was supported in part by a grant from the Bristol Laboratories, Syracuse, NY.

TABLE 1.—*Principal Preoperative Diagnoses of Patients Developing Staphylococcus Enterocolitis*

		No. of Patients
Carcinoma of gastrointestinal tract		9
Esophagus	3	
Colon	5	
Rectum	1	
Arteriosclerosis obliterans		2
Laennec's cirrhosis of liver		2
Regional enteritis		1
Carcinoma of urinary bladder		1
Gastric ulcer		1
Ulcerative colitis		1
Pancreatitis		1
Total		18

ylococcal enteritis and with *M pyogenes* in the stools in pure culture may have no pseudomembrane. Other authors [10-12] state that the two illnesses are identical in etiology, differing only in the virulence of the staphylococcus. The causative agent of both is the enterotoxin produced by the staphylococcus growing uninhibited in the stool. For the purpose of this presentation we consider the two conditions as identical. Antibiotics are considered an important cause.

Material

Eighteen patients with staphylococcus enterocolitis were seen from January, 1959, to July, 1962. Hemolytic coagulase-positive *S aureus* (*M pyogenes*) was present in large numbers in the stools of all patients. The bacteria were resistant to penicillin in all except four cases. Organisms resistant to erythromycin were found in nine instances and to chloramphenicol in one patient, although high concentrations of chloramphenicol in six other cases were necessary to demonstrate sensitivity. Resistance to sodium oxacillin or methicillin was not encountered. Five of the patients had a positive blood culture of this organism. Ages of the patients ranged from 38 to 72 years and averaged 56.4 years. Fourteen of the patients were in the immediate postoperative period. One patient was not operated upon, one patient had an emergency portacaval shunt 22 days after recovering from staphylococcus enterocolitis, and two patients were operated upon, discharged from the hospital, and had staphylococcus enterocolitis at a subsequent hospital admission. The principal diagnoses and the operative procedures are given in Tables 1 and 2. The patients received a variety of antibiotics prior to the onset of staphylococcus enterocolitis, as indicated in Table 3. Eleven patients received a preoperative bowel preparation of neomycin sulfate and succinylsulfathiazole. Two patients received no antibiotics preoperatively or before the onset of the staphylococcus enterocolitis. In two patients an antibiotic bowel preparation was started, stopped, and then restarted. All except two were debilitated as a result of severe chronic illnesses. Thirteen of the patients had lost 15 to 40 lb (6.8-18.1 kg) of weight over a period of two to eight months. In 14 patients in whom the condition occurred immediately postoperatively, the time of onset of the staphylococcus enterocolitis ranged from the second to the sixteenth postoperative day. The mean was on the fifth postoperative day. Fever and diarrhea consisting of profuse liquid greenish-white stomal or rectal discharges occurred in all patients. Usually the illness began with fever which lasted for a day or two before the start of the diarrhea. Vomiting, which occurred in five patients, probably was avoided in some by the presence of a nasogastric tube at the onset of the illness. Three patients complained of abdominal pain. Distention was observed in three and abdominal tender-

TABLE 2.—*Operative Procedures on Patients Developing Staphylococcus Enterocolitis* *

	No. of Patients
Colon resection	6
Lower extremity amputation	2
Portacaval shunt	2
Gastric resection	1
Open coagulation of bladder tumor	1
Esophagectomy	1
Colon bypass of esophageal carcinoma	1
Gastrostomy	1
Ileotransverse colostomy	1
Excision of perineum	1
No operation (pancreatitis)	1
Total	18

* One portacaval shunt was done after recovery from staphylococcus enterocolitis. In the remainder of the operated-on cases staphylococcus enterocolitis occurred postoperatively.

TABLE 3.—*Antibiotics Given Preoperatively to Patients Developing Staphylococcus Enterocolitis* *

Antibiotic	No. of Patients
Neomycin sulfate	11
Succinylsulfathiazole	11
Penicillin	5
Streptomycin	3
Chloramphenicol	2
Tetracycline	2

* Two patients received no antibiotics preoperatively or before the onset of the staphylococcus enterocolitis.

TABLE 4.—*Antibiotics Used in Treatment of Staphylococcus Enterocolitis* *

Antibiotic	No. of Patients
Erythromycin	9
Chloramphenicol	4
Ristocetin	3
Novobiocin	2
Kanamycin	1
Vancomycin	1
Sodium oxacillin	4
Methicillin	2

* Most patients received more than one antibiotic.

ness in two. Seven patients had an infected wound, seven had oliguria, and three developed acidosis.

Results

Treatment consisted of fluid and electrolyte replacement, corticotropin (ACTH) or cortisone, and one or more of the antibiotics listed in Table 4. Fecal enemas were given to five patients. Before February, 1961, the antibiotics preferred for treatment were erythromycin or chloramphenicol. Since then preference has been for sodium oxacillin or methicillin, and six patients have been so treated. The dose was 4 to 6 gm per day. No toxic reactions attributable to these antibiotics were noted. The treatment of these 6 patients differed in no significant fashion from that of the other 12 except for the use of the antibiotics.

All patients were treated intensively with full realization of the seriousness of the illness. It has been emphasized to the resident staff of the hospital that when a greenish-white diarrhea appears postoperatively a fecal smear and culture are indicated. If a preponderance of Gram-positive organisms is seen on the smear, treatment with corticotropin or corticosteroids and antibiotics is started at once without awaiting a report of the stool culture. The clinical response to erythromycin and chloramphenicol was seldom satisfactory. The diarrhea, fever, and toxicity persisted, and a downward course ensued. This lead to frequent changes of antibiotics to ristocetin, vancomycin, kanamycin, or novobiocin as the situation became desperate. In contrast the clinical response to either sodium oxacillin or methicillin was quite dramatic. Fever and abdominal distention were relieved in 48 hours and the diarrhea in 72 hours in all cases. It is a striking feature of this series that all 6 of the patients treated with sodium oxacillin or methicillin survived, whereas only 4 of the other 12 patients survived. The appearance of staphylococcus bacteremia was an ominous sign. Four of 5 patients who had a blood culture positive for the organism died.

Comment

In 1959 a hospital epidemic of penicillin-resistant staphylococcus wound infections occurred on the surgical service of the Veterans Administration Research Hospital. It was at this time that the first cases of staphylococcus enteritis were seen. It is unlikely that the disease had existed in the hospital and had been overlooked prior to this time. We were aware of the disease in other hospitals and had used a media for stool cultures suitable for growing Gram-positive organisms since 1953. Evidently a considerable period is necessary for an antibiotic-resistant staphylococcus to become established in a hospital. During this period hospital personnel and patients become carriers of the organism in the nose, throat, and on the skin.[3] Under normal conditions the *S aureus* is seldom present in large numbers in these individuals, but, if the usual intestinal flora is suppressed, the organism may proliferate rapidly to produce staphylococcus enterocolitis. On a surgical service this may occur in the early postoperative period. Dearing[5] has advised the routine oral use of bacitracin as soon as the postoperative patient can take liquids by mouth so that growth of staphylococcus in the intestine will be discouraged until the usual bacterial flora has returned. The early postoperative feeding of milk or lactobacillus has also been advised to accomplish this purpose.

Prohaska[10-12] and his associates have produced the typical lesions of staphylococcus enterocolitis in chinchillas by the administration of antibiotics for 9 to 15 days followed by the feeding of cultures of resistant strains of *S aureus*. If the antibiotics were administered for five days or less before the organisms were given, the resulting superinfection was not fatal, but if the antibiotics were administered again after the organisms had been fed to the animals, a fatal enterocolitis resulted. In all fatal cases the *S aureus* could be cultured from the animal's stools. Prohaska was also able to reproduce the lesions of staphylococcus enterocolitis by feeding the enterotoxin extracted from the *S aureus* and to correlate the potency of the enterotoxin with the severity of the enterocolitis.

Clinically there is fever, abdominal distention, diarrhea, and ileus. Characteristically one sees a blood pressure drop sometime during the course of the illness. It occurs at varying times, is of varying degrees of severity, and has been suggested as a factor in the etiology. In this series six patients had a fall of the systolic blood pressure to 90 mm of Hg or below before the onset of diarrhea, and three survived; of the eight patients who sustained a hypotensive episode of this degree after the diarrhea began, five survived. Hypotension appeared to be a manifestation of fluid loss into the lumen of the gut rather than an etiologic agent.

The lesions of staphylococcus enterocolitis are characterized pathologically by severe inflammatory changes in the bowel wall. They are most commonly found in the ileum and colon, but they also occur in the esophagus, stomach, duodenum, and jejunum.[7] Autopsies were performed on five of the eight patients in this series who died. A pseudomembrane was found in only one. This patient was operated upon for a carcinoma of the colon. As in other series,[9] all involvement was proximal to the point of obstruction. It is our impression that ileus or mechanical obstruction makes a patient more susceptible to the disease. In two instances an intestinal suture line leak was discovered at autopsy. It may be that staphylococcus enterocolitis predisposes to such leaks.

The treatment of staphylococcus enterocolitis consists of the use of corticotropin or corticosteroids to combat the potent enterotoxin elaborated by the *S aureus,* immediate and accurate replacement of fluids and electrolytes lost into the bowel lumen, and antibiotics effective against the offending organism. Methods of restoring normal intestinal flora such as the use of fecal enemas appear to be of some help.

It is widely appreciated that, as new antibiotics are introduced, resistant *S aureus* strains do not appear for some months, then appear sporadically, and finally become predominant in a hospital depending upon the usage of the antibiotics. At present, erythromycin- and chloramphenicol-resistant staphylococcal strains are being encountered more frequently. Strains of *S aureus* resistant to sodium oxacillin and to methicillin were not encountered in this group of cases and have been encountered extremely infrequently among the strains from other sources cultured in the hospital laboratory. Other laboratories have had a similar experience.[1,2,6] At present sodium oxacillin or methicillin are the antibiotics of choice for the treatment of staphylococcus enterocolitis. Allen and associates[1] and Dickinson and Pride[6] have found methicillin to be the antibiotic of choice for the treatment of severe penicillin-resistant *S aureus* coagulase-positive infections. In order to delay the appearance of resistant strains, sodium oxacillin and methicillin should not be used generally but should be reserved for serious cases.

The problem of control of hospital-acquired staphylococcus infections is a continuous one. Control cannot be maintained by the use of new antibiotics alone. Infections in clean surgical wounds in the majority of instances can be traced to hospital personnel or to patients who act as carriers. The majority of serious wound infections result from implantation of bacteria in the wound at the time of operation. A different situation prevails with staphylococcus enterocolitis. In this case the patient already has the organism preoperatively in his nasopharynx, having acquired it while in the hospital. Rigid isolation techniques for patients with infected wounds have their greatest usefulness here.

Summary

An experience with 18 cases of staphylococcus enterocolitis seen between 1959 and 1962 is presented. All had positive stool cultures for *Staphylococcus aureus,* coagulase positive. Fourteen patients were in the immediate postoperative period. Debility and weight loss resulting from chronic illness were common denominators in most patients. Before February, 1961, the antibiotics used to treat the disease were erythromycin, chloramphenicol, and occasionally ristocetin, novobiocin, kanamycin, and vancomycin. This group consisted of 12 patients. The mortality was 66% (8 patients). Since February, 1961, as broad-spectrum antibiotic-resistant strains of *S aureus* became more frequent, treatment was changed to include sodium oxacillin or methicillin. Four patients treated with sodium oxacillin and two treated with methicillin survived.

Frederick W. Preston, MD, Veterans Administration Research Hospital, 333 E Huron St, Chicago 11, Ill.

REFERENCES

1. Allen, J. D.; Roberts, C. E.; and Kirby, W. M. M.: Staphylococcal Septicemia Treated With Methicillin, New Eng J Med 266:111-116, 1962.

2. Artz, C. P., and Grogan, J. B.: Staphylococcal Infections: Incidence, Environmental and Laboratory Studies, Ann Surg 154:573-584, 1961.

3. Cairns, H. J. F., and Summers, G. A. C.: Penicillin-Resistant Staphylococci: Incidence in Relation to Length of Stay in Hospital, Lancet 1:446, 1950.

4. Dearing, W. H.: Micrococcic Enteritis and Pseudomembranous Enterocolitis as Complications of Antibiotic Therapy, Ann NY Acad Sci 65:235-241, 1956.

5. Dearing, W. H.: Current Status of Preparation of the Intestine for Operation: A Critical Appraisal, Surg Clin N Amer 39:1223-1242, 1959.

6. Dickinson, J. M., and Pride, M. B.: Treatment of Staphylococcal Infections With Methicillin, Brit Med J 1:432-436, 1962.

7. Dixon, C. F., and Weismann, R. E.: Acute Pseudomembranous Enteritis or Enterocolitis: A Complication Following Intestinal Surgery, Surg Clin N Amer 28:999-1023, 1948.

8. Gardner, R. J., and Preston, F. W.: Staphylococcal Enterocolitis, Quart Bull Northwest Univ Med Sch 35:20-27, 1961.

9. Pettet, J. D.; Baggenstoss, A. H.; Judd, E. S., Jr.; and Dearing, W. H.: Generalized Postoperative Pseudomembranous Enterocolitis, Proc Mayo Clin 29:342-349, 1954.

10. Prohaska, J. V.; Jacobson, M. J.; Drake, C. T.; and Tan, T.-L.: Staphylococcus Enterotoxin Enteritis, Surg Gynec Obstet 109:73-77, 1959.

11. Tan, T.-L.; Drake, C. T.; Jacobson, M. J.; and Prohaska, J. V.: The Experimental Development of Pseudomembranous Enterocolitis, Surg Gynec Obstet 108:415-420, 1959.

12. Warren, S. E. ;Sugiyama, H.; and Prohaska, J. V.: Correlation of Staphylococcal Enterotoxins With Experimentally Induced Enterocolitis, Surg Gynec Obstet 116:29-33, 1963.

DISCUSSION

On papers by Drs. Nora and Laufman, and Gardner, Henegar, and Preston.

Dr. John V. Prohaska, Chicago: The most important step in staphylococcus enterocolitis, as far as therapy is concerned, is a vigorous replacement of water, electrolytes, and colloids. The second and simultaneous step in therapy should be the eradication of the agent causing the disease. In this instance the agent is the enterotoxin elaborated by the staphylococci now growing successfully in a man's intestine.

Thus, one may choose to destroy the enterotoxin by destroying the microorganism elaborating it, or one may neutralize the enterotoxin effect with corticotropin (ACTH). Corticotropin cannot be expected to remain effective in the face of overwhelming continuous supply of enterotoxin. It is like an ice cube: it cools the water but does not freeze it.

The use of antibacterial agents to which staphylococcus is known to be sensitive may be a life-saving procedure. Staphylococci are known not to retain their sensitivity to antibiotics indefinitely. Therefore, sensitivity tests often have to be conducted in order not to use an antibiotic which would further enhance the growth or regrowth of staphylococci by continuous destruction of *Escherichia coli.* This is important because staphylococci and *E coli* do not grow together.

In our series of 50 patients, we had 54% mortality in those patients not receiving corticotropin but receiving vigorous supportive therapy and chloramphenicol, and we had 5% mortality in those patients who received the same treatment but with corticotropin. If you use corticotropin, use it early.

The reimplantation of normal stool provides *E coli* and makes the survival of staphylococci difficult.

Dr. Edward S. Judd, Rochester, Minn: We have tried to reduce the indiscriminate use of antibiotics throughout our hospitals, and I believe it has had a very telling effect in the last several years. I am certain we have reduced the staphylococcus enterocolitis problem drastically, and we think this is one of the reasons that we have a satisfactory report to make in that regard.

In fact, some of us in our group who are interested in surgery of the colon have gone so far as to eliminate all antibiotics in the preoperative period. Perhaps many of you have reached the same conclusion. Perhaps you are accepting an occasional Gram-negative infection as a result of that change. It will be interesting to discuss this problem with you.

Dr. Dearing, my co-author in several earlier papers, says we are now finding a new strain of staphylococcus in some cases which originally were listed as "no type."

Thus far we are referring to the new strain as the "UC 18." He tells me that we have about 25 cases. Unfortunately, however, all of them have been resistant to most of the antibiotics at the present time. Fortunately none of them has terminated fatally.

Dr. Prohaska and I have previously debated whether all of these cases are due to staphylococcus, because we have gone on record as recording an occasional case with severe pseudomembranous ileocolitis, almost always fatal, in which we have been unable to recover any staphylococci from the gastrointestinal tract in spite of the most modern and most elaborate culture methods.

This is a photograph taken at the autopsy table. Those are not postmorten changes. This is just one little segment of the entire intestinal tract revealing an extreme membrane, as you can see. It has sloughed off from most of the intestine. This is seen in staphylococcus enterocolitis also—in fact, the changes are indistinguishable according to our pathologists. We are still seeing an occasional case of so-called "idiopathic enterocolitis."

The study presented by Dr. Gardner and associates, is a very important one and reminds all of us once again that the problem still exists. It can be detected early by an alert clinician and an alert surgeon, and there are measures available to us so that lives can be saved.

Dr. William A. Altemeier, Cincinnati: The *Clostridium perfringens* has many exotoxins, probably seven. The most important one is the alpha-toxin, or lecithinase, which is also known as the lethal toxin. Unfortunately, it has not been purified as yet, but standardization has been possible for reproducible results.

The similarity of some of the results obtained by Dr. Nora and Dr. Laufman with exotoxin shock compared with those of others working with endotoxin shock suggested to me a common interphase or secondary mechanism initiated by both types of toxins.

In our experimental work with the alpha-toxin of *Clostridium perfringens* and more recently with the alpha-toxin of *Staphylococcus aureus,* we have recorded blood pressure, pulse, electrocardiogram, and urinary output continuously by means of the physiograph. We have noted the same type of double curve of blood pressure response after the intravenous injection of the alpha-toxin of *Clostridium perfringens* and the hemolytic *Staphylococcus aureus* with one exception. Often there has been an immediate, but temporary, rise in the blood pressure after the intravenous injection followed by a precipitous fall, a secondary rise, and a secondary and terminal fall.

It has been interesting to us to determine that exotoxin cannot be demonstrated in the blood after its intravenous injection. This has also been true when the exotoxin has been inoculated in vitro, suggesting immediate binding. Nevertheless, the double curve phenomenon will follow, and death will be the result.

Their demonstration of the protective effect of chlorpromazine when used prophylactically is interesting. Of greater interest to me, however, has been our observation that the injection of a sublethal dose of exotoxin from which the animal survives appears to have some protective effect for a subsequent injection of the same material. Since much higher doses are required to produce the terminal fall in pressure and death, the amount of lethal toxin needed under these circumstances may increase as much as 4 to 20 times.

Much more is known about endotoxin shock than exotoxin shock, and I would like to encourage the investigators to continue their work in this important and intriguing field.

I would also like to discuss briefly the paper on staphylococcal enterocolitis. I believe this condition is much more prevalent than most of us realize. It should be emphasized again that the laboratory methods used for the identification of enteric pathogens actually suppress the growth of staphylococci; consequently, a negative report for enteric pathogens may be misleading.

During the last four years, we have seen a total of 155 patients with staphylococcal enterocolitis. We became intrigued with the fact that, in 107 of these patients, the infecting staphylococci were untypable, using the international series of bateriophages. In a smaller series of 55 patients, 65.4% had untypable staphylococci. Phage type 80-81 were not found in any of the 55 cases.

Using two new bacteriophages isolated in my surgical research bacteriology laboratory, it was possible to analyze 25, and 4 strains of the 36 untypable staphylococcal isolates. Bacteriophage type UC 18 was found to be the most important.

In the 12-month period during the 1962 calendar year, 24 of 33 isolates of staphylococci from patients with enterocolitis were UC 18 type-specific. An additional two isolates were typable by the UC 13 and UC 18 phages. Thus in 26 out of 33 cases, or 80%, the staphylococci associated with enterocolitis were typable by UC 18 phage.

We agree that sodium methicillin (Staphicillin) is by far the agent of choice. The preoperative preparation of the gastroenteric tract with neomycin may predispose to staphylococcal enterocolitis, according to our studies, and I have discontinued its use for that purpose during the past year .

I would also like to point out that the UC 18 type-specific strain of staphylococcus with which we are working appears to be identical with the SD strain used by Dr. Prohaska in his experimental studies. The latter is typable by UC 18 phage, and the former has been shown to produce exterotoxin. I hope that the authors will continue their work in this very important field.

Dr. Paul Nora, Chicago: With reference to the possible clinical application of the use of chlorpromazine in shock, I think it is worthy of note that there is a recent report by Dr. Collins, of Cook County Hospital, in which he used a combination of blood and chlorpromazine and found it superior to blood alone for use in hemorrhagic shock.

Dr. Frederick W. Preston, Chicago: Dr. Judd's associates ten years ago reported 44 cases of staphylococcic enteritis and showed that oxytetracycline (Terramycin) and chlortetracycline (Aureomycin) given for 2 to 18 days so altered the bacterial flora of the intestine that resistant strains proliferated and produced gastrointestinal and systemic symptoms so severe that in some cases death resulted. In most of these cases the drugs were given orally, but in eight cases oxytetracycline was given intravenously, and in one case it was given intramuscularly. Thus the drug is excreted in such high concentration in the bile that it markedly alters the intestinal flora.

These antibiotics were discontinued, and, when erythromycin was given, the symptoms promptly disappeared, the micrococci disappeared from the stools, and there were no deaths in this series.

Thus, the response in their patients to erythromycin was similar to those we achieved with methicillin and oxacillin. Erythromycin was no longer effective in the management of our patients because the staphylococcus was resistant to this antibiotic.

I think we can anticipate that the same chain of events will occur with methicillin and oxacillin, and therefore it probably will be necessary to develop new antibiotics or to reintroduce old ones after they have been shelved for several years, in order to have available effective therapy for the hospital staphylococcus.

There are some unanswered questions. We wonder about the fact that our last fatal case of this disease was in March, 1962, and we wonder if this happy turn of events is related to an awareness on the part of our staff of this entity and its seriousness or whether we are dealing with a staphylococcus of waning virulence.

Also, we wonder if our results in these few cases with oxacillin and methicillin are related to the effectiveness of these antibiotics or whether this is also related to the fact that the staphylococcus is less virulent than it was when the fatal cases were encountered.

Studies of Fibrinolytic Activity After Hepatectomy

THEODORE DRAPANAS, MD; WALTON K. T. SHIM, MD; AND JOHN D. STEWART, MD, BUFFALO, NY

The occasional occurrence of spontaneous fibrinolysis following major surgical procedures resulting in altered blood coagulation and bleeding has been noted with increasing interest.

Numerous investigations recently reviewed by Astrup,[3] Albrechtsen,[1] Cooper,[6] and

Presented at the 20th Annual Meeting of the Central Surgical Association, Chicago, Feb 21-23, 1963.

Present address: Army Chemical Research Center, Edgewood, Md. (Dr. Shim).

From the School of Medicine, State University of New York at Buffalo, and the Department of Surgery, Edward J. Meyer Memorial Hospital.

This project was supported by grant A-2937 from the United States Public Health Service.

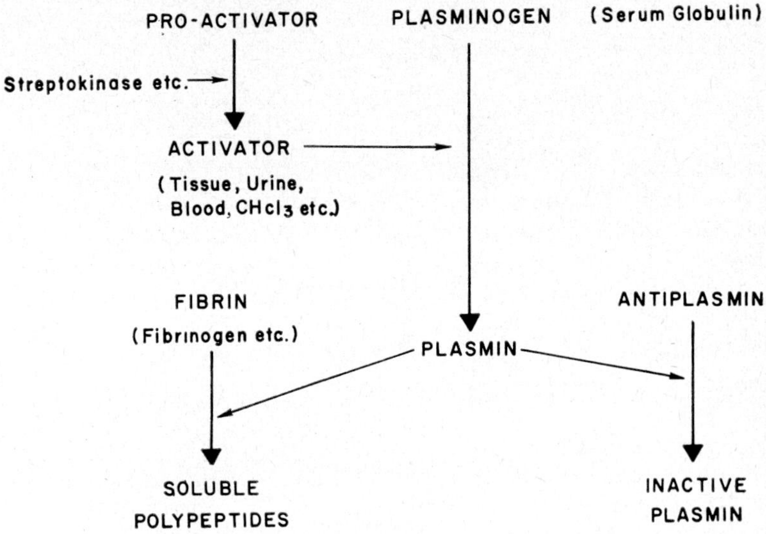

Fig 1.—Components of fibrinolytic system.

Cohen and Warren[5] have established that normal human blood contains an inactive proteolytic globulin termed plasminogen (profibrinolysin) (Fig 1). In the presence of certain activating substances in the blood, tissues, urine, or of bacterial origin, eg, streptokinase, staphylokinase, this globulin is converted to the active enzyme plasmin (fibrinolysin). This enzyme is capable of hydrolyzing the internal peptide bonds of the fibrin in the blood clot or other proteins containing structural sites suitable for activation by plasmin.[12] Free plasmin in the blood is neutralized by various inhibitors (antiplasmin).[17] Similarly, inhibitors of plasminogen activation are also known to exist.[5]

A significant observation by many surgeons has been the presence of excessive oozing in patients with advanced obstructive jaundice,[8] various forms of liver disease including Laennec's cirrhosis,[7,9,14] or after major surgery.[18] Although altered blood coagulability resulting from abnormalities in prothrombin, factor V and factor VII production, and hypofibrinogenemia has been shown to accompany extensive hepatic surgery,[19] relatively little is known about the primary relation of the liver to the fibrinolytic mechanism in the body.

Throughout the course of a continuous study during the past ten years of the metabolic alterations in the experimental animal following total extirpation of the liver, it was noted that the liverless dog when supported only by glucose infusion, with rare exceptions, died of hemorrhage. This hemorrhage is due to a failure in the coagulation mechanism accompanied by fibrinogen, prothrombin, and platelet depletion.[15,16]

The present study was undertaken to investigate the role of fibrinolysis in the coagulation defect following hepatectomy and to define the relationship of the liver to the aberrations in the fibrinolytic mechanism reported to accompany liver disease.

Methods

Total hepatectomy was performed in 42 adult mongrel dogs by the two-stage method of Markowitz and Soskin.[11] All dogs were supported after hepatectomy with a continuous intravenous infusion of 10% glucose sufficient to prevent hypoglycemia. With the exception of a transfusion of fresh canine blood given during hepatectomy to replace operative blood loss, no further transfusions were administered in the postoperative period in order to avoid any alteration in the blood constituents under study.

Serial samples of whole blood, plasma, serum, and prepared euglobulin fraction were assayed for plasminogen (profibrinolysin), plasmin (fibrinolysin), antiplasmin (antifibrinolysin), and antitryptic activity at regular intervals before and after hepatectomy. All studies were continued until death of the animals, and a similar assay was performed on any blood removed from the wound or the peritoneal cavity immediately after death. Analyses

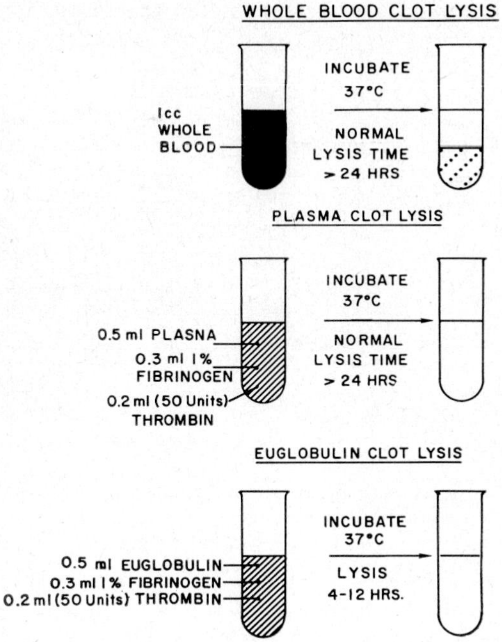

Fig 2.—Schema of clot lysis studies.

of the components of the fibrinolytic mechanism were performed as follows (Fig 2):

Whole Blood Clot Lysis Time.—Lytic activity of whole blood was determined by incubating 1 cc of clotted whole blood in a test tube for 24 hours at 37 C and checking for lysis of the clot at 4, 12, and 24 hours.

Serum or Plasma Clot Lysis Time.—This was recorded as the time required for complete lysis of a standard fibrin clot formed by mixing of 0.5 ml of serum or plasma to be tested, with 0.3 ml of a standard 1% bovine fibrinogen solution in barbital buffer and 0.2 ml of bovine thrombin (50 units).

Euglobulin Clot Lysis Time.—The method used was essentially as described by Milstone involving preliminary precipitation of the euglobulin fraction by acid extraction at a pH of 5.8. The resulting precipitate (euglobulin), which contains plasminogen and plasmin spontaneously formed with the removal of inhibitors, was dissolved in 1 ml of barbital (Veronal) buffer (pH 7.8). Lysis of a standard fibrin clot was then determined in the same manner as the whole serum or plasma clot lysis method by the addition of fibrinogen and thrombin to 0.5 ml of the euglobulin solution.

Fibrin Plate Lysis.—The fibrin plate technique as described by Astrup and Müllertz[4] was used: Stock bovine fibrinogen solution was prepared to a purity of 85%-95% clottable protein and dissolved in diethyl barbiturate buffer (ionic strength of 0.05, pH 7.8). In clean Petri dishes (10 cm diameter) 9.0 ml of diluted stock fibrinogen solution (0.3%) was clotted with 0.3 ml of thrombin solution containing 200 units/ml. In order to destroy all plasminogen, plasmin, and antiplasmin activity present in the fibrin substrate, the clotted plates were then heated to 80 C for 30 minutes in a constant-temperature oven according to the method of Lassen.[10] Assay for the various components of the fibrinolytic system was then performed on the heated fibrin plates as follows (Fig 3):

(*a*) Spontaneous Total Fibrinolytic Activity of Serum and Plasma: Exactly 0.03 ml of fresh serum or fresh oxalated plasma to be tested was placed

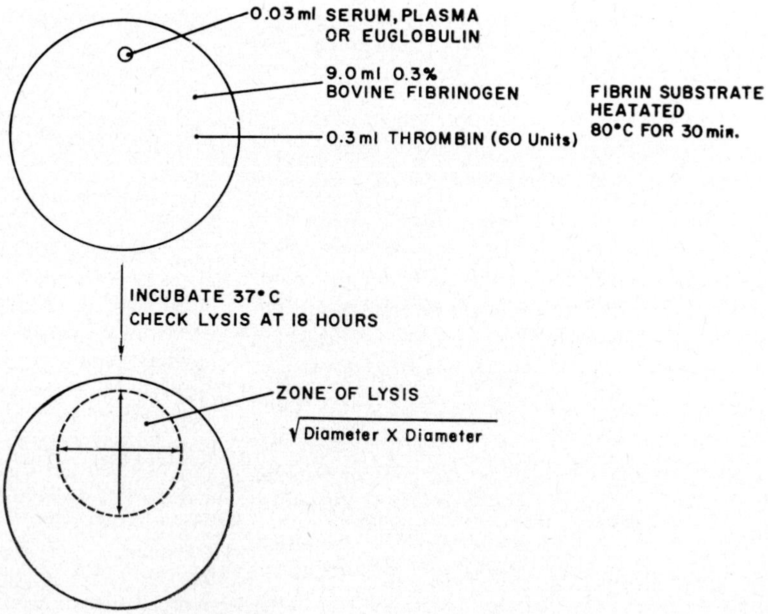

Fig 3.—Fibrin plate lysis method.

as a small drop on the surface of the fibrin plate which was then incubated at 37 C for 18 hours. The relative size of any zone of lysis produced was determined by measuring two perpendicular diameters with calipers and calculating the square root of their product.

(*b*) Plasminogen Activity of Serum or Plasma: To evaluate plasminogen activity, equal amounts of plasma were incubated for one hour with streptokinase (Lederle) as an activator containing 10,800 units/ml, and 0.06 ml of this solution was added to the heated fibrin plate prior to incubation.

(*c*) Euglobulin Plasmin Activity: To test plasmin activity of the euglobulin fraction, 0.03 ml of euglobulin solution, prepared as previously described, was added to the heated fibrin plate as the test material.

(*d*) Euglobulin Plasminogen Activity: This was obtained by activating the plasminogen in the euglobulin fraction with streptokinase in the same manner as described for plasma and adding 0.06 ml to the plate followed by incubation.

(*e*) Antiplasmin Activity of Plasma and Euglobulin: To study antiplasmin (inhibitor) activity of plasma, equal amounts of plasma and commercially prepared plasmin (Lederle) containing 25 mg/ml were incubated for one hour and then plated. The antiplasmin activity of euglobulin was similarly determined as a control in order to test the efficiency of removal of all inhibitors in the precipitation of euglobulin. In each instance, no antiplasmin activity was demonstrated in the euglobulin fraction.

(*f*) Antitryptic Activity of Plasma: The ability of plasma to inhibit lysis caused by a standard commercially prepared trypsin solution was tested. Equal amounts of plasma and freshly prepared trypsin (Tryptar, Armour) containing 400 units/ml were mixed, incubated for one hour, and plated.

(*g*) Plasmin Activity of Peritoneal Fluid: In order to test for any fibrinolytic activity present in the peritoneal fluid, an aliquot was removed immediately after death, centrifuged, and 0.06 ml of the supernatant was plated and incubated. Any lysis at 18 hours was considered evidence of abnormal lytic activity.

Finally, as a check of the effectiveness of the heating method in removing all residual plasminogen activity in the fibrin plate substrate, streptokinase was added as an additional test drop (0.06 cc) to each plate. If any lysis occurred beneath the streptokinase following incubation, this was indicative of plasminogen activity remaining in the substrate, and the plate was therefore discarded. In only one or two instances did this occur, testing to the efficiency of the heating method in removing substrate activity.

Results

Survival of dogs following complete removal of the liver averaged 17 hours, the longest survivor living 36 hours. No animal surviving less than 12 hours was included in this study. In almost every instance, death was related to hemorrhage into the peritoneal cavity with hypotension being a constant preterminal phenomenon.

Clotting times remained normal, and, despite prolonged survival in some animals, they were not appreciably altered from pre-

Fig 4.—Results of fibrin plate lysis. *A,* normal preoperative serum from a single experiment. The dark spots indicate areas of lysis on a fibrin plate (stained with methylene blue for illustrative purposes) after incubation for 18 hours at 37 C. Beginning at the top of plate and proceeding clockwise are tests for serum plasmin activity (no lysis), serum plasminogen activity activated with streptokinase, antitryptic activity of serum (no lysis), euglobulin plasmin activity, euglobulin plasminogen activity activated with streptokinase, euglobulin antitryptic activity, and control residual plasminogen activity of fibrin plate substrate activated with streptokinase (no lysis). In center of plate is a large zone of lysis produced by a standard trypsin solution as a control. *B,* studies in the same animal 24 hours after hepatectomy. *C,* studies of the free peritoneal blood at autopsy reveal no significant changes from the control preoperative results (4*A*).

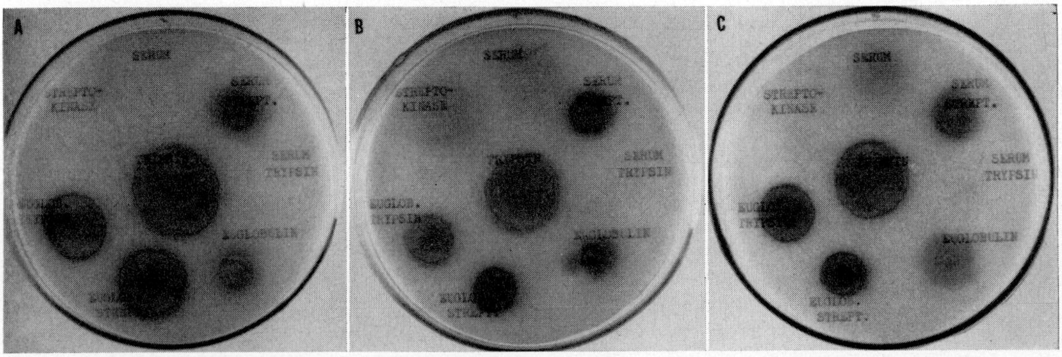

operative values. The strength of the clot produced, however, became progressively poorer with increasing survival. Inasmuch as this could be corrected by the addition of small amounts of fibrinogen to the test tube, it was apparent that this was related to depleted fibrinogen.

Whole Blood Clot Lysis.—No consistent spontaneous lysis of the clotted whole blood occurred in the postoperative period. In a few scattered samples, a small amount of lysis was evident between 12 to 24 hours, but this was not a constant finding and was not considered particularly significant.

Plasma Clot Lysis.—Spontaneous lysis of a standard clot by plasma following hepatectomy did not occur, and lysis times appeared in the normal range. The serum from these same animals showed identical results.

Euglobulin Clot Lysis.—In the dog, spontaneous activation of fibrinolysin normally occurs after precipitation of the euglobulin fraction at pH 5.8, presumably due to the removal of inhibitors, resulting in a clot lysis time of 8 to 12 hours. Any change in amount of circulating fibrinolysin would be expected, therefore, to cause an alteration in the normal lysis time. After hepatectomy, however, no significant alteration from normal in euglobulin clot lysis time occurred, regardless of the length of survival.

Fibrin Plate Lysis.—Results from a typical study utilizing the heated plate technique are shown in Fig 4. No plasmin activity occurred with whole oxalated plasma or serum before or after hepatectomy. Plasminogen and antiplasmin activity were unaltered from control values. Results utilizing serum or euglobulin also showed no change from control or prehepatectomy values. Interestingly, however, it was noted that normal dog serum or plasma shows significant antitryptic activity but very little antiplasmin activity indicating a specific inhibitor activity against each of these proteolytic enzymes.

It was also apparent that spontaneous residual plasminogen activity remained in the euglobulin fraction after precipitation which could be activated by streptokinase. Per se, this was indirect confirmation, when found in samples from the liverless dog, that no excessive lytic activity had been produced which would have used up all available plasminogen.

Finally, studies of the free peritoneal fluid similarly showed no significant lytic activity either by the clot-lysis or fibrin plate methods.

Comment

Astrup [3] has pointed out that "the quantitative estimation of most of the fibrinolytic agents and their inhibitors still awaits its ultimate solution. This applies especially to the important physiologic problems of the amounts contained in blood, where the simultaneous presence of active, activating and inhibitory agents presents a really puzzling problem." The clot lysis activity of whole blood plasma and serum in a sense reflects more accurately the potential situation existing in vivo because it represents the total expression of a complex series of reactions occurring under the limitations of inhibitors. Plasmin occurs predominantly in the euglobulin fraction of the plasma proteins; consequently this fraction was commonly used in assaying the fibrinolytic activity of plasma. No spontaneous fibrinolysis was discovered by utilizing these techniques.

The fibrin plate studies appear particularly significant in that, even by this sensitive method, no alterations from preoperative values were encountered. Plasminogen, plasmin, and antiplasmin activity remained essentially unchanged in all of the animals studied.

Consideration must be given to the concept that although no fibrinolytic activity of a general character is present in the blood stream of the liverless dog, a local process may be active, consisting of an interaction between plasminogen and activator released from injured tissue. Indeed, Müllertz [13] has indicated that plasmin may be specifically adsorbed to fibrin clots, the adsorption thereby allowing a high local plasmin concentration whereby fibrin can be split and removed in the continuing general process of body repair. This phenomenon can, therefore, occur locally, despite normal plasmin and antiplasmin blood levels, by the selective adsorption of plasmin from the blood stream by the fibrin clots. In our experiments, however, no fibrinolytic activity was measured even in the unclotted peritoneal fluid which was always present terminally in the liverless animal. The additional demonstration of normal plasminogen levels in the blood stream of animals following hepatectomy gave further confirmation that no excessive fibrinolytic activity had occurred which could cause depletion of plasminogen.

On the basis of these experiments it becomes clear that spontaneous fibrinolysis does not occur after total extirpation of the liver in dogs. The explanation of the abnormal bleeding tendencies following hepatectomy, therefore, rests on the other highly complex derangements of the blood coagulation mechanism, most of which are dependent entirely on hepatic production, including the availability of fibrinogen, the immediate precursor of the clot.[16]

It becomes difficult to reconcile the results of these experiments to the spontaneous fibrinolytic activity reported in patients with severely deteriorated liver function. However, these results indicate that tissues other than the liver may be the source of the spontaneous fibrinolytic activity when it occurs. Grossi, Moreno, and Rousselot[7] were able to demonstrate that a structural analog of lysine, ε-aminocaproic acid, administered intravenously interfered regularly with the spontaneous fibrinolytic activity noted in some patients with cirrhosis. They postulated that the inhibition of spontaneous fibrinolytic activity by this substance, a known inhibitor of plasminogen activation,[2] would indicate that an activator rather than free plasmin was circulating in the blood of these patients. Because of the abnormal extrahepatic globulin production in severe liver disease states, it would seem reasonable, therefore, to speculate that an excess of activator was also being produced. Similarly enhanced fibrinolysis with excessive bleeding has been reported in patients following pulmonary, prostatic, or uterine surgery presumably due to the large amounts of plasminogen activator present in these tissues[1] which was being released into the blood stream during surgical manipulation. Further investigation into these mechanisms and their inhibitors seems indicated.

Summary

Studies of the fibrinolytic mechanism were performed in 42 liverless dogs supported only by glucose. An average survival period of 17 hours was obtained. A progressive bleeding into the peritoneal cavity occurred in all animals after hepatectomy.

By using both the clot lysis and the heated fibrin plate techniques with whole blood, plasma, serum, or euglobulin fraction, no alteration in plasmin, plasminogen, antiplasmin, or antitryptic activity could be demonstrated. Peritoneal fluid following hepatectomy showed no abnormal fibrinolytic activity.

On the basis of these experiments, there appears to be no evidence of any aberrations in the fibrinolytic mechanism after total hepatectomy in the dog by utilizing the commonly accepted techniques of measurement. These studies indicate that in the dog the liver is not an essential organ in the maintenance and support of the fibrinolytic mechanism.

The significance of these results and their relation to the reported incidence of spontaneous fibrinolysis in patients with liver disease were discussed.

Theodore Drapanas, MD, School of Medicine, State University of New York, 462 Grider St., Buffalo, NY.

REFERENCES

1. Albrechtsen, O. K.: Fibrinolytic Activity in the Organism, Acta Physiol Scand 47:1, 1959.

2. Alkjaersig, N.; Fletcher, A. P.; and Sherry, S.: Epsilon-Aminocaproic Acid: Inhibitor of Plasminogen Activation, J Biol Chem 234:832, 1959.

3. Astrup, T.: Fibrinolysis in the Organism, Blood 11:781, 1956.

4. Astrup, T., and Müllertz, S.: The Fibrin Plate Method for Estimating Fibrinolytic Activity, Arch Biochem 40:346, 1952.

5. Cohen, S. I., and Warren, R.: Fibrinolysis, New Eng J Med 264:79, 1961.

6. Cooper, J. F.: Surgical Aspects of Fibrinolysis, Int Abstr Surg 108:417, 1959.

7. Grossi, C. E.; Moreno, A. H.; and Rousselot, L. M.: Studies on Spontaneous Fibrinolytic Activity in Patients With Cirrhosis of the Liver and Its Inhibition by Epsilon Amino Caproic Acid, Ann Surg 153:383, 1961.

8. Harrington, W. J.; Manheimer, R. H.; Des Forges, J. F.; Minkel, H. P.; Crow, C. B.; and Stohlman, F.: The Bleeding Tendency in Hepatocellular and Obstructive Jaundice, Bull Tufts New Eng Med Cent 12:121, 1950.

9. Kwaan, H. C.; McFadzean, A. J. S.; and Cook, J.: Plasma Fibrinolytic Activity in Cirrhosis of the Liver, Lancet 1:132, 1956.

10. Lassen, M.: Heat Denaturation of Plasminogen in the Fibrin Plate Method, Acta Physiol Scand 27:371, 1953.

11. Markowitz, J., and Soskin, S.: A Simplified Technique for Hepatectomy, Proc Soc Exp Biol Med 25:7, 1927.

12. Müllertz, S.: The Action of Plasmin on Fibrin and Fibrinogen in Blood, Acta Physiol Scand 28:29, 1953.

13. Müllertz, S.: Formation and Properties of the Activator of Plasminogen and of Human and Bovine Plasmin, Biochem J 61:424, 1955.

14. Ratnoff, O. D.: Studies on Proteolytic Enzyme in Human Plasma: Rate of Lysis of Plasma Clots in Normal and Diseased Individuals, With Particular Reference to Hepatic Disease, Bull Johns Hopkins Hosp 84:29, 1949.

15. Schenk, W. G., Jr.; Fopeano, J.; Cosgriff, J. H.; and Gray, J. G.: The Coagulation Defect After Hepatectomy, Surgery 42:822, 1957.

16. Schenk, W. G., Jr.; Schreiber, M.; Leslie, M. B.; Portin, B. A.; Mesmer, R. E. G.; and Stewart, J. D.: The Alteration in Plasma Proteins Resulting From Total Hepatectomy. Ann Surg 148:401, 1958.

17. Tsitouris, G.; Bellet, S.; Eilberg, R.; Feinberg, L.; and Sandberg, H.: Effect of Major Surgery on Plasmin—Plasminogen Inhibitors, Arch Intern Med 108:208, 1961.

18. Zucker, M. B.; Siegel, M.; Cliffton, E. E.; Bellville, J. W.; and Howland, W. S.: Generalized Excessive Oozing in Patients Undergoing Major Surgery and Receiving Multiple Blood Transfusions, J Lab Clin Med 50:849, 1957.

19. Zucker, M. B.; Siegel, M.; Cliffton, E. E.; Belleville, J. W.; Howland, W. S.; and Grossi, C. E.: The Effect of Hepatic Lobectomy on Some Blood Clotting Factors and on Fibrinolysis, Ann Surg 146:772, 1957.

Hereditary Pancreatitis

The Role of Surgical Intervention

BERNARD C. GERBER, MD, ABERDEEN, SD

The occurrence of hereditary pancreatitis was first suspected by Comfort and Steinberg [5] in 1952. They reported the appearance of chronic relapsing pancreatitis in four members of a single family, possibly affecting two others. Since that report, an additional four kindreds with hereditary pancreatitis have been reported.[7,8,10] Several other families have been studied in which the evidence is suggestive that hereditary pancreatitis is present.[8,12] In the five kindreds reported to date, 22 definite pancreatitis cases have been detected along with 16 suspected cases. We have studied an additional kindred with hereditary pancreatitis.

Presented at the 20th Annual Meeting of the Central Surgical Association, Chicago, Feb 21-23, 1963.

The clinical course of this disease is similar to that of the usual variety of chronic relapsing pancreatitis. Recurrent episodes of pancreatitis occur at varying intervals, with the onset of the usual sequelae of chronic pancreatitis as the disease pursues its course. Pancreatic calcifications have been observed in approximately half.[12] These calcifications are usually in the main pancreatic ducts, rather than in the gland parenchyma,[5] as is the case in the usual form of pancreatitis. Diabetes mellitus and steatorrhea have been frequent complications. Upper gastrointestinal bleeding and pancreatic pseudocysts also occur. A noteworthy feature of the disease is the early age of onset, the average being 11.8 years in the five kindreds described. In 18 of the cases listed by Gross

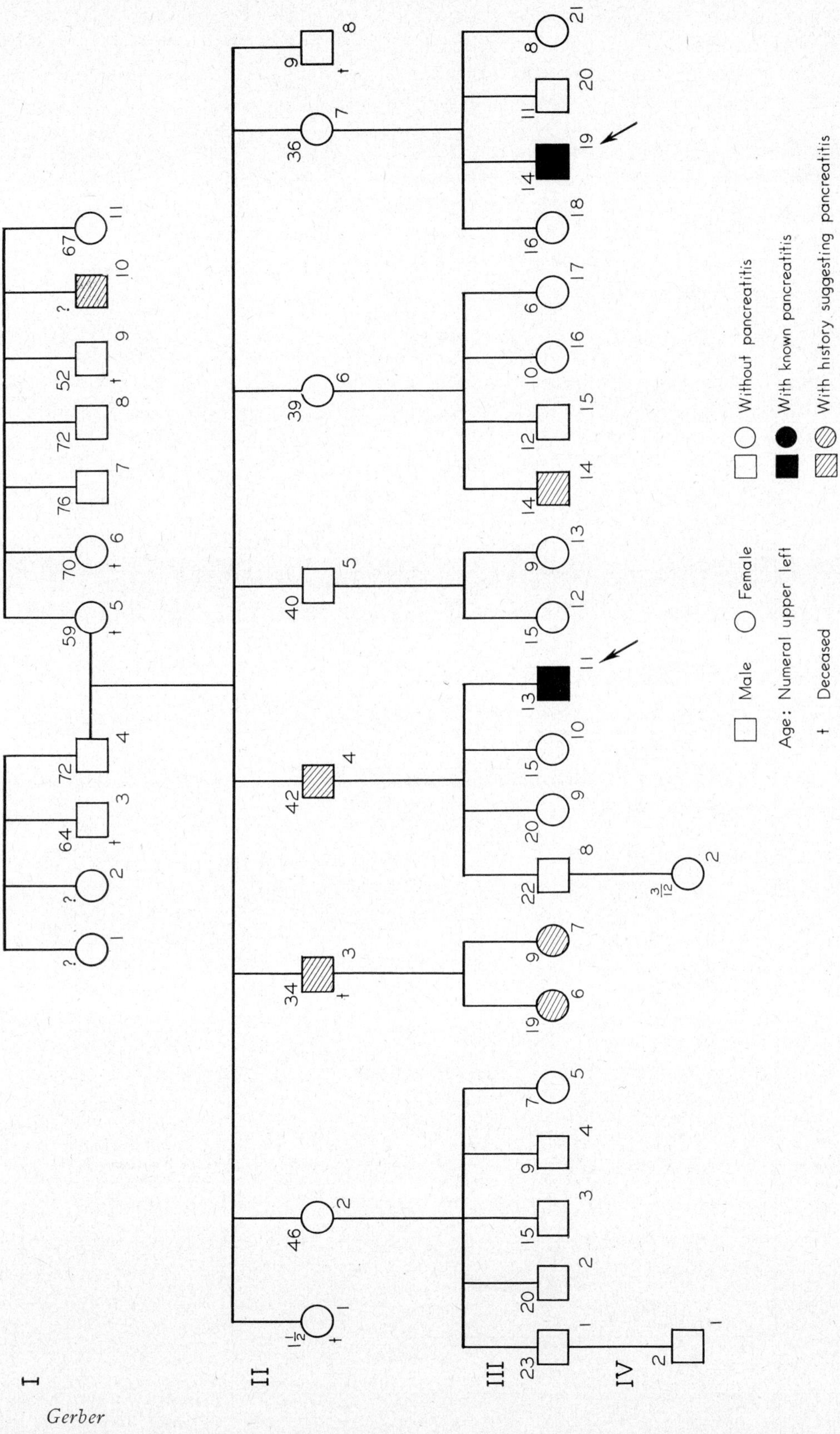

Fig 1.—Pedigree of the subject kindred.

et al[12] the patients were 5 years old or less at the time of the initial attack of pain. There has been no predilection for either sex, and all persons thus far observed have been Caucasians.

Gallstones have been discovered in only 1 of 22 of these patients. Values for serum calcium have been determined in only four persons previously reported and were normal in each instance.[12] Probably this disease is not related to the recurrent pancreatitis associated with hereditary hyperparathyroidism as reported by Jackson.[14]

Hereditary pancreatitis appears to be transmitted as a mendelian autosomal dominant trait. At present it is possible to rule out sex-linkage and complete recessiveness. The possibility of a gene with poor penetrance cannot be excluded.[12] Gross and co workers have had difficulty obtaining adequate medical information about many members of these families not definitely affected. We have encountered a similar problem.

Gross et al, in 1957[9] and subsequently,[10-12] have reported the excretion of excessive amounts of lysine and other amino acids in the urine of 15 of 30 persons (with or without pancreatitis) studied from their five kindreds with hereditary pancreatitis. They

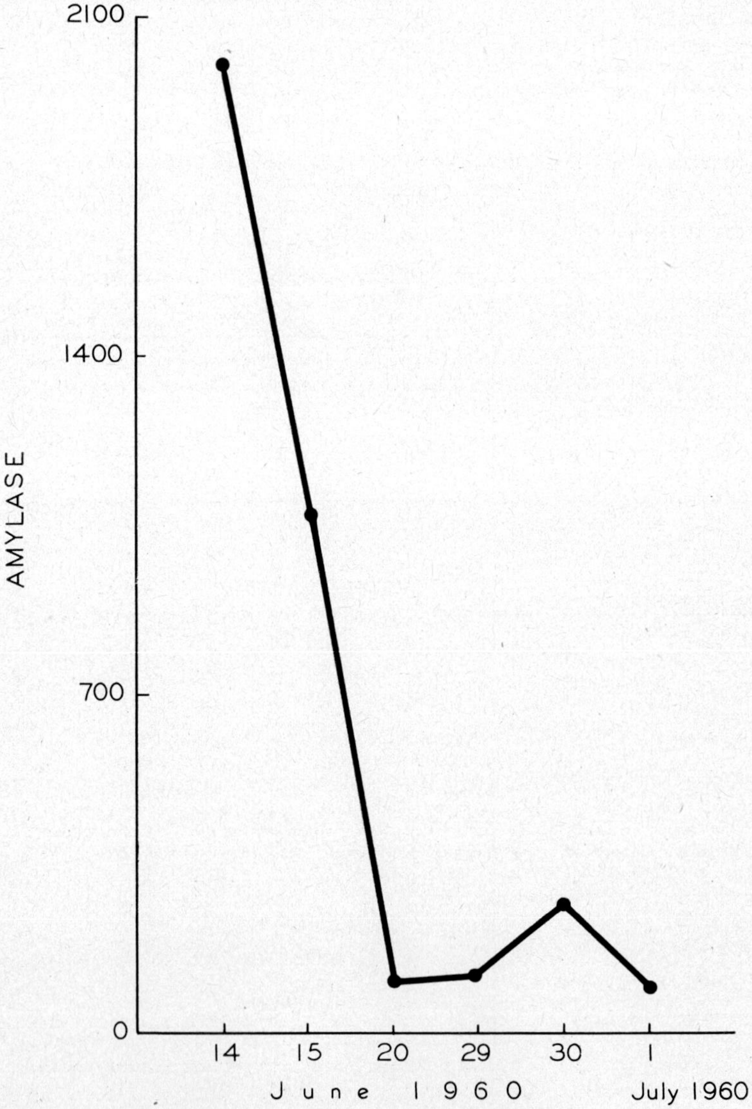

Fig 2 (Case 1).—Serum amylase (Somogyi units).

report that the biochemical and genetic features of the aminoaciduria closely resemble those described as the incompletely recessive form of "cystinuria." Gross believes there is no evidence to link the aminoaciduria and the pancreatitis etiologically or pathogenetically. This may merely represent the inheritance of multiple unrelated biochemical abnormalities.

The Subject Kindred

General Description.—In three generations of this kindred, two persons are definitely affected and six others probably have chronic relapsing pancreatitis (Fig 1). The first generation of this family emigrated from Germany and settled in North and South Dakota. There is no evidence of intermarriage.

Definite Pancreatitis

CASE 1 (III, 19).—This 12-year-old boy was first seen by us on June 14, 1960, because of abdominal pain which had started two days before. The pain began in the left upper quadrant and progressed to become more severe and extend to the midabdomen. The pain continued across the upper abdomen intermittently.

The child's parents stated that he had been having attacks of pain similar to this since before the age of two years. In the past two or three years these attacks had been occurring at least every month. He was hospitalized on Feb 16, 1953, and April 7, 1953, because of abdominal pain and vomiting. White blood cell count and differential were normal at that time. He was operated upon at that time for appendicitis. A normal appendix was removed, and the physician noted that there was serous fluid present in the abdomen. He continued to have recurrent attacks of pain and vomiting and was readmitted on May 25, 1958 at the age of ten for diagnostic studies during one of these episodes. At that time the physical examination was reported as normal except for midepigastric tenderness. His abdomen was soft. His white blood cell count and differential were normal. A chest x-ray was normal. Upper gastrointestinal series was normal except for mild pylorospasm. No abdominal calcifications were seen. A spina bifida of L-5 was seen on the roentgenograms.

On examination on June 14, 1960, he had considerable epigastric and left upper quadrant tenderness with marked muscle guarding and rigidity. No masses were felt at any time. Serum amylase (Somogyi units) was 2,000 (Fig 2). Numerous

TABLE 1.—*Laboratory Data*

	Case 1	Case 2
Serum bilirubin, mg %		
Total	0.6	0.5
Direct	0.2	0.1
Indirect	0.4	0.4
Calcium, mg %	9.4 & 10.3	10.1 & 9.6
Phosphorus, mg %	4.9 & 4.0	5.4 & 4.8
Alkaline phosphatase, King-Armstrong units	17	19
Serum lipase, units (normal 0-1.0)		5.5
Thymol turbidity	1.0	2.6
Total proteins, gm %	5.6	6.0
Albumin, gm %	3.8	3.9
Globulin, gm %	1.8	2.1
Blood sugar, mg %	110	86
Leucine aminopeptidase, Goldberg and Rutenberg units	205	
Lipemic serum	No	No
Total lipids, mg % (Natelson)	200	
Phospholipids, mg % (Youngberg)	5.1	
Fatty acids, mg % (Peters)	82.2	
Stool examinations		
Ova & parasites	Neg	Neg
Trypsin	++++	++++
Meat fibers	Absent	Absent

other laboratory tests were within normal limits (Table 1). A palm sweat test was normal. X-ray studies on this admission revealed numerous pancreatic calcifications (Fig 3). Cholecystograms were normal, and upper gastrointestinal series at this time showed some deformity of the duodenal cap due to extrinsic causes. His course in the hospital on this admission was one of rapid subsidence of symptoms.

His parents stated that he had never experienced abdominal trauma. He had apparently grown and developed normally. His appetite between attacks was fair, and he had no selective food intolerance. His stools had always been normal. He has three siblings, a sister 14, a brother 9, and a sister 6; they have all been in good health. Both his parents (ages 34 and 33) are of German extraction and in good health. In view of the pancreatic calcifications, and the frequent severe attacks of pancreatitis, he was readmitted on June 28, 1960, and surgery was performed. At surgery the positive findings were confined to the pancreas.

The pancreas was of about normal size but very firm and of irregular and nodular consistency. An incision was made across the tail of the pancreas about 3 cm from its tip. The pancreatic duct was exposed in this area and measured about 1 cm in diameter. Using probes and common duct scoops, several areas of strictures were encountered. Operative pancreatography (Fig 4) was performed which revealed multiple strictures and dilatations ("chain-of-lakes"). There was a severe stricture in the head of the gland, with practically no dye

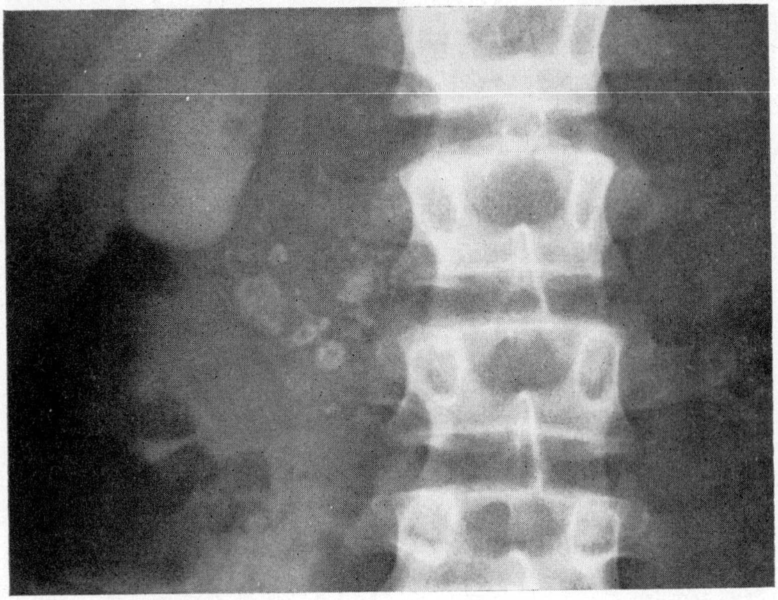

Fig 3 (Case 1).—Calcifications throughout pancreas.

entering the duodenum. Large stones were seen within the duct.

In view of the multiple strictures, the pancreatic duct was opened longitudinally to the head of the gland. Calculi in the main duct were removed. A side-to-side Roux en Y pancreaticojejunostomy was performed. The antimesenteric border of the jejunum was split for a distance equal to the length of the split in the pancreas. A side-to-side pancreaticojejunal anastomosis was constructed using a two-layer interrupted 4-0 silk technique. No attempt was made to suture jejunum to pancreatic duct wall. The area of the pancreas was drained with a Penrose drain.

The resected portion of pancreatic tail measured 4 cm in length and grossly showed patchy areas of fibrosis and calcification. A 3 mm stone was present in one of the larger pancreatic ducts. Microscopic examination (Fig 5) revealed moderate interstitial fibrosis which distorted and infringed upon the lobules. There was moderate infiltration into the fibrous stroma by mononuclear leukocytes and plasma cells. Some of the pancreatic ducts were dilated and partially filled with eosinophilic material. The epithelial lining of the ducts was relatively normal. His postoperative recovery was benign.

In the more than 2½ years since surgery, this boy has had no further attacks of abdominal pain. He has felt well, his appetite has improved, and his weight has gained from 98 lb (44.5 kg) to 129 lb (58.5 kg) when last seen. A recent x-ray of his abdomen shows almost complete clearing of the pancreatic calcifications.

Case 2 (III, 11).—This 11-year-old boy (a first cousin of the previous patient) was first seen on Aug 16, 1960, because of severe upper abdominal pains which had been present intermittently since infancy. His mother related that his pains dated back to about the age of 2 years and occurred intermittently and without apparent cause, lasting from several hours to a few days. The onset was usually sudden, and the pains might subside slowly

Fig 4 (Case 1).—Operative pancreatogram. Note multiple strictures and severe distortion of the duct.

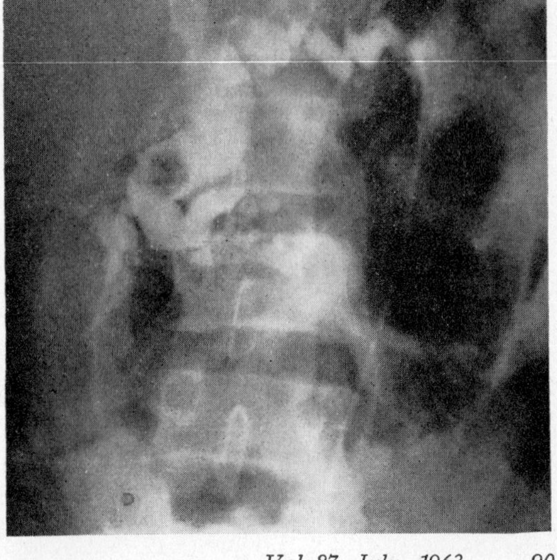

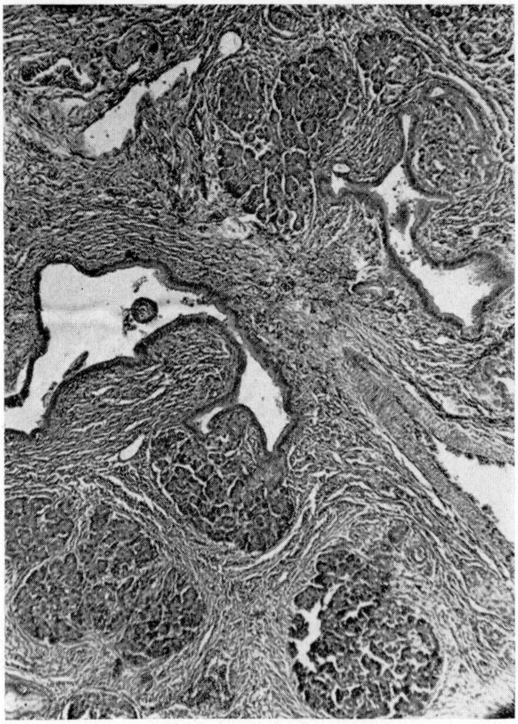

Fig 5 (Case 1).—Photomicrograph of pancreas Broad zones of fibrosis replace islet and acinar tissue. Reduced 38% from mag × 160.

or suddenly. An appendectomy was performed when he was 8 years old (normal appendix) with no influence on his distress. During the month prior to admission, these attacks of pain were occurring nearly every day.

At the time he was first seen, hereditary pancreatitis was suspected (Fig 6). On Aug 22, 1960, his pain was a little worse, and the urinary amylase was 800 Somogyi units (normal 0-300 units). A glucose tolerance test was normal. Except for the amylase, numerous other laboratory tests were normal (Table 1).

In the period between August, 1960, and March, 1962, he was seen on six occasions because of this same type of abdominal pain.

A chest x-ray was normal. Upper gastrointestinal series in 1960 was normal except for hypertrophic gastric rugae and some pylorospasm.

On March 29, 1962, surgery was performed. The gallbladder and common bile duct were normal. The stomach and duodenum were normal. The pancreas, which was exposed through the gastrocolic omentum, was normal size, firm, diffusely nodular, and fibrotic. A splenectomy was performed and the pancreatic duct was exposed through an incision in the tail. The duct at this point was dilated and admitted a 5 mm dilator with ease. The dilator could not be passed more than 1 cm cephalad in the duct. Operative pancreatography (Fig 7) revealed moderate dilation of the duct with several areas of narrowing. There was a stricture of the duct extending distally from the ampulla for over 2 cm. Dye entered the duodenum readily.

In view of the multiple areas of narrowing in the duct and the success achieved in treatment of his cousin, the anterior surface of the pancreas was split from the tail to the head to lay the main pancreatic duct open. Several strictures and dilatations were encountered; there were no calculi in the main pancreatic duct. A side-to-side Roux en Y pancreaticojejunostomy was performed, using a one-layer silk anastomosis between the jejunum and the anterior capsule of the gland. The resected portion of the pancreatic tail weighed 8 gm. Microscopically, there was interfollicular fibrosis present (to a lesser degree than in the previous case). Acinar tissue was abundant, and few islands were present. The small ducts and their lining cells were not unusual. In some areas considerably increased numbers of eosinophils were noted within the stroma and glandular tissue.

His postoperative recovery was uncomplicated. He has been seen at frequent intervals since his surgery and has suffered no attacks of abdominal pain in the 11 months since. He has gained from 79 lb (35.8 kg) to 95 lb (43.1 kg), whereas in the preceding year he gained only 5 lb (2.3 kg). He is eating better than preoperatively, and in general he is an apparently healthy boy at the present time.

Admittedly, at times, these patients will reach a plateau with a spontaneous marked regression of attacks which may last for extended periods of time. However, especially in the first child, the tempo of the disease appeared to be rapidly increasing, and surgical intervention with an adequate definitive drainage procedure appears to have dramatically altered the course of his disease. Both patients have obtained symptomatic relief, and the pancreatic calcifications have shown marked clearing in the first child. The course of these patients over the next 20 or 30 years will be interesting to observe.

Suspected Pancreatitis

CASE 3 (I, 10).—This man, a great-uncle of the two patients presented, is about 60 years of age and has suffered from recurrent attacks of abdominal pain for many years.

CASE 4 (II, 3).—This uncle of the proposita was killed in an accident at age 34, but the family relates that he suffered from attacks of "terrible" abdominal pains for years before his death.

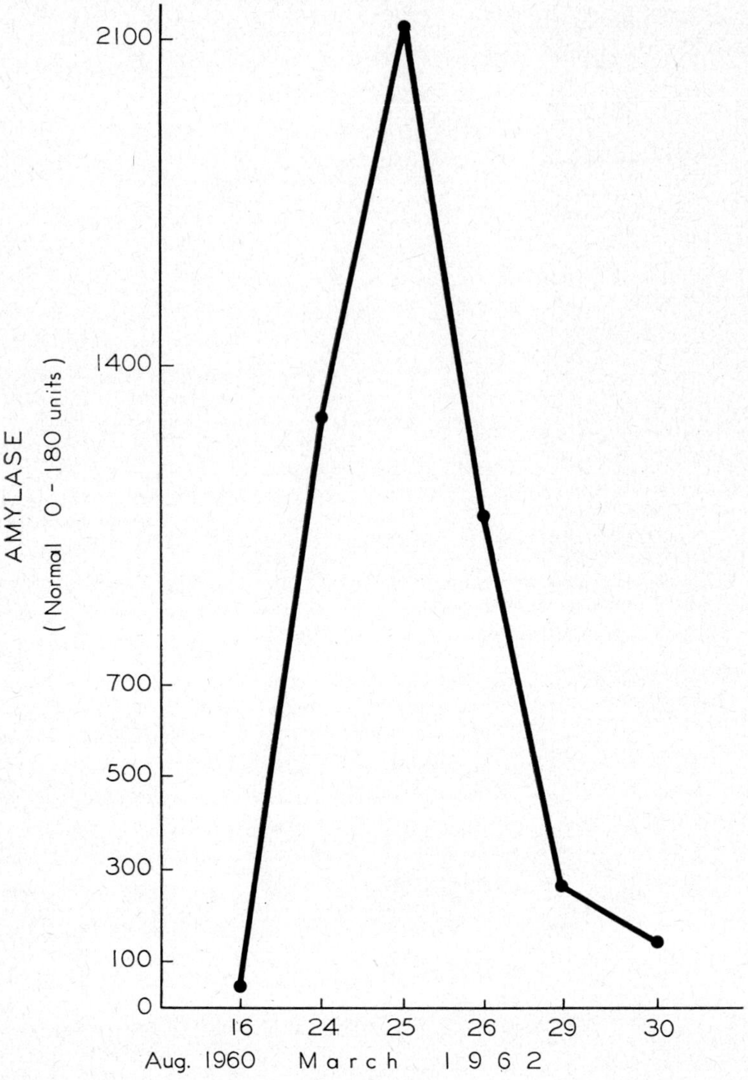

Fig 6 (Case 2).—Serum amylase (Somogyi units).

CASE 5 (II, 4).—This man, the father of III, 11, has had recurrent stomach pains for years. He has had three abdominal operations with no improvement. Inspection of the two operative reports available to us fails to reveal an adequate explanation for the cause of his pain, although there is no mention of the state of the pancreas in either report. X-rays of his abdomen two years ago did not show any calcifications. A single amylase 24 hours after an attack of pain was normal.

CASES 6 and 7 (III, 6 and 7).—These two daughters of II, 3, ages 19 and 9, both have had intermittent stomach pains. No diagnostic studies have been done.

CASE 8 (III, 14).—This 14-year-old first cousin of the proposita suffers from recurrent upper abdominal pain similar to that of III, 11 and III, 19, according to an uncle. No diagnostic data are available on this child.

Although strict criteria for the diagnosis of hereditary pancreatitis are not available at the present time, we believe these two cases represent hereditary pancreatitis because of the onset in early childhood, the absence of gallstones and trauma, and also a lack of alcoholic excesses.[12]

Role of Surgery

There are no reports available of a planned primary surgical attack upon the pancreas in patients with hereditary pancreatitis. All operative procedures thus far reported have been either abdominal explorations or indirect attacks upon the disease or its sequelae (sphincterotomy, common

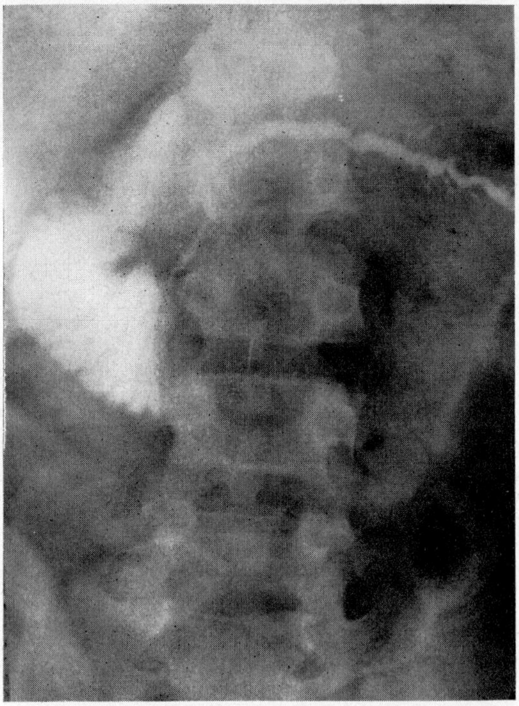

Fig 7 (Case 2).—Operative pancreatogram. Note long stricture in proximal duct and multiple short strictures.

duct drainage, or drainage of a pseudocyst). Three cases are reported in which sphincterotomy alone was the primary mode of treatment. It is significant that none of these three has had lasting relief of pain.[8,10] In relieving the recurrent pain, pseudocyst drainage seems to have offered the only success,[10] probably because it afforded indirect drainage to the ductal system. That a direct approach to the pancreas is warranted may be evidenced by the incidence of sequelae reported by Gross et al [12] (Table 2). Among 22 persons with definite pancreatitis, diabetes mellitus was diagnosed in 8 cases and steatorrhea in 9. Upper gastrointestinal bleeding complicated 5 cases, and a pseudocyst was found in 4 patients. Three of 22 persons with definite hereditary pancreatitis have died of pancreatic disease, 2 of these of carcinoma of the head of the pancreas at ages 48 and 52. It must be remembered that most of these patients are still relatively young, the mean age at diagnosis or death being only 33.8 years. The incidence of

Table 2.—*Complications of Hereditary Pancreatitis (24 Patients)* *

Pancreatic calcifications	18
Diabetes mellitus	8
Steatorrhea	9
Upper gastrointestinal bleeding	5
Pseudocyst of pancreas	4
Carcinoma of pancreas (ages 48 & 52)	2

* Gross et al plus present series.

complications, and deaths, can be expected to increase as this group of patients grow older. Thus far there does not appear to be an unduly high incidence of peptic ulcers, and no cases of severe ulcer diathesis, a possibility suggested by Zollinger [21] in patients with chronic recurrent pancreatitis with pancreatic fibrosis.

There are no reports of operative visualization of the pancreatic ductal system in patients with hereditary pancreatitis. Both the patients whom we have reported exhibited strictures in the main pancreatic ductal system. Whether these strictures are primary or secondary is problematical. However, we believe, on the basis of the long stricture in the duct demonstrated in case No. 2 and the lack of visualization of the most proximal portion of pancreatic duct in the first case, that there is a distinct possibility that these patients are born with an abnormally long narrowing of the pancreatic duct in the head of the gland. This narrowing may predispose to intermittent obstruction of the duct by inspissated secretions,[3] or ductal metaplasia,[13] with resultant pancreatitis. A vicious cycle of obstruction, inflammation, calculosis, stricturings, pseudocyst, fibrosis, etc, is thereby established. We realize that this may be a mechanical oversimplification of what may, in reality, be a complex metabolic disease. However, Gross [8] lends some support to the possibility of an anatomic defect as the basic underlying cause of the chronic pancreatitis in these patients.

Several studies [2,3,15] of normal pancreatic ductal anatomy have been conducted. Most authors report some incidence of a short area of narrowing in the region of the papilla of Vater, but not to the extent seen in these patients. Birnstingl[3] has described histological partial blockage of the main pancreatic duct and complete blockage of the accessory duct with an inspissated material resembling dental tartar. Ductal metaplasia has been described by others[1,13] as causing partial obstruction of the pancreatic duct. Operative pancreatograms in chronic relapsing pancreatitis often show that the major duct is strictured in the head or elsewhere.[18-20]

Thal[20] has reported evidence of ductal obstruction in the "vast majority" of a study of 42 fatal cases of acute pancreatitis. Hermann and Davis[13] have experimentally created changes similar to chronic pancreatitis in dogs with incomplete ductal obstruction. The evidence available suggests that the development of pancreatitis in either its acute or recurrent form is frequently dependent upon obstruction to pancreatic outflow from an actively secreting gland.

Carnevali et al[4] have experimentally produced multiple ductal obstruction in dogs and subsequently demonstrated the efficacy of side-to-side pancreaticojejunostomy in the treatment of the resultant pancreatitis. They have shown in dogs a marked improvement in the histologic picture with return of essentially normal acinar architecture and nodular regeneration of injured acinar tissue.

Puestow and Gillesby[6,18] have adequately demonstrated the feasibility of this procedure in humans. In their personal and collected series they report only 5 poor results out of 54 cases. The relief of all areas of obstruction which this procedure affords prevents increased intraductal pressure, which is believed to be responsible for the pain of chronic relapsing pancreatitis. It also should allow the greatest opportunity for regeneration of pancreatic tissue. Further, there should be no opportunity for recurrence of strictures.

It was with these facts in mind that in June, 1960, we operated upon the first child. It was our intent to attempt to relieve his symptoms by means of an appropriate drainage procedure. Operative pancreatography

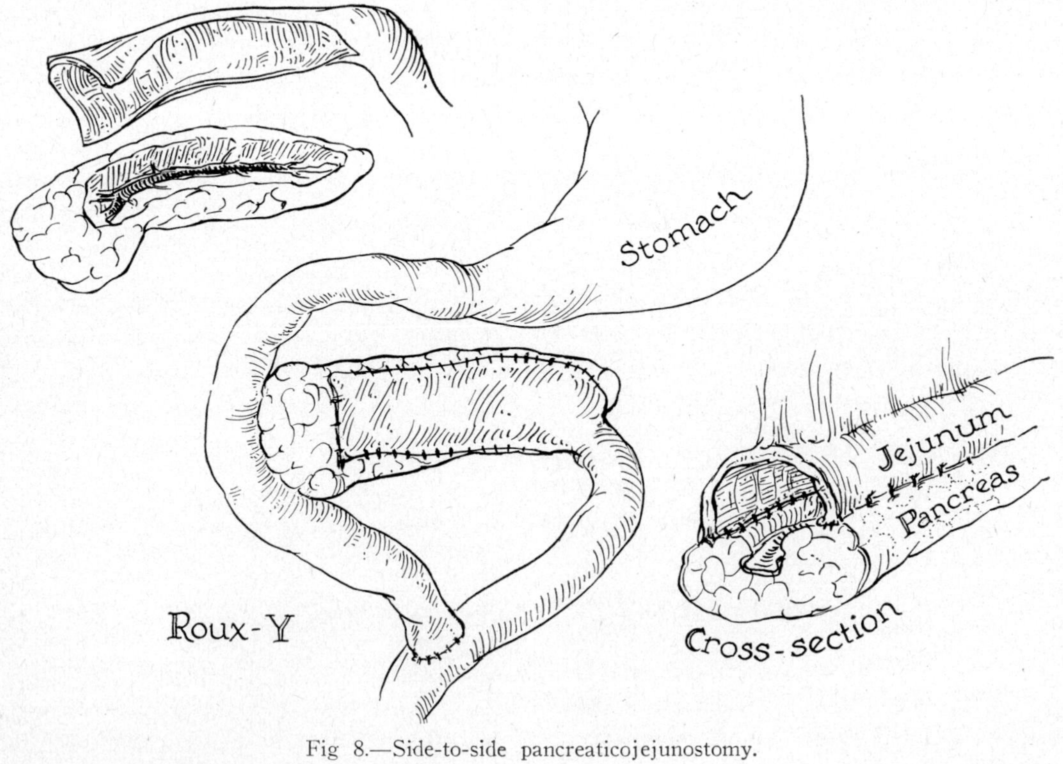

Fig 8.—Side-to-side pancreaticojejunostomy.

revealed that the best method to insure long-term adequate drainage of the ductal system would be side-to-side pancreaticojejunostomy. In the nearly three years since his operation he has not had any attacks of abdominal pain. His cousin has now gone almost a year since his operation without an attack of pancreatitis.

Summary

The sixth kindred with hereditary pancreatitis has been presented. There are two persons with definite pancreatitis and six with suspected pancreatitis in this kindred, which still has a relatively young mean age. Operative pancreatography in the two cases detailed revealed long strictures of the proximal pancreatic duct in addition to multiple short strictures. Side-to-side pancreaticojejunostomy in both these patients has resulted in complete remission of symptoms to date (32 months and 11 months, respectively).

It is proposed that the basic inherited defect may be an anomalous ductal narrowing, predisposing to obstruction and development of chronic relapsing pancreatitis and its serious sequelae of calculus formation, diabetes mellitus, steatorrhea, cyst formation, and possibly carcinoma.[16] It is further proposed, on the basis of this defect and the successful results in these two cases, that earlier and frequent definitive surgical attack on the pancreas may be warranted in hereditary pancreatitis in an effort to prevent development of these sequelae.

The encouragement and advice of Dr. Thomas W. Shields, Chicago, Ill. is gratefully acknowledged.

Bernard C. Gerber, MD, 310 Professional Arts Building, Aberdeen, SD.

REFERENCES

1. Berens, J. J.; Baggenstoss, A. H.; and Gray, H. K.,: "Ductal Changes in Chronic Pancreatitis," in Transactions of the Western Surgical Association, Chicago: American Medical Association Press, 1953, pp 225-235.

2. Berman, L. G.; Prior, J. T.; Abramow, S. M.; and Ziegler, D. D.: A Study of the Pancreatic Duct System in Man by the Use of Vinyl-Acetate Casts of Postmortem Preparations, Surg Gynec Obstet 110:391-403, 1960.

3. Birnstingl, M.: A Study of Pancreatography, Brit J Surg 47:128-139, 1959.

4. Carnevali, J. F.; ReMine, W. H.; Dockerty, M. B.; Bollman, J. L.; and Grindlay, J. H.: An Experimental Study of Side-to-Side Pancreaticojejunostomy After Ductal Obstruction, AMA Arch Surg 80:774-787, 1960.

5. Comfort, M. W., and Steinberg, A. G.: Pedigree, of the Family With Hereditary Chronic Relapsing Pancreatitis, Gastroenterology 21:54, 1952.

6. Gillesby, W. J., and Puestow, C. B.: Pancreaticojejunostomy for Chronic Relapsing Pancreatitis: An Evaluation, Surgery 50:859-862, 1961.

7. Gross, J. B.: Some Recent Developments Pertaining to Pancreatitis, Ann Intern Med 49:796-819, 1958.

8. Gross, J. B., and Comfort, M. W.: Hereditary Pancreatitis: Report of Two Additional Families, Gastroenterology 32:829-954, 1957.

9. Gross, J. B.; Comfort, M. W.; and Ulrich, J. A.: Abnormalities of Serum and Urinary Amino Acids in Hereditary and Non-Hereditary Pancreatitis, Trans Ass Amer Physicians 70:127-139, 1957.

10. Gross, J. B.; Gambill, E.E.; and Ulrich, J. A.: Hereditary Pancreatitis, Amer J Med 33:358-364, 1962.

11. Gross, J. B.; Ulrich, J. A.; and Maher, F. T.: Aminoaciduria in a Family With Hereditary Pancreatitis, presented at Meeting of American Gastroenterological Association, 1962.

12. Gross, J. B.; Ulrich, J. A.; and Maher, F. T.: "Further Observations on the Hereditary Form of Pancreatitis," in Ciba Foundation Symposium: Normal and Abnormal Functions of the Exocrine Pancreas, London: J & A. Churchhill, Ltd., 1962, pp 278-305.

13. Hermann, R. E., and Davis, J. H.: The Role of Incomplete Pancreatic Duct Obstruction in the Etiology of Pancreatitis, Surgery 48:318-329, 1960.

14. Jackson, C. E.: Hereditary Hyperparathyroidism Associated With Recurrent Pancreatitis, Ann Intern Med 49:829-836, 1958.

15. Millbourn, E.: Calibre and Appearance of the Pancreatic Ducts and Relevant Clinical Problems, Acta Chir Scand 118: 286-303, 1959-1960.

16. Paulino-Netto, A.; Dreiling, D. A.; and Baronofsky, I. D.: The Relationship Between Pancreatic Calcification and Cancer of the Pancreas, Ann Surg 151:530, 1960.

17. Pollock, A. V.: Pancreatography in the Diagnosis of Chronic Relapsing Pancreatitis, Surg Gynec Obstet 107:765-770, 1950.

18. Puestow, C. B., and Gillesby, W. J.: Retrograde Surgical Drainage for Chronic Relapsing Pancreatitis, AMA Arch Surg 76:898-905, 1958.

19. Thal, A. P.; Goott, B.; and Margulis, A. R.: Sites of Pancreatic Duct Obstruction in Chronic Pancreatitis, Ann Surg 150:49-56, 1959.

20. Thal, A. P.; Perry, J. F.; and Egner, W.: A Clinical and Morphologic Study of 42 Cases of Fatal Acute Pancreatitis, Surg Gynec Obstet 105:191-202, 1957.

21 Zollinger, R. M.; Elliott, D. W.; Endahl, G. L.; Grant, G. N.; Goswitz, J. T.; and Taft, D. A.: Origin of the Ulcerogenic Hormone in Endocrine Induced Ulcer, Ann Surg 156:570-578, 1962.

Pancreatic Abscess

A Study of 32 Cases

W. A. ALTEMEIER, MD, AND J. WESLEY ALEXANDER, MD, CINCINNATI

Abscesses developing as sequelae of acute pancreatic inflammation are infrequent and serious surgical complications [11,12] which usually present a confusing clinical picture. In addition, their successful management is beset by many problems in diagnosis, localization of the abscess, selection of the correct type of surgical operation, and recognition and treatment of a variety of complications.

The sparse number of published reports of patients with pancreatic abscess and the absence of any comprehensive review of this subject in the literature were both surprising. The first successful treatment of this condition was apparently reported by Davis in 1917.[5] Beller and Nach reported a case in 1942 and reviewed five previously reported cases.[3] Eleven years later Welborn reported three more cases,[13] but the remainder of reports have dealt with only one or two patients. A thorough clinical review and study of the subject have been made after several patients with pancreatic abscesses were recently seen at the Cincinnati General Hospital.

Material

During the period between 1936 and 1962, a total of 32 patients with proven pancreatic abscesses have been seen on the Surgical Services of the Cincinnati General Hospital and University of Cincinnati. They have represented approximately 4.5% of the total number of admissions for pancreatitis during this same period, excluding pancreatitis complicating mumps. A higher incidence was found in the white population, and males were involved significantly more than females (2.1). The youngest patient was 26 years of age, while the oldest was 86. A fairly even distribution was found between these extremes, but with peaks during the fourth and seventh decades.

Acute pancreatitis preceded the formation of an abscess in all but three cases. One abscess was related to a deeply penetrating duodenal ulcer, and the other two developed as complications of an established pancreatic pseudocyst. One of these followed a marsupialization procedure. There were the usual predisposing conditions contributing to the development of pancreatitis (table 1).

Disease of the biliary tract was proved in 18 patients (56%), chronic alcoholism in 7 patients (22%), periarteritis nodosa in 1, and abdominal trauma in 1. Although 7 patients gave no history of alcoholism or cholecystic disease, only 2 of these had had adequate studies for its demonstration. Information concerning the presence or absence of alcoholism was also often inadequate.

Symptoms and Physical Findings

The delay in diagnosis until the time of autopsy in one third of the patients em-

TABLE 1.—*Predisposing Conditions (32 Cases)*

Gallbladder disease	18
Chronic alcoholism	7
Periarteritis nodosa	1
Trauma	1
No demonstration of above	7 *

* Of these seven patients only two had been studied for gallbladder disease; two had both chronic alcoholism and gallbladder disease.

Presented at the 20th Annual Meeting of the Central Surgical Association, Chicago, Feb 21-23, 1963.

From the Department of Surgery of the College of Medicine, University of Cincinnati, and the Cincinnati General Hospital.

TABLE 2.—*Symptoms and Physical Findings (32 Cases)*

Abdominal pain	32
Tenderness over abscess	30
Fever	29
Nausea	29
Vomiting	28
Palpable mass	17
Abdominal distention	14
Weight loss	9
Shock	5
Jaundice	4
Stupor	3

phasized the obscure nature of these infections. The important symptoms and physical signs have been tabulated in Table 2.

Abdominal pain was present in every instance, and the pain frequently, but not always, radiated to the back. Nausea and vomiting were nearly always present (90%), and tenderness over the abscess was invariably present in the absence of stupor. A tender palpable mass was found in 17 (53%) of the cases. In the typical patient there was a daily spiking elevation in temperature to 101-102 F, but the degree of fever varied considerably. In three cases the temperature was not elevated above 100 F, and the highest temperature was 108 F. Jaundice, weight loss, abdominal distention, shock, and stupor occurred less frequently. The symptoms and physical findings associated with abscess formation usually appeared one to three weeks after the onset of acute pancreatitis but in a few patients were the initial complaints.

Laboratory Findings

The laboratory studies, although never conclusive, were frequently helpful in making a diagnosis. Leukocytosis was the rule with an average white blood cell count of 18,000, but a wide variation from 5,000 to 50,000 was seen. The serum amylase determination done at the time of admission was normal in 8 patients, elevated in 16, and unknown in 8. In 5 patients, representing 22% of those studied by this test, there was a prolonged and significant elevation of the serum amylase level for a period of two to six weeks. In these patients the amylase usually remained elevated until the abscess was drained and the inflammatory process had subsided (Case 1). The urinalysis and blood urea nitrogen were usually unremarkable.

TABLE 3.—*Bacterial Etiology (32 Cases)*

Polymicrobial	13
Monomicrobial	10
Staphylococcus	12
Escherichia coli	8
Streptococcus	6
Proteus	3
Miscellaneous coliform	6
Incompletely identified	3
Unknown	9

Cultures were taken from the abscesses in 25 of the 32 cases. Thirteen of the infections were polymicrobial and 10 monomicrobial. In two instances the initial culture showed no growth, but the lesions and their contents were typical in appearance of an abscess. The etiologic agents found most frequently were the *Staphylococcus aureus, Escherichia coli, Streptococcus,* and *Proteus* (Table 3).

Roentgen Findings

The roentgenographic studies showed significant changes which should have been helpful in arriving at a diagnosis in 86% of these patients. Displacement of intra-abdominal viscera was found in most patients in whom a barium enema or an upper gastrointestinal series had been done. Gas within the abscess cavity was evident in only two patients but, when found, was considered to be a pathognomonic sign.[6] Roentgenograms of the chest frequently showed elevation of the diaphragm, often with decreased motion as demonstrated by fluoroscopy. Injection of a sinus tract after drainage or spontaneous rupture of the abscess often revealed a communication with the pancreatic duct or the abscess cavity (Cases 2 and 3).

Complications

The complications associated with these abscesses are varied and severe (Table 4). Eight patients (25%) either had diabetes

TABLE 4.—*Complications (32 Cases)*

Extension to adjacent anatomical spaces	12
Diabetes mellitus	8
Recurrent abscess	6
Septicemia	4
Perforation into the peritoneal cavity	3
Arterial erosion with exsanguination	3
Gastric or duodenal ulcers	3
(with bleeding)	(2)
Persistent pancreatic fistula	3
Pancreatobronchopleural fistula	1
Wound abscess	2
Metastatic abscess	1
Incisional hernia	1

mellitus at the time of their admission to the hospital or developed it subsequently, one patient as long as 11 years postoperatively.

Perforation of the abscess into the free peritoneal cavity occurred in three (9%) of the cases, and only one patient survived this complication. Dissection and extension of the abscess directly into the subdiaphragmatic, subhepatic, or anterior retroperitoneal space occurred in one third of the patients. A thorough knowledge of the anatomical relationships of the pancreas is important in understanding the pathways of extension (Fig 1-4). Recurrence of the abscess developed in six (19%). The presence of proteolytic enzymes within the abscess led to erosion of a major blood vessel with hemorrhage and exsanguination of three pa-

Fig 1.—Anterior views showing the anatomical relationships of abscesses located (*A*) in the head, (*B*) in the body, and (*C*) in the tail of the pancreas.

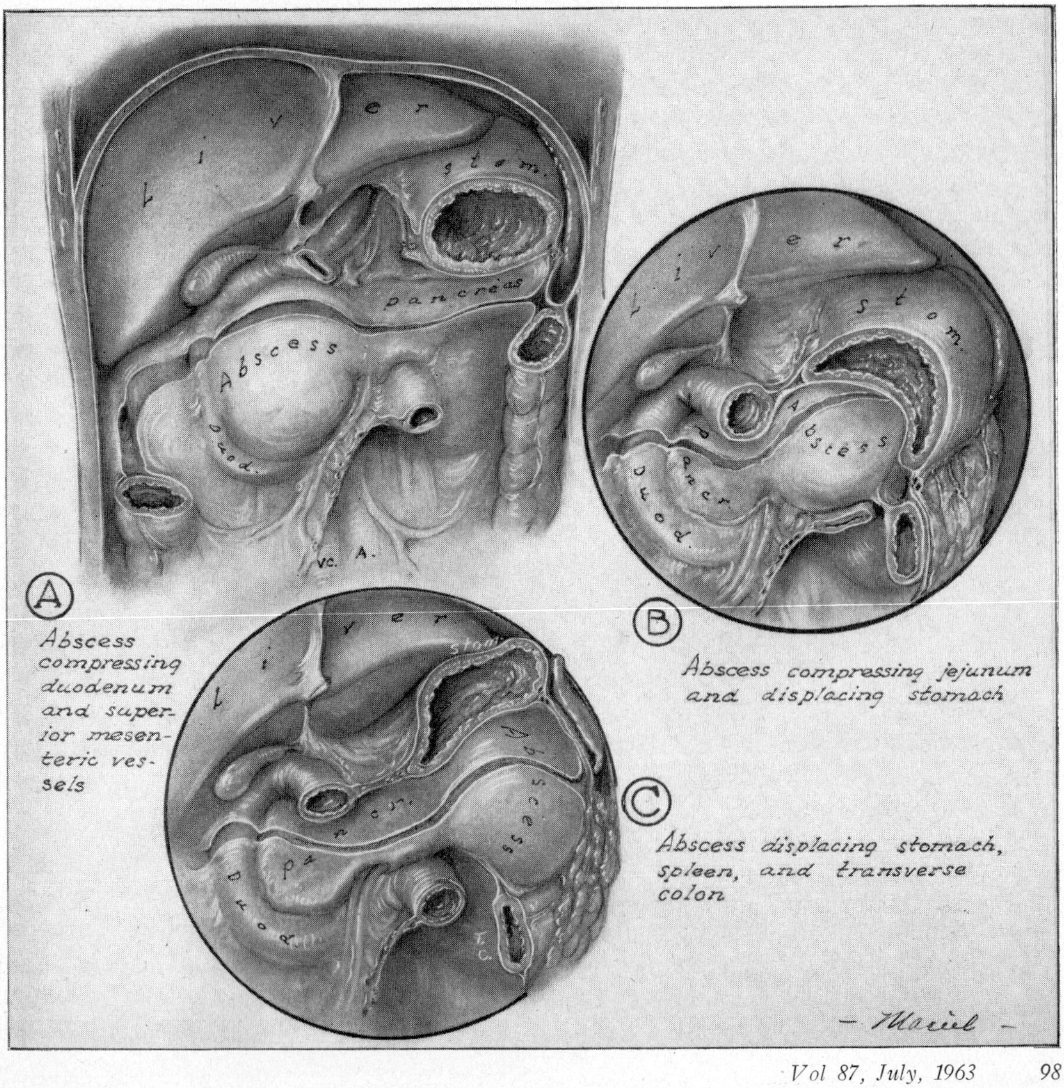

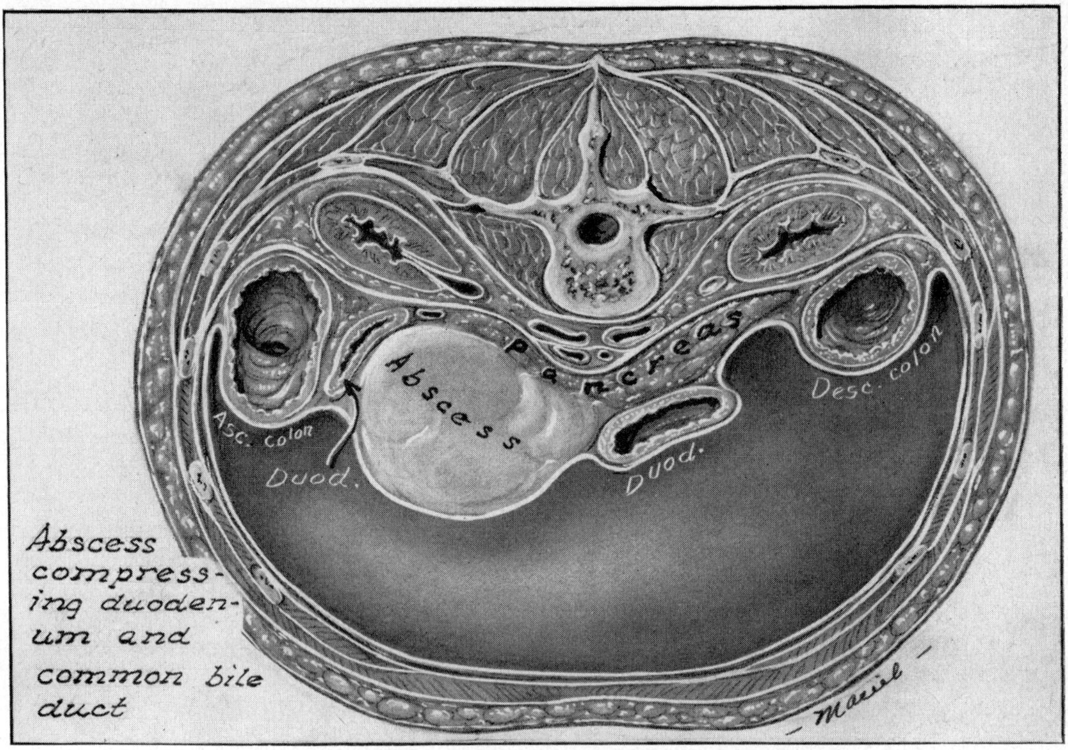

Fig 2.—Cross-sectional drawing at the level of second lumbar vertebra. An expanding abscess within the head of the pancreas may displace and compress the duodenum and common bile duct.

tients. Septicemia was proved in four patients, and gastric or duodenal ulcers were noted in three, two of whom had gastrointestinal bleeding. In one patient (Case 2) a pancreatobronchopleural fistula developed. No previous report of this complication was found in the literature.

Treatment

The necessity for early diagnosis and prompt surgical drainage is emphasized by reviewing the mortality factors. In the 21 patients in whom a correct preoperative or operative diagnosis of pancreatic abscess was made, 18, or 86%, recovered. Of the 3 remaining patients, one died from exsanguination when the abscess eroded into the splenic artery during a delay in treatment (Case 4); another had recurrence of his abscess after initial drainage with resultant rupture into the free peritoneal cavity and overwhelming peritonitis; and a third who also had a recurrent abscess refused another operation. The latter developed diabetic coma and subsequently died. None of the remaining 11 patients were correctly diagnosed, none had surgical drainage, and all died, emphasizing the primary importance of early diagnosis and adequate drainage.

The recommended treatment as determined from this study is external drainage of the abscess through a separate stab wound made in the flank with adjunctive antibiotic therapy. If large enough, the abscess may be marsupialized. Drainage into a Roux en Y loop or into the posterior wall of the stomach [4] has not been generally advocated, but drainage into the stomach may have great value in those cases where there is firm adherence of the abscess to the posterior gastric wall. Drainage through the working incision may lead to wound infection and is associated with a higher incidence of recurrent abscess formation.

Should a persistent external pancreatic fistula develop, it may be treated successfully by intestinal implantation using the Roux en

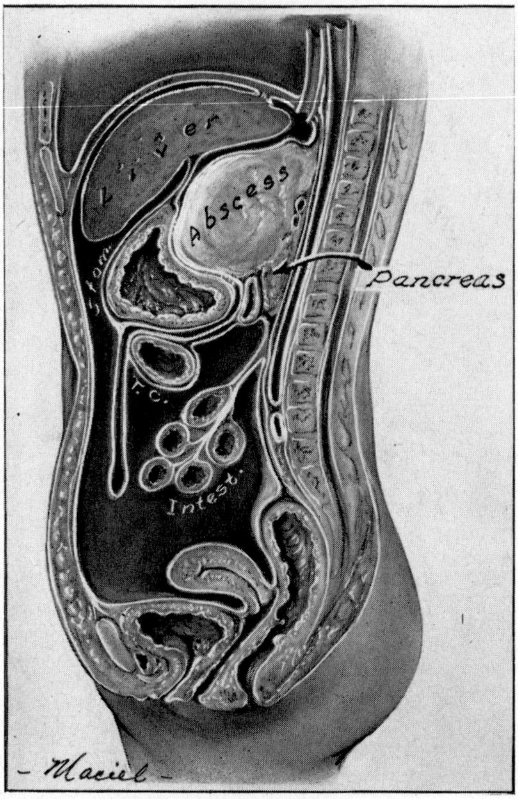

Fig 3.—Midline sagittal drawing of an abscess of the body of the pancreas. Dense adherence to the posterior gastric wall makes drainage into the stomach possible in selected cases.

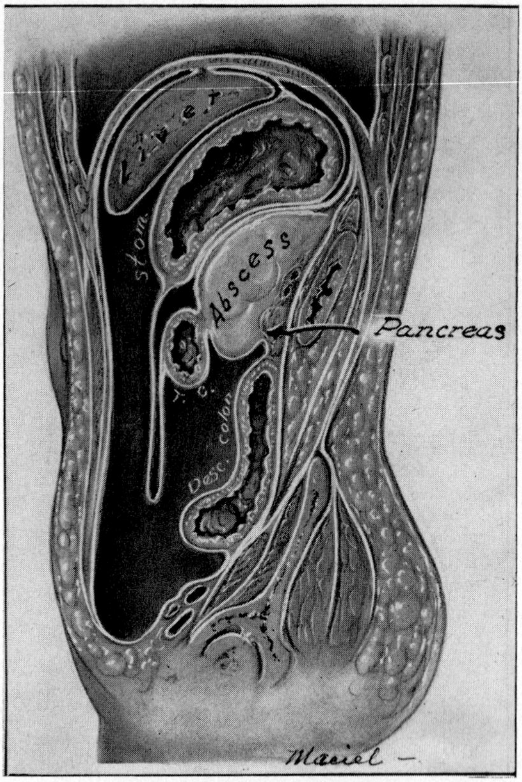

Fig 4.—Left sagittal drawing showing an abscess that has arisen in the tail of the pancreas. Note how dissection has occurred between the leaves of the transverse mesocolon.

Y anastomosis with a defunctionalized loop of jejunum.

Report of Cases

Four interesting and illustrative case reports have been selected to demonstrate the protean manifestations and complications of this serious condition.

CASE 1.—A 61-year-old Negro man was admitted to the Cincinnati General Hospital on Dec 14, 1950. He had been seen ten years previously because of a palpable, nontender, epigastric mass which had been associated with widening of the duodenal curve on roentgenographic examination. He was advised to have an exploratory laparotomy because of the clinical impression of pancreatic carcinoma, but he refused. He remained apparently asymptomatic until four days prior to this admission when he developed nausea, chills, fever, and epigastric pain radiating to both flanks. The initial examination showed abdominal tenderness without a palpable mass, and he was afebrile. The pain and tenderness subsided after two days of conservative therapy. During the following week, a slowly enlarging, tender, epigastric mass was felt, and he developed a spiking, daily fever of 101-102 F. A gastrointestinal series showed anterior and lateral displacement of both duodenum and stomach. He was given parenteral penicillin and streptomycin therapy, and on Jan 24, 1951, a large abscess of the body of the pancreas was discovered at operation which was drained through a separate stab wound. His postoperative course was uneventful although he developed an incisional hernia at the drainage site. This was repaired on April 25, 1952. He was followed for four years with no evidence of recurrence of either acute pancreatitis or pancreatic abscess.

Serial amylase determinations were done and were found to be persistently elevated, although decreasing, until the abscess was surgically drained (Fig 5). This finding in association with his clinical picture could have alerted his clinicians to the probability of an abscess of the pancreas.

CASE 2.—A 33-year-old Negro male who was a chronic alcoholic was admitted to the Medical Service of the Cincinnati General Hospital on

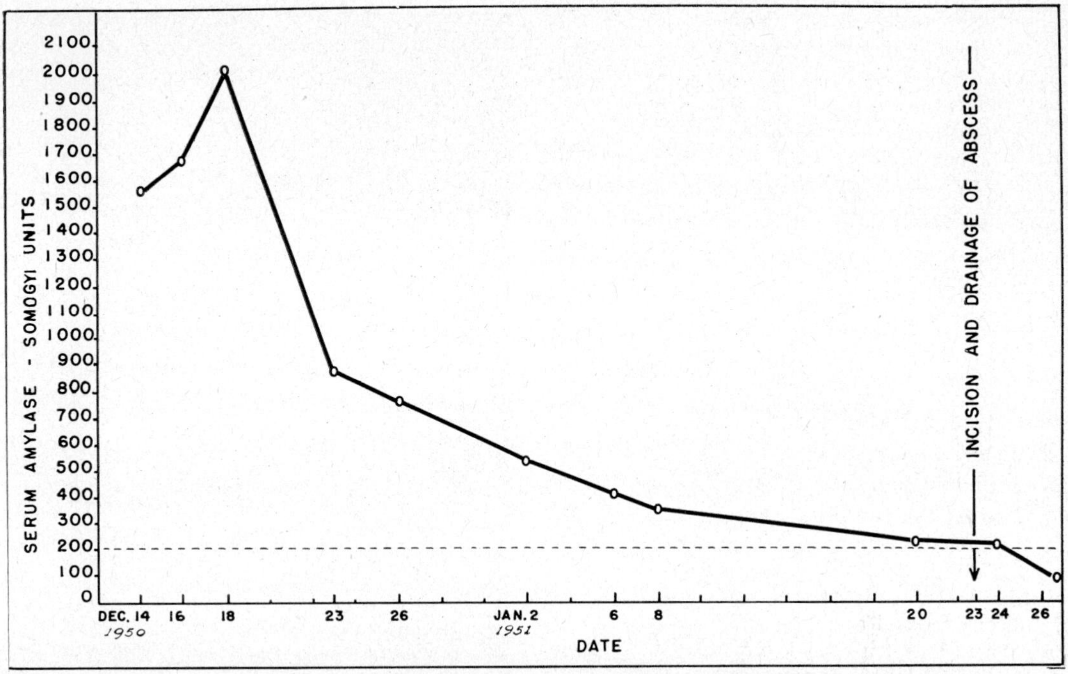

Fig 5 (Case 1).—Graphic representation of serum amylase levels. There was a significant and persistent elevation of the serum amylase until surgical drainage of the abscess was established.

March 9, 1960, because of bilateral bloody pleural effusions. Numerous studies failed to show a definite cause, and he was discharged on March 30, 1960, with a diagnosis of probable bilateral pulmonary emboli. He was admitted again Aug 9, 1960, with right pleuritic chest pain, fever, chills, dyspnea, hemoptysis, and a weight loss of 50 lb (22.7 kg). He developed a changing cardiac murmur, and penicillin and choloramphenicol (Chloromycetin) were administered after ten blood cultures were taken. Five of these yielded a paracolon bacillus. The development of a bronchopleural fistula necessitated treatment with tube thoracotomy. On Sept 10, 1960, he was transferred to the Surgical Service when tenderness and fullness were noted in his epigastrium, interpreted as being an enlarging tender mass secondary to pancreatitis. On Sept 22, 1960, an exploratory laparotomy was done and a large mass was found in the lesser omental sac with communications with both chest cavities. It contained about 500 cc of a greenish-brown purulent fluid and blood clots. Drainage was instituted through a separate stab wound. Erosion into a large blood vessel had occurred with resultant

Fig 6 (Case 2).—Roentgenograms. *A*, injection of a contrast medium demonstrated communication between the pancreatic duct and the sinus tract that formed following external drainage. *B*, the communication between the pancreatic abscess and the right pleural space was demonstrated by a contrast study of the empyema cavity. *C*, communication with a lower lobe bronchus was shown during the same study.

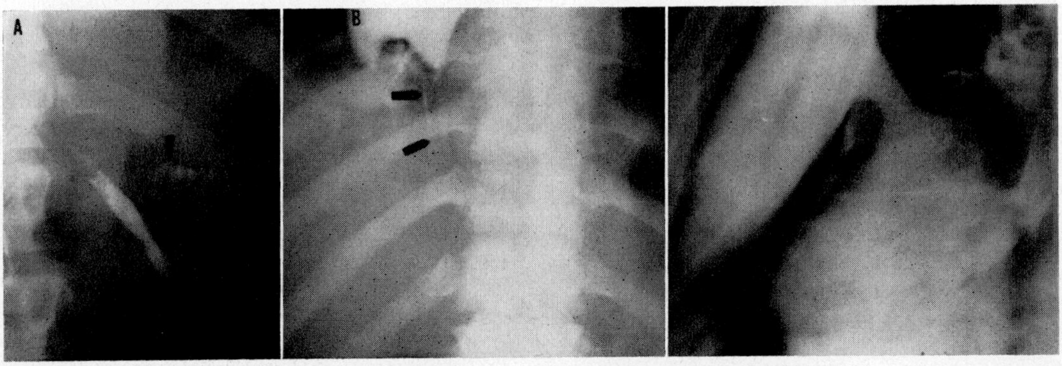

bleeding. Cultures from the abscess showed *Staphylococcus epidermitis* and an anaerobic streptococcus. Subsequent radiographic studies showed communication between the pancreatic duct, the abscess cavity, both pleural spaces, and the right tracheobronchial tree (Fig 6). By Jan 3, 1961, the sinus tract had healed, and the patient left the hospital against medical advice. He was without complaints, and all wounds had healed when he was last seen Jan 27, 1961.

This complication of pancreatobronchopleural fistula was undoubtedly caused by the prolonged existence of this obscure abscess before diagnosis, and it apparently was the first recorded case of its kind. Erosion into a large blood vessel has been noted before, and it has usually caused death of the patient.

Case 3.—A 34-year-old white man was admitted to Cincinnati Veterans Administration Hospital on Oct 20, 1958. He had been seen several times previously because of chronic alcoholism, duodenal peptic ulcers, and acute pancreatitis. While on an alcoholic binge ten days before admission, he developed left upper quadrant and epigastric pains with associated anorexia, vomiting, and left shoulder pain. At the time of admission his temperature was 102 F, the abdomen was distended, and he had left upper quadrant abdominal tenderness with a positive psoas sign on the left. The serum amylase was 102 Somogyi units, and the white blood cell count was 21,900. He was believed to have a perinephric abscess, but surgical exploration through the left flank showed only an encapsulated hematoma which was drained. One week later an enlarging, tender epigastric mass became palpable, and a roentgenographic study later showed marked anterior and medial displacement of the stomach (Fig 7). An oral cholecystogram and an intravenous cholangiogram both failed to show evidence of function. He continued to have a septic course from the time of admission, with *S aureus* being recovered from blood cultures.

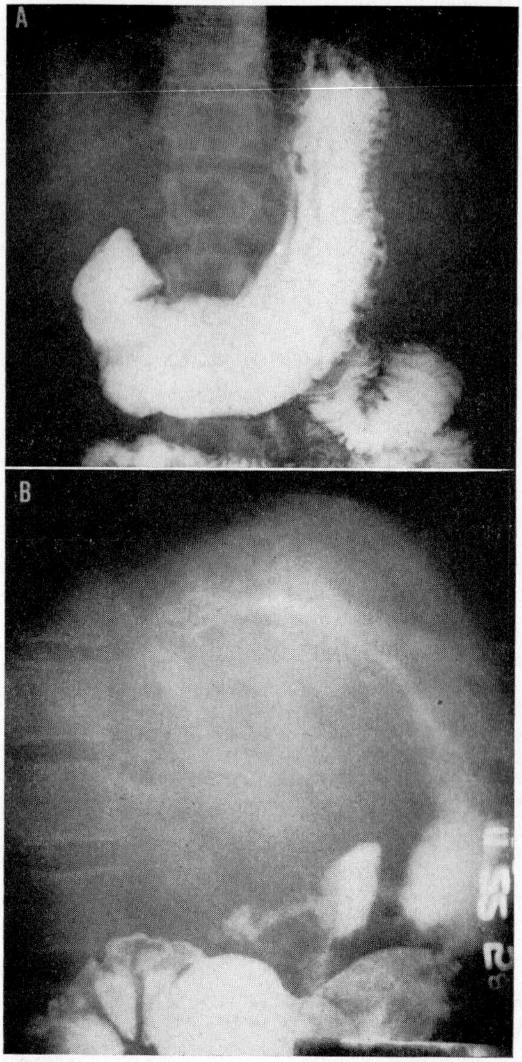

Fig 7.—*A,* the stomach is displaced medially by a pancreatic abscess in the body of the pancreas. *B,* a lateral view shows anterior displacement.

On Nov 22, 1958, one month after admission, the abdominal cavity was explored, and two abscesses were found. The larger was located in the body of the pancreas and contained 100 cc of pus. It was drained internally into the stomach through a posterior gastrostomy wound. The other abscess, containing 75 cc of pus, was located in the lesser omental sac and was drained through a stab wound in the right flank. Cultures from the abscesses were positive for *S aureus* and *E coli.*

His postoperative recovery was satisfactory, but he had intermittent minimal drainage from the left flank incision for two years. He also developed overt diabetes.

This patient had chronic biliary tract disease and chronic alcoholism, both of which were frequently found to be associated with the development of a pancreatic abscess in the series. The development of septicemia and extension of the abscess were serious complications in this case as in others in which the diagnosis has been delayed for four or more weeks.

Case 4.—A 73-year-old woman was admitted to the Cincinnati General Hospital on Feb 4, 1955, complaining of severe epigastric pain, nausea, and vomiting. She had had an intolerance to the ingestion of fatty foods for many years. Epigastric tenderness, hypoactive bowel sounds, and a temperature elevation to 101.4 F were noted at the time of her initial examination. Her serum amylase was

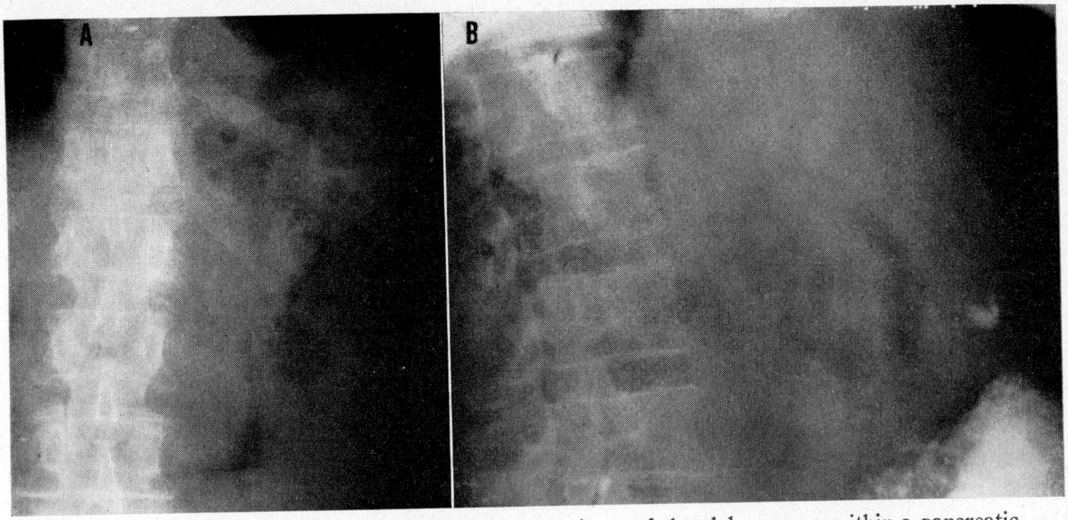

Fig 8.—*A*, the gas shadows in the left upper quadrant of the abdomen are within a pancreatic abscess. B, a slightly oblique view taken a few days before shows that the abscess lies posteriorly.

determined to be 628 Somogyi units. Nasogastric suction, anticolinergic medication with methantheline (Banthine) and antibiotic therapy with oxytetracycline were instituted and followed by gradual improvement. On the fifth hospital day she developed acute parotitis which was treated with chloramphenicol, erythromycin, and Lugol's solution with complete resolution. Her initial chest film showed fluid in the right costophrenic angle which progressed to a bilateral pleural effusion during the ensuing two weeks. A cholecystographic study failed to show visualization of the gallbladder. She still had a low-grade fever and slight leukocytosis on March 6, 1955, but her abdominal complaints had subsided. She was then discharged. When her abdominal films, taken shortly before discharge, were reviewed by a staff radiologist, however, he felt that a gas-containing abscess was present in the left upper quadrant (Fig 8). She was contacted and readmitted on March 14, 1955. An upper gastrointestinal roentgenographic examination demonstrated a forward and slight downward displacement of the stomach with numerous gas bubbles seen posteriorly outside of the gastrointestinal tract. Although the abscess was demonstrated radiographically, a mass was never palpated. Multiple transfusions and antibiotics were administered in preparation for operation, but the patient's family made arrangements for private surgical care at another hospital, and her transfer was planned for March 23, 1955. On the evening preceding the scheduled transfer, she developed upper abdominal pain which was followed by a massive upper gastrointestinal bleeding. An emergency laparotomy was performed, and a large abscess within the head and body of the pancreas was found to have eroded into the splenic artery with subsequent perforation into the fourth portion of the duodenum. The hemorrhage was uncontrollable, and she died on the operating table.

It seems obvious that this death could have been prevented by earlier operation with adequate drainage of the abscess. Abscesses of the pancreas, just as other retroperitoneal abscesses, have shown the propensity of dissecting for great distances, and this has often occurred before their discovery. The proteolytic action of contained pancreatic enzymes, furthermore, has contributed to the erosion of large blood vessels as demonstrated again in this case. It is important to note that this abscess developed during the systemic administration of antibiotic agents which tended to mask the symptoms of fever and tenderness usually associated with an abscess.

Comment

Although a large volume of information is available concerning pancreatitis and other diseases of the pancreas, it is curious that relatively little attention has been given to the study of pancreatic abscesses. In a study of 32 patients with pancreatic abscesses these lesions have been shown to be serious surgical infections which occurred in approximately 4.5% of over 600 patients with pancreatitis seen on the surgical services of the University of Cincinnati during the past 26 years.

The predisposing and complicating diseases significant to acute pancreatitis were also present in these patients with pancreatic abscesses and in a similar but slightly higher incidence. Ivy and Gibbs[7] reported that 55% of their patients with acute pancreatitis had biliary stones while 20% had a history of alcoholism. In the series of Paxton and Payne,[9] 40.7% had biliary tract disease and 18% alcoholism. These figures were very similar to those found in our series of patients with pancreatic abscess, biliary tract disease having been found in 56% of our cases and chronic alcoholism in 22%. The factors responsible for the development of an abscess as a complication of the pancreatitis, however, were obscure.

The evidence suggested that pathogenic organisms may reach the pancreas by a variety of routes. Infected bile may enter the pancreatic duct initially, or microorganisms may enter from disease processes in adjacent organs or along with the introduction of a foreign body.[2] Hematogenous spread from a distant focus and lymphogenous spread from the intestinal tract are also possibilities.

The clinical course considered to be typical was seen in the minority of our patients. They were admitted with the clinical syndrome of acute pancreatitis and seemed to improve after a period of conservative therapy. One to three weeks after this improvement there was a recrudescence of fever, abdominal pain, and evidence of toxicity. A tender mass usually became palpable in the epigastrium, and roentgenograms showed displacement of the intra-abdominal organs by a retroperitoneal mass. There was an increase in the leukocyte count, and not infrequently a prolonged elevation of the serum amylase was noted.

This last finding should strongly suggest the development of a pancreatic abscess when seen in a patient with the above history. It should be remembered, however, that a continued elevation of the serum amylase level may also be seen occasionally in patients with pancreatic carcinoma and pancreatic pseudocyst. It may even occur in patients having no demonstrable pancreatic disease. Pinkham[10] reported ten patients with "pancreatic collections" in 1945 and found a prolonged elevation of serum amylase levels in six. A review of his cases showed that two were frank abscesses and six others were probably abscesses with positive cultures reported in four. One unequivocal pseudocyst was described in which a prolonged elevation of the serum amylase was recorded.

Although the diagnosis was quite apparent in a few patients, it was more often enigmatic and elusive. The presence of signs and symptoms of obscure sepsis in patients who had a history compatible with recent pancreatitis should have led more frequently to a thorough search for a pancreatic abscess including a laparotomy if necessary. A correct diagnosis was less frequently made in patients having smaller abscesses, and fatal complications developed more frequently in this group. It is significant that in this series a correlation could be made between the size of the abscess and the survival rate.

The combination of bacterial inflammation and pancreatic proteolytic enzymes resulted in erosion of a major blood vessel in three patients, a complication uncommonly seen with other retroperitoneal abscesses.[1] Extension of the abscess to contiguous anatomical structures and spaces was seen with over one third of the patients. Spontaneous dissection of the abscess has been found to have extended to the abdominal wall, pleural cavity, retroperitoneal spaces, mediastinum, and even to the scrotum.[8] Whenever an otherwise unexplained abscess occurs in these regions a site of origin within the retroperitoneal structures must always be suspected.[1]

Recovery of the patient was primarily dependent upon prompt diagnosis and adequate and early drainage of the abscess. Only 3 of the 21 patients treated by incision and drainage in this series died, whereas all 11 patients died who had abscesses which had not been drained surgically. Moreover, in the case of each of the 3 patients who died after incision and drainage of the abscess, there was a delay in treatment or refusal for another indicated operation when a recurrent abscess developed. Our experience also indicated that operative complications and recurrent abscess formation were minimized by drainage through separate and adequately large stab wounds made in the flank. Internal drainage into the adherent stomach or intestine proved to be valuable in some of the cases, and marsupialization was used in a few of the larger ones.

Summary

A study has been made of 32 patients in whom a pancreatic abscess was proved by operation or postmortem examination. These infections have generally been obscure and severe. Failure to recognize the abscess was all too frequent, and the true nature of the disease was not clear until the time of autopsy in 11 of our 32 patients. On the other hand, recovery followed a correct diagnosis and adequate and prompt surgical drainage of the pancreatic abscess with few exceptions.

The great majority of these infections followed acute pancreatitis, and in most patients a period of improvement for one to three weeks after the initial episode was seen before the signs and symptoms resulting from the abscess became apparent. An intensive search must be made for a pancreatic abscess whenever a patient with a history of recent pancreatitis develops signs and symptoms of obscure sepsis. Roentgenographic studies were often of significant help by demonstrating displacement of intra-abdominal organs by a pancreatic mass. A prolonged elevation in the serum amylase level was noted after acute pancreatitis in five of our patients.

Treatment should be directed toward early diagnosis and operative drainage supported by appropriate antibiotic therapy. Delay or failure to drain can be expected to lead to a variety of serious secondary complications including retroperitoneal dissection, perforation into the free peritoneal cavity, extension to adjacent anatomical structures, septicemia, erosion into a major blood vessel, or death.

W. A. Altemeir, MD, Department of Surgery, College of Medicine, University of Cincinnati, Cincinnati, Ohio.

REFERENCES

1. Altemeier, W. A., and Alexander, J. W.: Retroperitoneal Abscess, Arch Surg 83:512-24, 1961.

2. Baldwin, R. S.: Foreign Body Abscess of the Pancreas, JAMA 104:1990-1991, 1935.

3. Beller, A. J., and Nach, R. L.: Chronic Pancreatic Abscess With Unusual Complications, Amer J Surg 57:539-543, 1942.

4. Bruckschwaiger, O.: Neues zur operativen Behandlung der Pankreas-abszesses, Wien Klin Wschr 61:227-229, 1949.

5. Davis, C. B.: A Case of Pancreatic Abscess: Result One Year After Operation, Surg Clin Chicago 1:561-564, 1917.

6. Felson, B.: Gas Abscess of Pancreas, JAMA 163:637-41, 1957.

7. Ivy, A. C., and Gibbs, G. E.: Pancreatitis: A Review, Surgery 31:614-642, 1952.

8. Mallory, T. B.; Castlemen, B.; and Parris, E. E., Editors: Case Records of the Massachusetts General Hospital (Weekly CPC): Case 35051, New Eng J Med 240:189-193, 1949.

9. Paxton, J. R., and Payne, J. H.: Acute Pancreatitis: A Statistical Review of 307 Established Cases of Acute Pancreatitis, Surg Gynec Obstet 86:69-75, 1948.

10. Pinkham, R. D.: Pancreatic Collections (Pseudocysts) Following Pancreatitis and Pancreatic Necrosis: Review and Analysis of Ten Cases Surg Gynec Obstet 80:225-235, 1945.

11. Raker, J. W., and Bartlett, M. K.: Acute Pancreatitis: The Fate of the Patient Surviving One or More Acute Attacks, New Eng J Med 249:751-757, 1953.

12. Siler, V. E., and Wulsin, J. H.: Acute Pancreatitis: A Clinical Study, JAMA 142:78-84, 1950.

13. Welborn, M. B.: The Surgical Management of the Sequellae of Acute Pancreatitis, J Indiana Med Ass 46:961-65, 1953.

Lateral Pancreaticojejunostomy

ROBERT E. LEMPKE, MD; ROBERT D. KING, MD; AND GEORGE C. KAISER, MD, INDIANAPOLIS

Operations upon the biliary tract and sphincter of Oddi have not proved to be effective in the treatment of chronic pancreatitis not associated with gallstones. Howard and Jordan [3] reported 69% recurrence in 16 such patients within five years of cholecystectomy and sphincterotomy. We have observed failure of sphincterotomy alone to protect against progression of the disease in 39% of 18 similar patients within one year of the operation. A characteristic common to most of the patients in this group is a grossly distorted main pancreatic duct with multiple areas of dilatation and stenosis. Without entering into the controversy concerning the etiologic implications of this observation, it is readily apparent that a procedure designed to relieve obstruction at one end or the other of the pancreatic duct will not suffice to drain adequately the entire duct in this situation. For this reason the procedure of lateral drainage of almost the entire length of the pancreatic duct as introduced by Puestow and Gillesby,[5] and modified by others, would seem to have merit. Our experience with this operation is presented to indicate some of the problems encountered and the short-term results.

Presented at the 20th Annual Meeting of the Central Surgical Association, Chicago, Feb 21-23, 1963.

From the Surgical Service, Veterans Administration Hospital, and the Department of Surgery, Indiana University School of Medicine.

Patient Material

Since September, 1960, ten patients with chronic pancreatitis have been treated by anastomosing the longitudinally incised main pancreatic duct to a jejunal Roux-Y limb. The preoperative data are summarized in Table 1. All were men from 33 to 56 years of age (mean 42.1 years) and had a history of recurrent abdominal pain compatible with pancreatitis of 3 months' to 14 years' duration (mean 5.3 years). In four patients the process had become chronic and unremitting. In seven, weight loss of from 4 to 47 pounds had occurred. All patients either admitted to or were otherwise known to have had an excessive alcohol intake; portal cirrhosis was diagnosed in six on the basis of hepatic function tests, liver biopsy, or both. At the time of operation none had gallbladder disease. Two patients had had cholecystectomy performed five years previously without altering the course of the pancreatitis, although small

TABLE 1.—*Preoperative Status* *

Patient No.	Age (Yr)	Duration (Yr)	Weight Loss †	Alcoholism	Cirrhosis	Gallbladder Disease	Diabetes	Calcification	Sphincterotomy	Pancreatic Duct: Diam. (Mm.)	Pancreatic Duct: Obstruction
1	37	6	9.5 (21)	+	0	(0)	0	0	(+)	10	+
2	34	2	18.1 (40)	+	0	0	0	++	+	?	?
3	38	5½	?	+	+	0	0	0	(+)	9	+
4	47	3	15.0 (33)	+	+	0	±	++	(+)	13	0
5	38	5	21.3 (47)	+	+	0	0	0	(+)	9	+
6	50	14	11.3 (25)	+	+	0	±	0	0	7	?
7	33	6	12.7 (28)	+	0	0	+	++++	+	8	+
8	48	¼	?	+	0	0	+	0	+	12	+
9	40	4	?	+	+	0	0	+	0	6	+
10	56	7	1.8 (4)	+	+	(+)	±	0	+	6	+

* In this table and Tables 2 and 3 the following symbols are used: +, present; 0, absent; ±, subclinical; ?, unknown; ( ), prior; not applicable.

† Number given first is weight in kilograms; number in parentheses is weight in pounds.

TABLE 2.—*Operative Technique and Complications*

Patient No.	Type *	Incision †	Adequate Exposure	Blood Replaced (Liters)	Drain	Postoperative Complications
1	P-G	BSC	0	3.5	+	Gastrointestinal bleeding, pancreatic fisutla.
2	P-G	BSC	0	4.5	+	Wound infection, homologous serum jaundice.
3	P-G	T-A	+	2.5	+	Wound infection, dehiscence, empyema.
4	P-G	T-A	+	1.0	+	Pulmonary embolism.
5	P-G	T-A	+	1.0	0	Incisional pain.
6	P-G	T-A	+	2.0	+	Wound infection and pain, pancreatic fistula.
7	T	O	+	1.5	0	0
8	P-R	O-C	+	0	0	0
9	P-G	K	+	1.0	0	0
10	Mod P-R	O-C	+	2.0	0	Wound infection, ileus, gastrointestinal bleeding.

* P-G indicates Puestow-Gillesby; T, Thal; P-R, Partington—Rochelle.
† BSC indicates bilateral subcostal; T-A, thoraco-abdominal, left; O, oblique abdominal; O-C, oblique, crossing costal margin; K, Kehr, left.

calculi had been present in the gallbladder of one of them. Five patients exhibited a diabetic response to the glucose tolerance test preoperatively, but only two required insulin. Pancreatic calcification was present in four patients. This varied from a single calculus in the main duct to multiple areas of calcification uniformly distributed throughout the gland.

Section of the sphincter of Oddi had been performed previously in four patients. Recurrent pancreatitis appeared two weeks to 17 months later, and pancreaticojejunostomy was performed from 14 weeks to 20 months postoperatively.

One patient (patient 6) had a vagotomy and pyloroplasty for duodenal ulcer 14 years previously and a subtotal gastrectomy for recurrent ulcer one year later. None of the others had evidence of duodenal ulcer by history or inspection at operation, and seven had normal barium-contrast radiographic studies of the upper gastrointestinal tract.

Selection of Patients

Initially, for the most part, patients with chronic noncalculous pancreatitis in whom section of the sphincter of Oddi had failed to control the disease were selected for this operation. As experience was gained with the favorable response of these refractory patients, the operation was used as the initial procedure in patients with noncalculous pancreatitis whose operative pancreatogram demonstrated a widened duct with areas of obstruction, usually multiple, due to stenosis, calcification or both (Table 2). The pan-

Fig 1 (Patient 1).—Operative pancreatogram showing dilatation and multiple areas of stenosis of the pancreatic ducts.

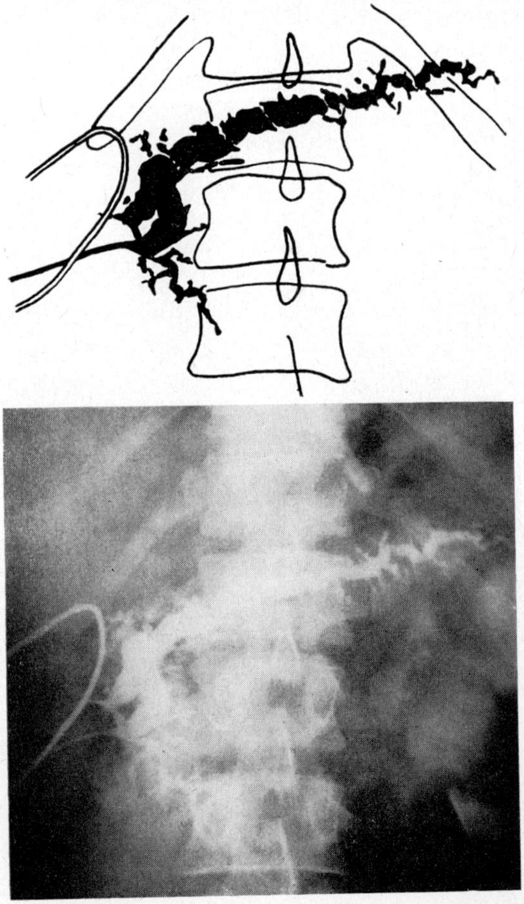

creatogram in Fig 1 shows the multiple areas of stenosis of the main duct typical of most of the patients.

Pancreatography was performed by cannulation of the duct of Wirsung after transduodenal sphincterotomy in eight cases, cannulation of the transected duct in the tail of the pancreas after excision of a pseudocyst in one case, and by direct needle puncture of the duct in one case. In four instances the sphincterotomy and pancreatography had been performed at a prior, supposedly definitive, operation, while in the other four these procedures were done as a prelude to pancreaticojejunostomy. If the dilated pancreatic duct is palpable, as it frequently is, direct needle puncture and injection currently is considered the preferred method, since it obviates the need for duodenotomy. We are unwilling at the present to incise the pancreas to locate the duct or otherwise commit ourselves to a pancreaticojejunostomy until ductal dilatation has been demonstrated. The maximum diameter of the duct, meas-

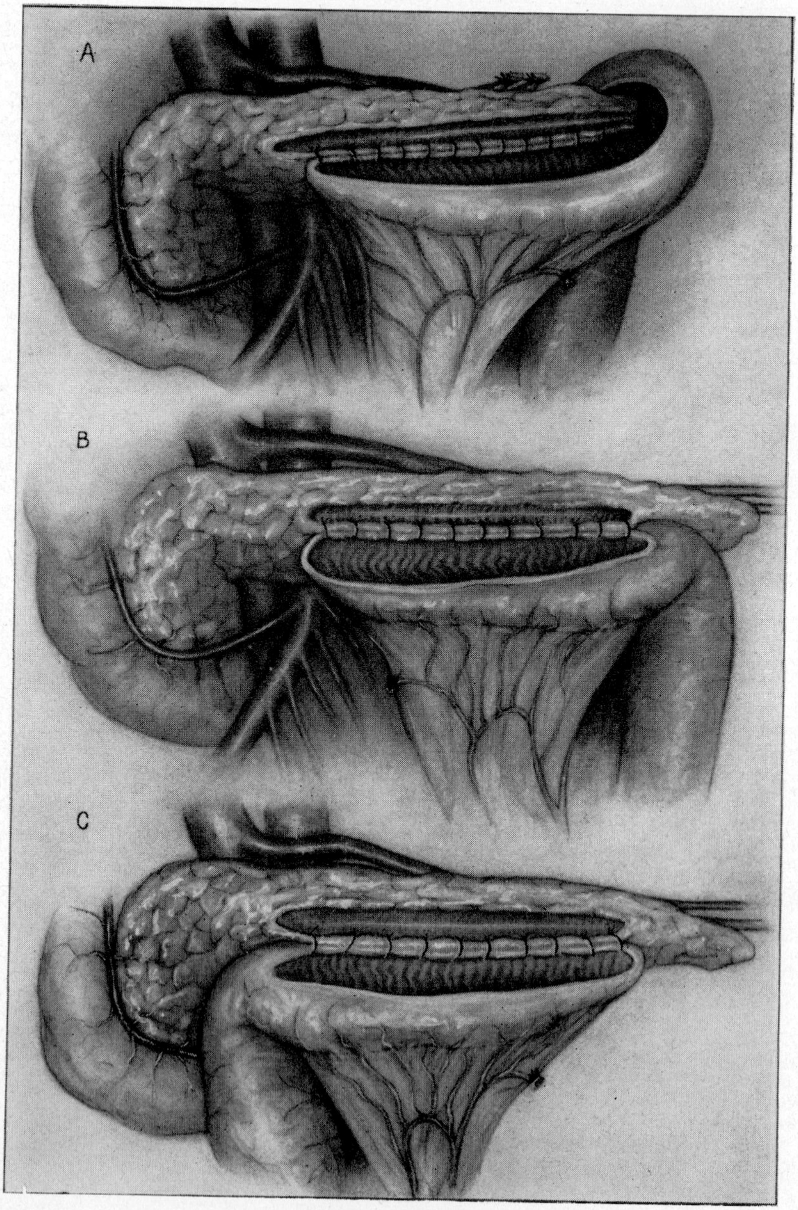

Fig 2.—Variations in the technique of pancreaticojejunostomy as described by (*A*) Puestow and Gillesby, (*B*) Thal, and (*C*) Partington and Rochelle.

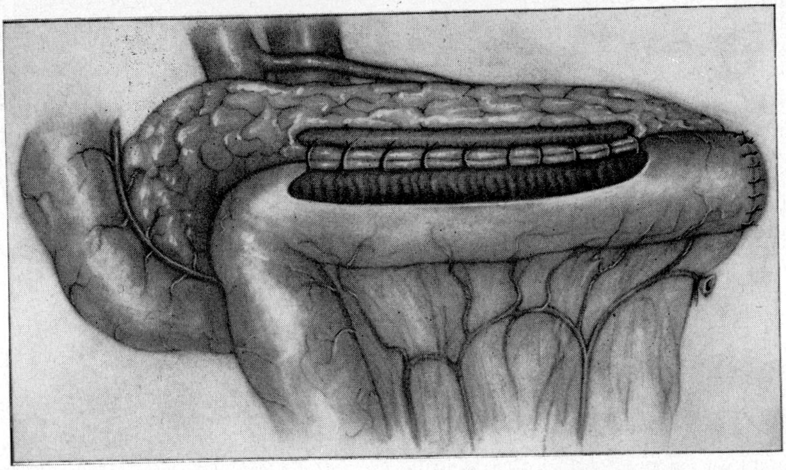

Fig 3.—Modification of pancreaticojejunostomy used in patient 10.

ured on the roentgenogram, varied from 6 to 13 mm. Obstruction by either calculus or stricture was demonstrated in seven of the eight studies adequate for evaluation.

The Operation

The first six patients and one later patient were treated by the technique of pancreaticojejunostomy evolved by Puestow and Gillesby.[5] The spleen and tip of the pancreas were excised, the main pancreatic duct incised longitudinally, and a long oblique anastomosis between the pancreatic capsule and a Roux-Y jejunal limb performed (Fig 2*A*). In the next two patients the procedure was modified as suggested by Thal[6] and by Partington and Rochelle[4] who demonstrated that the pancreaticojejunostomy could be performed safely and adequately without excising the tail of the pancreas and the spleen. Their techniques differ only in the direction in which the jejunal limb is anastomosed to the pancreas; the free end of the jejunum is anastomosed to the proximal end of the incised duct by the former (Fig 2*B*) and to the distal end by the latter (Fig 2*C*). An additional minor modification of the procedure was made in the tenth patient. The end of the jejunal Roux-Y limb was closed and a true side-to-side pancreaticojejunostomy performed (Fig 3).

Variations in the surgical procedure and the operative and postoperative complications encountered are summarized in Table 2. Al-

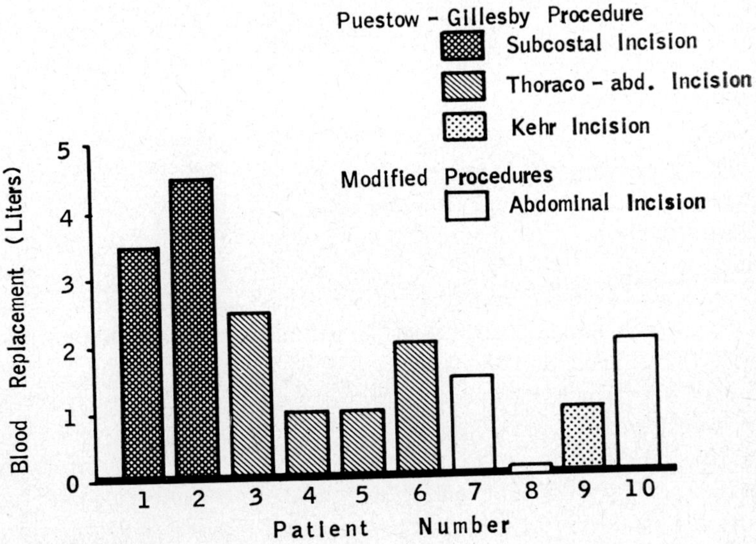

Fig 4.—Blood replacement during operation by type of pancreaticojejunostomy and incision.

though the numbers are small, a relationship is noted between the type of pancreaticojejunostomy, the incision, and the adequacy of the exposure it afforded on the one hand and the operative blood loss and postoperative complications on the other.

Adequate surgical exposure of the pancreas is necessary to control blood loss. The loss was exceptionally high in the first two patients (3.5 and 4.5 liters, respectively) in whom bilateral subcostal incisions were used (Fig 4). This choice was unfortunate, since both patients were obese, and the resulting exposure was poor. Consequently, the succeeding four Puestow-Gillesby procedures were performed through left thoracoabdominal incisions. The execution of the splenectomy and pancreaticojejunostomy was facilitated and blood replacement reduced from a mean of 4.0 to 1.4 liters. Much of this reduction undoubtedly was due to increasing skill with the technique and a generally more favorable bodily configuration of the patients. However, the third patient was the second most obese, but with adequate exposure required 2.5 liters of blood compared with the 3.5 and 4.5 liters of the preceeding two. The three patients upon whom the modified drainage operations were performed through abdominal incisions required replacement of 0 to 2.0 liters (mean 1.2 liters) of blood. The fact that the last three patients treated by the original procedure required the same amount, on the average, suggests that the adequacy of the exposure is more important in this respect than the incision used to achieve it or the type of pancreaticojejunostomy.

A preference for the operation as described by Partington and Rochelle [4] has developed because of the greater ease with which it can be performed in addition to the advantages accruing from the preservation of the spleen and all remaining functional pancreatic tissue. In every case it has been possible to perform this operation through an abdominal incision paralleling the right costal margin and extending to or through the left costal cartilages without entering the left thorax. The thoracoabdominal incisions were followed by incisional pain severe enough to require intercostal nerve blocks in two patients and an empyema secondary to a wound infection and dehiscence in another. Although not necessary in every case in which the Puestow-Gillesby procedure is performed, such an incision would probably be required more often with that than with the other types of pancreaticojejunostomy. This is particularly true if the modification used on Patient 10 is employed. Closing the end of the Roux-Y jejunal limb facilitates the anastomosis by avoiding the difficulty of inverting the jejunum at the distal end of the pancreatic incision, particularly when the pancreas lies high under the thoracic cage.

One other complication, that of homologous serum jaundice, must be attributed indirectly to the choice of incision and the subsequent excessive blood loss.

The incidence of wound infection was exceptionally high. This complication developed in four instances but was of significance only in patient 3 in whom it was followed by dehiscence and empyema.

Two patients experienced gastrointestinal bleeding during the early postoperative period. This occurred on the third and fourth day after the operation. It was manifested by a sudden change in vital signs, and a drop in hemoglobin concentration in each case, by the appearance of blood in the nasogastric and choledochal drainage tubes in one case, and subsequent melena in both instances. The bleeding was self-limited and required no therapy other than blood transfusion. Neither of these patients, nor any of the others, have subsequently demonstrated subjective or radiographic evidence of duodenal ulceration.

Thal [6] has raised the possibility of the occurrence of duodenal ulcer following pancreaticojejunostomy because of the diversion of alkaline pancreatic secretion away from the duodenum. To avoid this he suggested that the pancreas be drained by a jejunal loop interpolated between it and the duodenum rather than by a Roux-Y. Determination of the exocrine pancreatic secretion after stimulation with secretin was done before and after operation in one of the patients who bled. Preoperatively the maximum bicarbonate concentration and volume of secretion was 72 mEq/liter and 1.9 ml/kg/30 min (normal: 90 mEq/liter and 1.1 ml/kg/30 min), respectively. After pancreaticojejunostomy, these values were 35 mEq and 2.1 ml. One other patient, who did not bleed, has been studied postoperatively. The secretion in this case was 40 mEq/liter and 0.8 ml/kg/30 min. These values are not considered to differ significantly from each other or from those observed preoperatively in other patients with advanced pancreatitis. The bleeding seen in these two patients probably arose from the margins of the incised pancreas or jejunum. As yet we have no evidence that patients treated for chronic pancreatitis by pancreaticojejunostomy are more likely to develop duodenal ulceration than other patients with the same basic disease.

Gillesby [2] has reported that he places a Penrose drain down to the area of the pancreaticojejunostomy, whereas Puestow does not. In view of the extensive traumatization to the pancreas involved in this procedure it was elected to drain the area of the anastomosis in the first four cases. Subsequently drains were not used except in the case of one patient in whom the pancreatic capsule was not thickened and the suture line appeared less secure than usual. This patient and one other with a drain developed a leak of pancreatic secretion persisting for 34 and 15 days, respectively. The fistulae closed spontaneously and presented no problem in management. None of the five patients treated without drainage of the anastomotic area developed a pancreatic fistula. One patient, however, experienced segmental ileus which delayed resumption of oral alimentation for 20 days. This was attributed to an anastomotic leak, although no direct evidence of this was obtained.

Results

Relief of pain due to pancreatitis has been immediate and the most gratifying result of pancreaticojejunostomy. This was particularly noticeable, of course, in those patients who had been having constant or nearly constant pain. However, two patients have experienced recurrence of pain (Table 3). One has had two definite relapses of pancreatitis documented by serum and urine amylase determinations at 21 and 25 months after operation. The other patient developed epigastric pain which radiated through to the back 12 months postoperatively. The pain was constant and did not respond to the usual medical treatment for pancreatitis, nor was it accompanied by elevation of the serum concentration or urinary excretion of amylase. The psychologic constitution of this patient renders it difficult to evaluate his complaints, but for the purpose of this report they are considered to represent a recurrence of pancreatitis.

The clinical course of all ten patients before and after pancreaticojejunostomy is depicted in Fig 5. Relapses of pancreatitis for which objective documentation is available

TABLE 3.—*Results*

Patient No.	Last Seen (Mo)	Recurrence (Mo)	Alcoholism	Death (Mo)	Weight Gain * 2 Mo	Weight Gain * Later
1	26	21	+		1.3 (3)	10.4 (23)
2	2		?		2.3 (5)	?
3	12		0	13	3.6 (8)	6.4 (14)
4	19		0		?	8.2 (18)
5	4		?		0.5 (1)	16.8 (37)
6	12	12	+		5.9 (13)	7.3 (15)
7	9		+		?	1.3 (3)
8	2		?		3.6 (8)	
9	2		?		?	
10	2		0		0.5 (1)	

* Number given first is weight in kilograms; number in parentheses is weight in pounds.

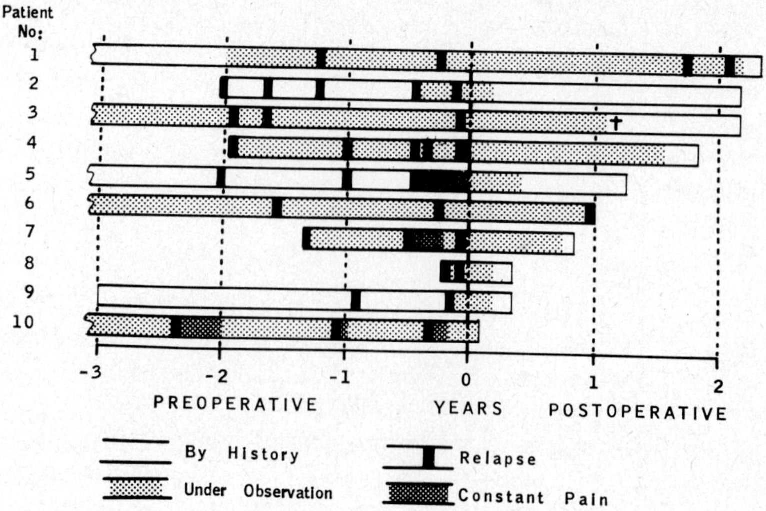

Fig 5.—Frequency of relapses of pancreatitis before and after operation. Also indicated is the duration of pancreatitis preoperatively, time since operation, and duration of personal observation.

are shown. In many instances patients reported episodes preoperatively in addition to those shown. After operation there have been no recurrences other than those indicated, at least while the patient remained under observation. The operation has reduced the number of relapses from 2.0 to 0.4 per patient-year (Table 4). The period of observation since operation varies from 2 to 26 months (mean 9.1 months). This is too short to permit any conclusion as to the ultimate effect of the procedure on the course of the disease. Actually the data suggest that the recurrence rate will increase with the passage of time.

Examination of the two cases in which recurrence has developed for factors which may have contributed to this result yields inconclusive information. Both patients resumed ingestion of alcohol postoperatively, and in one this was related temporally with his two relapses. One other patient is known to have continued drinking, and four others are suspected of it but have not experienced relapses yet.

DuVal[1] has emphasized the greater incidence of recurrence following his operation among patients who had neither diabetes nor pancreatic calcification and to a lesser degree among those with only one of these complications of the disease as compared to those with both. Neither of the two patients with recurrence of pain had calcification. One had an abnormal glucose tolerance but not overt diabetes.

In addition to the reduced frequency of relapses of pain, evidence suggestive of benefit derived from pancreaticojejunostomy has been afforded by postoperative weight gain (Fig 6). Most of the patients had been obese before the onset of pancreatitis. At the time of admission they had lost from 1.8 to 21.3 kg (4 to 47 lb) in weight, mean 12.9 kg (28.3 lb). During the hospitalization for pancreatitis and operation they lost an additional 3.6 to 14.5 kg (8 to 32 lb), mean 7.9 kg (17.4 lb). From this postoperative minimum all patients have shown a gain in weight. By the second month this has amounted to 0.5 to 5.9 kg (1 to 13 lb). Only

TABLE 4.—*Relapse-Rate of Pancreatitis Before and After Operation*

	Year Before Operation				Year After Operation			
	3	2	1	Total	1	2	3	Total
Number of relapses	2	11	19	32	1	1	1	3
Patient-years	1.0	6.0	9.1	16.1	5.7	1.7	0.2	7.6
Relapse-rate	2.0	1.8	2.1	2.0	0.2	0.6		0.4

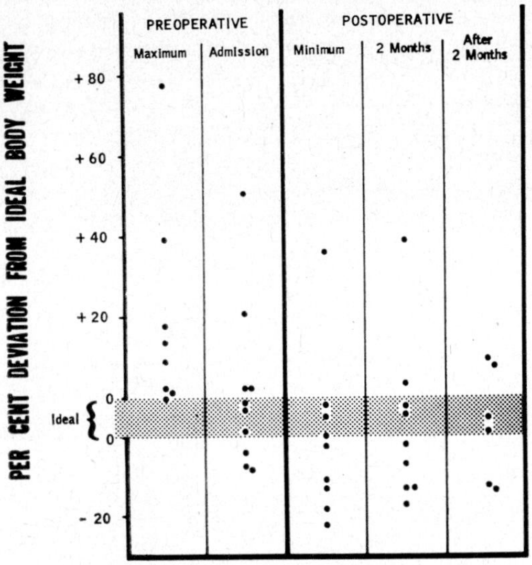

Fig 6.—Relation of actual to ideal or desirable body weight based on actuarial tables before and after operation.

six patients have been weighed after this time. They have gained from 1.3 to 16.8 kg (3 to 37 lb), mean 8.3 kg (18.3 lb), since operation. Among these, four have retained or regained a weight equal to or above that recommended as desirable on the basis of actuarial tables. Two patients with weight gains of 5.9 and 1.3 kg (13 and 3 lb) at 12 and 9 months, respectively, are still below their weight on admission and their desirable weight. The first of these (patient 6) had a previous subtotal gastrectomy and a fecal fat excretion of 33% before pancreatic surgery. He has mild symptoms of the "dumping syndrome" and a continued fecal fat loss of 17% on one determination postoperatively. This patient also is presumed to have had recurrence of pancreatitis. The other (patient 7) had severe steatorrhea preoperatively with a fecal fat excretion of 23% and 37% on two occasions. This has continued unaltered for nine months since operation; fecal fat losses of 42% and 41% have been observed on two determinations.

No conclusion concerning the effect of lateral pancreaticojejunostomy upon the exocrine and endocrine functions of the pancreas can be made on the basis of the data collected to date.

There has been no operative mortality, but one patient has died since operation. After a long, complicated postoperative course resulting from wound infection and dehiscence and empyema, he appeared well and satisfied with the results of his treatment. He had had no recurrent pain and had gained 6.4 kg (14 lb) in weight. He committed suicide 13 months after operation.

Summary

Ten male patients with chronic, alcoholic pancreatitis have been treated by a lateral anastomosis between the longitudinally incised main pancreatic duct and a jejunal Roux-Y with no operative mortality. Selection for the operation was based on recurrence of pancreatitis after sphincterotomy in four of the earlier patients and the demonstration by pancreatography in all patients of a widened pancreatic duct with one or more areas of obstruction by stricture or stone not amenable to decompression from either end of the duct.

Several variations in technique were used and a comparison made of the related morbidity. The modification of the procedure which preserves the spleen and tail of the pancreas requires less extensive exposure, is easier to accomplish, and has been associated with fewer operative and postoperative complications.

The operation has reduced the frequency or relapses of pancreatitis but has not prevented them. No conclusive evidence for change in pancreatic function after operation is available from this study as yet.

Robert E. Lempke, MD, Veterans Administration Hospital, 1481 W Tenth St, Indianapolis 7, Ind.

REFERENCES

1. DuVal, M. K., Jr., and Enquist, I. F.: The Surgical Treatment of Chronic Pancreatitis by Pancreaticojejunostomy: An 8-Year Reappraisal, Surgery 50:965, 1961.

2. Gillesby, W. J., and Puestow, C. B.: Surgery for Chronic Recurrent Pancreatitis, Surg Clin N Amer 41:83, 1961.

3. Howard, J. M., and Jordan, G. L., Jr.: Surgical Diseases of the Pancreas, Philadelphia: J. B. Lippincott, 1960, p 231.

4. Partington, P. F., and Rochelle, R. E. L.: Modified Puestow Procedure for Retrograde Drainage of the Pancreatic Duct, Ann Surg 152:1037, 1960.

5. Puestow, C. B., and Gillesby, W. J.: Retrograde Surgical Drainage of Pancreas for Chronic Relapsing Pancreatitis, Arch Surg 76:898, 1958.

6. Thal, A. P.: A Technique for Drainage of the Obstructed Pancreatic Duct, Surgery 51:313, 1962.

Discussion

On papers by Drs. Gerber, Altemeier and Alexander, and Lempke et al

Dr. William J. Gillesby, Chicago: Dr. Gerber's paper is an important one. We have seen no such cases, but this is an interesting paper and we will see what the function of the pancreas is after a few years as far as getting up off the floor is concerned.

Dr. Altemeier and Dr. Alexander's concept is interesting, but I suspect that many of these cases are pseudocyst, or at least we have classed them as pseudocyst with secondary infection amenable to internal drainage.

Both Dr. Gerber's and Dr. Lempke's groups have supported our thesis that adequate and complete drainage of the pancreas will give good results in these cases. The method of reconstruction is not so important.

Dr. Lempke and his associates have rejected those cases without dilated ducts. Some cases have marked sclerosis with ducts that are not dilated. We have incised the fibrotic pancreas with four longitudinal incisions to about two thirds of the depth of the pancreas, and then inserted the pancreas into the defunctionalized segment of the jejunum with Roux en Y reconstruction. About 6 to 12 cm of intraintestinal pancreas is thus produced. The pain has been relieved in these cases as well. Dr. Reynolds told me yesterday of a similar experience. We are not doing pancreatograms in every case at the present time.

I suspect that this implanting of open pancreas into the lumen of the jejunum prevents the leakage problem of the side-to-side procedure, as any slough or necrosis will be intraluminal and will act as any other intraintestinal refuse.

Dr. Thal's idea is a good one, and we have considered it; but the pancreatic juice was not reaching the duodenum before the procedure anyway, and routing it into the jejunum does not change the duodenal pH very much.

I remain addicted to the use of drains in these cases. I think you will feel safer with drains, despite Dr. Puestow and Dr. Lempke's abandonment of them.

When pancreatic pseudocyst has been internally drained we have had six cases of recurrence of cyst or evidence of chronic pancreatitis. Five have had longitudinal or lateral pancreaticojejunostomy. This is not difficult to understand if one accepts the concept that drainage of the pseudocyst probably adequately drains only one small duct dilation. Pseudocysts communicate with one lake in the chain of lakes, and other lakes must also be drained; we have had to go back on some pseudocyst-jejunostomy or other internal drainage situations.

Dr. William H. ReMine, Rochester, Minn: I had the opportunity of working with Dr. Gross at our institution on some of the cases that he has reported. The concept that Dr. Gerber has brought forth today should be pursued aggressively in order to get these patients operated upon as early as possible and determine just how much hereditary deformity of the pancreatic duct may be present and how much of it is due to changes attributable to chronic pancreatitis. Dr. Gerber's procedure certainly ought to be the answer to the problem, if indeed there is such an answer in chronic pancreatitis.

Dr. Carnevali and I reported on work we did on experimental animals about three years ago, using the side-to-side pancreaticojejunostomy of Puestow and Gillesby. Some of these animals are still alive and are being followed to determine just how extensive the disease may continue to be, or how much regeneration of pancreatic function may take place.

We have observed in patients what might be loosely called an inborn error of metabolism. Sixteen patients have been found to have aminoaciduria, characterized by an excess amount of lysine, cysteine, and arginine in the urine. Just what importance this may have, we do not know, nor do we know what part it plays in the picture of chronic pancreatitis of a hereditary type, but we hope to follow up the condition and to report on it later.

One additional patient who has not been reported upon is a girl that I operated on about 15 months ago. According to her history, five or six other people in the family have a problem similar to hers. She had had abdominal pain for the first time at about age 12. She was 21 years old at the time of operation. Exploration disclosed a pseudocyst at the head of the pancreas. We drained this into the duodenum with an internal drainage type of procedure and performed sphincterotomy at the same time. She has not had any further difficulty yet, but I think it highly possible that she may; she has a considerable number of pancreatic calculi. If she does have further trouble, I think Dr. Gerber's procedure would be an excellent one for her.

Dr. Charles B. Puestow, Chicago: Among women we know there is a frequent association between pancreatitis and biliary tract disease. In men this is not true. Of 216 patients with pancreatitis in our series, only 16 had associated biliary tract disease.

We know there are certain hereditary factors and certain psychosomatic factors that are difficult to explain. I read in the literature just recently that identical twins, age 31, living in separate cities, were admitted to different hospitals within two or three days of each other, each dying of acute hemorrhagic pancreatitis. There must be a hereditary factor because of a marked similarity of symptomatology and results of a rare disease occurring in identical twins at the same time.

The concept of the congenitally narrow pancreatic duct is not borne out by the pancreatograms we obtained in many patients with chronic pancreatitis, as we found that a long narrowing of the duct extended from the ampulla of Vater for a distance of 2 to four cm in almost all cases. None of these patients gave a history of hereditary disease. The patients reported by Dr. Gerber must have all had advanced pancreatitis, because 18 of 24 had calcification which is about twice as frequent as we have found in adults.

The disease in his cases began early in life and there was not an alcoholic factor. I think we have overemphasized the importance of alcohol in this disease, because I am sure all of us have friends who consume some alcohol and we seldom see pancreatitis among them.

I believe a thorough investigation of hereditary factors in pancreatitis may reveal interesting and as yet unknown information. The patients we have treated for this disease have all been adults and none have had their disease begin at the age of five, six, or eight, as is recorded in this series.

Dr. Gillesby said we had not decided on a name for the operation we have been doing. We have talked it over and decided we will call it a longitudinal pancreaticojejunostomy. We hope that any of you who have been doing this procedure and are getting good results will let us know. If you are getting bad results, we are more anxious to know.

Dr. Bernard C. Gerber, Aberdeen, SD: We did not encounter the difficulties at surgery that Dr. Lempke encountered. Both of these patients were out of the hospital 10 or 11 days postoperatively.

The gland is very easy to work with and is readily mobilized. We feel that it is important that these children be operated on early, before the severe complications ensue.

Dr. William A. Altemeier, Cincinnati: For a disease which has such a high mortality rate and which has presented so many problems in diagnosis and treatment, we have been very surprised to see so few reports in the surgical literature. Most are limited to one or two cases, and the largest series we have found consisted of five cases.

Dr. Gillesby is correct in his assumption that many of our cases represented infected pseudocysts of the pancreas. Most pseudocysts are sterile and have been shown to have negative cultures. When they are complicated by infection with the production of purulent contents, the combination of the pseudocyst and abscess formation is a particularly serious and lethal one, in regard to both morbidity and mortality. Moreover, abscesses of the pancreas are often small and very obscure and may show no other manifestations except general signs of sepsis.

The prolonged elevation of the serum amylase found in 22% of the cases studied by this test was of interest. It must be remembered, however, that similar elevations have been found in patients with pseudocysts of the pancreas, carcinoma of the pancreas, and other conditions with pancreatitis.

I would particularly like to emphasize the importance of early diagnosis and adequate drainage of pancreatic abscesses as the essential plan of management. In the 21 patients in whom the diagnosis was made correctly and drainage instituted, 18 survived. All other patients died as the result of extensive dissection, free perforation into the peritoneal cavity, septicemia, or exsanguinating hemorrhage.

Drainage usually has been served best by extraperitoneal drainage through flank stab wounds. In a few cases marsupialization of large abscesses was effective. More recently, during the past five years, however, internal drainage of those abscesses adherent to the posterior wall of the stomach has been used effectively and safely. The procedure is done through an anterior gastrotomy incision allowing approach to the posterior wall of the stomach and the underlying adherent wall of the abscess. An adequate opening is made through the posterior wall of the stomach and the cyst wall to establish the internal drainage.

At first we undertook this type of drainage for abscesses with some trepidation because of the concern over the healing of the anterior gastrotomy wound. Fortunately, however, this concern was not well founded and healing occurred without difficulty, probably under the adjunctive therapy with antibiotics. All patients on whom this procedure has been done have recovered and without serious complications.

Dr. Robert E. Lempke, Indianapolis: Many of the difficulties we had with this procedure were related to a very unusual circumstance, namely, that the first three patients were extremely obese. This is something not ordinarily seen in patients with severe chronic pancreatitis and is something we have not seen since.

Intestinal Complications Following Irradiation for Gynecologic Cancer

DAVID G. ASHBAUGH, MD, AND J. CUTHBERT OWENS, MD, DENVER

Despite the great advances and refinements of technique in radiation therapy, the treatment of gynecological cancer by irradiation remains a two-edged sword. Roentgen dosage sufficient to eradicate the malignancy carries the hazard of injury to normal tissue. This damage is usually minimal and resolves promptly, but it may be so extensive that, despite cure of the malignancy, prolonged morbidity and even mortality may result. Intestinal complications of radiation therapy can be extremely vexing problems for both patient and physician. The general surgeon is frequently called to see these patients at a time of crisis; unless he is familiar with the pitfalls involved, errors are likely to occur which can further complicate the course and outcome of this iatrogenic disease. Our recent experience with two fatal cases and several others that came to surgery has prompted us to review our own experience and some of the literature pertinent to the subject.

Material

From the records of the Colorado General Hospital and the Bonfils Tumor Clinic, we have been able to find 49 cases of intestinal injury following irradiation for pelvic cancer. Since these cases include women treated at this hospital and others who were referred after radiation elsewhere, we cannot state accurately the incidence of these complications. Additional patients who probably represented milder forms of intestinal damage were not included because insufficient objective evidence was found in reviewing the charts.

It seems both expedient and proper to divide these cases into three groups based on the severity of the damage: group I, those with mild injury and little or no residual damage and symptoms; group II, those with moderate injury and some permanent changes with or without symptoms; and group III, those with severe injury who were incapacitated or required surgery. Group III includes seven patients who were cured of their malignancies but who died of the complications of radiation injury and the subsequent attempts to correct this damage.

Of the entire series, 33 patients had radiation therapy at this hospital and 16 were treated elsewhere.

Representative Cases

Group I (8 Cases).—Symptoms consisted mainly of rectal pain, diarrhea, tenesmus, and constipation. There were two instances of mild rectal stricture. All patients became asymptomatic with nonoperative management.

Case 1.—This 62-year-old white female was treated for a League of Nations (LON) stage II squamous cell carcinoma of the cervix. She received 6,800 mg hr of radium in two applications, followed by 3,550 r from a 250 kv machine over a 36-day period. Two months after treatment, the patient noted tenesmus and constipation and was given suppositories (type not stated) and cod liver oil enemas. Six months after therapy, she complained of rectal pain and tenderness, with slight rectal bleeding. Sigmoidoscopy at this time showed a friable atrophic mucosa. The patient was hospitalized and treated with cortisone and olive oil enemas, and her symptoms rapidly disappeared. She is alive and well four years after treatment and has no symptoms referable to her rectum or bowels.

Comment: This is a mild case where the patient's symptoms cleared rapidly and where the patient has remained asymptomatic.

Group II (9 Cases).—The initial symptoms of this group were also pain, diarrhea, constipation, tenesmus, and rectal bleeding, persistent in varying degrees. Five patients developed stricture or narrowing of the rec-

Presented at the 20th Annual Meeting of the Central Surgical Association, Chicago, Feb 21-23, 1963.

From the Department of Surgery and the Bonfils Tumor Clinic, University of Colorado Medical Center.

tum and sigmoid, but none required operation.

CASE 2.—This 49-year-old white female was treated for an LON stage I squamous cell carcinoma of the cervix. She received 8,850 mg hr of radium in two applications and 3,419 r via a 250 kv machine. Six months after therapy, she began to have pain, tenesmus, intermittent diarrhea, and constipation. She was treated with a bland diet, cortisone and opium suppositories, and a stool-wetting agent, with some relief. One year after therapy, she began to have rectal bleeding on defecation. Proctoscopy at this time revealed an atrophic friable rectal mucosa, which bled easily on manipulation of the proctoscope. Her previous regimen was continued, and her symptoms improved somewhat. She is alive without evidence of disease five years after treatment. She has occasional bouts of cramping and diarrhea, which are controlled with Kaopectate (kaolin and pectin).

Comment: This represents a case of moderate injury occurring at the usual time, six months after therapy, and leaving the patient with residual symptoms. It was managed quite well with nonoperative therapy.

Group III (32 Cases).—All had severe disease with permanent incapacitating damage. Nineteen bowel strictures and 32 fistulas were found in this group, and 84 operations were performed in attempts to correct these problems. In this group are the previously mentioned seven patients who died from complications of radiation therapy and in whom no tumor was found at postmortem examination.

CASE 3.—This 42-year-old white female had an LON stage III squamous cell carcinoma of the cervix. The diagnosis was established by biopsy in December, 1947, and the patient was treated with 2,000 r to each of four ports over a period of one month. This was followed by 4,768 mg hr of radium in two applications one week apart. The patient had previously received three "treatments" at another hospital; the dosage of this is unknown.

One month after treatment was completed, the patient developed rectal bleeding, and in the course of the next three months a rectal stricture became evident. A biopsy done in July, 1948, was reported as proctitis presumably secondary to radiation. She was treated with dilatations until February, 1949, when a transverse colostomy was done for impending obstruction. In April, 1949, the stricture was excised, and a "pull-through" operation was done. She promptly developed a rectovaginal fistula, and in May, 1949, she was again taken to surgery where a hysterectomy and repair of the rectovaginal fistula were performed. No tumor was found at either operation. Shortly after operation her rectovaginal fistula recurred, and she developed a stricture at the site of her anastomosis. In May, 1950, the rectovaginal fistula was successfully closed, and rectal dilatations were begun daily. In August, 1951, the colostomy was closed. The patient is alive and well as of March, 1962, but has required weekly rectal dilatations for her persistent rectal stricture.

Comment: This case represents a more radical approach to treatment and illustrates some of the problems and complications associated with surgery of irradiated tissues.

CASE 4.—This 37-year-old Spanish-American female was admitted with an LON stage II adenocarcinoma of the cervix. A biopsy and exploratory laparotomy were performed in February, 1956, and no evidence of nodal metastasis was found. She was treated with 3,372 r tumor dose from a 250 kv machine over a period of 29 days. After this, she received 9,560 mg hr of radium in three applications.

One year after treatment, the patient began to have rectal bleeding, pain, and tenesmus, which proceeded to a stricture of the rectum. In May, 1957, a transverse colostomy and incidental cholecystectomy were performed. After this operation, the patient has done well and is satisfied with her colostomy. She has been admitted to the hospital several times for evaluation and consideration of a "pull-through" operation, but on each occasion no further operation was advised. As of March, 1962, she is alive and well.

Comment: This case represents a more conservative approach in the treatment of rectal stricture. This woman is in good health and has learned to manage her colostomy quite well. She has been spared the numerous hospitalizations and operations of the previous patient (Case 3).

CASE 5.—This 42-year-old white female was treated elsewhere for LON stage I squamous cell carcinoma of the cervix. She received 5,000 r to each of anterior and posterior pelvic ports and 5,600 r to the area of the aorta via telecobalt. After this, she received 3,000 γ-roentgens of radium to point A via a uterine and vaginal applicator. Treatments were completed in July of 1961. In December, 1961, she began to have severe tenesmus and diarrhea, but did not seek medical advice. In January, 1962, she had a spontaneous perforation of the sigmoid colon, and an exploratory laparotomy and pelvic drainage were performed at another hospital. She was then transferred to this hospital, and a transverse colostomy was done. Following this she improved temporarily, but soon developed enterocolic, enteroentero, and enterocutaneous fistulas. She was again taken to the operating room, where subtotal

TABLE 1.—*League of Nations Classification*

League of Nations Stage	Group I	II	III	Total
LON I	3	3	6	12
LON II	4	4	8	16
LON III		2	11	13
LON IV			1	1
Unknown			6	6
AdenoCa, uterus	1			1
Total	8	9	32	49

resection of the small bowel, closure of the small bowel fistulas, and an ileostomy were performed. At this operation, there was no evidence of carcinoma. The resected specimen showed severe radiation reaction. The patient's subsequent course was progressively downhill. She developed peritonitis and pneumonia, and despite vigorous supporting measures she died nine months after irradiation therapy. Autopsy revealed jejunocolic, jejunocutaneous, ileocutaneous, rectovesical, and vesicocutaneous fistulas. There was severe radiation reaction of the small bowel and colon along with peritonitis, cirrhosis, bronchopneumonia, and malnutrition. No tumor was found.

Comment: This case represents a severe, progressive, and fatal complication of radiation, in which the patient was cured of her disease but died from the treatment. Possibly a vigorous program of treatment initiated at the onset of her first symptoms could have prevented the fatal outcome.

All cases were carcinoma of the cervix except one, an adenocarcinoma of the uterus. League of Nations classification is shown in Table 1, and it is evident that stages alone played relatively little part in the subsequent course. However, there were no stage III or IV carcinomas in group I.

TABLE 3.—*Occurrence of Fistulas*

Fistulas	Group I	II	III
Enteroentero	0	0	1
Enterocolic	0	0	1
Enterouterine	0	0	1
Enterocutaneous	0	0	7
Colocutaneous	0	0	5
Rectovaginal	0	0	16
Rectovaginovesicle	0	0	1
Total	0	0	32

TABLE 2.—*Strictures of Rectum, Sigmoid, and Small Bowel Encountered*

Stenosis	Group I	II	III	Total
Rectal	2	4	11	17
Sigmoid		1	2	3
Small bowel			6	6
Total	2	5	19	26

A total of 26 strictures of the rectum, sigmoid, and small bowel were encountered. As expected, the great preponderance occurred in group III (Table 2).

Fistulas occurred 32 times in group III patients, but not all patients in this group had fistulas, as there were some with multiple lesions (Table 3).

The presence of recurrent cancer presents additional problems, both in diagnosis and in treatment. Of our 49 patients (Table 4), 14 had proved recurrent cancer, and 25 had no evidence of recurrence. In another group of nine patients, the diagnosis of recurrent carcinoma was suspected but never proved. These patients all died outside our institution, and records are insufficient to classify them further. In one patient, a carcinoma of the vulva developed eight years after radiation therapy for carcinoma of the cervix; it was thought to be an independent tumor.

The mortality for the series is shown (Table 5). Eighteen patients are alive with no evidence of disease for periods of time ranging from 2 years to 22 years. Ten patients succumbed to recurrent cancer, and four others died of the combined effects of cancer and radiation therapy. Seven patients died of the complications of radiation injuries to

TABLE 4.—*Recurrent Cancer*

Recurrent Cancer	Group I	II	III	Total
Yes	0	3	11	14
No	6	4	15	25
Unknown	2	2	5	9
Other			1	1
Total	8	9	32	49

TABLE 5.—*Mortality for Series*

Mortality	Group I	II	III	Total
Alive N.E.D.	5	3	10	18
Dead—cancer		4	6	10
Dead—Ca & radiation			4	4
Dead—radiation			7	7
Dead—other	3	2	5	10
Total	8	9	32	49

the bowel, and ten others died of unknown causes.

Comment

Various authors have reported an incidence of intestinal complications following pelvic irradiation ranging from 2.4% [11] to 17%.[1] Maas [6] even estimates that 50% to 75% of all patients treated will have some degree of rectal damage.

Etiology.—The problem with which we are faced is not simply an overdosage of radiation, although on occasion this undoubtedly does happen.

First and foremost, one is treating carcinoma, and the primary aim is eradication of the malignancy. Adequate dosage must be used or the patient will certainly succumb to her disease.

Second, individual sensitivity to radiation may differ tremendously, for reasons not completely understood. Sensitivity to radiation therapy cannot always be predicted, and this problem alone will probably insure a small but constant incidence of these problems.

Some factors, however, can be controlled, or at least foreseen. These are relatively self-explanatory: (1) improper application of radium or cobalt source; (2) slipping of uterine or vaginal application; (3) anatomical variations limiting accuracy of placement, eg, retroversion of the uterus, placing the applicator closer to the rectum; (4) previous pelvic surgery or infection with adhesions, fixing the bowel in the pelvis; (5) inaccuracy of calibration of machines and dosage calculations.

Clinical Course.—The complications of radiation manifest themselves in various ways, but they can be divided into the acute and chronic stages. The acute stage has its onset toward the end of radiotherapy or within a few weeks after treatment. Symptoms are diarrhea, constipation, and tenesmus. If the reaction is more severe, there will be blood and mucus in the stools. Maas [6] classifies this reaction as a part of radiation sickness and states that it occurred in 523 out of 600 cases. If the patient is proctoscoped at this time, the mucosa of the rectum will appear engorged and edematous and may bleed easily with manipulation of the proctoscope. The patient will usually complain of pain during this procedure.

Ordinarily these symptoms will subside after cessation of treatment, and the rectal mucosa will show only minimal signs of atrophy. This acute reaction is well known to radiologists and gynecologists, but is generally not considered significant.[13] However, Maas [6] states that every one of his patients who subsequently developed permanent pathology had gone through this initial acute phase.

The chronic phase of the disease usually becomes evident between 6 and 18 months after therapy, although it may occur as early as 20 days [6] and as late as 9 years. In the majority of our patients, it occurred within one year of treatment. The presenting symptoms in the chronic phase are likely to be constipation and rectal bleeding with diarrhea and tenesmus. If the small bowel has been injured, the presenting complaint may be intermittent bouts of abdominal cramps and distention, indicating a partial small bowel obstruction. Proctoscopy at this time may show severe atrophy of the rectal mucosa with ulceration, most commonly located opposite the cervix on the anterior rectal wall. The mucosa bleeds easily, and there may be fixation and narrowing of the bowel. The lesions are usually in the rectum, rectosigmoid, and sigmoid colon. Small bowel injuries are less common and usually occur when loops of small bowel are bound down into the pelvis by adhesions from previous surgery and infection. Some cases progress no further and, in fact, will heal, leaving some residual scarring and/or stenosis which may or may not cause symptoms; others, if left untreated, will develop severe stenosis, fistulas, intestinal obstruction, and perforation, with all the concomitant physiological and metabolic disorders.

Todd[14] divides chronic rectal and sigmoid lesions into two groups which he calls the *intrinsic* lesions and the *extrinsic* lesions. The intrinsic lesion is limited to the bowel wall and is caused by direct radiation damage to the mucosa; it will usually heal with little or no therapy. The extrinsic lesion, on the other hand, is a generalized thrombosis of the pelvic vasculature, leading to fibrosis, chronic granulation, pain, and a "frozen pelvis." It is this "frozen pelvis" that sometimes leads to the impression that the patient has recurrent cancer and is beyond help when in reality she has been cured of her malignancy and could get marked relief from her symptoms if appropriate therapy were undertaken. Two of our patients with radiation damage were followed for many months with the mistaken clinical diagnosis of recurrent carcinoma. It should be stressed that the diagnosis of recurrent carcinoma is a histological diagnosis, and all efforts should be made to obtain a positive biopsy. In the absence of a positive biopsy, one must assume that he is dealing with radiation damage. The previous case reports have shown that the damage is sometimes so severe and extensive that all attempts at correction are doomed to failure, and the patient proceeds steadily downhill and dies.

Prevention.—In the discussion of etiology, the need for an adequate dose of radiation to cure tumor and a variable individual sensitivity are pointed out as two ever present factors which are probably responsible for most of the damage that is seen. Foreseeable and preventable variables, however, can be minimized by the following measures:

1. A thorough history and physical examination should be performed, with special attention to previous surgery and pelvic inflammatory disease; the position of the uterus and extent of the tumor should be recorded. Proctoscopy and sigmoidoscopy should be done for baseline reference and to rule out invasion by tumor. If indicated, a barium enema and small bowel series may demonstrate fixed loops in the pelvis. With this information, the radiologist and gynecologist can plan and modify treatment as necessary.

2. The internal applicator should be carefully positioned, and its position should be checked by x-ray not only after insertion but also during therapy, to see that it has not become disloged.[13] A rectal tube will help keep the rectum empty and away from the radium source. Frequent changes in the position of the patient may dislodge loops of small bowel and sigmoid from the pelvis.[1] If vaginal packing is too tightly placed, it may cause rectal ischemia.[11]

It is hardly the place of a surgeon to prescribe the type and amount of radiation, but some points from the literature deserve mention. Corscaden et al[15] emphasize the importance of time in radiotherapy and believe that by reducing the amount of radium and roentgen rays given at any single dose and increasing the length of the treatment they were able to reduce their complications to almost nil. Strickland[12] has measured the rectal dose in patients with carcinoma of the cervix and carcinoma of the uterus. Although the cervix group received a higher dosage than the uterine group (55 r/hr $\pm$ 13 with a mean dose of 3,620 r $\pm$ 860 for cervical carcinoma versus 45 r/hr $\pm$ 8 with a mean dose of 2,160 r $\pm$ 384 for uterine carcinoma), the incidence of rectal damage was 5% in the cervical carcinomas versus 10% in the uterine carcinomas. The most notable variable was that the dosage in uterine carcinoma was given in one application, whereas the patients with cervical carcinomas received their doses in three applications.

3. The patient's bowels should be kept moving during the course of therapy. Mineral oil, bulk agents, and mild laxatives have been recommended. If the patient develops diarrhea, a bland low-residue diet, antispas-

modics, and intestinal antibiotics will help diminish local reaction and inflammation.

Treatment

It is our feeling that, with prompt recognition and early, vigorous treatment, many of the more severe cases could probably have been greatly modified.

Recognition depends on the physician's awareness of the problem. It is not necessary to alarm the patient, but she should be told what signs and symptoms may occur and should be instructed to report these as soon as possible.

In acute proctitis, it is important to put the bowel at rest. A low-residue, high-caloric, bland diet, along with intestinal antibiotics, will help minimize local reaction and inflammation. Diarrhea should be controlled. Cornstarch, olive oil and mineral oil enemas, potassium permanganate irrigations (1:2,000), and opium and cortisone suppositories may be of some value. Strickland [11] hospitalizes patients and puts them at bed rest until their bowel habits have been normal for two weeks.

Proctoscopy should be performed at this time to evaluate the extent of the disease and serve as a baseline for future observations.

When the patient is seen in the chronic stage, these nonoperative measures can be tried again. If there is a good and rapid response, with a decrease in symptoms and objective improvement as seen via the proctoscope, the patient will probably do fairly well. If there is no immediate response and the disease shows signs of progression, a diverting colostomy should be done without delay. Once a perforation or fistula has occurred, it may be too late for a colostomy or any other treatment. The colostomy, if done early enough, will allow the local inflammatory reaction to subside.

In a few patients the local reaction will subside and, although they may have some residual scarring, it will later be possible to close the colostomy and restore relatively normal bowel habits and function. Nothing is lost by waiting six months or longer to determine the extent of the resolving lesion. A thick cereal or gruel can be instilled into the distal loop of the colostomy to determine whether the patient's symptoms will flare up and is a fairly good test of the patient's readiness for colostomy closure.

A second group of patients may have severe but localized disease that will respond to resection and anastomosis. White and Finn [17] advocate primary resection and anastomosis, but caution against operating in a field where blood supply may be inadequate. It is our feeling, however, that a diverting colostomy should always be done first and all reaction allowed to subside for at least six months before the patient is re-evaluated for corrective surgery. The lesions most amenable to therapy are the strictures high in the rectum and sigmoid with relatively little damage to the distal rectum. Surgery in a previously irradiated field is fraught with much danger and possible tragedy, and frequently a stable and bearable situation is made much worse by inadvisable and ill-planned surgery. Such operations should be avoided if there is any doubt about the viability of the tissues involved. In some instances, biopsies of the distal rectum before surgery or frozen sections during surgery [13] may give helpful clues to the extent of radiation damage. Sigmoidoscopy and appropriate x-ray studies should certainly be done before any intervention is planned.

We have done four "pull-through" operations for radiation-induced rectal stricture or fistula. One patient required four subsequent operations for complications arising from the "pull-through" and still has a rectal stenosis that requires daily dilatations. The second patient also has residual stenosis and takes daily enemas for relief. The third patient has had five subsequent operations as a result of complications of her "pull-through" and now has another colostomy with a permanent and tight rectal stricture. The fourth patient had a successful "pull-through" operation, but subsequently developed recurrent cancer which necessitated another colostomy. As a result of these experiences, the "pull-through" operation has been largely abandoned as a part of our armamentarium. Conversely, three resections for sigmoid strictures have all been successful.

A third group of patients will have to be satisfied with permanent colostomies. In fact, several of our patients, perhaps remembering their previous troubles and fearing further surgery, have elected to keep their colostomies. When the risks and dangers of closure or other procedures are weighed and explained to the patient, the colostomy becomes considerably more acceptable and less of a nuisance. We have come to rely more and more on the colostomy as a permanent form of treatment in the more severe cases.

The management of small bowel injuries almost always requires operative intervention. When the lesion is fibrosis and stenosis resulting in complete or partial obstruction, the treatment is resection and end-to-end anastomosis, or a double-barreled ileostomy, whichever is more feasible at the time of surgery. Of seven patients with small bowel fistulas secondary to radiation, only two survived the immediate postoperative period. One patient is alive, but is a nutritional cripple with five feet of small bowel remaining; the other died of carcinoma six months after her last surgery. Frequently the problem is one of multiple fistulas and multiple segments of damaged bowel that present insurmountable problems to the surgeon attempting resection. In two of our most severe problems, the small bowel fistulas developed spontaneously after sigmoid perforation and pelvic abscess. Before perforation, both of these patients had had sufficient symptoms to indicate colostomy. Possibly in these two cases, colostomy done at the appropriate time would have prevented the fatal outcome.

A wide variety of other radiological lesions along with recurrent cancer can complicate the over-all therapy. As can be seen in Table 6, the incidence of these lesions increases with the severity of the radiation damage. Frequently involved is the lower urinary tract, where vesicovaginal fistulas and ureteral obstruction are not uncommon.

TABLE 6.—*Nonintestinal Complications*

Nonintestinal Complications	Group I	Group II	Group III	Total
None	8	5	15	28
Vesicovaginal fistula			7	7
Cystitis		1	2	3
Ureterovaginal fistula			1	1
Hydronephrosis		1	2	3
Narcotic addiction			3	3
Femoral neck fracture		1		1
Urethral stricture		1		1

Four of our patients have had to have permanent nephrostomies, two had construction of ileal bladders, and one has a permanent suprapubic cystostomy. Three cases of narcotic addiction resulted from attempts to relieve severe pelvic pain. One patient had bilateral fractures of the femoral neck secondary to radiation.[10] It is evident that the physician responsible for the care of these patients will need all the help he can get from the various specialties in surgery and medicine.

Summary

A total of 49 cases of intestinal injury following radiation for gynecological cancer are presented and discussed.

Precautions taken before, during, and after treatment can eliminate some injuries, but individual patient sensitivity and the necessity of eradicating cancer will probably provide a continuing source of intestinal damage.

The injury may present in the acute or chronic form. The chronic form may simulate recurrent cancer, misleading the physician in his subsequent therapy. Treatment is generally nonoperative in the acute stage, which is best managed by supportive measures and the cessation of radiation therapy. The chronic stage frequently requires operative intervention for the relief of stricture or fistula, and an initial diverting colostomy is the operation of choice. Subsequently, additional procedures may be performed, but these sometimes lead to increased morbidity and even mortality. Ill-advised and ill-planned operations are often catastrophic in these patients, and permanent colostomies will frequently be the procedures of choice. Small bowel injuries are less common than rectal or sigmoid injuries, but carry a higher mortality. Operative intervention is almost always required. A wide variety of nonintestinal injuries complicates the care of these patients and requires the combined efforts of almost all the surgical and medical specialties.

J. Cuthbert Owens, MD, Department of Surgery, University of Colorado Medical Center, Denver, Colo.

REFERENCES

1. Aldridge, A. H.: Intestinal Injuries Resulting From Irradiation Treatment of Uterine Carcinoma, Amer J Obstet Gynec 44:833, 1942.
2. Baud, J.: Carcinoma of the Cervix (Stage I) Treated Intracavitarily With Radium Alone, JAMA 138:1138, 1948.
3. Chanin, I. F., and McElwain, J. W.: Management of Advanced Radiation Proctitis, Ann Surg 150:890, 1959.
4. Colcock, B. P., and Hume, A.: Radiation Injury to the Sigmoid and Rectum, Surg Gynec Obstet 108:306, 1959.
5. Corscaden, J. A.; Kasabach, H. H.; and Lenz, M.: Intestinal Injuries After Radium and Roentgen Treatment of Carcinoma of the Cervix, Amer J Roentgen 39:871, 1938.
6. Maas, J. M.: Intestinal Changes Secondary to Irradiation of Pelvic Malignancies, Amer J Obstet Gynec 56:249, 1948.
7. McIntosh, H. C., and Hutton, J. E.: Clinical and Roentgen Aspects of Irradiation Stricture of the Rectum and Sigmoid, Its Course and Treatment, Amer J Roentgen 52:647, 1944.
8. Mulligan, R. M.: The Lesions Produced in the Gastro-Intestinal Tract by Radiation, Amer J Path 18:515, 1942.
9. Requarth, W., and Roberts, S.: Intestinal Injuries Following Irradiation of Pelvic Viscera for Malignancy, AMA Arch Surg 73:682, 1956.
10. Stampfli, W. P., and Kerr, H. D.: Fractures of the Femoral Neck Following Pelvic Irradiation, Amer J Roentgen 57:71, 1947.
11. Strickland, P.: Damage to the Rectum in the Radium Treatment of Carcinoma of the Cervix, Brit J Radiol 27:630, 1954.
12. Strickland, P., and Gregory, C.: Rectal Dose and Rectal Damage in the Intracavitary Treatment of Uterine Cancer, Acta Radiol (Stockholm) 56:289, 1961.
13. Sugg, W. L.; Lawler, W. H.; Ackerman, L. V.; and Butcher, H. R., Jr.: Operative Therapy for Severe Irradiational Injury in the Enteral and Urinary Tracts, Ann Surg 157:62, 1963.
14. Todd, T. F.: Rectal Ulceration Following Irradiation Treatment of Carcinoma of the Cervix Uteri, Surg Gynec Obstet 67:617, 1938.
15. Twombly, G. H.; Caceres, E.; and Corscaden, J. A.: The Cause, Incidence, and Treatment of Irradiation Injuries in the Female Pelvis, Amer J Roentgen 68:779, 1952.
16. Warren, S. L., and Whipple, G. H.: Roentgen Ray Intoxication: I. Bacterial Invasion of the Blood Stream as Influenced by X-Ray Destruction of the Mucosal Epithelium of the Small Intestine, J Exp Med 38:713, 1925.
17. White, W. C., and Finn, F. W.: Complications Following Irradiation of Pelvic Viscera, Amer J Obstet Gynec 62:65, 1951.

Villous Adenoma, a Surgical Dilemma

RICHARD D. LIECHTY, MD, AND LEO RATERMAN, MD, IOWA CITY

Introduction

The dilemma of radical versus conservative treatment ultimately confronts every surgeon who treats a patient with a villous adenoma (Fig 1). These friable, velvety, often extensive tumors defy precise diagnosis. They may grow to encompass the entire circumference of the bowel. Despite multiple biopsies without evidence of malignancy, the question often remains whether malignancy actually exists but has not been biopsied. Compounding this dilemma is the increased operative risk in the advanced age group in which this lesion commonly occurs. Is the surgeon justified in performing local excision of these tumors when multiple biopsies and gross appearance reveal no evidence

Presented at the 20th Annual Meeting of the Central Surgical Association, Chicago, Feb 21-23, 1963.

From the Deartment of Surgery, the State University of Iowa College of Medicine.

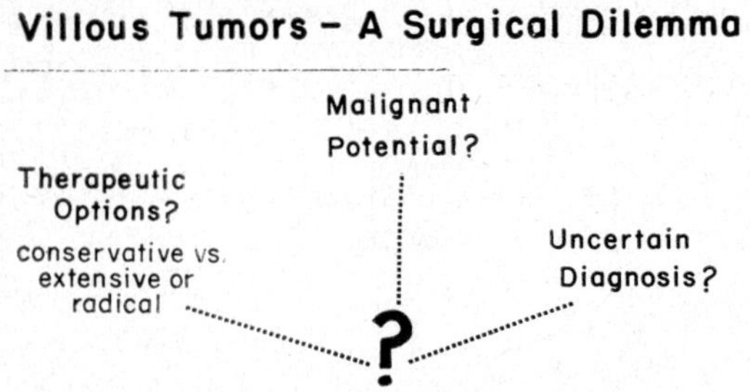

Fig 1.—The dilemma of villous adenomas.

of malignancy? Or should all villous tumors be treated by more extensive resection?[5] This study offers support for the conservative approach in the management of these tumors.

Materials and Methods

Grossly malignant lesions *histologically* confirmed as such were excluded from this study. Only sessile tumors were included which could not be diagnosed clinically as invasively malignant. Induration, fixation, and ulceration were used as the criteria of gross malignancy. Two villous tumors included in this series had indurated bases but on repeated biopsies were considered benign on histologic examination. The case records of 69 patients (70 tumors) were reviewed in which a diagnosis of villous or papillary tumor of the colon or rectum, meeting the above criteria, had been made. These patients were seen at the University of Iowa Hospitals in the period 1952 to 1962.

The incidence was almost equal in both sexes; there were 36 males and 33 females. The mean age was 68.8 years in all patients and 67.1 years in those with malignant change.

The size of the tumors averaged 4 × 4 cm (Fig 2). Sixty-three tumors (90%) occurred in the rectum and lower sigmoid colon. One (1.4%) occurred in the cecum, and the other six (8.6%) were found in the upper sigmoid, descending, and transverse portions of the colon. Sixteen (23%) of the tumors contained evidence of focal malignant change on histologic examination. Premalignant changes were very common. Over 80% contained one or more such atypical signs at loss of cellular polarity, stratification of epithelial cells, hyperchromatism, or scanty mucin production.

Clinical Data and Follow-Up

The most common symptom was diarrhea; rectal bleeding and tenesmus followed. Although discharge of excess mucus was common, no severe electrolyte disturbances were encountered in our patients.[4] All but four of these 69 patients were followed on sub-

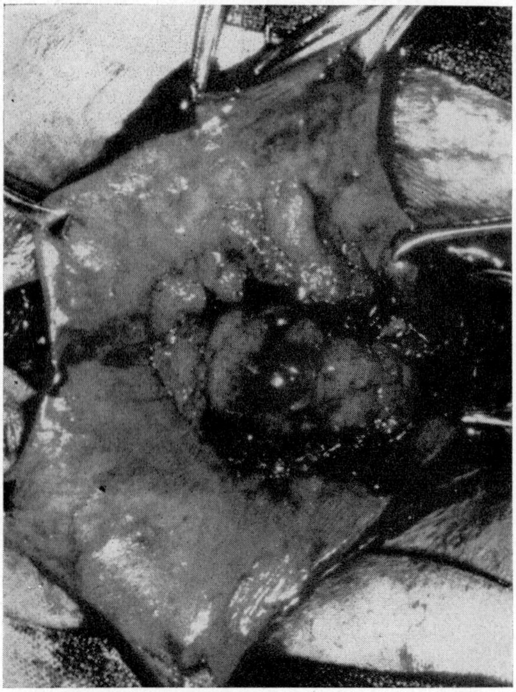

Fig 2.—Villous adenoma of rectum exposed by posterior proctotomy.

sequent postoperative visits. The average length of follow-up was 2.5 years; the longest follow-up was 8 years.

Of the 69 patients, 16% had malignant neoplasms elsewhere in the body (Table 1). This association has been reported by others.[1,2]

Treatment

Sixty-six primary operations were performed on 65 patients. The other four patients either refused operation or were denied operation because they were considered to be such poor operative risks. The operative procedures are listed in Table 2. Extensive

TABLE 1.—*Association of Other Malignancies With Villous Adenomas in 69 Patients*

Stomach		3
Colon		
Rt colon	2	
Sigmoid	1	3
Bronchus		2
Gallbladder		1
Basal cell		1
Alveolar ridge		1
Totals		11

TABLE 2.—*Surgical Procedures Used in the Treatment of Villous Adenomas*

	Benign	Malig. Change	Total
Transanal			
Excision 21			
Cautery 12	33	4	37
Posterior rectotomy	3	2	5
Colotomy and excision	2	0	2
Colon resection	7	7	14
A-P resection	4	2	6
Pull-through	1	1	2
No treatment	4	0	4
Totals	54	16	70

resections included: colon resections, combined abdominal-perineal resections, and pull-through operations. Local or conservative measures included: transanal excisions or cautery, posterior proctotomy with excision, and colotomy with excision.

Results

Benign Tumors.—Excellent results were obtained from local excision or cauterization of 39 benign tumors. Only two recurred, and these recurrences were also benign (Table 3). These were successfully treated by repeat local excision. Ten of these patients have died of intercurrent diseases, free of villous tumor. One patient (age 88) died postoperatively of a myocardial infarction.

Two postoperative deaths and one very complicated postoperative course marred the results in the 11 patients with benign tumors treated by extensive resection. In the nine surviving patients there have been no recurrences.

Malignant Tumors.—All ten of the patients in this group who had extensive resection have survived with no recurrences.

Six of these patients (average age 74) were considered such poor risks that temporizing local resections or cauterizations were performed. Two of these have recurred and have received additional treatment. Four patients have survived without recurrence.

Comment

Villous adenoma is a disease of the aged as reflected by the average age of the patients

TABLE 3.—*Treatment, Recurrences, and Mortality; 70 Villous Tumors*

	16 Malignant		54 Benign		
	Extensive	Local	Extensive	Local	None
Treatment	10	6	11	39	4
Recurrences	0	2 *	0	2 †	—
Mortality	0	0	2	1	0

* Malignant.
† Benign.

in this study. The incidence of this disease appears to be increasing. With life expectancy constantly on the rise, it is probable that villous tumors will be seen with increasing frequency.

Inexact diagnosis, fear of malignancy, and the increased hazard of extensive operations in elderly patients keynote the dilemma facing the surgeon who must deal with villous adenomas.

Diagnosis.—Most of these tumors occur in the rectum (80% in this series) and can be evaluated preoperatively both grossly and microscopically. However, the extensiveness of these lesions often prevents a precise preoperative histologic diagnosis. Even after multiple fractional biopsies the question often remains to plague the surgeon, "Did I make a biopsy in the right place?"

Fractional preoperative biopsies were made in the 62 patients in this series with accessible villous tumors. We believe they are useful if material is obtained from the margin as well as the deep portions of the lesion. Of the tumors of the rectum and lower sigmoid accessible to biopsy, 85.5% correlated with the final sections. One patient had four separate biopsy attempts before the diagnosis of malignant change was made.

If the lesion appears grossly benign (ie, no ulceration, fixation, or induration) and no malignant change is histologically apparent, we believe that conservative excision should be carried out. Diagnosis can then be carried a step further by frozen section or by serial permanent sections from the whole specimen. Induration in the base of these tumors does not, in itself, indicate malignancy. Two histologically benign tumors had underlying induration; this proved to be the result of secondary inflammatory change. Both of these lesions were removed by local resection with satisfactory results.

These lesions may be multiple as illustrated by one patient with large villous tumors of the rectum and cecum, both of which were benign on microscopic examination.

The association of other malignant neoplasms with villous adenoma (16%) is illustrated by one patient who had a large, benign villous adenoma removed by posterior proctotomy. Six months later he returned with melena and anemia. A malignant gastric polyp was removed. Complete diagnostic evaluation, especially of the gastrointestinal tract, probably should precede therapy for this tumor in most instances.[1]

Malignant Potential.—In all, 77% of the tumors in our series of 70 villous tumors proved to be histologically benign. Some of the largest tumors are included in this group. Size alone does not decide malignancy. The subsequent benign course of these patients has confirmed this impression. Of the grossly benign villous adenomas in Bacon's series,[5] 35.7% revealed evidence of adenocarcinoma as compared to 23% in our patients. Welch et al [8] have demonstrated malignancy in 22% of their villous tumors. Ewing [9] described malignant degeneration in 10%-20% in his series. We are left with the inescapable conclusion that grossly benign villous tumors are benign on microscopic examination in about three out of four instances. This knowledge should temper our approach to the treatment of villous adenomas.

Treatment.—Emphasis of the malignant potential of villous adenomas coupled with the large size these tumors often present on examination have induced some surgeons to recommend extensive or radical procedures for benign lesions.[5] Inconclusive histologic diagnoses were an important factor in deciding for extensive or radical operations in our series. We agree with Turell, Dreese, and Hayes that villous tumors should not all be treated by extensive or radical operations.[6,7,10]

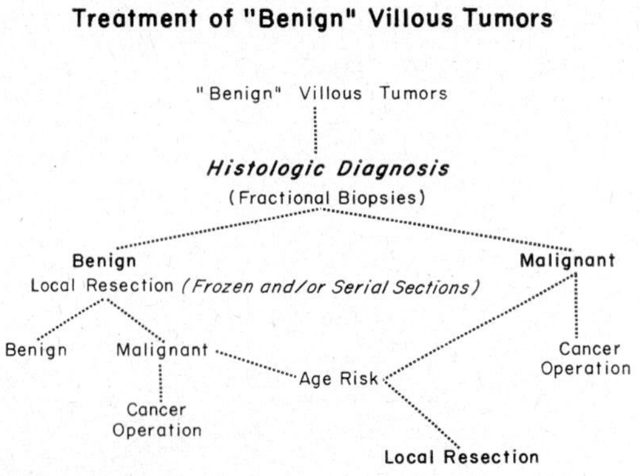

Fig 3.—Schematic plan for management of benign villous adenomas.

With a definite plan of diagnosis and the basic understanding that grossly benign villous adenomas can be and usually are benign, a more rational approach to treatment can be followed (Fig 3).

The benign lesions may be treated conservatively, as our data indicate, with excellent results. Although cautery was used to ablate villous adenomas in 12 patients, we believe that complete excision is more satisfactory since more accurate diagnosis is possible with the complete specimen. The posterior proctotomy approach has been most helpful in exposing the large rectal villous adenomas.

The villous tumor that is invasively malignant should, of course, be treated by a cancer type of operation. But the factors of age and operative risk in the elderly patient must temper the therapy in some patients with focal carcinoma. When the risk of extensive operation exceeds the probability of successful management by local ablation, conservative excision may be the treatment of choice. Although there were two recurrences (33%) in the six patients treated conservatively in whom malignant changes were demonstrated in the villous tumors, we believe our mortality with a radical operation would have exceeded this figure in these extremely poor-risk patients.

The two deaths in the 11 patients (18%) with benign disease treated by extensive operative procedures serve as a grim, yet essential, reminder of the consequences of radical operations in elderly and often debilitated patients.

The three horns of the dilemma of villous tumors, uncertain diagnosis, fear of malignancy, and therapeutic options (conservative vs extensive operations), will probably continue to confound surgeons. The results of this study should help lessen the dilemma.

Summary

A total of 70 cases of grossly benign, villous tumors of the rectum and colon have been reviewed. Of the tumors, 23% showed evidence of focal malignant changes on microscopic examination.

Local excision or cauterization was highly successful in the treatment of the histologically benign villous tumors. Of the patients who showed evidence of malignancy on microscopic examination in whom local resections or cauterizations were performed, no recurrence has been noted in four of six patients. Conservative excision is probably the treatment of choice in the poor-risk patient even when focal malignant changes are found within the villous tumor.

Richard D. Liechty, MD, Department of Surgery, State University of Iowa College of Medicine, Iowa City, Iowa.

REFERENCES

1. Enterline, H. T.; Evans, G. W.; Mercado-Lugo, R.; Miller, L.; and Fitts, W. T., Jr.: Malignant Potential of Adenomas of Colon and Rectum, JAMA 179:322-330 (Feb 3) 1962.

2. Wheat, M. W., Jr., and Ackerman, L. V.: Villous Adenomas of the Large Intestine, Ann Surg 147:476-487 (April) 1958.

3. Sunderland, D. A., and Binkley, G. E.: Papillary Adenomas of the Large Intestine, Cancer 1:184-207 (July) 1948.

4. Shnitka, T. K.; Friedman, M. H.; Kidd, E. G.; and MacKenzie, W. C.: Villous Tumors of the Rectum and Colon Characterized by Severe Fluid and Electrolyte Loss, Surg Gynec Obstet 112:609-621 (May) 1961.

5. Bacon, H. E.; Lowell, E. J., Jr.; and Trimpi, H. D.: Villous Papillomas of the Colon and Rectum, Surgery 35:77-87 (Jan) 1954.

6. Turell, R.: The Cancer Potential of Colorectal Adenomas, Editorial, Amer J Surg 103:529-530 (May) 1962.

7. Dreese, W. C.; Gradinger, B. C.; Hellwig, C. A.; Welch, J. W.; and McCusker, E. N.: Villous Tumors of the Rectum and Sigmoid, Surg Gynec Obstet 115:182-186 (Aug) 1962.

8. Welch, C. E.; McKittrick, J. B.; and Belringer, G.: Polyps of the Rectum and Colon and Their Relation to Cancer, New Eng J Med 247:959-965 (Dec) 1952.

9. Ewing, M. R.: Villous Tumors of the Rectum, Ann Roy Coll Surg Eng 6:413-441 (June) 1950.

10. Hayes, M. A.: Panel Discussion: Adenomas of Large Intestine and Their Malignant Potential, Amer J Surg 101:91-99 (Jan) 1961.

Duhamel's Operation for Hirschsprung's Disease

WILLIAM K. SIEBER, MD, AND WILLIAM B. KIESEWETTER, MD, PITTSBURGH

Abdominal-perineal resection of the aganglionic rectum and colon by the technique described by Swenson[1] in 1948 is the standard operation for the definitive surgical treatment of Hirschsprung's disease. Swenson emphasized that this is a "difficult operation that must be performed with careful attention to detail to assure satisfactory results."[2] The operation is difficult, long, and may result in serious operative complications. The morbidity and the mortality of the procedure are apparently related to removal of the rectum and the retroperitoneal suture line.

Presented at the 20th Annual Meeting of the Central Surgical Association, Chicago, Feb 21-23, 1963.

From the Department of Surgery, Children's Hospital of Pittsburgh, and the School of Medicine, University of Pittsburgh.

Modifications of Swenson's procedure have been sought. Hiatt's intussusception[3] procedure was designed to avoid intra-abdominal contamination. Later, State[4] suggested radical anterior resection of the left colon and proximal transverse colon leaving the rectum largely untouched, the anastomosis being just at the peritoneal reflection of the rectum. In 1959, commenting on the Swenson procedure, Potts[5] summed up the situation in advising that "the operation, not a simple one, nor without danger, is the best available."

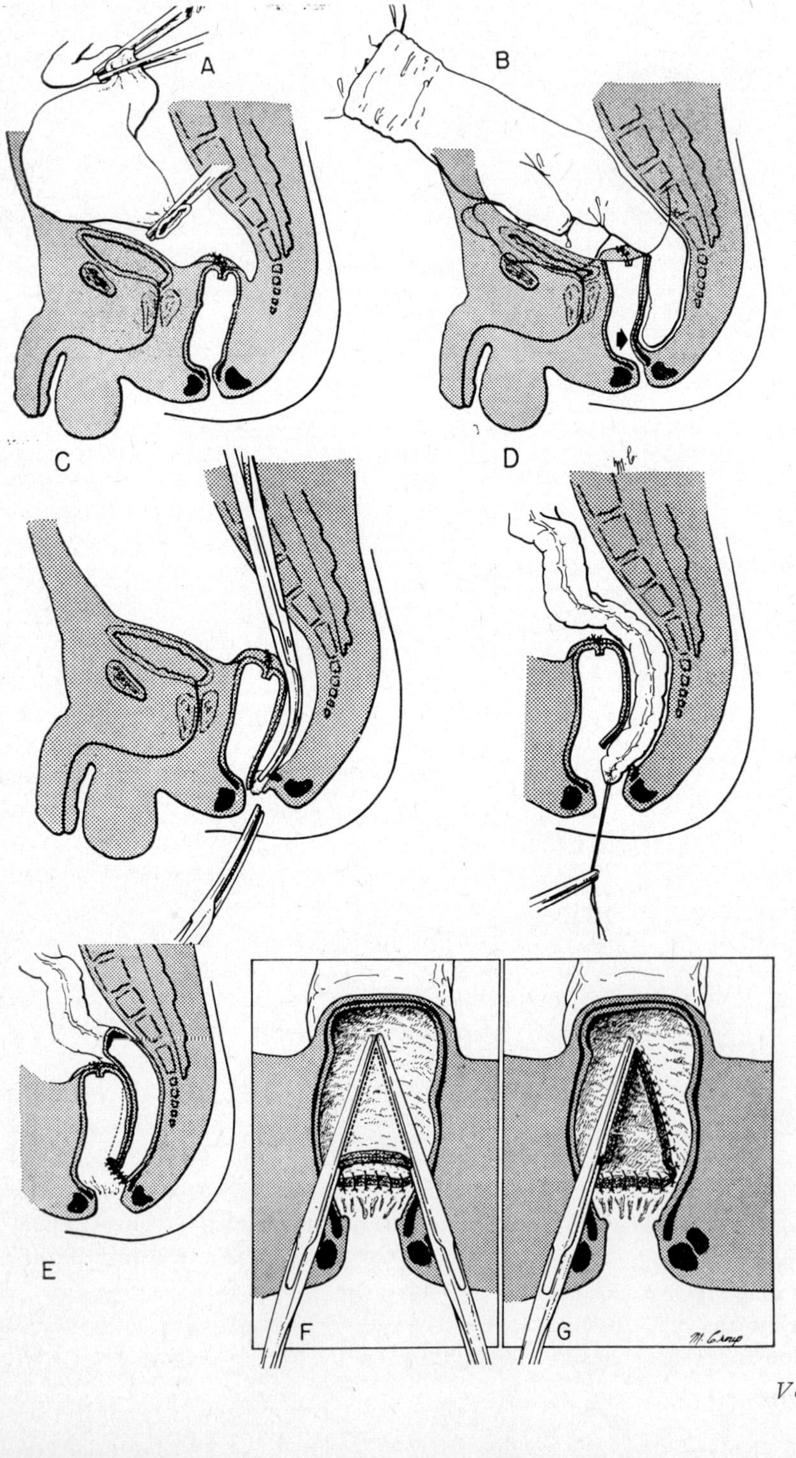

Fig 1.—*A,* the dilated distal colon is resected and the rectum closed at the level of the pelvic floor; *B,* a retrorectal channel is developed; *C,* the posterior rectal wall is incised 0.5 cm above the pectinate line; *D,* the proximal colon is pulled through the retrorectal channel; *E,* the relationship of the rectum and the pulled-through colon at the conclusion of the procedure; *F,* details of the application of the application of the clamps to the common wall formed by the posterior wall of the rectal pouch and the anterior wall of the pulled-through colon; *G,* alternate procedure used in older children. The clamps are replaced by through-and-through suturing.

In 1957 the French surgeon, Duhamel,[6] described a procedure which he emphasized as not a new concept in the treatment of Hirschsprung's disease, but rather a modification of Swenson's procedure, in which the rectum remains in place and an abdominal-perineal pull-through of the functioning colon is accomplished with minimal pelvic dissection.

This report described the Duhamel modification of the Swenson procedure as used at the Children's Hospital of Pittsburgh and assesses the immediate operative and postoperative result in 18 patients.

Operative Procedure

The patient is placed in lithotomy position with his thighs and knees flexed and abducted to allow simultaneous exposure of his lower abdomen and perineum. A venous cutdown is placed in either antecubital space, and an indwelling Foley urethral catheter is inserted into the bladder.

The peritoneal cavity is entered through a transverse suprapubic skin incision. The anatomical arrangement of the viscera and the associated pathology are assessed. With traction on the delivered sigmoid colon, the peritoneal reflections are outlined and the peritoneum incised semicircularly on either side of the rectum and anteriorly at the cul-de-sac reflection from the bladder. The ureters are identified and directed laterally. The rectum is freed from surrounding vascular attachments posteriorly and divided between clamps at the level of the peritoneal reflection (a large Mixter or renal pedicle clamp distally and proximally is most satisfactory for this maneuver. In larger children a Stone or Martel clamp is suitable). The distal rectal stump is securely closed by a continuous inverting catgut suture reinforced by interrupted 4-0 black silk sutures. The silk sutures remain long for traction at a later stage.

The proximal rectum and sigmoid colon are evaluated and the point of proximal resection located. This may require frozen section studies to verify the presence of ganglion cells. The colon is freed of mesenteric attachment in this area and divided between clamps. Division of the mesentery completes the resection. The proximal colon is closed with a continuous inverting catgut suture reinforced with interrupted 4-0 black silk sutures left full length.

Tension on the long sutures on the closed rectal stump permits easy access to the retrorectal space, where a long curved forcep easily develops a channel close to the posterior rectal wall.

The perineum is then cleansed and the rectal stump irrigated and cleansed with benzalkonium (Zephiran) and alcohol sponges. A tonsil sponge on a curved sponge forceps is passed from above to widen the channel and to evert the posterior rectal wall through the dilated anus. With this exposure an incision is made in the posterior rectal wall 0.5 cm above the pectinate line. Interrupted 4-0 black silk sutures are placed in the anal side of the rectal wall so as to include the full thickness of the wall exclusive of the mucosa. This incision is developed to include the posterior half of the circumference of the rectum.

At this point a uterine dressing forceps grasps the sponge in the rectal incision and with this as a guide is brought retrogradely through the retrorectal channel into the abdomen. The sutures on the proximal colon are grapsed by this forcep, and the colon is thus directed into place in the posterior rectal channel. The perineally placed rectal wall sutures are now sutured to the posterior half of the pulled-through colon. The colon is incised along this suture line and a second mucosa-to-mucosa suture line placed with continuous lock stitch of catgut. The opposed posterior wall of the rectal stump and the anterior wall of the pulled-through colon are now examined, and Ochsner clamps are applied from the lateral aspect of the suture line to the apex of the rectal pouch. The position of these clamps is checked by direct intra-abdominal inspection. The redundant wedge of rectal and colonic wall is removed.

The long sutures on the rectal stump are used to anchor the rectal stump to the pulled through colon. The peritoneum of the pelvic floor is sutured to the pulled-through colon leaving the rectal stump in retroperitoneal position. A one-fourth-inch Penrose drain is placed beneath the peritoneal closure behind the pulled-through colon into the left side of the retrorectal channel. This drain is brought out through the left side of the incision as the abdominal wall is closed.

In older children a continuous through-and-through lock stitch of 3-0 chromic catgut replaces the clamps. This is done by everting the tip of the clamp and beginning the suture distally. In infants and young children this maneuver is too difficult, and the clamps are permitted to remain in place until they fall off.

The catheter inserted at operation is usually removed from the bladder on the third postoperative day, but it may be removed earlier. The drain is removed on the fifth to seventh postoperative day, and the sutures are removed on the sixth postoperative day.

Although various incisions have been used, the present preference is for a transverse suprapubic skin incision followed by division of the anterior rectus sheath in the line of the skin incision and separation of the recti muscles and peritoneum in the midline. These procedures provide excellent exposure for low lesions where the length of the proximal colon is not a problem. The left pararectus incision is appropriate when mobilization of the splenic flexure is anticipated.

Recently when a preliminary colostomy has been necessary in the newborn period, and the infant has been in reasonably good general condition, the colon has been transected above the area of demarcation and a terminal colostomy constructed. The distal colon has been resected as close to the peritoneal reflection as is consistent with technical ease; the rectal stump has been closed and returned to the abdomen.

In newly born infants the colostomy has been constructed just proximal to the site of transition to normal colon whenever that site can be readily appreciated. Thus, the second procedure is definitive. In those infants where the site of transition is in doubt, or where the infant's precarious condition demands the simplest procedure, a transverse colostomy is done. Preliminary transverse colostomy has been necessary in chronically ill older children where the huge dilatation of proximal colon precluded a more distal type of colostomy. Colostomies have been closed four to six weeks after the Duhamel procedure has been done.

Material and Results

The Duhamel procedure was first performed at Children's Hospital of Pittsburgh on a 26-month-old female infant on June 7, 1960. The very small diameter of the colon distal to a transverse colostomy that had been performed in the newborn period, the delicate general health of this child, and her poor response under anesthesia prompted use of the Duhamel modification of the Swenson procedure. The ease with which this was done stimulated an extended trial of the operation.

Since June 7, 1960, a total of 18 children ranging in age from 9 months to 14 years have been operated upon by this technique. Six patients were female and 12 were male. There were no operative or postoperative deaths.

The operative time varied from 1 hour 30 minutes to 2 hours 45 minutes, contrasted with an average of 3½ to 4 hours for other pull-through procedures. No anesthetic problems were encountered.

Immediate postoperative complications included evisceration of the colostomy site in one patient and postoperative colonic inertia in a patient with a low aganglionic segment. The evisceration was repaired surgically, and the subsequent course was uneventful. The colonic inertia was successfully treated by surgical exploration and appendicostomy. Wound infections occurred in two patients. Pelvic abscesses were not encountered, but temperature elevations to 100 to 101 F (37.8 to 38.3 C) for the first two to three postoperative days were not unusual.

When clamps were used, they fell off as early as the third day following surgery, but usually remained in place for five to eight

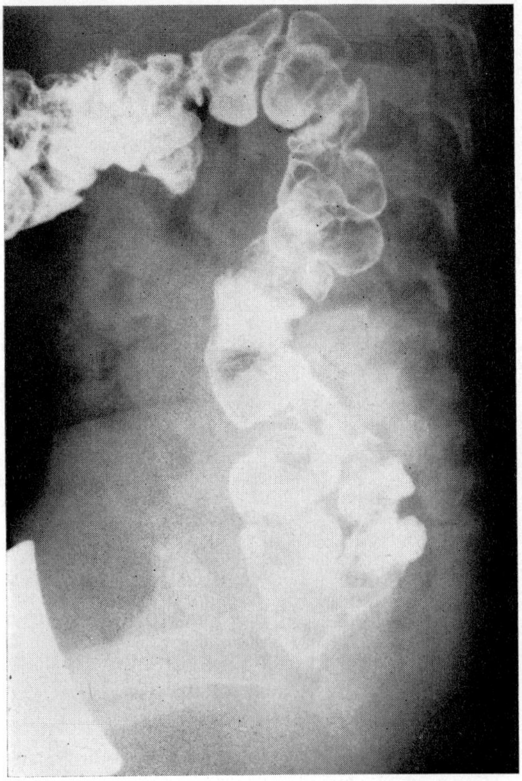

Fig 2.—Postoperative barium study illustrating the rectal pouch and the normal caliber of the colon.

days. In one instance it was necessary to remove the clamp on the 12th postoperative day. All patients were ambulatory and on full diet by their seventh or eighth postoperative day.

Because the longest follow-up period is 2½ years, few conclusions can be drawn. All 18 patients were evaluated in January of 1963. One child with familial megacolon continued to have abdominal distention and diarrhea. Neither more extensive division of the rectocolic septum nor transverse colostomy has corrected these symptoms. A second patient was readmitted to the hospital because of occasional impactions in his rectal pouch. He has had no episodes of impaction after the common wall between rectal pouch and colon was more widely divided. This patient continues, however, to require occasional enemas. A third patient, whose early postoperative result was excellent, developed diarrhea with impactions. He responded well to division of the rectocolic septum. The remaining patients (15) have been well for periods ranging from two years and eight months to six months. Follow-up x-ray studies reveal the expected rectal pouch with the proximal colon returned to normal caliber (Fig 1). There have been no urinary tract problems.

Comment

This experience confirms that of others. The original procedure as described by Duhamel involved perineal dissection between the internal and external sphincter. Because of the high incidence of incontinence, Grob [7] modified the procedure by incising the posterior rectal wall above the sphincter, thus avoiding sphincter injury and preserving continence.

Available reports concerning the use of this procedure are listed in Table 1. In each report the lack of complications is stressed.

TABLE 1.—*Reports of Procedure*

Author	Yr Reported	No. Cases	Mortality	Complications	Results
Duhamel (6, 8)	1957	(7)			
	1960	11	None	None	Good
Grob (7)	1950	15	None	None	Good—no complications
Louw (9, 10)	1961	15	None	None	Excellent
		30	None	None	2 require resection of pouch
Eek and Knutrud (11)	1962	13	None	None	12 cured, 1 much improved
Ehrenpreis (12)	1961	8	None	None	Good
Menghetti (13)	1960	2	None	None	Excellent
Martin and Altemeier (14)	1962	7	None	None	Excellent
Forshall (15)	1962	12	None	None	Well
Kostia (16)	1962	26	1	Postop. intussusception (1)	Well 4 required division of rectal septum

TABLE 2.—*Summary of 18 Patients With Hirschsprung's Disease Treated by Duhamel's Procedure at the Children's Hospital of Pittsburgh, 1960—1962*

I. Procedure		
A. Preliminary colostomy		10
1. 3-stage procedure	(6)	
2. 2-stage procedure, terminal colostomy used for "pull through"	(4)	
B. Primary pull through		8
Total		18
Suture anastomosis		6
Clamps used		12
II. Ages: 9 mo to 14 yr		
III. Complications		
A. Immediate: evisceration of colostomy site		1
B. Wound infection (minor)		2
Long term:		
A. Persistent diarrhea with distention		1
B. Persistent constipation improved by septal division		2

Martin [14] and Louw [9] have used this procedure with success in cases of total aganglionosis of the colon. In Martin's case a wide long anastomosis of the ileum with the colon provided an excellent result.

Fretheim [17] used the procedure in two patients who had previously had standard Swenson operations. In one of these patients necrosis of the rectal pouch occurred, and pelvic sepsis required emergency colostomy and drainage. Although Duhamel, Louw, and Kostia have recommended this procedure for reoperation when the Swenson procedure has failed, this experience supports the theoretical argument against its use, since the blood supply to the upper part of the rectal pouch comes from the colon to be resected or pulled through and can be interrupted by the procedure.

Louw [10] reports that two patients operated upon as babies had impactions in the rectal pouches as they became older. This was not a problem in those operated upon at a later age. From this experience he suggests a more radical and lower excision of the rectum in younger patients. Since one of the outstanding features to commend the procedure is the fact that it can be performed in young infants, this may be an important consideration.

What will be the long-term fate of the rectal pouch; will it be a source of fecal stasis, of ulceration, of lower urinary tract problems secondary to pressure? Louw's observation indicates that the rectum will continue to grow and the pouch become sizable. Martin and Altemeier,[14] and Kostia [16] make note of this problem and have attempted complete division of the septum, avoiding the pouch or at least making the pouch less prominent than in the usual Duhamel procedure. This has been an endeavor in the group of cases reported here, but follow-up barium enemas reveal a surprisingly consistent residual pouch even though digital examination is normal and the patient's septum is barely palpable. It does appear that the more completely the septum is divided the better the result.

The question may well be asked as to why modifications of the accepted Swenson procedure are needed. Duhamel argues that, because Hirschsprung's disease is essentially a benign disorder, any treatment should be as simple, conservative, and complication free as possible.

To commend the procedure are: (1) pelvic dissection is minimal, thus making injury to nerves to the bladder unlikely; (2) the rectum is left in place, thus making the procedure simple: (3) the anastomosis may be a simple nonsutured one, making leakage unlikely and therefore allowing it to be used in young infants. Indeed, the procedure has been used in infants as young as two weeks of age.

The major points of concern in this procedure are the startling appearance of the rectum in postoperative barium enema studies, the uncertainty of the ultimate fate of the rectal pouch, and the long-term results.

From the limited experience presented here and in the literature, caution is advised in accepting this modification of the Swenson procedure as a replacement for the standard Swenson operation. It seems advisable at this time that the procedure continue to be evaluated before it is universally accepted. There may be contraindications to the procedure in those patients who had unsuccessful standard Swenson pull-through operations. Necrosis of the rectal stump may occur. Technical considerations contraindicate its use in those patients with large rectums.

Summary

Experience with the Duhamel modification of the Swenson operation has demonstrated that it is a safe and effective surgical treatment for Hirschsprung's disease. Of 18 patients operated upon by this method, 16 patients are well. One patient has continued to have persistent abdominal distention and diarrhea, and a second has continued to have mild constipation.

This procedure has merit because it does not require the removal of the rectum with its associated extensive pelvic dissection and possible complications. The uncertainty of the fate of the rectal pouch provides a note of caution to the general acceptance of this procedure.

William K. Sieber, MD, 3500 Fifth Ave, Pittsburgh 13, Pa.

REFERENCES

1. Swenson, O., and Bill, A. H.: Resection of Rectum and Recto-Sigmoid With Preservation of the Sphincter for Benign Spastic Lesions Producing Megacolon, Surgery 24:212, 1948.

2. Swenson, O., and Fisher, J. H.: Resection of the Colon for Hirschsprung's Disease, Surg Clin N Amer 36:821-829, 1956.

3. Hiatt, R. B.: The Surgical Treatment of Congenital Megacolon, Ann Surg 133:321, 1951.

4. State, D.: Physiologic Operation for Idiopathic Congenital Megacolon (Hirschsprung's Disease), JAMA 149:350, 1952.

5. Potts, W.: The Surgeon and The Child, Philadelphia: W. B. Saunders Company, 1959.

6. Duhamel, B.: Technique chirurgicale infantile, Paris: Masson & Cie, 1957.

7. Grob, M.; Genton, N.; and Vontobel, V.: Experiences With Surgery of Congenital Megacolon and Suggestion of a New Surgical Technique, Zbl Chir 44:1781-1789, 1959.

8. Duhamel, B.: A New Operation for the Treatment of Hirschsprung's Disease, Arch Dis Child 35:38-39, 1960.

9. Louw, J. H.: The Duhamel Operation for Hirschsprung's Disease, S Afr Med J 35:1033-1036, 1961.

10. Louw, J. H.: Personal communication to the authors.

11. Eek, S., and Knutrud, O.: Megacolon Congenitum Hirschsprung, J Oslo City Hosp 12:245-270, 1962.

12. Ehrenpreis, T.: Long-Term Results of Rectosigmoidectomy for Hirschsprung's Disease With a Note on Duhamel's Operation, Surgery 49:701-707, 1961.

13. Menghetti, L.: Considerations on the Duhamel Operation for Treatment of Aganglionic Megacolon and of Other Surgical Diseases of the Rectosigmoid, Acta Chir Ital 16:107-115, 1960.

14. Martin, L. W., and Altemeier, W. A.: Clinical Experience With a New Operation (Modified Duhamel Procedure) for Hirschsprung's Disease, Ann Surg 156:678-681, 1962.

15. Forshall, I., and Brown, J. J. Mason: Surgery of Childhood, London: Edward Arnold (Publishers) Ltd., 1962.

16. Kostia, J.: Results of Surgical Treatment in Hirschsprung's Disease, Arch Dis Child 37:167-168, 1962.

17. Fretheim, B.: Personal communication to the authors.

DISCUSSION

On papers by Drs. Ashbaugh and Owens, Liechty and Raterman, and Sieber and Kiesewetter

Dr. Clifford Benson, Detroit: The paper presented by Dr. Sieber is a very valuable contribution because he has evaluated the Duhamel procedure purely as trying to find a less complicated and less major procedure for a satisfactory surgical treatment of Hirschsprung's disease.

In his experience with 18 patients you will note there has been no mortality and very few complications, but time will tell what will happen in the future to these children because of the occasional remaining rectal stump, which I think may show that some of these stumps can enlarge and probably will give rise to inertia of the rectal stump itself.

I think the results of the Swenson operation have been so satisfactory in experienced hands that it behooves the surgeon not to give up the Swenson operation at this time, because I think the follow-up studies of these children as they grow older may show that we will still retain the Swenson procedure.

Dr. George W. Dorman, Dallas: I do not rise to laud or recommend this operation to replace Dr. Swenson's procedure in the treatment of Hirschsprung's disease. However, like Dr. Sieber and others, I have found certain dissatisfactions inherent with the use of the Swenson operation, there being an occasional anastomotic leak, the loss of sensation of rectal fullness imparting conscious knowledge of the need of defecation, even though the child is continent, and the lengthy time necessary to perform the procedure even in accomplished hands. There is also the occasional patient with recurrence of the original disease symptoms such as distention, fecal impaction, and, more alarming, recurrence of diarrhea or enterocolitis, after a seemingly adequate resection of the rectum; the very short cuff of aganglionic sphincter remaining still may act as a partially obstructing agent. Dr. Swenson had advocated the use of sphincterotomy in these infrequent instances, and in my experience this has been a satisfactory solution to the problem.

I became interested in the Duhamel principle with Grob's modification while visiting in Western Europe and the Scandinavian countries in the fall of 1961. Performance of this procedure seemed quite atraumatic, rapid in time, and there was preservation of the intact innervation of the entire rectum which, according to my hosts, allowed the patient to retain a normal sensation of need for defecation. Considering their relatively short period of follow-up the Scandinavians were quite enthusiastic about the functional results obtained, seemingly very satisfactory.

Since September, 1961, we have utilized the Duhamel principle in nine children ranging from 11 weeks to 3 years of age. If the results of this procedure prove satisfactory I can see the possibility of elimination of the major dissatisfactions I have previously mentioned with the Swenson operation. I find the procedure is still a difficult one in the smaller babies and would recommend leaving an infant with a satisfactory enterostomy until he has reached sufficient size (approximately 20 lb [9.1 kg]) before undertaking the definitive procedure. We have adopted this procedure temporarily in the spirit of research to accumulate a series of perhaps 20 to 25 patients and then critically to evaluate the results in comparison with those patients who have received treatment by the Swenson procedure.

I congratulate Dr. Sieber for the content and spirit of his presentation. I believe our views are very similar in that he, as well as I, will base our future recommendations upon the results of the work we are doing today.

Dr. Walter Gerwig, Clarksburg, W Va: I think it was McKittrick and Wheelock who in 1955 attracted our attention to another phase of villous adenoma, namely, that of hypersection of the tumor with a terrific amount of sodium loss from the surface of the tumor, resulting in severe electrolytic imbalance. Some of these individuals have died in a very short period of time.

In those cases that are being reported with increasing frequency it is now advocated that possibly they should be treated as emergency measures, establish their fluid and electrolyte balance to a correct level as rapidly as possible, and operate on them immediately.

Dr. Sidney E. Ziffren, Iowa City: As all of us are aware, a massive villous adenoma can be a very trying problem, especially in the aged. These tumors may look very dangerous on superficial gross examination. Even on microscopic examination small foci may suggest malignancy. But I do not believe we should fall into the trap of being so fearful of the appearance that we jeopardize a patient's life to remove radically what is essentially a very low-grade lesion which does not have the potential, in the vast majority of instances, to kill. These are the types of lesions Dr. Liechty has been discussing.

Most of us, without hesitation, say that a patient with such a tumor must be operated on even if multiple biopsies report the lesion as benign. Personally, I have never seen one of these lesions change from benign to malignant character. If the patient is a very poor risk, as so many in the extreme age group are, why must such a lesion be operated on? In the series Dr. Liechty presented there were four who were not operated on. In other words, Dr. Liechty, what are the indications for operation in such a patient?

Secondly, it was not clear to me if merely cauterizing the lesion is as effective as excising it. There were 20 patients listed on the slide in the series presented. If the former is adequate to handle the lesion, that is, by merely cauterizing the epithelium, is it then replaced by scar tissue, and does this completely handle the problem? If cauterization does cure villous adenoma, this would solve the problem in the poor risk patient and answer my previous question.

Lastly, since 16% of the patients had tumors elsewhere, does this mean that any patient with a villous adenoma should have complete studies of the chest, stomach, lower bowel, gallbladder, and genitourinary tract? This seems to be a very high figure for associated neoplasms. Perhaps the villous adenoma is merely a manifestation of something more serious occurring elsewhere in the body.

Dr. Eugene M. Bricker, St. Louis: I would like to emphasize two or three points regarding the technical features of operation for this very serious complication of irradiation therapy.

The problem, of course, is precipitated by the fact that irradiated bowel is notoriously poor in its healing and the chance of breakdown of an anastomosis is very great. The factors decreasing the risk of such a complication include: (1) the preoperative preparation, both mechanical and bacteriological, to get the bowel in optimal condition. (2) Of great importance is an adequate resection of the involved bowel if this is possible and practical. It must be remembered that what may seem to be an adequate resection of all obviously irradiated bowel does not mean that the remaining bowel is normal. (3) A meticulous technique of resection and anastomosis is of utmost importance. (4) Finally, a point that is perhaps of greatest importance must be emphasized because it is not generally recognized, and that is the prolonged defunctionalization that is necessary after anastomosis of overly irradiated bowel. This is quite easy, of course, when the resected bowel is the sigmoid or rectum and the anastomosis is done in an area where a proximal colostomy can be carried for several months. We believe three or four months of defunctionalization is not too long for these low colonic anastomoses after resection for irradiation damage.

The problem of how to handle the small intestine is not as simple. I would like to hear Dr. Owens comment in this regard.

We believe that prolonged decompression and defunctionalization is important here too, but it is not so practical to carry it to such an extent as one can for the low colon. The case presenting only localized small bowel damage is really no problem, but the case treated by intraperitoneal radioactive gold and/or extensive external irradiation to the abdomen may be extremely difficult to manage.

You might be interested in the way we provide for decompression at the operating table in the severe cases. This is done by the insertion of a long intestinal tube which can be carried by the patient for two, three, or four weeks if there are any symptoms that warrant it. The tube is inserted from the normal jejunum down past the anastomosis or anastomoses for continuous and effective decompression during the immediate postoperative period, which is the most critical period for healing of the damaged bowel. We have found this long-tube jejunostomy to be most helpful.

Dr. J. Cuthbert Owens, Denver: This patient, our 50th, was recently seen and therefore was not included in this paper. Her history of radiation therapy for cervical carcinoma was similar to those previously reported. A diagnosis of intestinal obstruction due to metastatic carcinoma was entertained. At operation, the bowel was markedly hyperemic and thickened and presented the gross appearance of fibrinous peritonitis. No carcinoma was found.

In view of our experience and a recent report of Suggs et al from Barnes Hospital, we did a massive resection of the involved small bowel, leaving about seven feet of small intestine. A frozen section was examined distally and proximally to be sure our anastomosis was not in an irradiated area. We believe this is very important, to lessen the possibility of complications when intestinal surgery is necessary because of tissue damage from radiation therapy.

We wish to repeat that our purpose in presenting this paper is not to be critical of the roentgenologist. We desire only to alert the general surgeon to the possible pitfalls involved when he is called in consultation or to treat these patients.

Dr. Richard D. Liechty, Iowa City: In answer to Dr. Gerwig, we had no instances of electrolyte imbalance in our patients. However, as for indications, mucous diarrhea was the No. 1 complaint of these patients, with bleeding and tenesmus following. These patients were almost all symptomatic in one form or another.

As far as cautery is concerned, this has been effective in the 12 cases in which it was employed. It was usually limited to the smaller lesions, or some larger lesions in the very old and debilitated patient. One of those that recurred, as a matter of fact, was in a 92-year-old man treated by cauterization.

We found that 23% of these grossly benign lesions were malignant. Therefore, I think in the younger patient or anyone who can stand a local procedure these should be removed, even if they do not cause symptoms.

As far as investigative studies are concerned, yes, we believe the complete gastrointestinal tract should be evaluated. We had one patient in whom we removed a villous adenoma who did not have an upper gastrointestinal tract series. He returned to the hospital with massive gastrointestinal bleeding three months after his procedure, with a large, malignant gastric polyp which had suddenly bled.

Dr. William K. Sieber, Pittsburgh: This paper was presented because vague descriptions of this procedure in the literature and extreme points of view concerning its status in the treatment of Hirschsprung's disease have produced confusion. We hope that these remarks have to some extent clarified our position in advising that this is the safe procedure for the surgical treatment of Hirschsprung's disease. Caution is advised in recommending the total acceptance of this procedure until the question of the ultimate fate of the rectal pouch is determined. I believe that it is clear that we will be hearing more about the long-term results of this procedure in Hirschsprung's disease.

Esophageal Strictures After Anastomosis in Esophageal Atresia

LOYD R. SCHULTZ, MD, AND H. WILLIAM CLATWORTHY, JR., MD, COLUMBUS, OHIO

Congenital atresia of the esophagus occurs once in every 3,000 births.[1] In approximately 90% of these anomalous infants the upper esophageal segment terminates blindly and the lower segment forms a fistula into the trachea at or near the carina. Division of the fistula and end-to-end anastomosis of the esophagus is the treatment of choice. With prompt surgical treatment, the survival rate has steadily increased since the first successful case was reported by Haight and Towsley.[2] A collected series of 967 patients reported from 11 separate institutions since 1956 yields a mean operative survival rate of 52%.[3]

The commonest complication in the infants who survive esophageal anastomosis is stricture formation. Gross,[4] Swenson,[5] Holinger,[6] and, more recently, Morrison[7] have noted that significant difficulty due to post-anastomotic stricture was observed in 35% to 50% of their patients. Although dysfunctional swallowing may mimic stricture, for the purpose of this paper, a stricture is defined as a radiographically demonstrable persistent narrowing at the site of anastomosis associated with feeding difficulties.

In order to investigate the factors operable in the genesis and treatment of postoperative esophageal strictures we have reviewed our experience with 61 consecutive cases of esophageal atresia admitted to the Columbus Children's Hospital between 1951 and 1961.*

Summary of Case Material

Three of the 61 patients were moribund at the time of admission and died shortly thereafter. Cervical esophagostomy, gastrostomy, and a division of the tracheo-esophageal fistula were performed in seven because of extreme prematurity, associated other anomalies, or absence of the distal esophageal segment. Fifty-one of the infants were subjected to a primary one-stage retropleural division of the tracheo-esophageal fistula and a two-layer 5-0 or 6-0 silk end-to-end anastomosis of the esophagus. Gastrostomy was routinely performed. Forty-five (88%) of these patients so treated survived the immediate postoperative period and were discharged from the hospital.

Significant radiographic and clinical strictures developed in 23 of these patients. A recurrent tracheo-esophageal fistula also developed in two of these. Of the 23 strictured patients, 21 became symptomatic in the first ten weeks following surgery. Dysphagia with chronic cough and choking during feedings was the dominant symptom. In some cases the child was unable to swallow even his own saliva. Aspiration pneumonia was commonly observed on the radiographs.

Twenty-two of the 45 patients in this series did not develop symptomatic strictures, although 7 were found to have a 50% or more constriction at the site of anastomosis on at least one radiographic study. These children were continued on oral feedings without dilatations. Radiographic studies four months to several years following surgery showed only minimal narrowing at the anastomosis (Fig 1). Four of these patients have subsequently experienced difficulty with foreign bodies, ie, coins, orange peel, carrot pieces, lodging at the anastomotic site. Six infants have experienced significant dysphagia without any radiographic evidence of stricture. Cinefluoroscopic studies on these children suggested a neuromuscular incoor-

Presented at the 20th Annual Meeting of the Central Surgical Association, Chicago, Feb 21-23, 1963.

From the Department of Surgery, The Ohio State University College of Medicine, and The Children's Hospital.

* Forty-nine previously reported.[3]

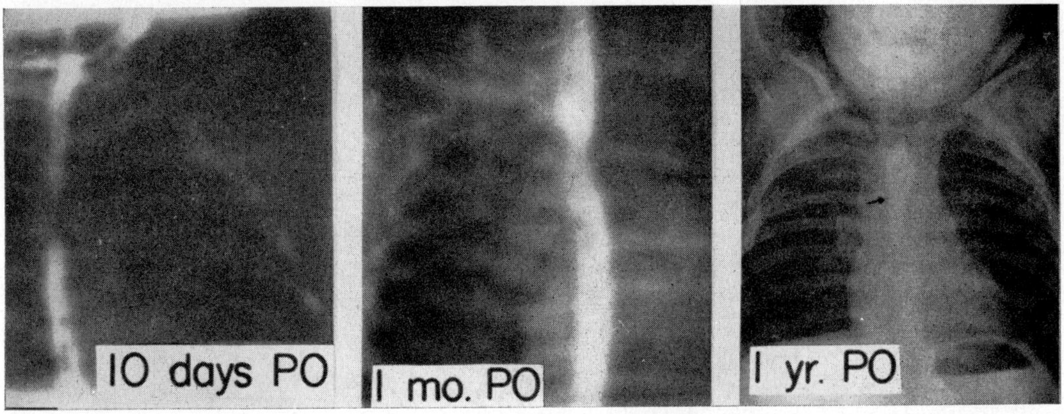

Fig 1.—Typical serial esophagrams of an infant with asymptomatic narrowing of esophagus. The caliber of the anastomosis improved with growth. No dilatations were needed.

dination of the upper esophageal segment. Similar findings have been recorded by Haight [8] and Haas [9] in patients after the repair of esophageal atresia.

Only 12 of the 45 patients have been totally free of deglutitory difficulties.

Treatment of Strictures

Esophageal dilatation was performed on each of the infants who developed a symptomatic stricture. In 13 of the patients, symptoms were controlled by this treatment. Eight required less than 12 dilatations, 2 required between 12 and 24, and 4 required more than 24 dilatations to alleviate their symptoms (Fig 2).

The technique of dilatation varied. When a gastrostomy tube was in place dilatations were accomplished by using a nasogastric string tied in a circle. Soft rubber Tucker type dilators were first used in retrograde manner (Fig 3). In most instances the dilatations were begun between two and three weeks after surgery if the child had significant dysphagia and the stricture was demonstrable on the radiograph. Dilatations were begun with a size 10 or 12 French catheter and normally increased to a 20 French in infants within a year. While in the hospital, dilatations were carried out two or three times weekly and, after discharge, once every week or two. As soon as oral feedings were well tolerated the gastrostomy tube was removed and the Tucker dilators were drawn through the mouth. When an adequate esophageal lumen could be maintained between dilatations the string was removed. Infrequent subsequent dilatations were carried out with fluoroscopic control using metallic-tipped filiform followed by a woven urethral dilator. No esophageal perforations occurred with these two methods of dilatation.

Fig 2.—Serial esophagrams of severe symptomatic stricture successfully treated by dilatations over one-year period.

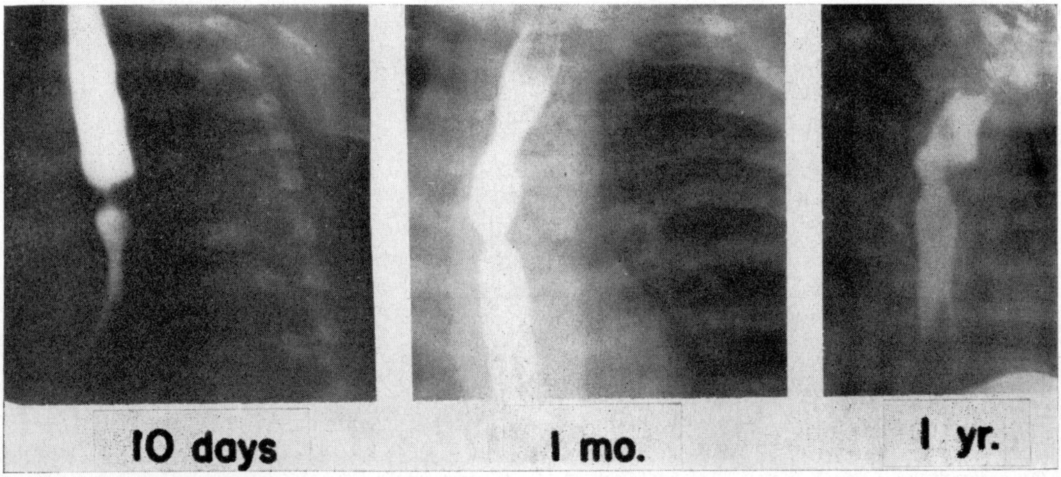

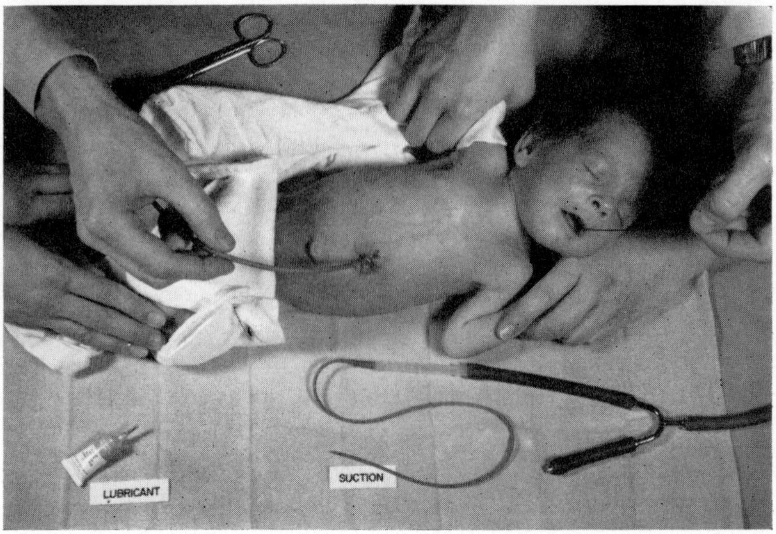

Fig 3.—Retrograde dilatation of postoperative stricture of the esophagus is safely accomplished with Tucker dilators (8-28 F) in a three-week-old infant.

Dilatations with the esophagoscope and bougie were used in older children. Hurtz mercury weighted dilators have been useful in a few patients. Unfortunately perforation of the esophagus occurred in two children being subjected to an esophagoscopic dilatation. Thoracotomy tube drainage controlled the subsequent empyema and pneumothorax in each case.

Transpleural reoperation and resection of the stricture with an end-to-end anastomosis was carried out in five children. Two of these were operated upon at four weeks of age because of complete functional obstruction at the anastomosis; two were resected from three to ten months of age; and one at three years because of recurring stricture in spite of periodic dilatations. In a single case it was necessary to revise the second anastomosis because of recurrent stricture.

Comment

In spite of what appeared to be a rather reasonable approach to the problem of esophageal stricture, seven of these patients have died. One patient died of an unrecognized tracheo-esophageal fistula associated with a recurrent stricture and four of recurring aspiration pneumonia. In addition there were two deaths in the group of patients who had dysfunctional deglutition, both of whom also had intraventricular septal defects and recurrent pulmonary infection.

The mortality associated with swallowing difficulties, usually due to stricture in this group, has, therefore, exceeded the immediate operative mortality. The factors which appear to contribute to postoperative stricture formation following esophageal anastomosis are: (1) type of anastomosis, (2) tension on the suture line, (3) leakage at the site of anastomosis, (4) extensive mobilization of the esophagus, (5) tissue reaction to suture material, and (6) infection.

Several different techniques have been devised for reconstruction of the esophageal continuity to minimize the incidence of stricture at the site of anastomosis. In the construction of the anastomosis, Haight recommended an anastomosis whereby the smaller, thinner, distal segment was telescoped into the proximal esophagus. The entire thickness of the wall of the lower segment was joined by interrupted sutures through the mucosal and submucosal portions of the upper segment. The muscularis of the upper segment was then lapped over the first suture line to the adventitia of the lower segment.

In 1946 Gross [10] described an end-to-end oblique anastomosis in which a slit was made in the thin portion of each esophageal segment. Since this proved to be the anterior wall of each, the distal esophagus required a 180 degree rotation.

An end-to-side anastomosis was described by Sanderud in 1960.[11] With this technique the blind proximal esophagus is sutured to the side of the distal fistula. In ten reported cases, no strictures developed during the follow-up period of 1 to 15 months. Anatomical limitations, namely the distance between the proximal pouch and the distal esophageal segment, lead to tension which is difficult to alter in any individual patient without extensive mobilization of the distal esophagus. In many instances the distances between the dilated proximal esophagus and the distal narrow segment will not permit the latter type of anastomosis, and indeed considerable tension must be placed upon the suture line in order to accomplish any type of primary anastomosis. The factor of tension appears to be a most important one in stricture formation, since in our series 60% of the patients in whom the anastomosis was done under marked tension (2½ or 3 cm gap) developed strictures. When no tension was placed on the suture line strictures occurred in but 10% of the cases.

The effect of operative manipulation and tissue reaction to suture material on the formation of esophageal strictures is difficult to determine. In a limited number of animals, we have shown that the tendency for stricture formation varies with different suture materials. A two-layer anastomosis was accomplished in puppies after resection of 3 cm of esophagus. The following sutures were used: silk, cotton, Dacron, chromic catgut, and wire. During a follow-up period of three months, strictures developed in two of four animals sutured with chronic catgut and none with Dacron or wire. Newer suture materials including a braided polyester fiber, Tefdac,† are currently being tried in our laboratory.

Infection and/or breakdown of the anastomosis associated with the development of an extrapleural esophagocutaneous fistula occurred in six patients, three of whom subsequently developed severe strictures. In each instance the esophageal leak closed spontaneously, and there were no fatalities as a result of this complication.

Because of the high mortality associated with recurrent aspiration pneumonia in the presence of a very tight or persistent stricture a segmental re-resection of the esophagus was done in five patients. There were no deaths in this group, and a much more satisfactory anastomosis could be accomplished particularly in the infants in whom the original anastomosis was done under marked degrees of tension.

† Manufactured by J. A. Deknatel and Sons, Inc.

Summary

Fifty-one of 61 patients admitted to the Columbus Children's Hospital for esophageal atresia have been subjected to a primary single-stage division of the fistula and end-to-end anastomosis of the esophagus. Forty-five of these patients survived and were discharged from the hospital. Twenty-three of the 45 survivors developed a symptomatic stricture at the site of anastomosis. These strictures developed in the first ten weeks following surgery in 21 of the infants and were always associated with dysphagia, chronic cough, and aspiration pneumonia. Five of these patients and two patients with dysfunctional esophageal disease who did not have strictures demonstrable at autopsy have subsequently died of aspiration pneumonia.

The major factors which contribute to the formation of strictures appear to be the tension on the suture line, type of suture material, and leakage at the suture line. Of these, the amount of tension appeared to be the most important. Because of this 22% mortality from aspiration pneumonia in patients who developed strictures, the more liberal use of routine postoperative dilatations and occasional reoperation and resection of very tight or persistent strictures is recommended.

Loyd R. Schultz, MD, Department of Surgery, Ohio State University College of Medicine, Columbus, Ohio.

REFERENCES

1. Sulamaa, M.; Gripenberg, L.; and Ahvenainen, E. K.: Prognosis and Treatment of Congenital Atresia of the Esophagus, Acta Chir Scand 102: 141, 1951.

2. Haight, C., and Towsley, H. A.: Congenital Atresia of the Esophagus With Tracheoesophageal Fistula: Extrapleural Ligation of Fistula and End-

to-End Anastomosis of the Esophageal Segments, Surg Gynec Obstet 76:672, 1943.

3. Minton, J. P., and Clatworthy, H. W., Jr.: Congenital Esophageal Atresia: A Report of Improved Survival of Infants Through Prompt Recognition and Surgical Correction, Ohio Med J 58: 1262, 1962.

4. Gross, R. E.: The Surgery of Infancy and Childhood, Philadelphia: W. B. Saunders Company, 1953, chap 6, p 99.

5. Swenson, O.: Pediatric Surgery, New York: Appleton-Century-Crofts, Inc., 1958, p 172.

6. Holinger, P. H.: Clinical Aspects of Congenital Anomalies of the Larynx, Trachea, Bronchi and Oesophagus, J Laryng 75:1, 1961.

7. Morrison, L.: Experience With Dilatation of the Esophagus Following Surgery for Esophageal Atresia, Ann Otol 68:580, 1959.

8. Haight, C.: Some Observations on Esophageal Atresias With Tracheoesophageal Fistulas of Congenital Origin, J Thorac Surg 34:141, 1957.

9. Haas, L., and Sturridge, M. F.: Congenital Tracheo-Oesophageal Fistula, Proc Roy Soc Med 54:329, 1961.

10. Gross, R. E., and Scott, H. W.: Correction of Esophageal Atresia With Tracheo-Esophageal Fistula by Closure of Fistula and Oblique Anastomosis of Esophageal Segments, Surg Gynec Obstet 82:518, 1946.

11. Sanderud, A.: Treatment of Oesophageal Atresia: A Modification in Technique, Acta Chir Scand 119:339, 1960.

DISCUSSION

DR. CAMERON HAIGHT, Ann Arbor, Mich: I appreciate very much being asked to discuss the paper of Dr. Schultz and Dr. Clatworthy because they have presented a problem which needs considerably more clarification. They have emphasized one of the important complications in the postoperative management of infants with esophageal atresia and it is one which has been glossed over a bit too lightly in the literature.

Several of the deaths in our earlier cases were the result of esophageal stricture. Not only may the deaths be due to aspiration pneumonitis, but they may occur very quickly, in a patient who is apparently doing well, because of sudden distention of the esophagus proximal to the stricture with secondary pressure against the rather soft posterior wall of the trachea. Two of our earlier cases died very suddenly and within a matter of only a few minutes, apparently as a result of respiratory obstruction from this cause.

Our attitude regarding esophageal strictures has changed considerably within the past few years. Formerly we dilated the esophagus only if a stricture was causing symptoms. More recently we have dilated the esophagus of almost all of the infants after primary repair of esophageal atresia, merely to prevent the development of true strictures subsequent to their discharge from the hospital. It is recognized that in all the patients the area of the anastomosis is narrow in the immediate postoperative course.

The method which I use differs somewhat from that employed by Drs. Schultz and Clatworthy. It consists of the standard filiform and followers such as are used for urethral dilatation. It is done without benefit of fluoroscopic control, and as yet we have seen no perforation as a result of this method.

The plan that is employed is to test the size of the anastomosis approximately two to three weeks after operation by the passage of small catheters of size No. 8 F, 10 F, and 12 F. This allows an estimation of the caliber of the lumen at the anastomosis, and unless even larger size catheters can be readily passed, dilatations are then started with a filiform and followers. The dilatations are begun at an interval of two or three days and they are repeated at gradually increasing intervals. Ordinarily the sizes of the dilators that are used are advanced one size at each sitting so that the increase in the caliber of the stricture is brought about gently and gradually. Otherwise if one dilates a stricture too abruptly it is readily possible to cause a tear which will result in a stricture of even tighter caliber. After discharge of the patients from the hospital they return on an outpatient basis until the size of the follower has been increased gradually to No. 28 F. They then return at infrequent intervals merely to be certain that the lumen has not contracted in the meanwhile. The dilatations are done without the use of fluoroscopy and in this manner it is often possible to gain an estimation of the caliber of the esophagus without the need to subject the infants to fluoroscopy or roentgenograms.

DR. LOYD R. SCHULTZ, Columbus, Ohio: We, too, have seen sudden deaths with strictures. In one instance, a child was seen in the clinic and returned four hours later, dead on arrival, with the sudden death related to the stricture, probably from aspiration.

We have not had perforations with our dilations using the Tucker Dilators or the urethral sounds. We have, however, had two perforations in the older children while they were undergoing dilatation with an esophagoscope.

Cancer Chemotherapy by Arterial Infusion

JERREL W. BENSON, MD; CLIFFORD L. KIEHN, MD; AND WILLIAM D. HOLDEN, MD, CLEVELAND

The most disquieting feature common to all forms of effective cancer therapy is that they are injurious to the patient. The significance of this factor diminishes as the probability of cure increases with respect to a specific therapeutic method. A valid measurement of the balance between these two opposing factors continues to be particularly elusive in the field of cancer chemotherapy. A comprehensive search for agents with a relatively specific action against cancer during the last decade has met with limited success. Perhaps because of this fact, increasing interest has developed in techniques for improved utilization of agents with limited specificity of action and partial effectiveness against cancer. Most of these methods are designed to enhance tumoricidal effects while still controlling the level of host toxicity by establishing a differential in the dose of the drug between tumor and patient which favors the patient. Perfusion and infusion methods currently in use are so designed to attain this end. The exploratory development of these methods has resulted in the evolution of two important concepts in chemotherapy: (1) the in vivo titration of paired agents consisting of a cytostatic compound and its natural metabolic antagonist, and (2) the fact that rate and route of administration of various drugs may be critical determinants of their biologic effects to a degree not previously appreciated. The simultaneous use of amethopterin (methotrexate) and folinic acid, first reported by Sullivan and associates,[1] is the best known example of increased drug versatility based on the first concept. The unique quality of 5-fluorouracil to produce treacherous systemic toxicity when given by rapid intravenous injection is most difficult to reconcile with its relatively innocuous systemic effects when given by slow continuous infusion. This is the currently best known example of the second concept.

The direct intra-arterial injection of drugs for the treatment of cancer was first reported independently by Klopp [2] and Bierman [3] in 1950. Sullivan et al [1] reported the intermittent use of a metabolic antagonist to counteract the systemic toxicity of a continuously administered drug nine years later. The first series of patients treated with some measure of success by this method was described in this report in 1959. The methodology of arterial infusion has subsequently captivated the interest of an increasing number of investigators. Tarr [4] reported the first small series of patients treated with protracted intra-arterial administration of 5-fluorouracil in November, 1961, after the observations of Sullivan et al [5] that this and other pyrimidine analogues elicited variable tolerance patterns when administered at slow rates for prolonged intervals.

We began using methotrexate * and folinic acid in combination during 1960 in an attempt to reproduce Sullivan's results. In a preliminary report [6] our initial experiences with this type of chemotherapy for tumors of the head and neck were briefly described. This report is a summation of our collective experiences during the last 2½ years accumulated from patients treated with chemotherapeutic agents for a variety of lesions by

Presented at the 20th Annual Meeting of the Central Surgical Association, Chicago, Feb 21-23, 1963.

From the Departments of Surgery, Western Reserve University School of Medicine, University Hospitals, and Highland View Hospital.

Supported in part by a grant from the American Cancer Society, Cleveland Chapter.

* Methotrexate and leucovorin were obtained from Dr. J. M. Ruegsegger, Lederle Laboratories Division of American Cyanamid Company.

arterial infusion at University Hospitals of Cleveland and the Highland View Unit of Cuyahoga County Hospital. Since the greater number of patients to be reported upon were treated in Highland View Hospital, factors of selection imposed by circumstances bear special emphasis in the interpretation of results to be presented. Standard criteria for admission of a patient with cancer to this hospital has been a life expectancy of approximately one month and medical requirements which exceed those provided by a nursing home. The only criterion of patient selection within the County Hospital was that the patient to be treated must exhibit at least one index lesion with unicentric blood supply accessible to catheterization. As may be concluded from the above description of circumstances, the majority of patients were clearly beyond hope of benefit from conventional therapy. Extended survival was therefore not a primary therapeutic objective for the majority of patients. Most patients had carcinomas of the oropharynx or neck which had necessitated either tracheotomy, feeding tube, or both. A proportionately smaller group of patients with extensive pelvic metastatic disease which had become refractory to conventional methods of palliation was also treated with arterial chemotherapy. After the relative safety of methods and expected frequency of tumor response had been determined from this cumulative experience, a more selective group of patients was infused prior to definitive resection of their tumors at University Hospitals.

Observations based on 121 arterial catheterizations in 74 patients who received 125 courses of infusion chemotherapy provide the background for this report.

Technical Aspects of Protracted Arterial Infusion Chemotherapy

Exacting technical standards are no less critical in assessing the merits of regional chemotherapy than technical consistency is to the evaluation of an operative method for tumor removal. Lack of tumor response may occur because the infused drug is not effective. This becomes a valid conclusion only when there is reasonable certainty that drug has been delivered adequately to the tumor. If degree of tumor response is related proportionally to sustained drug concentration within its total fluid content, then a number of variables which collectively determine the general circulatory status of the infused field might be manipulated to the disadvantage of the tumor. As will be subsequently described, the existing vasculature of areas to be infused has been altered by various technical means. The dispersal patterns of dyes (5% fluorescein, 1% methylene blue, 2% lissamine green) resulting when they were arterially infused have been noted visually under changing conditions. These observations are presented because they appear to lend special significance to minor variations in method of chemotherapy. In addition, an attempt has been made to standardize the methodology of arterial infusion with respect to equipment, techniques, and precautionary routines. The principle objective has been to identify and control various factors which may limit the efficiency, safety, and reliability of infusion systems designed for continuous drug transport to arterial systems. Detailed technical aspects of the methods we employ will be described in relation to anatomical regions. Certain observations and related concepts which appear to be pertinent to all anatomical areas will first be presented.

Local Factors Which Modify Delivery and Distribution Via Arterial Systems.—

1. Collateral Blood Supply: If the major collateral vessels other than the artery receiving the infusate are ligated, a more uniform distribution of infused dye is obtained, particularly in lesions which encroach upon the midline of the body, where a double blood supply prevails. Ligation of contralateral arteries results in immediate crossover of circulation from the side infused. The reciprocal situation prevails when a ligated artery is infused distal to the ligature. Although one might suppose this to be a highly efficient mechanism for tumor infusion, this result was not obtained. The contralateral

arterial system perfuses the major portion of the field previously supplied by the ligated vessel. The distribution of the infusate is restricted to a small area which subsequently undergoes changes suggestive of ischemic necrosis. Faster rates of infusion eventually result in local edema.

2. The Size of the Lesion: It has been observed by other investigators[7,8] that as certain tumors undergo progressive enlargement, the distribution of blood flow changes in favor of the more actively growing periphery. The central mass of such tumors is frequently devoid of direct circulatory contact with the host. Our observations with respect to distribution of injected dyes in patients with multiple metastatic surface nodules are consistent with these reports. The observed effects of infusion chemotherapy upon such nodules are usually inversely proportional to their size and most evident at their periphery.

3. Associated Inflammation: It has been observed that edema associated with tissue breakdown and regional inflammation results in an irregular distribution of injected dyes. In addition, the time required for their disappearance after injection is markedly prolonged. When infusion chemotherapy results in accelerated tissue necrosis with marked regional edema, increasingly large amounts of dye must be injected to achieve the same degree of color change. It is assumed that under such circumstances the infused drug is not being delivered with desired efficiency. When such infusions are discontinued for a few days to allow regression of inflammatory changes, intra-arterial dye injection carried out preliminary to reinfusion usually demonstrates a more satisfactory distribution of infusate, unless vessels have become thrombosed.

4. Thrombosis of Vessels: Extensive thrombosis of arterial systems being infused has occurred in our experience. It is desirable to do angiography when this is suspected, for continued infusion of occluded vessels may result in emboli.

5. Previous Irradiation: Previously irradiated large tumor masses have not regressed to a degree comparable to nonirradiated tumors of similar size and type. Ulcerating lesions which have escaped from radiotherapy control often show an accelerated inflammatory response to regional chemotherapy, attended by marginal necrosis. The circulatory status of the previously irradiated tumor field is certainly altered. The disappearance time of injected dye is usually prolonged. The distribution of dyes is irregular and patchy, and the incidence of previous occlusion of major arterial branches is higher in such patients. Arterial elasticity and lumen size are diminished, and the tendency toward complete occlusion secondary to the presence of indwelling catheters is greater. A reduction in local tissue resistance to trauma incidental to direct catheter insertion is clearly evident. Edema is more easily elicited by infusion effects in previously irradiated fields. Some investigators[9] describe a high correlation of negative infusion responses with antecedent radiotherapy when tumors were infused with 5-fluorouracil. Reports of other investigators[10-12] differ with respect to results of methotrexate infusion administered to previously irradiated lesions. Our experiences in this regard suggest that although local complications may be of greater incidence in irradiated patients, some favorable responses to regional chemotherapy can be obtained in this group. It is suspected that extensive fibrosis, residual inflammation, and related changes in the circulatory status of the field are important factors in determining response rate to infusion among these patients.

6. Incidental Ligation of Veins Draining the Infused Field: Although one might presume that venous ligation could enhance regional chemotherapy through the mechanism of retarded drug escape, our observations suggest that this is not a prudent measure. Ligation of superficial veins draining tumor areas was attempted as a possible means of potentiating drug effects in a few patients. The apparent results were an increased tendency toward edema and inflammation which was slow to subside, more irregular distribution of arterially injected dyes in the area,

plus more pronounced inflammatory changes in normal tissues without evidence of increased tumor destruction. We therefore do not believe this approach has merit.

7. The Importance of Catheter Size and Bore: For infusate volumes not to exceed 2,000 ml in 24 hours while being impelled by a mechanical pump system, very small bore catheters (0.015-0.02 inches) afford greater reliability and potential for reuse. Since resistance is inversely proportional to bore size, the reflux of blood with variations in blood pressure is less, and the incidence of clot occlusion at the tip is reduced. Furthermore, the increased velocity of infusate through small bore catheters tends to protect their patency when extremely low volumes of infusate are being delivered. Independently of these factors, a more important reason for using catheters of minimum size appears to be related to changes which occur within the arterial lumen after they are inserted (Fig 1). A number of arterial specimens examined at autopsy in which polyethylene catheters had been present for periods of four days to one year showed that these catheters had become completely excluded from the blood stream by a circumferential sheath of fibrin thrombus. Through this mechanism, the catheter had become fixed to the arterial wall at all points within the lumen. Whether this intra-arterial thrombus should be regarded as an expected consequence of all intra-arterial catheter insertions cannot be stated until more specimens are examined. If it occurs only occasionally, however, this still constitutes a significant reason for minimizing catheter size whenever possible. This is particularly true on those occasions when the subject is elderly, with a probability of already existing partial atheromatous occlusion of the vessel which will retain the catheter.

Types of catheters which have been found encased in fibrin within human arterial specimens are polyethylene and polyvinyl. Silastic tubing † is capable of eliciting a similar response in the rabbit aorta.[13] Whether silicon offers a means of preventing these deposits in human arteries is currently being investigated. The use of Silastic catheters for infusion purposes in the common and external carotid arteries of six patients has not been attended by complications. Excessive pliability of this material and its affinity for foreign particulate matter are two disadvantages to its use for arterial catheters.

† Made available through the courtesy of Dow Corning Center for Aid to Medical Research, Midland, Mich.

Fig 1.—Aortic specimen and thrombus. *A*, fibrin thrombus completely encircling polyethylene catheter within the aortic lumen; *B*, photomicrograph of cross-section showing fibrin tunnel occupied by catheter which was firmly attached to intima of artery.

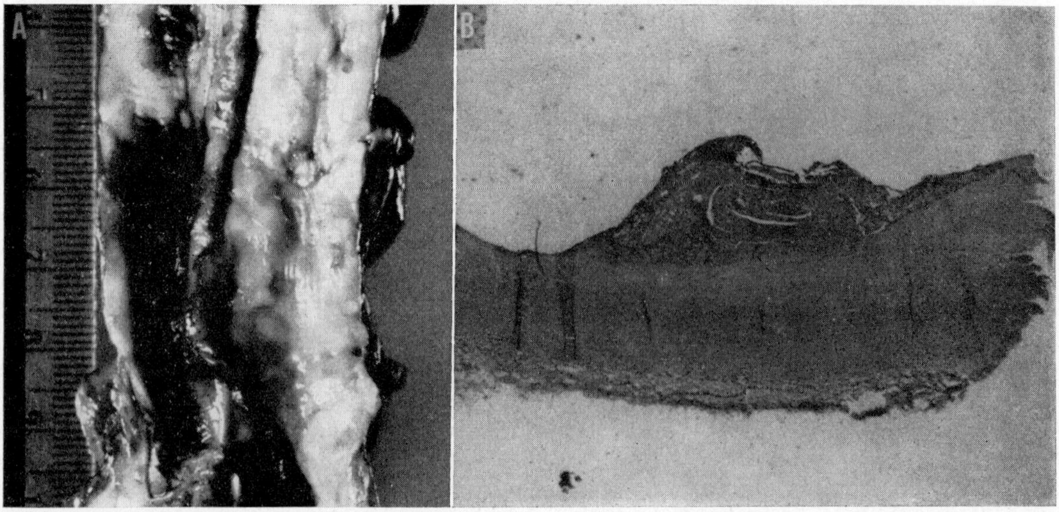

The factors which have been described above are generally pertinent to the application of regional infusion chemotherapy without special regard to site of tumor. Other technical considerations which are related specifically to body regions will now be discussed.

Technique of Infusing Tumors of the Head and Neck.—The methods which have been employed have not been essentially different from those previously described by other investigators.[10,11] The selection of arteries for catheter insertion must be based on the distribution of disease and its relationship to the dominant sources of blood flow in the individual patient. Such features are not uniform among patients with primary tumors in the same anatomical location and must be evaluated by specific measures. The majority of lesions in the head and neck are accessible to infusion via the external carotid artery by retrograde insertion of the catheter through the superficial temporal artery under local anesthesia. Among the 45 patients who received external carotid artery infusions in our series, the catheter was placed by this method in 35. We began using this approach after early experiences with the direct technique employed below the mandible yielded a high wound complication rate in patients with advanced disease. Failures with the superficial temporal approach are to be expected when the artery has been obliterated by radiotherapy, tumor encroachment, or atheromatous changes. As others observe,[14] no single maneuver is reliable in achieving success in all patients, but this approach has been 95% effective in our hands. We use a tapered polyvinyl catheter which conforms at body temperature to the contours of the artery. Failure on the first attempt can usually be attributed to one of several factors: (1) excessive tortuosity of the vessel which will yield to further dissection; (2) arteriospasm which will yield to 2% procaine through the catheter; (3) disruption of the intima due to excessive force which can be circumvented on occasions by proximal re-entry. Altering the position of the head is sometimes helpful. When an obstruction is met within or below the parotid gland (beyond the internal maxillary branch), persistent attempts to advance the catheter are not advisable. This often means that partial thrombotic occlusion has occurred at a level which poses a threat to the internal carotid system if promulgation of a thrombus is encouraged by the presence of a catheter. In such instances, direct submandibular exposure of the external carotid artery is performed if the neck structures are not severely deranged by tumor or the effects of previous radiotherapy. If one or both of the latter circumstances prevail, the common carotid artery can be approached well below the area of disease and a fine bore catheter inserted through its medial wall for a maximum distance of 5 mm. Dominant flow from such catheters, if optimally placed, is into the external carotid system. Although this approach is technically feasible, extreme caution is advised with respect to drug dose, the necessity for continuous infusion of such catheters with heparinized solution, and altered drug distribution which may occur with changes in neck position. Attempts to advance catheters from this site into the external carotid artery via the common carotid are particularly ill advised because of instability of the catheter tip and risk of emboli. In certain patients who demonstrate no palpable pulsations in the face on the involved side, the external carotid artery may be ligated proximally and the catheter for infusion may be inserted in the contralateral artery. This alternative approach has been used effectively in treating some lesions in the oropharynx. Where such disease has also encroached upon the larynx, the thyrocervical trunk on the involved side has been ligated in addition to the external carotid artery.

Technique for Direct Catheter Insertion and Fixation: Although we have tried a variety of methods, including those described by Sullivan[10] and associates, we prefer techniques of maximum simplicity. No one method is universally acceptable for all arteries, but the following alternative methods are useful and reliable.

1. Needle insertion is accomplished with the catheter inside the needle. The only significant disadvantage in this method is that the resulting defect in the arterial wall is larger than necessary to accommodate the catheter.

2. A Rochester type needle (16 G) may be inserted into the artery and the catheter (PE-20) passed through the plastic sheath after the needle is withdrawn. This technique allows more flexible direction of catheters when they must be inserted under conditions of limited wound exposure. The Rochester needle sheath is subsequently withdrawn from the artery, leaving the catheter in place.

3. A curved round needle which is swaged on to a length of polyethylene tubing may be passed in and out of the arterial lumen after which the needle is amputated and the catheter tip positioned within the artery. This method, which was devised by Ulm, appears to be more satisfactory in our experience if both needle and tubing are smaller in diameter than was originally described.[10] This item ‡ has been modified to our specifications and is quite useful when arteries cannot be ideally exposed.

4. A miniature arteriotomy may be performed with a No. 11 Bard-Parker blade which permits catheter introduction without the necessity for arresting blood flow through the artery. When the artery is suspended by traction on a single mastoid drain, the resultant compression of the arterial wall prevents bleeding while a single suture is placed adjacent to the catheter.

The method of catheter fixation at the arterial wall which we utilize differs significantly from that which has been described by Sullivan et al.[10] The "tight-bite" ligature about the catheter which he proposes is difficult to apply with controlled degrees of lumen constriction. In addition, the placement of sutures within the lumen of the artery entails considerable manipulation and distortion of the arterial wall which we believe should be avoided. A 2 mm collar of Silastic tubing can be placed over the catheter as it emerges from the artery (Fig 2). This affords security through friction when a ligature of average tension is applied and subsequently sutured to the arterial wall. The Silastic collar need not be circumferentially intact and may be slit longitudinally to expedite placement. This is the only positioning suture required with our technique. The incidence of retrograde leaking of infusate along the catheter tract has been negligible in our experience. This has been true despite interrupted use of the same catheters for infusion over protracted periods. We suspect the frequency of this complication is related inversely to the length of catheter within the artery and directly to the amount of trauma to the vessel which accompanies catheter placement. The fibrin thrombus (Fig 1) which is found to encircle these catheters apparently undergoes little organization in the absence of trauma or suture material. Retrograde leaking has been seen least frequently when a small branch of the major artery is chosen for catheter introduction.

Maintenance and Final Disposition of Catheters: Catheters which are not greater

Fig 2.—Method of catheter fixation to arterial wall. Ligature tied with moderate tension over Silastic collar secures catheter with single suture to outer wall of artery.

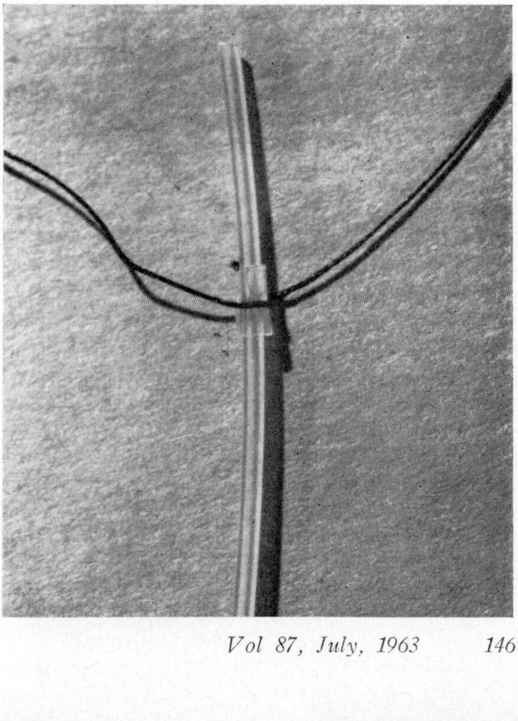

‡ Courtesy of Mr. R. J. Semple, Ethicon, Inc.

than 0.020 inches inside diameter will remain patent for long intervals of disuse if care is taken to prevent blood reflux and the outlet is kept tightly closed. When infusions are terminated, such catheters are filled once with heparin, clamped securely, and the ends are sealed with heat distal to the clamp. If early resumption of the infusion is contemplated, the catheter is not amputated, but the distal end is kept closed with a three-way plastic stopcock which has a self-sealing rubber stopper. Heparin is introduced by needle puncture through this stopper at 48-hour intervals. When such catheters are positioned in the common or internal carotid arteries, heparinized infusions are continued until the catheters are withdrawn, with finger compression being the only hemostatic mechanism which has been required.

The tapered polyvinyl catheters (Baxter Cut-Down pediatric size) which are used in the superficial temporal artery approach will usually retain patency for four days or more after one injection of heparin. This property is probably related to a very small distal orifice in combination with a proximal reservoir of increasing diameter and capacity. Hemolyzed blood is aspirated each time heparin is replenished. Such catheters are easily extracted without need for special precautions against bleeding.

Techniques for Outlining the Therapeutic Field: Direct Visualization With Dyes injected Arterially. Five per cent fluorescein is quite effective for use without the refinement of ultraviolet fluorescence since it stains tissues visibly in ordinary light. From 1 to 10 ml is injected slowly as may be required to determine the position of the catheter. For positioning of catheters introduced through the superficial temporal artery, where complete external carotid artery infusion is desired, staining of the tongue without staining of the eye is the objective. We prefer to use methylene blue dye, 1%, however, since it will fade instantaneously from the tissues when used in 2 to 3 ml amounts. Serial observations may be accomplished repeatedly in the same area without delay. We have found this technique particularly suitable for photography. Edema, the result of excessive use of either of these dyes, has been seen to linger in the face for 24 hours. This has been observed only in patients who received antecedent radiotherapy and only after amounts greater than 10 ml were used. When dyes are to be used in the retrograde placement of catheters in any artery, injection is best done before the catheter is fully advanced. Initial flooding of the entire field from an advanced position obscures the zonal pattern of individual branch filling which is the best guide to accurate final placement.

Angiography. Fifty per cent sodium diatrizoate (Hypaque) solution is employed to outline major arterial patterns when there is reason to suspect unusual distortions by tumor or occlusion of one or more major branches. When it is anticipated that angiography will be desired, a catheter of larger bore than PE-20 is desirable, since the necessary rate of injection cannot usually be achieved through tubing with this diameter. Frequently, a percutaneous carotid arterio-

Fig 3.—Infusion assembly. Consists of two disposable plastic units with simple, inexpensive rotary pump.

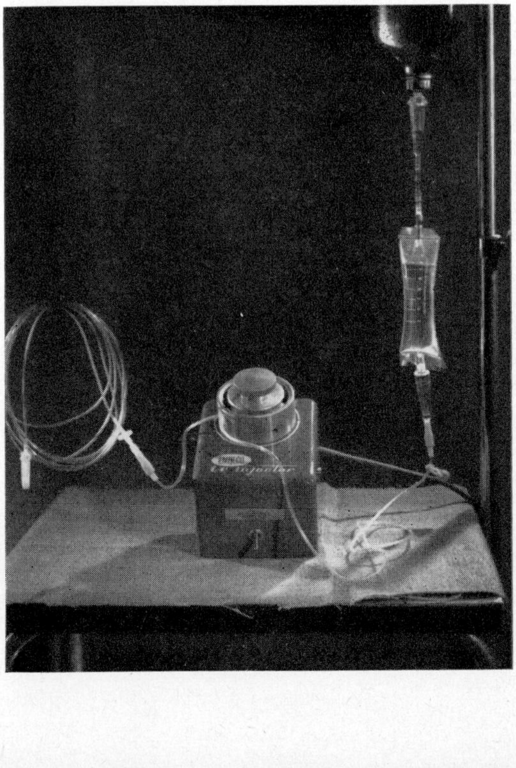

gram will be the most expedient means of outlining the vascular tree.

Design and Maintenance of Infusion Assembly: The component parts of a very reliable and relatively inexpensive infusion assembly are pictured in Fig 3. Certain factors of importance pertain to each unit of the system.

The Volume and Rate of Infusate to be Administered. It has been found that a minimum volume and rate of fluid (approximately 1,000 ml per 24 hours) has certain advantages. All infusates other than blood tend to produce varying degrees of arteriospasm, thereby diminishing the capacity of the vascular bed being infused. Certain patients who experience pain or develop excessive edema with arterial infusions are usually relieved when the rate of infusion is reduced. Since the drug effects upon tumor tissue are not known to be otherwise related to volume of infusate used, the smallest amount of fluid which is consistent with maintaining the system in continuous operation would seem desirable. Heparin in the amount of 20 mg (2,000 units) is added to each liter of fluid.

The Infusate Reservoir. A single liter bottle appears sufficient despite the fact that multiple bottles connected in series have been advocated as a means of preventing air embolism.[10] This problem is circumvented in the system described by the use of a 100 cc capacity plastic bag beneath the bottle which requires two hours to empty at the rate suggested. Under circumstances where reasonable attention to the system by the nursing staff cannot be guaranteed, a more definite safeguard may be introduced. If a short segment of one-quarter inch Penrose drain tubing is inserted at any point in the system between the reservoir and the pump, this tubing will collapse with minimal vacuum effect when the fluid is expended. This device is illustrated in Fig 4. A deformed paper clip applied in the manner shown ensures contact of the opposing walls of the drain.

Choice of Pumps. Experience has been gained with the performance characteristics of a number of commercially available pumps, including the Bowman, Sigmamotor, Barron, and I-V Injector models. All models tested were adequate for the purpose; however, the I-V Injector and Barron models are the least expensive. Greater variability in rate control is the major advantage offered by the more expensive models. The I-V Injector § model which is illustrated is priced under $100 and performs reliably at a fixed rate which will deliver 1,000 cc per 24 hours. Special tubing is not required, and it offers the advantage of being able to propel fluid through standard intravenous plastic tubing of the disposable type. Some flexibility in rate is

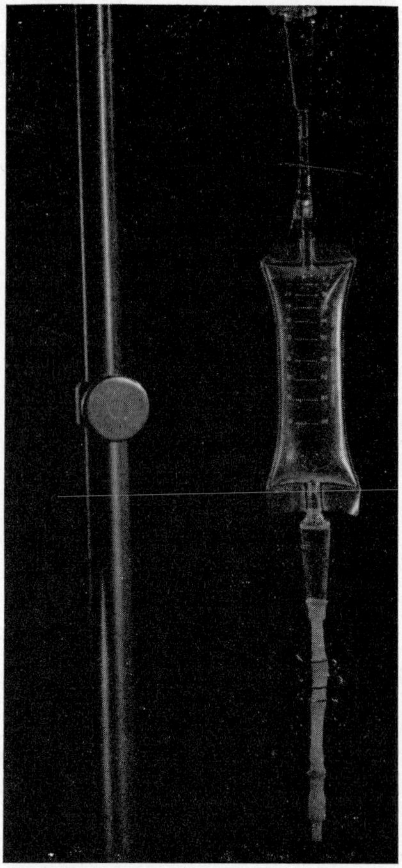

Fig 4.—Air-trap tube. Penrose drain section of infusion line collapses to prevent air embolism when fluid in reservoir is expended. Bent paper clip insures contact of opposing walls in absence of liquid flow by gravity.

§ I-V Injector pump obtained from Electro-Mechanical Development Co., Houston, Texas.

achieved by using tubing of varying diameters. All pumps have limitations with respect to their performance against excessive resistance in that they will allow partial regurgitation of fluid at one or more points in the cycle. When this occurs noticeably, occlusion of the catheter by blood clot should be suspected.

If simultaneous radiotherapy is to be given in conjunction with infusion therapy, the use of electromechanical pumps is cumbersome. Prolonged confinement in the hospital room also becomes intolerable to certain patients who are being infused. To circumvent these problems, a completely portable system has been devised by one of us (J.W.B.) which consists of a plastic bag (plasma type) as the infusate reservoir, sealed within a semirigid (polyethylene) container, which is in turn pressurized with carbon dioxide. The power source is a small refillable carbon dioxide cylinder equipped with an adjustable regulating valve which permits rate control without constant supervision. A one-way valve in the fluid line prevents retrograde flow in the event of pressure loss or change. The fluid reservoir is refilled every 24 hours by gravity flow after gas is allowed to escape. Rate of infusion may be otherwise supervised by weighing the container at intervals and by regulating the manual control proximal to the drip chamber. This apparatus (Fig 5) may be used quite safely by any patient who can be trusted to refrain from tampering with the controls.

Tubing Between Pump and Patient. The length of tubing interposed between the pump and the patient can be arbitrarily extended to suit the patient's convenience until the relationship between distance and resistance to fluid flow becomes dominant. In our experience, 10 ft of tubing length allows the patient moderate freedom but does not seriously compromise uniformity of rate of flow. Tubing which is too easily distensible yields the widest rate fluctuations with increasing length, changes in patient position, and blood pressure. This length of tubing may be created by joining several

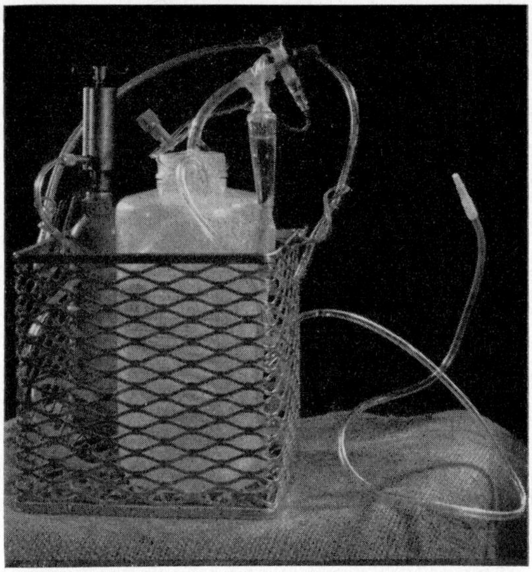

Fig 5.—Portable infusion assembly. CO_2 pressure, controlled by regulating valve, compresses plastic bag within polyethylene bottle to propel infusate. System operates for 24 hours without need for special attention.

extension tubes of the type used for anesthesia or may be fashioned from stock polyethylene or polyvinyl tubing. The item || depicted in Fig 3 is a single unit with Luer adapters constructed for this specific purpose.

Techniques for Infusing the Blood Supply to the Pelvis and Lower Extremities.—The same technical principles have been utilized for infusion chemotherapy in these areas as have been described for treatment of disease in the head and neck region. Generally, the choice of method has been based on whether there is need for a laparotomy other than for placement of infusion catheters.

Where metastatic disease to be treated is largely confined to the central pelvic region and laparotomy is being performed for other reasons, the internal iliac artery on the most involved side is catheterized while the contralateral internal iliac artery is ligated at its origin. This permits delivery of infusate through one catheter system to pelvic disease not supplied by the external iliac arteries. The catheter is usually inserted through the

|| Courtesy of Pharmaseal Laboratories, Glendale, Calif.

lumen of a needle. Frequent ligation of collateral arteries has been resorted to in the treatment of pelvic disease. For example, when the principal area of involvement is about the rectum in a female patient, both ovarian arteries and the superior hemorrhoidal plus one internal iliac artery are ligated. A proximal colostomy is usually established in such patients prior to infusion.

In patients for whom laparotomy seems unjustified because of general condition or stage of disease, pelvic infusions may be accomplished through catheters inserted by simpler means. Percutaneous placement of catheters via the femoral artery in a retrograde direction is easily accomplished. This is done by insertion of a needle into the artery at the level of the inguinal ligament. A length of catheter estimated to reach a point below the patient's umbilicus is advanced. Position of the catheter tip is checked by angiography in addition to the injection of 1% methylene blue dye. The moderate irritation of the dye elicits sufficient pain to permit the perceptive patient to describe the location of discomfort as to whether it is in the pelvis or one or both of the extremities. The reason why catheters inserted in this manner deliver the bulk of the infusate to the pelvic structures is not entirely clear. Examination of autopsy material has revealed that such catheters are usually positioned along the anterior surface of the aortic wall. The proximity of the outflow tip to the bifurcation apparently accounts for bifid flow which distributes itself predominantly along the medial walls of the iliac arteries. Several trials may be necessary in order to achieve the desired catheter position. Rotation of the catheter will usually alter its position effectively, unless the tip is quite high above the bifurcation.

If the above approach does not prove technically satisfactory, bilateral retrograde femoral catheters may be placed with the tips short of the aortic bifurcation. The superior gluteal branch of the internal iliac artery can also be exposed under local anesthetic as it emerges posteriorly near the iliac spine. Retrograde insertion of catheters is feasible from this location; however, the susceptibility of debilitated patients to pressure ulceration in this area is a disadvantage. The transfemoral single catheter approach to bilateral pelvic infusion has been used principally for 5-fluorouracil administration when the catheters are allowed to remain in situ for repeated use. Some patients have remained out of the hospital with these catheters in place for several weeks, and no attendant complications have yet resulted.

Technique for Infusing the Extremities and Other Areas.—Lesions of the shoulder may be infused via catheters placed through a branch of the axillary artery beneath the clavicle. Tumors of the elbow, forearm, or hand are infused by inserting a catheter into the brachial artery above the elbow through a needle.

Neoplasms of the lower limb have been infused via catheters placed in the femoral artery below the inguinal ligament. It is not deemed advisable to place catheters within major arteries below this level, unless a small branch is available for sacrifice as the recipient artery.

The technical accessibility of other regions for the application of regional chemotherapy is being explored, and infusions have been accomplished via the celiac axis or its branches, including the hepatic artery. Infusion of breast lesions via the axillary artery has been tried. Our experience with these approaches is insufficient at the present time to justify specific comment.

Selection of Patients for Arterial Infusion Chemotherapy

A retrospective examination of our experiences from the standpoint of frequency of complications as compared with incidence of beneficial responses prompts us to suggest the following categories of patients which appear to be most favorable:

1. Patients with operable squamous cell carcinoma of the oropharynx in whom the probability of regional lymph node involvement is high.

2. Patients with more advanced, but regionally confined neoplasms of the oropharynx and neck

which have not been previously irradiated or otherwise treated.

3. Patients with persistent or recurrent localized disease who have previously undergone definitive surgical resections and are still capable of independent ambulation although hospitalized for their disease.

Current belief is that all patients in category 1 should have complete surgical removal of the lesion without modifying conventional resection technique shortly after infusion is completed. Resection should be carried out soon after the signs of local inflammation and tissue reaction have subsided within the treated field, providing the bone marrow elements reflected by blood cell and platelet counts are within normal range. It appears that certain patients selected from category 2, whose lesions have extended only recently beyond the resectable stage, may respond to infusion sufficiently to justify surgical resection with hope of cure.

Among those patients who have far advanced disease which has already been subjected to conventional measures of palliation, including radiotherapy, those who may be expected to achieve significant benefit from regional infusion chemotherapy are classified as follows:

1. Patients with advanced inoperable, but regionally confined, oral cancer not involving the larynx.
2. Patients with squamous cell carcinoma of the middle face, which may or may not involve the retro-orbital tissues and adjacent skull.
3. Patients with locally extensive carcinoma of the distal colon and rectum.
4. Patients with progressive obstructive uropathy owing to regionally confined pelvic metastases.
5. Patients with intractable pain due to metastatic cancer in the head or neck, lumbar spine, pelvis, or lower extremities.

Patients for whom palliative regional infusions have produced a high complication rate in our experience are classified as follows:

1. Dehydrated, malnourished patients who have deeply ulcerating oral cancer persisting after radical removal followed by radiotherapy.
2. Preterminal cancer patients with one or more of the following features in their history:
   - A. The maximum tolerated dose of pelvic irradiation.
   - B. One or more courses of systemic chemotherapy previously.
   - C. Chronic renal disease.
   - D. Liver metastases.
   - E. Pronounced anemia with cachexia.

The type of patient referred to in category 1 usually has anatomical derangements within the area of the lesion related to previous therapy and advancing disease which preclude the use of reliable technical approaches to infusion therapy. There is also an associated high incidence of complications such as local hemorrhage, hemiplegia owing to thrombosis, tracheobronchitis, and pneumonia. The patients referred to in the second category appear highly susceptible to drug toxicity. There is often a tendency among these patients to present with delayed evidence of severe bone marrow depression.

Choice and Dose of Drugs.—All patients having squamous cell lesions which are presumably contained within the area infused are treated with 50 mg of methotrexate intra-arterially per 24 hours, accompanied by the intramuscular administration every 6 hours of 6 mg of folinic acid. This regimen is continued for 6 to 12 days, the exact duration being determined by the individual responses as reflected by serial blood counts and degree of local reaction. Patients with squamous cell carcinoma not completely contained within the area infused are treated similarly with not more than 5 mg of methotrexate daily without folinic acid being given concomitantly. Contiguous disease which is not being infused will occasionally respond in patients on the latter regimen although not to the same degree as that which is directly infused. This regimen is also used whenever the site of catheter insertion is the common or internal carotid artery.

Patients with tumors located in the extremities or pelvis are infused each 24 hours with 5-fluorouracil in the amount of 10 mg per kg of body weight for periods of 6 to 14 days. This drug is also used in a lesion which hase failed to respond to methotrexate infusion. The drug 5-fluorouracil appears to be more effective than methotrexate for infusion into vascular fields of larger size such as may exist if an attempt is made to treat widely disseminated pelvic disease. At least, more pronounced evidence of local tissue reaction may be achieved under such circumstances prior to the onset of systemic toxicity than is seen with methotrexate effects. For this reason, if poor risk patients are selected for adjunctive chemotherapy trials prior to attempted tumor resection, 5-fluorouracil is preferred. When given by slow infusion in the amount specified for periods not exceeding ten days to patients without previous radiotherapy or chemotherapy, no evidence of bone marrow depression has been detectable. Local tissue reaction within the treated field may be quite violent and may not reach its peak until 48 to 72 hours after the infusion is terminated. Here again, the time of onset and degree of reaction appear to be related inversely to the size of the infused field. These phenomena are presumably related to the level of sustained tissue concentration of the drug. For reasons which will be cited in the section under *Complications* the wisdom of using this drug in doses exceeding 10 mg/kg of body weight for regional infusion is questioned.

Among certain patients with squamous cell carcinoma which was initially susceptible to methotrexate infusion but showed a diminished response to the second course, retreatment of these patients with 5-fluorouracil infusions has produced another remission. The subsequent reuse of methotrexate in a few of these patients has yielded some evidence of a return of susceptibility to the drug. The possibility of altering tumor susceptibility to regional chemotherapy by the alternate use of two or more drugs is currently being explored.

When methotrexate infusions of four to five days' duration are followed immediately by 5-fluorouracil administered through the same system, a quite severe reaction of local tissues ensues within 48 hours which prohibits further treatment. The relationship of this phenomenon to the relative degree of tumor regression obtained has not been determined. The average duration of tumor regression seen after methotrexate infusion appears to be longer than that which follows 5-fluorouracil. No remission of longer than two months' duration has been seen with single infusion courses using the latter drug.

We are currently of the opinion that the simultaneous use of any two potentially toxic compounds for cancer therapy poses a more incalculable risk to the individual patient than the sequential use of the same agents.

Definition of Remission.—Patients are classified as having demonstrated a remission following infusion chemotherapy if one or more of the following criteria have been satisfied:

1. A reduction in the size of lesions by 50% sustained for a period of two months.
2. Restoration of functional capacity through changes such as:
   - A. Return of cranial nerve function.
   - B. Restoration of swallowing ability.
   - C. Closure of oral or perineal fistulas and sinus tracts.
   - D. Resolution of ulcerating draining lesions which are incapacitating.
   - E. Relief of obstructed ureters.
   - F. Control of leg edema due to pelvic disease.
3. Relief of intractable pain when evidenced by a sustained reduction of narcotic requirements by 50% or more.

Categories of Patients Treated by Infusion in this Series.—Group 1. Preoperative Adjunctive Infusions Followed by Tumor Resection: The infused resected group were 18 in number, 13 of whom had squamous cell carcinoma of the oropharynx.

Group 2. Palliative Infusion to Ambulatory Patients With Advanced Disease: This group of patients had been hospitalized with advanced residual disease late after surgery and x-ray therapy. Many had sequentially received conventional and supravoltage radiotherapy. Their disease was progressive, but not totally bed confining, and most could ambulate without assistance. Twenty-two of 25 patients in this group had lesions about the head and neck.

Group 3. Palliative Infusions to "Terminal" Patients With Cancer: Many of these were patients with an estimated life expectancy of three weeks or less. Most of these

TABLE 1.—*Current Results*

	Total Patients	Alive	With Tumor: Yes	With Tumor: ?	With Tumor: No	Remission	Death By: Ca	Death By: Therapy	Unknown or Lost
Infused resected	18	14	2		12	16	2	1 *	1
Advanced ambulatory	26	13	9	1	1	18	6	4	1
"Terminal"	30	3	3		0	21	15	9	3
Total	74	30	14	1	13	55	23	14	5

* Not due to infusion.

patients were with considerable disease outside the treated area.

Results

Group 1. *Infused Resected.*—Among 18 patients who were subjected to resection following infusions, one is lost to follow-up after four months, three are dead of their disease, and two alive with disease. The remaining 12 are clinically free of disease for follow-up periods ranging from 1 to 26 months (Table 2). It is of interest that all patients who are dead of disease or who have developed recurrences were classified as unresectable because of extent of disease prior to infusion except two. Details of treatment of these two patients merit special comment. Both patients had squamous cell carcinoma of the oral cavity, were infused with methotrexate, and then underwent radical composite resections. One tumor was resected on the fifth day of infusion at a time when inflammation and edema were maximal. Three months later, widespread tumor recurrence appeared at the line of wound closure. Subsequent courses of infusion with methotrexate produced short remissions, as did x-ray therapy. When the patient died one year later with extensive local disease, no distant metastases were found at autopsy. The second patient underwent tumor resection seven days after termination of methotrexate infusion of nine days' duration. The infused external carotid artery had been ligated at the time of catheter insertion, and fluorescein dye failed to stain the area of disease when injected during the course of infusion. This patient died one year later with widely disseminated metastases, although no recurrence appeared

TABLE 2.—*Resected Cases—Post Infusion*

Patient	Organ	Drug *	Follow-Up Interval, Mo	Current Status †
1	Tongue, local excision	MTX	26	ND
2	Tongue	MTX & 5-FU	12	D
3	Tongue, local excision	MTX & 5-FU	8	ND
4	Tongue	MTX	15	ND
5	Tongue bilaterally and mouth	Unilat. MTX	6	ND
6	Mouth	MTX	7	ND
7	Mouth, local excision	MTX	12	ND
8	Mouth	MTX	1	ND
9	Mouth	MTX	1	ND
10	Tonsil	MTX	16	ND
11	Neck	MTX	8	D-Rec 4 mo postop
12	Neck	MTX	8	?
13	Oropharynx	MTX	12	D (lung metastases)
14	Colon	5-FU	12	Rec
15	Leg (osteogenic sarcoma)	MTX & 5-FU	6	ND
16	Leg (osteogenic sarcoma)	MTX	14	ND
17	Arm	5-FU	1	ND
18	Arm	5-FU	4	Rec

* MTX indicates methotrexate; 5-FU, 5-fluorouracil.
† ND indicates no disease; Rec, recurrence; D, dead.

in the lines of wound closure about the neck. The relationship of postoperative recurrence in these patients to the antecedent use of chemotherapy by infusion remains conjectural. It appears unlikely that the second patient's tumor was within the treated field. A third patient who had bilateral cervical nodes metastases from squamous cell carcinoma of the nasopharynx is dead as a result of ill-advised systemic chemotherapy by others which produced hematologic depression followed by septicemia. This was administered when a single supraclavicular lymph node biopsy obtained three months after bilateral neck dissection showed residual squamous cell carcinoma. Metastases in posterior cervical lymph nodes had been encountered at surgery. A fourth patient with adenocarcinoma of the colon had extensive disease which yielded a positive biopsy from the bladder wall obtained by cystoscopic manipulation. After infusion and resection, this portion of the bladder which was excised with the colon contained no identifiable tumor. One postinfusion specimen obtained by radical resection of squamous cell carcinoma of the oral cavity initially proven by superficial biopsy yielded no evidence of residual tumor when examined histologically. This patient had been infused with methotrexate. Rupture of the common carotid artery occurred on the 16th postoperative day, requiring ligation. No neurological deficit resulted. The destructive changes in residual squamous cell carcinoma which followed methotrexate infusion of another patient are illustrated in Fig 6.

When resections were performed on these patients, some technical difficulties which could be attributed to the recent infusions were encountered in most. Edema and inflammation obscured tissue planes in the operative field in some instances. Postoperative cervical wound complications have been much less frequent when the temporal ar-

Fig 6.—Photomicrographs of tumor before and after infusion. *A,* squamous cell carcinoma of the alveolar mucosa overlying mandible; *B,* minimum residual tumor present in resected specimen after infusion chemotherapy. Disruption of tumor structure, multiple giant cells, and granulomatous type of inflammation have developed in area of primary lesion.

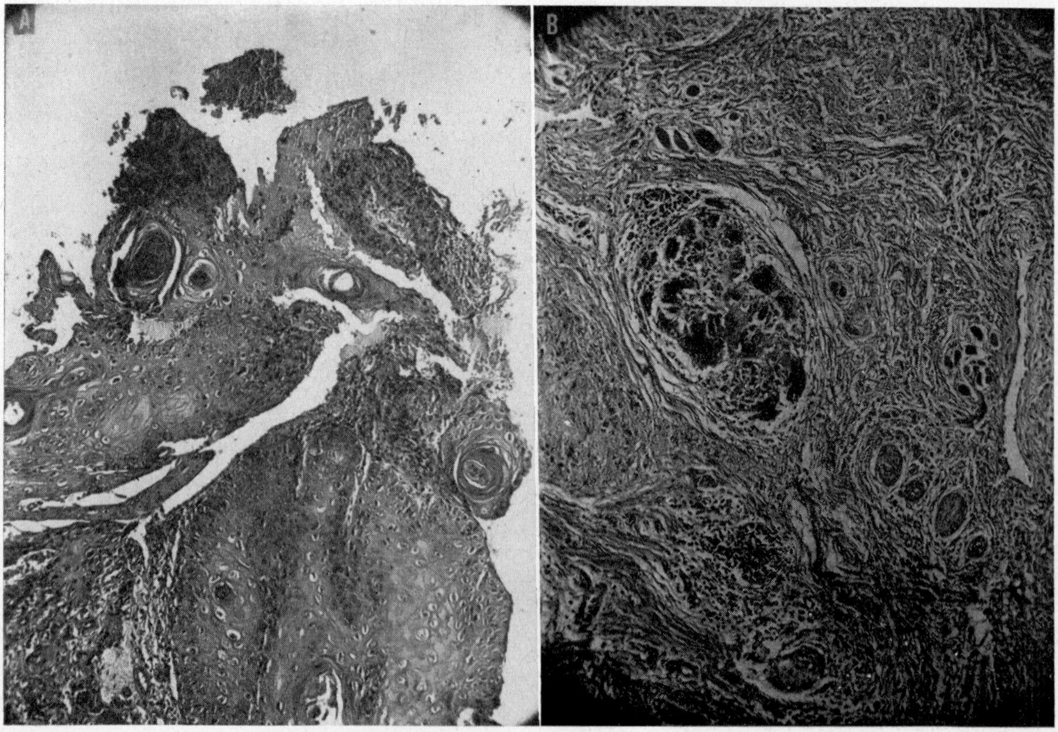

tery has been used for infusion. Three patients in this series who are clinically free of disease at 26, 12, and 8 months, respectively, had squamous cell carcinomas of the oral mucosa which were subjected to very conservative local resections following infusion responses, because they declined a more radical approach (Fig 7). The lesion of one of these patients yielded serial negative biopsies for three months after infusion with methotrexate. The area of the primary tumor was subsequently removed, and a final diagnosis of intraepithelial carcinoma was made, although an invasive malignancy had been clearly evident in sections of the original biopsy. Two osteogenic sarcomas of the femur were encountered in children who were subjected to immediate hip disarticulation following infusion. A final patient who is currently living with disease underwent palliative amputation of an arm after infusion because of destruction of the humerus owing to metastatic breast cancer.

Fig 7.—Carcinoma of the tongue excised post infusion. *A*, squamous cell carcinoma of tongue before infusion; *B*, local excision of residual lesion four days after methotrexate infusion via external carotid artery terminated; *C*, surgical scar in lesion area two years later showing no evidence of tumor. No cervical adenopathy noted after 26 months.

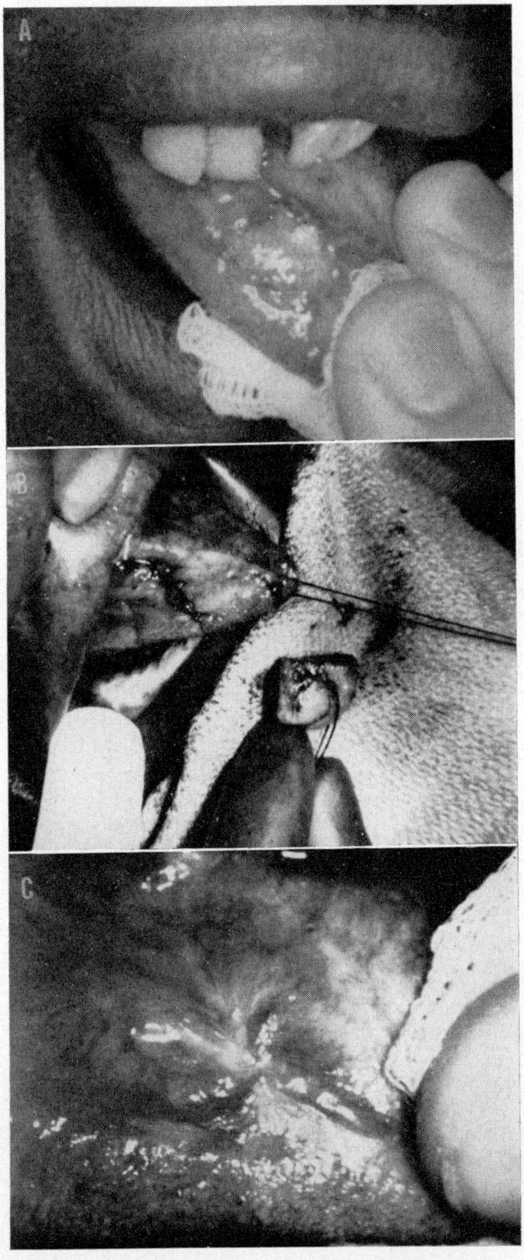

No infusion-related deaths occurred among this group. No life-threatening complications of combined therapy were observed, except for the one instance of delayed carotid artery rupture, which was preceded by wound infection.

Group 2. Ambulatory Patients With Advanced Recurrent Disease.—The patients in the advanced ambulatory category all had tumors of the head and neck, or metastatic pelvic carinoma of genitourinary origin. There were four infusion-related deaths. Two patients had cerebral vascular accidents related to carotid infusion. One patient had a vasculitis of cerebral arteries and veins which developed during 5-fluorouracil infusion. A fourth exsanguinated from the carotid artery after tumor slough in an area well removed from the site of catheter insertion. Thirteen patients of 26 are currently alive in this group. The longest survivor has lived for one year after a single methotrexate infusion for recurrent irradiated carcinoma of the tongue. Residual disease is not in evidence by recent biopsy.

Of special interest in this group is a patient with a very large anaplastic carcinoma of the thyroid which responded transiently to radiotherapy. He subsequently required tracheotomy for a rapidly enlarging tumor mass extending from the hyoid bone to the clavicle. Methotrexate infusions were given through the superior thyroid artery, using the following approach. The external carotid artery was ligated inferior to the lingual branch, and a catheter was placed in the residual stump which then supplied only the superior thyroid artery. The inferior thyroid artery was then ligated. Methotrexate was then infused for five days, and the lesion underwent 60% regression in size with evidence of marked necrosis of tumor substance. Valid assessment of this local therapeutic result has been thwarted by the unchecked progress of tumor elsewhere and infection about the tracheostomy stoma. This technical approach to infusion of thyroid tumors seems worthy of consideration if the efficacy of chemotherapy for such lesions can be established with further experience.

All patients in this group had been previously irradiated and/or resected except five. These five all responded favorably to therapy, as did 13 of the remainder. One treatment failure occurred in a patient with bilaterally extended sebaceous cell carcinoma of the neck. Four patients with metastatic lesions not accessible to repeat biopsy or inspection were treated, but results were not objectively assessible. Remissions of disease lasting from two to ten months coincided with infusion therapy in the responding group. Two of the infusion-related deaths in this group occurred on the second and fourth courses of treatment in patients who had previously responded well.

Group 3.—Prolonged extension of survival was not a primary objective of treatment in the majority of patients classified as "terminal." A large number had metastatic disease outside the areas infused, and second courses were not given as a rule, despite favorable responses to the first course of treatment. An extended series of courses was attempted in a few patients to determine the maximum capabilities of the method. In most instances, we were ultimately dissuaded from pursuing this plan with individual patients. Familial and economic considerations relevant to excessively prolonged hospitalization by noncurative therapy in patients without rehabilitation potential could not be disregarded.

As might be expected, deaths occurred frequently in this group as did complications. Nine patients died within three weeks of a course of infusion. One died after hemiplegia which was associated with infusion via the external carotid artery. The entire external carotid system thrombosed within a previously irradiated, ulcerating, tumor-laden field. Two patients exsanguinated when tumor slough developed about major arteries as a result of infusion. Two patients died of pneumonia which ensued after severe leukopenia resulted from methotrexate infusion which had produced extensive tumor necrosis. Three patients died because of thromboembolic complications to heart or lungs. Two of these patients demonstrated at autopsy thrombotic occlusion of multiple veins and/or arteries suggesting a generalized thrombotic state. Both were receiving 5-fluorouracil at the time of death. Only three patients are now living in this entire group of "terminal" subjects.

Among 30 patients who were classified as terminal prior to infusion, there were 21 remissions and 9 therapeutic failures. The longest survivor in this group was a female with widely recurrent adenocarcinoma of the rectum within the scar of a combined abdominoperineal resection and also involving the inguinal lymph nodes. Her lesions responded favorably to alternate infusions of methotrexate and 5-fluorouracil for a period of 15 months during which time on two separate occasions ureteral obstruction was relieved by 5-fluorouracil infusions delivered to the terminal aorta. She died of her disease four months after her last infusion after she and her family had declined further treatment. The longest survivor to date in this category with advanced squamous cell carcinoma of the oropharynx was a patient who on admission had already lost swallowing function owing to extensive bilateral disease. He became ambulatory and without specific need for hospital care during a three-month interval after infusion. He received three infusions of methotrexate with less

TABLE 3.—*Complication List*

Leukopenia	18
Technical	13
Local	13 *
Systemic	12 †
Skin eruptions	14

* Six deaths.
† Seven deaths.

effective remissions after each course. He died two months after his last infusion, having survived for ten months after initial chemotherapy.

Complications

The complications which are listed in Table 3 refer to events which can be more specifically classified as follows:

Leukopenia denotes a fall in white blood cells below 4,000 and was observed in 18 patients. White blood cell counts below 2,000 were infrequent except among those in the "terminal" patient group who are also listed as having other systemic complications. The infusion of 5-fluorouracil was associated with leukopenia in only one patient who also had pneumonia and obstructive uropathy.

Technical complications include: (1) catheter displacement, (2) leaks resulting in a loss of catheter patency which was not reparable, (3) any mechanical difficulties requiring termination of therapy, and (4) extravasation around catheters. There were 13 patients who sustained one or more such problems. Most were incurred among the first 20 patients treated.

Local complications include: (1) necrosis and suppuration at the catheter site, (2) tumor slough leading to exsanguination, (3) stroke due to embolus, and (4) airway obstruction due to edema necessitating tracheotomy. The number of patients in whom these problems occurred was 13. These appear to be least preventable except through better case selection.

Systemic complications include: (1) pneumonia, (2) myocardial infarction, (3) pulmonary embolus, (4) chills and high fever, and (5) gastrointestinal disorders.

Skin eruptions occurred in 14 patients and receded after methotrexate-folinic acid therapy was discontinued. These were usually assumed to be due to methotrexate and often preceded early leukopenia by 24 hours.

Comment

We first attempted to explore the potential capabilities of chemotherapy by arterial infusion when used as a last resort in terminal cancer patients. Our early experiences with this type of patient were rife with frustration but were also productive of certain accomplishments in methodology. It became apparent that technical complications incurred with the method were largely avoidable if certain principles were adhered to in the choice of techniques and materials. Local wound complications at the site of catheter insertion also became a rarity as we tended more and more to avoid the immediate vicinity of tumors and to choose sites of entry more distant from the center of irradiated fields. One complication which seems as yet unavoidable, however, is arterial blow-out and exsanguination following tumor slough when all supporting structures of a major artery have been invaded by tumor. Prophylactic ligations are of partial benefit, but retrograde bleeding may still be lethal.

It is perhaps noteworthy that we have been able to avoid serious incidents of hemorrhage around the sites of catheter insertion. This we attribute to two factors: (1) We insert smaller catheters (<0.04 inches in diameter) than other investigators have reported using. This minimizes the defect in the arterial wall and facilitates spontaneous closure upon withdrawal. (2) The absolute minimum in dissection around arteries is employed, and no intra-arterial suture fixation of catheters is ever attempted, as advocated by Sullivan et al.[10] Emphasis on maximum simplicity of technique and minimum size of the arteriotomy is maintained in all areas.

If the true merits of any form of chemotherapy for cancer are to be determined, it would appear that at least three primary conditions must be met. First, the drug must arrive at the tumor site in sufficient quantity and concentration to be effective. Second, the patient must be capable of detoxifying that portion of the drug administered which is not incorporated into the tumor. Third, the patient being treated must at the same time be capable of sustaining the accelerated catabolism imposed by tumor destruction in situ. For meeting the first condition, it is indeed difficult to conceive of a more rational approach than protracted intra-arterial delivery. By this method, the first named condition is the most easily controlled of the three. The second condition, control of systemic drug toxicity, is somewhat more difficult to achieve but can be standardized within limits which are currently acceptable. The third condition which relates to the patient's tolerance for accelerated tissue necrosis has never been clearly defined even under circumstances far less complex than those attending the use of cytotoxic chemicals for cancer. The overlapping effects of drug toxicity plus massive tissue autolysis in vivo present a problem which is completely unexplored. That both factors have a collective impact of marked proportions upon the homeostatic mechanisms of the total organism can hardly be doubted.

Our experience with infusion therapy in a large number of patients with advanced disease who obtained good local responses to therapy only to succumb to systemic complications such as pneumonia have caused us to question the therapeutic merit of precipitous tumor destruction in these patients. Because of our earlier suspicion that the amount and rate of tissue destruction might be contributory to these complications, we began to treat certain patients with large tumor masses more slowly. Continuous infusion periods were shortened to four or five days and then resumed for a similar period after four days or more of rest. Although this altered routine has been followed in only a small number of patients, our experience to date indicates that tumor regression proceeds to a similar degree, but with fewer complications both locally and systemically. Some patients who were treated with a single protracted course of methotrexate initially have later been given a second divided course using a similar amount of drug. Leukopenia and pneumonia encountered during the first course did not appear with the altered regimen.

Could it be that the most immediate objective of chemotherapy should not be rapid tumor regression? If rapid and massive tumor necrosis does occur during a course of chemotherapy, should the lesion not be at least partially removed surgically if therapy is to be continued?

Surgical reduction of tumor size in conjunction with chemotherapy was shown by Martin et al [15] to be definitely beneficial with respect to cure rates in mice bearing spontaneously occurring tumors. Such studies tend to emphasize the role of immunological and mechanical processes in determining the outcome of cancer therapy and suggest that certain combined therapies may have additive effects through mechanisms other than increased rate of tumor destruction. Other evidence recently reported by Wolberg et al [16] suggests that the dose schedule of 5-fluorouracil may be altered in favor of less toxicity for debilitated patients without significant compromise of potential antitumor effects.

Certain general concepts of chemotherapy should perhaps be modified to stress the following points:

1. Time-dose relationships in chemotherapy should be made more flexible according to individual patient response as well as tumor response after therapy has been initiated.

2. The optimal drug dose used for initial courses in chemotherapy infused through a regional artery should be inversely proportional to tumor size if no ancillary means of tumor removal from the patient is contemplated.

3. Forms of combined therapy which are expected to produce rapid extensive necrosis of large tumors in debilitated patients should be approached with extreme caution.

Summary and Conclusions

Experiences are summarized which relate to the treatment of 74 patients with protracted arterial infusion chemotherapy using methotrexate with and without folinic acid, or 5-fluorouracil. Techniques for placement of catheters and maintenance of infusion assembly which have been found most reliable in our hands are described. Patients were classified into three groups for assessment of results: (1) resected postinfusion, (2) ambulatory patients with advanced nonresectable disease, and (3) patients hospitalized for terminal care.

The incidence of complications, both local and systemic, was lowest in patients resected postinfusion and highest in the terminal group.

Objective evidence of therapeutic benefit was most prevalent in the resected group. Several advanced classically inoperable tumors responded sufficiently to permit removal. In one resected specimen from a patient with histologically proven squamous cell carcinoma, no tumor could be found. Histological evidence of tumoricidal effect was observed in most specimens resected. No clear evidence that infusion chemotherapy may result in accelerated dissemination of disease when followed by surgery has been observed. Twelve of the 18 patients in this group remain without evidence of residual tumor for periods of 2 to 26 months since resection. Only one patient of 26 in the advanced ambulatory group has been and is presently without clear evidence of residual disease for more than a ten-month period, after receiving one or more courses of infusion therapy. Regression and retardation of tumor growth could be documented in approximately 70% of patients in this group.

There were also regression and retardation of neoplastic activity in approximately 70% of the patients classified as terminal. Prolongation of survival was not sought as a primary objective in treating this group, however, and single index lesions only were infused as a rule.

It is from experiences gained in treating the latter group of terminal patients that we conclude the following: Precipitous destruction in situ of large tumors in debilitated patients carries a high morbidity and mortality rate. On this basis, we propose that two alternative approaches be evaluated clinically in patients who receive regional infusion chemotherapy directed at large tumors:

1. Use divided courses and flexible dosage related inversely to rate of visible tissue response.

2. Consider serial debridement or fractional removal of necrotic tumors after reliable evidence appears that the agent used is locally effective.

Jerrel W. Benson, MD, Chief of Surgery, Highland View Hospital, Cleveland 22.

REFERENCES

1. Sullivan, R. D.; Miller, E.; and Sikes, M. P.: Antimetabolite-Metabolite Combination Cancer Chemotherapy: Effects of Intra-Arterial Methotrexate-Intramuscular Citrovorum Factor Therapy in Human Cancer, Cancer 12:1248-1262 (Nov-Dec) 1959.

2. Klopp, E. T., et al: Fractionated Intra-Arterial Cancer: Chemotherapy With Methyl Bis Amine Hydrochloride; Preliminary Report, Ann Surg 132:811-832 (Oct) 1950.

3. Bierman, H. R.; Shimkin, M. D.; Byron, R. L., Jr.; and Miller, E. R.: "Effects of Intra-Arterial Administration of Nitrogen Mustard," in Proceedings of the Fifth International Cancer Congress, Paris, 1950 (Abstract of Papers), pp 186-187.

4. Tarr, N.; Sensenbrenner, L. L.; Fletcher, R.; and Griffing, J.: Intra-Arterial Infusion of Malignancies With 5-Fluorouracil, Cancer Chemother Rep 14:23-37 (Oct) 1961.

5. Sullivan, R. D.; Young, C. W.; Miller, E.; Glatstein, N.; Clarkson, B.; and Burchenal, J. H.: Clinical Effects of the Continuous Administration of Fluorinated Pyrimidines (5-Fluorouracil and 5-Fluoro-2′-deoxyuridine), Cancer Chemother Rep 8:77-83 (July) 1960.

6. Kiehn, C. L.; DesPrez, J. D.; and Benson, J. W.: Chemotherapy for Tumors of the Head and Neck, Plast Reconstr Surg 30:577-580 (Nov) 1962.

7. Goldacre, R. J., and Sylven, B.: A Rapid Method for Studying Tumour Blood Supply Using Systemic Dyes, Nature (London) 184:63-64 (July) 1959.

8. Cataland, S.; Cohen, C.; and Sapirstein, L. A.: Relationship Between Size and Perfusion Rate of Transplanted Tumors, J Nat Cancer Inst 29:389-394 (Aug) 1962.

9. Johnson, R. O.; Kishen, W. A.; and Curreri, A. K.: The Response of Squamous Cell Carcinoma to Intra-Arterial Infusion With 5-Fluorouracil, Cancer Chemother Rep 24:29-31 (Nov) 1962.

10. Sullivan, R. D.: Continuous Arterial Infusion Cancer Chemotherapy, Surg Clin N Amer 42:365-388 (April) 1962.

11. Espiner, H. J.; Vowles, K. D. J.; and Walker, R. M.: Cancer Chemotherapy by Intra-Arterial Infusion: A Preliminary Report Concerning Tumours of the Head and Neck, Lancet 1:177-181 (Jan) 1962.

12. Nahum, A. M., and Rochlin, D. B.: Regional Arterial Chemotherapy of Cancer of the Head and Neck, Surg Gynec Obstet 115:478-483 (Oct) 1962.

13. Benson, J. W.: Unpublished data.

14. Ramsden, C. H., and Duff, J. K.: Continuous Arterial Infusion of Head and Neck Tumors: Improvements in Technique by Retrograde Temporal Artery Catheterization, Cancer 16:133-135 (Jan) 1963.

15. Martin, D. S.; Fugmann, R. A.; and Hayworth, P.: Surgery, Cancer Chemotherapy, Host Defenses, and Tumor Size, J Nat Cancer Inst 29:817-834 (Nov) 1962.

16. Wolberg, W. H.; Johnson, R. O.; and Curreri, A. K.: Controlled-Dose Chemotherapy as an Adjunct to Surgery, Cancer 16:5-7 (Jan) 1963.

Hyperbaric Oxygenation and Mechlorethamine Effectiveness

ROBERT P. LEATHER, MD, AND CHARLES ECKERT, MD, ALBANY, NY

In order to test one of the possible radiomimetic qualities of alkylating agents, we have studied the influence of hyperbaric oxygen on the tumoricidal action of mechlorethamine (nitrogen mustard) in spontaneous mammary tumors of heterozygous, randomly bred Swiss-Webster mice.

Since the initiation of this study, two reports have been published relating to it. In a similar test, Krementz and Knudson,[6,7] using the Ehrlich ascites tumor, sarcoma 180 and sarcoma 37, demonstrated a significant decrease in cell counts and mortality in the Ehrlich ascites tumor, but they were unable to show any change in the sarcoma 180 or sarcoma 37. Back,[3] working with sarcoma 180, leukemia 1210, and Gardiner lymphosarcoma, found no change in the mechlorethamine sensitivity in environments of 100% oxygen at up to four atmospheres absolute pressure. In both of these studies, transplanted tumors were used, in contrast to the spontaneous tumor used in the present report.

Presented at the 20th Annual Meeting of the Central Surgical Association, Chicago, Feb 21-23, 1963.

From the Department of Surgery, Albany Medical College of Union University.

This project was supported by Grant CY6354 of the USPHS.

Methods and Materials

The heterozygous, randomly bred Swiss-Webster mouse with spontaneous mammary cancer was chosen for the test tumor for two reasons: first, any spontaneous tumor eliminates the problem of homograft rejection response inherent in transplanted tumors; and second, because the growth characteristics of the tumor selected had been extensively studied by others in our laboratory.[5] The latter studies demonstrated that the most predictable range of growth was a tumor volume of 2 to 4 ml observed over a two-week period. This, then, was the size of the tumor used in all animals studied.

All animals were anesthetized with ether, and the tumor was examined and measured with calipers graduated in millimeters in three planes at right

Fig 1.—Measurement of tumors with calipers.

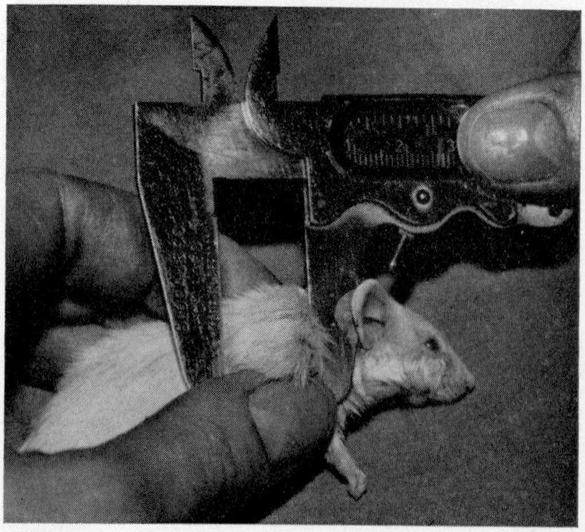

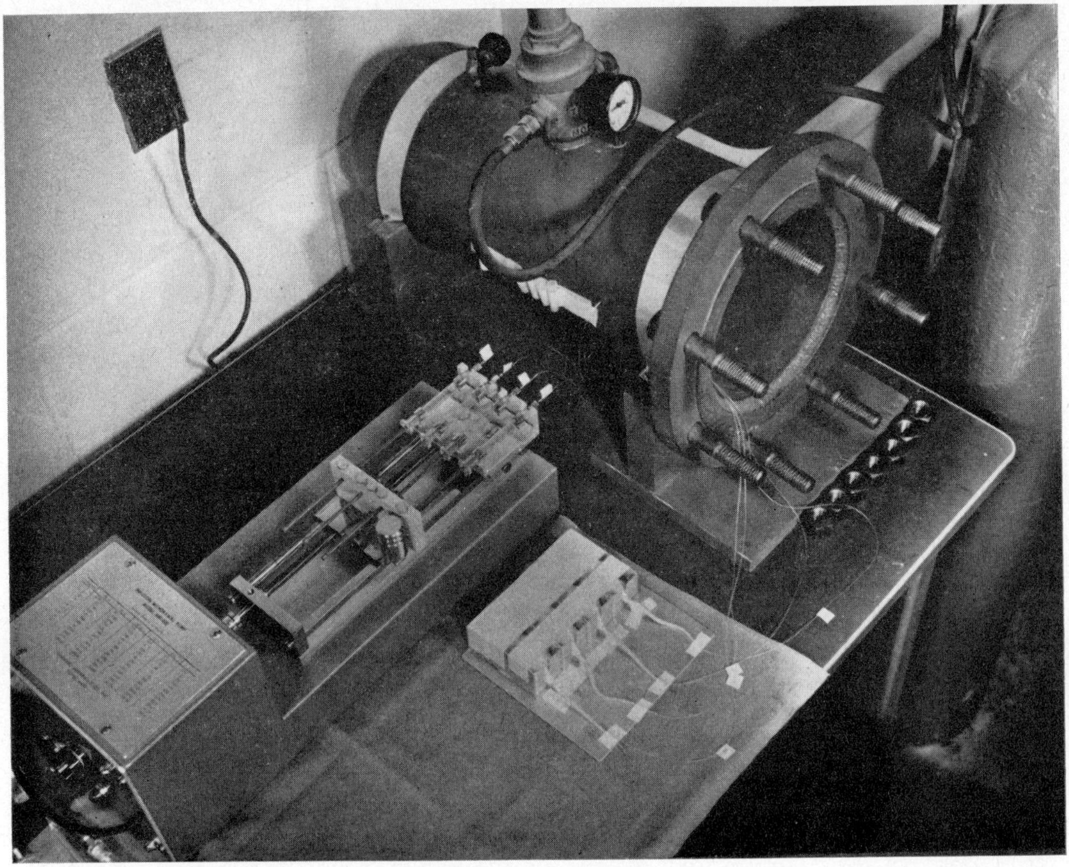

Fig 2.—Anesthetized mice with IV infusion running immediately prior to placement in pressure chamber.

angles to each other (Fig 1). The product of these three measurements was designated as the tumor volume. All animals were then anesthetized with intraperitoneal pentobarbital sodium (Nembutal), 30 mg per kilogram body weight prior to treatment. Both 0.9% saline and mechlorethamine were administered intravenously via the tail vein, 0.02 ml per kilogram body weight; the concentration of mechlorethamine was such that 1 mg per kilogram body weight was delivered. In those animals treated in the pressure chamber, the patency of the intravenous infusion was maintained by delivery of the drug at a minimum rate with a syringe pump, less than 5% of the total dose being delivered during the 20 minutes required for flushing pressurization and time, to attain tissue saturation (Table 1). The drug was then delivered and pressure maintained constantly for an additional ten minutes. Decompression was carried out over the following 15-minute period. The tumors were then measured at 7 and 14 days as described above, the animal sacrificed, the tumor excised and studied histologically. Only solid tumors were included. Any tumor containing cyst, hematoma, or abscess was discarded.

In order to properly control the study of mechlorethamine infused in an environment of hyperbaric oxygen three control groups were necessary. The experimental design is shown in Table 2. Group 1 (30 animals): All animals were given 0.9% saline intravenously while in an environment of room air. Group II (56 animals): All animals were given mechlorethamine intravenously while in an environment of room air. Group III (30 animals): All animals received injections of 0.9% saline while in the pressure chamber in 100% oxygen at three atmospheres absolute pressure. Group IV (50 animals): This was the study group in which mechlorethamine was injected while in the pressure chamber in 100% oxygen at three atmospheres pressure.

TABLE 1.—*Pressure Chamber Program*

Flush	3 min
Compression	3 min
Saturation	10 min
Drug administration	1-2 min
Drug utilization	10 min
Decompression	15 min

TABLE 2.—*Experimental Design and Results*

Treatment	Pressure Absolute: 1 Atmosphere Air	Pressure Absolute: 3 Atmosphere Oxygen
0.9% Saline	Group I 30 animals Median growth Index = +70%	Group III 30 animals Median growth index = +88%
HN_2	Group II 56 animals Median growth index = +75%	Group IV 50 animals Median growth index = +33%

Results

Fig 3 is a graphic representation of the population distribution of the groups treated. A statistical analysis using the rank-sum procedure of Mann and Whitney showed a significant difference ($P=<0.05$) in growth index to exist between animals treated with mechlorethamine at one atmosphere of air (group II) and those treated at three atmospheres of oxygen (group IV). There was no statistical difference between growth indices of those animals treated with isotonic saline at one atmosphere of air and those treated at three atmospheres of oxygen (groups I and III, respectively).*

Comment

These data indicated that the tumoricidal effect of mechlorethamine is enhanced by hyperbaric oxygenation. The effect of pressure alone has been studied in mice with transplanted tumors with data indicating that pressure per se can cause slower growth.[1] However, the magnitude of pressure exposure was many times greater than that used in this study, that is, 70 lbs per square inch gauge pressure gauge for two to six hours per day, five days per week for two to five weeks, or an average of 65 times the exposure used in this study. Furthermore, if pressure or oxygen alone was a significant factor in the observed results, it should have been reflected in the comparison of the growth indices of those animals treated with isotonic saline at one atmosphere of air and those treated in three atmospheres of oxygen.

Of prime importance in the chemotherapy of solid tumors is the concentration of drug delivered to the tumor. Isolated perfusion and infusion have been the direct means of accomplishing this. However, other variables, namely flow, temperature, pressure, and oxygen tension appear to have a distinct influence on the utilization of drug made available. It has been shown in isolated per-

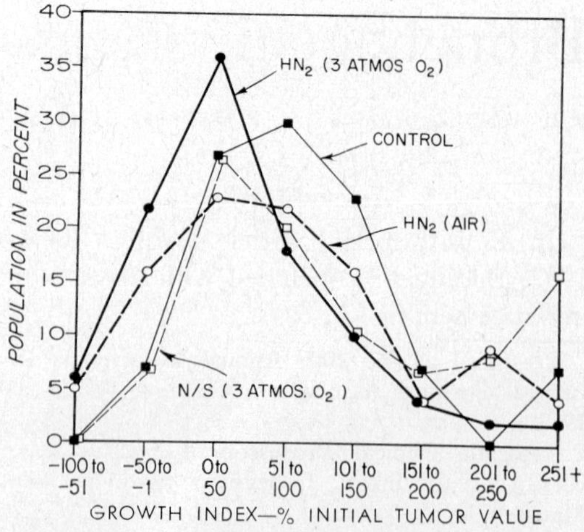

Fig 3.—The influence of hyperbaric oxygenation on HN_2 effectiveness.

* Utilizing the growth index as a measure, comparison of groups II and IV or I and III was on the basis of the rank-sum procedure of Mann and Whitney. This is a two sample test of the hypothesis that both have been drawn for the same population. In the present case, $n_1=50$ and $n_2=56$, the distribution of statistic Z approaches the normal distribution.

$$Z=\frac{U-\frac{n_1 n_2}{2}}{\left[\frac{n_1 n_2 (n_1+n_2+1)}{12}\right]^{1/2}}$$

For groups II and IV, $Z=2.08$. The probability of obtaining a value of Z as great as 2.08 under the null hypothesis is 0.039.

For groups I and III, $Z=1.508$. The probability of obtaining this value is $>15\%$, and therefore the difference is not significant.

fusion studies that increases in temperature, relatively small flow, and reduced oxygen saturation resulted in increased drug utilization.[2,8] However, it is likely that the flow and oxygen saturation effects observed in these studies are the result of their effects on the vascular bed and therefore on blood flow, rather than a direct effect on drug utilization or alteration in cellular sensitivity. It is also notable that the rapid increase in tissue oxygen tension under hyperbaric oxygenation of tumors can be prevented by giving serotonin [4] which also diminishes blood flow to the tumor bed. Hence, the pressure and concentration of ambient oxygen is only one factor upon which tumor tissue oxygen tension depends; and whatever the means used to attain it, increases in oxygen at the cellular level would appear to enhance the effectiveness of mechlorethamine.

Summary

The tumoricidal effect of mechlorethamine (nitrogen mustard) is increased by hyperbaric oxygenation in solid spontaneous mammary carcinomas of Swiss-Webster mice.

Robert P. Leather, MD, Department of Surgery, Albany Medical College of Union University, Albany, NY.

REFERENCES

1. Antopol, W.; Chryssanthou, C.; and Kooperstein, S.: Effect of Air Pressure on Carcinoma 755 and Sarcoma 180 in C57B1 Mice, Proc Amer Ass Cancer Res 3:205, 1961.

2. Ausman, R. K., in discussion of paper by Krementz et al: Perfusion Conference, Chemother Rep 10:125, 1960.

3. Back, N.: Effect of Oxygen Tension on the in Vitro and in Vivo Sensitivity of Normal Tissues and Tumor Cells to Alkylating Agents, Proc Amer Ass Cancer Res 3:207, 1961.

4. Cater, D. B.; Schoeniger, E. L.; and Watkinson, D. A.: Effects on Oxygen Tension of Tumors of Breathing Oxygen at High Pressures; Lancet 2:381. 1962.

5. Garb, S.; Stein, A. A.; and Sims, G.: Observations of Spontaneous Mammary Carcinomas in Heterozygous Random Bred Mice, unpublished data.

6. Krementz, E. T., and Knudson, L.: The Effect of Increased Oxygen Tension on the Tumoricidal Effect of Nitrogen Mustard, Surgery 50:266, 1961.

7. Krementz, E. T.; Harlin, R.; and Knudson, L.: The Enhancement of Chemotherapy by Increased Tissue Oxygen Tension, Chemother Rep 10:125, 1960.

8. Shingleton, W. W.: Selective Heating and Cooling of Tissue in Cancer Chemotherapy, Ann Surg 156:408, 1962.

Effect of Chemical Agents on Bronchogenic Cancer

F. L. MENDEZ, JR., MD; E. R. P. MAURER, MD; AND HERMAN A. FRECKMAN, MD, CINCINNATI

Introduction

In an informative article written during 1957, Budinger [2] concluded with the following statement:

That such a large series of terminal patients is easily accumulated testifies to the subtlety of bronchogenic carcinoma and perhaps to the failure of patient education in this group. At present, the great majority of patients with lung cancer at Boston City Hospital are seen too late to permit an attempt at definitive therapy.

Hayward [5] made the following observation:

. . . if a hint that surgical successes are few creeps in [the literature], it is fashion to counter it by a call for earlier diagnosis, thus creating the impression that this will correct the position. I . . . do not believe that earlier diagnosis [of lung cancer]

Presented at the 20th Annual Meeting of the Central Surgical Association, Chicago, Feb 21-23, 1963.

Associate Clinical Professor of Surgery University of Cincinnati, College of Medicine (Dr. Maurer).

Director of Chemotherapy, Christ Hospital and Bethesda Hospital (Dr. Freckman).

will increase surgical "cures" to a really significant percentage. . . . surgery of carcinoma of the lung is depressing. . . . The idea that more extensive operations or more powerful X-ray machines will go an appreciable way towards the solution of the problem seems to me absurd.

Yet other authors have published information suggesting the five-year over-all survival rate varies from 33% to 10%.[7,8] Certainly it is increasingly difficult to reach dependable conclusions concerning proper therapy for bronchogenic carcinoma when one is bombarded from all points with such varying remarks and statistics. Our personal experiences with bronchogenic carcinoma have forced us to conclude that our present methods, regardless of what they may be, are quite inadequate. If one includes all cases, operated upon and not operated upon, one is forced to accept a five-year survival rate, a figure little better than that for carcinoma of the stomach.

We do not intend to belabor the much-discussed point of the increase of bronchogenic carcinoma during the last decade. As to whether this increase is actual or relative, we are not prepared to say. However, our experience with the disease has forced us to search for other methods of therapy. As early as 1955, we began to utilize the available chemotherapeutic drugs in the treatment of bronchogenic carcinoma. It was not until about 1958 and 1959 that we joined efforts and began to treat these patients in earnest. One of us (H. A. F.) had been working with these agents for several years. Thus it was fortunate that the combination of individuals brought together both medical and surgical dicta. Since that period, we have engaged in treating bronchogenic carcinoma by the accepted modalities, and in addition to this, we have tried various techniques and chemotherapeutic drugs in an effort to increase the five-year survival rates. Thus we are reporting our experiences with this group of 117 patients.

Material and Technique

These cases were derived from the private practice of Drs. E. R. Maurer and F. L. Mendez, Jr. As such they represent the less satisfactory groups, since those patients in whom we felt a surgical cure was effected were withheld from the study. Our medical colleague, Dr. H. A. Freckman, having considerable experience in the use of the chemotherapeutic agents, was elected to give the therapy as he felt it was indicated. The type of drug, the amount, and the method of delivery were left in his control in order to establish, where possible, a constant mode of administration. During this effort, we utilized various techniques. Our early efforts were confined to the intravenous administration. However, as our experience grew, our approach became more bold. We utilized such techniques as surgical exposure and implantation of plastic catheters into the vessels of the tumor-bearing area: indwelling cardiac catheters were placed in the pulmonary artery, and some of these remained in situ for eight to ten days without complication. Gradually we recognized the value of intra-arterial medication over a long period of time. From this concept came our final and present technique. Much of this technique is directly attributable to Dr. Freckman.

At present we are utilizing a fine plastic catheter introduced percutaneously into the aorta via the femoral, radial, or carotid arteries. The catheter outlet is then adjusted to give maximum drug concentration into the tumor-bearing area. This technique is readily carried out in the average hospital without the benefit of special personnel or equipment. To date, it has been free of serious complications or infections in spite of the fact that such drugs as utilized often markedly depress the autoimmune mechanism. We have found that these catheters can be implanted at the exit site and reopened for use at a later date.

Realizing that chemotherapy depends for its effect on the interference of the cellular division, we felt that it was necessary to utilize certain of the drugs over the longest possible period of time. Since only a relatively small number of the tumor cells would be in fission at a given moment, it was recognized that it would be necessary to administer the drug on a constant basis whenever possible. Thus we arrived at our present technique. Likewise, we are engaged in the research laboratory in an effort to provide visual and radioactive proof of such drug concentration. This work we will report at a later date.

Basically, the drugs used in the treatment of these patients fell largely into two major groups: the polyfunctional alkylating agents such as chlorambucil and cyclophosphamide, or the antimetabolites such as methotrexate and fluorouracil. In cases where methotrexate was given, the calcium leucovorin (Citrovorum Factor) was prescribed in adequate amounts to prevent excessive drug toxicity. The dual antagonists series, such as uredepa (AB-100), benzodepa (AB-103), and meturedepa (AB-132) were given but without apparent success. In cases failing to respond to the previously mentioned drugs, we resorted to dihydro-E73 (NSC 33012, Pfizer), N-methyldihydro-E73 (NSC 48400, Pfizer), and dimethcylacetamide; again these failed to be of benefit to the patients to whom they were given.

In those cases where results were not forthcoming, and in more recent patients, we have resorted to the use of drug combinations such as the alkylating agents and the antimetabolite fluorouracil. It would be premature to discuss the results of such studies at this time.

As we have stated, the mode of administration varied while we searched for a simple, logical method. Frequently, several modalities were brought to bear in an all-out effort to produce tumor death or regression. Supervoltage irradiation was frequently combined with drug administration. Several cases received resectional surgery, irradiation, and chemotherapy simultaneously.

There is no need, at this time, to give details regarding drug amounts, etc. Suffice it to say that these agents were given in adequate dosages and as frequently as necessary, or as often as the human organism could tolerate them. The accepted published dosages were usually followed, except in certain cases where the technique differed or where we deliberately exceeded the accepted dosage level. Table 1 lists the various drugs given and route of administration to this group of patients.

TABLE 1.—*Specific Agents Utilized* *

Agent	Route of Administration
Nitrogen mustard	I.V. & I.A. & I.P.A.
Chlorambucil	Oral, I.V., I.A.
Cyclophosphamide	I.V. & I.A.
Methotrexate	I.V. & I.A.
Fluorouracil	I.V. & I.A.
Uredepa, benzodepa, & meturedepa	I.V.
Dihydro-E73	I.V.
Dimethyacetamide	I.V.

* Combinations of drugs were often utilized.

Results

A total of 117 patients suspected of having bronchogenic carcinoma were treated with the chemotherapeutic drugs. Of this number we accepted only 68 cases to report at this time. The remaining 49 cases were excluded for various reasons. Many were unsatisfactory from the standpoint of a proven diagnosis, and others were lost to adequate, authentic follow-up. Wherever there was any question whatsoever regarding diagnosis, treatment, or results, the case was excluded from the study.

In the group reviewed for study there were 59 males and nine females, 85% and 15%, respectively. The average age for the males was 58.7 years, while the average age for the female listed in the study was 53.5. Because of the small number of females appearing in the study, the average age is of very little significance. At present, there are ten patients surviving, six patients with known malignant disease and four patients apparently without known disease. Of the patients surviving without disease, one has lived 34 months, another 42 months, and a third 60 months. These patients have been exhaustively investigated to date, and no evident malignant disease is discernible at present. The patients who have not survived their disease lived an average of 8.2 months after the date of established diagnosis. This figure, of course, has very little significance, since it is exceedingly difficult to establish a time

TABLE 2.—*Data on Survival*

Total No. Treated		No. Reported
117		59 males (85%) 9 females (15%)
No. Reported	Dead	Alive
68	64	* 4

* 2 years plus.

interval in the course of the process wherein one case can be compared to another.

It would appear, therefore, that in the light of statistical analysis, only four patients in this group have survived to the present date without disease. In view of the various modalities of therapy employed, we would be exceedingly presumptious to claim these survivors for chemotherapy. The subjective changes which we have time and again observed do not lend themselves to a mathematical expression. Therefore, it becomes necessary for this audience to accept our statements regarding symptomatic relief in our patients without statistical proof. We have seen hemiplegia abate with resulting temporary discharge from the hospital. We have seen skin metastases disappear and radiographic evidence of improvement occur in others. We have seen the course of this disease temporarily halted with regression in liver nodules; several of these patients have returned to full employment. Again, we have many times observed the relief of pain and have been impressed with the temporary improvement in the appetite and the weight gain of these cases. We are certain that most workers in this field have been so impressed. However, we feel that these facets of chemotherapy are often overlooked in the light of the eventual mortality.

During this effort, we collected and reviewed the data related to the hemopoietic changes, total drug dosages utilized, and other such facts. Analysis of the data failed to present any clear trend, and this information has not been included in this report.

Comment

The surgical approach which can be successfully applied to the treatment of bronchogenic carcinoma has reached the limits of expansion. More aggressive or wider resection of the tumor-bearing area does not appear to be of value in extending the five-year survival rate. In addition to this, such radical excision must be viewed in the light of its increased mortality and morbidity. Tumor irradiation, likewise, has failed to produce substantial results regardless of how the rays have been produced. Therefore, we are faced with the necessity of seeking out new modalities to apply to these unfortunate patients of bronchogenic carcinoma. As to whether earlier diagnosis and resection would materially improve the five-year survival rate, we are not prepared to say. Efforts directed toward professional and lay education have failed to yield satisfactory results. Mass radiographic surveys have proven too expensive and have yielded too small a number of patients to be successful.

For these reasons, we feel that continued efforts should be directed at two main points. First and foremost, we should make all possible progress in the realm of prophylaxis. There is simply too strong a connection between the use of tobacco and bronchogenic carcinoma to be totally ignored. Regardless of whether this be cause and effect, if there is any chance whatsoever that tobacco adversely influences the rate of lung cancer, every possible step should be taken to control such adverse influence. The second point of attack centers around the continuation of research and the clinical trial of the various chemotherapeutic agents. To date, we have had precious little to work with, but we feel we have utilized this time to develop and expand the technique of administration. Our present technique of administration is a simple, safe, and effective method of producing drug concentration in the tumor-bearing area. Of course, additional efforts along this line are necessary and essential. However, we must await the development of more successful chemicals if we are to gain better results in the treatment of bronchogenic carcinoma. When such drugs are available, we believe that chemotherapy will become a more useful method of therapy. Until such time arrives, we must continue to explore the uses of such drugs and techniques as we now have available. Perhaps the judicious application of several modalities will be of benefit to these patients. Certainly we believe this to be the situation from our experiences to date.

Summary

During the past five years, we have endeavored to treat patients who have bronchogenic carcinoma with the available chemotherapeutic agents. A total of 117 patients have been analyzed and 68 cases critically reviewed. This group of individuals represents the far advanced, often hopelessly ill patients. Those patients in whom surgical cure was a possibility were not treated with such drugs and therefore represent more ideal cases. No comparison was made between these groups for the obvious reason that such selection would heavily favor the surgical approach. Of the cases reviewed, only four patients are known to be alive and without disease. These patients were treated by a combination therapy which included limited resection, chemotherapy, and often irradiation. The remainder of the group survived on an average of 8.2 months following diagnosis. Some, however, were given chemotherapeutic agents only as a final effort and thus heavily load this figure.

The major contribution which we feel has been derived from this effort centers about the development of a simple technique of prolonged intra-arterial infusion. Various interesting techniques were utilized and abandoned as the work progressed.

Where bronchogenic carcinoma is concerned, there is no chemical agent available today which will yield satisfactory results over a five-year period. Temporary remission and/or improvement can at times be accomplished. However, this necessitates clinical trial and error with these patients. In conclusion, we would like to point out that the chemotherapy of bronchogenic carcinoma is palliative to a degree but not curative. Such therapy, however, is worthy of continued efforts. Palliation, in itself, is of value to these patients suffering the effects of lung cancer. Surgery, where indicated, in combination with other modalities, remains the present first line of defense in bronchogenic carcinoma.

F. L. Mendez, Jr., MD, 5 W Fourth St, Cincinnati, Ohio.

REFERENCES

1. Brock, R., and Whytehead, L. L.: Radical Pneumonectomy for Bronchial Carcinoma, Brit J Surg 43:8-24, 1955.
2. Budinger, J. M.: Untreated Bronchogenic Carcinoma: A Clinicopathological Study of 250 Autopsied Cases, Cancer 11:106-116, 1958.
3. Bignall, J. R., and Moon, A. J.: Survival After Lung Resection for Bronchial Carcinoma, Thorax 10:183-190, 1955.
4. Hall, T. C.: Present Status of the Chemical Treatment of Solid Tumors, Med Sci 11:3-48, 1962.
5. Hayward, J.: Some Observations on the Pathology and Treatment of Carcinoma of the Lung, Med J Aust 1:14-17, 1959.
6. Horn, D.: (Quoted on smoking and health), CA 11:70, 1961.
7. Kirklin, J. N.; McDonald, J. R.; Clagett, O. T.; Moersch, H. J.; and Gage, R. P.: Bronchogenic Carcinoma: Cell Type and Other Factors Relating to Prognosis, Surg Gyn Obstet 100:429-438, 1955.
8. Paulson, D. L.: Survival Rates Following Resection for Bronchogenic Carcinoma, Ann Surg 146:997-1010, 1957.
9. Watson, W. L.: Radical Surgery for Lung Cancer: Evolution of the Operation of Radical Pneumonectomy and 5-Year End Results, Cancer 9:1167-1172, 1956.

DISCUSSION

On papers by Drs. Benson et al, Leather and Eckert, and Mendez et al.

Dr. Anthony Curreri, Madison, Wis: In a group of approximately the same number we have obtained about the same results as Dr. Benson and Dr. Holden. However, in all of our patients, where there was complete healing of the neoplastic ulcer, when we obtained biopsies one month later we were able to find nests of cancer cells, and because of this we are presently utilizing x-ray therapy at the end of one month in the hope that we may control the lesion completely. I should remind you that all of these patients were treated with 5-fluorouracil, not with methotrexate.

In lesions such as anal carcinomas and squamous cell carcinomas, again we were able to reduce the lesion better than 50% and make an unresectable lesion now a resectable lesion. Thus, by the use of chemotherapy we are able to convert an inoperable lesion to one that may be treated by x-ray therapy or surgery.

I would also like to point out that in another series of 17 cases we did, who had had previous radiotherapy, the picture is totally different. In this group, only one patient responded and only with a 25% response, indicating that with such involvement from x-ray therapy, usually somewhere between 6,000 to 9,000 r into the tumor, one has either changed the bed, because of fibrosis, or probably changed the cells so that the enzyme systems are not quite the same.

However, I would like to remind you that chemotherapy is here to stay with lesions of the oral pharynx. We had an idea that 5-fluorouracil would be effective in this group of cases because early studies that we did with 5-fluorouracil some seven or eight years ago taught us that with doses which produce tremendous toxicity, one could find regression of the tumors, but it was too hazardous and dangerous, and it was lethal in some instances. One may say that in the group of cases studied by Drs. Mendez, Maurer, and Freckman there has been considerable response, but they have been utilizing agents either individually or in combination. They have shifted their modes of administration from one method to another, so one can only conclude that this has been a probing approach into the problem of chemotherapy, and from that standpoint it is excellent.

The burden of proof remains upon them to select one or two approaches and then establish a prospective protocol, adhering to a randomized study, and finally following this and comparing it with a standard method of treatment. In this manner we will know whether their approach is good.

Intra-arterial catheterization into the aorta at this high level brings to mind the fact that we may be in trouble, because the aortic stream may disperse the chemotherapeutic agent away from the bronchial arteries. They have had success with this method, and therefore I cannot argue against it.

In regard to the hyperbaric pressures, I think Dr. Leather and Dr. Eckert have done a splendid job. I think we should realize that by raising the oxygen tension in the cancer cell we may be burning out the tumor or helping it to burn itself out. Here, too, we make it possible to introduce chemotherapeutic agents. I can well see some antimetabolites, for example, utilized much more successfully in the presence of a high oxygen content such as they produce in this chamber.

Dr. Claude R. Hitchcock, Minneapolis: The field of chemotherapy, as I am sure Dr. Curreri and the others will attest, is a very new field, and certainly the field of chemotherapy with hyperbaric oxygenation is just sitting on our threshold at this point.

Since we became interested in the problem of hyperbaric oxygenation for cardiac surgical problems as well as for cancer chemotherapy about a year ago at the Minneapolis General Hospital, and pending the actual completion of our hyperbaric facilities (we hope later this year), we have instituted a study in humans with 5-fluorouracil, using supersaturation of the tissues by means of a very tight-fitting, high-altitude, Air Corps type of mask which permits us to run the pO_2's, or partial pressures of oxygen, in the blood of the patient as monitored in the femoral artery, from levels of 90 mm Hg partial pressure up to as high as 400 mm Hg during a four-hour period when the patient is receiving chemotherapy with 5-fluorouracil. These are patients all of whom have very serious internal visceral metastatic cancers.

We have been involved with this for only ten months, and we cannot tell you yet whether this is going to be beneficial on a statistical basis; but I can say that we are hopeful of success, on the basis of our initial observations of the patients at reoperation where we see the effects of the chemotherapy on the tumors and also in our assessment of what is happening as we give the therapy.

The patients, by and large, had an increased affinity for the 5-fluorouracil. I would assume all the tissues of their body have an increased affinity for 5-fluorouracil under these circumstances. We have had to reduce the dosage quite universally in these patients, sometimes to as little as half of what we ordinarily would have given in our previous group of 35 patients whom we treated without any supplemental oxygenation.

I think this is a tremendous new field. We may be on the threshold of some really solid advances in terms of improvement in the selective action of cancer chemotherapy agents on the cancer cells.

Among the things that have bothered us in this business of hyperbaric oxygenation so far is the fact that there is so much confusing data with regard to nitrogen narcosis and oxygen toxicity in the literature and also the fact that the sensors that are available for measuring oxygen tensions within tissues themselves (not the blood but the tissues) are inadequate and unreliable. We are going to have to see quickly, now, I think, some really solid work done in that area also.

Dr. J. W. Benson, Cleveland: Our experience with the use of 5-fluorouracil, although certainly not as extensive as Dr. Curreri's, is entirely consistent with his remarks. After the use of this drug by protracted infusion, maximum lesion regression persists an average of four to six weeks. Our results currently suggest that methotrexate, when used in the same way, yields somewhat more lasting effects upon tumor growth. The average duration of the so-called biopsy-negative state which occasionally follows the use of the latter drug has been between two and three months in our experience. An exception to this has been one patient whose tumor site remains biopsy negative after one year since methotrexate infusion. We therefore favor relatively early resection of those lesions which are infused adjunctively with these chemical agents before operation.

We concur with the thought that antecedent radiotherapy reduces the incidence of favorable responses to this form of chemotherapy. As previously stated, we believe inflammation, fibrosis, and diminished vascularity may account for this difference. The incidence of favorable responses among previously irradiated lesions has been approximately one third that which has occurred with similar lesions not irradiated.

Finally, I would like to stress that this method is not being proposed as a substitute for conventional forms of potentially curative therapy. Above all, it should not be regarded as a reasonable basis for compromise with conventional methods of tumor excision which are known to yield favorable results.

Dr. Charles Eckert, Albany, NY: I agree that the possibilities in the field of hyperbaric oxygenation in many areas are in their infancy and that a great many more studies are necessary to determine whether the effects observed are really due to oxygen saturation at the tissue level or whether they are due to other alterations resulting from pressure.

Whether this is really a radiomimetic quality, I think, is open to considerable question because, while both radiation therapy and alkalating agents appear to act on the DNA molecule, they appear to do this in different ways.

Dr. F. L. Mendez, Jr., Cincinnati: One thing that struck me was the fact that we were dealing with clinical patients and this was not set up originally as a research study, and therefore we had no way to compare these things one against another quite this simply.

At the present time we are using a combination of drugs, but we also have used other modalities. We have tried preoperative chemotherapy and then surgery. I would also remind you that in the days when we started this, there were very few places to turn to for advice, and, as Dr. Curreri said, it was really a probing operation. We have continued that, looking for a good drug or one we think will do the job. We think we have developed the techniques. When we have the drug available we will then go on with the rest of the study.

Clinical Manifestations and Treatment of Congestive Atelectasis

ROBERT E. L. BERRY, MD, AND CHARLES A. SANISLOW, MD, ANN ARBOR, MICH

As a complication of the clinical course of disease, injury, or operation, the sudden and unanticipated onset of dyspnea, tachypnea, and cyanosis has achieved a well-deserved respect for serious portent and need for immediate and effective treatment. It is unfortunate, therefore, that accurate diagnosis of the causative factor or factors responsible for such disasters can be considerably more difficult to achieve than simple recognition that "something has gone wrong," so dramatically manifested by the initial symptoms. For surgical patients, additional difficulty in diagnosis may be superimposed by the intangibles of anesthesia, operation, serious trauma, and errors in parenteral fluid administration. Also, the diagnostic problem is not made easier by the variety of complex disturbed physiologic processes responsible for the principal signs and symptoms of acute cardiopulmonary insufficiency: (1) cyanosis; (2) tachypnea; (3) dyspnea; (4) tachycardia; and (5) hypotension.

Congestive atelectasis is a descriptive term applied to an acute form of respiratory insufficiency characterized by intense dyspnea, cyanosis, tachypnea, and progressive hypotension secondary to a diffuse nonobstructive collapse of the pulmonary alveoli with

Presented at the 20th Annual Meeting of the Central Surgical Association, Chicago, Feb 21-23, 1963.

From the Department of Surgery, University of Michigan Medical Center.

Supported in part by grant 450 of the Horace Rackham School of Graduate Studies of the University of Michigan.

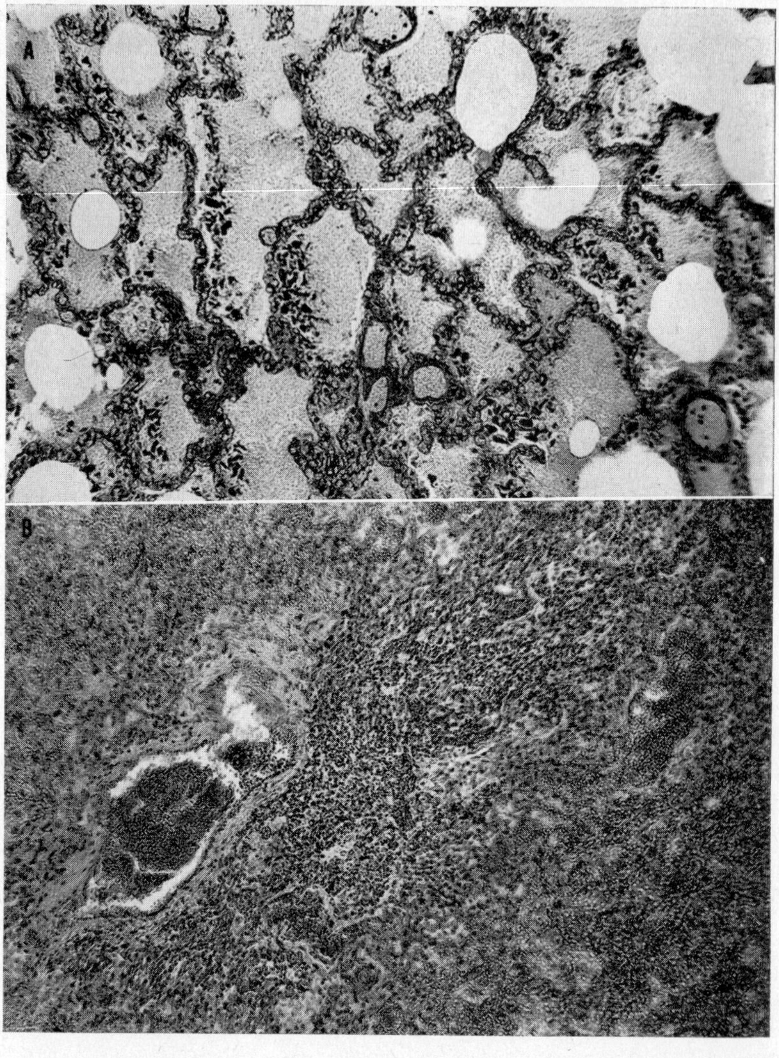

Fig 1.—Comparison of *A*, the microscopic appearance of transudative pulmonary edema and *B*, the atelectasis of congestion. There is sharp contrast between the distended fluid-filled alveoli of transudative edema and the solid pseudoangiomatous appearance of congestion. *B* is a photomicrograph of a tissue specimen obtained from autopsy in case 2.

intense interstitial plumonary capillary congestion (Fig 1). It is primarily a complication of parenteral fluids, and only with relative rarity has recovery been achieved. Certain facets of this problem are presented in the following case histories.

Report of Cases

CASE 1.—A 16-year-old girl was admitted two hours after an automobile accident.

Physical Examination.—A cut-down was functional, and 500 ml of blood had been given during transport. The patient was unconscious. Blood pressure was 90/60, pulse 120, and respirations 20. The following diagnoses were made: (1) cerebral concussion; (2) bilateral fractures of the maxillae; (3) compound fracture of right femur; and (4) multiple sutured lacerations of the scalp, face, chest, left arm, and right leg.

Subsequent Course.—Because of unconsciousness and audible rhonchi, an immediate tracheostomy was performed and oxygen administered by catheter. Within a short period of time, however, an episode occurred that was interpreted as a "cardiac arrest" and treated by the rapid infusion of 1,000 ml of whole blood and external cardiac massage. The blood pressure was restored and then rose to 156/100. Pulse rate increased to 140. Dyspnea, tachypnea, and cyanosis appeared and rapidly worsened. Apparently because of the "rapid pulse," blood transfusions were continued; the blood pressure reached a high of 166/110, and the pulse rose to 160 four hours after tracheostomy. Rapid deterioration followed, and death occurred seven hours after admission. *A total of 11 units of blood (5,500 ml) had been given.*

Autopsy.—Left lung: weight was 670 gm; marked engorgement with blood, dark red in color; no areas of normal aeration or crepitation palpable. Right lung weighed 780 gm, was dark red in color, firm consistency; only one small area of aeration and normal color was noted (at the apex). *The Heart was firm with no evidence of dilatation.*

Some serosanguineous fluid in the bronchi was noted. Microscopic examination showed intense pulmonary congestion and edema with intra-alveolar hemorrhage. Early purulent inflammation was present (aspiration).

Comment.—The obvious immediate cause of death was overtransfusion resulting in almost complete obliteration of the pulmonary air space. Anatomically the heart was "normal." Adequate warning was provided by an increasing blood pressure and worsening of dyspnea and cyanosis, but these were ignored as additional blood was given in an attempt to bring down the pulse rate and "improve her appearance." Under these circumstances, an increase in cardiac rate is not a pressor response to volumetric depletion (blood pressure 160/110). Tachycardia is the result of chemoreceptor stimulation by lowered oxygen and increasing carbon dioxide concentrations of mixed arterial blood.[20] The need is not for more blood but to correct arterial hypoxia and hypercapnia.

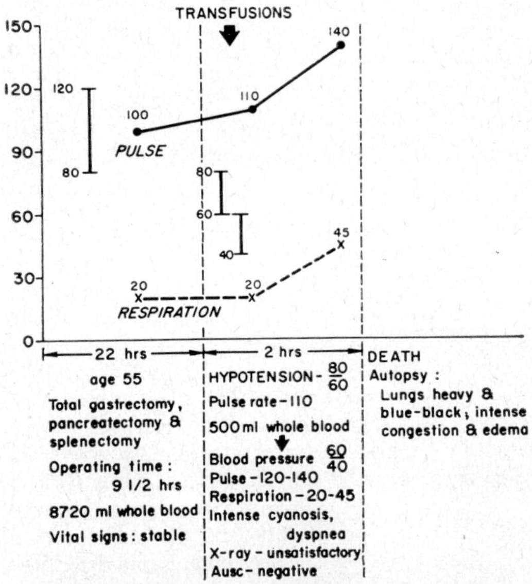

Fig 2. (case 2)—Lethal sequence of events following "supportive" transfusions given 14 hours after completion of a long operation with massive blood replacement. Death occurred two hours following onset of dyspnea, tachypnea, cyanosis, and progressive hypotension. Massive congestion of both lungs was found at autopsy (Fig 1 *B*).

CASE 2.—A 55-year-old male was operated on for an extensive adenocarcinoma involving the upper stomach and lower esophagus. Through a left thoracoabdominal incision partial esophagectomy, total gastrectomy, total pancreatectomy, duodenectomy, and splenectomy were done. Operating time was 9½ hours; parenteral fluids, 8,720 ml whole blood and 1,000 ml 5% dextrose and water. Excepting a transient fall in blood pressure to 80 systolic and some difficulty with anesthesia about midway, the operation was well tolerated. The immediate postoperative condition appeared satisfactory (Fig 2).

After about 14 hours, during which all seemed well, the blood pressure fell to 80/60, and 500 ml of whole blood was given. There was now rapid onset of progressive dyspnea, cyanosis, tachypnea, and tachycardia. Auscultation demonstrated the lungs to be "clear" bilaterally with no evidence of mediastinal shift. X-ray of the chest was unrevealing and reported as "unsatisfactory." There was no evidence of pulmonary edema or increased venous pressure. Positive pressure oxygen administration was attempted with the O.E.M.* meter mask with no response. Rapid deterioration followed, and death occurred two hours after onset of symptoms of respiratory insufficiency.

Autopsy.—Each lung was heavy (700 gm) and blue-black in color. Microscopically intense congestion (congestive atelectasis) and pulmonary edema were present (Fig 1).

Comment.—Simplicity has been emphasized in this protocol in order to demonstrate the lethal sequence of events. At a certain critical point of this insidiously progressive respiratory insufficiency, a fall in blood pressure was "logically" treated by transfusion with catastrophic results. The mechanics of this paradox remain incompletely understood, and certainly the physiological complexities of operations of this magnitude preclude identification of a single clearly culpable etiological factor. Cases 2, 3, and 4, however, do have one facet in common: loss or immobilization of considerable amounts of sodium-rich extracellular fluid, as witnessed by increased hematocrit, relative increase in hemoglobin mass in cases 3 and 4, or loss as could be reasonably anticipated from the magnitude of surgical manipulation and dissection in case 2. This concept will subsequently be discussed in detail.

* Oxygen Equipment Manufacturer.

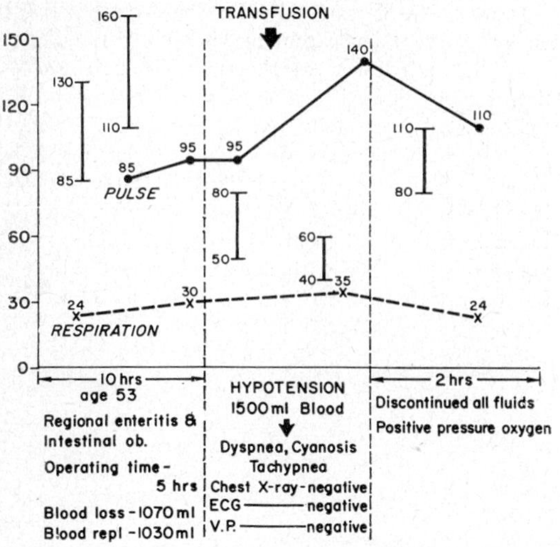

Fig 3 (case 3).—Successful recovery from acute respiratory insufficiency apparently due to congestive atelectasis. Onset of severe dyspnea, tachypnea, cyanosis, and hypotension after transfusion given for "hypotension" about five hours after completion of the operation. Despite administration of 1,500 ml of whole blood, recovery followed successful administration of positive pressure oxygen. X-ray of the chest was "normal" at the time her clinical condition was most critical (see Fig 6).

Case 3.—A 53-year-old female underwent a bypass ileotransverse colostomy for severe regional enteritis with partial intestinal obstruction. The operating time was five hours. Approximately 1½ hours prior to termination the blood pressure rose from 120/80 to 160/110. There was little change in pulse rate, and no difficulty was encountered with anesthesia. Parenteral fluids were given: 200 ml of 5% glucose in water in 0.2% NaCl and 1,030 ml of whole blood. Estimated blood loss was 1,070 ml. A third unit of blood was started at the end of the operation. Her condition appeared entirely satisfactory until about five hours after operation when hypotension was first noted (Fig 3).

Initial therapeutic effort was directed at the hypotension, and two units of whole blood (1,000 ml) were given. This was followed by progressive dyspnea, cyanosis, and tachypnea, and when the pressure fell to 60/40 and the pulse rose to 160 her condition was indeed critical. Venous pressure was normal as was an electrocardiogram. Auscultation was negative, and x-ray examination of the chest showed little change from a preoperative film (Fig 4).

Administered fluid now exceeded estimated losses as, in addition to 2,500 ml of blood, 500 ml of Hartmann's solution containing 12½ grams of serum albumin had also been given. A diagnosis of congestive atelectasis was made. Further administration of fluid was discontinued, and positive pressure oxygen was administered with the Bird respirator. Immediate improvement was noted. Within a period of two hours the systolic pressure rose to 110, pulse fell to 108, respiratory effort was markedly eased, color returned to normal, and the patient was alert and talkative (Fig 5 and 6). Five hours later the hemoglobin was found to be 17 gm% and the hematocrit 45%. This was interpreted as representing a probable absolute extracellular and plasma volume deficit. Serum electrolytes were normal. Serum proteins were not available.

Comment.—Because of the obvious serious respiratory insufficiency of congestion and refractoriness to conventional therapy, the "therapeutic book" is usually thrown at these unfortunate patients as clinical deterioration accelerates. Parenteral fluids, nasal oxygen, phlebotomy, bronchoscopy, adrenal steroids, and vasopressors are components of a diffuse therapeutic modality usually administered in a shotgun pattern as regards quantity and timing. In reality, none of these entities is effective. Furthermore,

Fig 4 (case 3).—*A*, normal preoperative appearance of the chest; *B*, portable examination of the chest taken during acute respiratory insufficiency. When this film was taken the blood pressure was 60/40, pulse 140; intense cyanosis and dyspnea were present. The patient appeared terminal. Despite intense cyanosis and dyspnea the appearance of the lungs is not strikingly different from the preoperative film. During the early phase of congestive atelectasis there may be little change in a scout chest film.

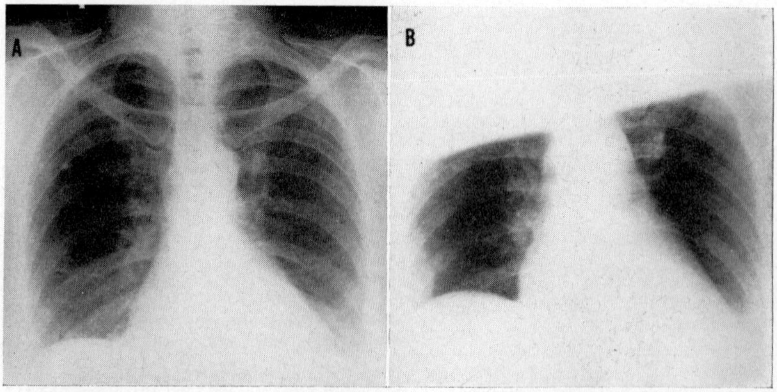

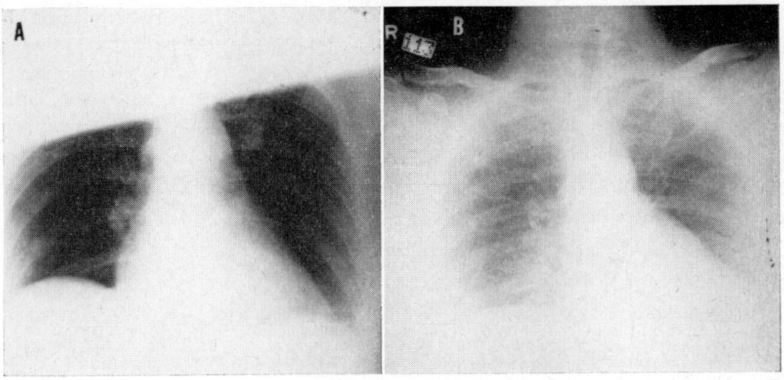

Fig 5 (case 3).—*A,* appearance of chest during acute respiratory insufficiency (this is the same film as Fig 4*B*). *B,* appearance of chest approximately eight hours after recovery from acute respiratory insufficiency. Diffuse haziness suggests a more significant exudative component. Clinical pulmonary edema did not develop, however.

parenteral fluids, phlebotomy, and vasopressors are not only contraindicated but may be deleterious. Attempts at conventional

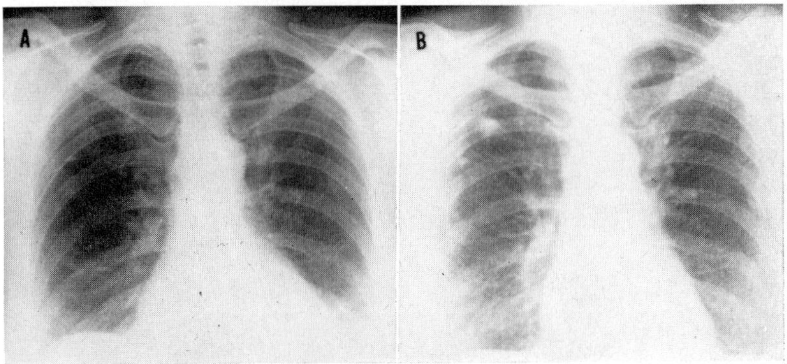

Fig 6 (case 3).—A comparison of the, *A,* normal preoperative appearance of the chest with appearance approximately 72 hours after recovery from an apparent episode of acute congestive atelestasis. There has been rapid clearing of the diffuse haziness observed in Fig 5*B*.

"tinkering" with blood volume and vascular resistance are ineffective and dangerous. Unless the hypoxemia and hypercapnia of arterial blood can be rapidly corrected, death ensues as the muscles of respiration become exhausted.

Case 4.—A 44-year-old female was operated on for severe regional enteritis accompanied by subacute peritonitis. After freeing an inflammatory mass occupying the lower abdomen, 2 feet of terminal ileum and the cecum were resected. Continuity was re-established by ileo-ascending colostomy. The sigmoid colon was inadvertently entered necessitating colostomy.

The operation required four hours. Estimated blood loss was 700 ml. Parenteral fluids given during the operation were 400 ml 5% glucose in water in 0.2% NaCl and 1,000 ml of whole blood. There was nothing of significance during the operation until toward termination when a moderate increase in respiratory rate accompanied by an increasing pulse and slowly falling blood pressure were noted (Fig 7). Blood pressure at the end of operation was 90/70. Because of this hypotension a third unit of 500 ml of blood was started. There was now onset of progressively severe dyspnea, cyanosis, and tachypnea. The pulse rose to 140, blood pressure fell to 60/?, and another unit of blood was started. The chest x-ray was grossly abnormal and

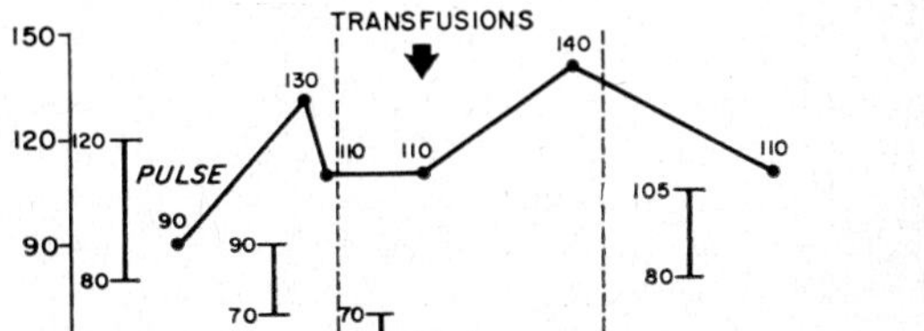

Fig 7 (case 4).—Successful recovery from acute respiratory insufficiency apparently due to congestive atelectasis. Onset of severe dyspnea, cyanosis, tachypnea, and hypotension in the immediate postoperative period after supportive transfusion given because of mild hypotension. Bronchoscopy negative at the time she appeared agonal. Successful response to positive pressure oxygen. However, frank pulmonary edema developed several hours after recovery from acute respiratory insufficiency.

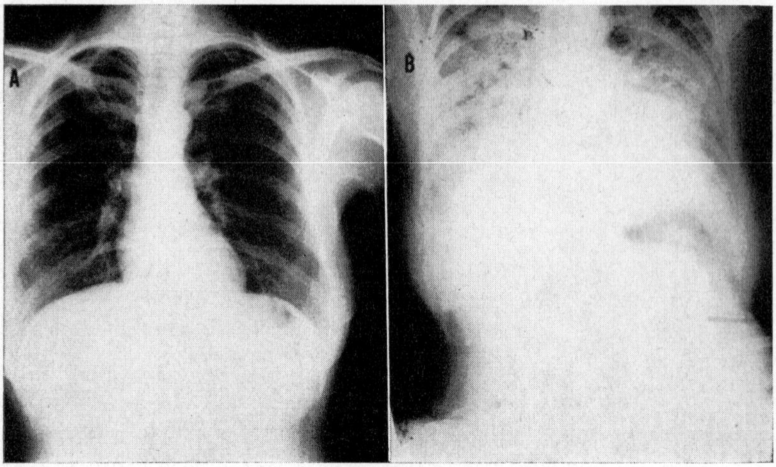

Fig 8 (case 4).—*A*, normal preoperative film of chest; *B*, appearance of the chest two hours after the onset of cyanosis, dyspnea, and a drop of pressure to 60/?. Despite the degree of diffuse pulmonary involvement and x-ray appearance of "pulmonary edema," bronchoscopy done at this time was negative, and there was no accompanying increase in venous pressure. It was several hours later (after recovery from acute respiratory insufficiency) that the exudative phase of pulmonary edema became clinically apparent. This necessitated tracheostomy and support with a respirator.

diagnosed as "pulmonary edema" (Fig 8). Bronchoscopy was entirely negative, however, and peripheral venous pressure was normal. Death appeared imminent. A diagnosis of congestive atelectasis was made, all fluids discontinued (BP 60/?), and positive pressure oxygen administered with the O.E.M. meter mask. Within 30 minutes the blood pressure increased to 100/70, pulse rate fell to 110, color markedly improved, and respiratory effort approached normal.

It is significant, however, that five hours after recovery from this episode of respiratory insufficiency, decompensation into frank pulmonary edema was observed necessitating tracheostomy and temporary support with the Morsch respirator. Within a period of eight hours previously normal venous pressures rose to 40 cm of water. At this time the hemoglobin was 22 gm%, the hematocrit 55%, serum electrolytes were normal, but proteins were not available. X-ray of the chest demonstrated considerable clearing despite the high venous pressure (Fig 9). A removal of 650 ml of blood by phlebotomy was well tolerated.

Comment.—A transudative pulmonary edema component in this instance cannot be ignored, yet there apparently was nothing wrong with this patient's heart, and fluid replacement during operation had done little more than balance the losses. *Furthermore, hypotension is not part of the usual syndrome of acute left heart failure.* The apparent precipitating factor of acute respiratory insufficiency was a single transfusion followed by aggravation as additional blood was given to correct the "low blood pressure." Hemoglobin and hematocrit levels again suggest a severe volumetric loss of extracellular fluid.

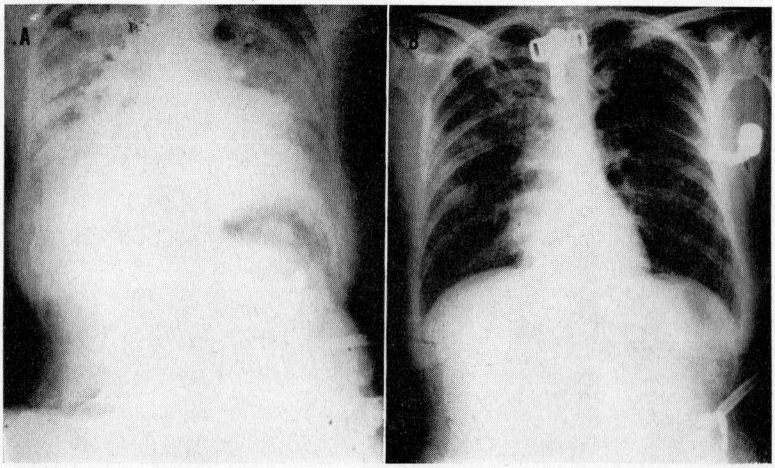

Fig 9 (case 4).—*A*, appearance during period of acute respiratory insufficiency (same as Fig 8*B*); *B*, appearance of chest 18 hours later demonstrating clearing of lung fields following tracheostomy and support with respirator.

Pathologic Anatomy

There has been adequate gross and microscopic description of the pathologic features of congestive atelectasis.[3,10,12,19] The term "congestive,"[12] as related to the atelectasis, has apparently not been widely used, however. Descriptive terms as "diffuse" and "nonobstructive" atelectasis have been suggested, but perhaps the most commonly used is "intense congestion of the lung." Regardless of terminology, the pulmonary pathology of congestive atelectasis is reasonably specific. There is considerably less specificity of associated clinical disease states, as this abnormality has been identified with excessive administration of parenteral water and electrolyte, excessive transfusion of blood, compression and blast injuries, and burns and shock.[1,5,17,18,19]

The essential findings are as follows:

1. Grossly the lungs present a reddish-blue to blue-black discoloration. Areas of normal aeration and crepitation may be entirely absent. Both lungs are always involved, and the tissues resemble a solid organ difficult to recognize as lung. Lungs are individually heavy, usually in the 600-850 gm range.
2. Microscopically the appearance may be that of gross hemorrhage, but areas of congestion disappear upon inflation of the lung. In miniature, this same phenomenon may be observed in the collapsed viable lung prior to "prophylactic" periodic inflation necessitated by open thoracotomy. The areas of blue-black discoloration are readily obliterated by inflation.
3. Microscopically there is engorgement of the uniformly dilated pulmonary capillaries, venules, and arterioles resulting in a pseudoangiomatous appearance.
4. Atelectasis of the pulmonary alveoli occurs with loss of normal alveolar arrangement. The epitheliod cells are closely packed together obliterating alveolar air spaces.

The difference in microscopic appearance between pulmonary edema and congestive atelectasis is demonstrated by comparing Fig 1, *A and B*.

Pathologic Physiology

Simply stated, the transport of oxygen from air to the tissues and carbon dioxide from tissues to the air is dependent upon three major systems:

1. The proper movement of air resulting in adequate alveolar ventilation.
2. Normal blood transport as a function of adequate cardiac output and perfusion pressures.
3. A normal transport zone between blood and air. This depends upon the thickness and available area of the alveolar membrane and the amount of blood shunted past nonfunctioning alveoli.

A decompensation of one or more of these systems is quite capable of producing any or all of the signs and symptoms of acute cardiopulmonary insufficiency. Detailed discussions of the movement of respiratory air and changes in cardiac output are not within the context of this paper and will be considered only as significantly related to the titled subject. Although to some degree harboring abnormal components of the other systems, the disturbed transport of oxygen and carbon dioxide resulting from congestive atelectasis appears primarily to be a disturbance of the normal transport zone between blood and air.[25]

There are two major considerations: (1) how does congestive atelectasis develop, and (2) what are the physiologic disturbances resulting in refractoriness to conventional treatment and high mortality rates? Knowledge of both remains incomplete.

The Cause of Congestive Atelectasis.—Change in Environmental Barometric Pressure: One of the first comprehensive experimental studies was made by Fegler and Banister.[12] Rabbits were subjected to controlled environmental barometric pressure (100-500 mm Hg) with variations in oxygen partial pressure (pO_2) and speed of decompression. The conclusions were:

1. Congestive atelectasis was not produced when environmental pressure was increased to 500 mm Hg and then reduced to a normal 300 mm Hg (ground level).
2. The most important component in the development of congestive atelectasis was rarefaction of air produced by low barometric pressure and followed by recompression. This could be prevented, even at low pressure, by a slight increase in intrapulmonic pressure.
3. The partial pressure of oxygen (and therefore the degree of anoxia) was of no etiological significance.
4. Forcible displacement of stomach and liver in a thoracic direction increased atelectatic areas, as did prolonged anesthesia, time duration of closed pneumothorax, and simultaneous tight bandaging of both abdomen and chest.

These data are of significance and demonstrate that: (1) the atelectasis of congestion may develop *without an obstructive component* in the usual clinical sense; and (2) if a "critical closing pressure" of the alveoli is a reality, it may be obviated by a small increase in intrapulmonic pressure. Because anoxia was apparently not a factor in these experiments, the physical factors may be examined by the LaPlace expression for a sphere which relates surface tension,* curvatures of the surface, and the resultant pressure difference across it:

$$P = \frac{T \times 2}{r}$$

where: P, indicates pressure in dynes per square centimeter; T, surface tension in dynes/cm; r, radius in centimeters; dyne, that force which acting continuously on a mass of 1 gm will impart to it an acceleration of 1 cm/sec.

Assuming that surface tension of the alveolar lining membrane does not change, by analogy a decreasing alveolar pressure will be followed by an equivalent decrease in radius and eventual alveolar collapse. As protection from complete collapse is provided by a small increase in intrapulmonic over ambient pressure, in these experiments the critical factor would appear to be small. It should be noted, however, that changes in surface tension of the alveolar lining membrane secondary to such higly unphysiologic environmental pressure cannot be excluded as a precipitating and/or sustaining entity.

Regardless of these observations, the realities of clinical congestive atelectasis appear to be more importantly related to other areas.

Changes in Surface Tension of the Alveolar Lining Membrane: Reference is again made to the LaPlace expression:

$$P = \frac{T \times 2}{r}$$

It would then follow that an increase in surface tension would double the pressure increment across the sphere and by analogous inference comparably increase the intra-alveolar pressure necessary to maintain normal expansion. The alveoli of the lung are lined by a layer of a substance demonstrated to be a liproprotein (predominantly a phospholipid) that, under normal circumstances, has a very low surface tension.[2,9,14] Any protein denaturing or other vitiation of the alveolar lining membrane resulting in increased surface tension could conceivably close the alveoli if a comparable increase in pressure were absent. An increase in the surface tension of alveolar lining material has been described after anoxia or extended extracorporeal perfusion with loss of the specific surface active substance.[14] Change in surface tension activity as a contributive and/or sustaining component of congestive atelectasis is of interest but requires considerably more proof.

The Humoral Factors: Attempts to evaluate humoral changes as an etiological consideration in congestive atelectasis have not been rewarding, as much remains to be learned in this field particularly as pertaining to man. Pulmonary artery pressure elevation, apparently due to pulmonary vasoconstriction, attends acidosis, hypercapnia, and acute anoxia.[4,11] The catecholamines apparently have a variable effect depending upon the degree of anoxia. With moderate hypoxia, epinephrine and norepinephrine apparently do not increase pulmonary artery pressure to that degree observed with greater oxygen want.[15] Changes in pulmonary vasculature produced by histamine are surprisingly small; infusion of acetylcholine into the pulmonary artery precipitates a fall in pressure which is greater if pulmonary vasoconstriction has been induced by anoxia.[7,13]

Humoral factors cannot be lightly shunted aside however. Hyperemia of the lungs after tourniquet release in tourniquet shock occurs before a fall in blood pressure can be recorded, thus suggesting an important humoral factor.[19] Serotonin (5-hydroxytryptamine) produces a marked increase in pulmonary vasoconstriction and pulmonary artery pressure.[7] Because serotonin is liberated by intravascular clotting, the demonstrated profound effect upon pulmo-

* Surface tension: The contractile surface of a liquid by which it tends to assume a spherical form and to present the least possible surface.

nary vasculature warrants further investigation in order to exclude any causative relationship with congestive atelectasis.

Although most investigators agree that the tone of the pulmonary vasculature can be changed by drugs, the physiologic importance of such changes has been challenged.[8] This does not include endogenous humoral response inherent to local tissues, however. As emphasized by Drinker, the effect of hypoxia and acidosis of mixed arterial blood upon lung capillaries and the capacity for contiguous lung bed capillaries to dilate and become congested as "anoxia begets anoxia" cannot be easily dismissed as of little importance.[10]

Parenteral Fluids: Congestive atelectasis *is a complication* of parenteral fluid administration. It is the "why" that remains elusive.

With the exception of hypotension, Jenkins et al were able to reproduce clinical manifestations of congestive atelectasis in dogs.[19] The results are summarized as follows:

1. In the absence of hemorrhage or hypoxia, rapid injection of 0.9% NaCl produced: (*a*) a rise in pulmonary artery pressure and a fall in systemic pressure; and (*b*) no change in jugular vein and left atrial pressure. After temporary recovery, further administration produced a second rise in pulmonary artery pressure simultaneously accompanied by falling left atrial pressure suggesting that left ventricular failure was not causative.

2. Concurrently, intrapleural expiratory pressure became positive and inspiratory pressure became more negative. Respiratory work was increased but tidal air moved changed little. The lungs were becoming "stiff."

3. The rate of oxygen consumption fell, cyanosis appeared, pulmonary and systemic pressure fell, and just before death the peripheral venous and left atrial pressures rose rapidly.

4. Tourniquet shock produced visibly hyperemic lung before saline injection. After infusion, there were pressure increases in the pulmonary artery, peripheral veins, and left atrium while systemic arterial pressure fell. This was compatible with backward heart failure.

5. Hemorrhage and controlled hypoxia remarkably increased the lung blood volume. Alteration in pressure relationship between the pulmonary artery and left atrium was again noted as was stiffening of the lung. Rapid injections of saline again produced vascular pressures comparable with acute heart failure, and the *severity of the shock was increased.*

It is indeed unfortunate that the clinical form of the disease does not lend itself well to these excellent investigative techniques. Symptomatic clinical disease, however, represents an advanced state of development, and necessity for saving the patient's life becomes overwhelmingly dominant.

A search for common denominators in cases 2, 3, and 4 reasonably permits certain observations:

1. These were long operations (four to nine hours), and at least 1,000 ml of whole blood was given in each instance.

2. All were operations of considerable magnitude requiring extensive dissection and manipulation of soft tissues. Important inflammatory components were present in cases 3 and 4.

3. All operations were apparently well tolerated.

4. Precipitating factors all followed the same pattern: mild hypotension thought to be due to "hypovolemia," then a single transfusion was given, followed by progressive cyanosis, dyspnea, tachypnea, hypotension, and tachycardia.

5. Intraoperative replacement of blood and administration of other fluids did not appear excessive. Respiratory insufficiency appeared to be "triggered" by a single transfusion suggesting a "straw that broke the camel's back."

6. Subsequent hematocrit and relative hemoglobin concentrations were all significantly elevated. Little change was observed in serum electrolyte concentrations. Preoperative serum protein determinations were normal, but no information is available regarding protein change during and following recovery from acute pulmonary insufficiency.

The increase in hematocrit and relative increase in hemoglobin mass, a common factor in all instances, infers that plasma water and sodium salt loss have exceeded that of red blood cells and probably that of plasma protein, resulting in relative acute increase in both plasma protein concentration and red cell mass. This would be compatible with extracellular water and salt sequestration expected to accompany soft tissue dissection and manipulation necessitated by these operations.

The precipitation of lethal pulmonary congestion following the intraperitoneal injection of a Tyrode's solution saturated with albumin has been demonstrated in the experimental animal (rat). Moyer and Nissan, as a part of studies on oxygen consumption during variables of sodium depletion, found significant increases in hematocrit and plasma colloid content as well as pulmonary and hepatic congestion, sanguineous pleural effusion, and cardiac dilatation after administration of 10 ml per 100 gm of body weight of the modified Tyrode's solution to rats by the intraperitoneal route.[24] These observations have suggested that the simultaneous occurrence of extracellular fluid depletion and an increase in intravascular colloid profoundly affects blood flow in small vessels. There is experimental evidence demonstrating the development of transudative pulmonary edema at significantly lower pulmonary vein pressure if the plasma colloid osmotic pressure has been reduced.[16] There is little information regarding the specific effects of increased colloid osmotic pressure on the pulmonary circulation. Working with fine glass tubes, Lawler has demonstrated a ratio reversal of the flowing/static hematocrit by the addition of serum albumin to human blood.[21] The flowing hematocrit now becomes greater, and the flow of blood is sharply reduced. Parallel occurrence in the capillaries of living animals would be significant but remains conjectural.

Cautious application of these experimental data to clinical cases is tenuous but not grossly unreasonable. Volumetric depletion of extracellular fluid produced by large exudating wounds, extensive dissection, and soft tissue trauma when accompanied by repeated blood transfusions is not without comparative analogy in clinical cases. The profound effects upon the cardiovascular system produced by salt depletion are probably more than those of decreased volume. Significant disturbance of capillary flow produced by colloid alterations and direct cellular effects may well attend salt deficits thus setting the stage for variable response to "corrective" parenteral fluids. As expressed by Moyer and Nissan:[24]

> The dependence on the quality of biologic response to sodium depletion upon the concomitant alteration in the concentrations of salts and colloids in the plasma suggests that use of colloid-containing solutions for the treatment of certain oligemic states could be a two-edged sword; beneficial one hour under particular circumstances and lethal another hour under only slightly different hydration circumstances.

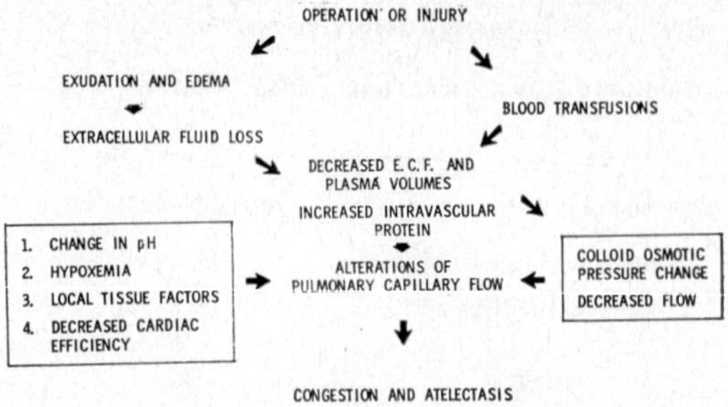

Fig 10.—Schematic demonstration of the many potential factors that must be considered as providing contributive components to the etiology of congestive atelectasis. No claim for clairvoyance is made, as the multiple biological variables defy accurate assessment.

The cause of congestive atelectasis remains unknown. As complex as the interrelated biologic variables appear to be, one simple truth emerges: low blood pressure is a sign and not a cause of problems, and every hypotensive episode is not due to the loss of blood Fig. 10).

The Resulting Physiologic Disturbances.—As progressive numbers of alveoli become atelectatic, the oxygen saturation of arterial blood delivered to the left heart falls, and the pCO_2 increases secondary to mixing normally oxygenated with venous blood shunted past nonfunctioning alveoli (Fig 11). The resultant hypoxemia and hypercapnia will therefore respond only to treatment directed at restoring function to the atelectatic alveoli. Osborn et al, in an extensive study of pulmonary insufficiency following cardiopulmonary bypass and open heart surgery, were able to observe the development of hypoxemia, hypercapnia, and acidosis in a syndrome comparable to or equivalent with congestive atelectasis.[25] The sickest patients and those who died demonstrated a marked increase in minute respiratory volume, normal or somewhat increased cardiac output, and a sharply increased pCO_2 of arterial blood compared to that of alveolar air. This was interpreted as arteriovenous shunting and diffuse alveolar atelectasis.

PULMONARY ARTERY BLOOD

↓

CAPILLARY FLOW OF PULMONARY ARTERY (Venous) BLOOD

↙ ↘

OPEN ALVEOLI
a. adequate increase pO_2
b. adequate reduction pCO_2

ATELECTATIC ALVEOLI
a. no change in pO_2
b. no change in pCO_2

↘ ↙

PULMONARY VEIN (Arterialized) BLOOD

↓

a. reduced pO_2
b. increased pCO_2

Pulmonary Arteriovenous Shunting as a Cause of Hypoxemia and Hypercapnia in Congestive Atelectasis.

Fig 11.—Because of the high ratio of the pCO_2 of arterial blood to that found in the alveoli, pulmonary arteriovenous shunting has been suggested as the cause of hypoxemia and hypercapnea in the congestive syndrome.[25] Blood flowing past atelectatic alveoli would remain unchanged and when mixed with oxygenated blood results in a net decrease in pO_2 and increase in pCO_2.

The physiologic effects of hypoxia, per se, are difficult to assess because of attendant changes in blood pH, pCO_2, lactic acid, and many other biochemical variables. In the experimental animal (dog), generalized systemic hypoxia results in an increase in venous return and a striking decrease in systemic blood volume.[20] These changes have been attributed to systemic venoconstriction. If this occurs in humans the severe hypoxia of clinical congestive atelectasis would theoretically establish the elements of a vicious circle.

Systemic hypoxemia in most mammalian species is accompanied by an elevation in the heart rate and a small increase in cardiac output. As the heart is perfused with progressively poorly oxygenated blood, the contractile force decreases. The effect upon the total vascular resistance is nonspecific.[20]

The stimulus for increased rate and amplitude of respiration provided by the proprioceptive reflex of pulmonary congestion and increasing arterial pCO_2 needs little emphasis; essentially this is a compensatory effort at reducing hypercapnia (hypercarbia) by lowering the pCO_2 of alveolar air. The effectiveness of this biological compensation appears severely limited in congestive atelectasis because of arteriovenous shunting.

Because of CO_2 retention and hypoxic depression of intracellular metabolism, an increased hydrogen ion accumulation is compounded by elements of a respiratory and metabolic "acidosis." [22,25,29] Biologic effects directly attributable to increasing hydrogen ion concentration become obscured by a multiplicity of complex variables. Decreased cardiac output, a falling blood pressure, and sudden death have been attributed to acidemia. There is general agreement, however, that the deleterious effects produced by hypoxemia are aggravated and possibly synergized by any significant increase in the hydrogen ion concentration.[22]

Diagnosis

Exclusion is important in the diagnosis of congestive atelectasis because *what is not present can be as important as the presenting signs and symptoms.* Experience has demonstrated that the most common erroneous clinical impressions are: (1) acute hypovolemic shock (this is the most frequent and serious mistake); (2) obstructive atelectasis; and (3) acute left heart failure. Significant differential points are shown in the Table.

The clinical considerations may be examined as follows: (1) the disease state and preoperative condition; (2) the conduct of the operation; (3) postoperative or posttraumatic decompensation into pulmonary insufficiency.

Disease State and Preoperative Condition.—Dogmatic statements outlining the disease state or type of injury that potentially could develop congestive atelectasis are not valid because of the nonspecific nature of reported [1,17,19] and observed cases and the obvious successful management of parallel clinical situations in which this complication did not occur. For the most part, however, the disease or injury component has been of considerable magnitude. Of the four included cases in this report, one was a severe trauma resulting from an automobile accident, one an advanced carcinoma of the stomach with pancreatic invasion, and two

Differental Features Between Congestive Atelectasis, Obstructive

	Cyanosis	Dyspnea	Hypotension	X-Ray of Chest
Congestive atelectasis	Deep and refractory to usual O_2 therapy	Severe, with limitation of expiratory phase; tachypnea begins early and is severe; no response to O_2 therapy	Progressive and severe; unresponsive to and aggravated by parenteral fluids, particularly blood; peripheral "cold" shock	Early: little change; late: diffuse patchy involvement
Obstructive atelectasis	Not as deep and more responsive to oxygen	Less severe; partial alleviation with O_2 therapy	Not necessarily attendant; if present, is not a dominant feature	Mediastinal and tracheal shift; unilateral involvement
Hypovolemia	"Cold" shock but color changes less marked	Uncommon	Dominates clinical picture; responds to administration of fluids	Noncontributory
Acute left heart failure	May be absent	Moderate to severe; expiratory phase has greater amplitude; some response to O_2; tachypnea may be severe	Is not a prominant feature although blood pressure fall may occur	Early onset of pulmonary "edema"

* All signs, symptoms, and responses to treatment vary considerably depending upon temporal relationships. There is no real specificity of any given sign or symptom, and any value so derived must depond upon integration into the total clinical picture.

were cases of advanced regional enteritis with appreciable inflammatory and obstructive factors. Successful recovery of these last two were the stimulus for this report.

Considerable anticipatory respect has been awarded surgical disease attended by: (1) a significant inflammatory component; (2) chronic anemia; (3) metabolic erosion produced by advanced disease or malnutrition; (4) severe trauma particularly if accompanied by significant hypotension; (5) periods of anesthesia in excess of six hours; and (6) excessive obesity.

Conduct of the Operation.—It is doubtful that the type of anesthetic or method of administration is a diagnostic consideration. Drinker, during studies of lymph flow in dog lungs under conditions of rigid control of respiration, observed that parts of the lungs dependent to the major orifices of the pulmonary veins slowly underwent changes compatible with congestive atelectasis.[10] These congested areas disappeared when variable amplitudes of respiration were permitted. A critical eye has been cast at the routine use of anesthetic bag compression as a rather unpredictable type of controlled respiration. Common sense, however, dictates that if this practice significantly contributed to pulmonary congestion more acute congestion should be seen. Regardless of the damping effects on respiration produced by anesthesia or controlled respiration, neither seems to be a primary etiologic factor although a contributory component cannot be ignored.

Certain signs may occur during operation which have been identified with the subsequent development of the congestion syndrome. These *signs are not diagnostic and do little more than suggest that the syndrome may be developing.* Their onset should initiate thoughtful consideration for the need to terminate the operation as expeditiously as possible.

1. It is usually an operation of considerable magnitude requiring repeated transfusion. The first hours go well, but it is soon apparent that the amount of blood necessary to achieve circulatory stability appears significantly greater than the estimated blood loss. The possibilities: is this an inaccurate estimate of blood loss, a manifestation of the instability of body fluid compartments, or is the blood starting its deadly entrapment in the lung?

2. The anesthetic is not going well. Attempts at "proper" depths of anesthesia are accompanied by undesirable fall of blood pressure and increase in pulse rate. Or, more importantly, "adequate" relaxation is accompanied by poor color or other evidence of oxygen want. Again: Is this poor pulmonary ventilation, excessive blood loss, instability of fluid compartments, or has blood entrapment in the lungs begun?

*Atelectasis, Hypovolemic Shock, and Acute Left Heart Failure.**

Auscultation	Venous Pressure	Bronchoscopy	Phlebotomy	Digitalization
Surprisingly few findings in early stage	No change in early stage; veins of neck not distended	Of no benefit; rules out pulmonary edema of acute left heart failure by exclusion	Of no benefit; may aggravate hypotension	Of no benefit
Rales and change in breath sounds	No pertinent change	Diagnostic and therapeutically beneficial	Of no benefit	Of no benefit
No change	No change	Of no benefit	Contraindicated	Of no benefit
Early onset of rales	Rapid increase as right heart failure ensues	"Pulmonary edema"	Of great benefit	Beneficial

3. The systolic pressure is drifting downward but is not accompanied by a parallel fall in diastolic pressure resulting in a narrowing of the pulse pressure. At the other end of the scale: significant increase of both systolic and diastolic pressure may be meaningful. Fluids should subsequently be used sparingly.

Decompensation Into Pulmonary Insufficiency. It is well recognized that significant depression of pulmonary function may occur without clinical symptoms.[26] The onset of symptomatic congestive atelectasis, therefore, is a most ominous warning of the magnitude of the pulmonary pathology, the advanced state of hypoxia and hypercapnia, and urgent need for effective treatment (Table).

Dyspnea. This comes on rapidly, is steadily progressive, is not alleviated by conventional oxygen administration, and quickly incorporates the energetic use of the accessory muscles of respiration. The initial attempts to move air are most vigorous, resulting in an increased minute volume although the tidal volume is unchanged or decreased.[25] The expiratory phase of the respiratory cycle becomes progressively less efficient as the lung stiffens. Inspiratory negative pressures increase, but the expiratory intrapleural pressure approaches zero or may become positive.[19]

Cyanosis. It is deep and refractory to conventional oxygen administration.

Tachypnea. This is severe and may reach rates of 35-45 per minute.

Tachycardia. Tachycardia is prominent; rates: 120-160 per minute. Elevated pulse rate is due to oxygen debt of arterial blood and not hypovolemia.

Hypotension. The blood pressure continues a relentless downward course and is most serious because of the fallaciously assumed need for the correction of "shock" by the administration of parenteral fluids. Whole blood given under these circumstances can literally be the "kiss of death."

X-ray of the Chest. Early in the process this may show little change (Fig 6). A chest film is of real value in excluding other intrapulmonary pathology, particularly obstructive atelectasis. Subsequent x-rays of the chest when positive for congestion tend to demonstrate diffuse parenchymal involvement.

Auscultation of the Chest. Despite symptoms of severe pulmonary insufficiency, early auscultation of the chest may demonstrate surprisingly few abnormalities.

Bronchoscopy. Therapeutically ineffective, when done early it's completely negative. Transudative pulmonary edema is absent at this stage but may subsequently occur and must be watched for.

Venous Pressures. Usually these are normal in the early stages. Neck veins are not distended.

Treatment

Mortality rates from congestive atelectasis are high. Among possible identifiable causes are: (1) advanced state of the congestive process by the time of recognition; (2) severe oxygen debt and acidosis; (3) inability to reverse the congestive process; and (4) continued administration of parenteral fluids because of "hypotension."

To date, the only effective treatment: (1) stop all parenteral infusions; and (2) effectively administer positive pressure oxygen.

The Hazard of Parenteral Infusion.—Repeated clinical experience has demonstrated that the falling blood pressure only too often captures the therapeutic imagination in these circumstances, and the intense cyanosis and dyspnea are relatively ignored. The result is continued infusions of fluids and administration of oxygen by nasal catheter. *This is not the Hypotension of Hypovolemia.* The cause of this hypotension is not known but probably is closely related to serious disturbance of the cardiovascular system initiated and sustained by hypoxia and acidosis.[20,24,25]

Administration of Oxygen.—The mechanics of corrective action and the value of positive pressure oxygen therapy in acute pulmonary edema have been well demonstrated.[6,23,27,28] Although congestive atelectasis is not an edema in the transudative context, it has been so considered because of the predominant interstitial space capillary congestion.[10] Conventional administration of oxygen by nasal catheter or tent is ineffective in congestive atelectasis. Survival has only followed the use of positive pressure oxygen when all other therapeutic measures have been ineffectual.

The Bird respirator, successfully used in case 3, permits administration of 100% oxygen up to pressures of 40 cm of water and flow rates of 80 liters per minute. The system must be as tight as possible if maximum pressures are to be obtained, particularly during the important inspiratory phase. Adequate cooperation from a cyanotic, gasping, and semiconscious patient may be impossible to obtain and render administration of oxygen by oronasal mask a farce. Recourse must then be taken to a cuffed intratracheal tube and, if this is also unsatisfactory, to tracheostomy. A tight-fitting tracheostomy is required if mediastinal leak of air is to be avoided.

Summary

Congestive atelectasis is a form of acute respiratory insufficiency characterized by nonobstructive, nontransudative, alveolar collapse and intense interstitial pulmonary capillary congestion. The cause is unknown and the mortality is high; it is a complication of parenteral fluid therapy.

The attendant clinical symptoms of severe cyanosis, dyspnea, tachycardia, and progressive hypotension may be triggered by a single transfusion given to "stabilize the circulation." The subsequent hypoxemia and hypercapnia are severe as are the respiratory and metabolic components of the accompanying acidosis.

The only effective treatment is efficiently administered positive pressure oxygen. Emphasis has been placed upon proper interpretation of the attending hypotension and tachycardia if fallacious and lethal administration of additional parenteral fluids is to be avoided.

Robert E. L. Berry, MD, Department of Surgery, University of Michigan Medical Center, Ann Arbor, Mich.

REFERENCES

1. Adwan, K. O., and Wilson, B. J.: The Effect of Treatment for Chronic Anemia on Respiratory Dynamics, Amer Surg 26:152, 1960.

2. Avery, M. E.: The Alveolar Lining Layer: A Review of Studies on Its Role in Pulmonary Mechanics and in the Pathogenesis of Atelectasis, Pediatrics 30:324, 1962.

3. Bergamini, H., and Shepard, A.: Bilateral Atelectasis of the Lung, Ann Surg 86:35, 1927.

4. Bergofsky, E. H.; Lehr, D. E.; and Fishman, A. P.: The Effect of Changes in Hydrogen Ion Concentration on the Pulmonary Circulation, J Clin Invest 41:1492, 1962.

5. Berry, R. E. L.: The Abuse of Parenteral Fluids During Anaesthesia and the Immediate Postoperative Period, Amer A Nurse Anesth J (Aug) 1954.

6. Bondurant, S., and Hickam, J. B.: Pulmonary and Circulatory Effects of Acute Pulmonary Vascular Engorgement in Normal Subjects, J Clin Invest 35:692, 1956.

7. Borst, H. G.; Berglund, E.; and McGregor, M.: The Effects of Pharmacologic Agents on the Pulmonary Circulation in the Dog, J Clin Invest 36:669, 1957.

8. Burton, A. C., in Pulmonary Circulation: International Symposium, 1958, edited by Adams, W. R., and Veith, I., New York: Grune & Stratton, Inc., 1959, pp 26-35.

9. Clements, J. A.; Brown, E. S.; and Johnson, R. P.: Pulmonary Surface Tension and Mucous Lining of the Lungs: Some Theoretical Considerations, J Appl Physiol 12:262, 1958.

10. Drinker, C. K.: Pulmonary Edema and Inflammation, Cambridge: Harvard University Press, 1945.

11. Duke, H. N.: Observations on the Effects of Hypoxia on the Pulmonary Vascular Bed, J Physiol 135:45, 1957.

12. Fegler, J., and Banister, J.: Congestive Atelectasis in Lungs of Rabbits and Other Animals Subjected to the Action of Low Barometric Pressure, Quart J Exp Physiol 33:291, 1946.

13. Fritts, H. W., Jr.; Harris, P.; Clauss, R. H.; Odell, J. E.; and Cournand, A.: The Effect of Acetylcholine on the Human Pulmonary Circulation Under Normal and Hypoxic Conditions, J Clin Invest 37:99, 1958.

14. Gardner, R. E., et al: Cited by Osborn et al.[25]

15. Goldring, R. M.; Turino, G. M.; Cohen, G.; Jameson, A. G.; Bass, B. G.; and Fishman, A. P.: The Catecholamines in the Pulmonary Arterial Pressor Response to Acute Hypoxia, J Clin Invest 41:1211, 1962.

16. Guyton, A. C., and Lindsey, A. W.: Effect of Elevated Left Atrial Pressure and Decreased Plasma Protein Concentration on the Development of Pulmonary Edema, Circ Res 7:649, 1959.

17. Hatch, H. B., Jr., and Carrera, G. H.: Congestive Atelectasis: A Fatal Postoperative Complication, J Thorac Cardiov Surg 37:257, 1959.

18. Holden, W. D.; Cole, J. W.; and Portmann, A. F.: Myocardial Intolerance to Excessive Blood Transfusion, Surg Gynec Obstet 90:455, 1950.

19. Jenkins, M. T.; Jones, R. F.; Wilson, B.; and Moyer, C. A.: Congestive Atelectasis: A Complication of the Intravenous Infusion of Fluids, Ann Surg 132:327, 1950.

20. Kahler, R. L.; Goldblatt, A.; and Braunwald, E.: The Effects of Acute Hypoxia on the Systemic Venous and Arterial Systems and on Myocardial Contractile Force, J Clin Invest 41:1553, 1962.

21. Lawler, W. H.: Cited by Moyer et al.[24]

22. Manger, W. M.; Nahas, G. G.; Hassam, D.; Habif, D. V.; and Papper, E. M.: Effect of pH Control and Increased O_2 Delivery on the Course of Hemorrhagic Shock, Ann Surg 156:503, 1962.

23. McGregor, M., and Becklake, M. R.: The Relationship of Oxygen Cost of Breathing to Respiratory Mechanical Work and Respiratory Force, J Clin Invest 40:971, 1961.

24. Moyer, C. A., and Nissan, S.: Alterations in the Basal Oxygen Consumptions of Rats Attendant Upon Three Types of Dehydration, Ann Surg 154 (suppl):51, 1961.

25. Osborn, J. J.; Popper, R. W.; Kerth, W. J.; and Gerbode, F.: Respiratory Insufficiency Following Open Heart Surgery, Ann Surg 156:638, 1962.

26. Schramel, R. J.; Cameron, R.; Ziskind, M. M.; Adam, M.; and Creech, O., Jr.: Studies of Pulmonary Diffusion After Open Heart Surgery, J Thorac Cardiov Surg 38:281, 1959.

27. Sharp, J. T.; Bunnell, I. L.; Griffith, G. T.; and Greene, D. G.: The Effects of Therapy on Pulmonary Mechanics in Human Pulmonary Edema, J Clin Invest 40:665, 1961.

28. Sharp, J. T.; Griffith, G. T.; Bunnell, I. L.; and Greene, D. G.: Ventilatory Mechanics in Pulmonary Edema in Man, J Clin Invest 37:111, 1958.

29. Weidner, M. G., Jr., and Simeone, F. A.: Physiology of Prolonged Oligemic Hypotension: Investigation of Pulmonary Function, Ann Surg 156:493, 1962.

Mechanisms of Fever in Pulmonary Atelectasis

A. M. LANSING, MD, PhD, FRCS(C), AND W. G. JAMIESON, MD, LONDON, ONT, CANADA

Pulmonary atelectasis, a common postoperative complication, is associated with high fever, tachycardia, and a rapid respiratory rate. The stimuli for these changes and the mechanisms whereby they are effected are the topics of this paper. An experimental method for production of the clinical syndrome will be described first and then the investigation of the physiological disturbances. The physiological studies consist of two aspects: the changes that cause fever, and the stimuli for these changes.

Methods

The experimental animals were mongrel dogs of both sexes, weighing 20 to 40 lb. They were devocalized and allowed to recover for one week in the animal house before use in the experiment. The diet consisted of standard animal chow with the addition of meat five days a week. Anesthesia was induced in most instances by the intravenous injection of hexobarbital (Evipal *) in a dose of 15 mg/lb. This gave a duration of anesthesia of 30 to 60 minutes at most, although the animals responded to bronchoscopic stimulation within five to ten minutes. Pentobarbital was not used because of the prolonged duration of anesthesia and marked depression of rectal temperature that it caused.

Temperature was measured by a Yellow Springs Instruments telethermometer, the animal being awake except when the effect of anesthesia on temperature was studied. The rectal temperature was measured by insertion of the probe at least three inches beyond the anus, skin temperature by a surface electrode on the ear and a needle electrode under the skin over the scapula, and room temperature by a mercury thermometer. The thermal circulation index (TCI) was calculated from these measurements.[1] Heart rate was counted from the femoral pulse.

Obstruction of the bronchus from within the lumen was carried out under a short intravenous anesthetic, one to four plugs of cotton being inserted through a No. 8 bronchoscope into the left main bronchus and packed in place with biopsy forceps (Fig 1). In the first experiments the cotton plugs were clean but not sterile, but later the plugs and bronchoscope were sterilized. The plugs were removed by bronchoscopy under anesthesia. When antibiotics were used, these consisted of intramuscular penicillin (400,000 units) and streptomycin (1.0 gm) once or twice daily.

Vagotomy was performed in the neck and was confirmed by the immediate occurrence on the same side of ptosis, paralysis of the nictitating membrane, and constriction of the pupil. A one-week period of recovery was then allowed before experimentation. Thoracic sympathectomy included removal of the entire sympathetic chain from the stellate ganglion to the diaphragm. At least ten days were allowed for complete recovery of the animal before its use in an experiment.

Three weeks elapsed after thyroidectomy before the animals were used for experimental purposes. No thyroxin replacement therapy was administered. One animal developed signs of hypoparathyroidism and was given 12.0 gm of calcium lactate by mouth daily with alleviation of the tetany.

Bilateral adrenalectomy was accomplished by the abdominal route. Replacement therapy consisted of

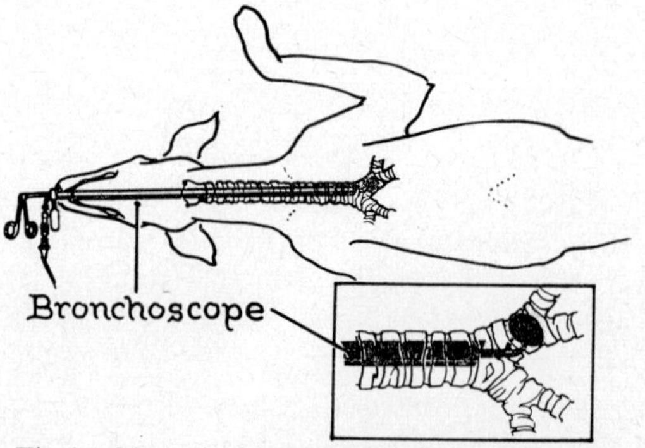

Fig 1.—Method of insertion of the bronchial plug.

Presented at the 20th Annual Meeting of the Central Surgical Association, Chicago, Feb 21-23, 1963.

John and Mary Markle Foundation Scholar in Medical Science, Assistant Professor of Surgery and Physiology, University of Western Ontario (Dr. Lansing); M.R.C. Fellow in Physiology, Resident in Surgery (Dr. Jamieson).

Contribution from the Departments of Surgery and Physiology, University of Western Ontario.

Research supported by an Ontario Heart Foundation research grant (H-22).

* Winthrop.

184

15 mg of cortisone acetate intramuscularly daily. Salt was added to the meat given to these animals, and at least ten days were allowed to elapse between operation and experiment.

Oxygen consumption was measured for five minutes by a Sanborn Metabulator connected to an endotracheal tube. The oxygen consumption was usually measured under a short hexobarbital anesthetic, although in a few animals with a tracheotomy this value was compared to the oxygen consumption when the animal was not anesthetized.

The sympathetic blocking agents employed during the experiments were hexamethonium bromide and reserpine. The hexamethonium was administered as a single dose of 5.0 mg/kg intravenously and reserpine in a dose of 0.02 mg/lb intramuscularly daily for five days.

The presence of atelectasis was confirmed in a few animals by chest x-ray, although this was somewhat unreliable because of the tendency for mediastinal shift to occur in the dog. Microscopic sections of the lung were obtained in a few animals and stained with hematoxylin and eosin. In another group of animals the presence of atelectasis was confirmed by measurement of the arterial oxygen saturation with a Kipp oximeter. The animals were anesthetized, an endotracheal tube was inserted, and they were artificially ventilated with room air for one to two minutes to overcome the respiratory depression caused by anesthetic agent. At the end of this time the arterial sample was drawn by percutaneous puncture from the femoral artery into an oiled syringe wet with heparin.

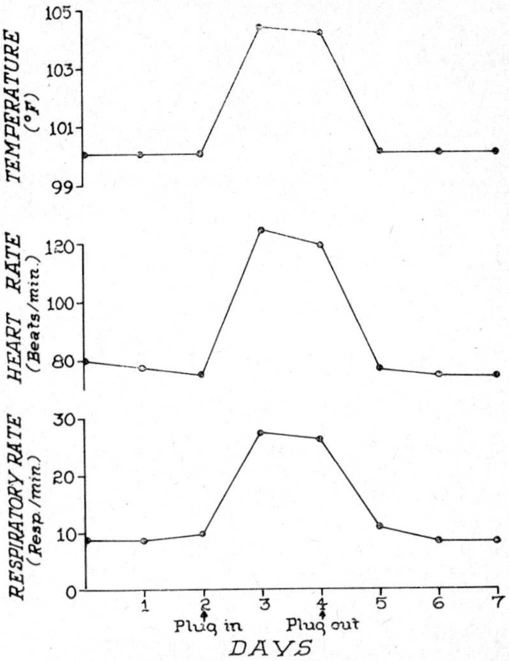

Fig 2.—Response to plug insertion and removal.

Results

Insertion of a cotton plug into the left main bronchus (30 dogs) resulted in the classical clinical picture of pulmonary atelectasis (Fig 2). Within 12 hours, the rectal temperature rose to 103-105 F, the heart rate increased to 110-160 beats per minute, and the respiratory rate was 25-50 per minute. This same course has occurred on each occasion regardless of whether the conditions used for insertion of the plug were merely clean or were sterile. The dogs seldom coughed the plug out and at the height of the response appeared to be very ill. Beyond the plug, the distal bronchial tree was filled with a thick mucopurulent exudate. Removal of the plug 24 to 72 hours later was always followed by a return to normal conditions within 12 hours.

The possible role of increased metabolic activity as a cause of the fever was investigated by measurements of oxygen consumption, thyroidectomy, and adrenalectomy. It was found that the oxygen consumption was identical when the animals were awake and when they were lightly anesthetized with hexobarbital, that is, an average of 10 ml/kg/min. In 12 dogs the oxgen consumption was measured before insertion of the plug, at the height of the fever, and after return of the temperature to normal. A representative experiment is shown in Fig 3: it can be seen that there is only a very slight increase in oxygen consumption at the height of the fever.

Thyroidectomy without thyroxin replacement was performed in two animals. The control values of temperature, pulse, and respiration were the same as in the normal animals. The oxygen consumption was, however, only 5 ml/kg/min, and the animals moved very slowly and appeared to be hypothyroid. Insertion of a bronchial plug in the thyroidectomized animals resulted in the same increase in temperature, pulse, and respiration as in the normal animals, without, of course, any increase in oxygen consumption.

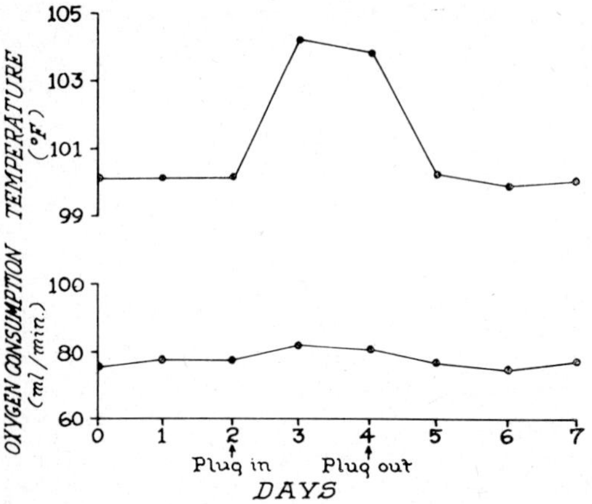

Fig 3.—Oxygen consumption during the fever of pulmonary atelectasis.

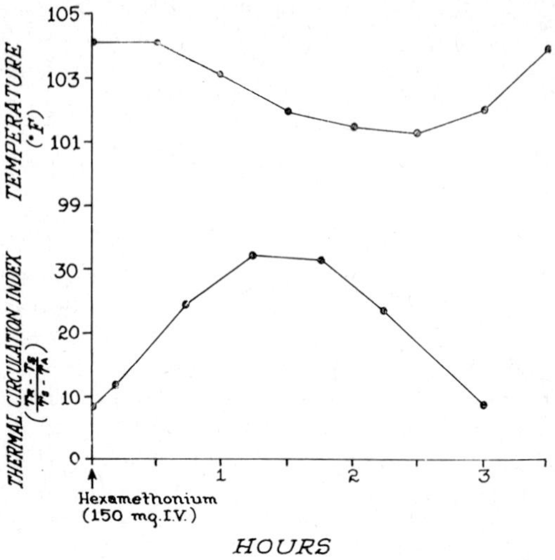

Fig 4.—Effect of intravenous hexamethonium on rectal temperature and thermal circulation index (skin blood flow) during atelectasis. T_R indicates rectal temperature; T_S, skin temperature; T_A, air temperature.

Adrenalectomy was carried out with cortisone replacement to rule out the possible metabolic effect of circulating epinephrine and norepinephrine released from the adrenal medulla (two dogs). The oxygen consumption of these animals before insertion of the plug was the same as in the normals, and it did not rise after atelectasis had been produced. The usual increase in temperature, pulse, and respiration occurred with atelectasis in the adrenalectomized animals.

The role of vasoconstriction of the skin blood vessels in the production of the fever was investigated by adrenalectomy, intravenous hexamethonium, and intramuscular reserpine. As has been mentioned, adrenalectomy did not prevent the fever despite the elimination of this source of circulating epinephrine and norepinephrine.

In another group of animals (seven dogs) a plug was placed in the bronchus, and at the height of the fever 5.0 mg/kg of hexamethonium bromide was injected intravenously without anesthesia. An immediate fall in rectal temperature occurred that reached its limit in 30 to 60 minutes (Fig 4). The temperature returned to its previous high value in three hours. At the same time, the skin temperature rose as did the thermal circulation index, indicating a marked increase in skin blood flow (Fig 4).

Administration of intramuscular reserpine for five days was carried out in one dog to block the peripheral sympathetic nerves and to exhaust the peripheral stores of epinephrine and norepinephrine. The general effect on the animal was to produce marked lethargy and weakness, a loose anal sphincter, and paralysis of the nictitating membrane. Under these conditions the rectal temperature was slightly below the usual basal value, the pulse rate was slightly increased, and the respiratory rate was normal. When the bronchus was occluded, the temperature rose slightly to normal levels, but a fever was not produced and only a very slight tachycardia was observed. The respiratory rate doubled, however.

The stimulus for vasoconstriction was investigated by interruption of the afferent nerve fibers from the lung. The following procedures were carried out: vagotomy on the same side as the atelectasis (three dogs), thoracic sympathectomy on the same side (two dogs), vagotomy and sympathectomy on the same side (two dogs), and bilateral vagotomy and sympathectomy (one dog). None of these measures prevented the changes in temperature, pulse, or respiration that occurred with atelectasis.

The role of bacterial infection was investigated by administration of intramuscular penicillin and streptomycin at the time of

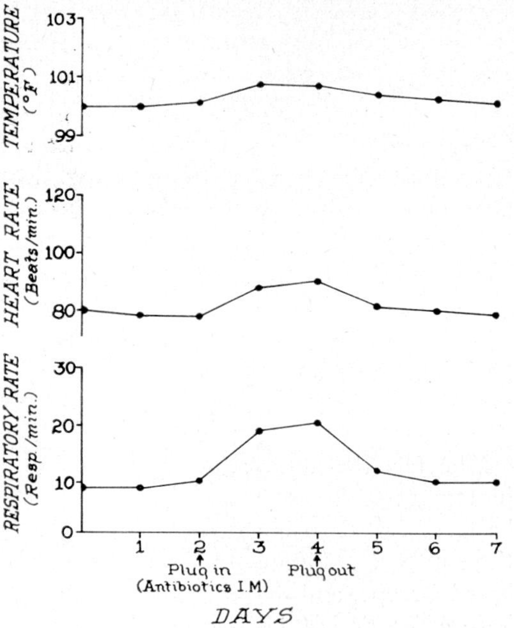

Fig 5.—Effect of antibiotics on the response to atelectasis.

insertion of the plug into the left main bronchus (six dogs). With this treatment, only very slight rises in temperature and pulse rate were observed, but once again the respiratory rate doubled (Fig 5).

The presence of atelectasis in the animals that had no fever with antibiotic administration was confirmed by measurements of the arterial oxygen saturation. The oxygen saturation was always 95%-98% before the insertion of the plug and fell to 85%-88% after insertion of the plug both in control animals with fever (five dogs) and in antibiotic-treated animals without fever. The chest x-rays showed some evidence of atelectasis, but these were not entirely convincing. Microscopic examination of the lung, however, showed complete atelectasis of the lung with inflammatory cell infiltration.

Bacterial cultures were obtained from ten clean cotton plugs before their insertion: nine were sterile, and one was found to contain an anaerobic Gram-positive bacillus. The sterile plugs, which also caused fever, were never found to have any bacterial growth before their insertion, and culture of the bronchus at the time of insertion of the plug was also sterile on each occasion. At the time of removal of the plug, however, culture of the mucopurulent exudate in the distal bronchial tree always yielded bacterial growth (14 specimens). This was a mixture of organisms including a Gram-postive anaerobic bacillus, probably a *Clostridium,* and occasionally *Staphylococcus aureus* or *Streptococcus viridans.* In four cases, *Escherichia coli* were found after multiple subcultures, but were considered by the bacteriologist to be contaminants. Blood cultures were carried out in four animals, and organisms were found at the height of the fever in three of these.

The final experiment consisted of insertion of a plug into the bronchus without the administration of antibiotics. After the usual fever had developed, 25 ml of blood from this dog was injected into a second animal. This produced in the recipient an immediate fever, rigors, tachycardia, and rapid respiratory rate, starting within five minutes and lasting about four hours. The plug was then removed from the experimental animal, and its temperature returned to normal. The next day another 25 ml of its blood was injected into the same recipient, this time without the production of any change in temperature, pluse, or respiration.

Comment

These experiments were begun to develop an experimental method for production of the clinical syndrome of postoperative pulmonary atelectasis, and then to investigate the physiological disturbances involved. A standard response was obtained by insertion of a cotton plug into the lumen of the left main bronchus. Even when completely aseptic conditions were used for its insertion, a high fever, tachycardia, and rapid respiratory rate resulted on each occasion. The immediate return of the animal to normal conditions within 12 hours of removal of the plug was equally dramatic.

With this preparation, an investigation of the mechanism of the fever became possible. The first concern was whether the fever was caused by an increase in metabolic rate with increased heat production or whether it was due to vasoconstriction and decreased heat loss. The fact that the oxygen consumption at the height of the fever was only slightly increased over control values ruled against increased metabolic activity as the cause of the fever. The slight increase in oxygen consumption could be accounted for by the effect of the fever alone.[2] The observation that hypothyroid animals also developed fever, tachycardia, and rapid respirations supported this conclusion, and adrenalectomy prevented the possible participation of the adrenal medulla in a metabolic response.

It was evident, therefore, that increased heat production was not involved in the fever and that the mechanism must be decreased heat loss. The experiments in adrenalectomized dogs ruled out circulating catecholamines as the cause of peripheral vasoconstriction, decreased skin blood flow, and heat retention. It seemed likely that the fever was caused by vasoconstriction mediated through the peripheral sympathetic nerves, and the dramatic response to intravenous hexamethonium confirmed this observation. Rectal temperature fell rapidly, while skin temperature and skin blood flow increased markedly after administration of this sympathetic blocking agent.

Intramuscular administration of reserpine, a drug that not only blocks the sympathetic nerves but also exhausts the stores of epinephrine and norepinephrine in the peripheral tissues, provided further confirmatory evidence of the importance of the role of sympathetic vasoconstriction. Under these conditions, no fever resulted from insertion of the plug in the bronchus, and only a slight tachycardia was observed. It is noteworthy, however, that the respiratory rate doubled even in the absence of any fever.

It has been proved, therefore, that the fever is caused by vasoconstriction of the skin blood vessels with decreased heat loss. This is mediated by the peripheral sympathetic nerves as is the tachycardia, but the respiratory rate is only partially controlled by these factors. About half of the increase in respiratory rate caused by atelectasis is brought about by factors other than fever and sympathetic nervous system action.

The stimulus for vasoconstriction was next considered. The importance of afferent reflex stimuli from the collapsed lung, conducted to the central nervous system through the vagus or sympathetic nerves, was investigated by vagotomy and sympathectomy, alone or combined, unilateral or bilateral. None of these measures prevented the changes in temperature, pulse, and respiration, so it is unlikely that the stimulus for their occurrence is reflex in origin.

The fact that antibiotics prevent the rise in temperature and heart rate proves that bacterial infection is an important factor in these changes. Although the cotton plug, the bronchoscope, and the bronchus were sterile before insertion of the plug, positive bacterial cultures were always obtained from the mucus that accumulated distal to the plug. Even though the antibiotic-treated dogs did not develop fever, the presence of atelectasis was confirmed by chest x-rays, arterial oxygen saturation, and, on occasion, microscopic examination of the lung.

The humoral nature of the stimulus for the changes in temperature, pulse, and respiration in pulmonary atelectasis was confirmed by the injection of blood from an animal at the height of the fever into a second animal. An immediate fever with rigors was produced and the heart rate and respiratory rate greatly increased. This effect lasted only about four hours, and the next day when the experimental animal's temperature had returned to normal after removal of the plug, injection of its blood into the same recipient had no effect.

The dual nature of the stimuli for the changes in respiratory rate has also been demonstrated. When fever and bacterial infection are present, the respiratory rate increases three- to fourfold. In the absence of fever and infection, however, the respiratory rate is doubled. This is not prevented by vagotomy or sympathectomy, so the stimulus must be carried in the blood stream. It is considered that this stimulus is likely the low arterial oxygen saturation.

Summary

An experimental method has been developed that routinely produces in dogs the clinical picture of pulmonary atelectasis with high fever, tachycardia, and rapid respiratory rate.

The mechanism of the fever is not increased production of heat through increased metabolic activity, but rather is decreased heat loss through vasoconstriction. This vasoconstriction is mediated by the peripheral sympathetic nerves, not by the adrenal medulla. Sympathetic blocking agents will release the vasoconstriction and return the temperature to normal.

The stimulus for fever is not an afferent reflex through the sympathetic or vagus nerves. Infection distal to the plug is always present, and antibiotics prevent the fever. Injection of blood from an animal with fever produces an immediate fever in a second animal. It is likely that an endogenous pyrogen produced by the action of the bacteria in the distal bronchial tree is responsible for the fever.

The tachycardia is also under sympathetic control, and the stimulus for tachycardia is the presence of bacterial infection distal to the plug. The respiratory changes are partly caused by the bacterial infection and increased body temperature and partly by the central effect of the decreased arterial oxygen saturation associated with atelectasis.

The clinical importance of the investigation is that antibiotics may mask severe atelectasis, whereas removal of the obstruction rapidly cures the condition. It is also significant that the temperature can be returned to normal by administration of an adrenergic blocking agent, a technique that may be useful in the treatment of high fevers associated with infections, particularly in children, and that may replace more cumbersome methods such as alcohol sheets, fans, and cooling blankets.

Dr. R. G. Passi actively participated in the technical aspects of this investigation. Dr. R. G. E. Murray, Professoı of Bacteriology, assisted with the bacterial cultures; and Dr. G. W. Manning, Associate Professor of Medicine with the arterial oxygen determinations. The illustrations were done by Mrs. D. M. Hutchinson.

A. M. Lansing, MD, Department of Surgery, University of Louisville, 311 S Floyd St, Louisville 2.

REFERENCES

1. Burton, A. C.: Temperature of Skin Measurement and Use as Index of Peripheral Blood Flow, Meth Med Res 1:146, 1948.
2. Kinney, J. M., and Roe, C. F.: Caloric Equivalent of Fever: I. Patterns of Postoperative Response, Ann Surg 156:610, 1962.

DISCUSSION

On papers by Drs. Berry and Sanislow, and Lansing and Jamieson.

Dr. Fiorindo A. Simeone, Cleveland: The paper by Dr. Lansing demonstrates and illustrates the mechanism of an important and common clinical problem. Dr. Berry emphasizes some most important points in the problem of shock.

Although the clinical appearance of patients in shock may be similar, with perhaps only minor differences, the mechanisms that cause shock can be very different. In order properly to treat such patients one must have an understanding of the mechanism that is bringing about the hypotension and other signs of shock. In emphasizing this matter, Dr. Berry has rendered a great service.

I would like to ask a question. In these patients, were the venous pressures monitored? Is there any information on either their peripheral or central venous pressures?

I hope Dr. Berry might comment on the possible usefulness of monitoring venous pressures in such patients. It might hereby be easier to keep people from persisting in sending fluid into the circulation when the right auricular pressure or the superior vena caval pressure is normal or elevated.

Dr. John R. Paine, Buffalo: Dr. McLachlin you and your colleagues have answered a questior that has intrigued many of us for many years Some 10 or 12 years ago, Dr. Adler and I tried to carry out the experiments which you have done so very nicely. We were not able to duplicate the fever. We endeavored to obstruct the bronchus with balloons. Perhaps it was because we did not wait long enough.

Dr. Lansing has any thought been given to the possibilty of what role mucus itself might be playing in this clinical entity? Is it possible that mucus is a foreign protein and in some way finds access to the blood stream, and serves as the trigger mechanism to set off this physiologic syndrome which resembles that of a chill so very, very nicely?

I will admit that the results you get with the use of antibiotics would tend to mean that this probably is not so, but I think it is another possible mechanism that one should look into with respect to this syndrome.

Dr. Harold Laufman, Chicago: Hemorrhagic atelectasis and infarction are very difficult to tell apart microscopically, and atelectasis might well lead imperceptibly to infarction.

The paper by Dr. Lansing reminded me of some work that Dr. David Roach and I did seven or eight years ago (Roach, H. D., and Laufman, H.: Relationship Between Pulmonary Embolism and Pulmonary Infarction: An Experimental Study, *Ann Surg* 142:82, 1955) in which we endeavored to draw a quantitative correlation between pulmonary embolism and pulmonary infarction. In the dog, quite aside from the standard bits of knowledge which we had at that time, we found that it takes three things to produce infarction.

The occurrence of infarction following decreased aeration and decreased blood supply is apparently dependent upon the degree of completeness of either or both these factors. A firm, bland pulmonary embolism is more likely to lead to infarction, decreased aeration, or congestion are present in the lung. When pneumonia exists prior to embolization, infarction usually results. Decreased aeration, infection, and congestion may be severe enough to result in infarction in the absence of pulmonary embolism.

We were able to separate these factors. If a bronchial artery was ligated, and if it was a large enough bronchial artery, we could produce atelectasis and infarction. If a smaller artery was obstructed it would not produce infarction unless large infection was produced, and this large infection could be produced by the instillation of bacteria or by retained mucus. Nonseration was produced by the insertion of cotton plugs.

This, I think, is very closely related to the work we have heard about today, which was much more all-inclusive inasmuch as it went into the mechanisms of fever production, and certainly has been very enlightening.

Dr. Robert E. L. Berry, Ann Arbor, Mich: In answer to Dr. Simeone's question about venous pressures, peripheral venous pressures measured in all cases were normal. Little change would be anticipated until right heart overload is initiated. Central venous pressures were not monitored, as one is so busy trying to keep the patient alive under these emergent circumstances that time was not taken for such desirable refinements.

Domination of the clinical picture by hypotension unfortunately masks the true state of affairs. The time apparently arrives when one more transfusion is literally the "kiss of death" because the hypotension is not the result of hypovolemia.

To apply positive pressure oxygen properly is not an easy thing to do. The Bird respirator is fairly easy to use but constant attention is required. If there is any leak in the system the administration becomes a total farce. If the face mask cannot be made to work, then the cuffed intratracheal tube will be necessary. This can be poorly tolerated, however. If the intratracheal tube cannot be used, then tracheostomy may be necessary, but unless this is relatively airtight, undesirable leak into the mediastinum may occur. I should like to leave Dr. Lansing the question of the mucus problem. There is some evidence suggesting that changes in the surface tension of the alveolar lining membrane may occur during period of severe pulmonary stress. If this is true and some denaturization of the lipoprotein lining of the alveolar membrane does occur, a significant contribution to the problem of congestive atelectasis is a possibility.

Dr. A. M. Lansing, London, Ont, Canada: In regard to the question about the mucus, I think this is a very worthwhile suggestion; but the response to antibiotics was so dramatic (and the mucus was still present in these patients) that it seems difficult to imply that this was the situation.

I would like to emphasize that the chill one sees is associated with the vasoconstriction. This is the time the temperature starts upward. Secondly, removal of the plug completely cures the condition, even without any antibiotics.

Another factor is that the rate of development of atelectasis depends on the gas that is present in the lung. If you use room air it takes several hours; if you use pure oxygen it occurs in a much shorter period of time; if you use CO_2, atelectasis occurs almost immediately. I think it is significant in the selection of the gas used to ventilate the patient at the conclusion of the operation. If the patient has a plug, he is far more likely to develop atelectasis if he is ventilated with oxygen than if he is ventilated with room air.

Severe Ischemia of Lower Extremity Due to Arteriosclerosis Obliterans

ALFRED W. HUMPHRIES, MD; JESS R. YOUNG, MD; VICTOR G. deWOLFE, MD; FAY A. LeFEVRE, MD; AND EDWIN G. BEVEN, M,D., CLEVELAND

In 1958, we[1] reported the early results of attempted arterial reconstruction in 137 limbs ischemic beyond simple claudication but not yet at the stage of fixed extensive gangrene. At that time, it seemed that apparently hopeless extremities often could be saved by sympathectomy, arterial reconstruction, or both. It is of interest that a similar study, reporting essentially identical results, was independently published at the same time by Roberts and Hoffman.[2]

Between 1958 and Jan 1, 1961, an additional 411 severely ischemic limbs were treated at the Cleveland Clinic, increasing the total to 548 lower extremities in 495 patients. This study was terminated on Jan 1, 1961, in order to obtain a follow-up period of at least one year on all patients studied. The maximum follow-up period is eight years after operation.

The etiology of the ischemia in all instances has been arteriosclerosis obliterans. Ischemic limbs resulting from embolus or trauma have not been included in this study.

We are presenting a review of these cases to confirm the validity of our original impression that surgical intervention can be of lasting rather than transient value in the treatment of the severely ischemic limb.

Definitions

Chronic Ischemia.—The term "ischemia" is relative, signifying a decrease in blood supply to a part. It may range in severity from asymptomatic narrowing of an arterial lumen seen only on arteriography to total loss of blood supply to the part. It is of practical value in this study to define arbitrarily several degrees of chronic ischemia in terms of the symptoms produced:

A. *Intermittent claudication* occurs when blood flow has decreased to the extent that the metabolic demand of an exercising muscle cannot be fulfilled, although the tissues are satisfied under resting conditions.

B. *"Rest pain"* is an ill-defined term representing a range of ischemia next in severity to intermittent claudication. In its less severe form, it occurs when the arterial supply to the limb is reduced to the point where gravity can make the difference between a blood supply equal to the metabolic demand at rest and one that is unequal to this demand. Under such circumstances, the increment supplied by gravity is lost when the patient assumes the recumbent position, and peripheral pain results. Dependency, acquired by hanging the leg over the side of the bed, or by sitting or standing, permits sufficient additional blood flow to meet the baseline metabolic need, and pain disappears.

In its more severe form, peripheral pain is not relieved by dependency but continues, unremitting, regardless of position or activity. Perhaps this stage, usually classified under the term "rest pain," should more accurately be defined as "persistent ischemic pain."

The quality of this "rest pain" may range in severity from simple numbness or tingling in the toes to pain of such a degree that the patient is forced to spend his nights sitting in a chair. Rest pain is a way-station along the course of progressing ischemia and is of significance in that it represents a convenient, diagnosable point beyond which further loss of blood supply will result in death of tissue, manifested by ischemic ulcers and finally gangrene.

C. A *nonhealing ischemic ulcer* may occur, usually the result of minor trauma, or bacterial or fungus infection of the foot or toes. Such an ulcer is usually associated with severe rest pain.

D. Areas of *local gangrene,* involving one or more toes or the skin of the foot or leg, may develop as blood supply further diminishes.

Presented at the 20th Annual Meeting of the Central Surgical Association, Chicago, Feb 21-23, 1963.

From the Department of Vascular Surgery and the Department of Peripheral Vascular Disease, Cleveland Clinic Foundation.

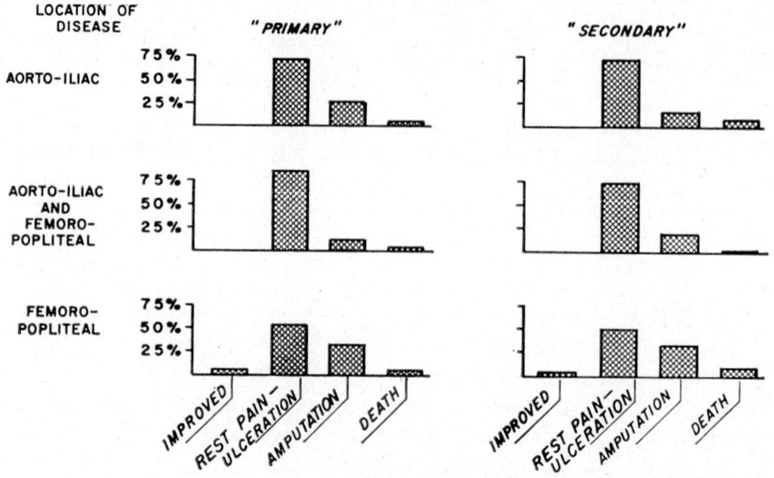

Fig 1.—Course following acute ischemia without specific vascular treatment.

E. *Extensive gangrene,* involving an entire foot or leg, represents the final stage of decreased blood supply to the extremity.

We consider the last four categories of "rest pain," "ischemic ulceration," "local gangrene," and "extensive gangrene" to be encompassed within the term "severe ischemia." Since extensive gangrene is treatable only by major amputation, patients presenting with this terminal phase have been excluded from this report.

These forms of chronic severe ischemia result from progressive loss of collateral pathways, generally occurring in small, stepwise episodes.

Acute Ischemia.—Any degree of ischemia, however, may occur cataclysmically by massive extension of a pre-existing occlusion, by the sudden development of a second significant occlusion, or by the onset of a primary thrombosis-in-situ occurring in previously patent arteries. Such acute ischemia may improve spontaneously or with the help of a good medical regimen, or it may result in rest pain, ulceration, or gangrene if time is permitted to pass.

Stages of Ischemia Represented in Series

Chronic ischemia		187
Rest pain	95	
Ischemic ulcer	72	
Minor gangrene	20	
Acute ischemia		361
Primary	144	
Secondary	217	
Total extremities		548

Acute ischemia may be divided into two groups, historically different, but clinically similar:

A. *"Primary" acute ischemia* is characterized by an unheralded thrombosis-in-situ occurring in patients who have had no previous ischemic symptoms,

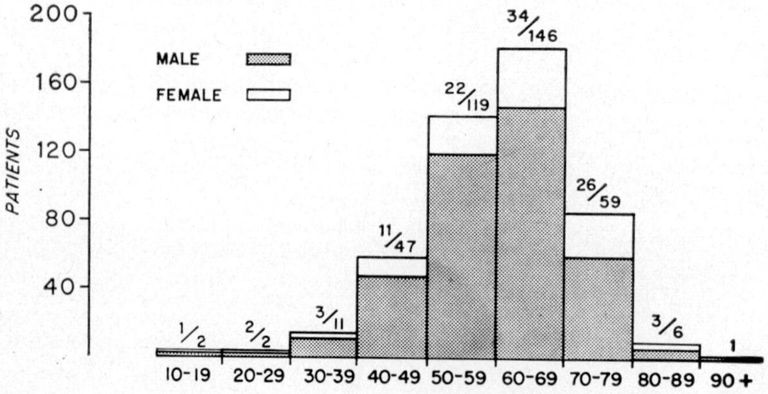

Fig 2.—Distribution by age and sex.

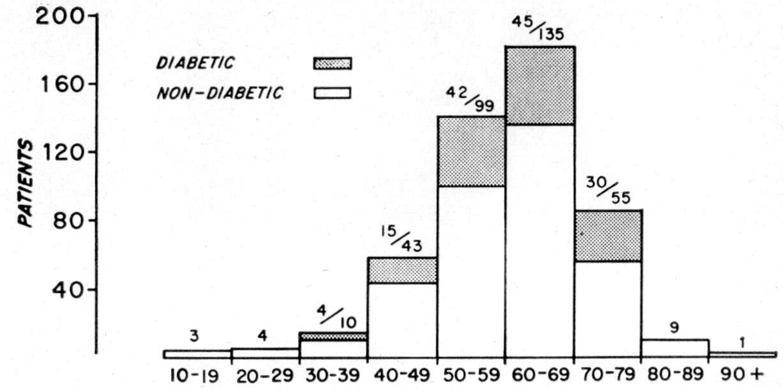

Fig 3.—Distribution of diabetes by age.

although some degree of atheromatous change undoubtedly pre-exists. Gangrene may not occur if collateral vessels are available to quickly supply sufficient blood to meet the basic metabolic demand. Collateral improvement may be spontaneous or it may be enhanced by sympathetic nerve blocks. Recovery may be complete, or only partial so that some degree of chronic ischemia may persist.

B. *"Secondary" acute ischemia* is characterized by a sudden significant diminution of blood supply in a previously claudicating extremity. This acute progression of the disease may occur as a result of sudden thrombosis superimposed on a previous occlusion or as a second occlusion in a different part of the arterial supply to the limb.

Reference to Fig 1 will show that (1) the incidence of improvement, (2) the persistence of rest pain and/or chronic ulceration, (3) the occurrence of amputation, and (4) the occurrence of death following an episode of acute ischemia are similar regardless of whether it was "primary" or "secondary" and regardless of whether the occlusion was in the aortoiliac vessels, the femoropopliteal vessels, or both.

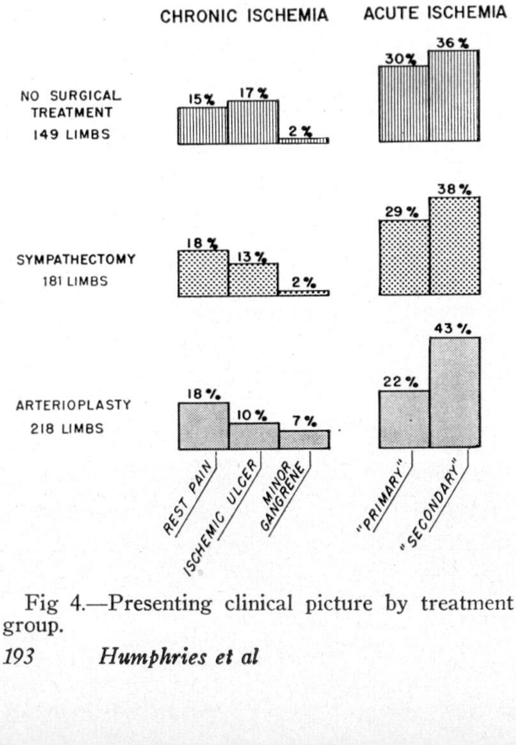

Fig 4.—Presenting clinical picture by treatment group.

Clinical Material

All stages of ischemia were represented in this group of limbs as indicated in the Table.

The age distribution and sex incidence are illustrated in Fig 2. The age follows a standard distributional curve centering in the 50- to 70-year zone. Twenty-one per cent of the patients were female, or approximately twice the female incidence in occlusive arteriosclerosis of all types.

As shown in Fig 3, the incidence of diabetes was 27%, somewhat higher than the diabetic incidence in occlusive arteriosclerosis in general.

Treatment

The 548 limbs reported here have been divided in retrospect into three "treatment groups": (A) no surgical treatment, 149; (B) sympathectomy, 181; (C) arterioplasty, 218.

The *presenting* clinical picture in each of these three treatment groups is illustrated in Fig 4. It should be noted that the distribution of symptom complexes as seen at the time of the first examination was so similar in each of these three groups as to make them clinically indistinguishable.

A. *No Surgical Treatment.*—No vascular surgery was employed in 149 limbs. Some of these legs were not seen until the ischemic changes had become irreversible. A few patients were not operated because of "poor risk." Certain patients refused treatment, allowing us to observe directly the course of

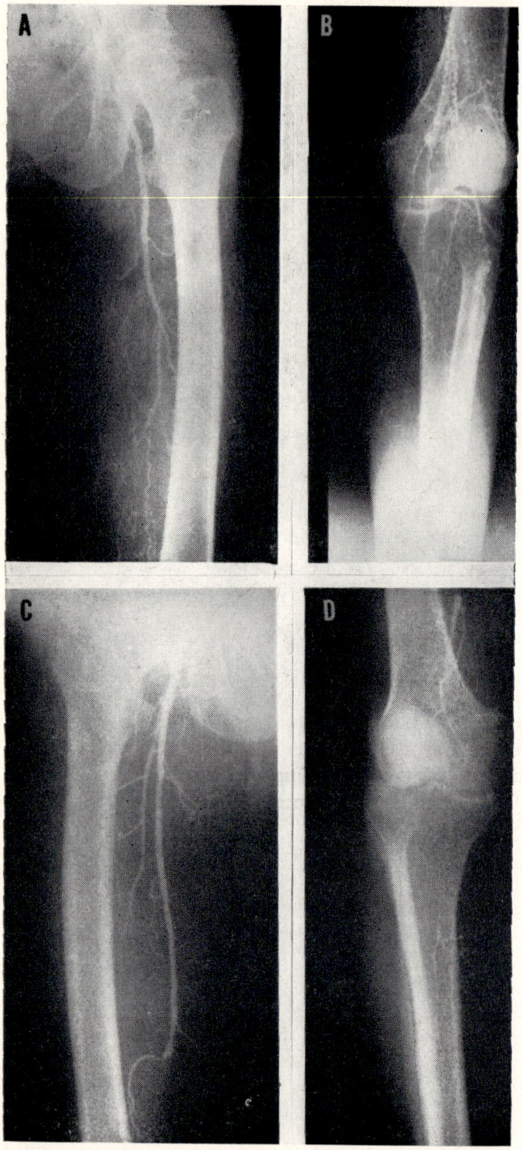

Fig 5, *A* and *B*.—Femoral arteriogram. The superficial femoral artery is completely occluded and shows no areas of patency anywhere along its course.

the non-surgically-treated severe disease through its various phases. The remainder occurred in patients in whom a newly diseased leg was currently under treatment. In these an accurate history concerning the previous course of the other limb could be obtained from the patient and frequently supplemented by the referring physician. We believe that the course of the disease in these limbs is historically accurate.

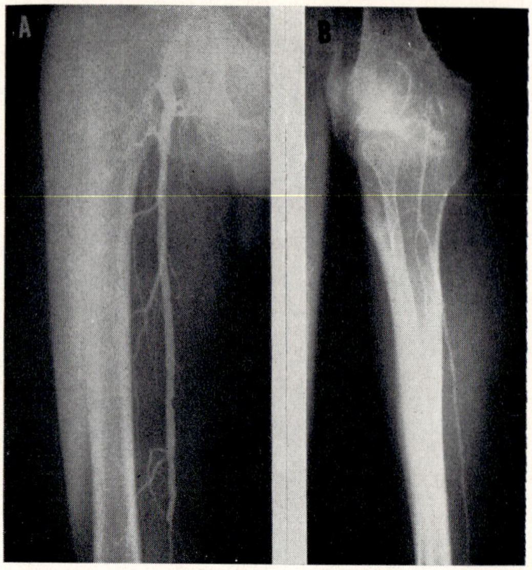

Fig 6.—*A* and *B*, femoral arteriogram. The superficial femoral artery shows patchy intimal disease in its course through the thigh and then is completely occluded in the region of the femoropopliteal junction, but regains patency in the midpopliteal area. Note associated occlusion of the deep femoral artery. *C* and *D*, femoral arteriogram. There is an occlusion of the superficial femoral artery in Hunter's canal, patency is regained for a short distance at the femoropopliteal junction, and then it reoccludes through the course of the femoropopliteal artery and the posterior tibial artery as far as the origin of the peroneal artery.

B. *Sympathectomy.*—In those limbs treated by surgery, the procedure employed was usually determined by arteriography. In 181 limbs the arteriogram revealed occlusion somewhere in the femoropopliteal tree, but at no point could refilling of the occluded artery be demonstrated—the so-called nonsegmental occlusion (Fig 5, *A* and *B*). These limbs were treated by sympathectomy or by sympathectomy combined with a fruitless popliteal exploration.

C. *Arterioplasty.*—In 218 limbs the occlusion was of varying length with refilling of the main stream at some more distal level—the so-called segmental occlusion (Fig 6, *A* and *B*). These legs were treated by direct arterial intervention. In occlusions involving the popliteal artery, reconstruction was attempted if as little as 1 cm of the artery refilled, and in spite of a poor outflow tract due to a second, more distal, occlusion (Fig 6, *C* and *D*).

In cases of combined aortoiliac and femoropopliteal occlusions, the initial procedure generally consisted of restoration of flow to the profunda femoris alone, by means of a suitable aortofemoral or iliofemoral arterioplasty. It was necessary to carry the arterial repair below the level of the profunda in only 20% of cases. Although a few endarterectomies were done, most of the procedures consisted of an arterial graft of either homologous artery (prior to 1958) or of plastic in the form of a woven Dacron tube (since 1958).

It should be stressed that the choice of treatment between sympathectomy and an arterioplasty was a factor of the anatomic extent of the disease as documented by arteriography.

Results of Treatment

Evaluation of the results of treatment is difficult, since results can be made to vary markedly by modifying the various frames of reference. For purposes of this paper, we have chosen certain criteria for evaluation, which are as follows:

1. "Better" is used to describe limbs which have unequivocally improved. In the case of arterioplasties this generally means complete relief of all symptoms of ischemia including claudication. The relief attained is a factor of the outflow tract as represented by the tibial and peroneal vessels. In most instances, we have found that if the outflow tract is sufficient to keep the graft open, it is also sufficient to relieve all symptoms.

2. "Unchanged" means no demonstrable changes occurred as a result of treatment. This occurred most frequently in patients who had undergone sympathectomy and in those instances where an arterioplasty has been attempted unsuccessfully.

3. "Minor amputation" (one or more toes or transmetatarsal) is classified as an acceptable result, since the legs remained of equal length.

The three categories defined above are considered as "good" results, since the involved leg remained viable and useful, even if not entirely normal.

4. "Major amputation" (below and above knee). This category has been subdivided into three groups based upon the time of amputation:

   A. "Immediate"—amputations occurring during the patient's initial ischemic episode or hospitalization for specific treatment.

   B. "Delayed"—amputations occurring *during* the first year following initial treatment.

   C. "Late"—amputations occurring at some time *after* the first year following initial treatment.

We believe this latter subdivision is important because, by observing these limbs for a minimum of one year, we avoid the pitfall of believing that early improvement necessarily implies continued improvement.

In terms of the above definitions, we have recorded the subsequent course of these limbs under the presenting stage of ischemia as shown in the Table, and each of these groupings is evaluated according to the type of

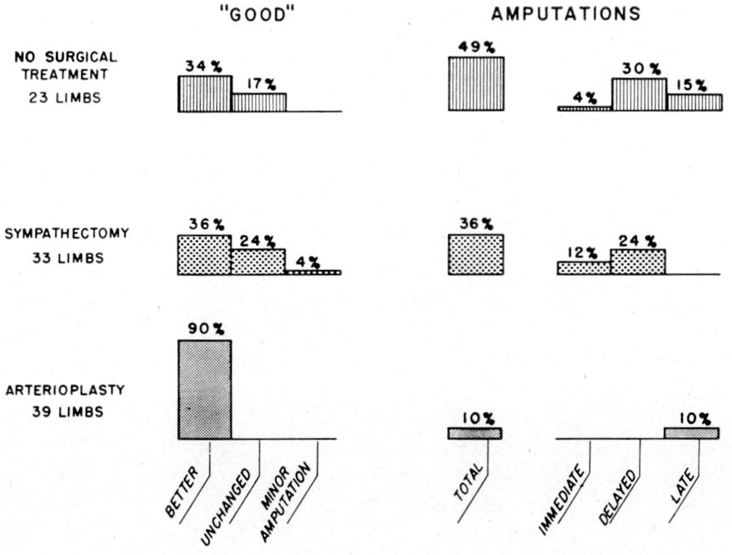

Fig 7.—Results of treatment in rest pain.

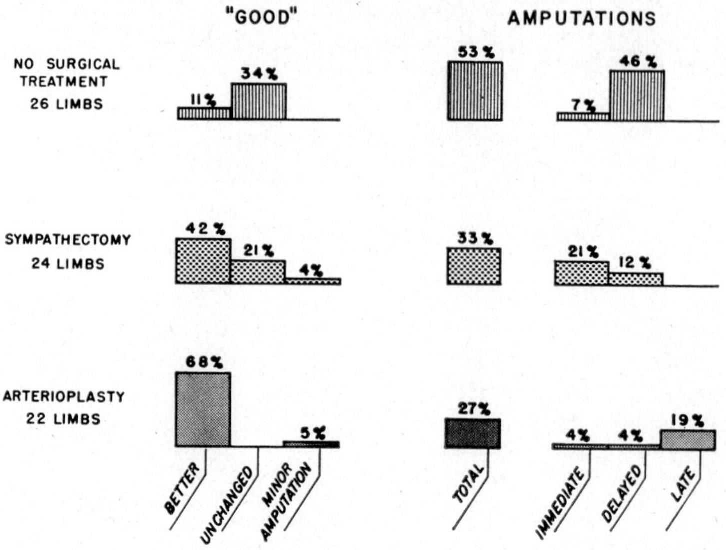

Fig 8.—Results of treatment in ischemic ulcer.

treatment employed: no surgical treatment; sympathectomy; or arterioplasty.

(Note: Among the patients treated by arterioplasty, 40 underwent concomitant sympathectomy. The results of treatment in these cases were identical to those treated by arterioplasty alone. For this reason these patients have not been considered separately but have been grouped with those treated by arterioplasty alone.)

1. *Chronic Ischemia.*—Ninety-five patients presented with *rest pain* (Fig 7). Of these, the total amputation rate was 49% in the non-surgically-treated group, 36% in the sympathectomy group, and 10% in the arterioplasty group. Sympathectomy reduced the total number of amputations a significant, but moderate, amount. Since sympathectomy was done in those instances in which arteriography showed a nonsegmental occlusion, only a moderate improvement over the untreated amputation rate should be expected. In those patients whose disease pattern was such that an arterioplasty could be attempted, the amputation rate was markedly reduced.

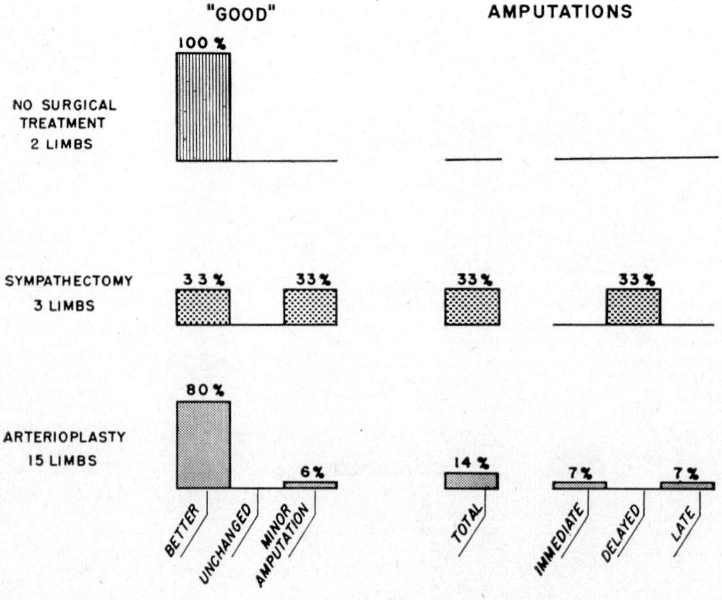

Fig 9.—Results of treatment in minor gangrene.

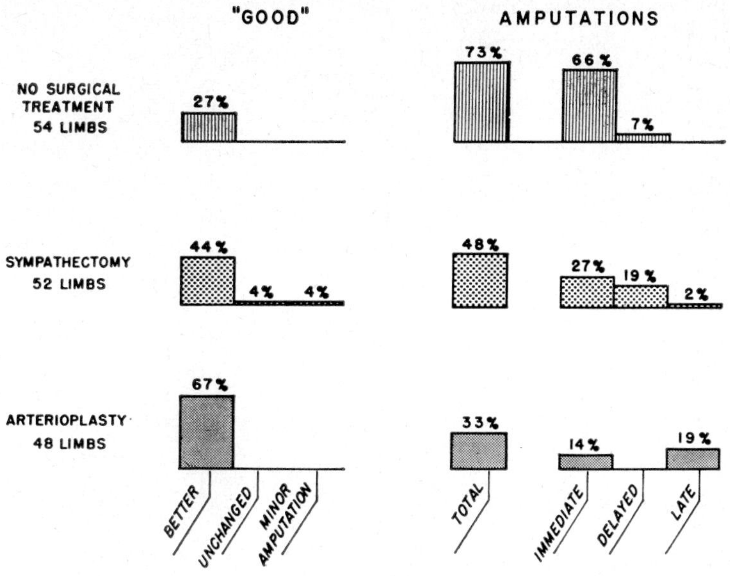

Fig 10.—Results of treatment in primary acute ischemia.

Seventy-two patients presented with *non-healing ischemic ulcers* (Fig 8). Of these, the total amputation rate was 53% in the non-surgically-treated group, 33% in the sympathectomy group and 27% in the arterioplasty group. In those patients whose disease pattern was such that an arterioplasty could be attempted, the amputation rate was not much better than in the sympathectomy group, although both were superior to the untreated group. We can find no apparent reason why these patients with arterioplasties did not fare better.

Since there were only 20 patients who presented with *minor gangrene* (Fig 9) in this series, undue emphasis should not be placed on the results in this group. It is interesting to note, however, that relatively few of these patients lost their limbs. We interpret this to mean that the remaining viable tissue had already attained an adequate blood supply and had already limited the extent of the gangrene to the toes.

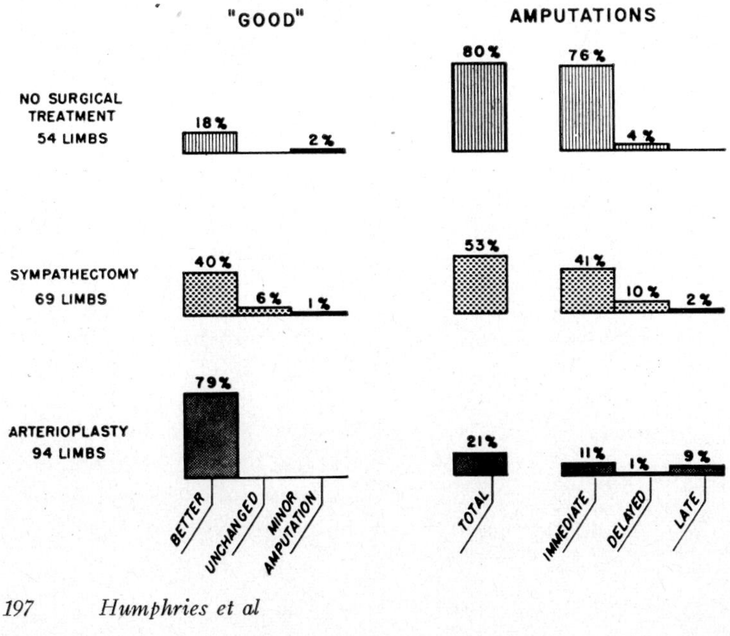

Fig 11.—Results of treatment in secondary acute ischemia.

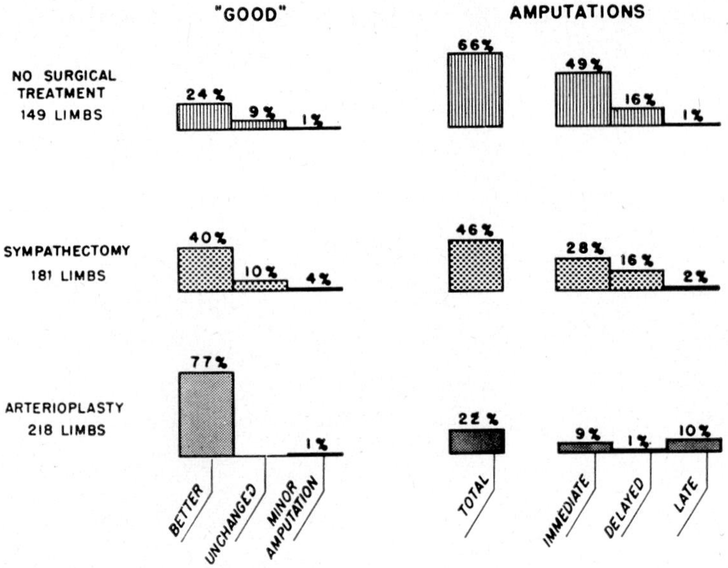

Fig 12.—Results of treatment in severe ischemia.

In all groups, it is significant that most of the amputations which eventually followed an arterioplasty occurred more than one year after treatment. Therefore, although an amputation may have finally ensued, the life of the limb was significantly prolonged.

2. *Acute Ischemia* (Fig 10 and 11).—There were 144 limbs in the "primary" and 217 in the "secondary" acute ischemia group. The course following treatment was essentially the same in each group.

As in the case of chronic ischemia, sympathectomy lowered the amputation rate a moderate amount and an arterioplasty lowered it a significant amount.

When amputation was necessary, it was necessary immediately in almost all instances in which no surgical treatment was employed. Sympathectomy delayed some of the eventual amputations for up to one year, but arterioplasty postponed about half of the eventual amputations for longer than one year. In the case of the acute ischemias, late amputation was usually associated with an additional episode of advancing disease.

3. *Combined Results.*—The subsequent course of all forms of severe ischemia, combined, is shown in Fig 12.

It can be seen that the eventual amputation rate of severely ischemic limbs treated by sympathectomy is approximately two-thirds that of non-surgically-treated limbs, while the eventual amputation rate of severely ischemic limbs treated by arterioplasty is approximately one-third that of non-surgically-treated limbs.

Most non-surgically-treated limbs that required amputation did so early; sympathectomy postponed many amputations into the ensuing year after operation, and an arterioplasty postponed about half of the eventual amputations to more than one year later.

Obviously, those patients in whom an arterioplasty could be done had less extensive disease than those in whom only sympathectomy could be employed. However, the degree of ischemia as judged by clinical evaluation was the same in all three groups, and evaluation of the extent of the anatomic lesion could be made only on the basis of arteriography.

Conclusions

Arteriography should, therefore, be done in all instances of severely ischemic limbs before a decision to amputate is made. If the arteries are amenable to vascular repair, an arterioplasty should be attempted, since the life of most of these limbs will be prolonged for a significant period of time.

Even if restoration of arterial flow can-

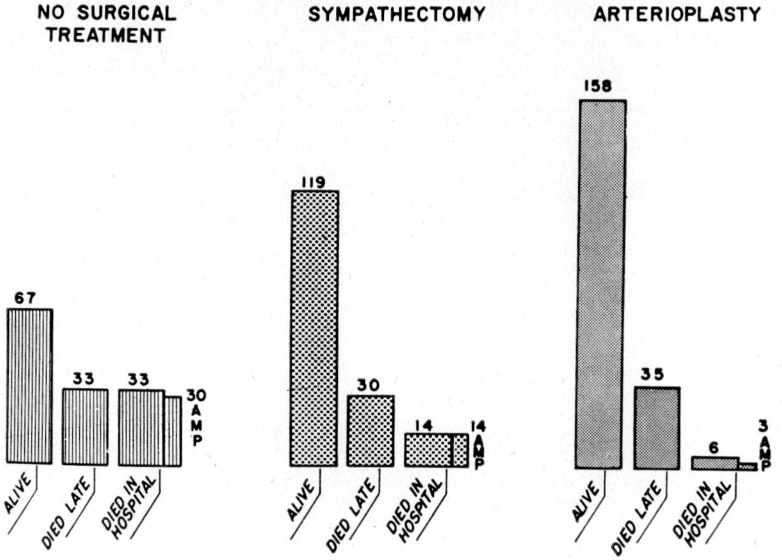

Fig 13.—Mortality and its relationship to major amputation.

not be accomplished, sympathectomy should be done, since some limbs will be saved by this procedure. Many of these, however, will be preserved for only a short while. Even if amputation is ultimately required, the sympathectomy will enhance skin circulation and so permit a certain number of successful below-knee amputations that otherwise would require an amputation above the knee.

Mortality

As an ancillary study, we became interested in the relationship of severe ischemia and amputation to the life of the patient as well as the life of the limb. A very interesting discovery was made during the course of this analysis. Fig 13 shows, in each treatment group, the total number of patients alive at the time of this report, those who have died from any cause since leaving the hospital, and those who died while in the hospital.

It will be noted that, after leaving the hospital, essentially the same number of patients have died in each of the three groups. This figure represents the normal mortality of this age group, the causes of death being legion.

In the "no surgical treatment" group, 30 of 33 patients who died during the initial hospitalization did so after a major amputation. Of those treated by sympathectomy all 14 who died in the hospital also had an associated amputation. Of the 6 patients who died in the hospital in the arterioplasty series, 3 also had an amputation. Thus, of the 53 patients who died during their initial hospitalization, 47 underwent a major amputation during the same period.

The statistical correlation of 89% between amputation and death seems too high to be coincidental. We are led, therefore, to the conclusion that the reduction in amputations which attends successful surgical treatment is also reflected in a reduction in mortality to a proportional degree. It appears that the added stress attending the toxemia of a dead limb, the strain of a major amputation, and the exertion involved in the attempt at rehabilitation of the amputee seem, in many instances, to be related to his sudden death. The specific cause of death is usually arteriosclerotic involvement of the coronary or cerebral arteries.

Summary

Five hundred and forty-eight limbs exhibiting symptoms of severe ischemia have been studied in regard to their subsequent course following treatment. Three groups of patients whose symptom complexes were essentially the same, but whose anatomic disease differed in pattern, have been comparatively analyzed as to the eventual outcome. The three groups were treated by no form of surgical treatment, by sympathectomy, or by arterioplasty. The number of amputations was significantly, but moderately, reduced in those patients treated by sympathectomy as compared with those receiving no surgical treatment. The number of amputations was markedly reduced in those patients treated by direct arterioplasty as compared to both the group of patients receiving no surgical treatment and those receiving sympathectomy alone.

The close statistical relationship between in-hospital amputation and death makes us believe that mortality has been reduced in direct proportion to the reduction in the number of amputations. Accordingly, any form of treatment which will lower the amputation rate will also lower the death rate.

Alfred W. Humphries, MD, Cleveland Clinic, 2020 E 93rd St, Cleveland 6, Ohio.

REFERENCES

1. Humphries, A. W.; deWolfe, V. G.; and LeFevre, F. A.: Reversibility of Pregangrene in the Severely Ischaemic Limb, J Bone Joint Surg (Amer) 40:983, 1958.

2. Roberts, B., and Hoffman, D.: Arterial Grafting in Severely Ischemic Legs, JAMA 166:1316, 1958.

Caval Ligation in Thromboembolic Disease

RAYMOND J. KRAUSE, MD; JOHN J. CRANLEY, MD; MOHEB A.S. HALLABA, MB, ChB; EDWARD S. STRASSER, MD; AND CHARLES D. HAFNER, MD, CINCINNATI

Over a century ago, Virchow suggested that pulmonary embolism was related to thrombophlebitis of the lower extremities, but it remained for Homans[6] in 1934 to conceive of ligation of the inferior vena cava as a physiologically sound procedure to prevent thromboembolic episodes in patients with venous thrombosis in the lower half of the body. Trendelenburg[15] had already accomplished a successful ligation of this vessel, in 1910, for pelvic thrombophlebitis complicated by puerperal pyemia, and earlier surgeons performed ligations (with fatal outcome) necessitated by inadvertent injury to the vena cava during operative procedures. In 1937, Krotoski[8] collected 48 instances of ligation from the world literature, and by 1958, when Dale[3] presented 16 cases and once more reviewed the subject, the total number of published reports had increased tenfold to 468. In 1951, Collins and his associates[2] recorded the largest individual series, 70 patients with ligation of the inferior vena cava.

This report comprises a ten-year experience with 55 cases of inferior vena cava ligation, which represents 6% of the patients we have treated for superficial or deep thrombophlebitis of the lower extremity over this same period of time. Forty-five of the patients with caval ligation are still living, and 32 have been examined and photographed in the past two months. The remainder have been contacted either by telephone or by letter. In preventing recurrent pulmonary embolism, vena cava ligation has been 100% effective, and the associated morbidity has been minimal, confirming the reports by Dale,[3] Miller,[10] Schauble,[12] and Kirtley.[7] The undesirable sequelae emphasized in earlier studies by Shea and Robertson[13] and Bowers and Leb[1] have been observed only

Presented at the 20th Annual Meeting of the Central Surgical Association, Chicago, Feb 21-23, 1963.

From the Peripheral Vascular Laboratory and the Department of Surgery, The Good Samaritan Hospital, and the Department of Surgery, University of Cincinnati College of Medicine.

TABLE 1.—*Inferior Vena Cava Ligation: Follow-Up Period (45 Patients)*

Years	Patients
<1	17
1-2	13
3-4	5
5-6	4
7-8	4
>9	2

once in this series, in a patient who had recurrent thrombophlebitis at least seven times and who finally died of carcinoma of the lung. In all other patients the disability has proved to be of minor consequence. As a matter of fact, the adverse effects of this procedure have been so minimal and the total over-all results so good, we have steadily broadened our indications for operation and now consider it the treatment of choice in a large percentage of patients with thromboembolic disease who are to be treated surgically. Thrombectomy has been added to vena cava ligation whenever warranted during the past 3½ years and has further reduced the postphlebitic sequelae. In phlegmasia cerulea dolens, the results of thrombectomy have been most dramatic.[5]

Analysis of Cases

Duration of Follow-Up.—The duration of follow-up is shown in Table 1. As indicated therein, most of the ligations have been done in the past two years, which reflects our increasing conviction, based largely upon observation of our earlier patients, that the late sequelae are minimal.

Age and Sex.—Of the 55 patients, 37 (67%) were males and 18 (33%) females. The average age of the males was 51 years and of the females, 48 years. The extremes were 21 and 85 years. A breakdown of the ages by decades is shown in Fig 1.

Site of Origin of the Thrombus.—On the basis of clinical findings, the site of origin of the phlebitic process was in the lower extremities in 49 (89%) of the patients. The limb involved was the left in 28 (57%), the right in 12 (25%), and both in 9 (18%). In 6 (11%) of the patients, the pelvis was

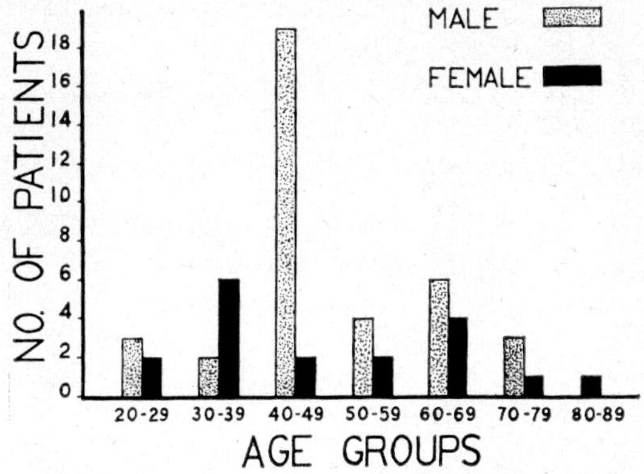

Fig 1.—Bar graph indicating breakdown of ages of males and females by decades.

the site of thrombosis. Judging by history and clinical evidence, embolization to the lung occurred as a single episode in 20 (48%), twice in 8 (19%), and three or more times in 14 (32%) of the patients.

Indications for Operation.—The indications were a diagnosis of pulmonary embolus in 42 cases and prophylaxis in 13 patients with acute ascending thrombophlebitis or phlegmasia cerulea dolens in whom thrombosis was encountered on exploration of the common femoral vein.

Diagnosis.—The clinical history and physical examination are believed to provide the most accurate information in regard to diagnosis, at least in the initial phase of the disease. Chest films in the early stages are frequently negative. In this series, radiologic confirmation was obtained in only 25 of the 42 patients with clinical evidence of pulmonary involvement. The electrocardiogram was of help only in patients with either multiple or massive pulmonary embolism, where it indicates right heart strain. Serum lactic dehydrogenase determinations have been in use too recently to be of value in our over-all series.

Operative Technique.—The operation is performed with the patient in the supine position. In most instances, spinal anesthesia is used. In the earliest cases, an oblique abdominal incision was used but was later abandoned in favor of a transverse incision approximately at the level of the umbilicus. This latter incision is used for lumbar sympathectomy and has been clearly described

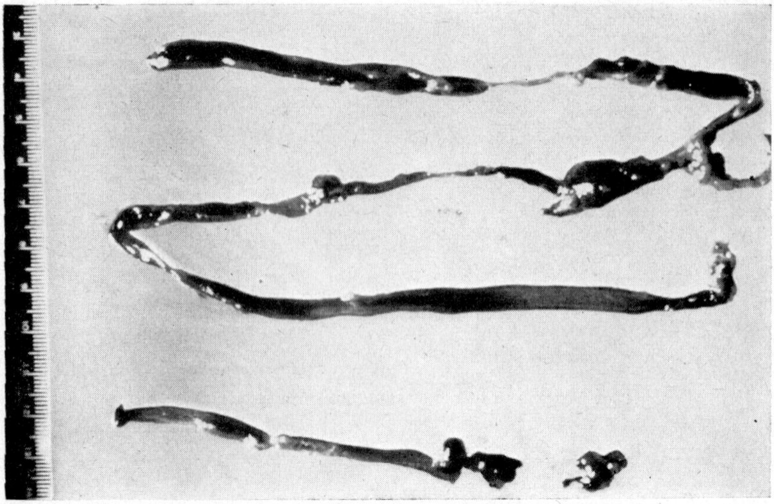

Fig 2.—Thrombus 47 cm in length extruded from femoral-iliac veins after vena cava ligation.

by Madden.[9] The only modification is the cutting of a small portion of the external oblique muscle. The internal oblique and transversus abdominis muscles are split and the retroperitoneal space opened. The inferior vena cava is inspected and palpated for intraluminal thrombus, then mobilized, particular attention being paid to the lumbar veins. A large blunt ligature carrier is used to pass an umbilical tape around the vena cava. With a little experience, this operation can be done quite simply and rapidly. The only real danger, tearing off a lumbar vein, can be avoided with due caution. This mishap occurred once in this series; approximately 2,000 cc of blood was lost and almost an hour was required to control bleeding.

Since 1958, thrombectomy has been added to vena cava ligation in patients with marked edema or with phlegmasia cerulea dolens, provided the operation is performed within 24 to 36 hours after onset of the massive edema. The combination of procedures was done in 14 patients in this series. Thrombectomy is carried out through a vertical incision in the common femoral vein after it has been mobilized and controlled proximally and distally. Thrombus can be removed from the pelvic veins by gentle milking with the finger or by pressure on the abdomen. Distally, massage and pressure over the superficial femoral vein with the fist in the thigh or vigorous dorsiflexion of the foot will usually cause the clots to extrude, at times in a very forceful manner. In one instance, a thrombus measuring 47 cm in length was removed (Fig 2).

Postoperative Management.—It is our conviction that the postoperative control of edema is the single most significant factor in determining the end results following ligation of the vena cava. In the immediate postoperative period the legs are wrapped with rubberized bandages. A 4-inch bandage is used below the knee and a 6-inch bandage on

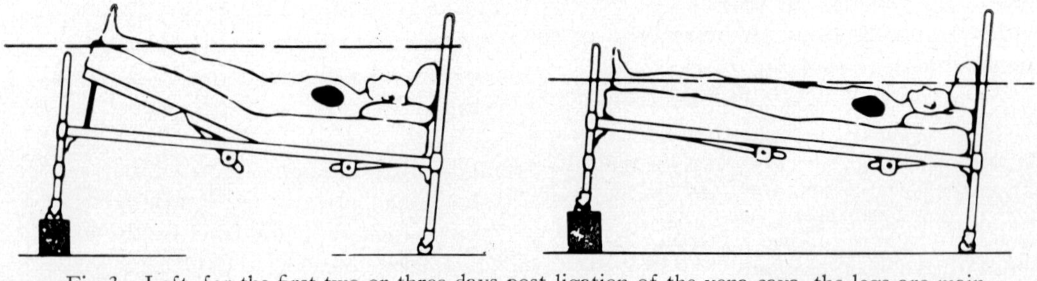

Fig 3.—Left, for the first two or three days post ligation of the vena cava, the legs are maintained in steep elevation. Right, after this, the foot of the bed is elevated 6 in off the floor.

the thigh. It is difficult to obtain good support with narrower bandages. For the first two or three days, the legs are maintained in steep elevation (Fig 3). Following this period, the most comfortable and most effective method of elevation has been found to be simple lifting of the foot of the bed 6 inches off the floor. Throughout the hospital stay the patient is encouraged to dorsiflex his feet forcefully "100 times each hour." When not contraindicated, heparinization is of value in preventing further propagation of the clot. In most instances, the first dose is administered 6 to 12 hours postoperatively. The patient is permitted to walk just as soon as he is able to do so; however, he is not allowed to sit in a chair more than five minutes at a time during the period of hospitalization. He is usually discharged wearing elastic bandages, but as soon as practical, heavy-weight elastic stockings are obtained. In some patients with excessive swelling of the thigh, a high-thigh stocking is used for the first two or three months postoperatively; subsequently, however, all patients wear below-the-knee stockings. In our experience, swelling of the thigh will almost always subside spontaneously. Furthermore, high-thigh stockings become uncomfortable and the patient refuses to wear them. In only one instance have we observed ulceration above the knee (see report of case). The importance of the weight of the stocking cannot be overemphasized. In addition to weight, two-way stretch characteristics are desirable, and the stocking should have a heel.*

All patients are given instructions as to how they can minimize their difficulties. They are advised to be as active as possible. It is explained to them that the muscles of the lower extremities act as a pump that forces the blood centrally and that standing still or sitting will produce the most swelling and the most discomfort. They are therefore instructed to avoid prolonged sitting. With few exceptions, however, the patients in this series have been able to resume their previous occupation and daily habits within a few months.

Mortality.—There were three operative deaths, a mortality rate of 5.5%. The first patient, a 64-year-old white male, had a cardiac arrest after ligation as the incision was being closed. Cardiac massage for an hour and a half failed to revive him. At autopsy, the lungs showed multiple pulmonary emboli with so much loss of lung parenchyma that the cardiac arrest was attributed to anoxia. The second patient, a 58-year-old white female, died of widespread carcinomatosis from carcinoma of the cervix two weeks postoperatively. The third patient, a 74-year-old white female, died of cardiac failure during the third postoperative week.

Late Deaths.—The late deaths are shown in Table 2. It is of interest that the patient with the retroperitoneal lymphoma had pelvic thrombophlebitis, probably precipitated by the malignant lesion.

Complications.—Of the patients who are now alive, none has a handicap of any significance. Specific questioning revealed the fact that twelve patients had exertional dyspnea, usually on climbing stairs; however, no patient complained of shortness of breath spontaneously. Eight patients stated their legs became tired if they walked fast and that this fatigue was relieved by rest (the major arteries in the lower extremities of all these patients were patent). Seven patients noted transient dizziness or lightheadedness on rising from bed. Five patients

TABLE 2.—*Inferior Vena Cava Ligation: Late Deaths (Seven Patients)*

Cause	Months Postop	No. Pts.
Ca. of colon	3	1
Lymphoma	4	1
Coronary occlusion	10	1
CVA	12	1
Ca. of prostate	12	1
Bronchogenic Ca.	87	1
Coronary occlusion	96	1

* The most effective stocking we have encountered is manufactured by the Tru-Form Division of the Surgical Appliance Industries, Cincinnati 37, Ohio, and is sold under the brand name "Formfit" or simply as No. 8345. When manufactured by Ohio Truss Co., another division of the same firm, the same stocking is called "Nu-Vein."

had recurrent thrombophlebitis. Three patients had transient hematuria. Cystoscopy revealed hemorrhagic prostatitis in two. Anticoagulant therapy is believed to be the cause of the bleeding in the third patient.

Three patients had ulceration of the extremity. In one, a small ulcer was present on the dorsum of the foot, thought to be caused by the stocking. When the stocking was omitted temporarily, the ulcer healed rapidly. Another patient developed ulceration of the skin above the medial malleolus. However, this patient also had occlusion of the aortoiliac arterial segment. After insertion of an aortofemoral bypass graft, the ulcer healed rapidly and has remained healed for four years. The third patient had uncontrollable edema and ulceration (see report of case).

Postligation Edema.—Heavy-weight elastic stockings were prescribed initially for all patients. It is noteworthy that one patient (who did not have thrombectomy) had no edema in the postoperative period and never has worn elastic stockings. At the present time, of 42 patients, 25 (60%) are still wearing elastic stockings bilaterally, 4 (10%) are wearing a stocking on one limb, and 13 (30%) are not wearing them at all (3 patients are excluded from these calculations because they state they wear elastic stockings occasionally).

One patient, who lived seven years after operation, could not be fully rehabilitated. Since his case presents some very unusual aspects, it seems worthwhile to report it in detail.

Report of Case

This patient was a 40-year-old white male first seen in January, 1954. At that time, a diagnosis of multiple pulmonary emboli was made (confirmed by chest films) and inferior vena cava ligation advised. At operation, large clots were found in the vena cava that extended up to the vicinity of the renal veins. This clot was removed and found to be partially fresh and partially organized. His initial postoperative course was difficult because of tremendous swelling. He was discharged on anticoagulant therapy (phenindione: Hedulin; 2-phenyl-1, 3-indandione). The patient was 76 in (193 cm) tall and, during the next few months, gained weight to 210 lb (95.2 kg). But with the heavy-weight elastic stockings he was able to return to work in May, 1954. From January to June, he had three attacks of thrombophlebitis, followed by four later on, making seven in all that we could document. We believe that he had other attacks while he was under the care of other physicians. Eleven months postoperatively, he developed pigmentation on the left ankle followed by ulceration two weeks later. It is to be borne in mind, all this was while the patient was on anticoagulant therapy. The ulcer healed within three months with pressure dressings. In March, 1955, a venogram was obtained. Since the patency of the femoral vein could not be demonstrated, the vessel was explored. However, both the superficial and common femoral veins, the external iliac vein, and the saphenous vein in this area were all patent. There was a fibrous cord along the wall of the common femoral vein which may have represented the original clot. Nothing further could be done in this area, and an incision was made in the vicinity of the previous ulceration, where some superficial veins were excised. No communicating veins could be found in the lowest fourth of the leg. No visible varicosities were present in the upper three fourths of the leg. Once more, the patient returned to work and was lost to follow-up for six months, when he entered the Veterans Administration Hospital for recurrent thrombophlebitis. At this time, his case was studied in a seminar. The consensus was to continue the anticoagulant therapy, upon which he had been maintained since discharge from the hospital approximately two years before. In August of 1957 he developed a new ulcer which again was healed with pressure after great difficulty. Three months later he was readmitted, and another venogram was obtained which showed patency of the vena cava up to the occlusion by the ligature and a huge internal spermatic vein. This time, the long saphenous vein was removed from the groin to the ankle, and subfascial ligation of four large communicating veins of the leg was performed. Postoperatively he did well and returned to work. He was maintained on anticoagulant therapy, the prothrombin concentration being kept between 30% and 35% most of the time. It is of interest that once he developed thrombophlebitis while taking 200 mg of phenindione a day. It is also to be noted that he regulated his prothrombin concentration himself and he was convinced he felt much better when it was down around 25% than when it was closer to 40%. During the next few years, he developed recurrent ulcerations and was seen on one occasion with multiple ulcerations of the left lower extremity, including one ulcer above the knee. All these ulcers had small engorged veins underneath them, and it was our opinion, therefore, that they were of venous origin—not excepting the one on the thigh. In all our experience, we have never seen another venous ulcer above the knee. His ulcers could always be

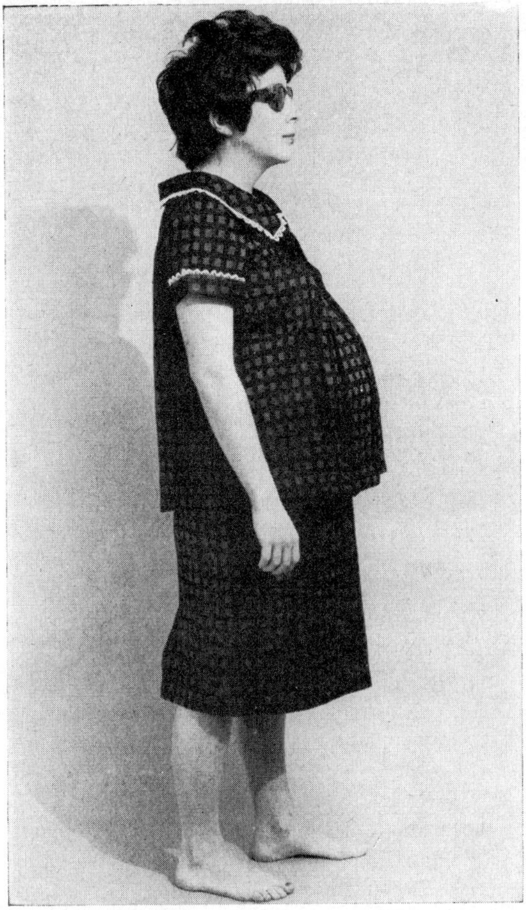

Fig 4.—Patient in the eighth month of her second pregnancy after vena cava ligation two years prior to this photograph.

healed, but it took a great amount of pressure to do so. He wore heavy-weight elastic stockings plus a 4-inch rubber bandage around the leg from toes to knee, and a 6-inch one from knee to groin. In 1959 he was admitted to the Veterans Administration Hospital, where he died of carcinoma of the lung in April, 1961.

In summary, this is a patient who had thrombophlebitis many times. Prior to vena cava ligation, he had multiple pulmonary emboli. After ligation, he had none, yet he did have at least seven attacks of venous thrombosis. He developed recurrent ulcerations of the legs, which, however, did not incapacitate him, since he continued to work. Despite removal of the diseased veins and the use of heavy-weight elastic stockings, the ulcers failed to remain healed. He ultimately died of carcinoma of the lung.

A second interesting patient is shown in Fig 4. At the time of this photograph, the patient was in the eighth month of her second pregnancy following vena cava ligation. There are no visible varicosities, no discoloration of the skin, and no swelling. She did not wear elastic support during either pregnancy. When photographed, she was two years postoperative and had worn elastic stockings for less than two months in the immediate post-ligation period.

Comment

There can be no doubt that ligation of the inferior vena cava is an effective method of preventing pulmonary emboli arising from the distal half of the body. Our experience supports that of Dale,[3] Schauble,[12] and and Miller[10] in that the sequelae of vena cava ligation can be managed and the patient rehabilitated in almost every instance. It is believed that most of the swelling which appears is explainable on the basis of the venous thrombosis rather than on the ligation itself. This swelling is controllable by elevation of the foot of the bed and the use of heavy-weight elastic stockings. In our experience all patients with this type of swelling have been controllable with the single exception described in the case report. A clear distinction must be made, however, between swelling due to venous insufficiency and that due to lymphedema or carcinomatous infiltration of the veins and lymphatics of the pelvis. In these latter instances, the swelling not infrequently may be impossible to control. Because the results in this series have been so satisfactory, we have not been eager to use temporizing procedures, such as ligation of the inferior vena cava with absorbable materials,[4] plication of the vessel[14] or temporary occlusion by means of clips.[11] The addition of thrombectomy following vena cava ligation in a smaller number of cases has given dramatic relief of swelling and, consequently, whenever it can be done, is considered the treatment of choice. The use of heparin in the immediate postoperative period is recommended to limit the extension of thrombosis.

Summary

A ten-year experience with ligation of the inferior vena cava in 55 patients is presented. Forty-five of the patients are still living, and with the exception of one with concomitant occlusive aortoiliac disease, their morbidity has been minimal. Indications, complications, and method of management are outlined.

Raymond J. Krause, MD, 311 Howell Ave, Cincinnati 20, Ohio.

REFERENCES

1. Bowers, R. F., and Leb, S. M.: Late Results of Inferior Vena Cava Ligation, Surgery 37:622-628, 1955.
2. Collins, C. G.; Norton, R. O.; Nelson, E. W.; Weinstein, B. B.; Collins, J. H.; and Webster, H. D., Jr.: Suppurative Thrombophlebitis: IV. Results; A Study of 70 Patients Treated by Ligation of the Inferior Vena Cava and Ovarian Vessels, Surgery 31:528-537, 1952.
3. Dale, W.: Ligation of the Inferior Vena Cava for Thromboembolism, Surgery 43:24-44, 1958.
4. Dale, W. A.; Pualwan, F.; and Bauer, F. M.: Ligation of the Inferior Vena Cava With Absorbable Gut, Surg Gynec Obstet 102:517-530, 1956.
5. Fogarty, T. J.; Cranley, J. J.; Krause, R. J.; Strasser, E. S.; and Hafner, C. D.: Surgical Management of Phlegmasia Cerulea Dolens, Arch Surg 86:256-263, 1963.
6. Homans, J.: Thrombosis of the Deep Veins of the Lower Leg Causing Pulmonary Embolism, New Eng J Med 211:993-997, 1934.
7. Kirtley, J. A.; Riddell, D. R.; and Hamilton, E. C.: Indications and Late Results of Ligation of Inferior Vena Cava, Ann Surg 141:653-661, 1955.
8. Krotoski, J.: Zur Venenunterbindung beziehungsweise Extirpation bei der puerperalen Allgemeininfektion von chirurgischem Standpunkt, Chirurg 9:425-439, 1937.
9. Madden, J. L.: Ligation of the Inferior Vena Cava, Ann Surg 140:200-205, 1954.
10. Miller, D. R.: "Inferior Vena Caval Ligation for Thromboembolism," in Current Surgical Management, Philadelphia: W. B. Saunders Company, 1960, vol 2, pp 255-261.
11. Moretz, W. H.; Naisbitt, P. F.; and Stevenson, G. P.: Experimental Studies on Temporary Occlusion of the Inferior Vena Cava, Surgery 36: 384-397, 1954.
12. Schauble, J. F.; Stickel, D. I.; and Anlyan, W. G.: Vena Caval Ligation for Thromboembolic Disease, Arch Surg 84:17-22, 1962.
13. Shea, P. C., and Robertson, R. L.: Late Sequelae of Inferior Vena Cava Ligation, Surg Gynec Obstet 93:153-158, 1951.
14. Spencer, F. C.; Quattelbaum, J. K.; Quattelbaum, J. K., Jr.; Sharp, E. H.; and Jude, J. R.: Plication of the Inferior Vena Cava for Pulmonary Embolism: A Report of 20 Cases, Ann Surg 155: 827-835, 1962.
15. Trendelenburg, F.: Über die chirurgische Behandling der puerperalen Pyaemie, Munchen Med Wschr, 1912, cited by Miller, C. J.: Ligation or Excision of the Pelvic Veins in the Treatment of Puerperal Pyemia, Surg Gynec Obstet 25:431-452, 1917.

DISCUSSION

On papers by Drs. Humphries, and Krause et al

Dr. Louis T. Palumbo, Des Moines, Iowa: Our experience and results are similar to those reported by Dr. Krause and associates. During the past 12 years, we have ligated 33 inferior vena cavas, 12 common iliac veins, two external iliac veins, and 12 superficial femoral veins in patients with the postphlebitic syndrome with or without pulmonary embolism and in a group of patients with pulmonary embolism from a "silent" phlebothrombosis.

During the past ten years all the ligations have been of the inferior vena cava. We found that ligation of the iliacs resulted in greater disability than vena caval ligation and with it, as well as those cases of ligation of the femoral veins, frequently did not prevent pulmonary embolism.

A high per cent had pulmonary infarction, and a number had a history of previous infarctions. Frequently, the thrombosis of the vascular tree had extended into the iliac vessels and to the lower segment of the vena cava. We, too, have removed a flagellate propagating thrombus extending superior to the renal veins.

Ligation at the proper level will prevent further pulmonary infarction, will arrest the process of recurrent phlebitis and propagating thrombosis. It is our opinion, too, that when thrombosis has occurred above the confluence of the femoral veins, superficial and deep, it is safer and more physiologic to ligate the inferior vena cava.

In addition, we prefer to perform an adequate lumbar sympathectomy at the time of vena caval ligation. This results in improvement of circulation, both arterial and venous. It eliminates sweating, which with the aforementioned change results in a warmer and drier extremity. This, alone, is an important consideration since it contributes immeasurably to reducing the incidence of cellulitis and recurrent infections, particularly those of fungus origin. By division of these nerve fibers, the vasosensory pathways are interrupted, thereby eliminating or reducing the severity of peripheral pain.

There were no deaths in this group, and the complication rate was low.

In our series, ligation of the inferior vena cava resulted in only slight restriction of the patients' activities, and with proper postoperative management the degree and extent of swelling of the extremities can be controlled.

Ligation of the vena cava is a lifesaving procedure, prevents recurrent episodes of pulmonary infarction and propagation of the thrombosis, and is usually not followed by enough disablement or impairment of function of the extremities to prevent the patients from returning to a gainful occupation.

Dr. D. Emerick Szilagyi, Detroit: The exceptional value of Dr. Humphries' paper lies in its approach to the comparative evaluation of the three possible forms of management of advanced arteriosclerotic disease of the limbs (conservative, direct surgical, and indirect surgical), notably their assessment in terms of amputation rates. In general, the results with respect to amputation rates in these three categories that I have observed are similar to those reported. As regards some statistical details, my observations differ. Time, of course, does not allow me to analyze these differences, and, what is more important, such an analysis would not affect the significant conclusion, namely, that the arterioplastic form of management has clear superiority. I might mention, however, that I have not been able to verify the capability of lumbar sympathectomy to improve appreciably the level of amputation, as suggested by Dr. Humphries and some other authors. Moreover, I do not find acceptable the statistical reasoning adduced by Dr. Humphries in support of the conclusion that arterioplasty lowered the mortality rate observed during the hospital management of these patients, all of whom had very severe arteriosclerosis.

I should, finally, like to call your attention to a fact that is implicit in Dr. Humphries' study and which deserves special emphasis. As you know, there is hardly room at the present time for argument with respect to the great benefits that reconstructive surgery has brought about in the treatment of aortoiliac occlusive disease of all grades. There is a good deal of doubt, however, about how much one can accomplish with these procedures in the management of femoropopliteal lesions. I myself have come to the conclusion that the most effective use of reconstructive methods in femoropopliteal disease is for advanced ischemia. In the large majority of these cases the surgeon's aim is to salvage the limb; and although the salvage is often only temporary, even a relatively short-lived success in achieving this goal makes surgical treatment worth while. Dr. Humphries has furnished further very valuable proof that this thesis is probably correct.

Dr. Rodman E. Taber, Detroit: One of the most important points that Dr. Krause made was that this procedure is essentially 100% effective in preventing pulmonary embolization if done at the proper level.

This is a rather sizable series of patients, and I think the only obvious exception at the present time is a patient with auricular fibrillation who may embolize from the right atrium and who must be excluded from observations of this sort.

Another point that Dr. Krause has made is that the close observation which this group has exercised in the use of stocking supports routinely in the first few years postoperatively will prevent stasis sequelae in the majority of patients. In a smaller series of patients but a group followed somewhat longer than his, from the Henry Ford Hospital, we have observed a much higher incidence of these stasis sequelae, and possibly this is because our management has not been as close as Dr. Krause's in the postoperative period.

We have designed a Teflon clip for nonocclusive caval control, which I should like to show. The clip with four serrations is the one we have found to be most satisfactory. This clip is held in place around the vena cava by nonabsorbable ligatures and by the two grooves that are on the end of the clip. Two residents working in our laboratory have done a considerable amount of work on this device and have found that it will trap emboli larger than 2 mm in diameter and yet will not produce obstruction to venous drainage, as demonstrated by a pressure gradient or evidence of occlusion by a cavogram.

When the clip is applied to the cava there is not too much difference in the size of the venous channel. Pressures were measured across both sides of the clip. A cavogram performed about six weeks after application of the clip is at about the same level. We see no evidence of obstruction as manifested by venous collateral supply.

The rationale for applying this device, of course, is that the patient who does not embolize further ends up with a patent vena cava, whereas the patient who does embolize and occludes the clip is no worse off than the patient who had a ligation.

Dr. John A. McLachlin, St. Thomas, Ont, Canada: Over the ten years that I have had the pleasure of attending the meetings of this Association, John Cranley and I have had a running skirmish regarding thrombo-embolism and very often have not seen eye to eye about our findings. However, today I would like to climb over to his side of the fence and support him strongly in inferior vena caval ligation for the prevention of recurrent pulmonary emboli.

Dr. Carroll and his group, from our center, recently reported 35 cases of ligation of the inferior vena cava for recurrent pulmonary emboli. The first case 15 years ago was my responsibility. We have reserved ligation of the inferior vena cava for recurrent cases, and personally I do not carry it out prophylactically.

In 1951, Dr. Peterson and I published a paper which was presented to this Society, in which we felt that ligation of the superficial femoral vein was inadequate because over 50% of the thrombi arose above the point where we usually ligate the superficial femoral vein. We feel very strongly that the lowest level of venous ligation to effectively block emboli is in the inferior vena cava.

I think it has been shown very well through anatomical studies that you have more bypasses with the ligation at the level of the inferior vena cava than if you ligate the superficial femoral vein or the common femoral vein.

In our 35 cases we had four deaths, one at seven days because of cerebral thrombosis, one at four weeks with coronary thrombosis, one at one month with the problem of the late sequela of carcinoma of the bladder, and the fourth case at three months with congestive heart failure.

None of our cases produced a further embolus. Twenty-one of the original 35 cases had edema preoperatively. Eighteen of the 35 cases showed no edema postoperatively. The remaining 17 showed edema postoperatively. Five of these had minimal edema, and 12 of them had moderate to severe edema in the postoperative phase. Of these 12, all were in the original group of 21 showing edema preoperatively. Nine of the 12 had some improvement in their edema, and none had any appreciable worsening of their edema.

We feel that edema arises only in the patient who has had previous damage to the deep veins in his legs and that the operation per se does not produce edema.

Dr. John J. Cranley, Cincinnati: In regard to Dr. Humphries' paper, we too have been interested in this subject and over the past ten years have examined, graded, and followed approximately 2,000 extremities with obliterative arterial disease, of which between 500 and 600 will fall into the category Dr. Humphries speaks of.

We, too, have used the amputation rate as a criterion of success or failure because it is logical and definitive. However, using this as a criterion of success, we are not able to demonstrate any significant difference between the patients treated conservatively and those treated surgically. Since there is overwhelming evidence of improvement in individual cases, this can only mean that our criterion is too severe, almost certainly because we find it impossible to select our patients at random.

In regard to our own paper, when we speak of prophylaxis, perhaps we were remiss in not explaining it. Almost all the patients who had a prophylactic ligation were patients in whom we explored the femoral vein and found the clots extending into the pelvis. Then we went ahead and tied the vena cava, and then went back and tried to clean out the clots in the groin.

The rest of the discussion comes down to two points: first, do you wish your ligation to be permanent? Second, does your ligation increase the swelling? In regard to the first question, we do wish our ligation to be permanent. We do not want to have to operate on these patients again. The second question I can answer best by showing two slides.

The patient shown is now 3½ years postoperative. She is not in this series because she did not have her vena cava ligated. She did, however, have one superficial femoral vein ligated and one common iliac vein ligated. Can anyone tell which extremity has had the common iliac vein ligated?

She was seen 3½ years ago with massive swelling due to postpartum phlebitis extending above the inguinal ligament. She was taken to the operating room, and clots were found extending into the common iliac vein. The common iliac vein was ligated and thrombectomy performed with the common iliac, external iliac, common femoral, and superficial femoral vein. Within 48 hours postoperatively she had no swelling whatever, has never had any since, and does not wear an elastic support. As you can see, her legs appear to be entirely normal.

This emphasizes the point that has become a conviction with us, namely, that the ligation of a major vein does not cause swelling; it is the venous thrombosis that causes swelling. If these patients have venous thrombosis they will have swelling no matter what you do. If you ligate the vein and take out the clots you will have a good chance of eliminating the swelling entirely.

Editorials

The Influence of Geography on Duodenal Ulcers

This editorial is prompted by my reading of the paper entitled "Peptic Ulcer in Africa" by Clarence A. Snyder and Merton J. Alexander in this issue of the ARCHIVES as well as by reflections on reported geographical factors influencing duodenal ulcer in India and in Norway.

While there have been many significant contributions in recent years dealing with the pathogenesis of duodenal ulcer, some factors still remain obscure. One of these is the high incidence of ulcer reported in certain areas, while neighboring regions inhabited by the same race of people remain relatively free from the disease. In my own view a hypersecretion of gastric juice of nervous origin has been established as the sufficient cause of duodenal ulcer in the overwhelming majority of patients in the United States and in Europe. These patients regularly display a hypersecretion of gastric juice in the empty stomach which, if reproduced in the same degree in experimental animals, regularly leads to the development of a similar progressive chronic ulcer in the duodenum. The fact that this hypersecretion is abolished if the vagus nerves to the stomach are divided or is markedly reduced by anticholinergic drugs indicates that it is of nervous origin. The final evidence is, of course, the rapid healing of duodenal ulcers which occurs when the vagus nerves to the stomach have been divided and the antrum is removed, or when stasis of food in the antrum is prevented. It would be of the greatest interest therefore to know if the increased incidence of duodenal ulcer in certain regions of Norway, India, and Africa is accompanied by a hypersecretion of gastric juice in the empty stomach which is returned toward the normal by anticholinergic drugs. If a hypersecretion of gastric juice in the fasting empty stomach is found, attention might then be directed to factors such as prolonged nervous tension, emotional and mental strain, and competitive effort as influences producing such hyperactivity in the vagus centers.

If hypersecretion in the fasting empty stomach is not found, the observations recorded in the paper by Snyder and Alexander that these duodenal ulcers occur frequently in people whose diets are deficient in animal protein and who habitually consume large amounts of alcohol are very significant. Experimental evidence is now adequate to indicate that diets low in animal protein and accompanied by the ingestion of alcohol produce often extensive fatty infiltration in the liver. This fatty infiltration can produce moderate to severe impairment of liver function and often leads to cirrhosis. The high incidence of peptic ulcer in patients with cirrhosis or following portacaval shunts now comes to mind. In these patients humoral agents such as histamine, absorbed from the intestinal tract and normally detoxified in the liver, may be shunted around the liver, fail to be detoxified, and consequently exert a stimulating action on gastric secretion. Liver function tests on patients in these areas where duodenal ulcer is frequent and where dietary inadequacies seem to be a factor might be very revealing.

It should also be borne in mind that the oral administration of alcohol provides a very effective stimulus for the release of gastrin but very little in the way of neutralization of the gastric juice secreted. For this reason, early in our work on vagotomy we chose to treat chronic alcoholics with duodenal ulcer by vagotomy and antrum resection rather than by vagotomy and a drainage procedure.

As a final comment I should like to point out that we still have no adequate explanation for the reported exacerbation of duodenal ulcer in the autumn and spring and its relative quiescence during the winter and summer months. It would be interesting and possibly worthwhile to find out if duodenal ulcer patients, and possibly also normal people, secrete more gastric juice in the fasting empty stomach during the autumn and spring months than they do during the winter and summer.

I have not touched on the factor of mucosal resistance in this disease because the evidence at hand is sufficient to show that a hypersecretion of gastric juice of the degree found in duodenal ulcer patients will destroy the normal mucosa of the duodenum and produce a typical ulcer. Nevertheless, it is probable that if a localized area of the mucous membrane of the stomach or duodenum is devitalized from any cause, such an area should break down more rapidly and thus determine the site of the ulcer. In this connection it should be emphasized that a local loss of resistance on the part of the mucous membrane will not result in a chronic peptic ulcer unless the corrosive properties of the gastric content are considerably greater than normal. The secretory hyperactivity of the gastric glands in ulcer patients does not make one suspect that a functional impairment of this membrane is present very often.

Lester R. Dragstedt, MD
Department of Surgery
College of Medicine
University of Florida
Gainesville, Fla

In Summary

As the number of new professional articles one must read each month increases by leaps and bounds much attention is presumably being given to making them more efficiently accessible to the reading public. Although digests, reviews, and collected abstracts play their important parts, a major accusation must still be leveled at us, the writing medical public. An intelligent, comprehensive, and succinct summary at the end of an article is all too unusual. Perhaps we are derelict in this regard because, blinded by an author's vanity, we assume that the reader will be so entranced by our style and lucidity that he will read the whole article word for word and a summary will be unnecessary. We then insert one merely as a genuflection to custom with little attention to its content.

Let us be undeceived! Gone are the days when doctors are expected to read papers written in the style set by the professors in the great German university medical schools who produced from 20 to 50 pages with no *Zusammenfassung* at the end. To be sure, seldom did such unassailable figures as Halsted, who derived his academic stimulus from that source, or Cushing, who inherited it from him, use a summary, and when they did they were never quite sure whether it was a summary, a summary and conclusions, or merely a discussion arranged under the head-ing of one of these. In those days there were fewer who were writing articles, and possibly readers' desks were not piled so high with important unread material.

The increasing need for an efficient summary, however, started to emerge in the surgical generation that was beginning near the end of Cushing's career. As an example witness the excellent one in the article on "Papillomas of the Choroid Plexus" by Davis and Cushing in the *Archives of Neurology and Psychiatry* (13:681, 1925):

1. Some twenty examples of true papilloma of the choroid are to be identified in the literature. They are to be found scattered under most varied titles and are generally confused with tumors of other sorts which project into the ventricles. In a series of 964 verified intracranial tumors, six of these papillomas have been encountered. Two arose from the lateral choroid plexus and four from the plexus of the fourth ventricle. In five cases the lesion was identified by tissues removed at operation; in one, at necropsy.

2. In three of the tumors, an accompanying cystic formation was a striking characteristic. In the other three, the tumor was a simple cauliflower-like papilloma. In all cases, however, the sections show villi with a central well vascularized core of connective tissue covered by cuboidal epithelium, usually in a single layer.

3. The epithelial cells of these papillomas contain round, darkly staining granules, which tend to be arranged perinuclearly, and which appear to be closely related to mitochondria. The tumors do not contain glia fibers, nor do their cells show "blepharoplasten". They are therefore not to be confused with the papillomatous ependymomas.

The value of this is that it summarizes the important information that the article covers. Most articles today provide a "summary" or a "summary and conclusions" at the end, but rarely does the section contain anything more than a statement of the motions that the author went through. We are left with a burning curiosity as to what he found out. Here is an example picked at random from thousands of others.*

An analysis is presented of . . . consecutive patients who suffered from primary sarcoma of the lung and were treated at the . . . Hospital during the . . . year period . . . to . . . .

A classification of mesenchymal tumors is given together with a discussion of their differential diagnosis, treatment and prognosis

Does this give one any more usable information than the title itself, which is "Sarcoma of the Lung"? Obviously all these things would be expected to be discussed in any article of worth that went under that title.

The article is otherwise a splendid one, beautifully written, and full of useful information. But the summary as it stands contributes nothing. It would have done so had it included such pertinent data from the body of the paper as that the diagnosis was made by x-ray in only 1 of 18, that only 1 presented with a massive hemorrhage, that frozen section was misleading in 2 of 8 cases, and that 5-year survival rate after resection was over 50%.

An orderly professional report has come to include (whether they appear as paragraph heads or not), an introduction, a description of methodology, results, a discussion, conclusions, and a summary. The summary should not be used to replace the discussion or conclusions but to summarize the paper as a whole for the exhausted reader and the harrassed abstractor. Let it consist then of a description of the type of work that is being reported, the pertinent results obtained therefrom, and the author's opinion of their significance.

Richard Warren, MD
Peter Bent Brigham Hospital
721 Huntington Ave
Boston 15

* For the purpose of disguising this material to make it unrecognizable (hopefully even to the authors) it has been paraphrased so that professionally it makes no sense. This does not detract from the point that is being made which has to do with the type and amount of information it provides.

Absent Left Pulmonary Artery and Right-Sided Patent Ductus Arteriosus

HENRY SWAN, MD, DSc; J. CUTHBERT OWENS, MD; PETER E. POOL, AB; JOHN H. K. VOGEL, MD; AND S. GILBERT BLOUNT, JR., MD, DENVER

Congenital absence of one pulmonary artery, while not a common anomaly, is nonetheless not rare. Over 100 cases of various modifications of this abnormality have been reported, and we have recently prepared a detailed analysis of 78 of these cases [1] in which an adequate amount of information was available for detailed study. Since an excessive pulmonary blood flow, because of associated shunts, is common, and since blood from the pulmonary artery in this anomaly all flows through one lung only, the development of pulmonary hypertension is a frequent occurrence and may result in the death of the patient in early childhood. For this reason it is impressive to recognize the lesion so that curative surgery may be undertaken early.

This report concerns what appears to be an almost unique modification of unilateral absent pulmonary artery in which absence of the left pulmonary artery is associated with a right aortic arch and a patent ductus arteriosus lying in the right side of the chest. Two such cases are presented, one of which also was associated with unrecognized ventricular septal defect. The purpose of the report is to call the attention of this entity to the profession and to discuss the surgical problems posed by the unusual location of the patent ductus arteriosus.

Review of Literature

Congenital absence of one pulmonary artery was first reported by Fraentzel in 1868.[2] A half century elapsed before a second case was reported by Doering.[3] However, it was soon apparent that the lesion was not as rare as was thought. In the decade 1950 to 1960, a total of 66 cases were reported in the literature, many of which were recognized before death. Terminology is somewhat confusing in this condition, as the word "hypoplasia" has been used in some case reports. We are concerned in this paper, however, only with those cases with complete absence of either the left or the right pulmonary artery, with an intact lung on the affected side. We are not concerned with agenesis of the lung. In our study of 78 reported cases including three of our own, it was apparent that the absence of a pulmonary artery is more frequently associated with other congenital anomalies of the heart and great vessels than not (Table). As can be seen from the Table, patent ductus arteriosus, the tetralogy of Fallot, septal defects, or multiple shunts are all commonly associated with the basic deformity. It is interesting, however, that the left pulmonary artery and the right pulmonary artery are involved in approximately equal numbers, that the tetralogy of Fallot is almost solely associated

Vessel Missing

	LPA	RPA
Isolated	14	18
Fallot	16	1 *
PDA	1	10
Septal defects	5	4
Other †	4	5
	40	38

* In a patient with dextrocardia.

† Cases with two shunts or a shunt and a vascular lesion in addition to an absence of one pulmonary artery.

Submitted for publication Jan 14, 1963.

Postdoctoral research fellow, National Heart Institute, US Public Health Service (Dr. Vogel).

From the Departments of Surgery and Medicine, University of Colorado School of Medicine.

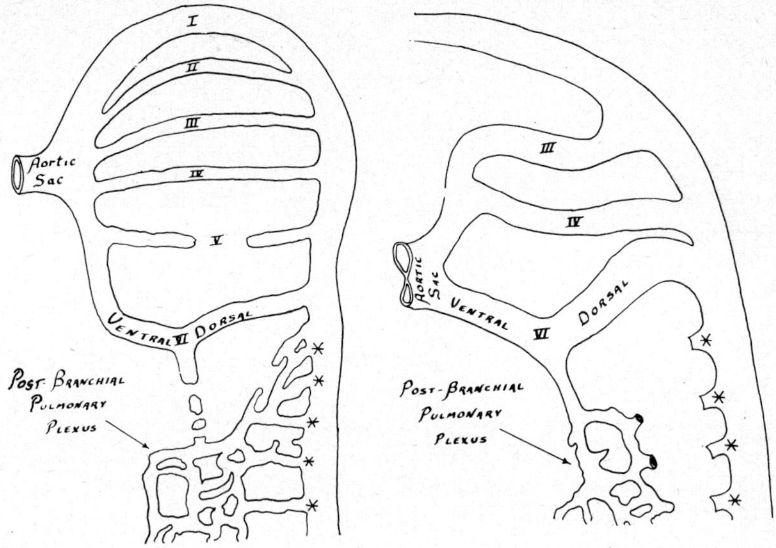

Fig 1.—The embryologic development of the pulmonary artery and the possible connections between the pulmonary vascular tree and the systemic circulation. (Reprinted by permission of the American Journal of Cardiology).

with absence of the *left* pulmonary artery, and that, conversely, patent ductus arteriosus, with the exception of the two cases reported herein, is almost always associated with the absence of the *right* pulmonary artery.

A number of theories as to the embryology of this defect have been proposed, based upon current understanding of the development of the aortic arches. This problem has been thoroughly reviewed in our previous publication, and we will simply summarize our analysis of the probable embryologic course of events as follows.[1] In most cases of absent right pulmonary artery, the vessel most often arose from the ascending aorta and was found to be the blood supply to the right lung. In the cases of absent left, and in the remaining cases of absent right, pulmonary artery the blood supply to the affected lung was found to derive from either bronchial vessels or a large vessel off the aortic arch. The latter is considered to be ductal in nature, both grossly and upon histological examination. It is our belief that the postbrachial pulmonary plexus, as seen in Fig 1, has three vascular channels leading to it: (1) the ventral blood from the aortic sac; (2) the dorsal bud from aorta (the precursor of the "ductal segment"), and (3) vessels from the dorsal aorta below the sixth arch, which are precursors of bronchial vessels. When the ventral bud fails to develop, the failure resulting in a unilateral absence of the pulmonary artery, the lung may then derive its blood supply from either of the other two dorsal connections noted above, and, in some cases, possibly from both. When the blood supply to the affected lung is via bronchial arteries, this probably represents persistence of the dorsal connections below the pulmonary arch (VI) to the postbrachial pulmonary plexus. Vessels from the aortic arch to the affected lung probably represent persistence of the dorsal or "ductal" portion of the pulmonary arch. The persistence of bronchial and ductal-like vessels are of approximately equal incidence for both left and right anomalies except for some very special cases.

In general, however, it would appear that when a patent ductus arteriosus is present, running between some portion of the aorta and the existing pulmonary artery, then the blood supply to the opposite lung must have been derived from the bronchial vessels.

We were able to come to no positive conclusion to explain why the tetralogy of Fallot is associated with absent left pulmonary artery only.

In summary, then, there is no evidence to indicate why one pulmonary artery should fail to develop or why only absence of the *left* pulmonary area is associated with tetralogy of Fallot. It is clear, however, that the blood supply to the affected lung can be explained in terms of embryonal development.

Physiologic Affects

It has been shown extensively by Cournand[4-6] and many other workers[7-9] that ligation of a pulmonary artery in the normal animal and in man does not cause pulmonary hypertension. It has also been extensively shown[10-14] that bronchial artery blood flow tends to increase significantly after ligation of the ipsilateral pulmonary artery.

Analysis of the 78 cases which we have studied revealed a marked difference between (1) those with unilateral absent pulmonary artery (UAPA) as the only lesion, and (2) those with absent pulmonary artery associated with shunts. In patients with isolated UAPA the over-all incidence of pulmonary hypertension was 19%, whereas in the group with combined lesions all of the patients with patent ductus arteriosus had evidence of pulmonary hypertension, as was also true of all the patients with septal defects. Of course, the patients with tetralogy of Fallot did not have pulmonary hypertension. Thus the over-all incidence of pulmonary hypertension in patients with a shunt in association with UAPA was 88%. Patients with multiple shunts showed a high spontaneous mortality rate. Four of six patients had evidence of pulmonary hypertension, and five of six were dead by the age of six months. This suggests to us that *an increased total pulmonary blood flow from the time of birth* may be an important factor in the development of pulmonary hypertension, since in the isolated cases where there was no reason to suspect increased pulmonary blood flow, only 19% have pulmonary hypertension.

It is interesting that those patients in our study who had pulmonary function studies all yielded results which were, essentially, within normal range. Occasionally, the vital capacity was somewhat decreased. In the few cases where bronchial spirometric studies were available, the oxygen uptake by the affected side was negligible, but, on the other hand, there was significant CO_2 output, explainable, perhaps, by the increased bronchial artery flow. Bronchoscopy and bronchograms generally revealed normal bronchial structure. Studies of one of our patients, together with two patients reported by Tabakin,[10] suggest significant increase in bronchial blood flow to the affected lung.

The Diagnosis

History.—There is no sex predilection or familial aspect to the disease. The chief complaint is usually cardiovascular and depends upon whether the lesion is isolated or combined.

When the lesion is isolated, the patient is usually asymptomatic, although 19% of such patients, as mentioned above, have pulmonary hypertension. When this occurs, it is usually at an early age and the patients die from right heart failure. If pulmonary hypertension does not develop at an early age, it is unlikely that it will develop later in life.

Patients with the combined lesions are generally young and have a very high intrinsic mortality. In fact, the oldest living patient with a combined lesion is our patient (Case 2), aged 25.

Physical Examination.—Certain findings are present in both the isolated UAPA and in the combined cases. The hemithorax on the affected side may be small with decreased breath sounds, and the heart and mediastinum tend to be shifted to the affected side; this shifting gives a false impression of an increase in the heart size. Auscultation of the heart in the patient with isolated UAPA is generally unremarkable. In those patients with pulmonary hypertension, however, an increased second sound at the base with an ejection click, a murmur of pulmonary insufficiency, and a right ventricular third heart sound may be heard. If patent ductus is present or if a shunt is present within the heart, the murmurs typically associated with these lesions are also audible.

Electrocardiogram.—The electrocardiogram is usually normal in the uncomplicated isolated case. In combined lesions, as also when pulmonary hypertension complicates the isolated case, there is almost always right ventricular hypertrophy.

X-Ray.—The chest x-ray is the most valuable clue toward the diagnosis of UAPA. Danelius,[15] in 1942, was the first to describe the absence of the hilar comma in UAPA. The most common radiologic feature is a difference in the vascular area of the two lung fields, found in virtually 100% of the cases. Indeed, this may be a misleading aspect of the x-ray, as these patients may masquerade with a diagnosis of hypoplasia or agenesis of the lung (as was true in our Case 1). The final diagnosis is confirmed by selective angiocardiogram. This technique, however, cannot distinguish between congenital absence and acquired obstruction of the pulmonary artery, but with the history, the marked difference in the lung fields, and the shift of the mediastinum, the distinction can be made with considerable presumption of accuracy. Thrombosis or embolism of a pulmonary artery is perhaps the most difficult lesion to distinguish radiologically from UAPA, for the angiograms may be identical. The differential here depends on the history of the acute episode.

In summary, then, a young patient, cyanotic or acyanotic, either asymptomatic or with progressive symptoms of dyspnea and fatigue suggesting diminished cardiac reserve, who shows on x-ray a significant difference between the two hemithoraces as regards the opacity of the lung, should call to mind the possibility of unilateral absence of the pulmonary artery with or without associated defects. Cardiac catheterization and angiocardiography should be undertaken to clinch the diagnosis.

Report of Cases

Of the four patients we have seen in our clinic in whom we have recognized the entity of UAPA, we wish to present two who have provided a surgical challenge which we think is unique, since both patients had absent left pulmonary artery, right aortic arch, and descending aorta and patent ductus arteriosus in the right chest. Our first patient is unique in the literature and is also the oldest living patient with a combined lesion. The second patient had, in addition, a ventricular septal defect, a combination previously reported once.

Case 1.—*History.*—A 25-year-old white male was admitted to Colorado General Hospital on June 30, 1961, from State Mental Hospital for evaluation of a murmur present since childhood. His only cardiopulmonary symptoms were mild fatigue and dyspnea on exertion. There was no known family history of heart disease.

Physical Examination.—The psychologically depressed patient was of thin body habitus. Blood pressure was 135/75 mm Hg, pulse 90; there was no clubbing, cyanosis, or edema. The chest was small and symmetrical with normal breath sounds throughout. The left border of cardiac dullness was in the sixth left intercostal space in the antero-axillary line, with a marked increase in ventricular activity. No thrills were felt; auscultation revealed a Grade 2 (on a 6 basis) systolic murmur, which was low pitched, nonobstructive, and maximal in the second left intercostal. Diastole was clear and an ejection click was noted at the left base.

Electrocardiogram.—The electrocardiogram revealed normal sinus rhythm with right axis deviation and right and left ventricular hypertrophy.

X-Ray (Fig 2).—The heart was shifted into the left chest, which was considerably smaller than the right. The right chest was obviously more radiolucent than the smaller left. The heart appeared moderately enlarged with definite right ventricular hypertrophy. The main and right pulmonary arteries were enlarged, and no left pulmonary artery could be seen. A right aortic arch was present. The vascular architecture was definitely increased in the right lung.

Bronchography.—The bronchograms were of good quality, and all major segmental bronchi were visualized and appeared normal.

Pulmonary Function Studies.—Arterial oxygen saturation and carbon dioxide content were normal. The vital capacity, maximum breathing capacity, and carbon monoxide diffusing capacity were essentially within normal limits.

Cardiac Catheterization.—The catheter followed a normal course to the pulmonary artery. A 2.2% rise in oxygen content was noted at the pulmonary artery level. Pulmonary blood flow was nearly two times systemic blood flow. Main pulmonary and brachial artery pressures were equal.

Angiocardiography.—A selective angiocardiogram from the main pulmonary artery (Fig 3) revealed complete absence of the left pulmonary artery. A late film showed a right aortic arch descending on the right at a time when there was re-opacification of the pulmonary artery.

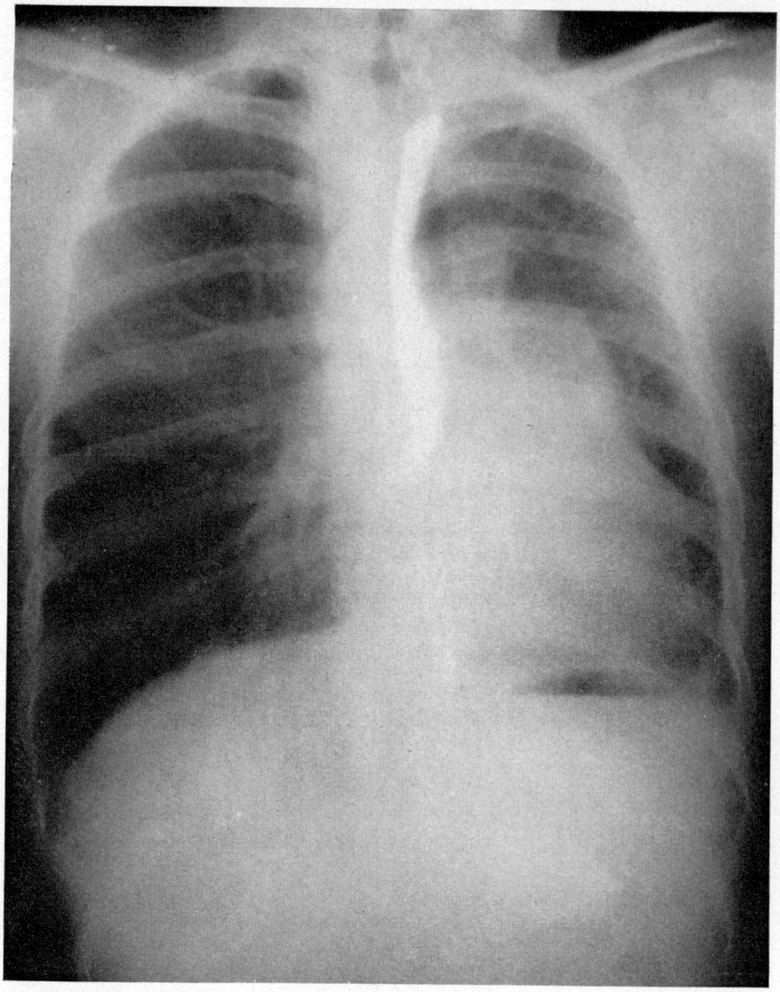

Fig 2.—The posteroanterior six-foot roentgenogram shows displacement of heart and mediastinum to the left and prominent radiolucency of the right lung with very prominent vascular patterns.

Retrograde Aortography.—A retrograde aortogram showed filling of the pulmonary artery from the dye injected into the right arch (Fig 4).

The diagnosis was absent left pulmonary artery, right aortic arch, and patent ductus arteriosus.

Hospital Course.—On June 19, 1961, the patient underwent surgical ligation of the patent ductus arteriosus, during moderate general body hypothermia (30 C [86 F]). The approach in this patient was anterior using a bilateral thoracotomy in the fourth interspace, transecting the sternum. The approach used revealed the difficulties of attacking a right patent ductus from an anterior direction. The dissection was very extensive, requiring mobilization of the thymus, opening the pericardium, and extensive dissection of the mediastinum behind the heart. The lesion lay directly behind the ascending aorta and the upper portion of the cardiac mass, slightly to the right of the midline. Eventually it was found that the patent ductus was a relatively long vessel, an inch and a half in length (3.8 cm) and 1.5 cm in diameter, originating from the descending aorta just below the innominate artery and entering the main pulmonary artery (the left pulmonary artery, of course, being absent). An operative photograph is seen in Fig 5.

Tapes were placed about the vessel, and the ductus was then doubly ligated with umbilical tapes and a No. 00 transfixing suture. This resulted in complete disappearance of the thrill palpable in the pulmonary artery. Biopsy specimen of both lungs was taken, and the operation was concluded by closure of the thoracotomy.

The biopsy specimens subsequently revealed very minimal medial hypertrophy of the small pulmonary vessels in the right lung, while those on the left showed extensive intimal thickening but normal media.

Postoperative Course.—The recovery from surgery was uneventful, and the patient was discharged after ten days. He noted a progressive increase in exercise tolerance. His heart became less active, but the murmurs found prior to operation were unchanged. On Aug 29 the patient was

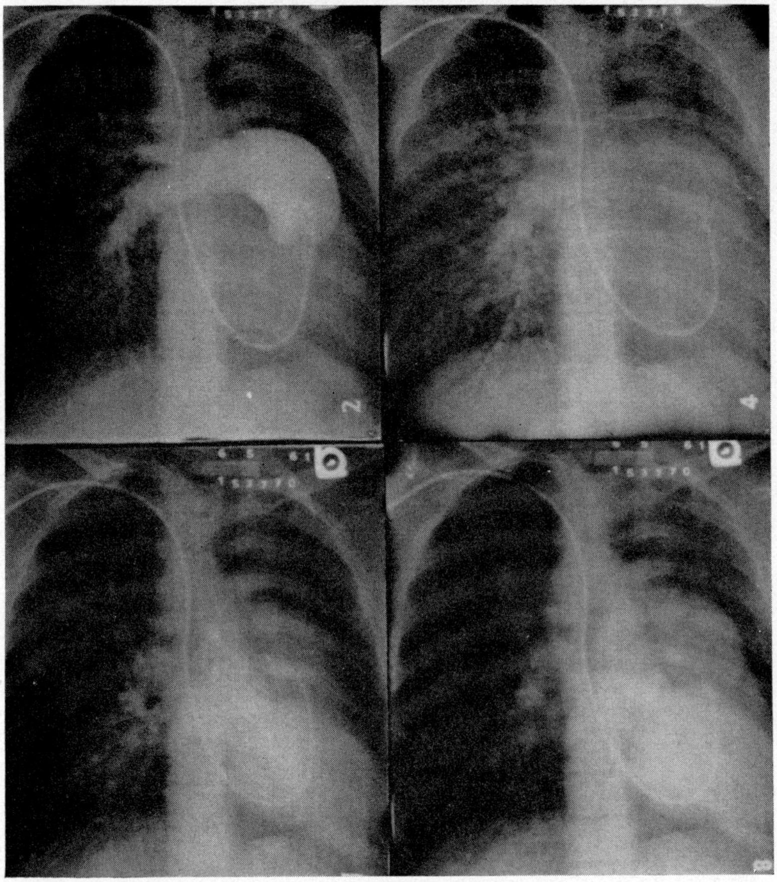

Fig 3.—The selective angiocardiographic series showed absent left pulmonary artery and late refilling of the pulmonary artery when the right-sided aorta became opacified. (Reprinted by permission of The American Journal of Cardiology).

recatheterized. There was no evidence of a left-to-right shunt, pulmonary blood flow was normal, but the total pulmonary resistance was unchanged (three times normal). The pulmonary artery pressure, which had been approximately 100/55 with a mean of 69 before surgery, now was 55/30 with a mean of 38. Thus, the patient had clear-cut objective evidence of improvement from the ligation of his ductus.

Case 2.—*History.*—A 17-year-old female was admitted to Colorado General Hospital on July 17, 1961, with the chief complaint of palpitation and increasing shortness of breath for three months. She had been first noted to have a murmur at the age of 18 months. There was moderate dyspnea on exertion, and over the past four years x-rays had revealed an increase in her heart size. There was no family history of cardiovascular disease.

Physical Examination.—The thin white girl was acyanotic; blood pressure was 110/70, pulse 88 and regular. There was slight scoliosis to the left, and the left chest appeared decreased in size. Lungs were clear to auscultation and percussion; the breath sounds were slightly diminished on the left.

Fig 4.—A retrograde aortogram outlines the pulmonary artery with dye injected into the aortic arch.

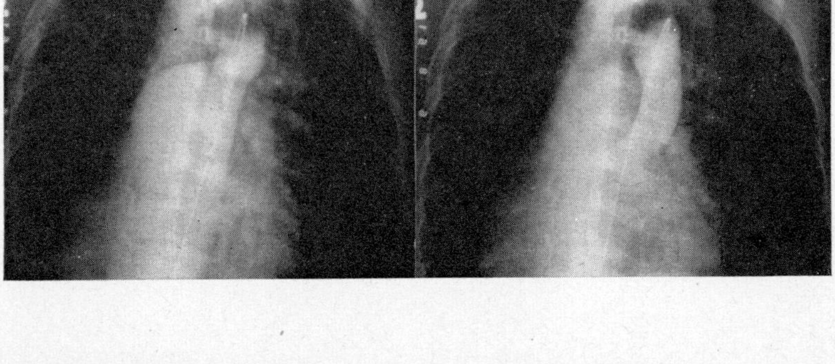

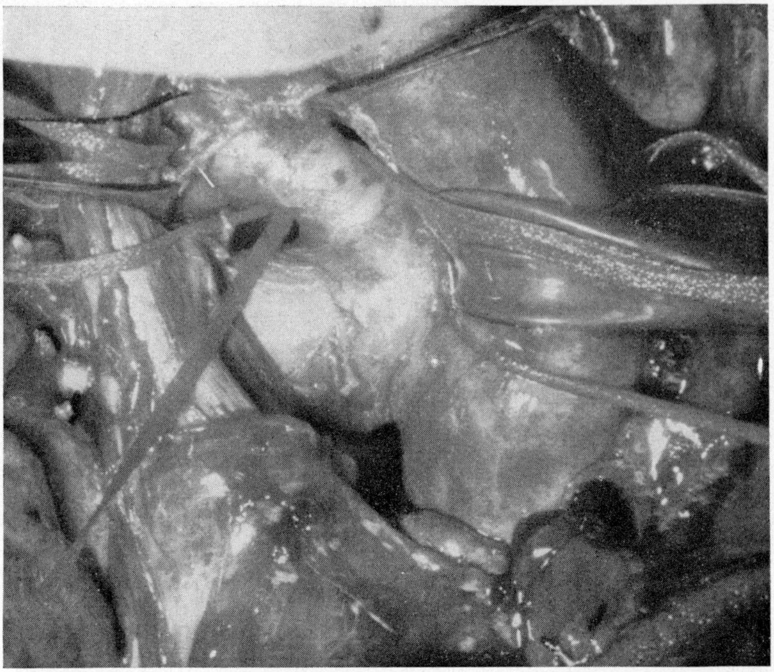

Fig 5 (Case 1).—Operative scene of patient showing tortuous patent ductus entering cephalad into the beginning of the large right pulmonary artery emerging under the ascending aorta. (Reprinted by permission of the American Journal of Cardiology).

Palpation over the heart suggested increased activity and a prominent lift along the left sternal border, which lay in the anterior axillary line. There was a widespread thrill over the entire precordium, and in the first left intercostal space a continuous machinery-like murmur was noted, Grade 5 (on a 6 basis). A harsh, obstructive systolic murmur was also heard along the left sternal border, maximum in the third intercostal space, and this murmur was transmitted to the aortic area. At the pulmonary area the second sound was split, accentuated, and followed by a high-pitched decrescendo diastolic murmur. A prominent ejection click was heard over the entire precordium.

Electrocardiogram.—Electrocardiogram revealed normal sinus rhythm, right and left ventricular hypertrophy, and possible right atrial hypertrophy.

X-Ray (Fig 6).—The left hemithorax was smaller than the right. The mediastinal structures were shifted to the left, and there was hyper-radiolucidity of the right hemithorax. The aortic arch appeared to be on the right with dilatation of the descending aorta. The heart seemed moderately enlarged, predominantly the left ventricle.

Cardiac Catheterization.—Cardiac catheterization was performed July 18. The catheter followed a normal course through the heart, but attempts to enter the left pulmonary artery were unsuccessful. Pressure in the right pulmonary artery was 75/37 with a mean of 50. A 1.5 vol% rise in oxygen content occurred high in the right ventricle with no further rise at the pulmonary artery level. Pulmonary blood flow was approximately twice systemic blood flow. The pulmonary total resistance was only slightly elevated at 480 dynes/sec/cm^{-S}/ Multiple dye curves, using the double catheter technique, confirmed the presence of a patent ductus arteriosus and pulmonary insufficiency. The presence or absence of a ventricular septal defect was not established. Selective angiocardiogram (Fig 7) revealed complete absence of the left pulmonary artery, pulmonary insufficiency, and nonfilling of the vessels of the left lung. Films late in the series showed a right aortic arch descending on the right with reopacification of the pulmonary artery.

Hospital Course.—On July 24, 1961, the patient underwent surgery. The incision was a right anterolateral thoracotomy in the sixth interspace. Exposure through this incision was somewhat more satisfactory than that which had been obtained with the anterior bilateral incision. (However, if the lesion were to be approached again, the incision we would suggest is a posterolateral incision on the right with resection of the sixth rib.) Dissection of the upper portion of the left lung root retropericardially revealed the right pulmonary artery which was a huge vessel measuring an inch and a half (3.8 cm in diameter and which divided into three large primary branches (Fig 8). The right recurrent laryngeal nerve curved around the arch of the aorta at the take-off point of a tortuous vessel 1½ cm in diameter and approximately 5 cm in length, running from the aorta at the level of the origin of the innominate artery to the upper border of the pulmonary artery. It appeared extremely friable. No continuous thrill was palpable in the pulmonary artery of this patient, and it was impossible to notice any change in the artery when

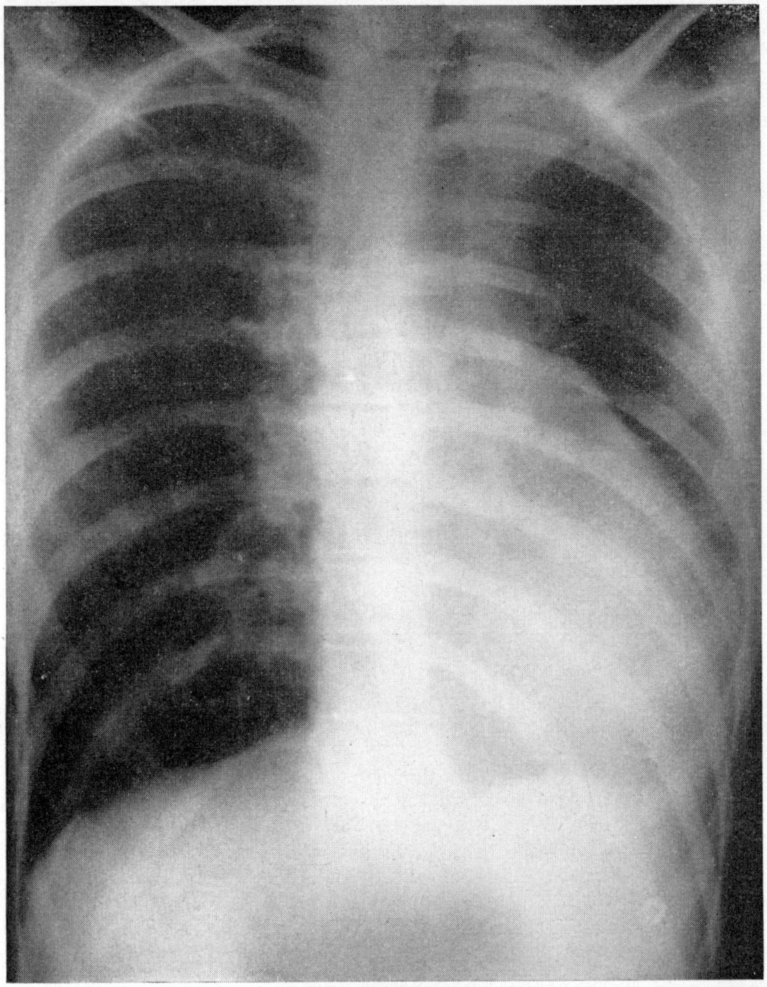

Fig 6.—Posteroanterior view of the chest reveals the radiolucency of the right thorax with the small left hemithorax and absent left hilar "comma."

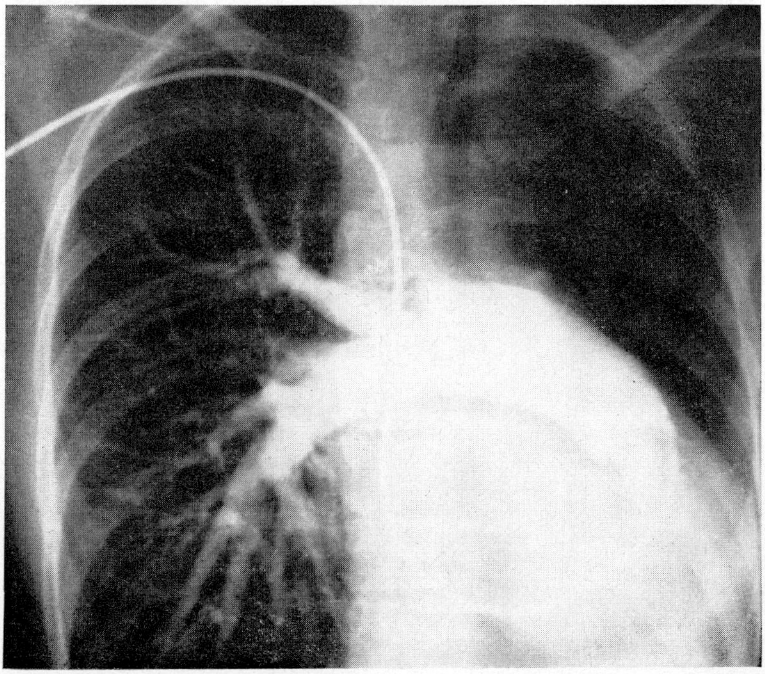

Fig 7.—The selective angiocardiogram showed absent left pulmonary artery and prominent pulmonary vessels on the right. A later film showed refilling of the pulmonary artery when the right-sided aorta became opacified.

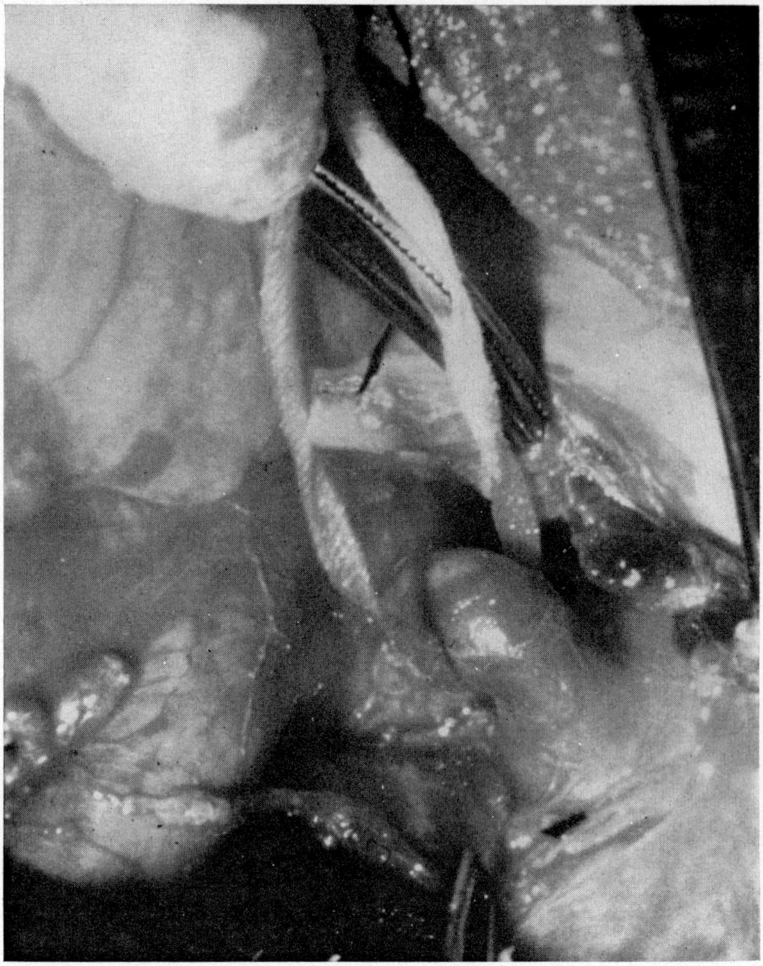

Fig 8 (Case 2).—Operative scene showing tortuous patent ductus coming from behind the lung root to enter the large right pulmonary artery.

the ductus was clamped. It was triply ligated with umbilical tapes and a transfixing suture of No. 00 silk. The anesthetist could still hear a systolic murmur through the esophageal stethoscope, and palpation of the great vessels was indefinite as to the vibrating structure. It was thought perhaps the root of aorta or even pulmonary vein on the right could have been the origin of the thrill. Hemostasis was completed, and a lung biopsy specimen was taken of the right lower lobe. The thoracotomy was closed, and the patient was returned to the recovery room. The biopsy specimen later showed mild dilatation of the pulmonary vessels without medical hypertrophy or intimal change.

The postoperative course was uneventful. The continuous murmur had disappeared as had the decrescendo diastolic murmur along the left sternal border. The systolic thrill and Grade 5 murmur persisted, maximal in the third left intercostal space, lateral to the left sternal border. Fluoroscopy revealed no change in heart size or in vascularity of the lung fields. Exercise tolerance was improved, and the patient felt better.

On repeat catheterization on Oct 6, a ventricular septal defect was demonstrated by hydrogen and oxygen techniques, and the pulmonary vascular resistance had risen to 880 dynes/sec/cm^{-5}/sq m with the pulmonary artery pressure still remaining elevated 85/40, mean of 56. It is thought that the patient remains a candidate for open closure of her ventricular septal defect.

Comment

The patient in case 1 is an instructive patient. Not only is he the first patient reported in the literature with absence of the left pulmonary artery associated with right patent ductus arteriosus and right aortic arch, but he is the oldest living patient with UAPA with an associated lesion. However, it is discouraging that his total pulmonary resistance has remained unchanged since surgery, at a very high level. One other patient, that of DuShane et al,[16] who had ligation of his patent ductus at the age of ten months, showed complete reversal of his pulmonary resistance to normal. This strongly suggests that the pulmonary hypertension and the vascular changes associated with UAPA and patent ductus are reversible only if the lesion is corrected at an early age.

Therapeutic results in our second patient cannot yet be assessed because a major anomaly, namely, ventricular septal defect, still remains uncorrected.

Summary

Unilateral absence of a pulmonary artery is an uncommon, but not rare, congenital anomaly. In over half of the cases it is associated with another anomaly of the heart or great vessels. In these patients pulmonary hypertension is frequent and the mortality rate is high.

The lesion can be diagnosed clinically and proved by selective angiocardiography.

Two patients are presented who are thought to be unique in that they combined absence of the left pulmonary artery with right aortic arch, right descending aorta, and right-sided patent ductus arteriosus. In one of these patients a ventricular septal defect was also present.

Surgical considerations relative to the ligation of the patent ductus are presented, and a posterolateral incision into the right chest with removal of the sixth rib is recommended.

Long-term follow-up will be necessary to evaluate the effectiveness of the therapy.

Henry Swan, MD, 303 Josephine St, Denver 6, Colo.

REFERENCES

1. Pool, P. E.; Vogel, J. H. K., and Blount, S. G., Jr.: Congenital Unilateral Absence of a Pulmonary Artery: The Importance of Flow in Pulmonary Hypertension, Amer J Cardiol 10:706, 1962.

2. Fraentzel, O.: Ein Fall von abnormer Communication der Aorta mit der Arteria pulmonalis, Virchow Arch Path Anat 43:420, 1868.

3. Doering, H.: Angeborener Defekt der rechten Lungenarterie, Studien zur Pathologie der Entwicklung, 2:41, 1914-1920.

4. Cournand, A.; Himmelstein, A.; Riley, R. L., and Lester, C. W.: A Follow-Up of the Cardiopulmonary Function in 4 Young Individuals After Pneumonectomy, J Thor Cardiov Surg 16:30, 1947.

5. Cournand, A.; Riley, R. L.; Himmelstein, A., and Austrian, R.: Pulmonary Circulation and Alveolar Ventilation: Perfusion Relationships After Pneumonectomy, J Thor Cardiov Surg 19:80, 1950.

6. Carlson, R. F.; Charbon, B. C.; Charbon, H. G. A., and Adams, W. E.: The Effect of Decreasing the Amount of Lung Tissue on the Right Ventricular Pressures in Animals, J Thor Cardiov Surg 21:621, 1951.

7. Harrison, R. W.; Adams, W. E.; Beuhler, W., and Long, E. T.: Effects of Acute and Chronic Reduction of Lung Volumes on Cardiopulmonary Reserve, AMA Arch Surg 75:546, 1957.

8. Adams, W. E.: Problems in Pulmonary Resection for Primary Lung Tumor in the Aged, J Amer Geriat Soc 2:440, 1954.

9. Harrison, R. W.; Beuhler, W.; Thompson, R. G.; Long, E. T.; Carlson, R.; Charbon, B., and Adams, W. E.: Cardiopulmonary Reserve 5 to 15 Years Following Fifty Per Cent or More Reduction of Lung Volumes, Surg Forum 7:209, 1957.

10. Tabakin, B. S.; Hanson, J. S.; Adhikari, P. K., and Miller, D. B.: Physiologic Studies in Congenital Absence of the Left Main Pulmonary Artery, Circulation 22:1107, 1960.

11. Fishman, A. P.: The Clinical Significance of the Pulmonary Collateral Circulation, Circulation 24:677, 1961.

12. Cudkowicz, L.; Calabresi, M.; Nims, R. G., and Gray, F. D., Jr.: The Simultaneous Estimation of Right and Left Ventricular Outputs Applied to a Study of the Bronchial Circulation in Dogs, Amer Heart J 58:732, 1959.

13. Cudkowicz, L.; Abelmann, W. H.; Levison, G. E.; Katznelson, G., and Jreissaty, R. M.: Bronchial Arterial Blood Flow, Clin Sci 19:1, 1960.

14. Fritts, H. W., Jr.; Harris, P.; Chidsey, C. A.; Clauss, R. H., and Cournand, A.: Estimation of Flow Through Bronchial-Pulmonary Vascular Anastomoses with Use of T-1824 Dye, Circulation 23:390, 1961.

15. Danelius, G.: Absence of the Hilar Shadow, Amer J Roentgenol 47:870, 1942.

16. DuShane, J. W.; Weidman, W. H.; Ongley, P. A.; Swan, H. J. C.; Kirklin, J. W.; Edwards, J. E., and Schmutzler, H.: Clinical-Pathologic Conference, Amer Heart J 59:782, 1960.

Peptic Ulcer in Africa

CLARENCE A. SNYDER, MD
AND
MERTON J. ALEXANDER, MD
BURUNDI, AFRICA

It is generally taught that peptic ulcer is a disease of civilization. It is believed to be much more common among the white race than among the dark races. Also it has been shown in the United States that peptic ulcer is much less common among the Negroes than the white population.[1]

However, there are reports in the literature revealing that there are localized areas in Africa and South India where duodenal ulcer is extremely common.

Bergsma reported in 1931 that gastric ulcers are very common among the adult male population of Ethiopia.[2] He considered their diet which is very rich in cayenne pepper as the agent responsible for the high incidence of ulcers among these people.

In 1948 Ellis published in the *British Journal of Surgery* a "Study of Peptic Ulcer in Nigeria."[3] He reported on 124 cases of peptic ulcer which he operated upon. Of these 123 were duodenal ulcers and 1 was a gastric ulcer. The vast majority of these were in males with various degrees of obstruction. They were treated with gastroenterostomy. There were 3 cases of acute perforation.

In 1954 Konstam published in *Lancet* an article "Peptic Ulceration In Southern Nigeria."[4] He showed as did Ellis that peptic ulcers are common in southern Nigeria and that these cases are among the more primitive Africans. He pointed out that peptic ulcer is rare in northern Nigeria and just as in India has a geographical distribution.[5] He felt that dietary differences accounted for the geographical differences.

Commenting on Konstam's paper Buxton wrote in *Lancet,* 1954:

> In the territory of Ruanda-Urundi, Belgian Congo, this condition is extremely common and my colleagues and I must have treated many hundreds of cases in six Mission Hospitals in the last 15 years. It is a mountainous area, some 6000-8000 ft. above sea level and average temperature about 70-80° F, with an agricultural and trading population. In this area peptic ulcer is much commoner in men than in women, and in the poorer classes. This may be related to the long intervals between meals. The men will often have only one meal in 24 hours. They are heavy smokers and drinkers and I have

Submitted for publication Feb 8, 1963.

always suspected these as contributory factors. The diet is deficient in animal protein, this deficiency being associated with a high incidence of kwashiorkor in children of 6 months to 2 years and of cirrhosis in adults. Infestation with ascaris is common. Although they are an agricultural people, free from the anxieties of civilization, they are animists by faith and this means that they are subject to intense fear—fear of evil spirits and fear of poisoning by their enemies. I have observed in many cases how fear results in digestive disturbance, and I believe that, if prolonged it is a factor in causing ulceration. As many of the cases have advanced to fibrosis and stenosis before coming for treatment, gastrojejunostomy has produced dramatic and satisfactory results. So much so that the simple folk demand operation as a cure-all for all types of abdominal pain, and it is difficult to persuade them that this is not the case! The ulcer is situated most frequently on the anterior surface of the first part of the duodenum . . . .[6]

The experience of my colleague and I in Ruanda-Urundi, in east Africa, confirms the report of Buxton. We found that peptic ulcer was extremely common among the male population. Since our work was done in a somewhat primitive mission hospital gastrointestinal x-rays were not available to us. However, we did confirm the presence of duodenal ulcer in many cases surgically. This report is concerned with 30 of these operated-on cases. Most of our cases were operated on for various degrees of pyloric obstruction.

The typical patient was a male between 20-40 years of age who came to the hospital complaining of midepigastric pain and vomiting. Symptom duration was from one to five years. Examination revealed a cachectic male with signs of weight loss. Examination of the abdomen often showed pyloric waves and a visibly dilated stomach. Passage of a Levin tube showed gastric retention of 300 ml or more. Some of these patients had to be put on gastric suction and given parenteral fluids immediately due to their severe debilitation.

When operated upon these patients were found to have a large dilated stomach and an ulcer on the anterior surface of the first part of the duodenum. There was often complete obstruction to the pylorus and extensive fibrosis and scarring about the first part of the duodenum.

Because the custom of these people is to eat just one enormous meal in 24 hours it was felt that gastroenterostomy was a better operation for them. A posterior gastrojejunostomy was therefore done, generally under spinal anesthesia, and occasionally under procaine infiltration. The impressive feature of these cases was that they complained very little of pain or discomfort postoperatively. They were usually started on small feedings on the third postoperative day and progressed up to full diets. Their weight gain was impressive, some gaining as much as 20 lb (9.1 kg) during the first month after surgery.

The patients were exceedingly gratified by the results of surgery, and for every patient so treated five more would show up at our dispensary begging for the same operation and offering to pay almost any price for it. Unless they had evidence of obstruction we scarcely dared admit ulcer patients to the hospital for medical treatment since they would often refuse to leave unless they were operated upon.

Of our 30 surgical cases, here reported, 23 showed various degrees of obstruction. There were 22 males and 1 female. There were 5 cases of acute perforation of duodenal ulcer; 4 of these were treated by simple closure. Among the 5 perforations there was one female, a 14-year-old girl, with a large amount of obstruction and enormous gastric dilatation in addition to the perforation. She was treated with closure of the perforation and gastroenterostomy. There was one case of perforation of a marginal ulcer in a man who had had a gastrojejunostomy almost two years previously for duodenal obstruction. This was treated by excision of the previous anastamosis and a new gastroenterostomy formed.

We had only one case of gastric ulcer. This was on the lesser curvature and was treated by partial gastrectomy. Pathological examination revealed it to be a benign gastric ulcer.

There were two deaths, both of these being among the acute perforations.

These findings as well as the reports from southern Nigeria, Ethiopia, and southern India reveal that peptic ulcer is not a disease limited to those living under the tensions and pressures of modern civilization as stated in many textbooks.

We found as in southern Nigeria and southern India that the incidence of peptic ulcer had geographical limitations. A neighboring mission hospital to the south of us in Tanganyika never saw peptic ulcer patients. Another mission hospital to the east of us in the Kivu province of the Belgian Congo also did not see ulcer patients.

Conclusions

Our conclusions are essentially the same as Ellis, Konstam, and Buxton.

The high incidence of duodenal ulcer among the peoples of Ruanda-Urundi is probably dietary in origin. The main stays of the diet are yams, cassava, and beans. The diet is deficient in animal proteins and vitamin B complex. The people consume large quantities of alcohol. They go long periods without eating and eat usually once a day in the evening.

As pointed out by Buxton these people are not free from anxiety. Many of them are primitive and live in great fear of evil spirits, poisoning, etc.

Also suggested is the role of heredity. These people have a tribal origin strictly limited to small geographical areas. The tendency toward this disease could be hereditary.

Further research into the etiology of peptic ulcer in these limited geographical areas could shed much light upon the pathogenesis of this disease.

Clarence A. Snyder, MD, 2463 College, SE, Grand Rapids, Mich.

REFERENCES

1. Sturtevant, M., and Shapiro, L. L.: Gastric and Duodenal Ulcer, Arch Intern Med 38:41 (July) 1926.

2. Bergsma, S.: Gastric and Duodenal Ulcer in the Black People of Abyssinia, Arch Intern Med 47:144 (Jan) 1931.

3. Ellis, M.: Study of Peptic Ulcer in Nigeria, Brit J Surg 36:60-65 (July) 1948.

4. Konstam, P. G.: Peptic Ulceration in Southern Nigeria, Lancet 2:1039 (Nov 20) 1954.

5. Somervell, T. H., and Orr, I. M.: Some Contributions to Causation, Pathology, and Treatment of Duodenal Ulcer and Its Complications, Brit J Surg 24:227 (Oct) 1936.

6. Buxton, K. L.: Peptic Ulceration in Tropical Africa, Lancet 2:1231 (Dec 11) 1954.

ERRATUM

The article, *Development of a Synthetic "Heart,"* by Drs. Hastings, Santos, and Potter (page 517, April, 1963, issue of the ARCHIVES) was received for publication June 13, 1961, not Jan 9, 1963, as given in the footnote to the article.

The Urine Sediment in Acute Appendicitis

LARRY H. KRETCHMAR, MD
AND
D. F. McDONALD, MD
ROCHESTER, NY

It is known that microscopic hematuria or pyuria may be associated with acute appendicitis. The present study was prompted by a review of the literature which indicated that little information is available correlating the urinary sediment with the signs, symptoms, and surgical findings in cases of acute appendicitis.

Material and Methods

One hundred twenty-nine patients underwent appendectomy for acute appendicitis at Strong Memorial Hospital in 1959. Ten had no admission urinalysis, and 6 had a preceding history of urinary tract infection. These patients were not included in the study. Of the 113 patients, 21 (19%) had a positive urinary sediment. All urine specimens were voided spontaneously. A centrifuged urine specimen with 5 or more white cells or red cells per high power field was considered positive. The patients were evaluated in regard to the admission urinalysis, sex, age, duration of symptoms prior to admission, urinary tract symptoms, fever, leukocyte count, and the findings at surgery.

Results

A. *Urinalysis.*—Twenty-one patients (19%) had microscopic pyuria ranging from 5 to 20 cells, occasionally with a few clumps. Four of these patients (5% of the entire group) also showed 5 to 30 red cells. No patient had a significant number of red cells alone.

B. *Sex.*—Seventy-two patients were males, and 41 were females. (Nineteen percent of the males and 17% of the females had a positive sediment.)

C. *Age.*—Figure 1 shows the number of patients with a positive sediment in each age group. (Significant pyuria was found in 40% of patients over 40 and only 14% under.)

D. *Duration of Symptoms Prior to Admission.*—Figure 2 shows the incidence of a positive urine sediment as it varied with the duration of symptoms. Patients with a brief history tended to have a negative urinalysis.

E. *Urinary Tract Symptoms.*—Five of the 21 patients with microscopic pyuria had complaints referable to the lower urinary tract. Three of these patients had frequency or dysuria. Two had right testicular pain, and 1 of these had microscopic hematuria in addition to pyuria. Seven of the 92 patients with a negative sediment complained of frequency or dysuria.

F. *Fever.*—Figure 3 shows an increasing incidence of a positive urinalysis in febrile patients. However, of 53 patients who were febrile (over 38 degrees), only 13, or 25% had pyuria.

G. *Leukocyte Count.*—Figure 4 shows the incidence of a positive urinalysis associated with elevation of the leukocyte count. Only 20% of the patients with counts of over 20,000 had a positive urinary sediment.

H. *Findings at Time of Surgery.*—Eleven of the 21 patients (52%) with microscopic pyuria were considered to have an abnormally positioned appendix. This includes retrocecal, retroileal, and pelvic appendices.

Submitted for publication July 30, 1962.

From the Division of Urologic Surgery, University of Rochester School of Medicine and Dentistry.

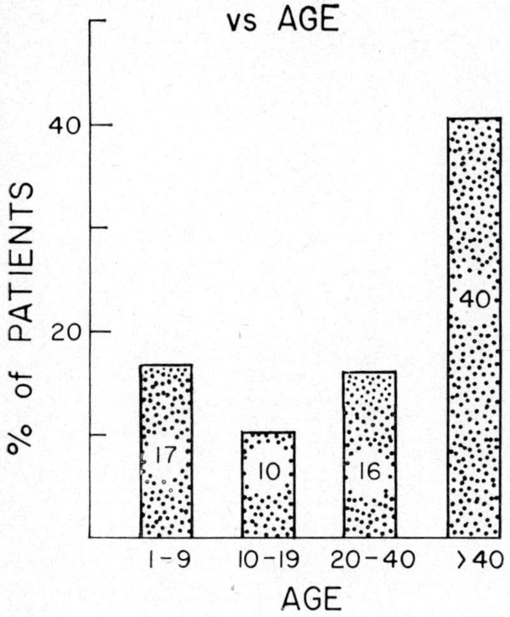

Fig. 1.—Percentage of patients with a positive urine sediment in different age groups.

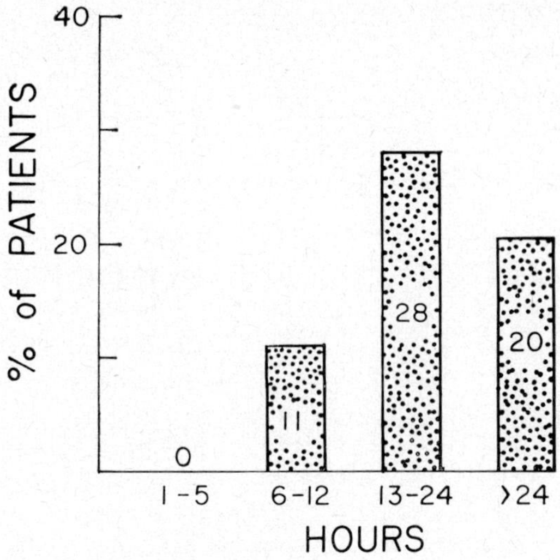

Fig. 2.—Percentage of patients with a positive urine sediment according to the duration of symptoms.

Four of these 11 patients also had significant microscopic hematuria. Twenty-four of 92 patients (26%) with a normal urine specimen had an abnormally situated appendix. Stated in another way, 31% of the patients with an abnormally positioned appendix had a positive urine sediment, whereas only 13% of the patients with an appendix in normal position had a positive sediment.

Three of 8 patients (38%) with abscesses and 4 of 18 patients (22%) with perforated

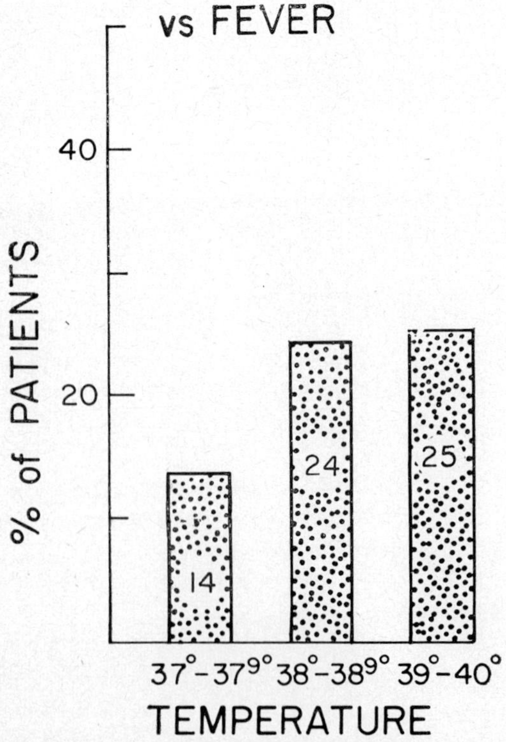

Fig. 3.—Percentage of patients with a positive urine sediment according to temperature elevation.

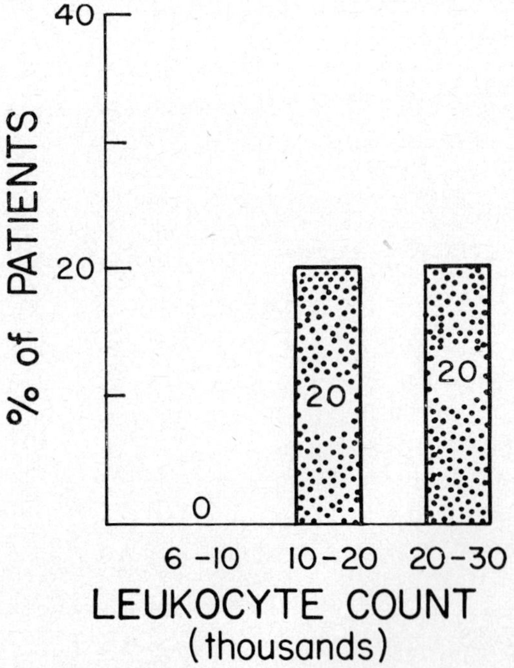

Fig. 4.—Percentage of patients with a positive urine sediment according to leukocyte count.

appendices had pyuria. Only 14 of 87 patients (16%) without abscess or perforation had a positive sediment.

Comment

The presence or absence of microscopic pyuria or hematuria in patients with acute appendicitis is variable and of little prognostic value. The greatest number of patients with a positive sediment falls into the older age group where unsuspected pyelonephritis or underlying prostatitis in males or vaginal discharge in females may contribute to a positive urinary sediment in any single, voided specimen.

Prolonged duration of symptoms, an elevated temperature, and an elevated leukocyte count all failed to be predictably associated with microscopic pyuria or hematuria. It is of interest that only 5 of the 12 patients with urinary tract symptoms actually showed a positive sediment.

The high incidence of patients with an abnormally located appendix in the group with a postive sediment (52%) suggests that ureteral proximity may be a factor. Furthermore, patients having an appendix in abnormal position had 2½ times the incidence of a positive urine sediment that patients with a normally placed appendix had. An inflamed retrocecal or retroileal appendix, or abscess, in close relationship with the right ureter may produce a localized inflammatory response in the ureteral mucosa with a secondary leukocytic infiltration. Presumably a pelvic appendix or abscess adjacent to the bladder can produce a similar response in that organ. The mere presence of an abnormally positioned inflamed appendix, however, does not consistently result in pyuria or hematuria, since only 11 out of 35 patients (31%) had a positive sediment.

No patient was found to have more than 30 red cells or 20 white cells with occasional clumps in a centrifuged specimen of voided urine. Therefore, the discovery of great numbers of white cells or red cells in the urine of a patient with equivocal signs of acute appendicitis should lead the observer to a more serious consideration of a diagnosis of urinary tract pathology such as pyelonephritis or ureteral calculus.

Conclusions

1. Microscopic pyuria was found in 19% of patients, without a previous history of urinary tract disease, who underwent appendectomy for acute appendicitis. Five per cent had microscopic hematuria as well.
2. There was a higher incidence of positive urine specimens in patients over age 40.
3. Patients with an abnormally positioned appendix may be more likely to develop microscopic pyuria or hematuria in the presence of acute appendicitis because of the close relationship to the baldder or right ureter.
4. Serious consideration should be given to a diagnosis of urinary tract pathology in patients with questionable signs of acute appendicitis if unusually large numbers of cells are found on urinalysis.

Larry Kretchmar, M.D., Strong Memorial Hospital, The University of Rochester, 260 Crittenden Blvd., Rochester 20, N.Y.

Mohs' Chemosurgery Technique for Basal Cell Carcinoma of the Chin and Cheek Areas of the Face

JOHN T. PHELAN, MD, AND JUAN JUARDO, MD, BUFFALO

Superficial basal cell carcinomas of the chin and cheek are currently treated by electrical and chemical dissection, surgical excision, and radiation therapy. Each of these methods has proved its usefulness in the management of basal cell carcinoma; however, each has certain limitations as attested by the number of reports that have been published concerning the management of recurrent lesions. In our opinion, the principal factor responsible for the recurrence of a basal cell carcinoma is the failure of the initial method of therapy to totally eradicate the tumor. Because of this problem, we began in 1960 to treat a selected group of basal cell carcinomas of the face by Mohs' chemosurgery technique,[1] as it was our belief that this method offered certain advantages of insuring total tumor removal that were not apparent in the more conventional forms of therapy.

Because collective experience with Mohs' chemosurgery technique is limited, it is the purpose of this report to review our experience with this method of therapy in treating basal cell carcinomas of the chin and cheek area.

Submitted for publication Jan. 2, 1963.

Departments of Surgery and Pathology, Roswell Park Memorial Institute, New York State Department of Health.

Material

During a two-year period, 16 patients, 4 females and 12 males, with basal cell carcinoma of the cheek and chin have been treated by Mohs' chemosurgery technique. The oldest patient in this series was 86, the youngest 38. The average age was 67. Of this group, 5 lesions were primary and 11 were considered recurrences in that other forms of management had been previously used in their treatment. The size of the lesions in this group varied from as small as 5 mm. to as large as 12 cm.; nine tumors were between 2-3 cm. in diameter (Figs. 1-4).

Each patient has been followed at three-month intervals, and over one-half of this group are one year post-treatment. To date, one patient has developed a local recurrence, and she was one of the first patients in whom chemosurgery was used.

Technique

The technique of chemosurgery as described by Mohs is presented below. The tumor and the surrounding skin are anesthetized with a suitable local anesthetic agent. A biopsy of the tumor is made and the tumor's histology established by frozen section technique. Next, dichloroacetic acid is applied to the surface of the tumor. The purpose of this chemical is to render the tumor more permeable to the zinc chloride

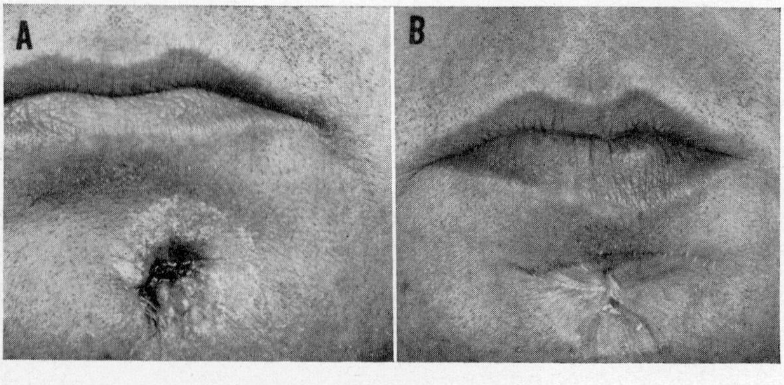

Fig. 1.—*A*, a recurrent basal cell carcinoma involving the chin. This lesion had been treated by surgical excision and radiation, and at the time of admission the tumor was fixed to the underlying bony mandible. *B*, the end-result following chemosurgery. No evidence of recurrent tumor one year after treatment.

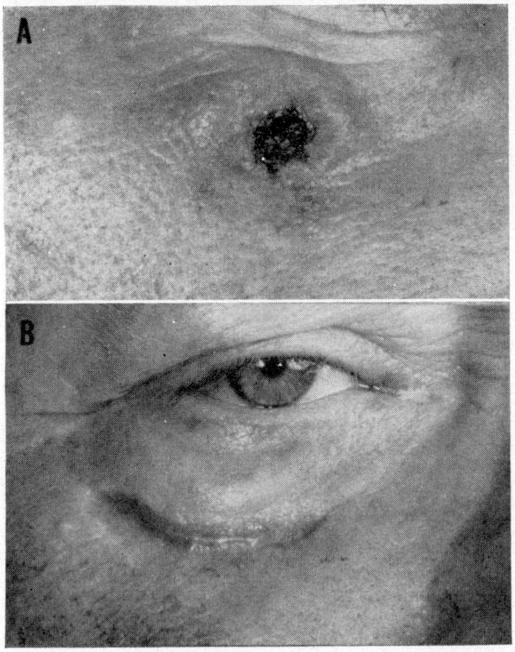

Fig. 2.—*A*, a basal cell carcinoma of the cheek. *B*, the results nine months later after chemosurgery.

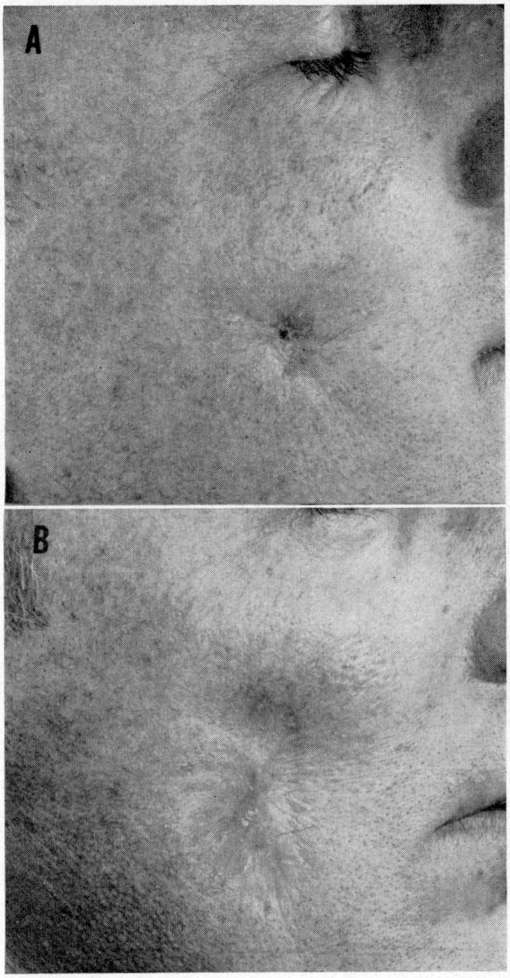

Fig. 3.—*A*, a recurrent basal cell carcinoma of the cheek that had been previously treated by electrical dissection, radiation, and surgical excision. The tumor clinically involved the entire confines of the cheek wall, except for the buccal mucosa. *B*, the end-result after 14 months. During the chemosurgery procedure, basal cell tumor was noted involving branches of the facial nerve, the parotid gland, and the masseter muscle.

fixative paste which is next applied in a thickness of about 1 to 2 mm. After 24 hours, the treated area is fixed sufficiently, and a 2-3 mm. thick layer is excised with a scalpel. The specimen is divided into segments measuring about 1.5 × 1.5 cm., a map of the tumor area is drawn, and each specimen is shown in its relationship to the tumor bed. The undersurface of each specimen is cut by a frozen section microtome and examined microscopically. If microscopic tumor tissue is present, the exact area is marked on the previously drawn map of the tumor and the zinc chloride paste reapplied to the corresponding area on the tumor field. This procedure is repeated at 24-hour intervals until a cancer-free surface is obtained. Five to seven days after the tumor has been excised, the eschar that has formed is easily removed leaving a clean, granulating wound. Scarlet red dressings are applied at daily intervals until wound healing is complete.

Comment

It is generally recognized that basal cell carcinoma is a locally invasive tumor and that the potential tumor field is much greater than the clinical appearance of the tumor would suggest. Not uncommonly, microscopic tumor foci extend beyond the main body of the tumor without visibly affecting the overlying skin. This growth feature of basal cell carcinoma is a point of considerable therapeutic importance, as most cancer therapists who treat basal cell tumors include in their fields of treatment an indeterminate margin of normal tissue. At the present time this margin of normal tissue has not been accurately defined in terms of specific dimen-

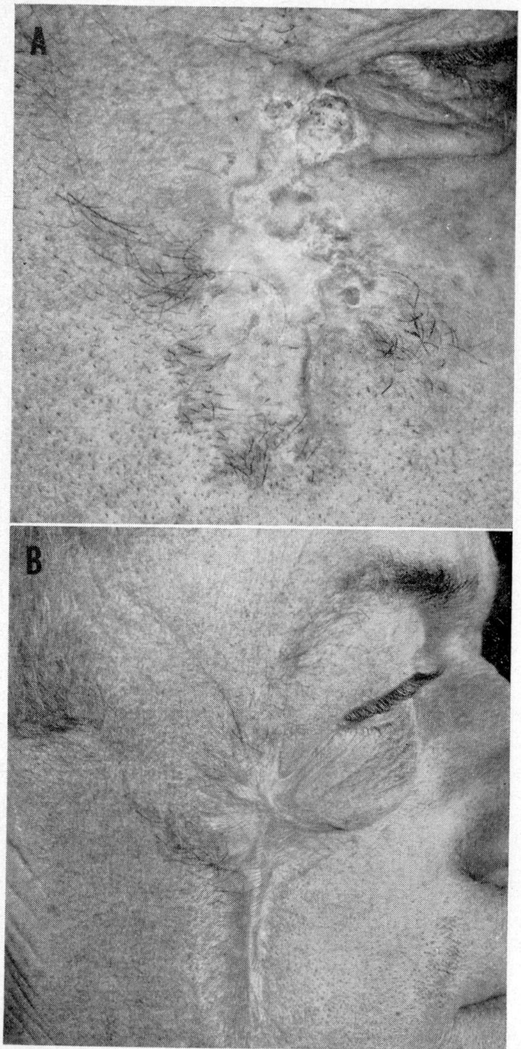

Fig. 4.—*A*, a basal cell carcinoma of the cheek treated primarily by Mohs' chemosurgery. *B*, the end-result after one year. There is slight lid retraction; however, this does not cause the patient any difficulty.

sion for a given tumor, and in our experience, we have been impressed by the marked growth variability of a basal cell carcinoma, not only in its peripheral extent but also in its depth of penetration. In this regard, we have observed microscopic tumor penetration extending well beyond what we considered cancer-free tissue. This tumor growth feature was most frequently encountered in recurrent basal cell carcinomas following radiation therapy.

In addition to tracking out the microscopic tumor growth, Mohs' chemosurgery embodies a certain degree of surgical conservation in that a minimal amount of normal tissue is sacrificed during the process of removing a given skin cancer. In the cases of chin and cheek lesions, where loss of normal tissue may present serious cosmetic defects, skin and soft-tissue conservation is important. Furthermore, if a plastic reconstructive procedure is contemplated, the skin and soft-tissue adjacent to a chemosurgically treated area is relatively normal and does not present the healing difficulties usually associated with irradiated tissue.

In this series, no patient required a plastic reconstructive procedure, and all wounds were permitted to heal by secondary intention. To some observers, a secondary healed wound on the face is to be avoided; however, we have been impressed by the pliability of the scar and the blending that takes place between the healed wound and the adjacent skin so that morbidity in this series has been slight.

From our experience, Mohs' chemosurgery technique is time consuming; it requires well-trained technicians for preparing frozen tissue sections and demands the service of a pathologist for their interpretation. Nevertheless, we are convinced that this procedure has a much wider application in the management of superficial cancer of the face and particularly of the chin and cheek area than is generally recognized.

Summary

A brief presentation of our experience with Mohs' chemosurgery technique in the management of carcinoma of the chin and cheek has been presented. Sixteen patients were treated by this method, and it was found to be a highly effective procedure of treating malignant superficial skin cancer in these areas.

John T. Phelan, M.D., Roswell Park Memorial Institute, Buffalo 3, N.Y.

REFERENCE

1. Mohs, F. E.: Chemosurgery in Cancer, Gangrene, and Infection, Springfield, Ill., Charles C Thomas, Publisher, 1956.

Out of the Past

The article by William Stewart Halsted that follows appeared in the April 12 issue of the *JAMA* fifty years ago. It is remarkable in many ways: as a model of literary style; as an example of vigorous and delightful exposition, including the charm conveyed by the careful use of the first person singular pronoun; and for its authoritative analysis and summary of the problems discussed. Many of his comments are as applicable today as a half century ago. For these reasons, it is reproduced now.

It also tells us much about the man himself and, by inference, his greater interest in the graduate training program and surgical technique of Theodor Kocher than in Lister's contributions to bacteriology, physiology, and physical chemistry. Halsted relates vividly the many troubles associated with the development of Lister's antiseptic sprays and dressings and with his other invention, chromic catgut. Halsted himself recognized that Lister's principles were sound but, in his desire to do "away" with Listerian sprays, dressings, and catgut, Halsted may have failed to foresee the development of other antiseptic measures (aerosols, detergents, etc.) and to recognize the role that industry was to play in the technical developments that resulted in the excellence of modern-day catgut. Whether fortuitously or in deference to Lister, Halsted did not publish this article until a year after Lister's death which occurred Feb 10, 1912.

The suggestion below about surgical gloves was written one year before Charles Goodyear obtained a patent for his vulcanization process for rubber; the same year that Oliver Wendell Holmes cautioned against the contagious nature of puerperal sepsis; five years before Semmelweis's initial insight and report on cross-infections; twenty-four years before Lister evolved his antiseptic technique; forty-eight years before the use of rubber gloves found its way into the operating room to prevent dermatitis; and fifty-three years before the routine use of gloves was advocated by Bloodgood to prevent infection in otherwise clean surgical cases.

> In these days of ready invention, a glove, I think, might be devised, which should be impervious to fluid, and yet so thin and pliant as not to interfere materially with the delicate sense of touch required in these manipulations. One such glove, if such shall ever be fabricated and adopted, might well be sacrificed to the safety of the mother in every labour. THOMAS WATSON, 1843.

Halsted's great forte in operative surgery was careful attention to all details, however minute: anatomic dissection, gentle handling of tissues, careful hemostasis. Lister was more interested in basic science, in which he was so admirably trained, and in its application to clinical problems, introducing careful experimental designs that changed a clinical art into a clinical science.

The paths of these men were divergent and possibly neither understood the driving philosophy of the other as well as Whitehead understood both:

> There can be no adequate technical education which is not liberal, and no liberal education which is not technical; that is, no education which does not impart both technique and intellectual vision. ALFRED NORTH WHITEHEAD, 1917.

J.G.A.

Received for publication Jan. 7, 1962.

LIGATURE AND SUTURE MATERIAL

The Employment of Fine Silk in Preference to Catgut and the Advantages of Transfixion of Tissues and Vessels in Control of Hemorrhage Also an Account of the Introduction of Gloves, Gutta-Percha Tissue and Silver Foil

William Stewart Halsted, M.D.
Baltimore

For a number of years I have had it in mind to call attention to the particular method of employing silk ligatures and sutures which has been practiced in the surgical clinic of the Johns Hopkins University since the opening of the Johns Hopkins Hospital in 1889, but have hesitated and also been eager to do so for the same reason, namely, that our school seems to be almost alone in its advocacy of the use of this material.

Theodor Kocher, however, has for many years employed silk quite to the exclusion of catgut and our position is greatly strengthened by the support of such eminent authority.

Surgeons, old and young, those who have been active and masterful in the marvelous period of development of antiseptic surgery, and the medical student who takes for granted the healing of wounds *per primam* and the achievements of modern surgery as he does the ability to speak his own tongue, will be interested to read the words of Kocher spoken in 1888. "Away with the spray!" cried Bruns some years ago—Bruns who achieved so much and who died, alas, so early—and gladly did one cast off this burden. 'Away with protective!' exclaimed Starcke in an admirable essay on the treatment of wounds. But with the elimination of spray and protective there are still many of the seemingly essential features of the antiseptic technic to be discarded before the physician in general practice can be placed in that happy state of mind which pertains to the consciousness of his ability to avoid making the famous seven errors of Nussbaum. The 'away' must resound still further, and we say, therefore, primarily, away with the catgut! and also: away with all the prepared gauzes, from the Lister gauze to the newest productions of the manufacturers of supplies for dressings.

"To what misfortunes catgut can give rise more than one communication in the medical journals of years ago has testified. In the first place von Zweifel called attention to the decomposition which took place when catgut was kept in phenolized oil as recommended by Lister. Other surgeons have confirmed the observations that one may infect wounds directly with catgut preserved in the manner mentioned and we also have at one time published the case of a woman whose death after the excision of a struma sarcomatosa was attributable to the employment of catgut which had decomposed in the phenolized oil."

Kocher proceeds to relate the disastrous experience he had with catgut from May to July, 1887. Of thirty-one operations performed in a period of seven weeks, serious infection of the wound occurred in twenty-nine.

In one of the two non-infected cases silk was employed. Hence in this particular "catgut period" only one operative wound, a small one in which were very few ligatures, healed *per primam.* Catgut being totally discarded and silk reinstated, the infections ceased. From that time until the present, except possibly for brief periods of experimentation with catgut, Professor Kocher has, I believe, employed silk. I have not heard him state his reasons for preferring silk in these days when catgut may be perfectly sterilized, but that they are sound we may be sure. I can testify to the admirable healing of his wounds.

Our method of employing silk differs quite essentially from Professor Kocher's. The silk which we use is much finer than his and we rely on transfixion to prevent the ligature from slipping.

I am unable to say precisely when it was that I definitely substituted silk for catgut. It must have been earlier than 1883, for in that year or in 1882 Warmbrum Quilitz & Co. of Berlin made for me, in glass, bobbins of my designing, to be held in the left hand of the operator during the act of ligating blood-vessels. A description and illustration of these spools is given in the Johns Hopkins Hospital Reports. I have employed them continuously from the time of their introduction

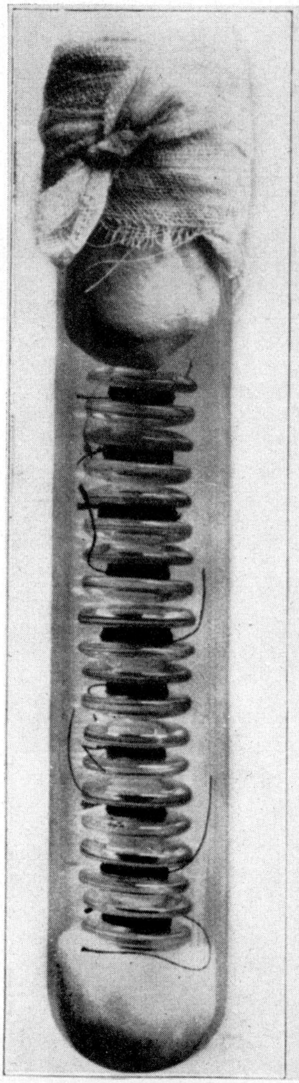

Fig. 1.—Ligature-spools of glass. A spool is held in the left hand while the right unwinds only so much of the thread as may be required for the ligation of one vessel.

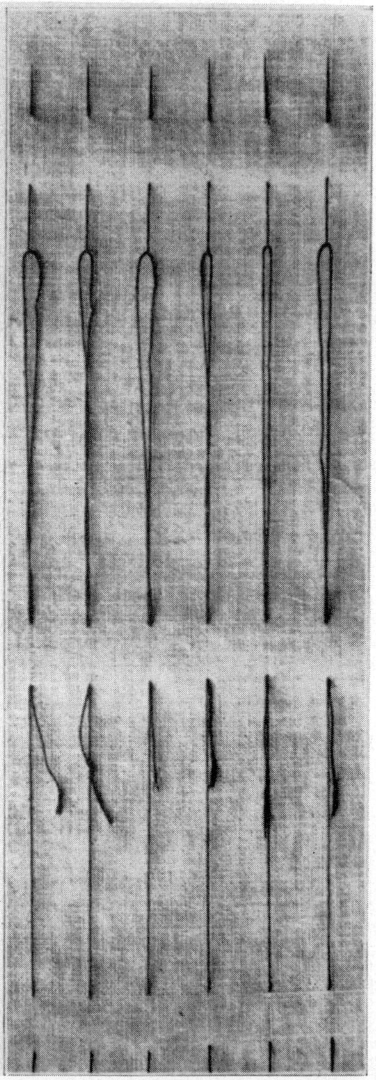

Fig. 2.—To show method of basting the threaded needles. Silk No. C. Needle No. 7. We usually employ silk two sizes finer than this. Reduced ⅗.

to the present. When the operator desires to tie a vessel without tissue-transfixion he is handed a spool—not a thread cut to the length desired for a ligature. With the right hand the silk is unwound, as required, from the spool held loosely in the left. Only two or three yards are wound on each spool, but enough for the tying off of many arteries; and for each operation the silk employed is sterilized only once. The armed glass spools are steamed in heavy glass test-tubes (Fig. 1).

In the winter of 1886 and 1887, experimenting on the subject of intestinal suture with Dr. Franklin B. Mall, I employed ordinary, fine black spool-silk as material for ligature and stitches. Black silk was selected in preference to white because it was easier to see it on the glass bobbins and in the fresh wound, and it was also more readily identified in the healed wounds. The little black loops of the mattress or Lembert stitches made a striking picture after a time, lying more or less free under the peritoneum along the line of the intestinal suture.

The following winters 1887-1889, in my experiments on the thyroid gland, I employed exclusively the black silk, just as we do to-day and have done ever since the opening of the Johns Hopkins Hospital twenty-four years ago.

The relatively high cost of catgut, its bulkiness, the inconveniences attending its use and sterilization, its inadequacy, the uncertainty as to the time required for its absorption, and the reaction which it excites in a wound, induced me to discard it completely for clean wounds in the surgery both of the human subject and of animals. From year to year and for various periods of time I have given the catgut, sterilized by the best known American purveyors of this material, a trial, but invariably with the results which we interpreted as being less perfect than with silk. Infection from pathogenic organisms can, of course, only rarely be ascribed, nowadays, directly to the catgut sterilized by our most reliable firms. With the fine silk in our wounds, which for twenty-three years have, as a rule, been closed without drainage, suppuration almost never occurs. But catgut, even that which we have no cause to believe is not sterile, irritates the wound for some reason, perhaps because it serves as culture medium for saprophytic organisms which are carried into it from the deep epithelium and follicles of the skin.

We have frequently observed this irritation and have occasionally had the opportunity to compare the reaction caused by catgut with that of fine silk in wounds symmetrically situated in the same patient and made at the same time.

Let the surgeon interested in making the comparison, when he has occasion to amputate both breasts for non-malignant disease, take a running subcuticular stitch on the one side with catgut, on the other with fine silk (No. A or AA) and observe the healing wounds from day to day; or when operating on two goiters on the same day, employ catgut for the platysma suture in the one case and very fine silk in the other. There is not only greater local reaction in the cases sewed with catgut but in them the wounds will occasionally open at one or more points to discharge a few drops of clear or cloudy fluid.

Wedded to the use of catgut, the operator develops, undoubtedly, a special technic which enables him to avoid procedures which would be likely to cause trouble or inconvenience, but on the other hand, he is deprived of very useful devices which become indispensable and a delight to the surgeon who has acquainted himself with the possibilities of silk threaded in the ordinary fine straight needle of commerce.

Straight needles of various sizes and lengths are threaded in great number with the silk corresponding in size, and are coarsely basted in rows into strips of thin muslin or gauze (Fig. 2). The loaded strips are folded and stored for subsequent use. The necessity for threading needles in the course of the operation is thus obviated in great measure. Occasionally more than one hundred of these needles are employed at one operation, since our ligations, for the most part, are made by transfixion of the tissues about the vessel or by piercing the vessel itself when it is large or sufficiently important, or by a combination (Fig. 5) of these methods. Figure 3 illustrates the usual method of controlling hemorrhage from the larger vessels which have been isolated. For the control of bleeding points when the vessels have not been isolated, the needle is passed first under or between the vessel or vessels to be ligated, and then a second transfixion is made, more superficially, close to the point of the clamp and in front of it; the clamp is now tilted in the opposite direction while the operator ties the knot behind it (Fig. 4). Piercing the tissues a second time in this manner eliminates the trouble of seeing to it that the ligature, in the act of tying, is carried over the tip of the artery clamp. This method enables one also to use to the best advantage the clamps with fine points which in my opinion have much to recommend them and which in our clinic are employed almost exclusively.

With the finest silk and needles one can perform feats in hemostasis which would be very difficult or impossible with catgut; for example, the control of small bleeding points over the trachea, of the pia mater, of the periosteum, and the suture of wounds of vessels.

In general terms ligatures taken in this way are drawn only with firmness sufficient to control completely the bleeding, and not so tight as to crush the tissues or interfere unnecessarily with their nutrition. The same tissues tied without transfixion would have to be crushed or strangulated by the ligature and thus, at best, be reduced to the condition of a graft with diminished chances of restitution and with increased danger of wound infection. Furthermore, ligation without transfixion necessitates the use of stronger silk for the reason that a transfixing ligature cannot slip.

The surgeon who has not tested the method will be surprised to find how large a vessel may be safely entrusted to a transfixion-ligature of the very finest silk. I have seen a ligature of coarse silk, tied with crushing force, blown off, as it were, from the aorta of a dog—a ligature which had been applied 12 mm. from

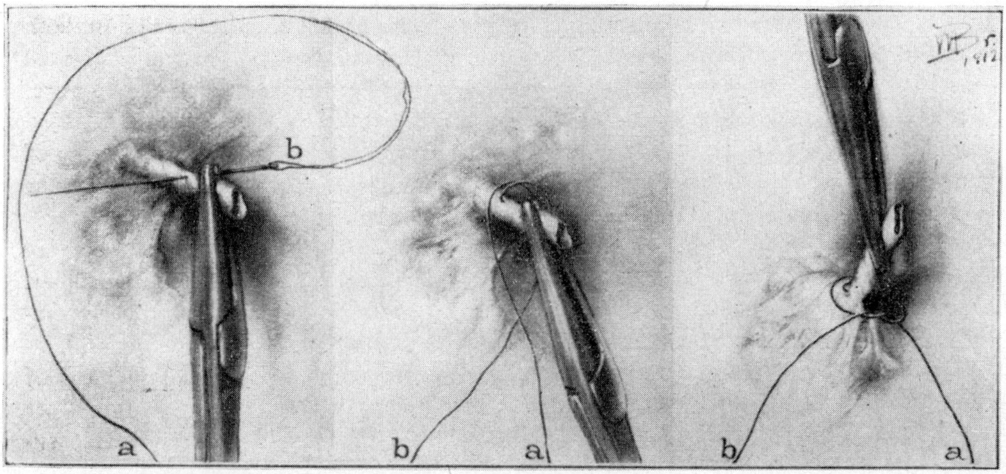

Fig. 3.—The ligation of an isolated vein or artery by transfixion. The vessel has been twisted to prevent bleeding from the needle-prick.

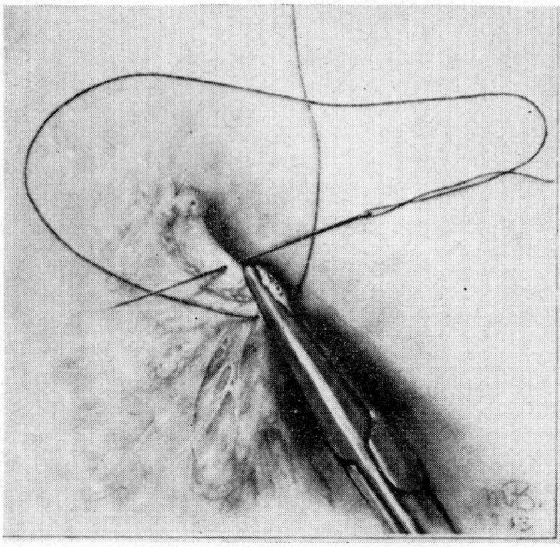

Fig. 4.—The usual method of controlling hemorrhage from one or more vessels by transfixion.

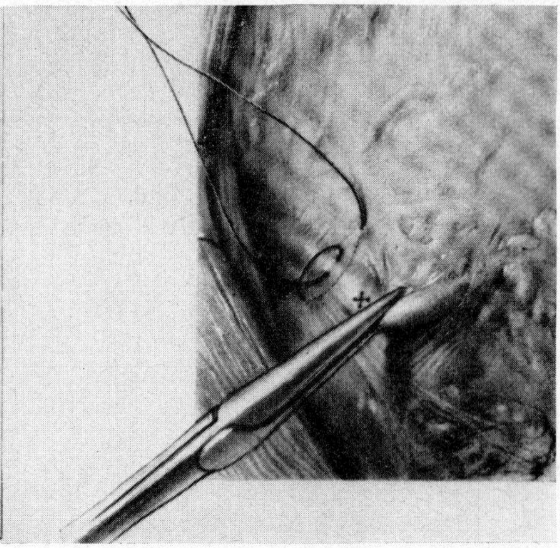

Fig. 5.—Ligation by transfixion of nonisolated vein, to be divided at *X*. The clamp is on the tumor-side of the vessel.

the proximal end of the divided vessel. This same artery was then safely obturated by a ligature of silk, No. A, which pierced it.

Repeatedly, he who uses catgut finds himself tying with a strand which is coarser than the vessel to be ligated.

Even for long abdominal wounds we rarely use a coarser silk than No. C (Fig. 2). Occasionally we reinforce with one or two sutures of silver wire which include skin and the anterior and posterior layers of the sheath of the rectus; otherwise fine silk (Nos. AA, A and C), is used throughout for sutures as well as ligatures. We seldom tie *en masse* in the ordinary sense of this term, and in clean wounds, I may say, never.

In the control of hemorrhage, parenchymatous or otherwise, we see to it that the thread is always well buried in the living tissue. It should not bridge over a dead space as a chord subtends an arc. In ligating the vessels of the superior pole of a thyroid lobe in the course of a lobectomy a fine, short, curved or straight needle, carrying one strand of fine silk is passed behind or between the vessels, and then through the twisted artery or vein, or both, and the thread is tied on both sides of the clamp. The ligation of the superior thyroid vessels is usually deferred until the end of the operation, these vessels being divided and entrusted to a reliable, fine-pointed clamp in the early stage of the operation.

The difficulty, the cost and the infeasibility of keeping on hand a large supply of needles threaded with catgut, as well as the size of the gut, almost preclude the extensive use of this material for the control of hemorrhage by transfixion.

That surgeons obtained excellent results with silk even when gloves were not worn one may convince himself by the papers of Kocher, Heidenhain and Hägler. Now that rubber gloves are invariably worn, the results with silk, properly employed, are so perfect that I believe its adoption will ultimately become general.

A few days ago, seeing a surgeon of great eminence and unusual fairness of mind burying sutures of catgut I inquired, "Why do you still employ catgut?"

"Because I cannot free myself of the prejudice against a non-absorbable suture. I believe," said he, "that it is foolish to use catgut; and every now and then when my wounds break down too frequently I discard it."

The catgut with which he was sewing was No. 2 chromicized; it was guaranteed by America's most reliable firm "not to absorb" for twenty-six days, but not guaranteed "to absorb" within as many weeks.

It should be borne in mind that during the greater part of the period of its disintegration the catgut suture is not only not serving its purpose but is playing the rôle of necrotic tissue, of a culture medium. I trust that I shall not be considered flippant in suggesting that the ideal absorbable suture-material might be a thread which would serve its purpose for, say, ten days and be absorbed in three.

Conceded that infection is less likely to occur with silk than with catgut, it would still be objected, and quite pertinently, that, in case is should occur, the buried silk might give endless trouble and have to be removed.

It is well within reason to expect that the technic may be at least so perfect when silk is employed that the wound will become infected not once in a hundred cases. If fine silk were used and the infection slight, probably none of the buried threads would be extruded, nor would healing be delayed demonstrably on account of their presence. When heavy silk has been used for any of the sutures and the suppuration is considerable, one or more or, perhaps, all of the threads would have to be removed. Even in such a case it is very unlikely that the ligatures and fine sutures would give trouble.

The Clamp Twist in the Control of the Hemorrhage

A vessel or bleeding point inaccurately caught by the artery clamps and requiring immediate ligation for any reasons may, as is undoubtedly well known, often be controlled by a half-twist or slight rotation of the clamp. The precise situation of the vessel may then be determined by cautiously untwisting the instrument to the degree necessary to permit the escape of a fraction of a drop of blood and then retwisting. Now, instead of removing the clamp and trying again to catch the vessel in a field which, in such case, might be more or less obscured by hemorrhage, one transfixes once or twice in a dry field at the proper place and ties on one or both sides of the forceps; or if there is indication and room for two clamps, a second may be applied when the exact situation of the bleeding point has been revealed by the untwisting of the first.

The surgeon can transfix accurately with one hand while he holds the clamp in the other, and, by pulling on the twice transfixing thread, check the hemorrhage before tying. The bleeding being arrested, both hands are freed for making the knot.

The Interrupted Stitch

We find ourselves using the interrupted variety of suture even more frequently than formerly. It is more accurate, reliable and convenient than the running stitch, and, with the long straight needles armed and conveniently arranged as I have described, can be taken about as quickly as the latter. The head nurse of the operating-room hands the threaded needles to the surgeon, presenting them to him pointward. The operator can take a stitch in the time required by the nurse to withdraw the next needle and thread from the cloth in which they have been basted. The knots are tied after all the stitches have been taken. With the aid of a good assistant very little time is consumed in the tying. A granny knot is adequate when fine silk is used. In some instances the granny is better than the reef knot, for in the tying of the former in the presence of tension the traction on the first turn of the knot can easily be maintained, and should the first turn loosen, in the taking of the second the slack can usually be taken up in the drawing home of the latter.

Undrained Wounds

Fine silk frequently enables one to close a wound which would have to be drained if catgut were employed. Bleeding points so fine as to be awkwardly or not at all ligable with catgut may be readily and quickly controlled by a transfixing suture of the finest silk tied sometimes with merely a half knot. When the ends of such a knot are cut very short the silk is barely visible.

I am taking for granted it will be conceded that unless the hemostasis is quite perfect and the likelihood of bleeding after closure of the wound negligible, drainage should usually be resorted to. Unfortunately catgut as material for ligature does not afford the security from hemorrhage that silk does, partly because its knots are not so dependable and partly because, as I have said, the former cannot so conveniently or so universally be resorted to for transfixion as the latter.

Faulty Technic

The surgeon who desires to use silk and who, after giving it a fair trial, finds that his results are not so good as with catgut may, I think, quite surely attribute his failure to himself—to faulty technic. By faulty technic I do not mean merely breaks in asepsis.

One should not of course use silk for ligating or suturing in the presence of infection. Nor should one bring parts together under such degree of tension as to cause necrosis or interfere greatly with the blood-supply, for nothing is gained by so doing and decided harm may result. Healing is menaced when the circulation of the tissues to be united is impaired.[1]

In operations made through healing tissues catgut may occasionally be used in preference to silk.

The silk employed should never be coarser than necessary and it is useless to employ a thread for suture which is stronger than the tissue itself. A greater number of fine stitches is better, as a rule, than a few coarse ones.

Avoid, if possible, the combined use of silk and catgut in a wound.

For sewing up an abdominal wound, when it is necessary here and there to take heavy deep stitches perforating skin and muscles, silver wire serves admirably. When the skin can be approximated without tension we usually employ interrupted perforating stitches of very fine silk. If the skin edges have to be brought together under considerable tension we recommend a subcuticular stitch of silver wire taken with the Hagedorn or Schnötter needle.[2]

I have presented this matter in such detail because so many have tried with indifferent or worse than indifferent success to substitute silk for catgut, and because I am told, as I have said, that the operators and pupils of the surgical clinic of the Johns Hopkins University are quite the only ones in this country who systematically employ the former.

I believe that the tendency will always be in the direction of exercising greater care and refinement in operating, and that the surgeon will develop increasingly a respect for tissues, a sense which recoils from inflicting unnecessary insult to structures concerned in the process of repair.

The Epithelial Stitch

In the toilet of wounds in animals we meet conditions different in some respects from those which obtain in the human subject. The long hair, the deep follicles of the skin of dogs and the inconveniences incident to subsequent dressings make it desirable to modify the technic of closing the wounds in these animals.

Stitching of the platysma muscle does not hold together sufficiently well the edges of the skin, and the subcuticular stitch taken close to the incised border is not so safe in the dog as in the human subject because the follicles are relatively deeper and more numerous in the former. Hence, in the dog, after suturing the platysma we place a running subcuticular suture a little further than usual from the free edge of the skin. Should now the approximation of the skin not be sufficiently perfect we add the "epithelial stitch." This is made with silk about 00 fine and with a needle to correspond. Hardly more than the epithelium is pierced by the needle, and the suture when completed describes almost a straight line (Fig. 6). The epithelial stitch produces no irritation and does not require subsequent attention, for it rubs off in the ordinary process of attrition, or it may be pulled off at any time like a plaster. Inasmuch as, in dogs, stitches which pierce the skin should be removed in two or three days lest the infection which they cause give rise to suppuration, and as it is undesirable and troublesome in the case of animals to remove stitches or to expose the wound so soon after operation, stitching in some such way as above described has decided advantages.

Celloidin-Batiste

In many of our operations, and always when it seems particularly indicated, we paste to the skin over a wide field a fine batiste (sometimes gauze, or silk) dipped in celloidin.

In amputations at or near the hip-joint, the actual field of operation may or may not be covered with the cambric. A liberal flounce-like sheet pasted along the side of the genitals from pubes to sacrum, along Poupart's ligament and from the anterior superior spine of the ilium along the outer side of the thigh to the tuberosity of the ischium, in other words a truncated hollow cone which encircles the thigh just above the line of amputation, suffices. This flounce should extend well up on to the abdomen and back and side, and down on the inside of the opposite thigh.

Gloves

Rubber gloves must, of course, be worn by all concerned in the operation.

In a letter of a few weeks ago the director of a famous German clinic asked me to give him references to articles that I might have written on the subject of rubber gloves. As response to his request and believing that a brief account concerning the introduction of gloves may eventually be of interest I will, in as few words as possible, relate the story.

In the winter of 1889 and 1890—I cannot recall the month—the nurse in charge of my operating-room complained that the solutions of mercuric chlorid produced a dermatitis of her arms and hands. As she was an unusually efficient woman, I gave the matter my consideration and one day in New York requested the Goodyear Rubber Company to make as an experiment two pair of thin rubber gloves with gauntlets. On trial these proved to be so satisfactory that additional gloves were ordered. In the autumn, on my return to town, the assistant who passed the instruments and threaded the needles was also provided with rubber gloves to wear at the operations. At first the operator wore them only when exploratory incisions into joints were made. After a time the assistants became so accustomed

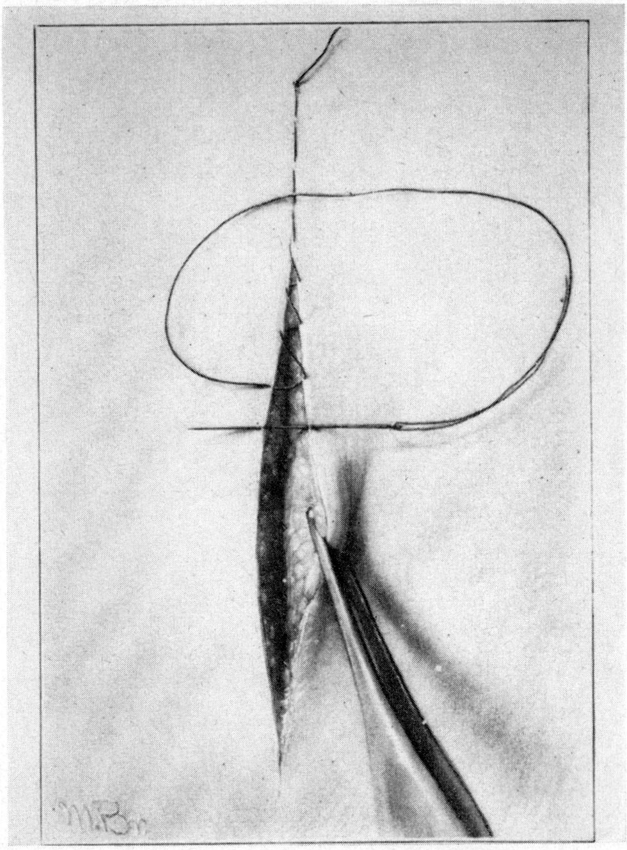

Fig. 6.—The epithelial stitch. The thread, needle and bite of skin should be much finer than the drawing indicates.

to working in gloves that they also wore them as operators and would remark that they seemed to be less expert with the bare hand than with the gloved hands.

I think it was Dr. Bloodgood, my house surgeon, who first made this comment and that he was the first to wear them, invariably, when operating.

In the report which I made of the first year's work at the hospital, written in November and December, 1890, and published in March, 1891, I stated that the assistant who passed the instruments wore rubber gloves. This assistant was given the gloves to protect his hands from the solution of phenol (carbolic acid) in which the instruments were submerged rather than to eliminate him as a source of infection. I do not recall having referred again, in my publications, to the employment of rubber gloves. Dr. Hunter Robb in 1894, in his book on aseptic technic recommended that the operator wear rubber gloves. Dr. Robb was, at that time, resident gynecologist of the Johns Hopkins Hospital and had frequent opportunities to observe the technic of the surgical clinic.

This incidental reference by Robb in 1894 to the wearing of rubber gloves, and the fact that a photograph of an operation for breast cancer taken late in the year 1893 shows that gloves were not being regularly worn by us at that time, serve to establish approximately the date of their definite introduction.

Dr. Joseph C. Bloodgood, in his elaborate report on Hernia makes the following statements with reference to the wearing of gloves:

The writer was the first as operator to wear gloves as a routine practice in practically all clean operations. He began to wear gloves invariably in December, 1896; before this date he had operated in twenty cases of hernia with four suppurations, all late infections; wounds were closed with silver wire. Since wearing gloves he has operated in 100 cases of inguinal hernia. In one case (recent) the wound suppurated.

Rubber gloves were introduced by Professor Halsted soon after the hospital opened in 1889. They were invariably worn by the assistant who handed instruments and by the assistant at the wound, usually the nurse in charge of the operating-room. The operator himself rarely wore gloves (*at that time*) except when clean joints were opened.

Thus the operating in gloves was an evolution rather than an inspiration or happy thought, and it is remarkable that during the four or five years when as operator I wore them only occasionally, we could have been so blind as not to have perceived the necessity for wearing them invariably at the operating-table.

It is also noteworthy that none of the many surgeons, foreign and American, who visited our clinic in those years should have recognized the desirability of eliminating the hands as a source of infection, by the wearing of gloves.

We did not realize how slightly the sense of touch is obtunded by the rubber covering,[3] or how unessential it is in most operations that the greatest delicacy of finger perception be preserved. Furthermore we were delighted with the results in healing already obtainable, so vivid were the memories of infections in the recent past.

Silver Foil

Since 1894 we have covered our fresh wounds with silver foil and are quite convinced that this dressing has appreciable chemical as well as physical values.

That various metals inhibit the growth of certain organisms has been proved by Miller, Nägeli, Behring, Uffelman, Meade Bolton and others.

Bolton's work interested me particularly because very kindly, in our behalf, he tested thoroughly the effect of silver on the growth of the common pyogenic microorganisms. For his experiments he used silver in various forms but particularly the silver foil with which we were at the time covering our wounds.

I had previously employed foils of copper, brass, gold and aluminum and had found that copper and brass irritated the skin. The silver foil had given, clinically, the most satisfactory results and I was pleased to find that its use had the support of Bolton's carefully conducted experiments. The admirable behavior of wire in wounds which has been commented on for centuries may, therefore, be attributed to its antiseptic properties.

Under the foil the stitches which perforate the skin may, it seems to me, be left undisturbed for a greater number of days than under the ordinary dressings. Thiersch grafts implanted on clean fresh surfaces and covered with silver foil need not be investigated for ten days or more. The foil, while it seals the dry wound hermetically, readily permits the escape of fluids.

We may, possibly, overestimate the value of silver foil as a dressing, but we are wedded to its use, and I know of nothing which could quite take its place, nor have I known any one to abandon it who had thoroughly familiarized himself with the technic of its employment. Moistening the skin and the applied foil with alcohol facilitates its application, but alcohol should not be employed in the laying on of the foil over skin-grafts.

Three or four layers of foil are usually placed on the closed incision, and over these is laid the thin paper between the leaves of which the foil is packed. We have occasionally covered the foil with strips of very thin, bibulous, Japanese paper. Foil without paper and covered with crêpe lisse and celloidin makes a particularly neat dressing for wounds of the face and scalp.

Gutta-Percha Tissue

Dr. Jacob Frank, in an interesting account of the discovery of gutta-percha and the uses of gutta-percha tissue in surgery stated that perhaps the first mention of this tissue is to be found appended to a report on gutta-percha submitted to the Académie de médecine, July 30, 1850, by a commission composed of Messrs. Chevalier, Poiseuille and Robert. It was called *tissu électro-magnétique,* approved by the National Academy of Medicine, tested in the various hospitals in Paris, and recommended as a sovereign remedy for gout, rheumatism, sciatica, migraines, neuralgias and gastralgias, for the resolution of varices, for the dressing of wounds, burns, etc.; also for pneumonia in its early stages. The tissue was relatively thick; it could be washed and used indefinitely, and was represented as being greatly superior to the medicated oiled papers which were not only inert but soiled the body and the linen and were altogether disagreeable in use. "To convince oneself of its magnetic properties, one had merely to rub it lightly on a piece of cloth and hold it above sawdust. Instantly particles of the sawdust would spring up and attach themselves to the tissue."

In the light of our experience with the gutta-percha tissue of the present day we can well believe that the *tissu électro-magnétique* was really serviceable at times in the treatment of the affections enumerated. Its disuse may have been due in part to its pseudonym.

Dr Manoury, six years later, recommended medicated plaques of gutta-percha.

> To apply a plaque one dips it in warm water, 40 degrees, in order that it may conform by its flexibility to the protuberances and anfractuosities of the ulcer; when it has been applied one covers it with a cloth wet with cold water, with view to preventing the adhesions of this cloth to the external surface of the plaque.

A. Cousin in 1872 wrote as follows:

> Gutta-percha, on account of its numerous and valuable properties, has for a long time attracted the attention of practitioners of medicine and surgery, and on consulting the instructive collection of the *Bulletin de thérapeutique* one finds not less than twenty-three papers devoted to the consideration of the diverse uses of this substance.
>
> It has been employed, in the solid state, in the fabrication of apparatus for fractures, of caustic pastes, of sounds and bougies, of prothesis, of various utensils; dissolved in chloroform it was at one time much vaunted in the topical treatment of certain skin affections as substitute for collodion.
>
> Every one knows to-day the excellent results obtained by the occlusive method in the treatment of a great number of medical and surgical affections (occlusive dressings, compressing or contracting, of collodion, swathing in impermeable cloths, pneumatic occlusion, wadded splints, etc.). It would take too long to study, comparatively, the indications for the various dressings or the advantages and defects that they present; I wish simply to make known to the readers of the *Bulletin* a method which I believe to be new and which is assuredly a simple and easy one for making occlusion.
>
> I employ for this purpose leaves of gutta-percha reduced by rolling to the thinness of waxed taffeta, and I take advantage of its extreme solubility in chloroform to give to this material adhesive qualities of considerable degree.
>
> I proceed in the following manner: Given a surface of skin to be covered, I cut a piece of flattened gutta-percha to dimensions two or three times as large as this area; I trace along the border of this variety of plaster, for an extent of 1 or 2 cm., a brush dipped in chloroform and apply it immediately to the skin; adhesion takes place with great energy at all the points touched by the chloroform, and so perfectly that the slightest irregularities of the skin are reproduced with remarkable fidelity in the impermeable material.

I have quoted at such length from the article of Dr. Cousin in order to make clear what were the uses which had been made of gutta-percha tissue to the year 1872, and because it may be interesting to others to read the original description of a clever and useful procedure—the pasting of the edges of a leaf of gutta-percha to the skin by means of chloroform.

Occasionally we paste with chloroform in this way a small scrap of gutta-percha tissue to a piece of old linen when the skin surrounding the granulating surface which is to be covered with gutta-percha tissue is likely to become irritated by the discharges from the ulcer. In such case the protective is cut to the precise size of sore, the skin about which being covered with an ointment of zinc oxid; the discharges are promptly absorbed by the linen and overlaid dressings. It is well, under these conditions, to cut a tiny hole through both protective and linen to permit the prompt escape of the secretions of the wound into the dressing.

Dr. Frank gave two references to the early employment by physicians of plaques or "sheets" of gutta-percha, but was unable to make any statement relative to its introduction in its present form and for its present purposes, and leaves unfilled a gap of perhaps a quarter of a century.

As I know of no one except myself who can tell the story I may be pardoned for a moment's indulgence in reminiscence.

As intern of Bellevue Hospital, New York, from 1876 to 1878, I had frequent opportunities to observe the pain and bleeding incident to the tearing out of gauze from large involucral cavities after sequestrotomy—gauze which had been stuffed into these cavities to arrest bleeding and into which the granulations had grown, often for a considerable distance. Wounds of the soft parts would also be packed with gauze, which from its adhesion to the skin would cause pain, sometimes very distressing, and the first removal of the gauze was an event anticipated with apprehension by the patients, who were quite sure to be advised by the ward-neighbors of its terrors.

During the two years of my study abroad the desirability of obviating this rather barbarous practice was repeatedly enforced on me by what I saw in the foreign clinics, and on my return to America in 1880 I promptly cast about for some sort of protective, non-adhering dressing. Oiled silk and the green protective of Lister were not sufficiently pliable. Finally a salesman in one of the surgical supply stores showed me a bed-sheet of gutta-percha as heavy as blotting-paper, remarking that it could be rolled out to any degree of thinness. I requested him to procure the thinnest tissue possible, and in the course of a few weeks he provided me with samples, none of which was sufficiently thin. After a month or two tissue of the desired thinness was obtained and from that day until the present, a period of nearly thirty-three years, gutta-percha tissue, usually referred to as rubber tissue or protective, has been one of the most prized and indispensable articles of my surgical armamentarium.

Accounts of the first employment of gutta-percha tissue to protect granulations from insult and to prevent them from growing into or adhering to drains, gauze packs and dressings and to promote healing under a moist scab can probably be found in the records of the Roosevelt Hospital Dispensary, New York, from 1881 to 1886, the term of my incumbency as director of this dispensary; and some of my assistants and students of those years will doubtless recall having employed it there as a dressing for wounds.

I have not searched for references to the use of gutta-percha tissue in its present form and for its present purposes subsequent to the time of its introduction in 1881, but I am quite sure that no mention of it will be found prior to 1884 or 1885, and that should there be any such it will have been made by surgeons of New York who might have learned of it from my students or seen it employed at one of the various hospitals with which, as attending surgeon, I was connected.

Its employment as drainage material for the abdominal cavity came about as follows:

At first we tucked it about the gauze drains at the surface only, in order to prevent adhesions to the skin. Then the protective was carried deeper and deeper into the wounds until finally the entire gauze drain or gauze pack, except at the very bottom, was enveloped in the gutta-percha tissue.

The experiments of Dr. Yates of my staff, made to determine the amount of time required for the formation about the protective of intestinal adhesions, were especially important and had their influence in emboldening the surgeon at times to dispense altogether with the gauze, placing his reliance on the gutta-percha.

Not very often do we venture to drain an abdominal wound with nothing but protective. Usually the cigarette form of drain is employed—gauze enveloped in protective—when we wish to know that a drain is precisely and promptly fixed in the desired position, as it is by the little tuft of gauze at the bottom of the cigarette.

For certain cases in which it seems desirable that adhesions should form more rapidly and firmly about the abdominal drain we make it as follows: Two squares, one of gauze (single sheet) and one of protective, are rolled together, the gauze outside, until a drain of the desired thickness is obtained. Granulations cannot pierce this drain deeper than the single layer of gauze, because they at once encounter the underlying protective. Such a drain is removed quite as easily as the cigarette drain and offers a little more security than the latter.

A moist scab, so-called, is better than a dry one. The surgeon has many opportunities to convince himself of this. When he has occasion to extract a toe-nail let him cover one-third of the raw surface with protective and allow the remainder to heal under the dry scab. The patient may have pain in the digit soon after the dry scab is well formed, and the surgeon will perhaps observe that the soft parts about the nail-bed on the side of the dry scab are inflamed. On covering the entire surface of the granulating wound with gutta-percha tissue the pain will promptly be relieved and the inflammation subside.

The dry scab imprisons secretion which in turn gives rise to tension, and the tension impairs the vitality of the tissues under and at the border of the dry scab to an extent sufficient to place them at a disadvantage in their combat with the micro-organisms, and to compel absorption of the toxins.

Even pimples and trivial wounds of, for example, the fingers behave best under the moist scab. For the healing of wounds under the moist blood-clot, particularly when the skin cannot be made to cover the cavity to be filled with blood, gutta-percha tissue is invaluable. It would be found useful in every household and should be included in the supplies provided for first aid to the injured. The value of the moist scab should be common knowledge for the layman, and gutta-percha tissue should replace for him the sticking-plaster as a covering for wounds.

A few months ago in reading one of Lister's first papers on the use of phenol in wounds I noted that he mentions having covered a wound with a tissue of gutta-percha. This interested me so much that I wrote at once to Sir William Watson Cheyne, being confident that no one could give me the desired information so well as he. From his kind reply I quote as follows:

> So far as I understand the matter, Lister tried various materials to cover the wound after an operation, so as to prevent the phenol in the dressing from penetrating in any quantity to the wound. Among other things he tried gutta-percha tissue, but he abandoned that because

the phenol easily passed through it so that it did not protect the wound from the irritation of the antiseptic, and the material he ultimately hit on was oiled silk, covered with a layer of dextrin, so as to allow it to be wet. The oiled silk itself did not prevent the phenol vapor from passing through it, but the combination of oiled silk and shellac, according to Lister's experiments, did. As regards any question of priority in using it, so far as any claim can be advanced on Lister's behalf, it would not hold, because he tried it and abandoned it as being unsuitable for his particular purpose.

From 1879 to 1889 I made frequent visits to England and the continent and was in close touch with the work of the surgical clinics of England, France and Germany, and not once in that period did I see gutta-percha tissue employed in Europe.

It is gratifying to me to observe the place in surgery which gutta-percha tissue has gradually won for itself. For the American surgeon it has become an indispensable appurtenance of his equipment.

---

[1] In operations for the oblique as well as the direct form of inguinal hernia we sometimes split vertically the sheath of the rectus muscle for the relief of strain on the stitches holding together the internal oblique muscle or conjoined tendon and Poupart's ligament.

[2] It is known only to a few surgeons that the late Dr. Schnötter, surgeon to the German Hospital, New York, devised and used the needle curved on the edge some years before Hagedorn described it.

[3] For example, in the early days of rubber gloves I removed the glove from one hand, not infrequently, to palpate the common bile-duct in search for stone.

Management of Juxtarenal Aortic Occlusions

JOHN J. BERGAN, MD, AND OTTO H. TRIPPEL, MD, CHICAGO

"... le traitement idéal consisterait évidement à reséquer la zône obliterée et à retablir la perméabilité arterielle si c'est possible ..."
—*Leriche,* 1923

While the syndrome of occlusion of the terminal aorta is frequently observed, the symptom complex caused by aortic obliteration at or above the renal artery level is seldom seen. Occlusion at this higher level usually results from slow proximal progression of a distal aortic thrombosis and insidiously threatens the blood supply to vital organs. The many years of development which this process entails notwithstanding, patients with this end-stage of the Leriche syndrome often remain undiagnosed until their surgical management poses very real problems.[9,11,19]

The incidence of the Leriche syndrome has not been ascertained but it has been shown that in patients with aortic occlusion who reach vascular centers, from 3% to 15% will have obstruction to flow at the level of the left renal artery.[15,28] That this represents the final stage of the Leriche syndrome in some cases is well recognized. It is known that the clinical course of such a patient is one of continued deterioration. Proximal progression of the occlusion not only blocks lumbar collateral vessels but encroaches upon the renal arteries.[20] Associated cardiac and cerebral arterial disease in these patients poses a constant threat to life.[6] Mesenteric infarction occurs with surprising frequency.[27]

Techniques for restoring distal blood flow in cases of aortoiliac occlusion have become standardized. From dos Santos' first report of thromboendarterectomy in 1947 through Oudot's description of aortic resection and homografting in 1951, the problems of main vessel reconstruction have largely been solved.[14,25] At present the two main schools of thought are represented by the advocates of endarterectomy and of bypass grafting using Teflon or Dacron prostheses.[7,12]

Although management of distal aortic occlusive disease is thus fairly uniform, methods of reconstruction of the aorta at or above renal artery level have attained no such degree of standardization. Suggestions in this regard have been proposed, but no single technique has evolved which has been entirely satisfactory.[10,28] This report attempts to clarify the place of a variety of technical aids including hypothermia, vasopressor agents, and osmotic diuretics as well as to suggest solutions to some of the problems encountered in restoring distal arterial flow.

The patients in this report were treated on the peripheral vascular service of the Veterans Administration Research Hospital and the Chicago Wesley Memorial Hospital. Each patient is presented to illustrate a method or to describe a technique. No attempt is made to detail the natural history of the disease or its total management.

Infrarenal Aortic Occlusion

Occlusion of the aorta which has ascended to the level of one renal artery may follow the proximal progression of thrombosis from an occluded aortic aneurysm or, more commonly, from a terminal aortic occlusion.

Presented at the 20th Annual Meeting of the Central Surgical Association, Chicago, Feb 21-23, 1963.

From the Departments of Surgery, Veterans Administration Research Hospital, Chicago Wesley Memorial Hospital, and Northwestern University Medical School.

This work was supported in part by a grant from the Chicago Heart Association.

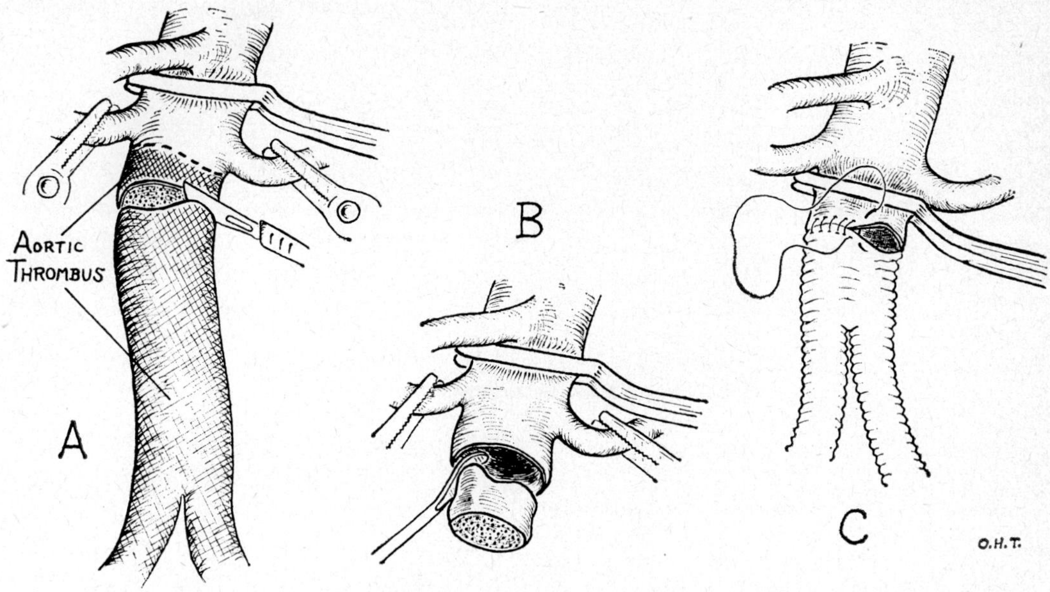

Fig 1.—Steps in the surgical management of infrarenal aortic occlusion designed to minimize the period of interruption of arterial flow to the kidneys.

Whether a bypass graft or an endarterectomy is used distally to restore flow to the extremities depends upon the nature of the lumbar aorta. However, more critical problems of management arise in dealing with the proximal portion of the reconstruction. It is here that particular techniques must be employed to preserve renal blood flow or lower renal metabolism to protect the kidneys from ischemic damage (Fig 1). The following cases illustrate revascularization with and without hypothermia.

CASE 1.—This 65-year-old male had known of his Leriche syndrome for 20 years. Increasing fatigue in his thighs and calves prompted him to seek therapy. He was found to have intermittent hypertension to 190/110. A left brachial aortogram revealed terminal aortic occlusion with encroachment upon the left renal artery. Operation was performed without hypothermia. A small, thrombosed aneurysm of the lumbar aorta was found. The aorta was clamped proximal to the renal arteries after each renal artery had been occluded at its origin from the aorta with a serrefine clamp. The aorta was transected below the renal vessels and above the aneurysm. Adherent thrombus was removed from the proximal aorta, and backflow was used to flush debris from each renal artery. An infrarenal clamp was then applied to the aorta and the suprarenal aortic clamp removed, thus re-establishing renal arterial flow. Total suprarenal clamping time was seven minutes. A Teflon aortofemoral bifurcated graft was interposed to restore distal blood flow. Postoperative urine volume and specific gravity were normal; no effects of renal ischemia were observed. No further hypertension was noted.

Rob has indicated a preference for the above technique with but a single modification.[28] After transecting the aorta below the renal vessels he displaces it anterior to the left renal vein before applying the suprarenal aortic clamp and performing thromboendarterectomy. After an infrarenal clamp is applied, he replaces the aorta posterior to the renal vein and completes the distal reconstruction. Rob believes that the 15 minutes necessitated by this portion of the operation produce no deleterious renal effects.

With Hypothermia.—The renal protective effect of hypothermia during aortic cross-clamping is adequately proved.[17] A comforting margin of safety is offered by its use during removal of infrarenal aortic occlusions.

CASE 2.—A 49-year-old male had exhibited progressively increasing intermittent calf claudication for three years. Aortography revealed aortic occlusion level with the left renal artery orifice (Fig 2). During hypothermia (32 C, 89.6 F) and under general anesthesia an aortic endarterectomy was performed. The suprarenal aorta was cross-clamped for 21 minutes. Distal blood flow was established

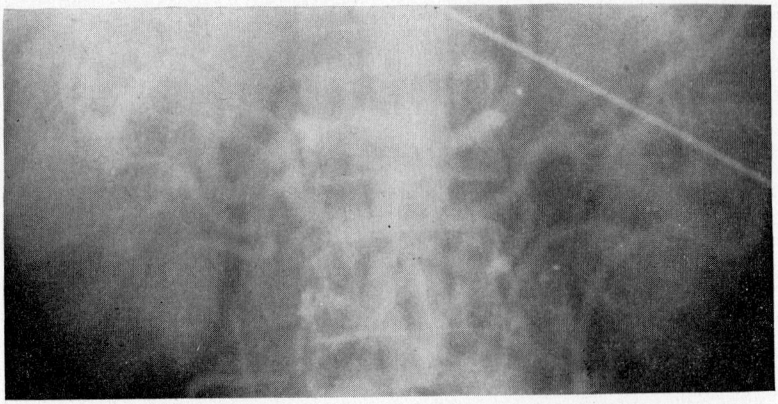

Fig 2.—A lumbar aortogram in a patient with infrarenal aortic occlusion shows the dye column ending abruptly after filling both renal arteries.

by iliofemoral bypass grafts after aortoiliac endarterectomy.

During surgery, 20% mannitol was infused as advocated by Barry.[3] No postoperative oliguria occurred; no depression of renal function was noted.

In this patient and in others in whom an infusion of mannitol has been utilized, the volume of urine excreted during and after surgery has been striking. A urine output of 60 to 120 cc per hour can easily be obtained. However, Beall has shown that such infusion of this osmotic diuretic does not increase renal blood flow and that within 24 hours renal function is comparable in patients who receive mannitol and in those who do not.[5] This agent certainly promotes diuresis but its true utility in patients undergoing aortic surgery remains to be determined.

Fig 3.—A lumbar aortogram in a patient with juxtarenal aortic occlusion shows the dye filling only the mesenteric artery and the stenotic right renal vessel.

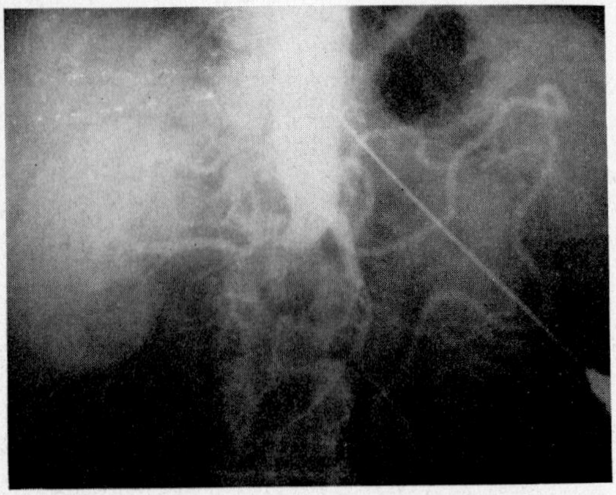

Aortic and Left Renal Artery Occlusion

As aortic thrombosis ascends, it gradually encroaches upon a renal artery orifice and produces increasingly severe hypertension. This hypertension is not the result of increased peripheral resistance.[29] In the past, nephrectomy was performed at this stage, and normotension was usually obtained for a variable period of time.[35] Inevitably further proximal progression of the aortic occlusion defeated this form of therapy.

The following case illustrates management of aortic and left renal artery occlusion.

Case 3.—This 62-year-old white male had a 15-year history of hypertension and was admitted with a blood pressure of 230/110. The radioisotope renogram showed no vascular spike and virtually no renal function on the left. Right renal function was markedly impaired. Aortography revealed aortic and left renal artery occlusion with stenosis of the right renal artery (Fig 3).

With the patient under hypothermia (30 C, 86 F), and utilizing an upper abdominal transverse incision, the juxtarenal aorta was exposed by reflecting the

Fig 4.—The specimen removed by aortic endarterectomy shows the thickened intima of the superior mesenteric and right renal artery as well as the totally occluded left renal artery.

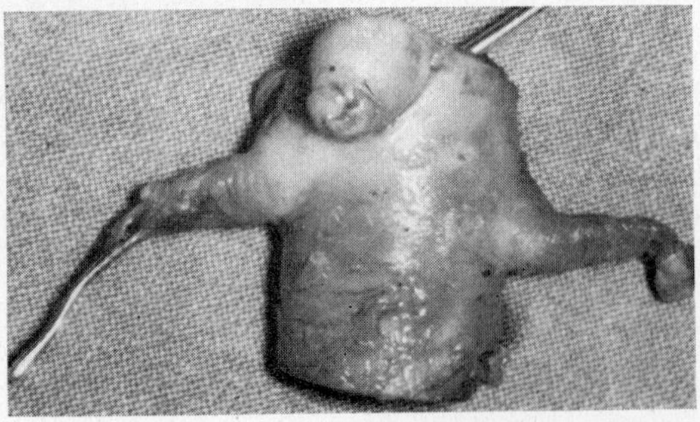

spleen, stomach, and left colon medially. An endarterectomy of the aorta, right renal, left renal, and superior mesenteric arteries was performed (Fig 4). After proximal aortic endarterectomy, it was necessary to terminate the operation rapidly. The endarterectomized aorta was oversewn distal to the renal vessels. No distal continuity was restored. A bilateral lumbar sympathectomy was performed, however.

The patient has been observed for three years. He experiences little difficulty in slow ambulation but has claudication on moderate exercise. His hypertension is now much less severe and is more easily controlled with medications.

Suprarenal Aortic Thrombosis

A number of patients will survive the slow, inexorable, proximal progression of aortic thrombosis.[8] As each renal artery orifice is gradually occluded, collateral vessels may arise from proximal lumbar arteries through ureteropelvic arteries to supply the main renal artery. While this occurs, severe hypertension usually supervenes. As congestive cardiac failure is added to the patient's disabilities, surgical risk increases. Nevertheless, no effective form of medical management for these patients has evolved. Surgery remains the patients' only hope for palliation or for cure.

Case 4.—This 63-year-old white woman had symptoms of an aortic occlusion for 14 years. Progressively deteriorating renal function was documented by serial radioisotope renograms. Severe sustained hypertension had been present for 4 years (Fig 5). Serial films exposed during aortography revealed a suprarenal aortic occlusion with obliteration of both renal artery orifices. Filling of the main renal artery was by way of the lumbo-ureteral collateral vessels (Fig 6,*A* and *B*).

Operation was performed using hypothermia to 31 C (87.8 F). A thromboendarterectomy of the aorta and both renal vessels was performed. After closure of this portion of the aortotomy, an infrarenal aortic clamp was applied and the suprarenal clamp removed. Reconstitution of flow to the lower extremities was accomplished using a Teflon bifurcated graft.

Immediately postoperatively hypotension could not be reversed by conventional means. A 500 cc blood volume deficit was replaced, but a continuous angiotensin infusion was required to maintain blood pressure at normal levels (Fig 7). As urine output fell, an infusion of mannitol was given. Urine output rose immediately and was sustained without further event. Slowly the angiotensin infusion was reduced and finally discontinued 24 hours after surgery. No subsequent hypotension occurred. Normotension was achieved and sustained.

The need for angiotensin infusion in this patient is not clear. It is known that the concentration of angiotensin in patients with malignant hypertension may be 20 times that of normal persons and that such patients may become dependent upon such high levels.[21] Nevertheless, it has not been necessary to use angiotensin in other hypertensive patients after correction of unilateral or bilateral renal artery lesions despite immediate reversal of preoperative hypertension.[33,34] It may be that this patient's vascular tone had become dependent upon a high level of autogenous angiotensin.

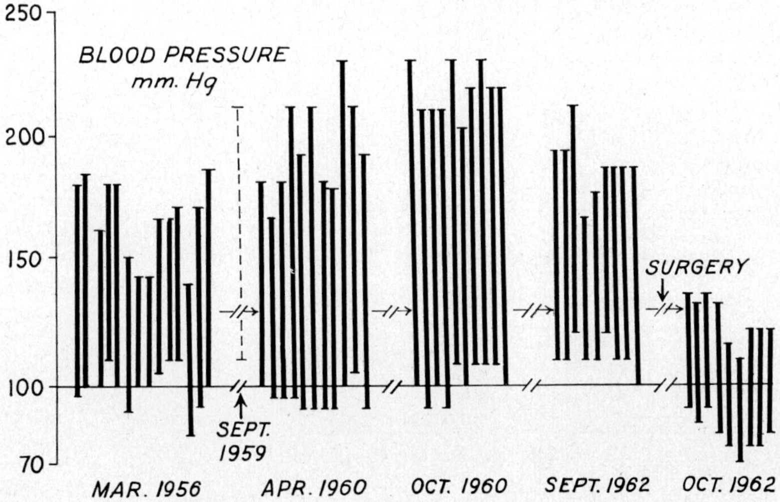

Fig 5.—This diagram indicates average daily blood pressure determinations obtained over a six-year period in a patient with ascending aortic thrombosis which occluded both the right and left renal artery.

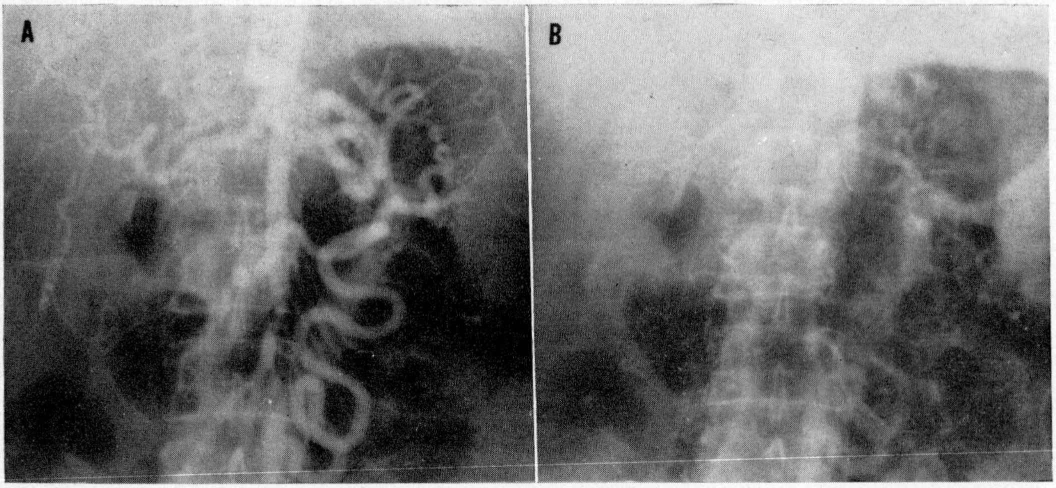

Fig 6, *A* and *B*.—Sequential films exposed during aortography reveal an abrupt occlusion of the aorta at the superior mesenteric artery level. As the dye column dissipates, retrograde filling of the main renal arteries is seen simultaneous with the nephrogram phase of kidney opacification.

Angiotensin has demonstrated itself to be highly useful in treatment of hypotension. Its potency allows use of minute quantities in a small volume of fluid, an important consideration in patients with marginal renal function.

The mannitol infusion in this instance was given in a small quantity of intravenous fluid rather than continuously.[2,4] Used in this manner, this agent is safe and effective. It is freely and quickly filtered by the glomerulus and is neither reabsorbed nor excreted by the tubules. An immediate response to this type of infusion is to be expected. Should no such response be obtained, an immediate isotope renogram may clarify renal functional status.[24]

Aortic, Renal, and Mesenteric Occlusion

This lesion is the most spectacular of those under discussion.

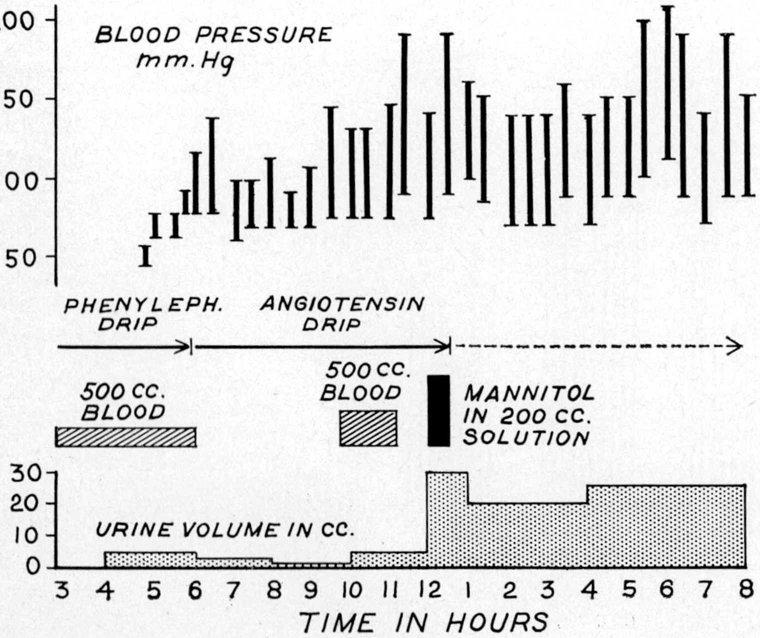

Fig 7 (case 4).—This diagrammatic representation depicts the immediate postoperative course. The place of vasopressor substances, solute diuretics, and blood replacement is indicated. Blood pressure effects and urine volumes are shown.

This case of a 62-year-old male has been previously reported in detail by Starzl and Trippel.[31] During operation utilizing a thoracoabdominal incision and hypothermia to 31 C (87.8 F) an extensive endarterectomy of the aorta, renal arteries, and superior mesenteric artery was possible. The endarterectomy was performed starting in the distal aorta and working proximally. A unilateral iliofemoral bypass graft combined with an opposite endarterectomy completed restoration of distal arterial flow. Preoperative malignant hypertension was reversed. Preoperative intestinal angina and malabsorption were eliminated.

An excellent result was obtained in this patient, but certain alterations in surgical technique arose from this experience. An extensive distal endarterectomy is more time consuming, technically difficult, and entails more blood replacement than an aortofemoral bypass graft. Therefore present technique involves performance of a proximal endarterectomy to clear visceral artery orifices followed by a swift restoration of distal aortic flow by bypass grafting.

Comment

As has been suggested, patients with aortic thrombosis at or above the renal vessels may have a prolonged history. Usually a rapid evolution of symptoms occurs during the first few months. Thereafter such symptoms remain unchanged or progress very slowly.[30] As thrombosis reaches arteries supplying kidneys or intestine, specific symptoms appear and demand surgical correction of the underlying abnormality. Renal hypertension in this connection is common,[25] and the nephrotic syndrome has been reported.[18] Mesenteric artery stenosis leads to abdominal angina, inefficient alimentation, and poor absorption in the gastrointestinal tract and is often the forerunner of catastrophic gangrene of the bowel occurring when complete arterial occlusion finally supervenes.

Correction of aortic obliteration by direct attack upon the offending lesion demands and presupposes medical-surgical cooperation. Preoperative and postoperative consultation between surgeons and internists is required. The decision for surgery in these patients with cardiac decompensation, severe hypertension, and the stigmata of chronic illness is difficult. Nevertheless, it is clear that aortic occlusion is a progressive condition the ultimate consequence of which is death. Surgical correction of the condition and arrest or cure of associated hypertension are largely predictable.

While patients with aortic occlusion just below the renal artery level are not expected to have profound renal impairment, some evaluation of kidney function is imperative. In this regard the radiosotope renogram is valuable. When combined with the aortogram, accurate estimation of renovascular status is possible. Should the renogram indicate an abnormality, differential renal function studies can be performed. These have not been necessary in cases of infra-aortic occlusion in our experience.

Split renal function studies are desirable, however, in patients with aortic occlusion involving one or both renal arteries. Accurate knowledge of renal capability aids in exercising surgical judgement during operation. In these hypertensive patients with some degree of myocardial impairment a planned operation may have to be abandoned or modified at the time of surgery. Such modification can best be made only with a maximum of preoperative information.

Choice of incision and approach to the aorta is of some importance. Thoracoabdominal incisions or extraperitoneal exposure of the proximal aorta are not now recommended. Transverse incisions must be utilized in treating aortic occlusive disease only after careful consideration. DeWeese has advocated such incisions for surgery of the aorta, and our experience has been most satisfactory using long transverse supra- or infraumbilical incisions for resection of aortic aneurysms.[13] However, in long-standing aortic thrombosis an important large collateral often exists linking the high-pressure subclavian circulation to the compromised femoral arteries through the internal mammary-epigastric inosculation. These collaterals should be preserved in patients with occlusive disease whenever possible. Therefore a midline or paramedian incision finds great utility in surgery of this condition.

The entire upper aorta is well exposed intra-abdominally by developing the retropancreatic fusion fascia. In doing this the spleen, stomach, and pancreas are turned from the left to the right upper quadrant. The renal arteries are well seen, and the superior mesenteric artery arises 1.4 cm above this level.[16]

Systemic hypothermia to 30-31 C (86-87.8 F) is recommended as an adjunctive aid in surgery for juxtarenal aortic occlusion because it protects the kidneys during total occlusion of renal arterial flow. It has been shown by Semb that normothermic deprivation of arterial flow to a human kidney for ten minutes produces little functional reaction. Doubling occlusion time produces reactive dysfunction which reverses.[22] Fatal cases of renal artery clamping for 105 and 110 minutes are reported.[1] While in the majority of cases, minimal renal artery clamping time can be expected, and hypothermia will prove unnecessary, the need for more prolonged clamping time will usually not be predictable preoperatively.

After exposure of the proximal aorta, it will be found useful to apply small arterial clamps to the renal arteries before cross-clamping the aorta. This will prevent atheromatous or thrombotic emboli from reaching the kidney.[32] A totally occluded renal artery needs no such protection, of course. Endarterectomy of this portion of the aorta will be found easy to perform, and residual adventita will be adequate to support aortic pressure. All ragged fragments of media must be excised, and assurance that no intimal flaps are present in the renal arteries must be concrete. If such assurances are obtained, the aorta can be closed to an infrarenal area, the renal arteries and proximal aorta flushed free of debris, an infrarenal clamp applied, and the proximal clamp removed so as to revascularize the kidneys.

At this point a decision can be made whether or not to progress with distal revascularization. The most important object, the clearing of renal artery orifices, has been accomplished. Existing hypertension is now either cured or controlled, and myocardial function can be expected to improve.

In most instances, the distal re-establishment of flow can proceed. A choice between endarterectomy or graft can be made. Endarterectomy will leave flexible, autogenous tissue in a normal location. No foreign body will be present; infection would be better tolerated. However, thromboendarterectomy is somewhat more difficult technically, is more time consuming, requires more blood replacement than a graft. The bifurcation graft can usually be placed quickly, can be tunneled to a distal open vessel with less retroperitoneal dissection and exposure, and can be expected to function well for many years. On the other hand, it is a foreign body, will tolerate infection poorly, and it will have to cross body flexion creases, since reconstruction to the femoral artery level is usually required in this type of patient. Therefore it is clear that each procedure has advantages and disadvantages. The decision for one and against the other must be made by the individual surgeon for his particular patient at the time and in the circumstances of the operation.

Reconstruction of flow below the femoral artery will rarely be necessary. The profunda femoris will act as a useful, if imperfect, autogenous femoropopliteal bypass which will work well in most cases if high-pressure arterial flow can be brought to it by proximal endarterectomy or graft.

Postoperatively, every effort is made to regain a normal physiologic state. Hypothermia is reversed, hypovolemia is corrected, and normotension maintained. Radioiodinated serum albumin (RISA) blood volume determination is rapid and accurate. Minor degrees of volume alteration can be discovered if the postoperative volume is compared to one obtained preoperatively. Appropriate blood fractions are administered in the amount required.

Since rigid regulation of fluid intake may be desirable, angiotensin is preferred if a vasopressor agent is necessary. Accurate minute-to-minute monitoring of blood pressure and regulation of the microdrip infusion is mandatory. However, the agent is otherwise safe, as it produces no tissue ischemia or slough. Renal blood flow is increased by this drug, a desirable feature of its actions.

The role of mannitol infusion in patients undergoing aortic cross-clamping is currently under investigation. As evidence accumulates, it is apparent that in patients with normal renal function and in the absence of renal artery occlusion or shock, solute diuresis is probably unnecessary. However, in other situations: in patients with renal impairment, during renal artery occlusion, and in patients in shock, such diuresis may exert a renal protective effect. This agent may be influsect continuously during surgery as a 20% solution at a rate of 5 ml per minute or it can be used as a rapid infusion of 25 gm in 100 or 200 cc of 5% dextrose in water. Either method tends to produce a rapid diuresis.

Summary

Juxtarenal aortic occlusion represents a late stage of the Leriche syndrome. Clearing of the aorta below the renal vessels can easily be performed with or without the renal protective effects of hypothermia. However, special technical problems are encountered if the occlusion involves one or both renal vessels and/or the superior mesenteric artery. Accurate preoperative renal function evaluation is necessary. This includes radioisotope renography and split function studies. Techniques of surgery under hypothermia involve use of endarterectomy alone or with distal prosthetic grafting. Osmotic diuresis may be utilized intraoperatively or postoperatively. The use of these agents and vasoactive substance is discussed.

John J. Bergan, MD, Chicago Wesley Memorial Hospital, Chicago, Ill.

REFERENCES

1. Bahnson, H. T.: Treatment of Abdominal Aortic Aneurysms by Excision and Replacement Homograft, Circulation 9:494, 1954.

2. Barry, K. G.; Cohen, A.; and LeBlanc, P.: Mannitolization: I. Prevention and Therapy of Oliguria Associated With Cross-Clamping of the Abdominal Aorta, Surgery 50:335-340, 1961.

3. Barry, K. G.; Cohen, A.; and LeBlanc, P.: Mannitol Infusion: II. Prevention of Acute Functional Renal Failure During Resection of Aneurism of the Abdominal Aorta, New Eng J Med 264:967-971, 1961.

4. Barry, K. G., and Malloy, J. P.: Oliguric Renal Failure, JAMA 179:510-513, 1962.

5. Beall, A. C.; Holman, M. R.; Morris, G. C., Jr.; and DeBakey, M. E.: Mannitol-Induced Osmotic Diuresis During Vascular Surgery: Renal Hemodynamic Effects, Arch Surg 86:34-42, 1963.

6. Beckwith, R.; Huffman, E. R.; Eiseman, B.; and Blount, S. G.: Chronic Aortoiliac Thrombosis, New Eng J Med 258:721-726, 1958.

7. Cannon, J. A.; Kawakami, I. G.; and Barker, W. F.: The Present Status of Aortoiliac Endarterectomy for Obliterative Atherosclerosis, Arch Surg 82:813-825, 1961.

8. Castillo, P. A., and Barrera, F.: Human Hypertension Due to Thrombotic Occlusion of Both Renal Arteries: Report of a Case Cured by Surgical Removal of the Thrombus, Amer Heart J 56:769-775, 1958.

9. Cooper, F. W., Jr., and McGarity, W. C.: Surgical Treatment of Insidious Thrombosis of the Aorta, Amer Surg 24:201-204, 1958.

10. Creech, O.: "Complications of Procedures on the Abdominal Aorta," in Artz, C. P., and Hardy, J. D.: Complications of Surgery and Their Management, Philadelphia: W. B. Saunders Company, 1960.

11. Day, S. M., and Terry, J. H.: Mesenteric Thrombosis Complicating Occlusive Disease of the Abdominal Aorta, Amer Surg 24:315-318, 1958.

12. DeBakey, M. E.; Crawford, E. S.; Cooley, D. A.; and Morris, G. C., Jr.: Surgical Considerations of Occlusive Disease of the Abdominal Aorta and Iliac and Femoral Arteries, Ann Surg 148:306-324, 1958.

13. DeWeese, M. S., and Fry, W. J.: Transverse Abdominal Incisions in Aortic Operations, Ann Surg 154(suppl):45-50, 1961.

14. dos Santos, J. C.: Sur la Désobstruction des thromboses artérielles anciennes, Mem Acad Chir (Paris) 73:409-411, 1947.

15. Erskine, J. M.; Gerbode, F. L.; French, S. W.; and Hood, R. M.: Surgical Treatment of Thrombotic Occlusion of Aorta and Iliac Arteries, AMA Arch Surg 79:85-93, 1959.

16. Feller, I., and Woodburne, R. T.: Surgical Anatomy of the Abdominal Aorta, Ann Surg 154 (suppl):239-252, 1961.

17. Grosskreutz, D. C.; Magee, A. C.; and Stephen, C. R.: Value of Hypothermia During Aortic Occlusion, JAMA 165:949-951, 1957.

18. Gubbay, S. S., and Beveridge, B. R.: Thrombosis in Abdominal Aorta Associated With the Nephrotic Syndrome, Brit Med J 2:1730-1731, 1962.

19. Johnson, J. K.: Ascending Thrombosis of Abdominal Aorta as Fatal Complication of Leriche's Syndrome, AMA Arch Surg 69:663-668, 1954.

20. Julian, O. C.; Javid, H.; Dye, W. S.; and El Issa, S.: Diagnosis and Surgical Approach to Aorticoiliac Arterial Disease, Amer J Cardiol 4: 622-631, 1959.

21. Kahn, J. R.; Skeggs, L. T., Jr.; Shumway, N. P.; and Wisenbaugh, P. E.: The Assay of Hypertensin From the Arterial Blood of Normotensive and Hypertensive Human Beings, J Exp Med 95:523-529, 1952.

22. Kerr, W. K.; Kyle, V. N.; Kerestrci, A. G.; and Smythe, C. A.: Renal Hypothermia, J Urol 84: 236-242, 1960.

23. Leriche, R.: Des Obliterations artérielles hautes comme causes des insuffisances circulatoires des membres inferieurs, Mem Soc Chir (Paris) 49: 1404-1406, 1923.

24. Libretti, J. V.; O'Conor, V. J., Jr.; and Grayhack, J. T.: Early Differential Diagnosis of Postoperative Anuria by Means of the Radioisotope Renogram, Surg Forum 11:492-494, 1960.

25. Oudot, J.: La Greffe vasculaire dans les thromboses du carrefour aortique, Presse Med 59: 234-236, 1951.

26. Palou, J.: Hipertension arterial maligna por thrombosis aortoiliaca ascendente, Angiologia 12: 95-100, 1960.

27. Palou, J.: Thrombosis aortoiliaca: evolucion y complicaciones, Angiologia 14:93-99, 1962.

28. Rob, C. G., and Downs, A. R.: Chronic Occlusive Disease of the Aorta and Iliac Arteries: Treatment and Results, J Cardiov Surg (Turino) 1:57-64, 1960.

29. Shucksmith, H. S., and Wilson, G.: Aortic Thrombosis Causing Hypertension, Lancet 1:75-76, 1959.

30. Starer, F., and Sutton, D.: Aortic Thrombosis, Brit Med J 1:1255-1263, 1958.

31. Starzl, T. E., and Trippel, O. H.: Reno-Mesentero-Aortic-Iliac Thromboendarterectomy in Patient With Malignant Hypertension, Surgery 46: 556-564, 1959.

32. Thurlbeck, W. M., and Castleman, B.: Atheromatous Emboli to the Kidney Following Aortic Surgery, New Eng J Med 257:442-447, 1957.

33. Trippel, O. H.: Surgical Management of Hypertension Due to Renal Artery Occlusion, Surg Clin N Amer 40:177-189, 1960.

34. Trippel, O. H., and O'Conor, V. J., Jr.: Renovascular Hypertension, Surg Clin N Amer 42: 109-130, 1962.

35. Wyatt, G. M., and Felson, B.: Aortic Thrombosis as a Cause of Hypertension: An Arteriographic Study, Radiology 69:676-683, 1957.

Comparison of Methods Used to Diagnose Renal Hypertension

Renal Arteriography Versus Individual Ureteral Catheterization

JAMES M. STOKES, MD; MARVIN J. FRIENDENBERG, MD; AND HERBERT SUNSHINE, MD, ST. LOUIS

The diagnosis of hypertension secondary to renal artery or kidney disease presently depends upon abnormalities detected by renal angiography, radioactive isotope renal scanning, and differential ureteral catheterization. The comparative accuracy of each of these techniques, however, and the role each should have in the examination of patients with high blood pressure, have not been clarified.[1-3] The purpose of this paper is to describe the application of these methods and their correlation in the evaluation of 130 hypertensive patients. On the basis of the data obtained, a diagnostic program has evolved for the evaluation of patients suspected of having hypertension of renal artery or kidney origin.

Material and Methods

A total of 130 patients with arterial hypertension were examined by percutaneous transfemoral retro-

Presented at the 20th Annual Meeting of the Central Surgical Association, Chicago, Feb 21-23, 1963.

From the Departments of Surgery and Radiology, Washington University School of Medicine.

Supported by a grant-in-aid from the St. Louis Heart Association.

grade catheter aortography on the basis of the following criteria: (1) sudden onset of hypertension, (2) hypertension refractory to medical management, (3) hypertension occurring below age of 40 years, (4) abnormal intravenous pyelogram, (5) history of trauma to a kidney, or (6) history of thromboembolic phenomena. Fifty of these patients had radioactive I^{131} orthoiodohippuran renal scans, and 29 of this group then had differential renal function studies by individual ureteral catheterizations. Diagnosis was confirmed by operation in 26 patients.

A. *Renal Angiography*.—The technique of percutaneous transfemoral retrograde catheter aortography has been described in detail.[4] All procedures were performed using 1% lidocaine (Xylocaine) local anesthesia, and each required about 30 to 45 minutes. A radiopaque (yellow Odman-Ledin) catheter * was used. Its tip was placed at the inferior cortical margin of T-12 because optimum visualization of the renal arterial systems and kidneys was most consistently obtained only when the superior mesenteric artery was opacified. If the superior mesenteric or splenic artery obscured part of a renal artery, it was examined by a second injection with the patient in a slightly oblique position. A dose of 30 to 50 ml of contrast medium † was injected with the Gidlund injector under 4-6 kg per square centimeter pressure while the patient performed the Valsalva maneuver. Fifteen 14 × 14 in films were exposed serially with the Shonander film changer at a rate of three per second for the first ten films and one every other second thereafter in order to demonstrate: (*a*) renal arterial inflow, (*b*) renal parenchymal nephrograms, and (*c*) venous return from the kidneys. At times, additional films were exposed at one and three minutes followed by routine pyelographic examination. Diagnosis was based upon: (1) the morphology and speed of "wash-out" of the main renal arteries and their subdivisions, (2) the appearance time, intensity, and disappearance time of the nephrograms, (3) the size and outlines of the kidneys, (4) the degree of opacification and speed of "wash-out" of the renal veins, (5) the appearance time and density of contrast material in the renal collecting systems, and (6) the morphology and speed of "wash-out" of the renal collecting systems (Fig 1).

B. *Individual Ureteral Catheterization*.—Differential renal function tests by individual ureteral catheterizations were performed by using standard constant infusion clearance techniques[5] to obtain the following data: urine inulin (U_{In}), *p*-aminohippuric acid (U_{PAH}), creatinine (U_{Cr}), sodium concentrations (U_{Na}), and urine flow/minute (UF). Osmolality (mOsm) of urine and plasma was meas-

Fig 1.—Bilateral medial fibrous hyperplasia. *A*, arterial phase; *B*, nephrogram (left kidney) and arterial lag (right kidney); *C*, venous phase.

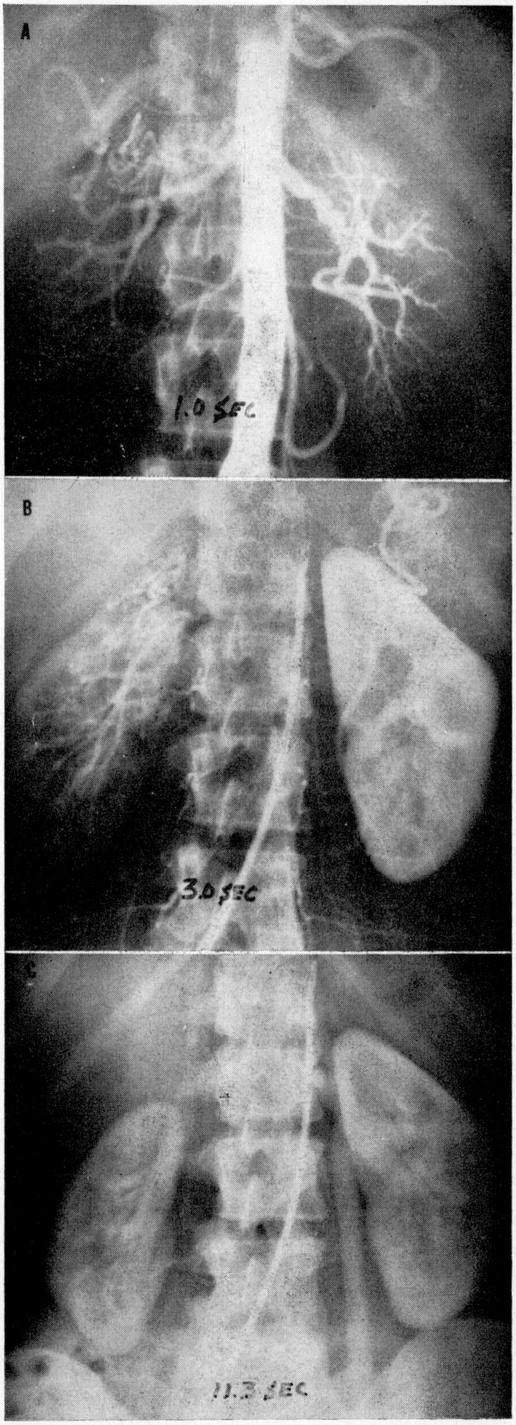

* KIFA Instrument & Equipment Co. of Sweden through Shick X-Ray Co., Inc., 205 W Wacker Dr, Chicago.

† Composed of 60% methylglucamine diatrizoate (Renografin, E. R. Squibb & Sons, New York) or 60% meglumine iothalamate (Conray, Mallinckrodt Pharmaceutical, St. Louis).

TABLE 1.—*Separate Kidney Functions in Renal Hypertension*

	UF, Ml/Min		U_{In}, Mg/100 Ml			U_{PAH}, Mg/100 Ml			GFR, Ml/Min		RPF, Ml/Min		OSM, mOsm/Kg H_2O	
Patient	D	O	D	O	D/O	D	O	D/O	D	O	D	O	D	O
1	1.4	4.7	45	12	3.8	411	98	4.19					560	462
2	2.4	3.6	262	170	1.56	170	97	1.75	57	54	242	227	600	533
3	1.4	7.2	820	232		278	88		45	61	216	300	550	400
4	0.52	10.9	575	128		809	217		16	70	102	353	580	385
5	2.0	4.8	730	320		230	85		54	66	291	296	636	458
6	4.0	5.9	217	168	1.29	122	101	1.2	40	46	150	184	418	400
7	0.4	9.5	51	5.6	10.7	848	67	15.3	4	55	45	315	304	345
8	1.6	2.5	13	16		121	141						474	499
9	1.25	3.98	10	23	0.43	124	197	0.62	12	88	40	201	427	520
10	1.62	2.26	280	367	0.76	182	202	0.90	10.2	20.3	52	87	215	216
11	6.1	2.2	304	225	1.35	59	43	1.37	83	30	429	140	454	419
12	4.6	7.6	15	9	1.67	201	105	1.91	45	50	243	226	389	327
13	2.8	13.7	4.2	2.5	1.75				12	34			136	96

Patients 1-8, unilateral arterial stenosis; patient 8, pyelonephritis; patients 9-13, bilateral arterial disease.
D indicates diseased kidney; O, opposite kidney; UF, urine flow; U_{In}, urine inulin concentration; U_{PAH}, urine *p*-aminohypurate concentration; GFR, glomerular filtration rate; RPF, renal plasma flow; OSM, osmolality.

ured by freezing point depression. Spinal anesthesia was used in all patients, and diuresis was obtained by intravenous infusion of hyperosmotic urea-vasopressin (Pitressin) solution. Glomerular filtration rate (GFR), renal plasma flow (RPF), excretion fraction of filtered water (EF_w), and excretion of filtered sodium (EF_{Na}) and urine solute (U_{osm}) were calculated for each kidney (Tables 1 and 2).

Preparation of Data: Derived clearances were calculated by standard methods. The excretion fraction (%) of filtered sodium excreted *:

$$EF_{Na} = \frac{\text{Filtration Rate} \times \text{Plasma Na Conc.}}{\text{Urine Sodium Conc.} \times \text{Urine Flow Rate}} \times 100$$

or

$$EF_{Na} = \frac{P_{Inulin} \times U_{Na}}{U_{In} \times P_{Na}} \times 100$$

The excretion fraction of filtered water (EF_w) is calculated:

$$EF_w = \frac{P_{In}}{U_{In}} \times 100$$

The variance of function (as % difference) for each kidney indicates the deviation of the function of one kidney from the mean function of both kidneys.[6,7]

* Where P_{NA} and P_{IN} are the plasma sodium and inulin concentrations.

C. *Radioactive Renograms.*—I^{131}-labeled *o*-iodohippurate (Hippuran) was used for simultaneous external renal uptake scanning by dual balanced scintillation counters which recorded the time-activity rate slope of individual kidneys. The labeled *o*-iodohippurate was administered intravenously in the amount of 0.5μc per kilogram of body weight, and the radioactivity over each kidney area was recorded for 20-30 minutes. The strip recordings were interpreted on the following features: (1) the time required to reach one-half maximum activity, (2) the slope of the time/activity curve to maximum, (3) the relation of individual renal activity at ten minutes with the counters repositioned for maximum counting rates, and (4) the slope of the excretory phase.

Results

A. *Renal Angiography.*—Renal angiography in 79 of the 130 patients was not

TABLE 2.—*Water and Sodium Excretion in Renal Hypertension*

	U_{Na}			EF_{Na}			EF_w		
Patient	D	O	% Diff.	D	O	% Diff.	D	O	% Diff.
1	88	91	3.3	0.74	0.65	13	1.2	1.0	2
2	83	111	30	2.5	5.9	81		6.7	5.1
3	15	94	138	0.4	9.9	184	3.7	12	106
4							3.3	15	133
5	66	98	39	1.5	5.9	118	3.6	7.0	155
6	122	122	0	16	21	26	18	24	26
9	95	88	7.6	7.3	2.9	86	10	4.6	74
10	52	50	4	4.1	4	<1	14	11	24
11	64	70	15	4.9	6.7	31	8.7	9.7	11
12	87	93	7	5.9	10	74	9.6	15	43

considered to be significantly abnormal. Twenty-six patients had hemodynamically significant disease confirmed by operation and/or separate kidney tests. Twelve patients had *parenchymal* disease of one kidney with normal renal arteries. Nine patients had bilateral renal artery and/or kidney disease including five with bilateral renal artery stenosis, two with bilateral renal artery aneurysms, and two with aneurysm on one side and renal artery stenosis and/or a contracted kidney on the other. In addition, three patients not included in this series had coarctation of the abdominal aorta with involvement of the renal arteries and two patients had polycystic kidneys.

Four examinations were unsuccessful. Occlusive arterial disease prevented passage of the catheter up the aorta in two patients; in another patient several side holes in the catheter became occluded prior to injection. In the fourth patient there was an intramural injection of contrast material into the abdominal aorta which was well tolerated and required no special therapy. There was no mortality and no serious complication. The only morbidity was the occasional development of a clinically insignificant hematoma at the puncture site. One aortogram was done in a patient with acute renal failure and uremia without apparent ill effect. None of the 79 patients with normal renal angiography subsequently was proved to have hypertension of renal origin, ie, there were no false negatives. After angiography, 16 of these patients had equal differential renal function studies by ureteral catheterization. In none of the remainder did the clinical course or routine re-examination from 6 to 24 months demonstrate further evidence of nephrogenic hypertension.

B. *Individual Ureteral Catheterization.*—Severe unilateral main renal artery occlusive disease produced a characteristic decrease in urine flow rate, glomerular filtration rate, and renal plasma flow in the affected kidney (Table 1) compared to the opposite normal one. Urine inulin and p-aminohippuric acid concentrations from the affected kidney were increased, reflecting relatively greater water reabsorption. A comparison of the inulin/PAH urine concentration ratios (Table 1, columns 6 and 9) of the diseased and normal kidneys showed similar directions of change and minor quantitative differences. Urine flow rates and urine inulin concentration in the urine of kidneys with arterial obstructions were altered to a much greater degree than were the filtration rate or renal plasma flow. Urine osmolality differences between the affected and normal kidney urine were less than were urine inulin concentrations and urine flow rates (Table 1, columns 14 and 15). Glomerular filtration rates of the two kidneys were nearly equal in five patients with renal disease, but total tubular water and sodium reabsorption were greatly increased in the kidney with renal artery stenosis (Table 2). One of these patients (Fig 2) had stenosis of the lower renal artery of a double kidney. The separate renal functions did not disclose significant differences in the two kidneys. Correction of the stenosis did not lower the blood pressure. The other patient had a nephrectomy for partial stenosis without improvement.

Fig 2.—Stenosis of lower left renal artery of double kidney.

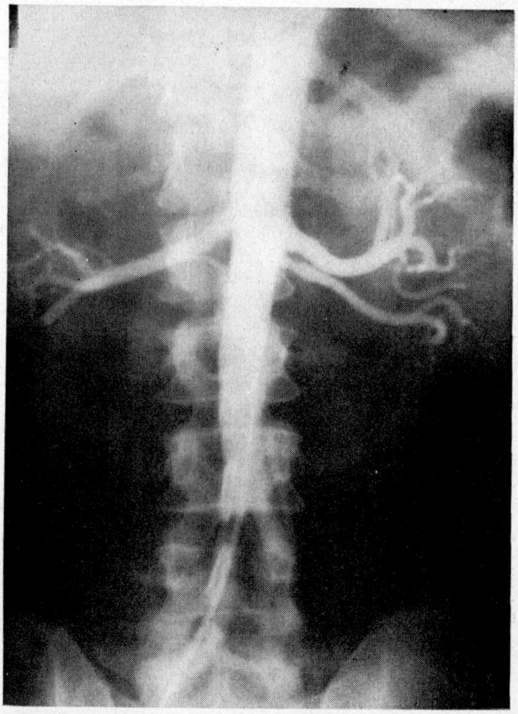

TABLE 3.—*Individual Kidney Functions With Unilateral Renal Artery Stenosis*

Function	Moderate R	Moderate L	Moderate % Diff.	Severe R	Severe L	Severe % Diff.
Urine flow, ml/min	2.4	3.5	37	1.4	7.2	135
Filtration rate, ml/min	53	59	11	45	61	30
Renal plasma flow, ml/min	242	227	6	226	300	—
Urine sodium, mEq/liter	83	111	30	15	94	140
% filtered sodium excreted	2.5	5.9	81	0.4	10	184
% filtered water excreted	4.0	6.7	61	3.7	12	106

The marked reduction in the per cent of filtered sodium (EF_{Na}) and water excreted (EF_w) was the most useful functional test for renal artery obstruction (Table 2). Data from two patients (Table 3) demonstrates the functional effects of moderate and severe renal artery narrowing. Fig 3 is an example of electrolyte and water excretion abnormalities even though filtration rates and renal plasma in the two kidneys are equal. Advanced narrowing of the renal artery effects a measurable decrease in filtration rate (Fig 4) accompanied by even greater reduction in the excretion fraction of filtered sodium and water. In contradistinction, the effects of unilateral pyelonephritis upon renal water and sodium excretion are an *increased* excretion fraction of the filtered water and sodium by the affected kidney (Table 4). The disparity between functions of the separate kidneys in renal hypertension is summarized in Table 5.

As a control comparison, the ureteral catheterization results in patients with essential hypertension are summarized in Tables 6 and 7. The highest individual kidney variation from the mean renal function‡ was 23% for urine flow per minute, 20% for urine inulin, 47.3% for urine *p*-aminohippuric acid, and 40% for glomerular filtration rate. The mean disparity indices for these functions are summarized in Table 8. Despite evidence of predominant unilateral reduction in filtration rate of two patients with essential hypertension (Tables 6 and 7, patients 2 and 9), the pattern of decreased urine flow rates and *decreased* sodium and water reabsorption indicated clearly that primary renal artery disease was not the cause of the hypertension.

After bilateral ureteral catheterization, two patients had transient evidence of renal infection and four had renal colic. One patient with minimal kidney function and aortic aneurysm had exacerbation of renal failure after catheterization. Individual renal clearances were incomplete in two patients because of bladder leakage and in two others because

‡ $\frac{2 \times (R - L)}{R + L} \times 100$

TABLE 4.—*Unilateral Pyelonephritis*

Function	Affected Kidney	Opposite Kidney	% Variance
Urine flow	1.25	4.0	D 104
Filtration rate	12	88	D 152
Renal plasma flow	39	201	D 160
Urine sodium, mEq/liter	95	88	I 7.6
Filtered load sodium, mEq/liter	1.66	11.9	
% filtered sodium excreted	7.3	2.9	I 86
% filtered solute excreted	14.6	7.8	I 61
U/P inulin	10	23	D 138
% filtered water excreted	10	4.6	I 74

D indicates decreased; I, increased.

TABLE 5.—*Functional Disparity of Separate Kidneys in Renal Hypertension: Per Cent Variance Between Right and Left Kidneys* *

Patient	UF	U_{In}	U_{PAH}	GFR	RPF
1	108	116	122		
2	40	43	54	5	6
3	44	9	14		
4	104	79	45	152	134
5	192	160	178	172	150
6 †	32	27	10	66	50
7 †	92	1	3	92	100
8 †	49	50	63	10	7
9 †	132	50			
10	258	126	107	125	110
11	124	97	92	30	33
12	38	25	19	14	20

* % variance = 2 (R—L)/R + L × 100.
† Bilateral disease by arteriography.

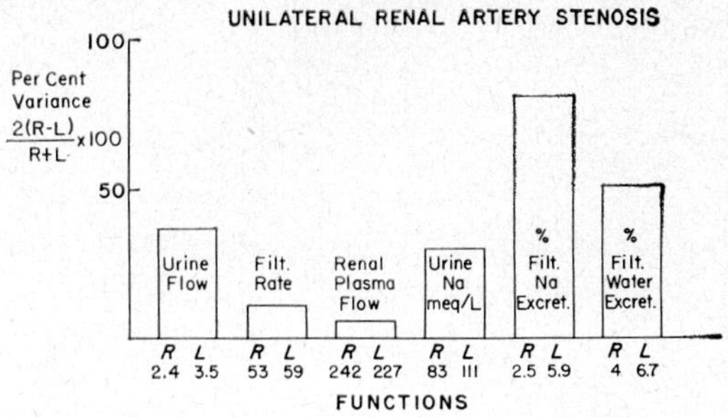

Fig 3.—Variance of separate kidney functions with unilateral renal artery stenosis.

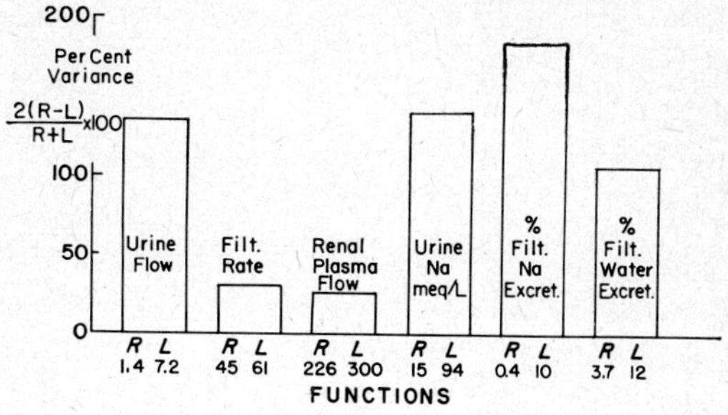

Fig 4.—Variance of separate kidney functions with right renal artery stenosis.

TABLE 6.—*Separate Kidney Functions in Essential Hypertension*

	UF, Ml/Min		U_{in}, Mg/100 Ml			U_{PAH}, Mg/100 Ml			GFR, Ml/Min		RPF, Ml/Min		OSM, mOsm/Kg		
Patient	R	L	R	L	R/L	R	L	R/L	R	L	R	L	R	L	R/L
1	0.82	0.90	128	123	1.04	522	415	1.25	84	87	362	310	628	669	0.94
2	1.5	1.3	283	223	1.27	162	100	1.62	15	10	89	39	435	422	1.03
3	1.2	1.2	55	59	0.93				66	68					
4	8.6	8.0	3.7	3.6	1.03				39	38					
5	2.0	2.1	523	363	1.44	181	132	1.37	81	50	297	290	217	178	1.22
6	2.5	2.6	25	20	1.25	135	139	0.97	54	55	259	278	456	445	1.02
7	1.9	2.4	37	37	1.0				63	66					
8	5.1	6.1				120	222	0.54					469	437	1.07
9	3.8	4.1	306	259	1.18	207	181		42	29	199	179			
10	1.3	10.8	65	76	0.85	44	56								
11	2.0	3.5	15	8.5	1.76				37	37					
12	2.1	2.3	29	29	1.0	293	285		69	66	246	231	551	546	1.0
13	5.9	4.6	200	200	1.0	90	82		63	54	293	235	403	408	0.99
14	5.35	4.87	227	185	1.23	106	85	1.25	37	31	272	199	372	370	1.0
15	3.43	4.02	313	320	0.94	119	101	1.18	19	22	96	96	361	358	1.0
16	2.0	2.2	557	517	1.08	230	224	1.03	26	26	120	129	435	440	0.99

of inability to catheterize one ureter of a double collecting system.

C. *Radioactive Renograms.*—Fifty radioactive I^{131} *o*-iodiohippurate renal scans were performed. One was interpreted as normal when a lesion was demonstrated by renal angiography and/or ureteral catheterization. Seven renal scans indicated unilateral vascular disease when none was disclosed by the other tests. Thus, there were 1 false nega-

TABLE 7.—*Water and Sodium Excretion in Essential Hypertension*

	EF_w			U_{Na}			EF_{Na}		
Patient	R	L	% Diff.	R	L	% Diff.	R	L	% Diff.
1	0.93	0.97	0						
2	10	13	26	72	73	1	5.3	7.0	27.6
3	1.3	1.29	0						
4	22	22	0	52	43	19	8.3	6.8	19.8
5	3.2	4.1	24	50	43		1.3	1.3	0
6	4.0	4.1	2.4						
7	2.7	2.7	0						
9	8.3	9.1	9						
12	3.1	3.1	0						
14	14	18	28	117	121		12.4	13	4.7
15	15.9	15.6	<1						
16	7.7	8.0	3						

EF_w indicates % filtered water excreted; U_{Na}, urine sodium concentration; EF_{Na}, % filtered sodium excreted.

TABLE 8.—*Functional Disparity of Separate Kidneys in Essential Hypertension*

Patient	% Difference UF	U_{in}	U_{PAH}	GFR	RPF
1	9.3	3.98	22.8	3.5	1.5
2	14.3	23.7	47.3	40	78
3	0	7.0		3.0	
4	7.2	2.7		2.6	
5	4.9	6.9		11.3	2
6	6.5	2.22	2.9	1.8	7
7	23.3	0		4.7	
8	17.9				
9	7.6	16.6	13.4	36	10
10		15.6	24		
11	54.5	140		0	
12	9.09	0	2.8	6.3	6
13					21
14	9.39	20.4	21.8	31.2	30
15	15.8	2.2	16.3	14.6	0
16	9.52	7.45	2.64	0	7

% Difference = 2 (R−L)/R+L × 100.

tive and 7 false positives among the 50 renal scans. There were no complications.

Correlation of Tests

Table 9 summarizes the correlation of renal angiography and radioactive isotope renal scanning. Differential ureteral catheterization studies were done in 29 patients, 13 with renal artery and/or kidney lesions and 16 with essential hypertension.

A. *Renal Angiography and Separate Catheterizations.*—None of the 79 patients with normal renal angiography subsequently was proved to have hypertension of renal origin; ie, there were no false negatives. After angiography, 16 of these patients had equal differential renal function studies by ureteral catheterization. In none of the remainder did the clinical course or routine re-examination studies from 6 to 24 months demonstrate further evidence of nephrogenic hypertension.

In two patients, renal angiography demonstrated renal artery or kidney disease which was considered to be hemodynamically significant but was shown subsequently not to be functionally significant by differential ureteral catheterization studies and by failure of operation to effect a reversal of the hypertension; ie, there were no false positives.

TABLE 9.—*Comparison of Renograms and Aortography*

Renogram		Aortogram
Pos	11	4 agreed with affected kidney by arteriography 1 identified opposite kidney 6 neg by arteriography
Neg	39	1 pos arteriogram 38 neg arteriograms
Total	50	50

7 of 11 positive renograms were wrong; 1 of 38 negative renograms was wrong.

Renal angiography and ureteral catheterization tests agreed perfectly in the separation of patients with nephrogenic hypertension from those with essential hypertension. These two procedures also indicated the affected kidney without fail in patients with unilateral disease. Renal angiography was particularly helpful in identifying the type of morphologic abnormality present. However, it did not always indicate the most affected kidney when bilateral renal artery disease was present. Neither did it disclose the etiology of the hypertension when both arterial and parenchymal cellular disease coexisted in the same kidneys.

The individual renal function tests differentiated obstructing arterial disease from parenchymal disease and often identified the particular type of parenchymal disease present. These tests were of great value in determining the functional significance of obstructing arterial lesions demonstrated by renal angiography. However, ureteral catheterization tests alone would not have been completely adequate for planning appropriate therapy in patients with bilateral arterial abnormalities (Table 1, patients 9 and 11) or in patients with a different disease in each kidney (Table 1, patient 10).

B. *Radioactive Renograms.*—Radioactive isotope renal scanning was unsatisfactory in terms of accurately recognizing renovascular hypertension and in the limited information that was provided about cases that were identified.

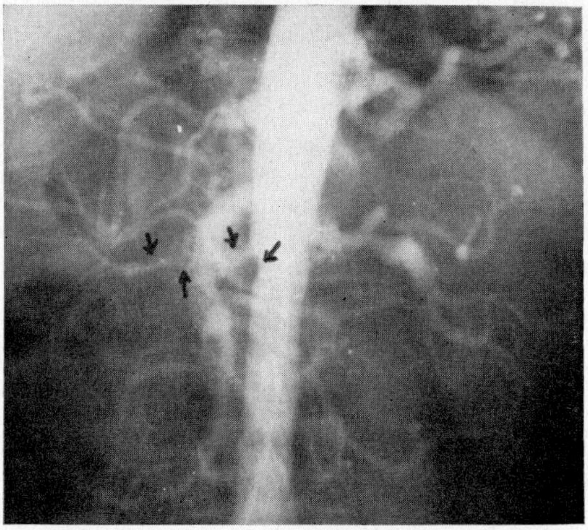

Fig 5.—Right renal artery disease.

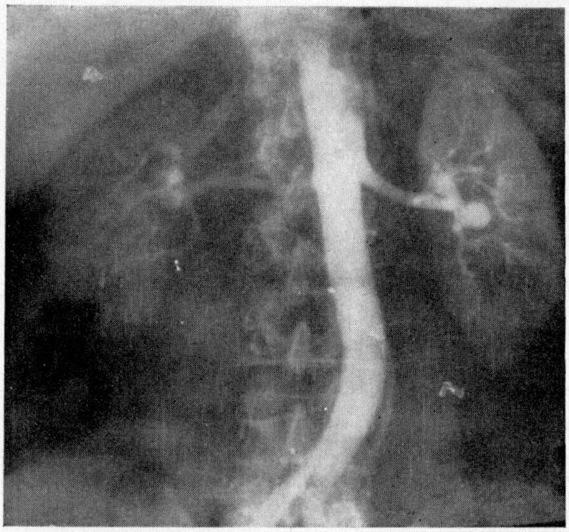

Fig 6.—Bilateral renal artery aneurysms.

Nephrogenic Hypertension Requiring Both Renal Angiography and Differential Renal Clearance Tests for Proper Evaluation

To demonstrate the necessity for renal angiography and differential ureteral catheterization function studies, the following types of renal disease are summarized and the corresponding renal angiograms are presented:

I. *Combined Arterial and Parenchymal Disease Affecting One Kidney.*—The renal angiogram for this 47-year-old male (Fig 5) showed obstruction of the inferior branch of the right renal artery, complete absence of circulation to the lower pole of the right kidney, and total reduction in the right kidney mass.

The clearance data showed a decrease in glomerular filtration rate, *p*-aminohippuric acid urine concentration, and urine flow rate, but an *increase* in urine sodium concentration. These functions (Table 4) are clearly indicative of parenchymal kidney disease even though arterial narrowing exists. The pathologic diagnosis was chronic pyelonephritis.

II. *Bilateral Arterial Disease With Unilateral Renal Ischemia.*—The patient was 45 years old and male. The renal angiogram (Fig 6) showed bilateral renal artery aneurysms but did not demonstrate a sufficient difference in the rate of intrarenal arterial filling or intensity of nephrograms to indicate which kidney was more significantly involved. Individual renal clearances (Table 10) showed a decrease in urine flow, filtration rate, urine sodium concentration, and decreased excretion fraction of filtered sodium and an increase in inulin concentration on the *right,* identifying the right kidney as the one causally related to the hypertension.

TABLE 10.—*Bilateral Renal Aneurysms*

Function	Affected Kidney	Opposite Kidney	% Difference
Urine flow, ml/min	4.6	7.6	D 49
Filtration rate, ml/min	45	50	D 10
Renal plasma flow, ml/min	243	226	I 7
Urine sodium, mEq/liter	87	93	D 7
% Filtered sodium excretion	6	10	D 50
U/P inulin	10	6.6	I 41

D indicates decreased; I, increased.

III. *Small Kidney of Undertermined Etiology.*—The renal angiogram for this 57-year-old female showed a small right kidney with no major renal arterial disease. Clearance data (Table 1, case 7) disclosed increased osmolality and *p*-aminohippuric acid concentration and decreased sodium concentration, urine flow, and filtration rate in the right kidney, changes consistent with primary renal ischemia. Blood pressure was significantly reduced by right nephrectomy. Pathological examination disclosed only arteriolar narrowing. The function data accurately indicated the type of renal disease in this patient in the absence of definitive information from aortography.

IV. *Bilateral Renal Disease of Different Etiology in Each Kidney (Right Renal Artery Aneurysm and Left Hypoplastic Kidney).*—The patient was a 45-year-old female. The renal angiogram (Fig 7) showed a poststenotic aneurysm of the right renal artery bifurcation and a very small left kidney. Arterial flow through the right kidney was slightly delayed. Clearance data (Table 1, patient 10) indicated the urine flow and filtration rate were reduced in the left kidney but urine inulin and solute concentration were slightly higher in the right kidney, and the excretion fraction of filtered sodium was reduced. Arterial pressure gradient measured in the right renal artery across the narrowed seg-

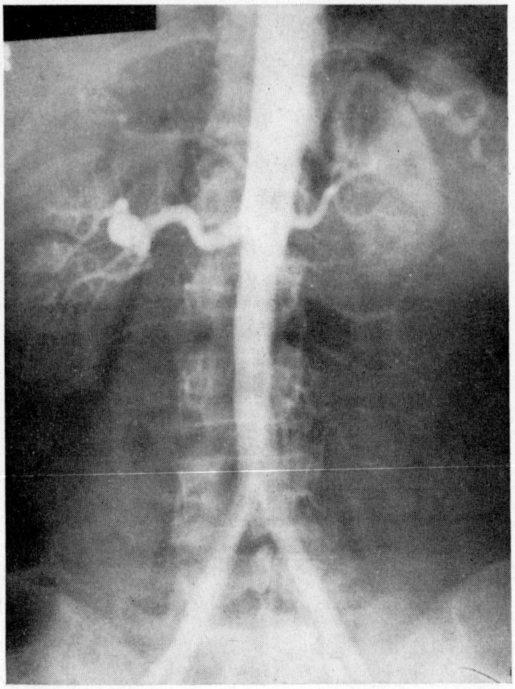

Fig 7.—Right renal aneurysm and left hypoplastic kidney.

ment was 40 mm Hg. Resection of the bifurcation aneurysm and reconstruction were performed using a free splenic artery autograft.

Both diagnostic methods were necessary for the proper therapy in this patient. The *left* renal mass was reduced, but the *right* exhibited functional criteria compatible with a primary renal arterial disease.

A Diagnostic Program for Hypertension of Renal Origin

If hypertension of renal artery or kidney origin is suspected after clinical history, physical examination, routine laboratory examinations for kidney disease, and intravenous pyelography, then percutaneous transfemoral retrograde aortography catheterization is performed. Preoperative individual ureteral catheterization is not considered necessary when renal angiography shows complete renal artery occlusion or when unequivocal unilateral renal artery stenosis is demonstrated (Fig 1*A*) which is associated with one or more of the following:

1. Delayed arterial "wash-out" beyond the stenosis (Fig 1*B*).
2. Delayed appearance time and/or diminished intensity of the nephrogram of the affected kidney (Fig 1*C*).
3. A 3 cm or more decrease in size of the affected kidney (Fig 1*C*).

Thirteen of our patients with unequivocal unilateral renal artery disease demonstrated by renal angiography had corrective surgery without differential ureteral catheterization studies. These patients had normal total renal capacity proven by routine laboratory tests of renal function.

If no lesion is demonstrable by a satisfactory angiographic examination, further examination is not done except in patients with strong clinical evidence of renal hypertension or malignant changes refractory to medical therapy. Individual renal clearance tests by ureteral catheterization are necessary in the latter group to recognize the rare type of intrarenal vascular disease not demonstrated by arteriography.

The routine use of differential renal function studies by individual ureteral catheterization following renal angiography is essential when:

1. The abnormality demonstrated by renal angiography is minimal or equivocal.
2. Renal angiography demonstrates bilateral renal artery and/or kidney disease.
3. Two diseases involve a renal artery and/or a kidney unilaterally.
4. No abnormality is demonstrated by angiography but there is strong clinical evidence of hypertension of renal origin, or malignant hypertension is present which is refractory to medical therapy.

Those patients whose renal angiograms show minimal unilateral disease or bilateral abnormalities require individual renal function studies to establish the diagnosis and to avoid surgical procedures upon lesions without causal relation to the hypertension. Reduction of the functional renal mass by nephrectomy is unwise in these patients. In addition, differential ureteral catheterization function studies are indicated when renal angiography shows renal artery and kidney abnormalities which do not appear to be related pathogenetically and the functional significance of each abnormality must be determined to plan the appropriate surgical therapy. In our hands, radioactive renal scanning served usefully neither as an adequate screening test nor as an entirely reliable procedure to evaluate the hemodynamic significance of a known lesion. Aortography invariably is needed when isotope renal scanning indicates a lesion is present in order to plan the appropriate type of corrective surgery. As an initial definitive diagnostic method serial renal angiography by the technique used provides the greatest amount of information with the least morbidity and is considered to be the method of choice for survey of patients suspected of having hypertension of renal origin. It is more reliable than isotope renal scanning. It avoids the need for anesthesia and the danger of renal infection associated with individual ureteral catheterization. In our experience, intravenous pyelography and renal angiography have demonstrated without fail all renal artery and kidney lesions responsible for hypertension.

Although no single diagnostic test can be relied upon to assess accurately *all patients* with hypertension of renal origin, the use of serial angiography as a primary diagnostic method and differential ureteral catheterization as a complementary procedure in selected patients for evaluation of the function significance of demonstrated lesions has proved to be the safest and most reliable plan of approach.

Summary

A total of 130 patients selected on the basis of clinical history, physical examination, routine laboratory tests for renal disease, and intravenous pyelography were examined for hypertension of renal origin by percutaneous transfemoral retrograde catheter aortography. Fifty of these patients had radioactive I^{131} *o*-iodohippurate (Hippuran) renal scans, and 29 had differential renal function studies by individual ureteral catheterizations. Twenty-six patients were operated on without fatality. At present, the safest and most reliable diagnostic program for evaluation of patients suspected of having hypertension of renal artery or kidney origin is renal angiography followed by differential ureteral catheterization as a complementary procedure in selected patients for evaluation of the functional significance of demonstrated lesions or for the detection of the rare lesion not demonstrated by angiography.

Mrs. M. Stubits and Mrs. A. Braitberg gave technical assistance. I^{131} Hippuran was donated by the E. R. Squibb Company.

James M. Stokes, MD, Department of Surgery, Washington University School of Medicine, St. Louis 10, Mo.

REFERENCES

1. Stamey, T. A.; Nudelman, I. J.; Good, P. H.; Schwentker, F. N.; and Hendricks, F.: Functional Characteristics of Renovascular Hypertension, Medicine (Baltimore) 40:347, 1961.
2. Spencer, F. C.; Stamey, T. A.; Bahnson, H. T.; and Cohen, A.: Diagnosis and Treatment of Hypertension Due to Occlusive Disease of the Renal Artery, Ann Surg 154:674, 1961.
3. Crawford, S., in discussion on Spencer et al.[2]
4. Stokes, J. M., and Carlsson, E.: The Use of Percutaneous Transfemoral Aortography to Diagnose Abnormalities of the Renal Arteries, Amer J Roentgen 87:276, 1962.
5. Smith, H. W.: The Kidney, London: Oxford University Press, 1951.
6. Baldwin, D. S.; Hulet, W. H.; Biggs, A. W.; Gombos, E. A.; and Chasis, H.: Renal Function in the Separate Kidneys of Man: II. Hemodynamics and Excretion of Solute and Water in Essential Hypertension, J Clin Invest 39:395, 1960.
7. Snedecor, G. W.: Statistical Methods, Ames, Iowa: Iowa State College Press, 1956.

DISCUSSION

On papers by Drs. Bergan and Trippel, and Stokes et al

Dr. Hushang Javid, Chicago: Lesions of the upper abdominal aorta present a challenging problem, as we have witnessed here. In our experience greater difficulty has been encountered in aneurysmal disease compared to occlusive lesions. This is particularly true in extensive aneurysms involving the renal arteries or in cases of disrupted proximal suture line. In these patients, one has to cross-clamp the aorta above the renals and occasionally above the superior mesenteric artery, and leave it clamped for the entire period of preparation and completion of the proximal suture line. Since one does not know the complications exist, usually hypothermia is not available.

We have had to cross-clamp the aorta at this level up to a period of 25 minutes with salvage of the patient and with no apparent damage to the kidney or the intestine.

We prefer to reserve endarterectomy to segmental occlusion of the superior mesenteric artery in its midportion. In patients who have occlusion of the origin of the superior mesenteric artery or renal arteries, we have accomplished restoration of circulation by a side-arm from the bifurcation graft, and we feel this can be done with less trauma, less bleeding, and less risk to the patient.

We have had no occasion to use angiotensin, and we have been impressed by osmotic diuretics in patients with more complicated lesions of the abdominal aorta.

Dr. Fletcher A. Miller, Minneapolis: It is obvious that these data are the end point of great deal of hard work. I would like to illustrate one brief case presentation.

This patient, a 42-year-old female, was admitted to our hospital in acute pulmonary edema. Blood pressure was 200/100. After medical management for treatment of the edema, a detailed work-up of the hypertensive status was carried out.

This slide shows the IVP that we obtained. You will notice there is a cobblestone effect in the pelvis of this kidney leading us to feel that something must be abnormal in this kidney, as opposed to the opposite kidney.

In going into her past history, it was found that she had had hypertension for ten years, and an IVP obtained ten years previously, when compared with this IVP, showed similar results. We felt that retrograde aortogram was in order. This showed multiple punctate areas out in the periphery of the kidney, as opposed to a more normal vascular distribution pattern in the left kidney. If one notes carefully the venous phase of this kidney fill, it stands out in marked contrast to the opposite kidney. We presupposed that this represented multiple arteriovenous fistulas in the right kidney, probably congenital in origin.

We proceeded with our work-up, which included differential occlusive catheterization of both ureters by our urologist. The data obtained were not too informative, but the postcatheterization results were frightening. She became anuric for 12 hours and bled, presumably from the right kidney, lowering her hemoglobin from 14 to 12 gm in a matter of 24 hours.

We subsequently have seen two other such instances of obstructive uremia, post differential catheterization, and in discussing it with various urologists I find it is not an uncommon complication; as a matter of fact, one urologist reports three instances in which nephrostomy had to be performed, and one of these patients died.

I bring this out not to detract from this paper, because I think the data presented are very important to our own basic knowledge. I think Dr. Stokes brought this out very well in pointing out the fact that these were indicated in only a certain number of patients.

I am sure that the amount of work he put into this investigation would prevent unnecessary, and perhaps dangerous, reduplication, because for most of us our uninhibited enthusiasm will not carry us over the barrier presented by such a work load.

Dr. Robert E. L. Berry, Ann Arbor, Mich: I was left behind on some of the data Dr. Stokes used demonstrating decreased excretion of filtered sodium and water as the renal defect under these circumstances. Does he attribute this to decreased renal medullary sodium concentration as proposed by the countercurrent multiplier theory of sodium excretion, a change in antidiuretic hormone effect, or possibly a combination of both?

Dr. James M. Stokes, St. Louis: Time did not permit discussion of the techniques of constant infusion or the characteristics of the excretion fraction of the sodium, but they simply represent the clearance of sodium divided by the clearance of inulin, and they have a nice advantage because they depend only upon the urine and plasma concentrations of sodium and the urine and plasma concentrations of inulin or any other substance used to measure glomerular filtration rate—that is, the collection of urine can be inaccurate but the ratios of concentration between the two kidneys is still a very useful index of function. So, errors are not introduced by errors in flow collections of urine.

Furthermore, there are some fascinating things about the kidney with a constricted main renal artery, in that it does excrete much less a proportion of the filtered sodium, and the reasons for this may be relevant to the so-called countercurrent multiplier theory of the kidney, and perhaps may depend upon the filtered load of urea delivered to the kidney tubules, because it has been well established that a kidney with a very low filtration rate can still concentrate urine more than the opposite kidney if the amount of urea delivered to the tubules is sufficient. This is a unique property of urea, and it is the reason we have chosen hyperosmotic urea infusions to carry out our clearance data.

Furthermore, as a diuretic it affords us urine flows between 4 to 10 ml of urine from each kidney during the clearance period, which makes it more accurate, and it reduces the post-ureteral-catheterization colic that is likely to occur with very low urine flows.

Surgical Treatment of Ventricular Aneurysm

Report of Ten Cases

DONALD B. EFFLER, MD; RICHARD N. WESTCOTT, MD; LAURENCE K. GROVES, MD; AND NIALL M. SCULLY, MD, CLEVELAND

Introduction

Aneurysm of the heart was described in 1757 when John Hunter[1] included a case report in "An Account of the Dissection of Morbid Bodys." For two centuries ventricular aneurysm has remained an interesting pathologic entity and has been displayed prominently in every major collection of postmortem oddities. Occasionally the diagnosis of ventricular aneurysm was established in the living patient,[2] an event of interest to the clinician but not helpful to the patient. The recent advent of open-heart surgery and its application in various types of acquired heart disease has made ventricular aneurysm a correctable lesion. This development removes ventricular aneurysm from the sole realm of the pathologist and makes clinical recognition now mandatory.

Presented at the 20th Annual Meeting of the Central Surgical Association, Chicago, Feb 21-23, 1963.

Formerly, Fellow in the Department of Thoracic Surgery; present address: The Straub Clinic, Honolulu, Hawaii (Dr. Scully).

From the Department of Thoracic Surgery, and the Department of Cardiology, The Cleveland Clinic Foundation.

Pathologic Features

Historically ventricular aneurysm was associated with syphilis, rheumatic myocarditis, tuberculosis, trauma, and a number of other etiologic factors. In light of present knowledge, however, it appears that ventricular aneurysm is the end result of myocardial infarction. Whenever ventricular aneurysm is recognized it can be assumed that the patient has significant coronary arteriosclerosis.

Ventricular aneurysm most commonly occurs in the anterior surface of the left ventricle and may involve the anterior aspect of the interventricular septum (Fig 1). Study in the living patient by selective coronary arteriography usually demonstrates obstruc-

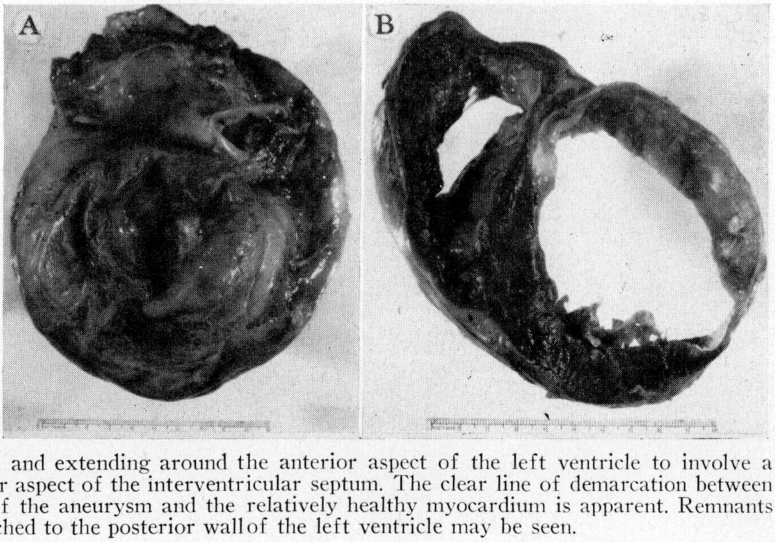

Fig 1.—Postmortem appearance of a heart with ventricular aneurysm. The patient died in uncontrolled left heart failure. *A* shows the gross appearance of the heart viewed from its anterior aspect. The thin fibrous wall of the huge ventricular aneurysm has become decompressed and, even in death, suggests paradoxic motion; *B*, sagittal section of both ventricles to illustrate the typical involvement by ventricular aneurysm. The fibrous wall may be seen extending from the lateral aspect of the left ventricle (lower right hand) and extending around the anterior aspect of the left ventricle to involve a limited portion of the anterior aspect of the interventricular septum. The clear line of demarcation between the attenuated fibrous wall of the aneurysm and the relatively healthy myocardium is apparent. Remnants of the papillary muscles attached to the posterior wall of the left ventricle may be seen.

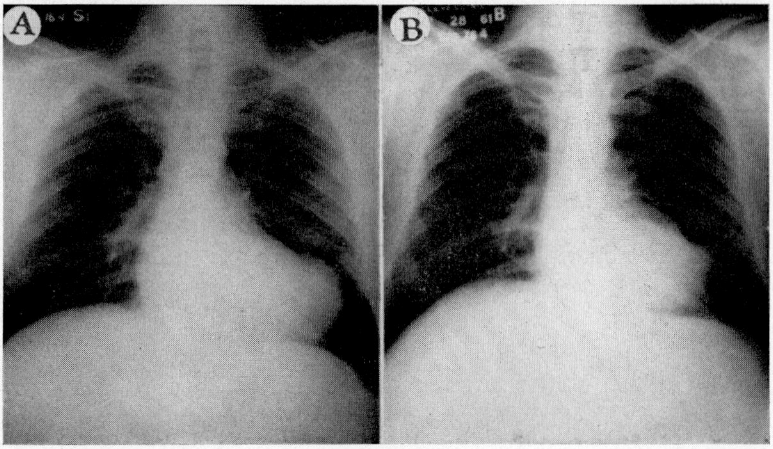

Fig 2.—Ventricular aneurysm may be quite obvious by radiographic examination and the paradoxic motion apparent by fluoroscopic examination. *A*, the typical appearance of ventricular aneurysm as demonstrated on this roentgenogram. *B*, progress film made six months after surgery demonstrates reduction in heart size and alteration in cardiac contour.

tion of the anterior descending branch of the left coronary artery; in addition, there is significant collateral supply from both the right coronary artery and the posterior aspect of the left circumflex artery. Occlusion of the anterior descending branch of the left coronary artery does not invariably produce ventricular aneurysm. There must be total replacement of muscle by fibrous tissue, and the area involved must be large. It is our belief that two other factors explain why in certain patients who survive massive myocardial infarction subsequent aneurysm of the left ventricle develops. These factors are: (1) availability of collateral circulation and (2) restriction of the infarction to the ventricular wall alone.

Consideration of these two factors gives one understanding of the development of ventricular aneurysm and its consistent localization to the anterior surface of the left ventricle (Fig 2). The ventricular myocardium is perfused by two coronary arteries, the right and the left, the latter dividing into the anterior descending artery and the circumflex artery. Coronary occlusive disease may be segmental or diffuse, and for this reason myocardial infarction may occur anywhere in the two ventricles and their common septum. Massive myocardial infarction that follows occlusion of a major arterial branch is only tolerated in an area protected by available collateral branches. The anterior wall of the left ventricle is supplied by the left anterior descending branch. In addition, this area is flanked on either side and posteriorly by vessels capable of collateral supply, provided that they are free of occlusive disease. No other major area of ventricular myocardium receives this degree of collateral

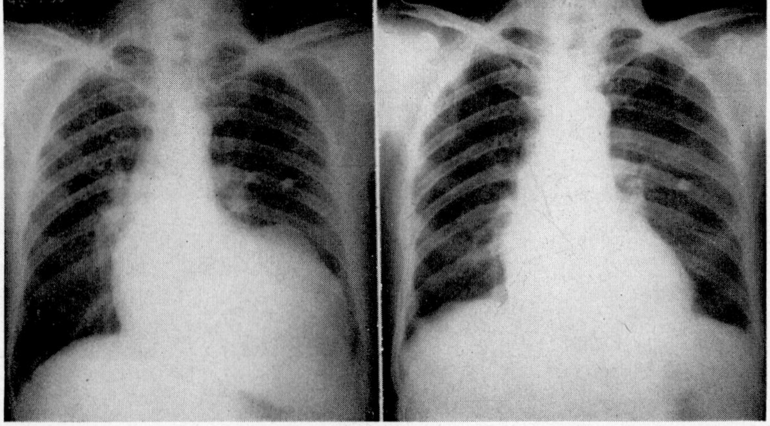

Fig 3.—Roentgenograms before and after ventricular aneurysmectomy demonstrate the striking improvement that may occur. The left-hand figure demonstrates the marked cardiac enlargement associated with the aneurysm and chronic congestive failure. The follow-up film on the right was made less than six months after surgical treatment.

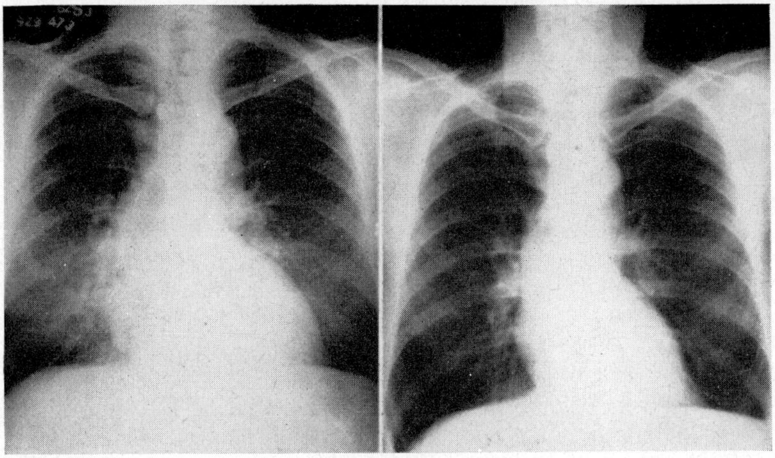

Fig 4.—The striking improvement that follows successful removal of ventricular aneurysm is illustrated here. Relief of left-heart failure and paroxysmal ventricular arrhythmia may be striking.

support. On this basis alone, it seems logical to assume that the initial insult of massive myocardial infarction is tolerated better when the anterior descending branch of the left coronary is involved (Fig 3).

The second factor of importance has to do with the dynamic responsibility of the infarcted area. Anatomically the anterior wall of the left ventricle contributes little to valve support or to major conductive pathways. Physiologically the anterior wall of the left ventricle has little responsibility except for its pumping action in ventricular output. This is quite unlike the posterior wall of the left ventricle where massive infarction would of necessity involve the papillary muscles supporting chordae tendineae of the mitral valve. Infarction of the posterior aspect of the left ventricle, sufficient to cause aneurysmal formation, affects mitral valve integrity. The added burden of acute mitral valve insufficiency greatly reduces the chance of initial survival. We have seen one patient who did have aneurysm of the posterior wall of the left ventricle and the typical feature of mitral valve insufficiency. This patient died soon after diagnosis was established; postmortem examination disclosed rupture of the chordae tendineae, involving the anterior leaflet of the mitral valve in addition to the aneurysm itself.

If our interpretations are correct and these two factors are of significance, this would explain why ventricular aneurysm is invariably found on the anterior wall of the left ventricle. Aneurysm of the right ventricle must be a rare lesion. Perhaps the lower intracardiac pressures of the right heart are a factor (Fig 4).

Clinical Features

The prognosis of ventricular aneurysm is only half as favorable as in myocardial infarction without aneurysm. The patients are chronically ill and require constant medical supervision and therapy. The inefficient ventricular contraction, with associated paradox, impairs cardiac output to such an extent that left-sided failure is a feature of this disease. Congestive failure and paroxysmal arrhythmias are the main reasons for the multiple periods of hospitalization these patients require. A review of 102 necropsy reports, by Schlichter, Hellerstein, and Katz,[3] suggests that 75% of the patients are dead within three years after initial infarction and that congestive heart failure, thromboembolic phenomenon, or recurrent infarction accounts for 83% of deaths.

Ventricular aneurysms are alleged to rupture with prompt loss of life. Perhaps this is true, but such an occurrence has not been reported in the records of The Cleveland Clinic Foundation. Inspection of nine ventricular aneurysms at the time of surgery suggests that fibrous replacement of the ventricular myocardium and reinforcement by the densely adherent pericardial sac make perforation unlikely (Fig 5).

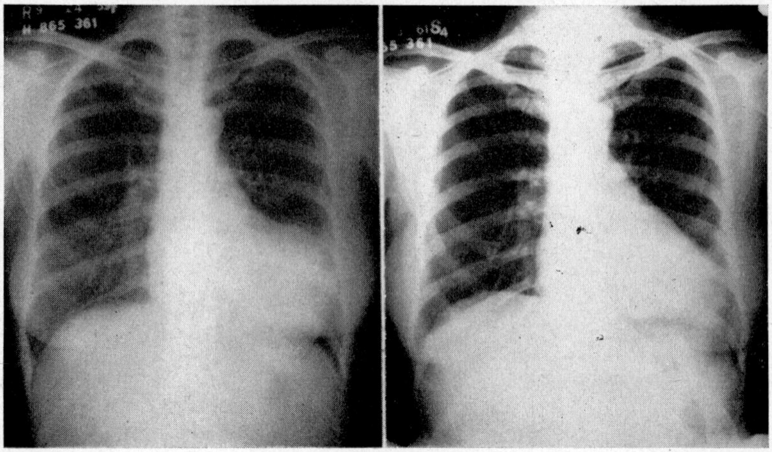

Fig 5.—Comparison of the roentgenograms before and after surgery in our first operation for ventricular aneurysmectomy is shown. Reduction in heart size almost two years after operation is not so striking as might be expected. This may be explained on the basis of incomplete resection because of surgical timidity. From a clinical standpoint this patient has done quite well with marked relief of symptoms and no radiographic evidence of residual ventricular paradox.

Perhaps the most important observation in the patient who presents ventricular aneurysm is demonstrable coronary arteriosclerosis. It is unlikely that the coronary occlusive disease will be restricted entirely to the site of the initial occlusion with its resultant infarction. That the patient is subject to subsequent infarction elsewhere in the coronary circuit cannot be disregarded. Evaluation of this clinical feature will be discussed later.

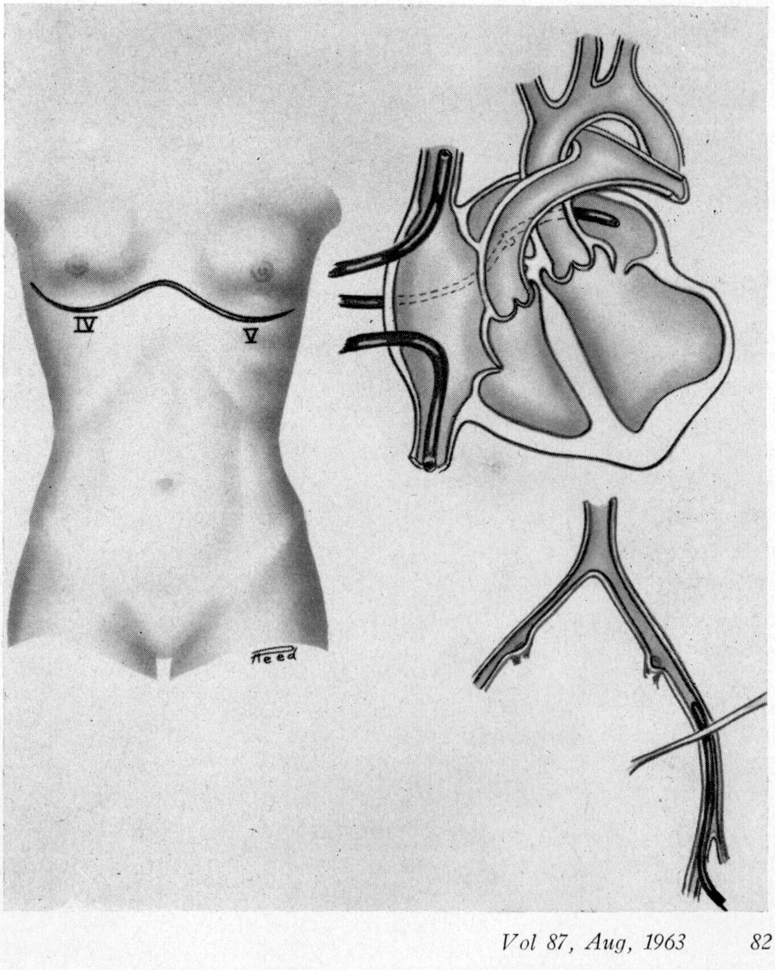

Fig 6.—Schematic illustration of the surgical incision and the basic pattern of cannulations utilized for extracorporeal circulation. A transverse sternotomy with bilateral thoracotomy is performed beginning in the fourth interspace, right, and entering the left fifth interspace. Arterial cannulation utilizes the left common femoral artery. The left-heart cannula is seen entering the left atrium via the right superior pulmonary vein.

Treatment

Evaluation of Patient for Surgical Treatment.—It is our belief that the diagnosis of ventricular aneurysm qualifies the patient for surgical consideration. Whereas the initial diagnosis may be made on the basis of history, physical findings, and radiographic study, information obtained by left heart catheterization and selective coronary arteriography is of value (Fig 6).

Injection studies within the left ventricle itself demonstrate paradoxic motion and resultant inefficiency of left ventricular contraction. Involvement of the anterior septum may also be apparent. These studies add much to our understanding of the basic problems but are not mandatory for diagnosis or evaluation. Likewise, cinematography and injections of the major coronary arteries with contrast medium provide graphic film records. Opacification of the coronary circuit by selective arteriograms identifies the site of the major occlusion and, more important, offers appraisal of the remaining coronary arterial circut.* We have had the opportunity to examine ten patients in whom the diagnosis of myocardial aneurysm was established (Fig 7). All of these patients were chronically ill, and several were in desperate straits because of poorly controlled left-heart failure. Operation was recommended in every instance regardless of the patient's status. It would seem, therefore, that the excellent studies undertaken before surgery were useless, as operation was predetermined. Actually this is not the case. Increasing experience and accumulation of detailed information will certainly lead to better understanding and clinical management.

Surgical Treatment.—In 1944, Beck operated upon a patient with ventricular aneurysm; an effort was made to reduce the volume of this aneurysm by circumferential sutures and plication. Likoff and Bailey [4] re-

* Each of the patients described in this series was studied by left heart catheterization techniques and selective coronary arteriography. These studies were performed by Dr. F. Mason Sones, Jr., and Dr. Earl K. Shirey, of the Cardiovascular Laboratory.

Fig 7.—Artist's conception of left ventricular aneurysm. It would be more correct if the aneurysm were lower in position. Usually the apex of the left ventricle is replaced by fibrous tissue, and healthy myocardium is found between the upper limits of the aneurysm and the circumflex coronary artery.

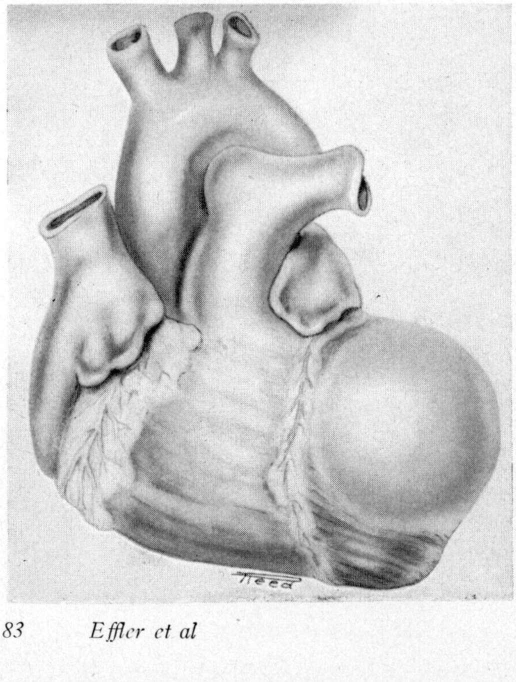

Fig 8.—Excision of the aneurysmal sac is a relatively simple surgical task. It is our usual practice to incise the center of the aneurysm in order to decompress the ventricle and to remove adherent clot. It might also be stated that the anterior descending branch of the left coronary artery is not apparent as depicted in this illustration.

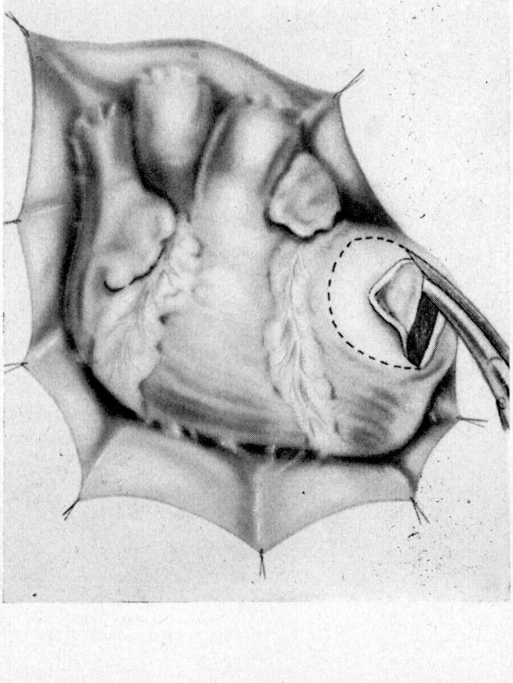

ported in 1955 on experience with ventriculoplasty; Bailey applied an occluding clamp to the base of the aneurysm and excised the redundant tissue (Fig 8). The operations of both Beck and Bailey were undertaken before the era of open-heart surgery that utilizes extracorporeal circulation.

When extracorporeal circulation made total bypass of the heart feasible, the definitive treatment for ventricular aneurysm was established. We believe that Cooley accomplished the first successful removal of ventricular aneurysm.[5] Published reports by Cooley et al,[5,6] Lillehei et al,[7] and our own clinical experience indicate that ventricular aneurysmectomy is tolerated remarkably well even by the patient who comes to the operating room in left ventricular failure.

The surgical mission is restricted entirely to excision of the aneurysm, removal of related thrombus, and reconstruction of the left ventricular chamber to re-establish an effective pumping unit. Relief of the paradoxic motion produced by the aneurysm may be followed by remarkable functional improvement and rehabilitation of the patient. However, a successful result does not alter the fact that the patient may well have significant residual coronary arteriosclerosis. This last point merits constant repetition (Fig 9).

Fig 9.—Photographs of the gross specimen obtained from removal of one ventricular aneurysm. The fibrous wall of the aneurysm is seen at the bottom of the illustration. Above are pieces of laminated clot found within the huge aneurysmal sac.

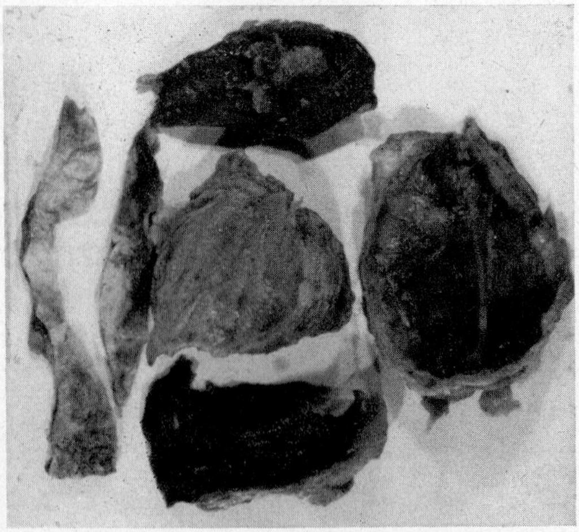

Technique.—The first operation in our series was performed in September, 1959. We are indebted to Lam [8] for valuable suggestions made before this surgical undertaking. After initial success we have not deviated from the original method. A transverse incision is made entering the right thorax through the fourth interspace, transecting the sternum, and entering the left pleural space through the fifth interspace. In all probability median sternotomy would suffice, but lateral deviation of the enlarged left ventricle has prompted us to stay with the transverse approach. The patient is heparinized, and routine cannulations are made preparatory to extracorporeal circulation. In addition to the two venae caval cannulae it is our practice to

Fig 10.—After removal of the aneurysm, inspection of the left ventricular chamber is possible. The competent aortic valve as seen from its ventricular aspect is readily apparent. The papillary muscle originating from the posterior and lateral aspects of the left ventricle as well as the intact chordae tendineae is evident. This illustration gives an incorrect impression, as the site of aneurysmectomy is high on the anterior wall of the left ventricle. Actually the diseased area extends invariably to the apex of the ventricle, and healthy myocardium is not found adjacent to the anterior descending branch of the left coronary artery.

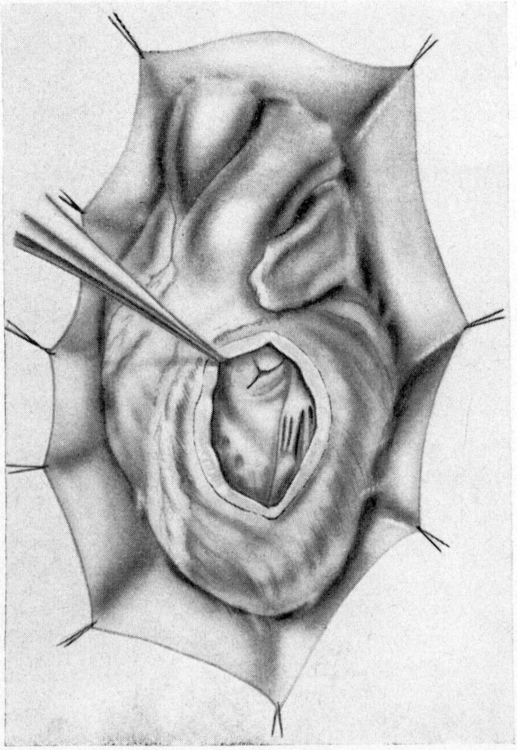

insert a left atrial cannula through the right superior pulmonary vein. This third venous cannula is used later to maintain decompression of the bypassed heart.[9] When total body perfusion has been established, moderate cooling (rectal temperature approximately 32 C [89.6 F]) is employed. Cardioplegia is not employed (Fig 10).

When on total bypass, the decompressed heart may be manipulated as needed to expose the region of disease. Usually the pericardium is densely adherent over the aneurysm, and the symphysis is divided by sharp dissection. After the heart is freed of pericardial adhesion, it is elevated by placing a large pad of gauze beneath the ventricles. This brings the aneurysm into better view and raises the apex of the left ventricle above the aortic valve; this position eliminates the hazard of systemic air embolus. A vertical incision is made in the central portion of the aneurysm itself. When clot is present, this may be dissected away from the fibrous wall by simple decortication and piecemeal removal by ring forceps. Any clot element that falls into the ventricular chamber is easily recovered, as the beating ventricle has

Fig 11.—Reconstruction of the left ventricular chamber is not difficult. The initial closure is made in a vertical plane and utilizes a continuous suture of nonabsorbable material. The second line of closure employs interrupted sutures placed at sufficient depth to incorporate the two closure planes.

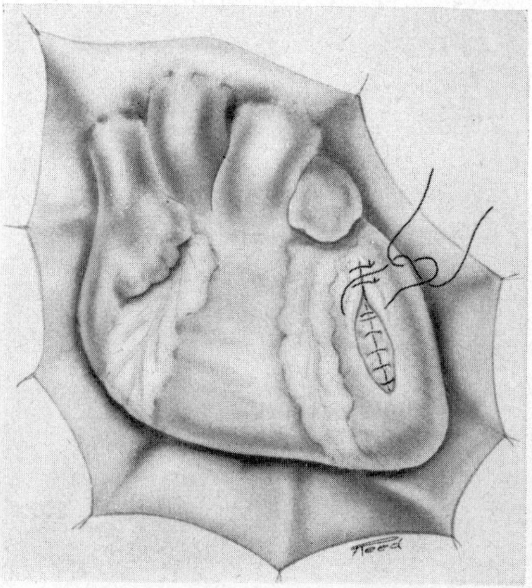

no output after it is opened and is decompressed. As long as satisfactory extracorporeal circulation is provided, there need be no hurry in performing aneurysmectomy; the surgeon should be as thorough and meticulous as he would be for any other form in intracardiac operation (Fig 11). At this stage of the operation ventricular arrhythmias are of no consequence, and the surgeon should not be disturbed by electrocardiographic gyrations.

After clot removal the extent of the aneurysm becomes obvious. There is usually a sharp line of demarcation between the fibrous aneurysmal wall and the adjacent healthy myocardium. An incision is made completely around this juncture until the entire fibrous sac is removed. When this has been accomplished, the interior of the left ventricle is open for inspection. The ventricular aspect of the aortic valve, the interventricular septum, and the underside of the mitral valve with its related chordae tendineae and papillary muscles are in view. Blood that enters the field by way of the mitral valve orifice and the thebesian veins is easily removed by a sterile sucker. That the left ventricle usually maintains its beat with this gaping incision and attendant manipulation is impressive t the surgical team. Ventricular fibrillation ha occurred once in our experience and was converted promptly by a single electric countershock.

We were concerned initially at the limits of excision, fearing that healthy myocardium might not support closing sutures. It seemed worthwhile to leave a small rim of fibrous tissue for suture support. We also visualized critical reduction in capacity of the reconstructed chambers. However, this has not been apparent thus far. As healthy myocardium is entered, active bleeding points from supporting collateral circulation and from terminal branches of the intact left and right coronary arteries are encountered. Remnants of the left anterior descending branch are usually lost in the fibrous reaction associated with the aneurysm itself. Closure of the surgical defect is accomplished in a vertical plane. It is our practice to use a two-layer closure, the first accomplished with a continuous running suture for initial approximation. Key sutures are placed at the extreme limits of the incision above and below to anchor the running suture. When initial closure has been accomplished, it is good practice to place a small catheter at the apical end of the incision to allow escape of air that may have been trapped within the left ventricle. It may be helpful at this juncture to release one of the vena caval tourniquets to allow more blood to enter the heart and to fill the left atrium and ventricle. The second layer of closure consists of carefully placed interrupted sutures. Each suture is placed at sufficient depth to incorporate with the initial layer of closure. Nonabsorbable suture material, particularly silk, has been employed in each instance. Reconstruction of the left ventricle has not required removal of the anterior portion of the interventricular septum. If significant paradox of the septum itself were encountered, it is likely that a plaque of reinforcing plastic cloth might be inserted from the left ventricular aspect. At the completion of the operation the elevating pad is removed; the heart is returned to its proper position within the pericardial sac, and the extracorporeal circulation is withdrawn. At this point, systemic blood pressure is frequently better than before operation, attesting to the improved efficiency of the left ventricle. If measurable vital signs are satisfactory, the routine decannulation process is undertaken, and the heparin effect is neutralized by an appropriate drug. As the pericardial sac is reconstructed, one or two counterincisions may be helpful for drainage purposes; then the thoracic incision is closed, and waterseal suction drainage for both pleural spaces is routinely used. The postoperative care is the same as that for any individual who has undergone open-heart surgery for acquired heart disease and who is known to have an element of residual coronary arteriosclerosis.

Results.—Ten patients have been considered for surgical correction of ventricular aneurysm. One of these had a posterior myocardial infarction and, as reported earlier, died before surgery was undertaken. The immediate cause of death was an uncontrolled ventricular arrhythmia. Of the nine patients who underwent surgery, two have since died: one of late wound infection and subsequent mycotic aneurysm of the ventricular incision; the other, of myocardial infarction sustained 2½ months after surgery. Postmortem examination in this latter late patient demonstrated excellent healing in the reconstructed left ventricle (Fig 12). The seven patients who have survived operation have shown uniform improvement and relief of the symptoms attributable to the aneurysm and its attendant paradoxic motion.

Comment

The need for surgical treatment in the patient who acquires a ventricular aneurysm is obvious. The life expectancy of the patient with ventricular aneurysm is shortened appreciably; once aneurysm has formed, the patient is rarely free of left heart failure or ventricular arrhythmia. Medical treatment

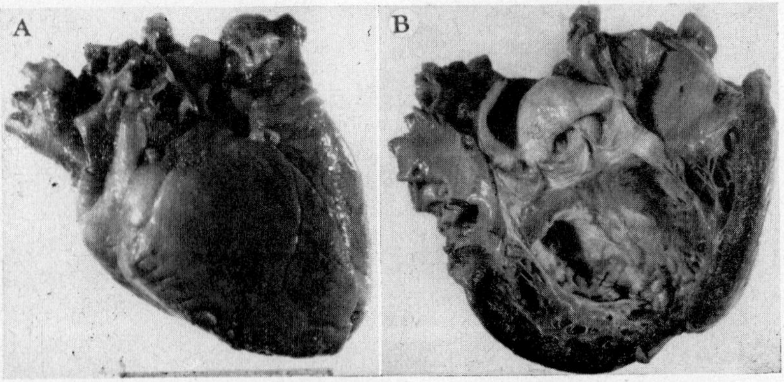

Fig 12.—Postmortem appearance of a heart 2½ months after ventricular aneurysmectomy. This patient died of myocardial infarction sustained several hours before death. *A*, the suture line on the anterior wall of the left ventricle is readily apparent; and in *B*, a surgical closure is viewed from the interior of the left ventricle. Primary healing had occurred, and there was no clot apparent on the suture line.

of ventricular aneurysm can only support the myocardium that was spared by the previous massive infarction. This medical regimen cannot be considered definitive therapy for the patient with ventricular aneurysm.

Surgical treatment of ventricular aneurysm is undertaken with the full knowledge that the patient has residual coronary arterial disease. The extent of this residual disease is the dominant factor in estimating the prognosis, even if initial success follows the operation. We believe that selective coronary arteriography is a worthwhile method of appraising the coronary arterial circuit.

Donald B. Effler, MD, Cleveland Clinic, 2020 E 93rd St, Cleveland 6, Ohio.

REFERENCES

1. Hunter, J.: An Account of the Dissection of Morbid Bodys, manuscript copy in Library of Royal College of Surgeons, No. 32, 1757, pp 30-32.

2. Sternberg, M.: Das chronische partielle Herzaneurysma, thesis, Erlangen University, Dresden, Germany, 1914.

3. Schlichter, J.; Hellerstein, H. K.; and Katz, L. N.: Aneurysm of the Heart: A Correlative Study of 102 Proved Cases, Medicine 33:43-86 (Feb) 1954.

4. Likoff, W., and Bailey, C. P.: Ventriculoplasty: Excision of Myocardial Aneurysm; Report of a Successful Case, JAMA 158:915-920 (July 16) 1955.

5. Cooley, D. A.; Collins, H. A.; Morris, G. C., Jr.; and Chapman, D. W.: Ventricular Aneurysm After Myocardial Infarction: Surgical Excision With Use of Temporary Cardiopulmonary Bypass, JAMA 167:557-560 (May 31) 1958.

6. Cooley, D. A.; Henly, W. S.; Amad, K. H.; and Chapman, D. W.: Ventricular Aneurysm Following Myocardial Infarction: Results of Surgical Treatment, Ann Surg 150:595-612 (Oct) 1959.

7. Lillehei, C. W.; Levy, M. J.; DeWall, R. A.; and Warden, H. E.: Resection of Myocardial Aneurysms After Infarction During Temporary Cardiopulmonary Bypass, Circulation 26:206-217 (Aug) 1962.

8. Lam, C. (Henry Ford Hospital, Detroit): Personal communication to the authors, September, 1959.

9. Effler, D. B., and Groves, L. K.: Open-Heart Surgery for Acquired Valvular Heart Disease; Present Techniques and Trends, Arch Surg 84:155-169 (Feb) 1962.

Direct Auscultation of the Heart

D. W. BUSSMANN, MD; V. REDDY, MD; AND C. R. HANLON, MD, ST. LOUIS

In 42 patients with congenital or acquired heart disease, we have recorded the heart sounds before and after operation together with direct auscultation of the heart exposed at operation. This was done to clarify certain poorly understood aspects of cardiac murmurs, such as their persistence after apparently adequate repair of the underlying defect. Our experience has provided some practical guides in surgical treatment of cardiac lesions.

Methods

Studies at operation involved the application of a sterile, special microphone to parts of the heart and great vessels before and after operative treatment of the lesion. These operative studies were compared with the preoperative findings and with those recorded after about a week when the chest dressings had been removed.

Heart sound recordings were made simultaneously on the Sanborn Twin-Beam and on the Cambridge heart sound magnetic tape recorder with oscilloscopic projection. Before entering the surgical field, the examiner was equipped with earphones connected to the recorders, permitting him to monitor the sounds and to decide which portions of the examination were to be recorded.

Presented at the 20th Annual Meeting of the Central Surgical Association, Chicago, Feb 21-23, 1963.

From the Heart Sound Laboratory, the Center for Cardiovascular Research, Department of Internal Medicine, and the Department of Surgery, St. Louis University.

Aided by USPHS Grant HE-0612 and a grant from the Missouri Heart Association.

It should be emphasized that the selection of areas of the heart and vessels for auscultation, the firmness of contact between the heart and the recording pickup device, and the assessment of significance of the sounds were at the discretion of the consultant phonocardiographer (D.W.B.) who was "scrubbed up" as a member of the team. Recording from a wet, moving surface which may be irregular or fibrinous can introduce sounds which do not originate within the heart. Identification of rubs and extraneous noises by study of the photographic paper alone is difficult, whereas the experienced ear can readily isolate them. By adjusting the firmness of application of the recording device and allowing it to move with the heart, the examiner can eliminate most artifacts from the recording.

Between the Sanborn dynamic microphone and the Cambridge tape recorder, a transformer is interposed to match impedances. To facilitate access to the heart at operation, we added 4-inch tubular nylon extensions to the microphone (Fig 1). These had pickup heads varying from one-half to one inch in diameter, some with the end opening at right angles to the shaft. The extensions prevented entry of pericardial fluid into the microphone itself but naturally modified the transmission of sound as compared to conditions with the microphone applied directly to the intact chest wall. The apparatus was sterilized by ethylene oxide, and no evidence of infection associated with the auscultatory study was seen in any case.

By interchange with the anesthesiologist's monitoring equipment, all electrocardiograms during operation are recorded as an inverted lead II.

Case Material

The patients studied represent a wide spectrum of operable heart disease with septal defects predominating (Table). We shall comment only on four entities, which illustrate certain theoretical and practical yields from the technique.

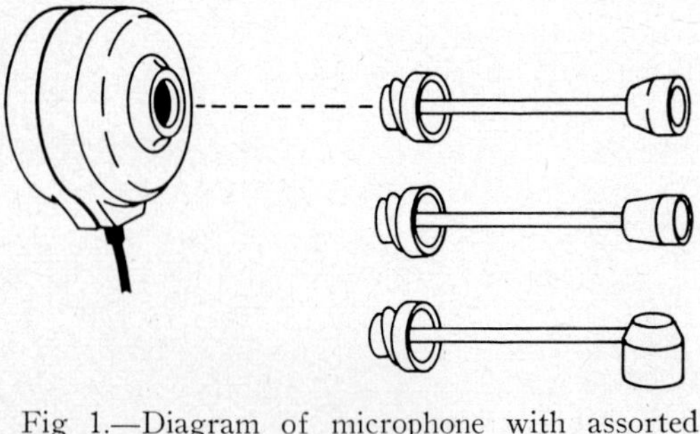

Fig 1.—Diagram of microphone with assorted pickup heads to permit access to remote areas. The heads also prevent entry of fluid into microphone structure.

Case Material (42)

Ventricular septal defect (VSD)		14
Atrial septal defect (ASD)		7
Mitral valve disease		4
Patent ductus arteriosus (PDA)		3
Aortic stenosis		3
Valvar	1	
Supravalvar	1	
Subaortic hypertrophic	1	
Pulmonic stenosis, valvar (PS)		2
Complex lesions		6
VSD + PS	3	
ASD + PS	1	
ASD + PDA	1	
ASD + Ebstein's anomaly	1	
Miscellaneous		3
Aortic insufficiency	1	
Coronary artery fistula	1	
Truncus arteriosus	1	

Patent Ductus Arteriosus.—Three patients with this entity were studied. The auscultatory phenomena were similar in all. Each had a continuous murmur at the pulmonic area. Fig 2 illustrates the striking rise in intensity when the recording is made directly over the heart as compared to the intact chest.

The modest continuous murmur on the chest wall is exemplified more strikingly by the tape recording than by the phonocardiographic tracing. With exposure of the heart, the continuous murmur was extremely loud on the pulmonary artery at the point of impact by the jet of blood from the aorta. Over the ductus itself the murmur was continuous but of only moderate intensity. Over the aorta one could hear only a minimal systolic murmur.

After division of the ductus, a modest murmur remained over the pulmonary artery and the aorta. Auscultation of the intact chest at a later date showed only a minimal, low-pitch systolic murmur at the pulmonic area.

These observations corroborate the known facts concerning propagation of murmurs. In an indeterminate lesion, the character and direction of flow through the ductus could be assessed to a considerable degree by direct auscultation.

Pulmonary Valvar Stenosis.—Two patients with pulmonary valvar stenosis were studied. They provided interesting data on

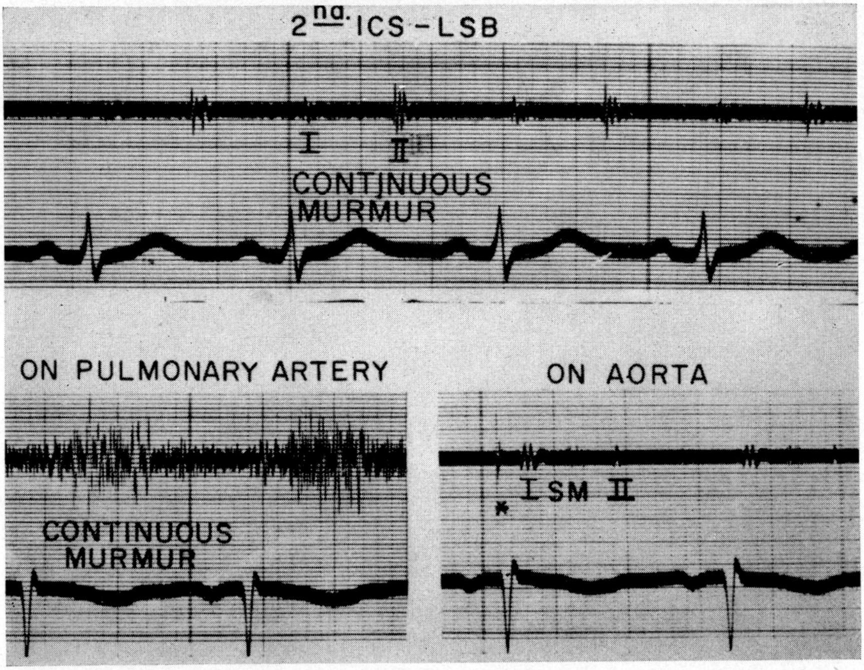

Fig 2.—Patent ductus arteriosus. Recordings directly from the pulmonary artery show much louder sounds than are heard over intact chest. However, systolic murmur (*SM*) on the aorta is inconspicuous. Asterisk before first aortic sound indicates artifact, detected by simultaneous tape recording.

the basic nature of the murmur in this lesion and on its alteration by valvotomy. In one patient with a gradient of 130 mm of mercury across the pulmonary valve, right ventricular systole lasted 0.14 seconds longer than left ventricular systole. Within the confines of its own systole, the murmur of pulmonary stenosis was a diamond-shaped, ejection type.

After valvotomy the gradient fell to 20 mm of mercury, but there was no diminution

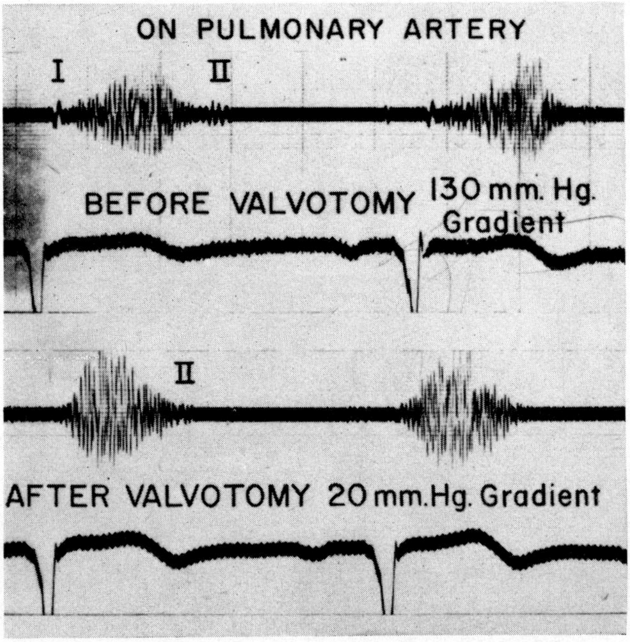

Fig 3.—Pulmonic stenosis. Phonocardiograms from the exposed pulmonary artery before and after valvotomy for valvar pulmonic stenosis. The loudness is not appreciably decreased despite a good lowering of the gradient. However, systole is shortened, and the shape of the tracing is altered.

in intensity of the murmur. By the criterion of intensity alone one could not have judged the gradient to be lower (Fig 3). However, certain other changes occurred after valvotomy. Right ventricular systole was shortened by 0.12 seconds, the peak of the murmur moved toward early systole, and the murmur was of a lower sound frequency. These three changes indicate a lower gradient.

After operation there was a significant residual systolic murmur over the chest. This murmur was placed in proper perspective by the knowledge gained from direct auscultation at operation.

Atrial Septal Defect.—Seven patients had an ostium secundum defect with pulmonary pressures up to 50 mm of mercury and a large left-to-right shunt at the atrial level. Each had the typical low-pitch systolic murmur at the second or third left intercostal space. All but one had a low-pitch mid-diastolic murmur at the lower left sternal border. The exception was a man with pulmonary emphysema. The second heart sound was persistently split in all, the range being 0.04 to 0.08 seconds.

On direct auscultation of the exposed heart, the systolic murmur in all cases was loudest over the pulmonary artery. The mid-diastolic murmur was best heard at the inflow area of the right ventricle. By recordings directly over the pulmonic and aortic valves, it was easily established that pulmonic valve closure followed aortic valve closure in every case.

Immediately after closure of the defect, recordings from the heart showed a persistent although diminished systolic murmur over the pulmonary artery. The diastolic murmur disappeared in every instance. The second heart sound remained widely split at this time (Fig 4).

Examination of the intact chest several weeks later showed that only four had a remaining systolic murmur, and only three had a persistently wide split of the second sound.

These observations indicate the origin of the systolic murmur from the dilated pulmonary artery and constitute a reassuring factor in those patients whose systolic murmur appears unchanged immediately after operation. This need not give rise to con-

Fig 4.—Atrial septal defect. Recordings at operation for closure of atrial septal defect showing systolic murmur (*SM*) over pulmonary artery in left upper panel and diastolic murmur (*DM*) over right ventricle in the right upper panel. After closure of defect, the diastolic murmur disappeared, but the systolic murmur persisted along with the split second sound (*A-P*) as seen in the left lower panel.

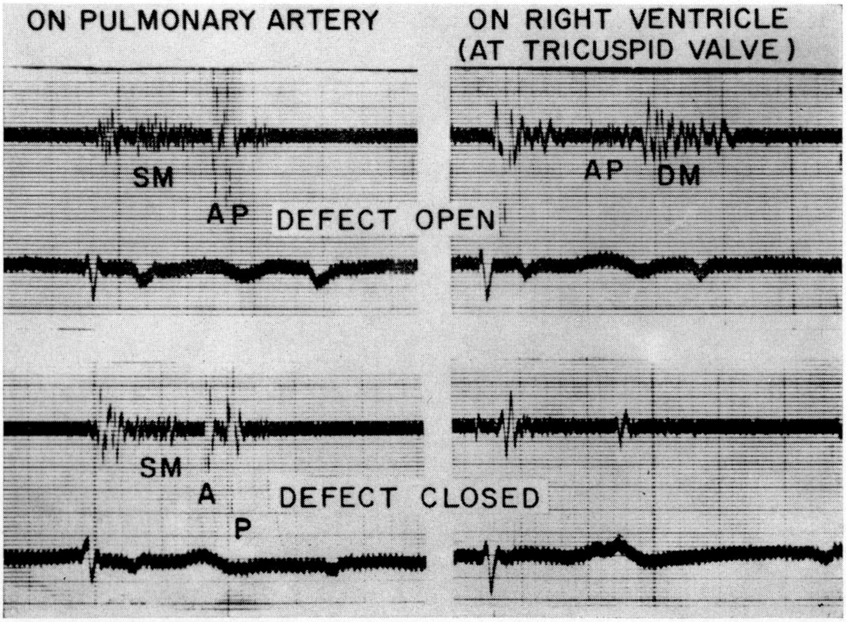

cern that the atrial defect is inadequately closed.

Ventricular Septal Defect.—Thirteen patients had a left-to-right shunt at the ventricular level. Preoperative recordings showed the classical findings of a loud, harsh systolic murmur at the third and fourth interspace to the left of the sternum.

Five had a very large shunt with significant excess flow through the lungs. These also had a low-pitch mid-diastolic murmur at the left ventricular apex. With the heart exposed, the maximal thrill was palpable over the right ventricle or its outflow tract. Direct cardiac recordings showed the harsh systolic murmur to be extremely intense over the right ventricle with rapid diminution of intensity as one moved away from this area. Recordings over other chambers showed only trivial systolic murmurs. The diastolic murmur could be heard over the apical areas of both the right and left ventricles.

At operation one patient with known incomplete closure had a persistent thrill over the right ventricle before chest closure was begun. In the remaining 12, the surgeon felt that closure was complete, since they showed no thrill and no rise in oxygen saturation of the blood in the right ventricle. The 12th had a moderately intense, high-pitch murmur over the right ventricle, with typical characteristics of a small ventricular septal defect (Fig 5). Months later, catheterization studies of the right heart showed no rise in oxygen saturation in the right ventricle, but cineangiocardiography revealed a small left-to-right shunt at the ventricular level.

These studies indicate that persistent shunts at the ventricular level too small to be detected as a palpable thrill or by rise in oxygen saturation may be revealed by direct auscultation over the right ventricle.

In the 14th patient with a ventricular septal defect and balanced pressures, the customary murmur due to systolic jet into the right ventricle was absent. A systolic murmur originating in the dilated pulmonary artery was not altered by closure of the defect. A murmur representing tricuspid incompetence was likewise unchanged after operation.

Fig 5.—Ventricular septal defect. Sound recordings from the exposed heart of two patients with ventricular septal defect, before and after repair. Both patients show prominent systolic murmurs (*SM*) before operation. After operation there is no murmur in *RS*, but a murmur is present in *MF* despite absence of thrill over right ventricle and lack of rise in oxygen saturation in right ventricle. Later cineangiocardiography showed small persistent shunt.

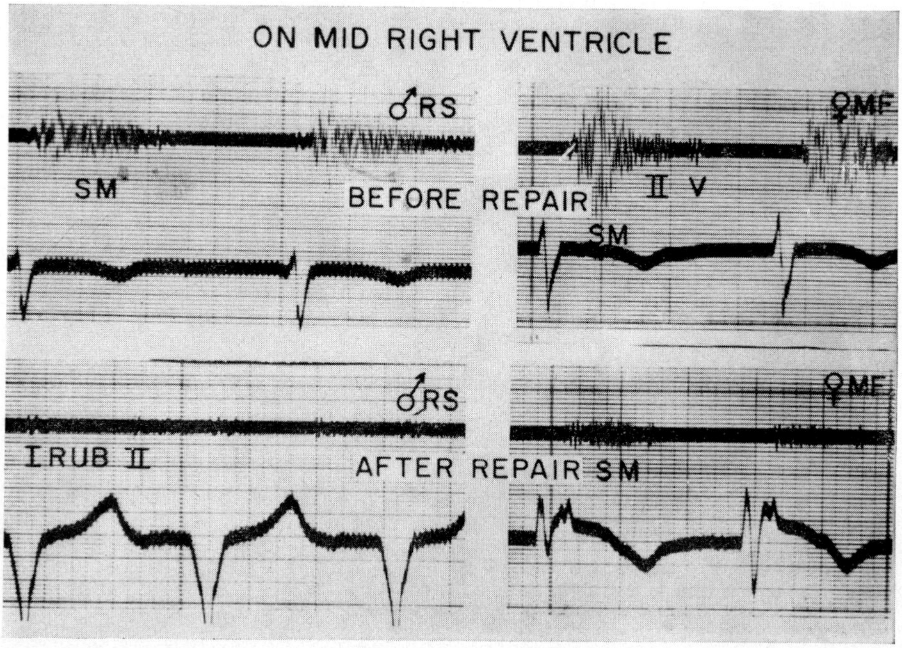

Comment

Our findings and those of others [1] confirm the logical supposition that murmurs recorded directly from the heart at operation are louder than the same murmurs recorded from the intact chest. Moreover, the intensity of the murmur over various parts of the heart gives valuable information on the origin and propagation of murmurs. A sound recording from the point of origin of a jet may give an inconspicuous murmur, whereas auscultation at the point of jet impact elicits a massive roar.

This principle is well demonstrated by the contrast between ventricular septal defect and mitral insufficiency. Sounds over the chest with ventricular defects are quite loud because the area of jet impact is close to the sound pickup. With mitral insufficiency one hears a less conspicuous murmur because he is listening at the origin of the jet.

The nongradient murmur of atrial septal defect and the obstructive gradient murmur of valvar pulmonic stenosis present different auscultatory situations. It is clear that the systolic murmur of atrial septal defect arises from the pulmonary artery, due to increased rate of flow into a vessel of increased caliber. Decrease in the flow leaves unchanged the dilated pulmonary artery. There remains a murmur of similar quality with slightly less intensity after the defect is closed.

The mid-diastolic murmur of atrial septal defect appears to originate at the tricuspid valve and in the right ventricle. With decrease in the flow this murmur totally disappears. The early persistence of a widely split second sound may be due to lack of resiliency of the pulmonary artery in the face of a lower pulmonary flow.

Significant relief of obstruction in a valvar pulmonic stenosis hardly alters the intensity of the murmur in the pulmonary artery, although the character of the murmur is considerably altered. This may be due to persistence of some gradient; even with a gradient reduced to zero, projection of the thickened valve into the stream may cause considerable turbulence. However, a lower gradient causes peaking of the murmur earlier in systole,[2] shortening of right ventricular systole, and a lowering of the pitch.

As indicated above, success of a surgical procedure on the heart is not necessarily related to abolition of murmurs. In the case of high gradient shunts, as with patent ductus and ventricular septal defect, persistent gradient murmurs suggest an incomplete operation. In ventricular septal defect a persistent murmur with direct auscultation over the right ventricle is an extremely sensitive indicator of incomplete closure.

Summary

Direct auscultation of the exposed heart has been carried out during operation in 42 patients with a variety of congenital and acquired heart diseases.

Comparison between the sound recordings at operation and those which were made before and after operation emphasizes certain theoretical and practical considerations.

From the theoretical standpoint, persistence of the systolic murmur after closure of an atrial septal defect confirms the origin of the murmur from the pulmonary artery rather than from flow across the septum.

From the practical standpoint, this technique can furnish reliable assurance of satisfactory relief of obstruction after valvotomy for pulmonary valvar stenosis. It also gives reliable evidence at operation regarding completeness of closure in ventricular septal defect.

These advantages recommend its use as a surgical adjunct in selected patients.

C. R. Hanlon, MD, 1325 S Grand, St Louis 4, Mo.

REFERENCES

1. Magri, G.; Jona, E.; Messina, D.; and Actis-Dato, A.: Direct Recording of Heart Sounds and Murmurs From the Epicardial Surface of the Exposed Human Heart, Amer Heart J 57:449, 1959.

2. Vogelpoel, L., and Schrire, V.: Auscultatory and Phonocardiographic Assessment of Pulmonary Stenosis With Intact Ventricular Septum, Circulation 22:55, 1960.

DISCUSSION

On papers by Drs. Effler et al and Bussmann et al

Dr. F. Henry Ellis, Jr., Rochester, Minn: I would like to commend Dr. Effler for again bringing to our attention the interesting and potentially lethal condition of ventricular aneurysms. It is a tribute to his skill that he was able to operate successfully on nine patients with this condition, for, as you all know, many of them are in a very precarious hemodynamic state.

Whether or not one should operate on asymptomatic patients is a point for discussion. I rather suspect we should only be operating on patients who are severely symptomatic, while those who have no symptoms should not be subjected to operation.

The February, 1963, issue of *Circulation* contains an article on ventricular aneurysms by Abrams and associates bearing on this particular problem. Their study involved 65 patients coming to postmortem examination. Contrary to what one might expect, it was their finding that patients with ventricular aneurysms rarely die from complications due to aneurysm. None of them died of a peripheral embolus. Only three deaths were due to rupture of the aneurysm; in fact, only 13.8% of the patients died of any condition related to the aneurysm, whereas about half died of another myocardial infarction.

This, then, would seem to indicate that patients with ventricular aneurysm should be operated on only if they have repeated emboli, congestive failure due to the aneurysm, or if there is evidence of progressive enlargement of the aneurysm.

I want to ask Dr. Effler if he would tell us what his indications for operation are in these patients. In view of the fact that so many of these patients ultimately die of myocardial infarction, then would it be wise to study them preoperatively with coronary arteriography to determine the status of these vessels before subjecting them to surgery?

Dr. Hugh E. Stephenson, Jr., Columbia, Mo: The comments I have to make can be illustrated by a short movie strip of a recently resected left ventricular aneurysm.

I would like to draw your attention to the very close approximation of this aneurysm to the interventricular septum and to the right ventricle. Dr. William Glenn has warned of the ease with which one can enter the right ventricle or interventricular septum in the resection of some of these aneurysms.

The induced fibrillatory arrest, we believe, lends itself ideally to this procedure. Not only is added insurance provided against peripheral embolization, but the myocardium is adequately and constantly perfused with oxygenated blood. Visualization is excellent. Suturing is easier.

Most of the clots are laminated. They are generally adherent, but pieces may break off and lodge in the crevices within the ventricular lumen behind the papillary muscles, in and around the mitral valve, and at the opening of the aortic valve. Therefore, I think careful irrigation and inspection at the conclusion of the procedure are indicated.

For several reasons, one should err on the side of not removing quite enough of the aneurysmal wall rather than too much. As will be shown later, one can utilize this extra tissue in suturing the ventricular wall. This is not similar to the ripe-banana-like tissue one sutures in some types of ventricular problem, but this is a very thick, scarred type of tissue through which it is difficult to place the needle, especially if a small cuff of tissue is left.

One mention about ventricular defibrillation. Reliable defibrillation attempts are associated with a well-decompressed ventricle, an evenly oxygenated myocardium, and properly placed electrodes. One must use large enough voltage. Postdefibrillation assist is of definite value.

Dr. Effler might comment perhaps on whether or not he has had any postsurgical embolization problems. We had one to the femoral artery, which I think possibly originated from the suture line.

The magnitude of the problems in coronary artery disease is quite apparent, but less apparent is the growing list of already at least a dozen surgically manageable complications of coronary artery disease. Drs. Effler, Scully, Groves, and Westcott have clearly illustrated that myomalacia with aneurysmal formation is, indeed, amenable to surgical resection with good subsequent results.

Dr. Egbert Fell, Chicago: Our experience is limited to six aneurysms, three congenital, which were resected (all are living normally); three acquired and secondary to coronary artery disease, two of which were encountered at reoperation for mitral stenosis (they were diffuse and inoperable), all three were in the posterior lateral portion of the left ventricle. None of the three gave electrocardiographic evidence of myocardial involvement. The one that was resected measured at its neck 8 cm across its diameter and 12 cm from its origin to the fundus. The patient is doing well two years after resection.

The transverse thoracic incision should be encouraged because of the adequate exposure it gives. The longitudinal, sternal-splitting incision is satisfactory for the small, anterior aneurysm but restrictive when dealing with a large heart having a larger aneurysm on the posterior lateral wall of the left ventricle.

There are patients who are debilitated because of their aneurysms, and it is wise to resect the well-localized aneurysm when diagnosed and before complications arise. We have all seen patients go along a number of years, with an aneurysm, in a semi-invalid state, so we believe the majority should be considered urgent, but not emergency, surgical problems.

Dr. Harris B. Shumacker, Jr., Indianapolis: I am thoroughly in agreement with Dr. Effler that ventricular aneurysms should be treated surgically. I have not as yet had the opportunity to read the paper just referred to. I do recall well, however, another very excellent paper from Chicago by Dr. Katz and his associates. They reviewed, as I recall, 102 cases some years ago. From this study they reached the conclusion that the prognosis was only half as good in the patient with ventricular aneurysm as in the patient with a myocardial infarction without an aneurysm. Most of the patients died of heart failure or thromboembolic difficulties. It is my feeling that it would be inadvisable to wait until symptoms are present.

I have had experience with the operative repair of only four ventricular aneurysms. I have liked the median sternotomy approach very well. One of our patients had an aneurysm which was a great deal larger than the remainder of the heart. We had no difficulty delivering it into the operative field. By holding the apex of the left ventricle up vertically from the horizontal position of the body, we could work upon the area of the aneurysm with ease.

We have been very much interested in the mechanisms responsible for the disability which accompanies so many ventricular aneurysms. My associates and I have investigated in the laboratory two possible explanations. One is the role of paradoxical filling. This, we have been able to show, is a very real factor. We have demonstrated that paradoxical filling of aneurysms produced in the experimental animal definitely depresses left ventricular function. The other, proposed by Dr. Burton of Canada and Dr. Burch of New Orleans, relates to LaPlace's law and certainly seems a logical explanation. We have not been able, however, to obtain any experimental confirmation of its importance in reducing the left ventricular function.

I feel that the repair of left ventricular aneurysms originating from myocardial infarction is a very satisfactory procedure. I hope that our medical colleagues will become more and more persuaded that this operation does indeed offer the patient a great deal. The patient who has been relieved of distressing complaints certainly testifies to its worth.

Dr. Donald B. Effler, Cleveland: As Dr. Ellis reported here, I think the cycle is complete. The first paper written on ventricular aneurysms was a report by John Hunter in 1753. There were a number of isolated reports from that time on by various pathologists. Then I think the first monumental paper was the one referred to by Dr. Shumacker, reporting on 103 cases at autopsy. If the number is wrong I will have to change my text.

The important thing was that throughout all of this the cardiologists decried completely this horrible disease for which there was virtually no treatment, and begged the surgeons for a way out. Now that we have a successful treatment, the cardiologists suggest that the disease is not so bad after all. So, I say, the cycle is complete.

The patients we have operated on have two or three different symptoms in common: (1) congestive failure—each of our patients was hospitalized repeatedly for this; (2) paroxysms of ventricular arrhythmia, again requiring frequent periods of hospitalization, and each time the patient is convinced he is going to die for sure this time. The last, of course, is the ominous threat of embolization.

As far as the selection of candidates is concerned, I think any patient who is shown to have a ventricular aneurysm, who has required hospitalization because of congestive failure or ventricular arrhythmia or embolus, certainly is a candidate for surgery, and to deny him this is inexcusable. All of our patients have been studied by left heart catheterization studies and selective coronary arteriograms. We know they have residual atherosclerosis in their coronaries, and we know they are likely candidates for myocardial infarction again, but we see no reason why this disease, which is in itself a crippling and usually fatal disease, should not be surgically corrected.

One last point. I enjoyed very much Dr. Stevenson's movie. By our current thinking, his aneurysmectomy is not complete. That is the way we started, too, but as we progressed and got a little bolder we are now removing the aneurysm in its entirety. Again, that is a detail.

Also, if you keep the heart elevated anteriorly, in the method Dr. Shumacker mentioned, and put a pillow or pad under it, there is no possibility of embolization because the open ventricle has no output and the competent aortic valve permits you to inspect it at your leisure. If the heart insists on stopping, then of course we complete the aneurysmectomy and defibrillate by direct current countershock.

Dr. D. W. Bussmann, St. Louis: I think that the cardiologist who attempts to interpret auscultation properly, if he keeps himself away from the catheterization laboratory, from the cineangiocardiogram, and from the operating room, is like the physician who stays away from the autopsy room. By the same token, I invite the surgeons to pick up their stethoscopes and join us.

Experimental Replacement of the Cervical Esophagus

DONALD M. HOPKINS, MD, AND PHILIP E. BERNATZ, MD, ROCHESTER, MINN

Replacement of the hypopharynx and cervical portion of the esophagus after resection for a malignant lesion has presented sufficient problems to justify a search for better methods. It has been more than 80 years since Czerny in 1877 first successfully resected a carcinoma from the cervical portion of the esophagus. Since then many ingenious methods of replacement have been devised, but no single method has found general acceptance. Impetus for the use of transplants of isolated segments of hollow viscera to accomplish replacement has been provided by reports of encouraging success with anastomoses of small vessels.

Jacobson and Suarez described excellent results with microsuturing techniques and demonstrated the feasibility of successfully anastomosing vessels as small as 1.4 mm in outside diameter. Good results have recently been reported [3,19,24] from use of the nonsuture method of Blakemore and Lord with cylinder prostheses. Holt and Lewis have devised a successful method using small rings and pins; their method has been modified and has been applied clinically by Nakayama and associates. New plastic adhesives have given encouraging results.[4,9,17] Circumferential stapling instruments developed independently by Androsov and Inokuchi [12,13] are ingenious devices which hold much promise for the future. Other workers have now developed similar instruments.[21,22,25]

Recent developments in the field of organ transplantation have stimulated consideration of free transplants of the hollow viscera to replace the esophagus in the neck. Seidenberg and co-workers in 1959 reported the first successful free transplants of jejunum in four dogs. They also reported the first clinical application. Unfortunately the patient died because of a cerebrovascular accident on the seventh postoperative day.[20] In the last three years, four other clinical cases in which jejunum was used have been reported. The two patients of Roberts and Douglass were doing well three months and six days after operation. Iskeceli attempted replacement in two patients, but both attempts failed because of venous thrombosis. Hiebert and Cummings reported a 3½-month follow-up on a free transplant of the antral portion of the stomach using the right gastroepiploic vessels for revascularization. Most recently Nakayama and associates reported the successful transplantation of a portion of the sigmoid colon in five patients, one of whom had a five-month follow-up. The feasibility of a free transplant of a segment of the gastrointestinal tract has been demonstrated by the authors mentioned. It therefore seemed pertinent to us to attempt to ascertain which portion of the gastrointestinal tract would be best suited for this purpose.

Materials and Methods

In our study we used 34 healthy mongrel dogs of both sexes ranging in weight from 12 to 25 kg. These dogs were divided into three groups: 7 for stomach-tube transplants, 11 for transplants of the terminal portion of the ileum, and 16 for colon transplants. Operations were carried out with the animals under intravenous pentobarbital anesthesia.

A segment of the cervical portion of the esophagus was excised. The external jugular vein (EJV) and the common carotid artery (CCA) were isolated and cleared of their adventitia in preparation for subsequent anastomosis with the vessels of the transplant. The abdomen was opened, and a segment approximately 10 cm in length was selected for transplantation. The gastric tube was con-

Presented as the 20th Annual Meeting of the Central Surgical Association, Chicago, Feb 21-23, 1963.

Fellow in Thoracic Surgery, Mayo Foundation (Dr. Hopkins), Section of Surgery (Dr. Bernatz), Mayo Clinic and Mayo Foundation.

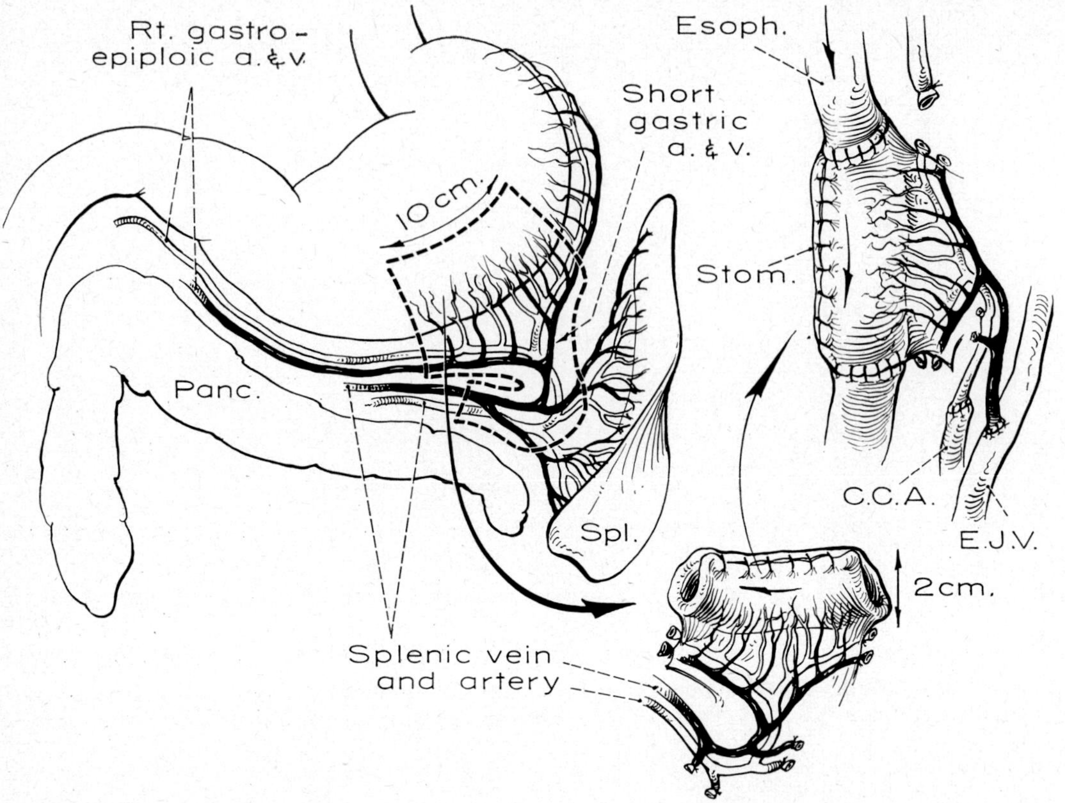

Fig 1.—Technique for creating and transplanting a stomach tube from the greater curvature. The greater omentum has been trimmed away.

structed by outlining it with clamps, excising the portion of the greater curvature and creating a tube as shown in Fig 1. The segment for the ileal transplants (Fig 2) was selected by the demonstration of vessels of sufficient size for anastomosis (outside diameter of 2.0 mm for the artery and of 3.0 mm for the vein). Vessels to the ileal transplants were, on the whole, significantly smaller than those supplying the other two types of transplant. In preparing the colon transplants, the sigmoid artery was isolated just distal to the branching of the superior hemorrhoidal artery, and the marginal vein was dissected out at a convenient location proximally so that a 10 cm segment of bowel could be resected (Fig 3). The segment was isolated by means of appropriate clamps. Neomycin (400 mg dissolved in 30 ml of saline solution) was then injected into the lumen and left for 15 minutes prior to resection. Prior to the surgical procedure, the bowel was prepared by fasting the animals for two days and giving each an ounce of castor oil. The colon was irrigated with tap water after the dog was anesthetized.

In each transplant, the artery was ligated first to prevent congestion. In 21 dogs, vascular anastomosis in the neck was accomplished by the Blakemore-Lord method as described by Urschel and Roth. Suturing technique with continuous No. 7-0 cardiovascular silk (Fig 4) was used for the remaining 13, with end-to-end anastomosis of the arteries performed by beveling the smaller artery to compensate for the disparity in size, and with end-to-side anastomosis of the veins. A caliper and a millimeter rule were used to estimate the outside diameter of the arteries and veins of each dog. The arteries of the transplanted segments averaged 2.5 mm in outside diameter (range, 2.0 to 3.0 mm); the veins, 4.5 mm (range, 3.0 mm to 6.0 mm). Flow was allowed simultaneously through both the artery and the vein. The dogs were then heparinized with 1 to 2 mg of heparin per kilogram of body weight. The revascularized segment was sutured end-to-end to the esophagus above and below. The stomach tube and ileum transplants were placed in the neck isoperistaltically (Fig 1 and 2); the colon segments, however, were placed antiperistaltically, largely because the vascular anastomoses could be accomplished more conveniently (Fig 3).

For the first week after operation all dogs were given 600,000 units of procaine penicillin and 0.5 gm of streptomycin intramuscularly twice daily, 1 to 2 mg of heparin per kilogram of body weight intravenously every six hours, and 500 to 1,000 ml

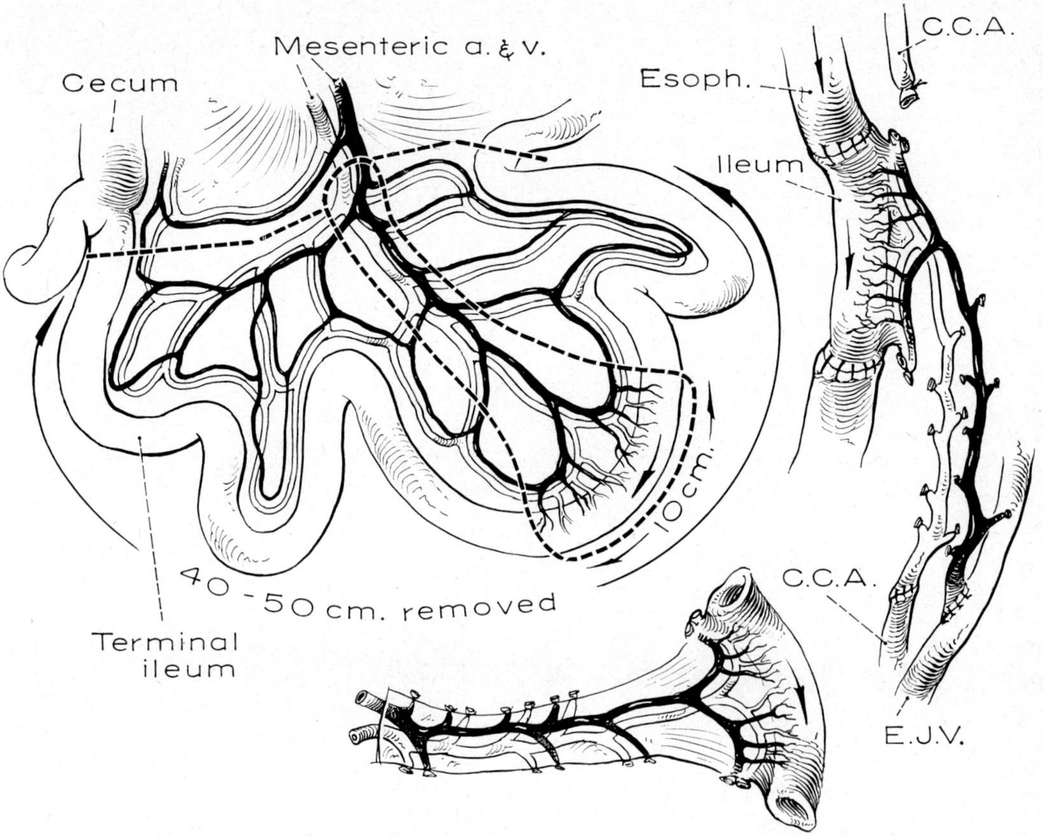

Fig 2.—Technique for transplanting a segment of the terminal portion of the ileum. To obtain vessels as large as possible for anastomosis, it is usually necessary to resect some of the adjacent bowel.

of fluids subcutaneously or intravenously every 24 hours. The survivors were given oral liquid feeding during the second week and were put on kennel rations thereafter.

The eating habits, weight and diet of the surviving dogs were studied subsequently. Esophagoscopic examinations were performed at periodic intervals, and specimens of mucosa from the transplant were removed for histologic study. The pH of the mucosal surface was determined by touching the mucosa of the transplant with indicator paper. Visualization of the segments was accomplished by cineroentgenography as the dogs swallowed milk or dog food mixed with barium. The motility of the transplants was studied by recording intraluminal pressures according to the method described by Carveth and associates.[5,6] Vessels supplying the transplanted segments were visualized by angiographic studies.

Results

Six dogs survived and were available for studies of esophageal function for periods of 6 to 17 months. Five others died in the early postoperative period. Necropsy showed viable transplants with patent anastomoses of vessels. In the remaining 23 dogs the transplants failed to take because of venous occlusion in ten, arterial occlusion in four, and occlusion of both veins and arteries in nine.

Two of the 21 dogs in which the Blakemore-Lord method of vessel anastomosis was used were long-term survivors. Better results were obtained in the 13 dogs in which vascular anastomoses were done by suture. Four of these became long-term survivors, and three others were in the group that died in the early postoperative period with viable transplants.

One of the seven dogs having stomach-tube transplants survived. Despite a troublesome early postoperative fistula at the site of proximal anastomosis, this dog has done well for 14 months. Cineroentgenography has

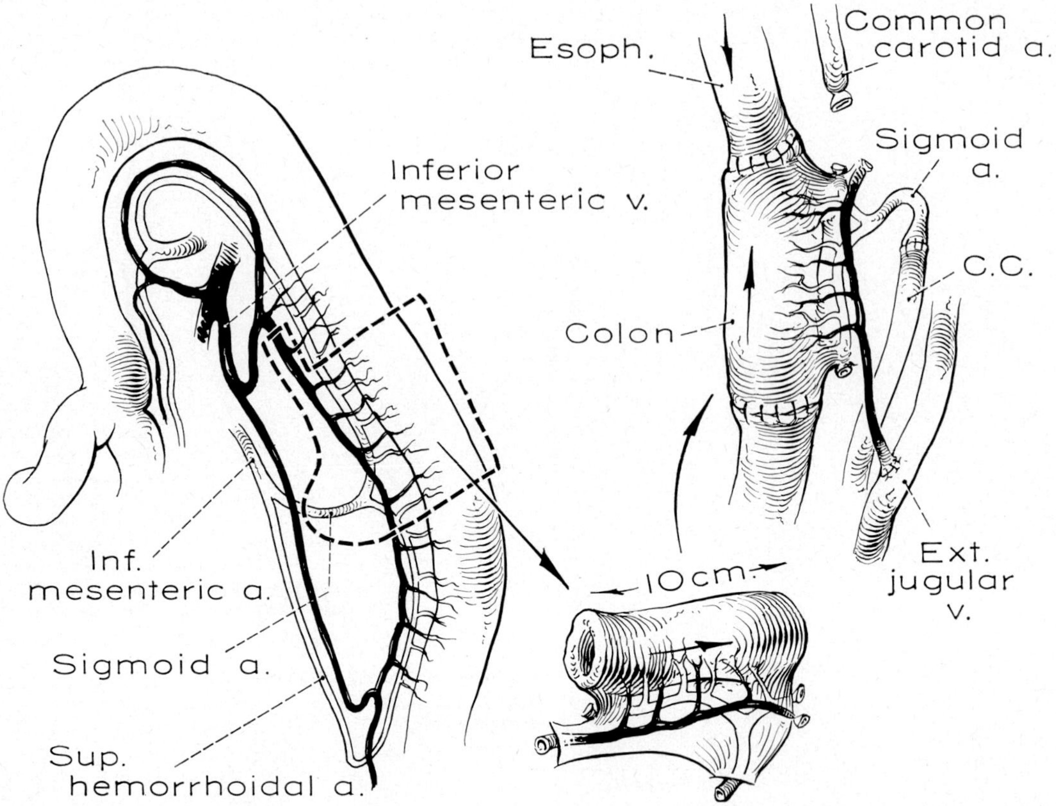

Fig 3.—Technique for transplanting a segment of the sigmoid colon. The superior hemorrhoidal artery is not disturbed. Note that the transplant is placed in the neck in the antiperistaltic direction.

shown good function with only minimal difficulty in swallowing solid foods. The dog's weight, although 20% below its preoperative weight, has remained stable on the regular kennel diet. While fasting a pH value of 5.0 was recorded at the mucosal surface of the transplanted segment 12 months after transplantation. On esophagoscopy the mucosa appeared like that of the normal stomach. Esophagitis was not noted. Biopsies showed normal gastric mucosa. Histopathologic changes were not seen in the parietal or chief cells (Fig 5*a*).

Fig 4.—Close-up of vessel anastomoses 10 months after operation in a dog with an ileal transplant with a continuous suture of No. 7-0 cardiovascular silk. The end-to-side anastomosis of the vein is shown below and the opened end-to-end arterial anastomosis is shown at the tip of the black arrow.

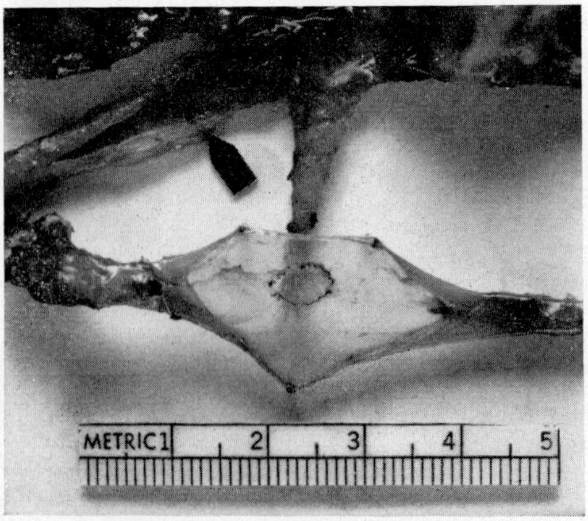

A segment of the terminal ileum was transplanted in 11 dogs; only two survived. In both survivors, swallowing of solid food was continuously difficult. Esophagoscopy and cineroentgenography demonstrated narrowing of the entire length of these segments. At the time of cineroentgenography study, solid food could not be seen to pass beyond the proximal anastomosis. On mechanical irritation caused by solid food, esophagoscopic manipulation, or, particularly, the removal of specimens of mucosa for biopsy, the segments demonstrated considerable spasm. Through the esophagoscope, the mucosa appeared reddened and bled easily on slightest trauma. Biopsy specimens showed moderate inflammatory changes with some fibrosis. There was fusion and loss of some of the villi with focal areas of mucosal ulceration (Fig 5*b*). One dog maintained its pre-

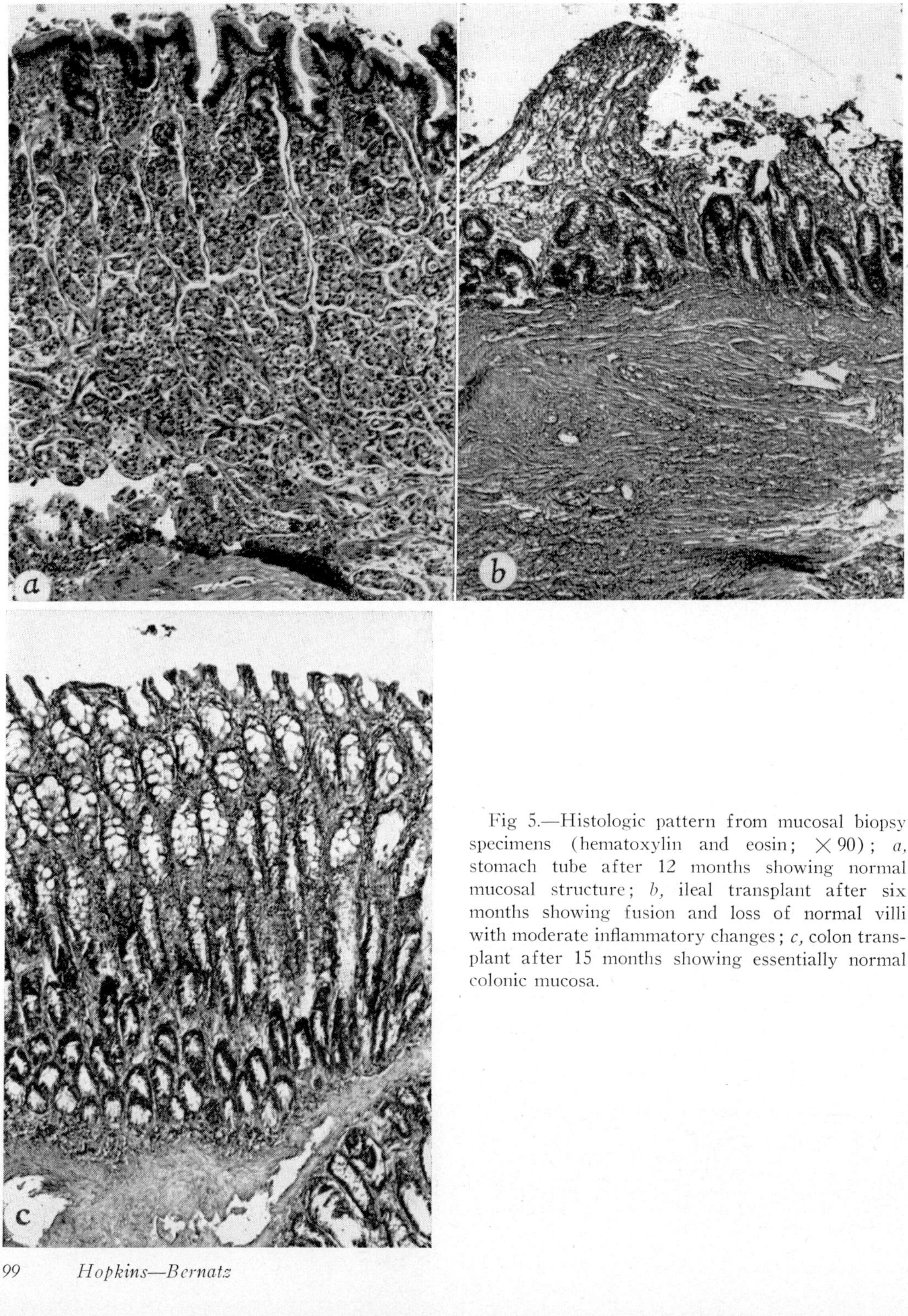

Fig 5.—Histologic pattern from mucosal biopsy specimens (hematoxylin and eosin; ×90); *a*, stomach tube after 12 months showing normal mucosal structure; *b*, ileal transplant after six months showing fusion and loss of normal villi with moderate inflammatory changes; *c*, colon transplant after 15 months showing essentially normal colonic mucosa.

operative weight, but a milk supplement was necessary. It died of indeterminate intrathoracic hemorrhage six months after operation. The other dog lost 40% of its preoperative weight despite supplements of milk. It died ten months after operation, and necropsy showed a mucosal prolapse protruding through the distal anastomosis. This prolapse had caused partial obstruction, and the dog had died of aspiration pneumonitis.

Three of the 16 dogs having colon transplants were long-term survivors. These three dogs had the least difficulty swallowing solid food. Cineroentgenography showed ready

Fig 6.—Esophageal motility in ileal replacement for cervical esophagus. Recording of intraluminal pressure made one month after operation. The three pressure detectors are located 5 cm apart and 24 cm, 29 cm, and 34 cm, respectively, from the upper incisor teeth. Note that in the three pressure detectors the swallowing complexes represented by the spiked waves occur simultaneously. This is characteristic of an inert tube. The normal progressive peristaltic pattern is lacking. Characteristic rhythmic ileal contractions, type I, occurring 16 times per minute, were recorded from the middle detector in the center of the ileal segment.

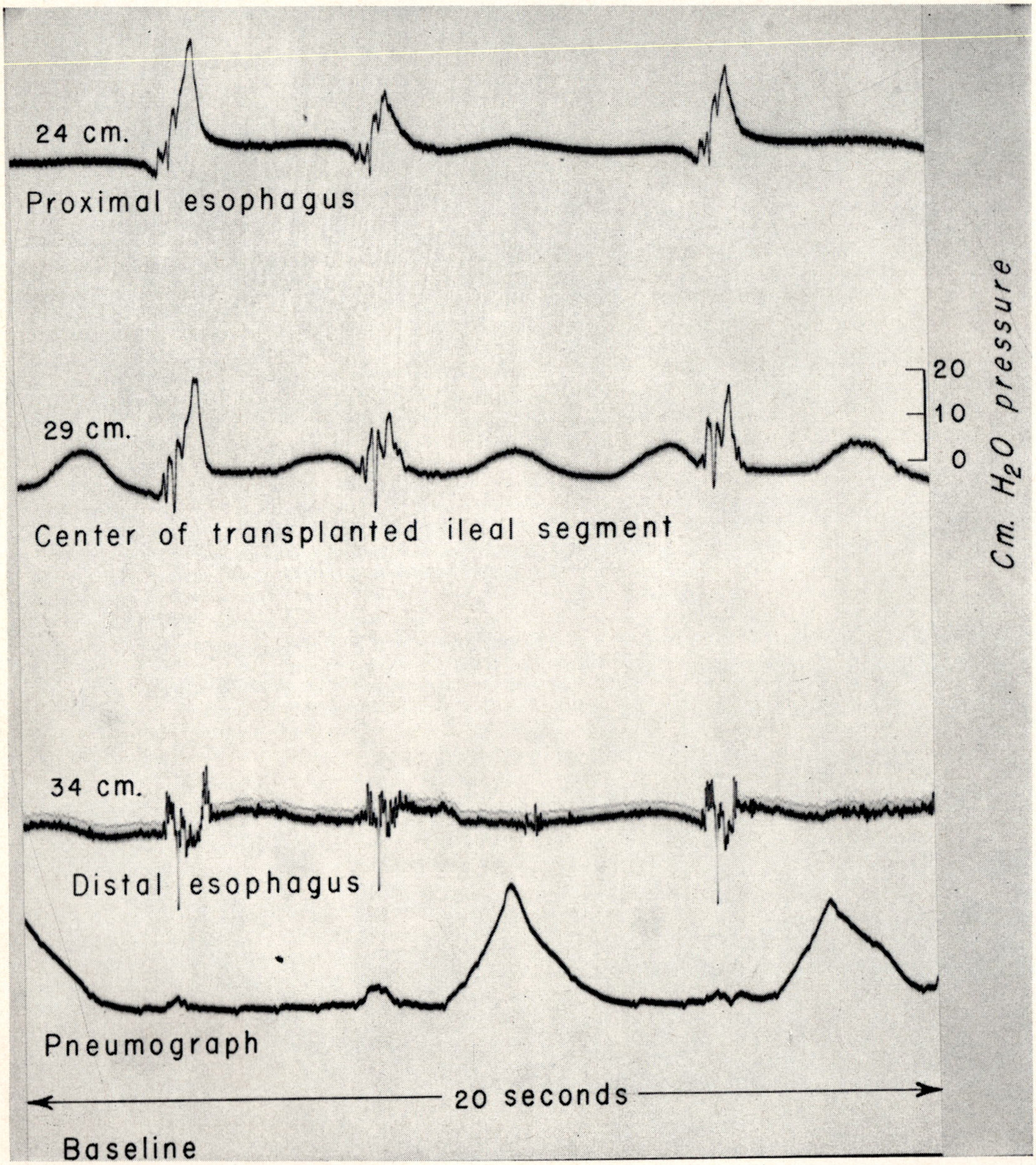

passage of barium mixtures through the transplanted segments. Anastomotic strictures developed in two dogs, but they were easily corrected by dilatation. Normal colonic mucosa was seen at esophagoscopy. The biopsy specimens showed no abnormalities (Fig 5*c*). Weight was maintained with the kennel diet alone except when a stricture was developing. One dog is doing well 17 months after operation. Although the other two dogs were doing well, they both died (nine months and one year after operation, respectively) as a result of technical difficulties during angiography.

Intraluminal pressure recordings of the segments and the remainder of the esophagus showed that in each dog the swallowing waves were not transmitted through the transplants in the normal peristaltic fashion; instead the deglutitory responses within the transplant occurred virtually simultaneously with those in the pharynx, as though these segments were inert tubes. The pressure responses of the pharyngoesophageal junction, the peristaltic deglutitory waves in the esophagus distal to the transplant, and the pressure profile of the esophagogastric junction were normal in all six dogs. As is characteristic of the normal ileum and colon, motility of these transplanted segments was sporadic and could be recorded infrequently when the dogs were in the fasting state.[7] In both dogs with ileal transplants, occasional periods of rhythmic waves were recorded from within the segments; these were characteristic of type I ileal contractions (Fig 6 and 7). The characteristic type II contractions of the pelvic colon [26] were recorded from the transplanted colon segment of one dog 12 months after operation (Fig 8). No motor activity was recorded from the stomach-tube transplant.

Angiography demonstrated the patency of the arterial and venous anastomoses of the transplants and showed some venous collateral drainage (Fig 9, *a* and *b*). These procedures were not without risk, as noted previously. In one colon transplant in which

Fig 7.—Esophageal motility in ileal replacement for cervical esophagus. Recording of intraluminal pressure made seven months after operation. *Left,* spontaneous ileal activity, type I, recorded from the center of the transplant (34 cm); *Right,* ileal activity, type I (34 cm), recorded ten minutes after the intravenous injection of 15 mg of morphine sulfate. In both instances the rate of contractions was 14 per minute.

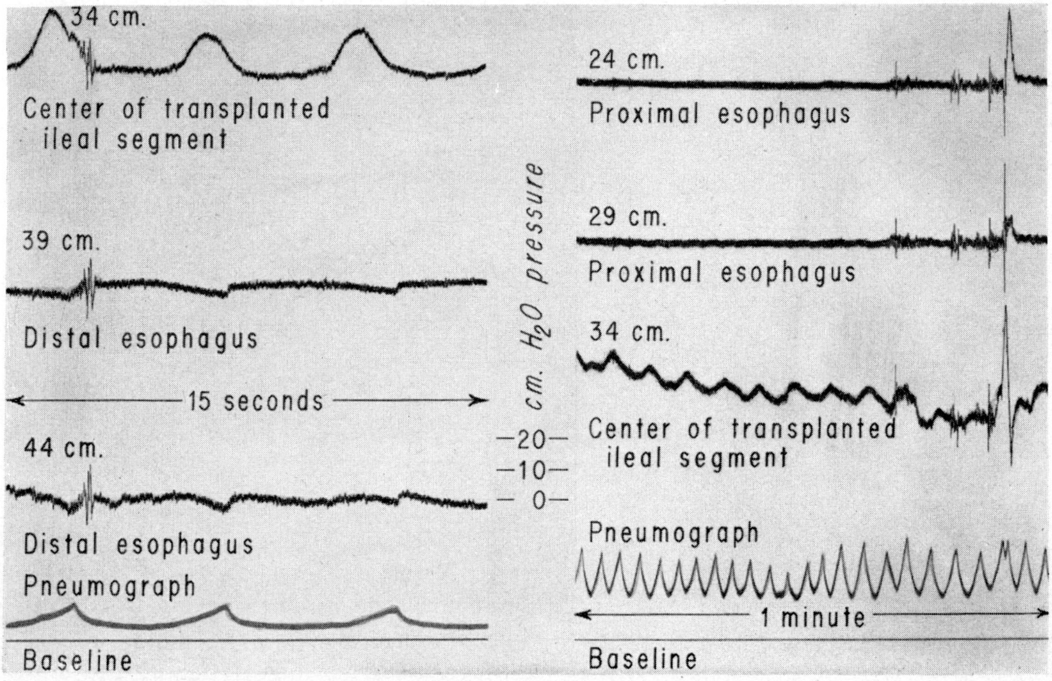

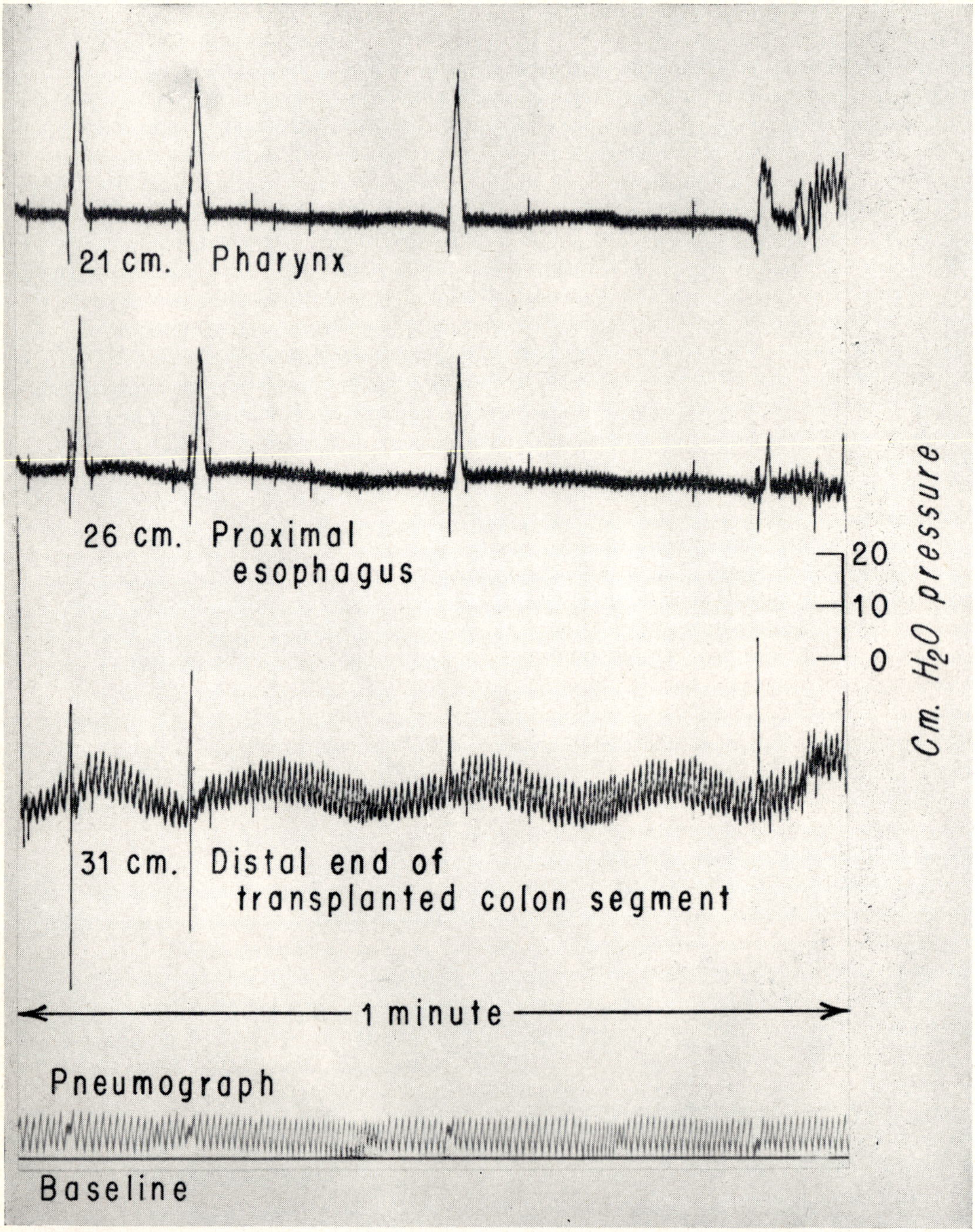

Fig 8.—Esophageal motility in colon replacement for cervical esophagus. Recording of intraluminal pressure four minutes after intravenous injection of morphine sulfate showing contractions from the center of the transplanted colonic segment (31 cm) at a rate of four per minute. These waves are similar to the type II waves detected from the pelvic colon of normal dogs, although their amplitude is not as high.

the angiogram was made during the injection of radiopaque dye directly into the common carotid artery, the artery subsequently thrombosed, resulting in slough of the mucosa in the central third of the transplanted segment and causing formation of a fistula, stricture, and death (Fig 10). Thus, even after one year, the viability of the transplant ap-

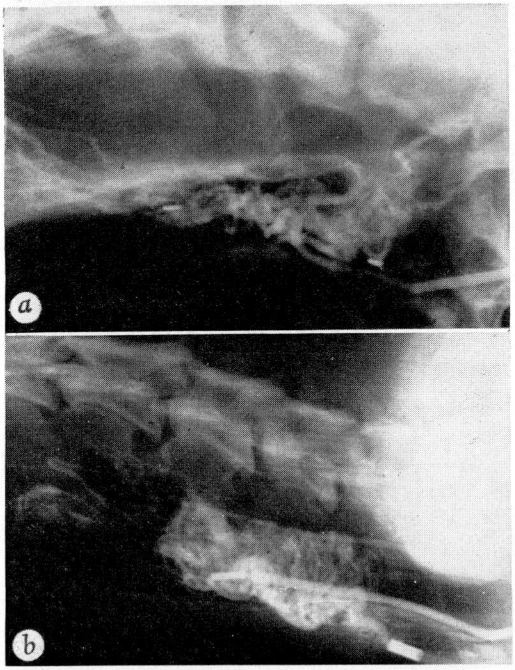

Fig 9.—Angiograms of dogs with colonic transplant. In both instances some venous collateral circulation was evident at both ends of the transplanted segment. The dye was injected through a catheter which had been threaded up into the carotid artery via a cut-down in the femoral artery. *a,* Transplant nine months after operation. The vessel anastomoses, performed by suturing technique, are both patent. The silver clips show the proximal and distal esophagocolic anastomoses (*left* and *right,* respectively). *b,* transplant 11 months after operation. Vessel anastomoses were done by the Blakemore-Lord method with stainless-steel cylinder prostheses. Contrast media is evident in the anastomoses of the artery (*left*) and the vein (*right*). The transplanted segment is outlined by the dense vascular pattern.

parently was dependent on the anastomosed vessel for its supply of arterial blood.

Comment

The feasibility of replacing the cervical portion of the esophagus with a transplanted segment of a hollow viscus has been demonstrated. The reliability of this technique depends largely on the consistent success of anastomoses of vessels considerably smaller than those commonly anastomosed in patients at the present time. Formidable problems will always be encountered in relation to this procedure, but experience with special methods of suturing, along with the availability of appropriate suture material, has moved the successful anastomoses of these small vessels from the realm of possibility to one where practical application is reasonable. The use of mechanical suture or nonsuture methods may result in more consistently successful anastomoses of such small vessels.

With respect to the ability of the individual segments of the gastrointestinal tract to act as conduits in the esophagus, spasm was encountered in the ileal transplants with resultant functional obstruction. A similar reaction has been recorded by Torbey and Waddell who noted obstructing spasm in short segments of denervated ileum interposed into the colon of the dog. From our observations, the ileum seemed poorly suited for use in replacing a portion of the esophagus. The stomach tube and colon transplants seemed to function as conduits without participating in the orderly motility usually associated with the act of swallowing.

Fig 10.—Specimen of colon transplant removed at necropsy (12 months after operation). The epiglottis, larynx, and a short segment of the trachea are shown at the upper right. The esophagocolic anastomoses are shown at the tips of the large arrows. The mucosa is denuded over the central third of the transplant. The small arrow shows the opening of the fistula, and stricture in this region is evident. The carotid artery was thrombosed as a result of introduction of the needle to obtain an angiogram two weeks previously.

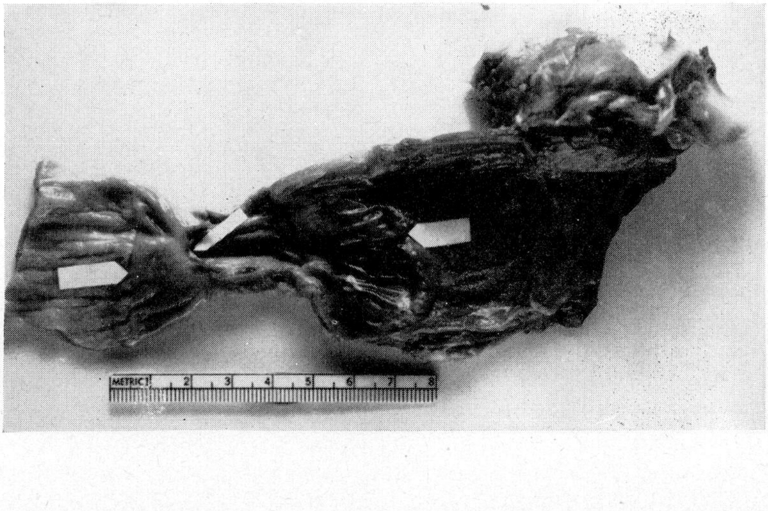

Our motility studies demonstrated that the transplanted segments retained the activity patterns inherent to the part of the gastrointestinal tract from which they originated. The colon segments were placed antiperistaltically, which seemed to make no practical difference; this has been true also of pedicle transplants of the left portion of the colon utilized to replace the entire esophagus.

It would be convenient if a plastic prosthesis could be used to bridge this defect in the cervical portion of the esophagus, but although our experience in the laboratory has included a variety of prostheses, we have been discouraged in our search for one which we could employ with reasonably consistent success.

The colon segments with vessels of convenient size provided the most successful transplants from all aspects. Although the stomach-tube segment functioned almost as well, the surgical procedure was more laborious and time consuming. More experience is obviously needed, but we have concluded from our limited studies that the clinical use of a free segment of colon, probably from the midtransverse or descending colon, is reasonable and offers good possibilities of becoming an accepted procedure in the replacement of the cervical portion of the esophagus and the hypopharynx. The recent report by Nakayama and associates supports this conclusion.

Summary

Free transplants of segments of stomach, ileum, and colon have been utilized successfully to replace the cervical portion of the esophagus in dogs. Experience in technique as well as studies of function in six surviving dogs indicate some advantage in the use of a transplanted colon segment over transplantation of segments from the ileum and stomach.

Mayo Clinic, Rochester, Minn.

REFERENCES

1. Androsov, P. I.: New Method of Surgical Treatment of Blood Vessel Lesions, AMA Arch Surg 73:902-910 (Dec) 1956.

2. Blakemore, A. H., and Lord, J. W., Jr.: A Nonsuture Method of Blood Vessel Anastomosis: Experimental and Clinical Study, JAMA 127:685-691 (March 24); 748-753 (March 31) 1945.

3. Carter, P. D.: Suture and Nonsuture Methods of Small Vein Anastomosis: A Comparison of Methods of Small Vein Anastomosis, Arch Surg 84:350-352 (March) 1962.

4. Carton, C. A.; Kessler, L. A.; Seidenberg, B.; and Hurwitt, E. S.: Experimental Studies in the Surgery of Small Blood Vessels: IV. Nonsuture Anastomosis of Arteries and Veins, Using Flanged Ring Prostheses and Plastic Adhesive, Surg Forum 11:238-239, 1960.

5. Carveth, S. W.: Motor Action of the Canine Esophagus and Gastroesophageal Sphincter After Muscle and Nerve Interruption Procedures, Thesis, Graduate School, University of Minnesota, 1961.

6. Carveth, S. W.; Schlegel, J. F.; Code, C. F.; and Ellis, F. H., Jr.: Esophageal Motility After Vagotomy, Phrenicotomy, Myotomy, and Myomectomy in Dogs, Surg Gynec Obstet 114:31-42 (Jan) 1962.

7. Code, C. F.; Wilkinson, G. R., Jr.; and Sauer, W. G.: Normal and Some Abnormal Colonic Motor Patterns in Man, Ann NY Acad Sci 58:317-335 (July 15) 1954.

8. Czerny: Neue Operationen, Zbl Chir 4:433-434 (July 14) 1877.

9. Healey, J. E., Jr.; Moore, E. B.; Brooks, B. F.; and Sheena, K. S.: A Vascular Clamp for Circumferential Repair of Blood Vessels, Surgery 51:452-455 (April) 1962.

10. Hiebert, C. A., and Cummings, G. O., Jr.: Successful Replacement of the Cervical Esophagus by Transplantation and Revascularization of a Free Graft of Gastric Antrum, Ann Surg 154:103-106 (July) 1961.

11. Holt, G. P., and Lewis, F. J.: A New Technique for End-to-End Anastomosis of Small Arteries, Surg Forum 11:242-243, 1960.

12. Inokuchi, K.: A New Type of Vessel-Suturing Apparatus, AMA Arch Surg 77:954-957 (Dec) 1958.

13. Inokuchi, K.: Stapling Device for End-to-Side Anastomosis of Blood Vessel, Arch Surg 82:337-341 (March) 1961.

14. Iskeceli, O. K.: The Use of Free Jejunal Segments in the Reconstruction of Cervical Esophageal Defects, Surgery 51:496-502 (April) 1962.

15. Jacobson, J. H., II, and Suarez, E. L.: Microsurgery in Anastomosis of Small Vessels, Surg Forum 11:243-245, 1960.

16. Nakayama, K.; Tamiya, T.; Yamamoto, K.; and Akimoto, S.: A Simple New Apparatus for Small Vessel Anastomosis (Free Autograft of the Sigmoid Included), Surgery 52:918-931 (Dec) 1962.

17. Nathan, H. S.; Nachlas, M. M.; Solomon, R. D.; Halpern, B. D.; and Seligman, A. M.: Nonsuture Closure of Arterial Incisions Using a

Rapidly-Polymerizing Adhesive, Ann Surg 152:648-659 (Oct) 1960.

18. Roberts, R. E., and Douglass, F. M.: Replacement of the Cervical Esophagus and Hypopharynx by a Revascularized Free Jejunal Autograft, New Engl J Med 264:342-344 (Feb 16) 1961.

19. Rohman, M.; Goetz, R. H.; and Dee, R.: Double Coronary Artery-Internal Mammary Artery Anastomoses: Tantalum Ring Technique, Surg Forum 11:236-237, 1960.

20. Seidenberg, B.; Rosenak, S. S.; Hurwitt, E. S.; and Som, M. L.: Immediate Reconstruction of the Cervical Esophagus by a Revascularized Isolated Jejunal Segment, Ann Surg 149:162-171 (Feb) 1959.

21. Sterling, J. A.: Experimental Use of an Apparatus for Stapling Small Blood Vessels, J Einstein Med Cent 7:192-193 (July) 1959.

22. Takaro, T.: A Simple Stapling Device for the Anastomosis of Blood Vessels, J Thorac Cardiov Surg 40:673-684 (Nov) 1960.

23. Torbey, K., and Waddell, W. R.: Function of the Colon After Removal of Anal Sphincters and Replacement by Denervated Ileal Segments: An Experimental Study, Ann Surg 154:424-431 (Sept) 1961.

24. Urschel, H. C., Jr., and Roth, E. J.: Small Arterial Anastomoses: I. Nonsuture, Ann Surg 153:599-610 (April) 1961.

25. Vogelfanger, I. J.; Beattie, W. G.; Brown, F. N.; DeVitt, J. E.; Scobie, T. K.; and Scobie, D. H: The Problem of Small Vessel Anastomosis, Surgery 52:354-361 (Aug) 1962.

26. Wilkinson, G. R., Jr.: The Influence of Morphine and Several Synthetic Non-Addicting Morphine-Like Substances on Pelvic Colon Motility in the Dog and Man, thesis, Graduate School, University of Minnesota, 1956.

Esophageal Prosthesis for Palliative Intubation

Further Evaluation of 378 Patients

THOMAS O'CONNOR, MD; RAYMOND WATSON, MD; DERWARD LEPLEY, JR., MD; AND WILSON WEISEL, MD, MILWAUKEE

What Homer wrote of the Lotus Eaters, he might as well have written of patients with carcinoma of the esophagus—"and the men waste day by day with slow disease and withering undelight."

Sweet, Garlock, MacManus,[18,6,7,12] and others have developed operations which, when applicable, have achieved gratifying results in this most ungratifying of diseases. Unfortunately, about one half of the patients with carcinoma of the esophagus have inoperable cancers when first seen by the surgeons. And of those explored, only about one half will have resectable lesions. Thus, for 75 out of 100 patients with this disease, we are faced with the grim reality that the best we can offer is palliation.

Presented at the 20th Annual Meeting of the Central Surgical Association, Chicago, Feb 21-23, 1963.

From the Division of Surgery, Department of Thoracic and Cardiovascular Surgery, Marquette University School of Medicine.

Gastrostomy, x-ray therapy, various bypass operations, and tube prostheses inserted through the carcinoma all are methods of palliation employed in the case of the inoperable or unresectable esophageal carcinoma. Since obstruction is the prime difficulty that must be overcome, any form of palliation should allow the patient to handle his salivary secretions and to maintain his nutrition in as near normal a fashion as possible. Of course, the method employed should not contribute to his discomfort or hasten his death. Gastrostomy is considered by most an undesirable palliative procedure. It does not solve the problem of the salivary secretations; it deprives the patient of the pleasure of normal alimentation; and in the debilitated patient with an advanced carcinoma it is associated with a mortality of over 30%. Bypass operations are associated with mortality rates reported to be in excess of over 40%. This seems to be an unreasonable risk when the objective is palliation.

X-ray therapy is unpredictable in its results, and the incidence of complications with this modality is better than 10%. In addition, x-ray therapy requires prolonged treatment during which a patient often can swallow neither saliva nor food. For these reasons, since 1948, the thoracic surgery service at Marquette University has employed polyethylene tube prostheses as a method of palliation in patients with inoperable or unresectable esophageal obstructions.

The total experience with this method up to January, 1963, is comprised of 388 patients. Seventy-three patients of this group were lost to follow-up after discharge from the hospital. Data are complete on the remaining 315 patients. There were 355 males and 33 females in this series. The patients ranged in age from 40 to 87 years. Ten of the patients had benign strictures that had not responded to periodic dilation. These patients were considered inoperable because of associated cardiac, renal, or pulmonary disease. The diagnosis in the remaining 378 patients was carcinoma.

The obstructions were located in the upper third of the esophagus in 48 patients, the middle third in 169, and the distal third in 171.

The prosthesis was positioned at the time of thoracotomy in 42 patients when an unresectable lesion was encountered. The remaining cases successfully treated with this method were intubated transorally without thoracotomy utilizing a method previously described. Initially, the majority of the transoral intubations were done under general anesthesia. It is a rare patient, now, that requires more than topical 4% cocaine anesthesia.

Complications occurred in 64 cases, an incidence of 16.7%. Postintubation temperature elevations above 100 F (37.8 C) were seen in 32 patients. This elevation of temperature was attributed to mediastinal contamination. None of these patients required more than conservative treatment. Eleven patients could not be intubated. Nine prostheses became dislodged and had to be repositioned. There were six postintubation obstructions. Five of these resulted from poorly masticated food particles, and one was the result of carcinomatous overgrowth. The esophagus was perforated in four patients. Complications of the esophageal perforation resulted in the patients' death in two cases. These two deaths were the only deaths directly attributable to this method of palliation. Two patients, whose lesions were in the proximal third of the esophagus, developed symptoms of moderate tracheal obstruction following intubation with acrylic tubes. In both, the obstruction was relieved when the acrylic tubes were replaced with less-rigid polyethylene prostheses.

Satisfactory palliation with respect to salivary secretion and oral alimentation was achieved in all of the patients successfully intubated. The average length of time of survival following intubation was eight months. The longest survival was 18 months.

Case 1.—This was a 68-year-old male with an obstructing squamous cell carcinoma of the upper one third of the esophagus. In addition to the almost total obstruction, the carcinoma had also eroded the trachea resulting in a tracheoesophageal fistula. A 13 cm polyethylene tube was inserted transorally through the lesion. Methylglucamine diatrizoate (Gastrografin) study following intubation demonstrated that the tube had not completely bridged the fistula. The tube was satisfactorily repositioned, and the patient was able to maintain a satisfactory nutritional status by oral alimentation without episodes of recurrent pneumonitis up to the day he died 18 months later. At autopsy, a malignant erosive lesion of the esophageal wall, 4-5 cm in length, was found to be bridged by the plastic prosthetic device.

Discussion

The technique of intubation and the method of fashioning the polyethylene tubes were described previously and will not be repeated.[20] To obtain the best function, we have found that the optimum length of the prosthesis is between 8 and 12 cm. However, we have used tubes up to 25 cm in length with satisfactory functional results. A properly placed tube will extend 2 cm proximal and 2 cm distal to the gross extent of the lesion, and this is taken into account when the length of the prosthesis is determined. This determination is made by directly measuring the extent of the defect seen on the esophagram, and it is verified immediately prior to intubation by means of endoscopic examination.

The position of the prosthesis may be checked via methylglucamine diatrizoate swallow the afternoon of intubation, and oral feedings may be begun the morning after the insertion of the tube.

With the exception of certain cases of scirrhous carcinoma, or patients with extensive postirradiation fibrosis, the thermolabile polyethylene tubes are rigid enough to be inserted through the obstruction without being compressed by it and resilient enough to accommodate to the slope of the obstruction. In these cases either a Mackler tube or an acrylic tube similar in design to the polyethylene prosthesis is used. In this group, it was necessary to use a Mackler [11] tube in three patients and an acrylic tube in four.

The problem of the tube dislodging or migrating has, in our experience, been infrequently encountered. When this occurs, the tube is easily repositioned. We have not found it necessary to utilize the "screw" tubes of Sachs [16] or the double-flanged tube designed by Mousseau-Barbin.[21] This latter tube has the disadvantage that it requires gastrostomy to position it satisfactorily. While most of the intubations in this group of patients were carried out without thoracotomy, this method can certainly be applied successfully, as it was in 42 patients, at the time of operation when a nonresectable lesion is encountered, and it can be done with less mortality than a palliative bypass procedure.

After the prosthesis has been satisfactorily positioned and oral alimentation begun, there are certain precautions which must be taken to assure continued satisfactory function of the tube. The patient must understand that although he can eat virtually any type of food he desires, the food must be very thoroughly masticated, and the bolus, when swallowed, must be accompanied by a generous quantity of liquid. If these precautions are not observed diligently, the lumen of the tube will plug. Occasionally, when this occurs, the obstructing food particle can be dislodged by the ingestion of an effervescent beverage. Most often, however, the particle must be removed through an esophagoscope. This need for complete mastication of food does not preclude the use of this method of palliation in those patients who have neither their own teeth nor a properly functioning set of dentures if their diet consists of pureed foods.

Conclusions

1. The results of the experience in this group of patients indicate that the use of a polyethylene tube inserted through an obstructing lesion of the esophagus is a satisfactory method of palliation.

2. The ease with which these tubes can be inserted under topical anesthesia makes this method readily available to anyone trained in endoscopy and eliminates the hazard of general anesthesia in debilitated, poor-risk patients.

3. The low incidence of mortality and morbidity would seem to recommend this method of palliation ahead of gastrostomy, bypass operations, and x-ray therapy in the treatment of inoperable or unresectable esophageal obstructions.

4. The objections to the insertion of a prosthesis via an esophagoscope, namely, that it is a blind procedure in an old patient, that perforation of the esophagus is a considerable hazard, and that the tube frequently migrates proximally or distally, have, in our experience, been found to be in a large measure unwarranted.

Thomas O'Connor, MD, Division of Surgery, Marquette University School of Medicine, Milwaukee, Wis.

REFERENCES

1. Allison, P. R., and Borrie, J.: The Treatment of Malignant Obstruction of the Cardia, Brit J Surg 37:1, 1949.

2. Berman, E. F.: The Experimental Replacement of Portions of the Esophagus by a Plastic Tube, Ann Surg 135:337, 1952.

3. Brown, A. L.: Carcinoma of the Esophagus: Use of Rigid Indwelling Esophageal Tube, J Thorac Cardiov Surg 18:493, 1949.

4. Carter, M. G., in discussion on Mackler and Mayer.[11]

5. Davidson, J. S.: Puncture of the Cervical Esophagus in the Palliative Treatment of Carcinoma of the Esophagus, J Thorac Cardiov Surg 30:348, 1955.

6. Garlock, J. H.: Combined Abdominothoracic Approach for Carcinoma of Cardia and Lower Esophagus, Surg Gynec Obstet 83:737, 1946.

7. Garlock, J. H., and Kline, S. H.: The Surgical Treatment of Carcinoma of the Esophagus and Cardia, Ann Surg 139:19, 1954.

8. Greening, W. P., and Ramsay, S. S.: Cancer of the Oesophagus, Palliation by Intubation, Lancet 2:1122, 1960.

9. Heimlich, H. J.: Two Palliative Operations for Cancer of the Esophagus Using Plastic Prosthesis, Amer J Surg 103:376, 1962.

10. Krishaber, M.: De la sonde oesophagienne à demeure, International Medical Congress Transactions, London: J. W. Kolckmann, 1881, vol 2, p 393.

11. Mackler, S. A., and Mayer, R. M.: Palliation of Esophageal Obstruction Due to Carcinoma With a Permanent Intraluminal Tube, J Thorac Cardiov Surg 28:431, 1954.

12. MacManus, J. E.: Esophageal Resections, Amer J Surg 84:61, 1952.

13. Parker, E. F., and Brockington, W. S.: Esophageal Resection With End-to-End Anastomosis: Experimental and Clinical Observations, Ann Surg 129:588, 1949.

14. Robertson, R., and Sarjeant, T. R.: Reconstruction of Esophagus, J Thorac Cardiov Surg 20:689, 1950.

15. Ravitch, M. M.; Bahnson, H. T.; and Johns, T. N. P.: Carcinoma of the Esophagus, J Thorac Cardiov Surg 24:256, 1952.

16. Sachs, L.: A Plastic Prosthesis for Palliating Carcinoma of the Esophagus, Surgery 45:377, 1959.

17. Souttar, H. S.: Treatment of Carcinoma of the Oesophagus: Based on 100 Personal Cases and 18 Post-Mortem Reports, Brit J Surg 15:76, 1927.

18. Sweet, R. H.: Carcinoma of the Midthoracic Esophagus, Ann Surg 124:653, 1946.

19. Symonds, C. J.: The Treatment of Malignant Stricture of the Esophagus by Tubage or Oral Catheterism, Brit Med J 1:870, 1887.

20. Weisel, W.; Raine, F.; Watson, R. R.; and Frederick, J. J.: Palliative Treatment of Esophageal Carcinoma, Ann Surg 149:207, 1959.

21. Waddington, J. K., and Bickford, B. J.: Use of Mousseau-Barbin Tube for Palliation in Carcinoma of Oesophagus and Cardia, Brit J Surg 49:522, 1962.

DISCUSSION

On papers by Drs. Hopkins and Bernatz, and O'Connor et al

Dr. Robert A. Mustard, Toronto: Drs. Hopkins and Bernatz presented some moderately encouraging evidence to indicate that it may be possible to replace the cervical esophagus by transplanted bowel segments. The key to the problem is small vessel anastomosis, the technique of which is far from a final solution. To this problem we should all give effort and consideration, for with its solution will come another great leap forward in surgical endeavor—transplantation of organs and tissues, direct attack on coronary artery and cerebrovascular disease, improved management of renal ischemia, and many other dividends.

I personally believe that the future lies with some mechanical device, possibly a stapling machine such as that originally devised by the Russians and since then modified and improved by many others. The suture technique is too slow, too traumatic, and too likely to leave foreign material exposed within the lumen of these tiny vessels.

My own experience has been with more conventional methods of reconstruction of the cervical esophagus.

The Wookey procedure utilizes a flap of neck skin, forming a groove at the first stage; in the second stage the groove is converted into a tube. After the first stage, the patient shows a deep skin-lined groove between the pharynx above and the esophagus below. The second stage is completed usually about six to eight weeks after the original operation.

Up to 1960, Dr. Wookey had done 30 of these operations, and I had done 14. Since then, I have done four others, two of whom are living and well, now, over two years later. We have had a gratifying number of five-year survivors, nine so far.

We have had little difficulty with closure except in postirradiation cases such as in one man who had heavy cobalt therapy and who required several plastic procedures to get the skin tube finally closed; but he is alive and well, eating everything and gaining weight now over two years. Even with these cases we have always eventually achieved success. In another recent case, a lady had her operation 2½ years ago. With few exceptions these patients eat almost a normal diet and maintain their nutrition without difficulty.

The Wookey procedure is a good one, and we have been pleased with its results. Nevertheless, when a one-stage operation becomes dependable we will certainly welcome it.

This photograph shows an example of one such method which can be used in a few selected cases. A roentgenogram of a 78-year-old woman with recurrent carcinoma of cervical esophagus after radiation therapy with cobalt is shown. In October, 1962, Dr. John Palmer and I resected this lesion and replaced her pharynx and larynx with a transplanted loop of terminal ileum and right colon here shown anastomosed to the oropharynx. The lateral view shows the entire transplanted bowel segment which is joined below to the stomach. A bulge on the anterior chest wall can be seen with the tube of bowel in the subcutaneous plane.

This photograph shows the same woman as she was three days ago, very well and able to eat everything, and showing the indomitable spirit which encouraged us to attempt on her this surgical tour-de-force.

Dr. William E. Neville, Hines, Ill: I believe that the method presented by Drs. Hopkins and Bernatz is ideal for reconstruction of the cervical esophagus if one could be assured of a long-term viable segment. For those who are adroit in vascular anastomosis of the small vessels this certainly could be the answer.

However, in spite of a satisfactory anastomosis of the artery it is invariably a venous thrombosis, which Dr. Hopkins did not allude to, which militates against a successful outcome of the transplant. At the moment, from our results with colon transplants, wherein a pedicle of the middle colic artery and vein is used for the blood supply to the interposed colon, this would seem to be the ideal manner to use with the transplant. One can obtain an extremely long segment of colon which can reach the hypopharynx and can be reassured of a continuing blood supply.

This photograph shows a rather long segment of right colon which is on the chest wall in anticipation of anastomosis to an esophagostomy in the neck. In deference to what Dr. Mustard has shown, we use an anterior mediastinal tunnel to transpose the colonic segment into the neck.

This photograph shows the colon transplanted through the anterior mediastinum in a retrosternal manner. This is the upper anastomosis. This man had a carcinoma at the thoracic inlet which was resected with the esophagocolostomy high in the neck. In many of these patients it is extremely easy to pull the colon up to the hypopharynx. Occasionally we have to actually take off a piece of colon so it is not too redundant in the thorax or in the neck.

Another maneuver which Dr. Mustard has already related to, leaving a segment of ileum attached to the colon and transposing this through an anterior mediastinal tunnel, is shown here. Notice the inoperable (or what we deemed inoperable) carcinoma of the middle third of the esophagus in this 79-year-old lady. For this reason, we used an ileal colonic segment to bypass the carcinoma. She lived comfortably for two years after this operation.

In spite of our successes with colon transplants we still believe the operation proposed by Dr. Bernatz and Dr. Hopkins gives great promise and may be the desired procedure in the future.

Dr. Rodman E. Taber, Detroit: It is difficult to discuss one of these papers and not to discuss the other because, of course, the indications have to be decided on as to whether to operate on the patient or to irradiate the patient, also whether to resect or put a tube through the tumor. Certainly Drs. Hopkins and Bernatz have demonstrated the anatomical feasibility of this sort of procedure. They have also shown the functional attributes of the procedure, because I noticed that one of those dogs was drinking uphill, which is a pretty good test of a segment such as this.

The question I want to put to Drs. Hopkins and Bernatz concerns the indications for this procedure in esophageal surgery, specifically whether they think it is preferable to transposition of the right colon and the terminal ileum, which Dr. Neville has been responsible for popularizing.

The other paper concerns the indications for operating on esophageal cancer. When the question of palliation of esophageal cancer comes up, one wonders a little about the palliation afforded by a procedure which requires you to drink and eat through a 1 cm lumen. I think that unless we are able to remove the cancer from the patient we cannot get him to eat, no matter how we might have opened up his esophageal lumen. So, we would try to make every possible effort to remove the neoplasm itself, even though in some cases there might be distant neoplasm or in some cases a small amount of local neoplasm left behind.

Dr. Philip E. Bernatz, Rochester, Minn: We feel the treatment of carcinoma of the proximal third of the thoracic esophagus and cervical esophagus is surgical, at least in the light of our present thinking. We admire a great deal the accomplishments of Dr. Mustard and his associates with the types of skin tube reconstructions that they have accomplished so successfully. We are a bit discouraged with the time involved in such procedures, and although we continue to employ them in selected cases we have utilized more one-stage methods using reversed gastric tubes or pedicle transplants of colon. It is this search for something we could do in one stage with better functional results that led us to evaluate the procedures presented by Dr. Hopkins.

Recently Dr. Nakiyama recorded the history of several patients in whom he had elected to do free transplants of the colon, successfully, as Dr. Hopkins demonstrated to you this morning experimentally.

We certainly concur with Dr. Mustard's comments that the future of the mechanical stapling devices is a big one in this area of surgery. We had an opportunity to use the Russian stapler in one of the dogs, and we were impressed with the potential of such a method.

Dr. Thomas M. O'Connor, Milwaukee: In answer to Dr. Taber's comment about the difficulty of patients eating after intubation, we have not had the experience that apparently he had had with cancer patients, namely, their being unable to eat after intubation. Our patients have all been able to maintain their nutritional status reasonably well until the date of their death.

Unilateral Thyroid Nodules With Lymphocytic Thyroiditis

Surgical Problems and Management

M. A. BLOCK, MD; R. C. HORN, JR., MD; AND J. M. MILLER, MD, DETROIT

In recent years the majority of operations on the thyroid gland have been carried out for the clinical finding of nodules because of the possible presence of carcinoma. Occasionally the surgeon encounters clinically unsuspected chronic lymphocytic thyroiditis in such patients at the time of surgery. We wish to call attention first to the fact that chronic lymphocytic thyroiditis may manifest itself clinically by localized enlargement which may be interpreted as a nodule or nodules, or, in some patients, it may represent another lesion associated with the thyroiditis, and secondly, that unless these patients are treated indefinitely with adequate doses of thyroid medication, many later return complaining of symptomatic enlargement of their remaining thyroid tissue.

Terminology

A clarification of certain terminology to be used in this paper appears appropriate. The term "chronic lymphocytic thyroiditis" is used as a general term to refer to the pathologic entity in which there is an abnormal infiltration of lymphocytes in the thyroid. It is acknowledged that chronic lymphocytic thyroiditis may not be an accurate term, inasmuch as the condition may not be an inflammation in the true sense of the word, but information to date does not provide a better or more accurate term. The histologic variations are discussed below.

"Clinical nodule" denotes a localized enlargement of the thyroid gland, the exact nature of which is unknown, palpated on physical examination or at the time of surgery. A clinical nodule may in fact be a specific pathologic lesion as an involutional nodule, adenoma, or carcinoma, or it may result from exaggerated lobulation or bosselation, an area of fibrosis, etc. "Pathologic nodule" will be used to refer to an involutional nodule, adenoma, or carcinoma in the thyroid.

Clinical Materials

The diagnosis of chronic lymphocytic thyroiditis has been established by microscopic study of the tissue removed at surgery in 95 patients seen at the Henry Ford Hospital from 1950 through 1962. In nine patients, the surgery was carried out in another institution, the patient being seen by us at a later date. There was no operative mortality in the entire group.

The patients followed the classic age and sex distribution, the typical patient being a female slightly over 40 years of age. The ages ranged from 16 to 80 years. Only six of the 95 patients were males.

The presence of a single or several nodules clinically in one lobe of the thyroid led to operation in 41 of the 95 patients (Table 1). In addition, there were ten patients for whom surgery was performed because of the presence of a clinical nodule of the thyroid isthmus.

TABLE 1.—*Chronic Lymphocytic Thyroiditis, Operations 1950-1962: Preoperative Configuration of Thyroid*

Unilateral enlargement or nodules	41
Nodule isthmus	10
Multinodular	44
Total number patients	95

Presented at the 20th Annual Meeting of the Central Surgical Association, Chicago, Feb 21-23, 1963.

From the Divisions of General Surgery, Pathology, and Endocrinology of the Henry Ford Hospital.

The remaining 44 of the total of 95 patients underwent operation because of the clinical presence of multinodular goiter. In many instances, the clinical nodule or nodules were predominantly unilateral. There were six patients whose thyroids were sufficiently large to produce significant pressure symptoms in the neck requiring surgery on this basis alone. Two of the patients were treated preoperatively for hyperthyroidism, one of the patients being considered as having toxic nodular goiter.

In 20 of the 95 patients, symptomatic enlargement of remaining thyroid tissue following operation resulted in their seeking medical attention at a later date (Table 2). The interval of time between their thyroid surgery and recurrent goiter varied from six months to seven years. Eight of the 20 patients had taken thyroid medication postoperatively, but five had discontinued the therapy, and three were taking only small doses. In all of these patients, at least the equivalent of one lobe of the thyroid remained after the operation carried out for nodular goiter involving the isthmus or primarily one lobe.

It is significant that three of the 20 patients were reoperated upon for recurrent enlargement of the thyroid gland due to chronic lymphocytic thyroiditis. The remaining 17 patients were managed satisfactorily with adequate medical therapy. In one of the three patients requiring reoperation, the second operation was performed for enlargement of remaining thyroid tissue three years after surgery for a clinical nodule in the isthmus which proved to be a carcinoma in a gland also involved by chronic lymphocytic thyroiditis. No evidence of malignancy was found in the tissue removed at the second procedure. A second patient was reoperated upon three years after excision of the isthmus containing a clinical nodule which proved to be an area of chronic lymphocytic thyroiditis. This patient refused to take thyroid, and a trial of steroid therapy was not of significant benefit. Reoperation was finally resorted to when the goiter produced increasing pressure symptoms. The course of the third patient is summarized as follows:

A 43-year-old housewife was first seen in 1952 with the finding of a hard, enlarged right lobe of the thyroid. Surgery was advised. The patient was operated upon elsewhere in 1952 and again in 1956 because of recurrent goiter. The thyroid tissue removed was reported to show thyroiditis. She was seen for the second time in our institution in 1957 because of an enlarged right lobe of the thyroid, producing tracheal deviation to the left with pressure symptoms. Surgery then was undertaken as her third thyroid operation, completing a right lobectomy. A 1 cm hard nodule was all that remained of her left lobe; this was not removed. The tissue removed showed chronic lymphocytic thyroiditis on microscopic study. The patient was continued on thyroid therapy subsequently and remains in satisfactory condition.

The microscopic study of the tissue removed showed one variety or another of chronic lymphocytic thyroiditis in all 95 patients. Carcinoma was found associated with the thyroiditis in five (Table 3). A total thyroidectomy was carried out for four of these patients. It is to be emphasized that the diagnosis of carcinoma may be especially difficult on frozen section study of the thyroid in which extensive Hürthle cell alteration of the parenchymal cells of the thyroid accompanies the diffuse lymphocytic infiltrate (lymphoepithelial goiter).

TABLE 2.—*Chronic Lymphocytic Thyroiditis, Operations 1950-1962: Recurrence of Goiter*

Total number patients operated on	95
Recurrence symptomatic goiter	20
Reoperations for recurrence	3

TABLE 3.—*Chronic Lymphocytic Thyroiditis, Operations 1950-1962: Associated Lesions*

Total number patients operated on		95
Associated carcinoma		5
Associated involutional nodules or adenomas		25
With diffuse lymphocytic thyroiditis	7	
With focal lymphocytic thyroiditis	18	

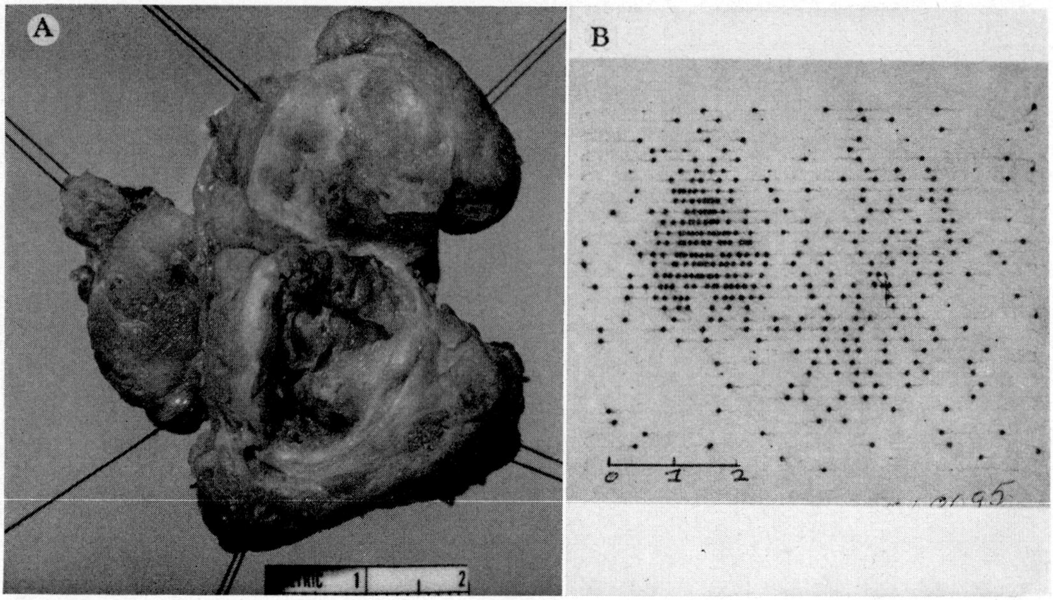

Fig 1.—*A,* Nodular goiter with chronic lymphocytic thyroiditis. Large involutional nodule in the left lobe of thyroid is seen in section of gross specimen. *B,* preoperative scintiscan illustrates reduced function in area of nodule.

Involutional nodules or adenomas were found to be associated with the chronic lymphocytic thyroiditis in 25 patients (Fig 1 and 2). Thus, in 30 of the 95 patients, or approximately 31%, the thyroid did contain a lesion (involutional nodule, adenoma, cancer) other than thyroiditis responsible for the nodularity detected clinically.

The operative procedures carried out varied considerably. In general, that procedure which would adequately remove the nodular tissue recognized clinically preoperatively and at surgery was removed. In seven patients a total thyroidectomy was performed for patients in whom the thyroid showed only chronic lymphocytic thyroiditis. In two of these seven patients, carcinoma was thought to be present on frozen section study done at the time of surgery.

Fig 2.—Adenoma with chronic lymphocytic thyroiditis. Cross-section of adenoma is seen within lobe of thyroid involved by diffuse lymphocytic thyroiditis.

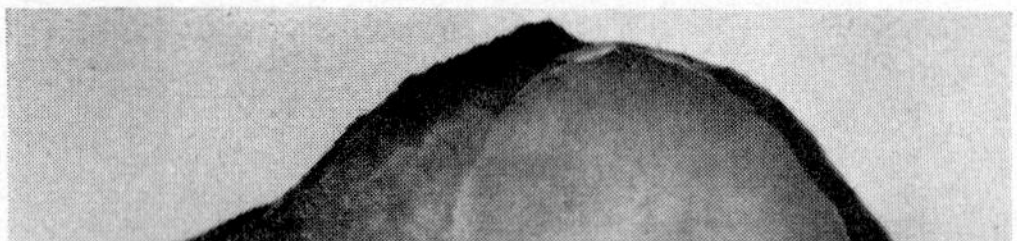

Of the total of 95 patients, 64 have not returned complaining of recurrent goiter, nor was a total thyroidectomy carried out (Table 4). Of this group of 64 patients, 27 have continued taking thyroid therapy. Of the remaining 37 patients, the follow-up period has been less than one year in 20.

Table 4.—*Chronic Lymphocytic Thyroiditis, Operations 1950-1962: Follow-up*

1. Recurrence goiter		20
Treated medically	17	
Reoperated	3	
2. Partial thyroidectomy, thyroid Rx postop., no recurrence		27
3. Total thyroidectomy (Carcinoma in 4)		11
4. Partial thyroidectomy, no thyroid Rx, no recurrence		17
5. Partial thyroidectomy, follow-up less than one year		20
Total number patients		95

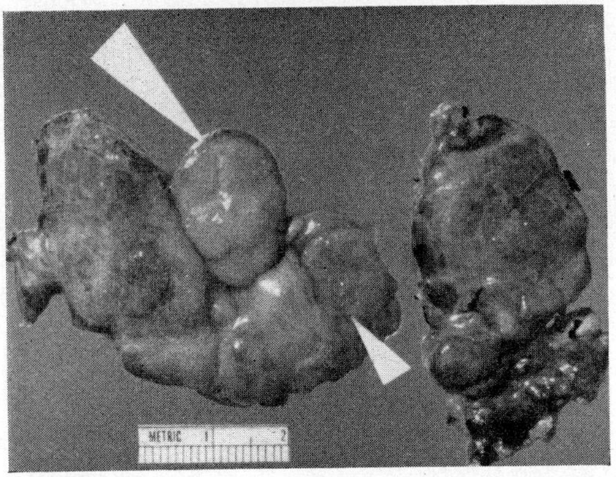

Fig 3.—Lobulation in chronic lymphocytic thyroiditis. Large arrow indicates lobule suspected on clinical examination of being pathologic nodule. Diffuse lymphocytic thyroiditis is present also in remainder of thyroid, not greatly enlarged, shown in cross-section.

Pathologic Classification

The thyroid glands of this total group of patients considered to have chronic lymphocytic thyroiditis could be arranged into two major categories based on gross and microscopic features. The majority were characterized by a diffuse lymphocytic infiltrate forming a quantitatively impressive (estimated 25% or more) part of the histologic picture. The infiltrate was usually, but not invariably, organized with prominent reaction centers. Plasma cells frequently accompanied the infiltrate, at times in large numbers and even predominating on occasion. The thyroid parenchyma itself might appear normal or resting with variations in infinite degree from minor deviations from normal (hyperplasia, involution, colloid storage, Hürthle cell alteration) to the full-blown picture of complete, or nearly complete Hürthle cell change, typically grouped in small follicles with little colloid or in solid clusters without evident lumina (lympho-epithelial goiter; Hashimoto's struma). The amount of colloid was more or less normal in the glands with parenchyma at the normal end of the spectrum, the amount of colloid tending to decrease progressively to the end of the spectrum characterized by complete Hürthle cell change.

Some degree of fibrosis occurred in some of these glands with a diffuse lymphocytic infiltrate accompanied by increasing parenchymal abnormality. On occasion the fibrosis was severe and accentuated the lobulations of the gland to simulate nodular goiter clinically. Although the fibrosis might be diffuse it was not necessarily symmetrical, and accentuated lobulations in areas of greatest change could simulate pathologic nodules clinically and even at operation (Fig 3 and 4). Metaplasia, usually epidermoid, occurred in some of the thyroid glands with extensive Hürthle cell change. In some specimens the heavy cellular infiltrate, with or without fibrosis, more or less obliterated the parenchyma, raising the question as to whether this represented the end-result of diffuse

Fig 4.—Extensive fibrosis in chronic lymphocytic thyroiditis. *A*, photo shows surface of gland involved by chronic lymphocytic thyroiditis with section of right lobe containing much fibrosis. *B*, preoperative scintiscan shows absent function in right lobe due to replacement fibrosis. The finding of a large, hard right lobe without function led to operation.

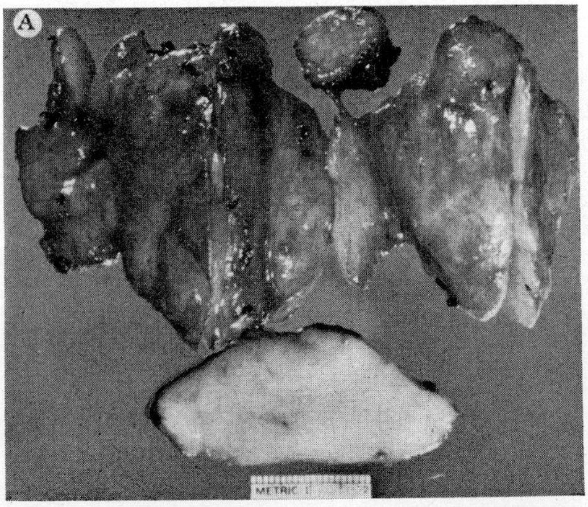

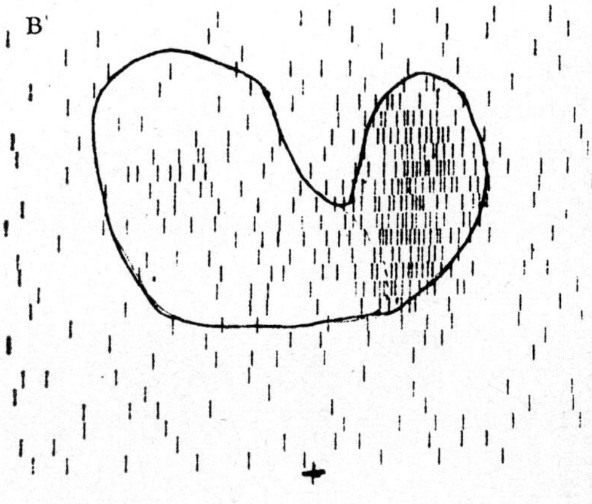

lymphocytic thyroiditis or possibly of a diffuse granulomatous thyroiditis.

Involutional nodules, adenomas, or even carcinoma were found as associated lesions in some of these glands in which the dominant picture was the diffuse cellular infiltrate with varying parenchymal change. In our total group of patients, seven of this category were found to have associated involutional nodules or adenomas.

The second major category of histologic change in the thyroids of this group of patients with chronic lymphocytic thyroiditis consisted of glands in which focal areas of a lymphocytic infiltrate with or without parenchymal cell change were present in a gland in which the dominant pathology appeared to be the presence of involutional nodules with adenomas or even carcinoma in a few. In this group it is sometimes difficult to be sure whether or not the "thyroiditis" aspect of the change is focal or diffuse because of the size and distortion of the gland. We classified 18 patients as having involutional nodules or adenomas associated with focal chronic lymphocytic thyroiditis.

Comment

This experience with chronic lymphocytic thyroiditis emphasizes certain problems in the surgical and medical management of the condition. Our current plans of management of some of these problems will be outlined.

Clinical Recognition of Chronic Lymphocytic Thyroiditis.—In many instances it is possible to recognize chronic lymphocytic thyroiditis by a combination of history, physical examination, and laboratory studies. The classic description is that of a diffusely enlarged, firm, or rubbery gland, often with scalloped edges, in a woman 20-60 years old. The differential diagnosis from sporadic goiter is accomplished by laboratory confirmation of the often scant clinical evidence of hypothyroidism. This disease, by virtue of its pathophysiology, involves all of the gland not previously affected by cancer or involutional nodules, but may be markedly asymmetric. Nodules may be present from the aforementioned causes, or the pronounced lobulation may be mistaken for them. Occasionally a history of mild tenderness in a rapidly enlarging gland may confuse the diagnosis with granulomatous thyroiditis.

Theoretically a positive diagnosis can be made only by needle biopsy, but practically this is a research and investigational tool. We make this statement because our program for patients selected for medical management does not depend on tissue diagnosis.

The determination of autoantibodies by any of several techniques separates chronic lymphocytic thyroiditis as a group by frequency of occurrence and height of the titer, but because of overlapping values with many other types of thyroid disease it is not recommended as a diagnostic procedure of high specificity. Elevation of γ-globulin is of greater specificity but of low sensitivity.

The demonstration of the important functional abnormality can be accomplished by the finding of a low PBI, a low BEI, or more important still, the characteristic low or absent thyroid reserve with the TSH test. The I^{131} uptake in the early stages may indeed be elevated in spite of the above.

In practice, when the clinical and laboratory features are present, thyroid feeding is instituted, and rapid disappearance of the goiter virtually substantiates the diagnosis. If only slight or no regression occurs, surgery is usually performed because of the difficulty of eliminating the diagnosis of cancer in a gland in which considerable replacement of thyroid tissue has taken place. The goiter itself is often objectionable to the patient. The prognosis for reduction of gland size by thyroid feeding can often be made by the I^{131} scintigram. Areas of diminished-to-absent function, incapable of stimulation by TSH, indicate that these areas are largely lymphocytes and fibrous tissue of pathologic nodule formation and unlikely to respond to TSH deprivation.

When Should Surgery Be Performed in Chronic Lymphocytic Thyroiditis?—If chronic lymphocytic thyroiditis is recognized unquestionably on the basis of the data listed above, we prefer to treat the patient medically with thyroid feeding. It will be possible to recognize and so manage most patients with this condition.

Surgery is indicated, in our opinion, in those patients with recognized lymphocytic thyroiditis if a clinical nodule requiring surgery on the basis of its features is present or if the thyroid mass itself is so large that serious pressure symptoms are produced and a satisfactory response to medical therapy has not been obtained. There are certain patients with lymphocytic thyroiditis for whom the diagnosis is not established until the time of operation. These patients are primarily those with clinically apparent unilateral or isthmic nodules of the thyroid. It is not always possible to differentiate pathologic nodules from lobulation or fibrosis (Fig 3 and 4). With increasing experience and alertness to the possibility of chronic lymphocytic thyroiditis, it should be possible to recognize those patients with this entity who are best treated medically. Others have reported the coexistence of actual or suspected pathologic nodules in significant numbers of patients with chronic lymphocytic thyroiditis and have commented on the problems in the evaluation of these thyroids on physical examination.[3-5]

The physician undertaking medical therapy for thyroiditis has a continuing and important responsibility to that patient. We have seen two patients treated for thyroiditis but eventually found to have carcinoma without microscopic evidence of thyroiditis. Therefore, the decision for therapy is critical, and if the decision is made to treat the patient medically, the patient must be followed closely.

As illustrated by our experience, patients with chronic lymphocytic thyroiditis may have associated carcinoma, involutional nodules, or adenomas. Carcinoma was present in about 5% and involutional nodules or adenomas in approximately 26% of our group for whom surgery was performed. Therefore, clinical nodules in the thyroid should be treated on the basis of their individual features, irrespective of the presence of associated thyroiditis. The low incidence of carcinoma associated with chronic lymphocytic thyroiditis does not, in our opinion, justify surgery for all patients with this form of thyroiditis.

It has not been our policy to utilize needle biopsy to prove the diagnosis of thyroiditis. In our opinion, the question in these patients is whether or not malignancy is present. If the findings indicate the possibility of malignancy, then we prefer to proceed with operation to adequately settle the issue. If the findings are unquestionably those of thyroiditis without nodule formation, we prefer to proceed with medical management and follow the patient closely.

What Operative Procedure Should Be Performed for Chronic Lymphocytic Thyroiditis?—Those patients undergoing surgery for clinical nodules associated with chronic lymphocytic thyroiditis should receive the proper operation based on the character of the nodules present, irrespective of the presence of thyroiditis. If we encounter a nodule suspected of being pathologic in one lobe, it is our practice to perform a lobectomy with excision of the isthmus and superficial portion of the contralateral lobe. A similar nodule in the isthmus is treated by resection of the isthmus and superficial portions of the adjacent lobes. Bilateral nodules are treated by total lobectomy on the side of a dominant nodule or predominance of nodules with contralateral partial lobectomy adequate to remove nodules on the opposite side. If nodulation is approximately equal on both sides, bilateral partial lobectomy may be the best procedure to carry out.

If the surgeon encounters only the exaggerated lobulation of thyroiditis but no discrete nodules at the time of operation, we usually remove the isthmus and superficial portions of each lobe, removing more on the side with greater mass. This is done inasmuch as a few patients may not respond well to medical therapy, and this procedure does remove excess mass of tissue. The likelihood of symptomatic enlargement of the remaining tissue in the future may thereby be reduced. This disease characteristically involves all of the thyroid tissue, even though it may not yet have resulted in enlargement of all the thyroid at the time.

If malignancy is found to be present, associated with chronic lymphocytic thyroiditis, the procedure indicated for the malignancy is performed without giving any special consideration to the associated thyroiditis.

The patient with chronic lymphocytic thyroiditis undergoing surgery to relieve pressure symptoms is treated by surgical excision of the excess bulk of thyroid tissue. The morbidity of total thyroidectomy does not justify this procedure for chronic lymphocytic thyroiditis, in our opinion. In some patients, the procedure can be technically difficult and result in hypoparathyroidism, vocal cord paralysis, and severe laryngeal edema.[6]

What Therapy Should Be Given Postoperatively for Chronic Lymphocytic Thyroiditis?—Patients with chronic lymphocytic thyroiditis should be treated indefinitely with thyroid whether or not surgery has been necessary. The dosage should be regulated by giving thyroid in some form to tolerance. The therapy is given whether or not myxedema is present. Although the efficacy of thyroid therapy in chronic lymphocytic thyroiditis has been long recognized, the need for continued therapy in sufficient dosage does not appear to be commonly appreciated.[7-10] Two patients for whom the diagnosis of chronic lymphocytic thyroiditis was established clinically tolerated thyroid in only small amounts; yet after total or near total thyroidectomy they were able to tolerate usual replacement doses.

Thyroid therapy is necessary to prevent continued enlargement of the thyroid in chronic lymphocytic thyroiditis. The pathologic changes in the thyroid produced by the disease are permanent, and progressive enlargement is produced frequently. Thus, 20 of 95 patients treated surgically were later seen with increasing enlargement of the thyroid. The enlargement may produce continuous or intermittent neck symptoms. Three patients reoperated upon illustrate the problem encountered by the surgeon seeing the patient with recurrent thyroid enlargement postoperatively. The patient may first undergo operation for unilateral thyroid enlargement, then later return with symptomatic enlargement of the contralateral side. Other reports have noted that reoperation has later been performed in patients with chronic lymphocytic thyroiditis because of enlargement of remaining thyroid tissue.[11-13] On the other hand, it is peculiar that in some individuals chronic lymphocytic thyroiditis does not produce any significant enlargement of thyroid tissue, and it may be an unexpected microscopic finding at autopsy.

Difficulty may be encountered in convincing patients of the need for continuous thyroid therapy and periodic examinations. Some patients have become discouraged with the lack of results when the dosage was inadequate. The dosage should be increased to tolerance if symptoms or the enlargement of the thyroid are not controlled. Even on therapy, some patients may occasionally experience transient soreness of the neck. Thyroid therapy may not produce complete disappearance of enlargement of the thyroid tissue, but residual diffuse palpable enlargement is usually minimal and not symptomatic. A few patients do not obtain help from thyroid feeding.

The patients should be reexamined periodically. It is possible, of course, for carcinoma to develop in remaining thyroid tissue at a later date.

Summary and Conclusions

1. Chronic lymphocytic thyroiditis appears as a unilateral enlargement in some patients. Surgery may be carried out because of the interpretation of this enlargement as due to pathologic nodule formation or because pathologic nodule formation actually coexists with the thyroiditis.

2. It is possible to recognize chronic lymphocytic thyroiditis in many patients by correlating the history, physical findings, and laboratory data.

3. Most patients with chronic lymphocytic thyroiditis are managed satisfactorily by therapy with thyroid.

4. Carcinoma was associated with chronic lymphocytic thyroiditis in approximately 5% of our patients who had undergone operation. Involutional nodules or adenomas were seen in about 26% of patients for whom surgery was performed.

5. Surgery is indicated in chronic lymphocytic thyroiditis when associated with pathologic nodule formation or in the occasional patient with pressure symptoms in the neck produced by huge enlargement of the thyroid gland.

6. The surgical procedure indicated in the patient with chronic lymphocytic thyroiditis will depend on surgical findings. Pathologic nodules should be managed without consideration of the thyroiditis. In others, the excess bulk of thyroid tissue is removed.

7. Total thyroidectomy is not justified as the procedure of choice for chronic lymphocytic thyroiditis.

8. Patients with chronic lymphocytic thyroiditis should receive thyroid therapy indefinitely. Relatively large doses may be necessary to prevent enlargement of the gland and control symptoms. This was emphasized in our experience by the fact that 20 of 95 patients previously operated upon for chronic lymphocytic thyroiditis returned later with symptomatic enlargement of their remaining thyroid tissue.

REFERENCES

1. Skillern, P. G.; Crile, G., Jr.; McCullagh, E. P.; Hazard, J. B.; Lewis, L. A.; and Brown, H.: Struma Lymphomatosa: Primary Thyroid Failure With Compensatory Thyroid Enlargement, J Clin Endocr 16:35-54, 1956.

2. Luxton, R. W., and Cooke, R. T.: Hashimoto's Struma Lymphomatosa: Diagnostic Value of Serum and Significance of Serum-Flocculation Reactions, Lancet 2:105-109, 1956.

3. Lindsay, S.; Dailey, M. E.; Friedlander, J.; Yee, G.; and Soley, M.: Chronic Thyroiditis: A Clinical and Pathologic Study of 354 Patients, J Clin Endocr 12:1578-1600, 1952.

4. Hendrick, J. W.: Diagnosis and Management of Thyroiditis, JAMA 164:127-133, 1957.

5. Woolner, L. B.; McConahey, W. M.; and Beahrs, O. H.: The Surgical Aspects of Thyroiditis, Amer J Surg 104:666-671, 1962.

6. Rudman, I.; Novota, O. J.; and Keener, R. L.: Complications of Hashimoto's Thyroiditis Surgery, Arch Surg 83:822-824, 1961.

7. Statland, H.; Wasserman, M. M.; Vickery, A. L.: Struma Lymphomatosa (Hashimoto's Struma), AMA Arch Intern Med 88:659-678, 1951.

8. Crile, G., Jr., and Schneider, R. W.: Diagnosis and Treatment of Thyroiditis With Special Reference to the Use of Cortisone and ACTH, Cleveland Clin Quart 19:219-224, 1952.

9. McConahey, W. M.; Woolner, L. B.; Black, B. M.; and Keating, F. R., Jr.: Effect of Desiccated Thyroid in Lymphocytic (Hashimoto's) Thyroiditis, J Clin Endocr 19:45-52, 1959.

10. Beahrs, O. H.; Woolner, L. B.; Engel, S.; and McConahey, W. M.: Needle Biopsy of the Thyroid Gland and Management of Lymphocytic Thyroiditis, Surg Gynec Obstet 114:636-639, 1962.

11. Chesky, V. E.; Hellwig, C. A.; and Welch, J. W.: Cancer of the Thyroid Associated With Hashimoto's Disease: An Analysis of 48 Cases, Amer Surg 28:678-685, 1962.

12. Marshall, S. F., and Meissner, W. A.: Struma Lymphomatosa (Hashimoto's Disease), Ann Surg 141:737-746, 1955.

13. Woolner, L. B.; McConahey, W. M.; and Beahrs, O. H.: Struma Lymphomatosa (Hashimoto's Thyroiditis) and Related Thyroidal Disorders, J Clin Endocr 19:53-83, 1959.

DISCUSSION

Dr. Oliver Beahrs, Rochester, Minn: In general, we agree with the comments Dr. Block has made. However, I think we would place a little more emphasis on establishing the definitive diagnosis by needle biopsy if one elects not to treat the lesion surgically.

We have found, in reviewing the needle biopsy specimens, that they substantiated the diagnosis in only 77% of cases. I wonder what Dr. Block's experience has been in regard to needle biopsy. I do not mean to imply that we would employ this method in all cases, but certainly we would in any case in which there is a question regarding the diagnosis.

If one accepts conservatism in the management of these lesions, it then becomes extremely important to continue seeing these patients clinically for a period of three to six months so that one may be completely satisfied that the lesion has regressed or disappeared entirely. In our experience, 18 among 605 patients treated surgically for Hashimoto's thyroiditis had a papillary carcinoma also present; this is approximately 3%. Though the incidence is not as great as has been reported by others, it is sufficient to warrant close observation of such patients—but not large enough to warrant prophylactic thyroidectomy for Hashimoto's thyroiditis. I believe this is the feeling expressed by Dr. Block.

I would like also to ask whether he has had any experience with lymphosarcoma occurring in patients with lymphocytic thyroiditis. In our experience with the same series of 605 cases we have encountered lymphosarcoma 16 times.

One other comment in regard to the type of surgical procedure that should be carried out when one operates on lymphocytic thyroiditis, suspecting that a nodular goiter might be present, but lymphocytic thyroiditis is diagnosed from gross examination or from pathologic study at the time of operation: we would be inclined to do a bilateral subtotal thyroidectomy, not a total thyroidectomy. We would do this—removing only a portion of the gland on either side of the neck—to reduce the mass of the thyroid tissue and also to reduce the chance of recurrence of a nodular enlargement on one side of the neck when none of the thyroid tissue is removed. I think this procedure reduces the chance of recurrence greatly.

DR. MELVIN A. BLOCK, Detroit: We have not used needle biopsy to establish the diagnosis of thyroiditis routinely nor very frequently in our institution. In general, we have felt that the question of microscopic diagnosis resolves itself into whether or not there is a possibility of a carcinoma being present in these thyroid glands. If the possibility does exist on the basis of clinical findings, we prefer to attack the problem surgically at the outset. If the clinical findings are unquestionably due to chronic lymphocytic thyroiditis alone, we have preferred to treat it medically. However, as Dr. Beahrs and his associates have pointed out, this requires frequent follow-up examinations of such patients. The needle biopsy has not been diagnostically infallible, either.

With regard to the problem of lymphosarcoma associated with chronic lymphocytic thyroiditis, we have encountered this problem in one patient not included in this study. This diagnosis may pose a problem for the pathologist.

I would like to re-emphasize that one of the problems we have encountered postoperatively in patients with chronic lymphocytic thyroiditis is that adequate doses of thyroid therapy have not been given. The patients later complain of neck symptoms. It is only when adequate thyroid therapy has been given, often necessitating doses to tolerance levels, that symptomatic enlargement of the neck has been controlled.

Aseptic Barriers

WILLIAM C. BECK, MD, AND WARNER W. CARLSON, PhD, SAYRE, PA

An aseptic barrier may be defined as a material placed between an aseptic area, such as an operative incision, and areas which harbor microorganisms with the purpose of preventing the spread of bacteria into the sterile zone. Examples of such barriers are rubber gloves, gowns, masks, drapes, as well as wrappers for materials which have been subjected to steam sterilization. Such barriers are in widespread use, yet criteria for their efficiency are barely existent. This study does not establish criteria but is intended to explore some of the methods by which barrier efficiency might be determined.

The motility of certain bacterial species has been studied by various investigators, but because of the experimental conditions usually employed, these studies are not significant in surgical bacteriology. In general, bacteria are transported from one area to another by some vehicle such as dust, water, or a human or other animate vector. When we consider bacterial transmission in relation to aseptic barriers, the transmission by a vehicle, rather than motility per se, is the factor of major importance. It is, therefore, imperative that a barrier material be impervious to bacterial vehicles if it is to be effective.

Presented at the 20th Annual Meeting of the Central Surgical Association, Chicago, Feb 21-23, 1963.

Water as Bacterial Conveyance

Not only are most of the usual barriers employed in surgical practice pervious to water, but because of their absorptive properties they diffuse liquid media over a wide area. This wicking action will diffuse aqueous fluids such as blood, serum, or amniotic fluid over wide areas, and if these fluids are contaminated the contained microorganisms will be transported to all of the moistened areas.

For example, if a bundle of sterile material is removed from a steam sterilizer while it is hot and placed upon a cold surface, the suddenly cooled area will form a condensate from the vapor which remains within the bundle even after use of conventional drying methods. This condensate will moisten the wrapper, permitting the passage of bacteria resident on the table top into the sterile zone within the bundle.[1]

The exact amount of moisture required to break through the cloth barrier is not known to us, but we are presently studying this subject. We feel certain that this is dependent upon the composition of the material rather than its thickness or the number of layers in which it is applied. The amount of moisture can be minimal with certain textiles which have a high sorptive quality, so that it is possible that, on days of extremely high humidity, many textile barriers may be quite useless.

We have previously demonstrated that an absolutely dry piece of cloth, such as is usually used for a gown or drape, is an efficient bacterial barrier.[2] This experiment is not easy to reproduce. Almost all attempts to demonstrate this barrier property are spoiled because it is so difficult to maintain the dry state of cloth. For example, if one places a dry piece of sterile surgical drape upon an agar medium which has a pattern of bacterial colonies growing upon it (Fig 1*A*), and then makes an imprint upon another agar medium from the opposite surface of the drape, the same bacterial pattern of growth will be reproduced (Fig 1*B*). There is sufficient moisture in the agar medium to vitiate the barrier effect of a textile drape. Placing several layers on top of one another will not enhance the barrier effect because of the wicking action of the cloth.

The conveyance of microorganisms by aqueous media is similarly the problem of other aseptic barriers. In previous investigations [3] we have shown that intact surgical gloves are splendid aseptic barriers. If, however, they develop even minuscule holes, then the entire barrier effect is lost. It might appear that a minute aperture would be an unimportant source of contamination. Yet as the finger moves within the rubber encasement it acts as a piston, pumping the patient's blood into the glove when the finger is flexed and the sweat of the surgeon into the wound when the finger is extended. Mute evidence

Fig 1.—*A,* the plate on the left, has been inoculated with a staphylococcus in a definite pattern. A swatch of surgical double drapes has been placed upon it, and the culture on the right, *B*, produced with a replicator. The drape was moistened only by the water contained in the agar medium.

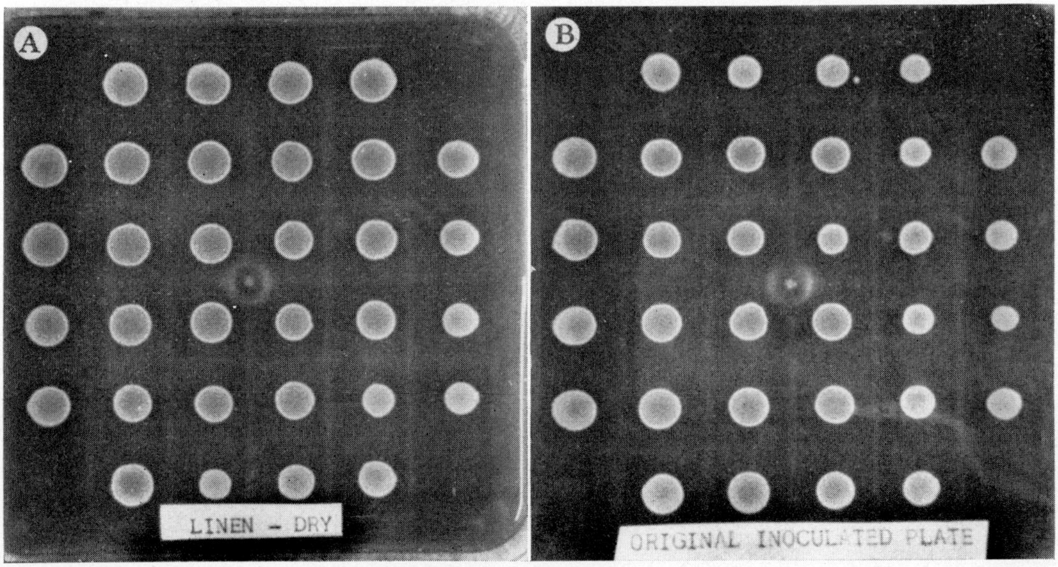

of this has been experienced by every surgeon who notices a smudge of blood on his index finger which has come through a minute pinhole in the glove tip. By routinely culturing gloves at the end of operations, Wise[4] has demonstrated that the inner surfaces of gloves have become heavily contaminated in a very high percentage of instances.

The surgeon's mask is another bacterial barrier in which water content becomes a problem. The surgeon does not breathe bacteria into the atmosphere. His breath contains droplets of water which are, in effect, bacterial suspensions. We could not breathe through a truly efficient bacterial filter. We can breathe with comfort through an efficient droplet filter.

Barrier Specifications

Because of the variety of functional elements which must be protected by barriers, simple and universal specifications are impossible to formulate. The barriers must permit the function of the part which is to be protected, as, for example, fingers must be capable of full mobility, and the mouth and nose of the surgical team must be permitted to pass in relative comfort the volume of air involved in normal respiration. On the other hand, the barrier must be as nearly impervious as possible to the passage of bacteria-transporting vehicles. In essence, this implies that the material must be waterproof.

Were waterproofness the only attribute needed, the problem would be a simple one. There are a multitude of plastic materials as well as rubber and rubber substitutes which possess this quality. But porosity is also needed in most areas. Were one to encase the human body in a nonporous material, it would soon become unbearably hot. Moreover, the heat accumulated because of the lack of skin evaporation may actually be dangerous. In testing for the accumulation of sweat in infants with supposed mucoviscidosis, encasement of the body in a plastic has resulted fatally in at least six instances, and only one of these in a child with proven pancreatic disease.[5]

This does not preclude the use of nonporous materials in smaller areas, such as the surgeon's hands, or the zone of the operative field. But it does deny the use of nonporous materials for surgical body drapes, surgeons' gowns, and, unless they are penetrable by steam, as wrappers for sterilized goods.

In addition to porosity, in surgical masks the water-trapping mechanism must be accompanied by a lack of resistance to the free passage of air if surgeons are to breathe in comfort. This, unfortunately, has been overlooked in certain mask designs which are completely air resistant so that the inhaled and expired air must go around the sides of the mask, without any lateral protection.

Flexibility sufficient to provide comfort during activity, as well as the ability to form the material into gowns, caps, and other accouterments must be possible. The word comfort is used advisedly, for it has been given too little consideration in the past. Comfort should be an essential, since the surgeon should be freed of the work necessary to overcome the limitations of his accouterments, if he is to expend his physical reserves in accomplishing the objectives of his activity.

The barriers must be strong enough to maintain their qualities for the duration of any single operative procedure, no matter what its length, and, if possible, breaks in barrier effect should come to the attention of the surgeon. They must be devoid of a tendency to produce static electricity, low in antigenicity, and should be of pleasing color. It is also desirable that they be within reason from the standpoint of cost, whether they be reusable or disposable. With reusable textiles it also would be worthwhile to have methods of determining age and wear.

Barrier Testing

Having set down certain criteria for barriers, there should be methods for evaluating specific materials to see whether or not they can conform to the specifications. If they cannot, then we must devise substitutes that will. With the diversity of materials, and of their applications, now in surgical use, the tests must necessarily differ so that the essential of "comfort-in-use" may also apply. A truly efficient barrier may be ideal from the standpoint of asepsis and yet be of no value as it will never be used by practical surgeons.

Unfortunately, there is very little background research in this general area. Definitions are generally lacking. One reads, for example, that a certain mask is "98.4% efficient by the accurate and reliable slit sampler method"; another mask is 94% efficient by an entirely different test. Until there is an accepted standardized test available by which all masks can be evaluated, the surgeon is just as lost as when a certain soap was advertised as being 99 44/100% pure.

Who should set up the testing criteria? In our opinion, this matter is of sufficient importance so that one of our major surgical societies should set up a special committee to determine standards and standard tests. The United States Pharmacopeia set standards for catgut, yet barriers are without definition. Testing methods are simple, but without standards.

If possible, testing methods should be performed upon barrier materials in use. This is not always feasible, but it should be employed wherever possible. Warning devices are available for many dangerous activities. Burglar alarms tell the police that the bank's barrier against thieves is being broken. Similar warning devices can and should be developed in surgery. We have devised one,[6] and the field could be much expanded.

Masks.—Most tests on masks are carried out on volunteers who utter certain test phrases while wearing the masks, the surrounding air then being sampled for bacterial content. We have employed the method described by Shooter et al,[7] modified by employing settling plates placed in front of and behind the test subject, as well as a slit sampler to enumerate bacteria in the circulating air (Fig 2). We have also used the modification of replacing the human test subject by a nebulizer, thus permitting a standard stream of bacteria to be applied to the mask. This approach removes the subjective element from the test. As a reference standard, we have used a double gauze mask (14 ply), this being the barrier in most widespread use today.

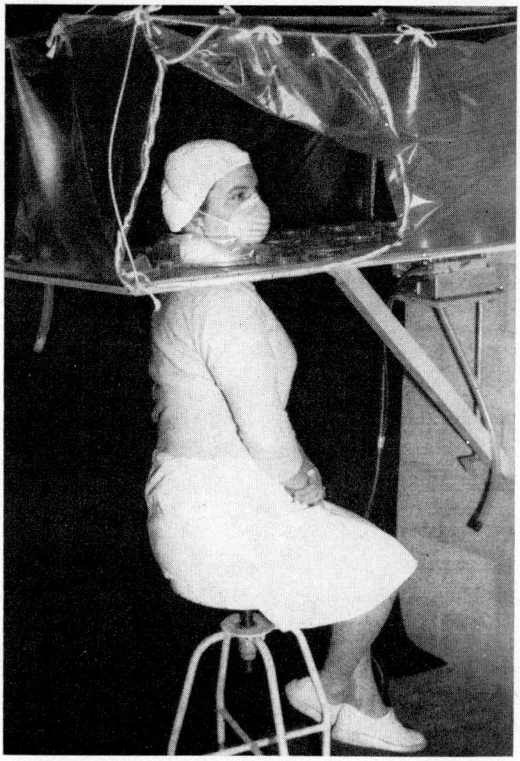

Fig 2.—Mask testing apparatus modified from the description by Shooter, Smith, and Hunter.[7] The test subject sits in the enclosed space repeating test phrases. Petri dishes are placed in front of *and* behind the subject. A slit sampler exhausts air for testing at the far end of the enclosure. The same technique can be employed substituting an atomizer dispersing specific-sized droplets into the enclosure, with far more accurate results.

After the bacterial barrier properties of the mask have been established, it is imperative that the mask be worn by test subjects for prolonged periods to evaluate the "comfort-in-use" factor. After being worn for a period of time corresponding to that of the longest operative procedure, the mask is again tested to determine whether it retains its barrier efficiency under conditions of use.

Gloves.—The testing of gloves falls into three categories: the new glove, the glove in use, and the reusable glove. The testing of the new gloves by manufacturers leaves much to be desired, as we have pointed out

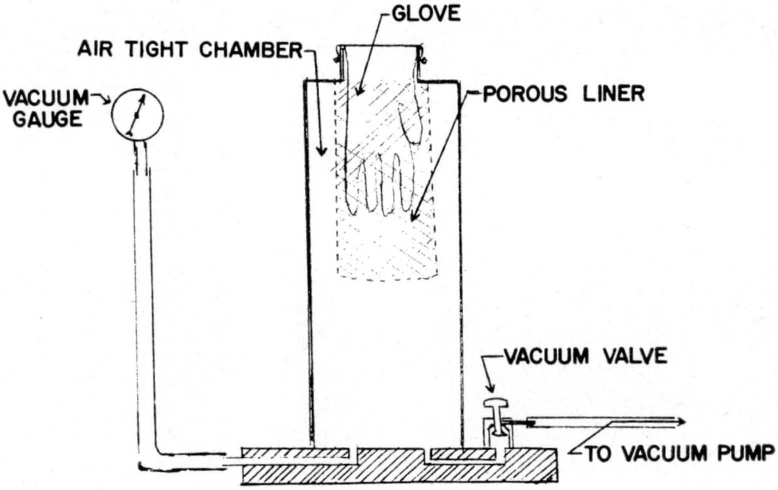

Fig 3.—Glove tester for central supply units. The glove is placed over the chamber supported by the everted cuff. Air is exhausted from the chamber by a vacuum pump activated by the valve. The glove distends to the limits of the porous liner which surrounds it. The vacuum gauge remains unchanged if the glove is devoid of holes. A few seconds suffice for the test.

previously.[8] Many new gloves contain minute holes. An adequate testing method should be available in the hospitals for evaluating new gloves before use. This method should not wet the glove, as this would imply too much work for the technician. We have devised a method for the testing of gloves either in the operating room or in the central supply area [9] (Fig 3).

While the glove is in use during an operation, it is possible to test it repeatedly by a very simple method based upon loss of electrical resistance if holes develop.[6]

Textiles and Other Draping Materials.—Whenever possible, tests should be carried out at the end of a period of normal use, as well as original testing before use. The bacteriologic efficiency of a material as a barrier can be determined in a simple manner. A standard pattern of growth of bacterial colonies upon an agar medium contained in a Petri dish is easily produced with a replicate inoculator (Fig 4*A*). A sterile swatch of the material is then placed over the growth pattern and the other surface of the material moistened with an aqueous solution. The swatch is then removed and an imprint of the outer surface made on a second agar medium. If the material is efficient as a bacteria barrier, no migration will be evident (Fig 4*B*). If the material is inefficient, the imprint will develop a pattern of growth identical with that of the original plate (Fig 4*C*).

Other tests for static accumulation, antigenicity, flexibility, and porosity can then be applied.

Barrier Materials

Having set up specifications and methods of evaluation, we can then appraise presently used materials. We can also speculate whether it will be necessary to relax specifications until new materials are devised which will more closely approach the ideal.

Again we must differentiate between the various uses of barriers, and discuss each separately.

Masks.—A variety of materials have been employed for masks. It is our personal opinion that, at present, we have no efficient and comfortable mask available for use. All of them are hot, difficult to breathe through (or around), and I know of no surgeon who does not remove one as soon as he is able to do so. At present we use a double gauze, 14 ply, washed mask and change masks frequently.

The future does hold out some hope. New materials are being devised for demisting atmosphere in air, which means the trapping of droplets of water. This may well be employed in future mask designs affording free breathing along with a true barrier effect.

Gloves.—The efficiency of the intact glove is undoubted. However, all holes must be discovered. If gloves were perfect we would not need to wash our hands, let alone scrub.

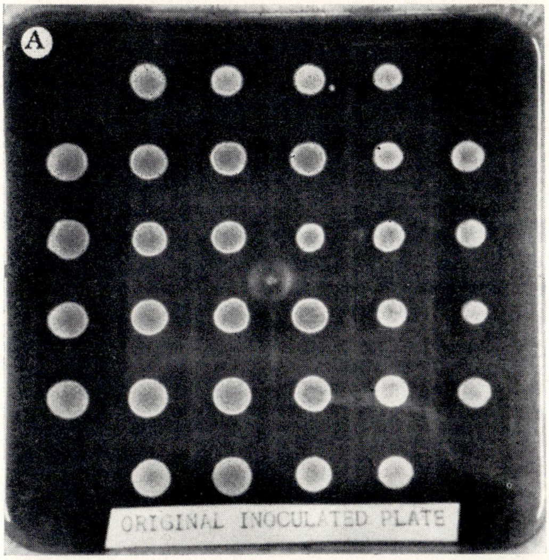

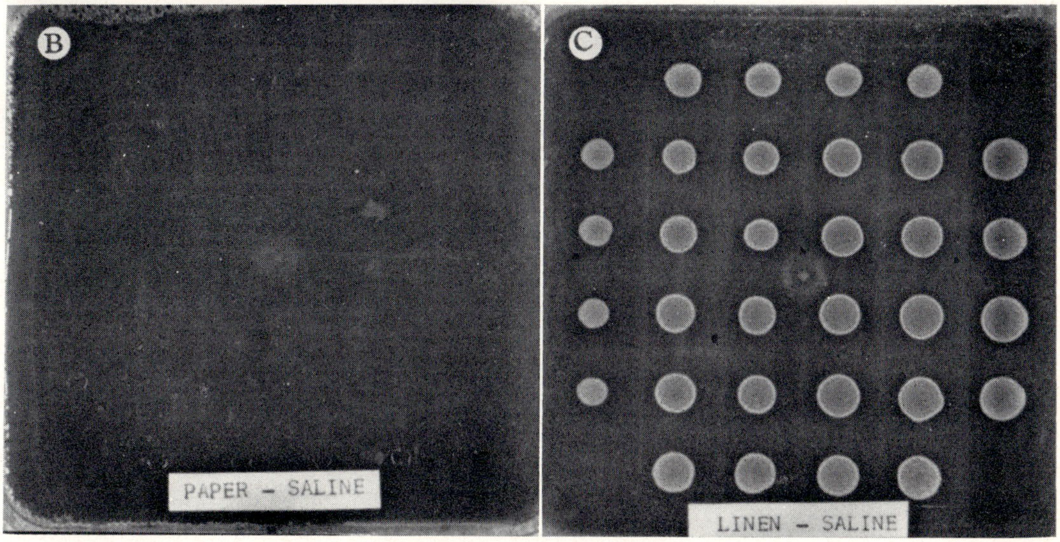

Fig 4.—Tests conducted as in Fig 1 for the comparative barrier effect of textile versus paper (Surg-O-Pac) drape material; *A,* the control or pattern plate; *B,* the paper drape moistened with saline; *C,* the textile drape moistened with saline.

Furthermore, we know that the scrub is not entirely efficient, or we would not need to wear gloves. At present, in our opinion, the combined use of a good surgical scrub coupled with a glove which has been adequately pretested and is continuously tested during use constitutes an efficient bacterial barrier. This holds true for all glove materials since they are all impervious to water while intact.

The Operative Field Barrier.—This subject should be discussed separately from the other zones of barrier activity, because in this area we now have excellent methods available. In the last few years, an old but effective principle has been revived. DeMartel [10] suggested the application of a skin varnish through which the incision was made. Now, plastic materials are available which can be sprayed on the skin, or affixed on the skin with an adhesive, and through which the incision is made. This technique is above reproach *if the area so prepared is confined and not too widespread.* The encasement of less than 10% of the body surface by a nonporous material is considered not to be harmful.

Surgical Drapes.—The drapes presently used over the remainder of the patient's body, and over instrument tables, basin holders, and other accouterments are not, by our criteria, acceptable as bacterial barriers. The use of multiple layers of towels or of textile sheets of varying plies is merely a subterfuge. A *single* sheet of a waterproof porous material can solve the problem.

So far, we have tested only one such material which is available for use. This is a treated paper material which is waterproof, moderately strong, and which can be made up in any shape or size.* As it is waterproof, a moistened, sterile towel can be placed upon it so that instruments will not slip nor sharp instruments perforate it. However, since it is waterproof, bacteria will not gain access to the towel from unsterile surfaces beneath it.

It is possible that certain textile materials will become available which will possess essentially the same attributes. There is a material manufactured in Great Britain which is a treated textile and which is waterproof. It is, as far as we have been able to learn, not available in this country. Tests as to an ability to withstand laundering, etc, would have to be made.

When the paper drape described above is employed, it is redundant to use the usual square of towels held in place with towel clips or layers of other material. One merely employs a plastic material glued to the skin of the operative site and a single aperture drape of this paper material.

Gowns.—The surgeon's gown poses a problem. The textile type now in use is *not acceptable.* The paper drape material referred to above is not available at present in the form of a gown. Until it does become available, or some other suitable material comes to hand, an expediency is to wear a paper apron, donned after the scrub and worn under the gown.

Sterile Goods Wrappers.—These should be made of a waterproof material, *or* placed within a waterproof envelope as soon as they come from the steam sterilizer. We are hoping to develop a tape of some type which will reveal not only that the bundle has been adequately sterilized, but that the bundle has not been exposed to moisture. This would give us a check on possible contamination from outside the bundle.

* Surg-O-Pac manufactured by Converters, Inc.

Summary and Conclusions

Aseptic barriers are materials which are placed between aseptic areas and zones of possible contamination, designed to prevent the migration of microorganisms into the sterile zone.

The migration of microorganisms is largely, if not entirely, effected by a vehicle; in surgical practice this vehicle is usually water or an aqueous solution.

Aseptic barriers, therefore, must be waterproof.

A set of specifications has been suggested for aseptic barriers, including waterproof structure, porosity, flexibility, lack of antigenicity and static accumulation, and most importantly "comfort-in-use" for the surgical team and for the patient.

A group of test methods have been described in brief. It has been suggested that one of our surgical organizations should set up a special committee to formulate specifications and standardized tests to insure conformity with these specifications.

The presently employed barrier materials have been discussed. A rating of satisfactory has been given to gloves, and to plastics limited to the operative field. Masks have been discussed briefly; present deficiencies have been indicated, along with the hope that the future will bring efficient and comfortable masks through the employment of new materials. Drapes have been reviewed in some detail. At present, the only drape which is given a satisfactory rating is one of a paper, waterproof, disposable type. Gowns also have been discussed. The only method presently available which affords at least partial protection against bacterial migration involves a waterproof apron under the textile gown.

William C. Beck, MD, Guthrie Clinic, Sayre, Pa.

REFERENCES

1. Perkins, J. J.: Principles and Methods of Sterilization, Springfield, Ill: Charles C Thomas, Publisher, 1960, p 113.

2. Beck, W. C., and Collette, T. S.: False Faith in the Surgeon's Gown and Drape, Amer J Surg 83:125-126, 1952.

3. Beck, W. C.: Exhibit shown at the American College of Surgeons, Chicago, October, 1956.

4. Wise, R. I.; Sweeney, F. J., Jr.; Haupt, G. J.; and Waddell, M. A.: The Environmental Distribution of Staphylococcus Aureus in Our Operating Suite, Amer Surg 149:30-42, 1959.

5. Gorvoy, J. D.; Acs, H.; and Stein, M. L.: The Hazard of Induction of Sweating in Cystic Fibrosis of the Pancreas, Pediatrics 25:977-982, 1960.

6. Beck, W. C.: Holes in Rubber Gloves: Description of a New Instrument to Detect Holes During Operations, Guthrie Clin Bull 29:14-18, 1959.

7. Shooter, R. A.; Smith, M. A.; and Hunter, C. J.: A Study of Surgical Masks, Brit J Surg 47:246-249, 1959.

8. Beck, W. C.: Holes in Rubber Gloves, Amer J Surg 100:363-364, 1960.

9. Reynolds, H. C., and Beck, W. C.: A Glove Tester for Central Supply Units, Guthrie Clin Bull 31:153-155, 1962.

10. DeMartel, T.: Personal communication to the authors, 1932.

DISCUSSION

Dr. James R. Watson, Pittsburgh: Dr. Beck has called attention to an operating room ritual which all of us go through daily during our professional lives, and which we have generally accepted as having a high degree of protection against infection in clean surgical wounds. Certainly there has been little in the surgical literature suggesting dissatisfaction with surgical gloves or with the commonly accepted methods of draping. The mask has obviously left something to be desired, but as yet there seems to be no improvement on the many-layered gauze filter without adding considerable discomfort to the surgeon.

These devices, which Dr. Beck has referred to as "aseptic barriers," can be breached, although the glove with the hole in it, or the mask which covers the mouth and nose of a surgeon or assistant who is harboring an acute upper respiratory infection, represents a break in aseptic technique rather than in failure of the aseptic barrier.

The barrier of greatest interest to me in Dr. Beck's presentation is the draping of the wound. I have always surrounded the edges of the wound with moist, sterile drapes, under the impression that this was a protective mechanism; now I have a concern as to whether or not this is a possible source of the occasional unexplained infection in what would be presumed to have been a clean surgical wound.

Knowing that infection is related not only to the virulence of the organism but also to the degree of contamination and to the resistance of the host, the latter being measured by the nutritional state of the patient and by the presence or absence of dead space, blood clot, and devitalized tissue in the wound, it is possible that all clean surgical wounds are contaminated at the conclusion of a major operation and that infection results only when the condition of the wound or the nutritional state of the patient favors it.

A better mousetrap, or maybe we should say a better bacterial trap, is always desirable; and if current methods of draping are shown to be a source of contamination, better methods should be sought. I have had no experience whatever with plastic skin sprays or paper drapes.

I would like to ask Dr. Beck what his routine method is today in draping his patients, after the study he has given to this particular subject.

Dr. Clarence W. Monroe, Oak Park, Ill: This is one of my favorite soapbox subjects, and I cannot resist the temptation to say what I often say to my residents. One of the things that annoys me most, when we start to prepare a patient for an operation, is to see the resident or the intern (and I have often seen my conferees who are beyond this stage do it too) get a lot of water and slop it all over the patient. When they get ready to drape, they lay the drapes right over the patient who is now lying in a puddle of soapy water.

I do not see how one can regard this as suitable preparation of the skin or draping of the patient. I think if the patient is washed with a lot of soapsuds and the suds washed off, then whatever magic —benzalkonium chloride (Zephiran) or anything else—is used, you are very likely to end up with dry drapes that do not have capillary action.

I think Dr. Beck's paper confirms work done about 20 years ago, when Neal Owens in New Orleans tried some of this same thing. He took 75 layers of moist toweling and was able to show that bacteria went through it very rapidly.

I think unless we get to the point of using some kind of impervious drapes, we will have this trouble. My own preference is to use the so-called underpad that Johnson & Johnson makes, covered with a single pillowcase that is on the margin of the wound, and any wet sponges or anything else are kept on this. It is very gratifying to come to the end of an operative procedure and find that as you lift off the heavy kraft paper drape everything beneath it is perfectly dry. You know you have not had any bacteria from the table come through your drapes and into the field.

Dr. William C. Beck, Sayre, Penn: Dr. Watson, the method that we will probably use, at least for the present, is to apply a plastic to the operative area using either the one with an affixed adherent or a spray adhesive and separate plastic. Over this we will use a single aperture drape made of waterproof paper. This drape is disposable; it is not excessively expensive; it is simple to apply; it needs only one layer. There is no square of towels. You may enlarge or refashion the aperture with a scissors. It can be adapted to any size or shape. There are several paper drapes on the market, but we have used only one of them. It must be waterproof. The one we have employed works well.

Dr. Lindon Seed once told me that he had made a long and expensive trip to Boston to observe a famous surgeon's thyroidectomy. He said that all that he learned was to use a wet towel between the incision and the instrument table. This prevented instruments from slipping when they had been discarded. Ten years ago, when we demonstrated the permeability of textile drapes to bacteria when wet, he had to abandon this technique, and his expense went for naught.

Now, Dr. Seed, using waterproof drapes, you may again use your wet towel and save your instruments.

Blood Ammonia Reduction by Potassium Exchange Resin

Experimentation in Eck-Fistula Dogs

GEORGE D. ZUIDEMA, MD; DAVID CULLEN; RICHARD S. KOWALCZYK, PhD; AND EARL F. WOLFMAN, JR., MD, ANN ARBOR, MICH

Introduction

Hepatic coma, a consequence of severe liver disease, is usually associated with elevated levels of blood ammonia and derangements of serum electrolytes and pH. Treatment of hepatic coma may be directed toward lowering of the blood ammonia level once this elevation has occurred or preventing the absorption of the products of protein digestion within the gastrointestinal tract.

Several methods have been employed to control blood ammonia. Neomycin is useful in removing urea-splitting organisms from the intestine, thereby limiting the amount of ammonia absorbed into the portal circulation.[1] The side effects of neomycin treatment, however, impair its usefulness. Hypothermia lowers blood ammonia, probably by limiting bacterial action.[2,3] Arginine and glutamic acid[4-6] enjoyed brief popularity because of the belief that they aided the metabolism of ammonia and its elimination via the Krebs urea cycle. Hemodialysis[7] is effective in clearing the blood of ammonia, but the technique is of transitory value and cumbersome to use.

It has been shown that an orally administered sodium-cycle sulfonated polystyrene cation exchange resin * is effective in lowering blood ammonium levels in Eck-fistula dogs.[8,9] Since this report the clinical effectiveness of this material has also been demonstrated.[10] Certain side effects of the sodium cycle resin, however, impose limitations in its usefulness. This resin exchanges sodium ions for ammonium and potassium ions. Consequently, potassium depletion may occur unless potassium supplements are provided. Many patients in hepatic coma are hypokalemic when first seen, and further potassium losses may potentiate the coma. Furthermore, patients with advanced liver disease often have ascites and sodium and

Presented at the 20th Annual Meeting of the Central Surgical Association, Chicago, Feb 21-23, 1963.

John and Mary R. Markle Scholar in Academic Medicine, USPHS Career Development Awardee (Dr. Zuidema).

Department of Surgery, University of Michigan Medical School.

Supported in part by grants from the US Public Health Service, National Institute for Arthritis and Metabolic Disease H4260 (C-3), and Career Development Award AM K3-13,702; US Army Contract DA 49-007-MD-1016.

* Kayexalate, product of Winthrop Laboratories, New York 18.

water retention. The addition of sodium ions from the resin may aggravate the condition.

The present study was carried out to determine the ability of a potassium-cycle exchange resin to lower blood ammonia in Eck-fistula dogs. This resin has the advantage of exchanging potassium ions for ammonium and sodium ions. Potassium depletion and sodium overloading would, therefore, be avoided.

The following experiments consist of two phases: an in vitro study to compare the abilities of sodium and potassium resins to bind ammonia; and in vivo observations on eight Eck-fistula dogs treated with potassium-cycle resin and these results compared with identical experiments using the sodium-cycle resin (Kayexalate).[9]

Methods

The potassium cycle cation exchange resin was derived from an ammonium cycle cation exchange resin† by heating with 6 N potassium hydroxide solution over a steam bath for 12 hours. The resin obtained in this way was of a coarse texture and could be readily reclaimed by filtration. It was air dried prior to use.

1. *In Vitro Experiments.*—Standard solutions containing 0μg, 100μg, 300μg, 500μg ammonia nitrogen per 100 ml were prepared using ammonium sulfate and distilled water. One hundred milliliters of each standard solution was agitated with sodium-cycle resin, 1.0 gm, in a covered beaker at room temperature for one hour. The solution was filtered and the filtrate titrated for residual ammonia. This process was repeated using the potassium-cycle exchange resins.

2. *In Vivo Experiments.*—Eight healthy mongrel dogs, weighing 9 to 18 kg, were anesthetized with sodium pentobarbital (25 mg/kg), end-to-side portacaval anastomoses performed, and one to two weeks were allowed for recovery. After fasting the dogs for 18 hours, venous blood samples were drawn and baseline determinations of ammonia, sodium, potassium, chloride, and blood urea nitrogen were made. A gastric tube was inserted, and stored human blood was administered (40 ml/kg). This was carried out in three equally divided doses over a one-hour period. Hourly blood ammonia determinations were obtained for eight hours. The individual and mean values are shown in Fig 2. Serum sodium, potassium, chloride, and blood urea nitrogen were determined by standard laboratory technique. Whole blood ammonia-nitrogen was determined by a modification of the Conway microdiffusion technique.[11,12]

Experiments using the potassium-cycle resin were identical to the control studies with the exception that, preceding each aliquot of blood, the powdered resin, 8.0 gm, was given by gastric tube. A final 8.0 gm of resin was administered with Sorbitol,‡ 30 ml. The total dose of potassium-cycle resin was 32 gm. The results obtained from this experiment are shown in Fig 3.

Fig 4 compares the mean curves obtained using potassium-cycle resin with the control studies and the results of a previously reported study using a sodium-cycle resin.[9]

† WIN-3000, Winthrop Laboratories, Special Chemical Department, 1450 Broadway, New York 18.

‡ Proprietary sugar solution for use as a cathartic.

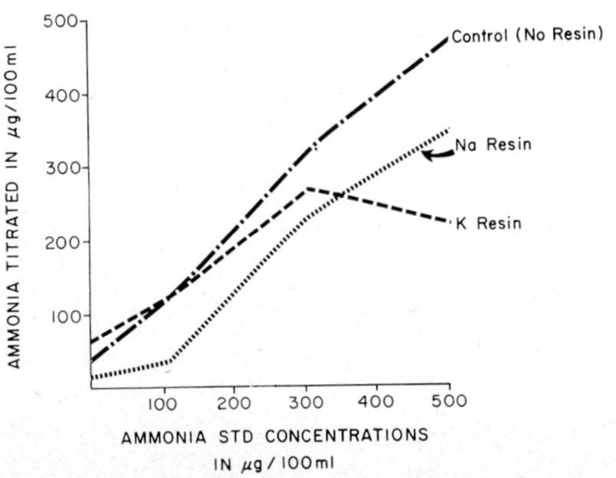

Fig 1.—Action of one sodium-cycle (Kayexalate) and one potassium-cycle exchange resins on standard solutions of ammonium sulfate containing ammonium ion concentrations of 100μg%, 300μg% and 500μg%.

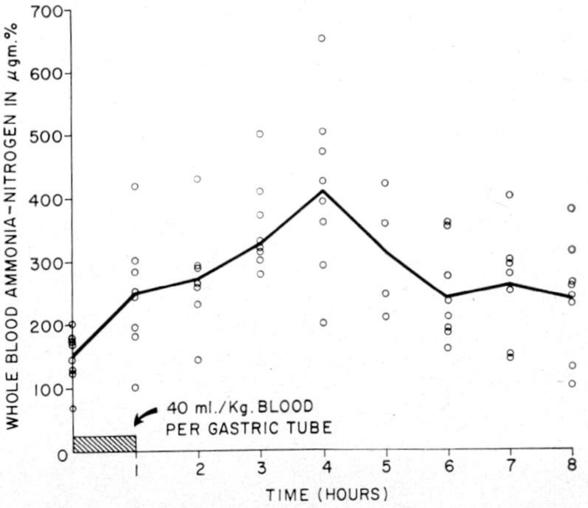

Fig 2.—Baseline blood ammonia curve: end-to-side portacaval shunts in dogs. Control study showing blood ammonia determinations and mean values obtained in eight Eck-fistula dogs given whole blood (40 ml/kg) by gastric tube.

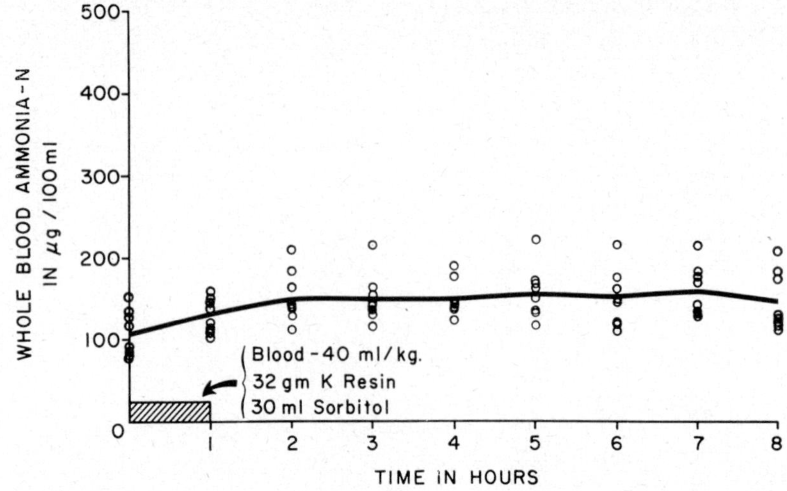

Fig 3.—The effect of a potassium-cycle exchange resin and Sorbitol on blood ammonia levels in eight Eck-fistula dogs given whole blood (40 ml/kg) by gastric tube.

Cation exchange resins in general have a constipating tendency which is troublesome. Sorbitol in 70% solution § prevents this side effect and was used for this purpose in these experiments.

Results

The in vitro experiment showed that both resins tested proved capable of binding ammonia (Fig 1). The potassium-cycle resin was slightly more effective than sodium-cycle resin in removing ammonia when agitated with the standard solution cotaining a higher concentration of ammonium sulfate. When it became apparent that the potassium resin was effective in binding ammonia, in vivo experiments were begun.

§ Sorbo, Courtesy of Biological Sciences Section, Atlas Powder Company, Wilmington, Del.

Control blood ammonia data obtained from eight Eck-fistula dogs given whole blood (40 ml/kg) show that peak blood ammonia levels of approximately 407μg/100 ml are attained about four hours after its administration (Fig 2). Experiments using the potassium-cycle exchange resin showed the efficacy of this substance in controlling ammonia levels. The mean blood ammonia level never exceeded 162μg%. The individual determinations and mean curve are shown in Fig 3. A comparison of the blood ammonia values four hours after administration of potassium resin and Sorbitol with control values from untreated dogs shows that the resin exerts a statistically significant effect ($P<0.001$).||

|| Determined by "student" *t*-test.

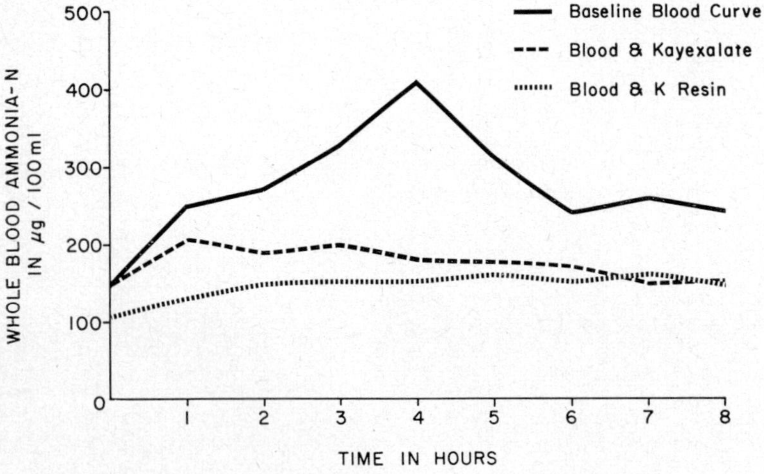

Fig 4.—Mean venous blood ammonia. Comparison of the sodium-cycle and potassium-cycle exchange resins with control curves. All data obtained from studies in eight Eck-fistula dogs given whole blood (40 ml/kg) by gastric tube.

TABLE 1.—*Effect of Potassium-Cycle Exchange Resin on Blood Ammonia: Statistical Analysis*

Time, Hours	0	1	2	3	4	5	6	7	8
Control blood NH_3, μg %	148±14	250±33	270±31	330±38	410±48	316±42	240±28	260±34	240±32
Potassium resin blood NH_3, μg %	110±9.8	131±7.5	151±11.7	153±10.6	152±7.6	159±11.5	151±12.3	162±11.3	148±12.9
Standard deviation	—	69	64	59	99	60	60	66	69
Relative deviate	—	3.4	3.6	5.9	5.2	4.3	3.0	2.9	2.4
P value		<0.01	<0.01	<0.001	<0.001	<0.001	<0.01	<0.02	<0.03

The statistical treatment of the data is given in Table 1. The electrolyte determinations from these experiments are listed in Table 2. It will be noted that little change occurred in serum electrolytes during the eight-hour experiment. Serum potassium levels rose slightly although they remained within normal limits. Blood urea nitrogen levels rose consistently during the experimental period.

Previous experiments using the sodium-cycle exchange resin (Kayexalate) had demonstrated its efficiency in controlling levels of blood ammonia.[9] A comparison of sodium- and potassium-cycle resins is shown in Fig 4 where the mean curves obtained with resin therapy and in control animals are displayed.

Comment

The metabolic derangements occurring with hepatic coma are often complex. Hypokalemia is frequently seen and is known to potentiate elevations of blood ammonia. Chlorothiazide, and related diuretics, may precipitate hepatic coma if potassium chloride supplements are not given to offset potassium losses.[13,14] Patients with advanced liver disease usually have an abnormal tendency to retain sodium and water, although this may remain latent at a subclinical level. Total body sodium may be increased although serum sodium values may be low. This is particularly likely in patients with cirrhosis and ascites.

TABLE 2.—*Results in Eight Dogs With Eck-Fistula Given Whole Blood (40 Ml/Kg), K-Resin (32 Gm), and Sorbitol (30 Ml)*

Blood Urea Nitrogen (Mg/100 Ml)			
Initial		Final	
Range	Mean	Range	Mean
7-13	9.1	18-48	28
Serum Potassium (mEq/Liter)			
Initial		Final	
Range	Mean	Range	Mean
3.9-5.2	4.6	4.1-6.2	5.6

Orally administered cation exchange resins have been used successfully in controlling hyperkalemia associated with renal insufficiency.[15,16] This work prompted Zuidema et al [8,9] to use exchange resins for ammonia intoxication. Work in dogs and later experience with cirrhotic patients [10] showed that a sodium-cycle resin was effective in lowering blood ammonia levels. Two problems were occasionally encountered. Some patients with ascites gained weight because of the sodium ions gained in the exchange for ammonium and potassium ions. Supplements of potassium chloride were necessary to avoid the development of hypokalemia which in turn may contribute to stupor and hyperammoniemia.

While careful management could control these side effects, the potential usefulness of other exchange resins was attractive. A potassium-cycle resin was selected for study because theoretically it would obviate both of the disadvantages of the sodium cycle resin. Since it would exchange potassium ions for ammonium and sodium ions it would help correct sodium retention rather than aggravate it. Furthermore, it would eliminate the tendency to deplete the body's potassium stores, help correct any pre-existing hypokalemia, and make the use of potassium supplements unnecessary. If one can be certain that renal function is good, potassium loads derived from the potassium-cycle resin would not be excessive.

These experiments, performed in Eck-fistula dogs, demonstrate that the potassium cycle resin is capable of easily controlling blood ammonia levels. Its effectiveness compares very well, in equivalent doses, with that of the sodium-cycle exchange resin (Kayexalate) reported earlier. Potassium intoxication was not encountered in these experimental animals. Clinical studies are now under way to evaluate its effects upon patients with hepatic coma and hyperammoniemia.

Summary

A potassium-cycle cation exchange resin and a sodium-cycle exchange resin were effective in binding ammonium ions in an in vitro study.

The potassium-cycle exchange resin was capable of preventing increased blood ammonia in eight Eck-fistula dogs given whole blood by gastric tube.

Serum electrolytes remained within normal limits during the experiment.

The effectiveness of the potassium cycle resin studied compares favorably with that of a previously studied sodium-cycle resin.

George D. Zuidema, MD, Department of Surgery, University of Michigan Medical School, Ann Arbor, Mich.

REFERENCES

1. Dawson, A. M.; McLaren, J.; and Sherlock, S.: Neomycin in the Treatment of Hepatic Coma, Lancet 2:1263, 1957.

2. Keirle, A. M.; McGloin, J. J.; Buben, R. W.; Altemeier, W. A.: Blood Ammonia: Experimental and Clinical Reduction by Hypothermia, Arch Surg 83:348-355, 1961.

3. Zuidema, G. D.; Gaisford, W. D.; Kowalczyk, R. S.; and Wolfman, E. F., Jr.: Effect of Whole Body Hypothermia on Ammonia Intoxication in Monkeys With Portacaval Shunts, to be published.

4. Walshe, J. M.: Glutamic Acid in Hepatic Coma, Lancet 1:1235, 1955.

5. McDermott, W. V., Jr.; Wareham, J.; and Riddell, A. G.: Treatment of "Hepatic Coma" With L-Glutamic Acid, New Eng J Med 253:1093, 1955.

6. Reynolds, T. B.; Redeker, A. G.; and Davis, P.: A Controlled Study of the Effects of L-Arginine on Hepatic Encephalopathy, Amer J Med 25:359, 1958.

7. Kiley, J. E.; Pender, J. C.; Welch, H. F.; and Welch, C. S.: Ammonia Intoxication Treated by Hemodialysis, New Eng J Med 259:1156, 1958.

8. Zuidema, G. D.; Fletcher, M. M.; and Burton, W. D.: Orally Administered Cation Exchange Resin-Sorbitol Regimen for Treatment of Ammonia Intoxication in Dogs, Proc Soc Exp Biol Med 109:732-734, 1962.

9. Zuidema, G. D.; Fletcher, M. M.: Burton, W. D.; and Child, C. G., 3d: Oral Cation Exchange Resin Therapy for Ammonia Intoxication in Dog, Surgery 52:117-126, 1962.

10. Zuidema, G. D.; Gaisford, W. D.; Kowalczyk, R. S.; and Wolfman, E. F., Jr.: Oral Cation Exchange Resins for Treatment of Ammonia Intoxication, to be published.

11. Reif, A. E.: The Ammonia Content of Blood and Plasma, Biochem 1:351:370, 1960.

12. Natelson, S.: Microtechniques of Clinical Chemistry: For the Routine Laboratory, Springfield, Ill, Charles C Thomas, Publisher, 1957, p 484.

13. Sherlock, S.; Read, A. E.; Laidlaw, J. L.; and Haslam, R.: Chlorothiazide in Liver Disease, Ann NY Acad Sci 71:430, 1958.

14. Read, A. E.; Laidlaw, J. L.; Haslam, R. M.; and Sherlock, S.: Neuropsychiatric Complications Following Chlorothiazide Therapy in Patients With Hepatic Cirrhosis: Possible Relation to Hypokalaemia, Clin Sci 18:409, 1959.

15. Scherr, L.; Ogden, D. A.; Mead, A. W.; Spritz, N.; and Rubin, A. L.: Management of Hyperkalemia With a Cation-Exchange Resin, New Eng J Med 264:115, 1961.

16. Flinn, R. B.; Merrill, J. P.; and Welzant, W. R.: Treatment of the Oliguric Patient With a New Sodium-Exchange Resin and Sorbitol: A Preliminary Report, New Eng J Med 264:111, 1961.

Pathogenesis of Esophageal Varix Rupture

A Study Based on Gross and Microscopic Examination of the Esophagus at the Time of Bleeding

MARSHALL J. ORLOFF, MD, AND H. STEPHENS THOMAS, MD, TORRANCE, CALIF

An understanding of the pathogenesis of esophageal varix rupture is of more than academic importance, since upon such knowledge depends the development of a rational approach to the prophylaxis and therapy of this highly lethal disorder. Although much is known about the mechanisms responsible for the formation of esophageal varices, considerable controversy exists regarding the exact cause of varix rupture. Two major factors have been implicated in the pathogenesis, namely, erosion of the varix due to reflux acid-peptic esophagitis, and bursting of the varix due to increased hydrostatic pressure in the portal venous system. The treatment of bleeding esophageal varices has consisted, in large part, of measures directed at counteracting one or the other of these two factors.

Much of the evidence cited to support the acid-peptic hypothesis has come from animal experiments of uncertain applicability to man,[1,2,15,16] from esophagoscopic examination of cirrhotic patients performed many days after bleeding had subsided,[13] and from autopsy examinations of the human esophagus conducted at varying periods of time after the onset of varix hemorrhage.[4,14,17] Furthermore, the autopsy and endoscopic studies in many cases followed clinical attempts to control the bleeding with therapeutic measures which may have altered the material upon which the studies were based.

During the performance of emergency transesophageal varix ligations over the past several years, it was our impression that esophagitis was a rare finding, an impression which conflicted with the autopsy observations of others and with the postulates of the acid-peptic hypothesis. To confirm or deny that impression, a study was undertaken in which the distal esophagus and proximal stomach were carefully examined grossly, and biopsies of the esophagus were obtained during operations which were performed shortly after the onset of varix bleeding. The opportunity to conduct such a study was afforded by another investigation, already in progress, which was aimed at evaluating the efficacy of early transesophageal ligation of bleeding esophageal varices in unselected patients with cirrhosis.[10] It is the purpose of this report to present the results of gross and microscopic examinations of the esophagus performed at the time of bleeding in 20 unselected cirrhotic patients with varix hemorrhage.

Presented at the 20th Annual Meeting of the Central Surgical Association, Feb 21-23, 1963.

Professor and Chief of Surgery and Markle Scholar in Medicine (Dr. Orloff); Resident in Surgery (Dr. Thomas).

From the Departments of Surgery, Harbor General Hospital and the University of California, Los Angeles School of Medicine.

Aided by United States Public Health Service grant A-5710 and The John and Mary R. Markle Foundation.

Materials and Methods

The study program for evaluating the efficacy of transesophageal varix ligation has been described in detail previously.[10] Briefly, every patient who entered the hospital with upper gastrointestinal bleeding and suspected or known cirrhosis of the liver was subjected to a series of diagnostic tests which were completed within six hours of admission to the hospital. In addition, cirrhotic patients who developed bleeding while in the hospital were included in the study and underwent the diagnostic procedures within six hours of the onset of hemorrhage. While the diagnostic studies were being completed, all patients received the same initial therapy which consisted of blood transfusions, parenteral vitamins and glucose, enteral cathartics and neomycin, neomycin enemas, and intravenous posterior pituitary extract (Pituitrin). A Levin tube was inserted in all patients and was used to lavage the stomach with cold saline and to instil cathartics and antibiotics. *None* of the patients received esophageal balloon tamponade.

The diagnosis of varix hemorrhage was based on the demonstration of esophageal varices on x-ray, the failure to demonstrate other lesions commonly responsible for upper gastrointestinal hemorrhage, and the presence of a history, physical findings, and laboratory results compatible with the diagnosis of cirrhosis of the liver. Histologic proof of cirrhosis was ultimately obtained in all but three patients by needle liver biopsy, liver biopsy at operation, or autopsy.

Transesophageal varix ligation was performed within eight hours of admission to the hospital, or in the case of those patients who developed bleeding while in the hospital, within eight hours of the onset of hemorrhage. One patient whose varices ruptured while in the hospital was not operated upon until fifteen hours after bleeding was detected, and this was the only case in which the planned time schedule was not followed. All operations were performed through a thoracic incision, and most of them were done under hypothermia. The varix ligation was accomplished through a 6 cm longitudinal incision in the distal esophagus which provided a clear view of the mucosa of the proximal 2 to 3 cm of the stomach and the distal 8 to 10 cm of the esophagus.

The appearance of the distal esophageal and proximal gastric mucosa was specifically noted at the time of operation. The point of varix rupture and bleeding was searched for, and its location in relation to the esophagogastric junction was recorded. A biopsy of the esophagus was obtained from a site within 2 cm of the esophagogastric junction. Sections of the biopsy specimen were stained with hematoxylin and eosin for microscopic study.

Results

The results of the study are shown in the Table. Twenty unselected patients with bleeding esophageal varices were included. On the basis of clinical and laboratory evaluations all patients had moderate to advanced cirrhosis of the liver, and in 17 of the 20 this was confirmed by liver biopsies. One of the patients had postnecrotic cirrhosis, and the others gave a long history of alcoholism. All of the patients had large esophageal varices which were demonstrated roentgenographically and at operation.

Nine patients ingested alcohol in sizable quantities up to the time when bleeding started, and five of these continued to drink

Characteristics of Patients Subjected to Varix Ligation,

Patient	Bleeding Episode	Admission Hgb, Gm %	Alcohol Ingestion Immed. Before Bleeding	Type of Cirrhosis	Liver Biopsy Proof of Cirrhosis	Varices on X-Ray	Onset Bleeding to Operation, Hr	Admission to Operation, Hr
1	1	6.2	Yes	Alcoholic	Yes	+	8	5
2	1	8.5	No	Alcoholic	Yes	+	12	6
3	2	9.8	?	Alcoholic	No	+	36	8
4	1	7.8	No	Alcoholic	Yes	+	14½	6½
5	1	9.4	?	Alcoholic	Yes	+	8	8 *
6	1	7.2	?	Alcoholic	No	+	16½	4½
7	2	8.9	No	Alcoholic	Yes	+	8	8 *
8	2	9.6	Yes	Alcoholic	Yes	+	13½	5½
9	2	9.1	Yes	Alcoholic	Yes	+	14	6
10	1	8.4	Yes	Alcoholic	Yes	+	10¾	5¾
11	2	8.1	No	Postnecrotic	Yes	+	5¾	5¾
12	1	4.9	Yes	Alcoholic	Yes	+	12	7
13	1	9.6	Yes	Alcoholic	Yes	+	8	5
14	1	4.3	No	Alcoholic	No	+	56	6
15	1	6.2	Yes	Alcoholic	Yes	+	13	5
16	2	5.0	No	Alcoholic	Yes	+	15	15 *
17	2	15.0	Yes	Alcoholic	Yes	+	12	8
18	2	10.3	No	Alcoholic	Yes	+	4¾	4¾ *
19	3	7.8	No	Alcoholic	Yes	+	14½	6½
20	2	5.4	Yes	Alcoholic	Yes	+	8¾	6¾

* Five patients developed varix bleeding while in the hospital.

for several hours after they vomited blood. Eight patients did not drink alcohol for at least several days prior to the onset of hemorrhage, and the remaining three patients were unable to provide this information.

Although the patients who entered the hospital with varix hemorrhage were operated upon within 8 hours of admission, they had been bleeding for a variable period of time before coming to the hospital. Thus, the time lapse between the onset of bleeding and operation ranged from 4¾ to 56 hours. Eighteen of the 20 patients were operated upon within 16½ hours of the time when they first became aware of bleeding.

All patients bled massively during the few hours prior to operation. The hemoglobin level on admission or at the onset of bleeding was below 10 gm% in all but two cases and ranged from 4.3 to 15.9 gm% in the group. Ten patients had not experienced a previous episode of hemorrhage, nine were bleeding for the second time, and one was bleeding for the third time.

In 16 of 20 cases a definite solitary point of varix rupture and bleeding was found. In 4 of these cases the bleeding point was located at the esophagogastric junction, and in the remaining 12 it occurred in the esophagus within 1.5 cm of the junction. In all but 1 of the 16 cases the bleeding point had the appearance of a clean tear or hole in the mucosa overlying a varix from which blood spurted under considerable pressure. The mucosal defects were approximately 1 to 3 mm in diameter and had none of the characteristics of chronic ulcers or erosions from without.

In 19 of the 20 cases, the distal esophageal mucosa down to and including the esophagogastric junction was smooth and glistening, and there was no gross indication of inflammation. The mucosa was obviously thinned by the bulging varices underneath, which could be seen clearly and gave the mucosa a bluish color (Fig 1). In one case, the mucosa of the distal esophagus was red, granular, friable, and contained many ulcers, and was obviously the seat of severe esophagitis. It is noteworthy that the patient who was found to have esophagitis had been drinking heavily up to the onset of bleeding and for several hours afterwards, and had been vomiting repeatedly for several days prior to rupture of his varices.

Biopsies of the distal esophagus were obtained from 15 of the 20 patients (Fig 2 and 3). In only one, the patient with gross esophagitis, was there microscopic evidence of inflammation. The remaining 14 specimens showed many dilated submucosal veins, and a few showed a minimal round cell infiltration which is known to accompany rup-

and Esophageal Findings

Distance of Bleeding Point From Esophagogastric Junction	Esophagitis	
	Gross	Microscopic
At junction	No	No
1 cm above	No	No
1 cm above	No	—
1 cm above	No	No
1 cm above	No	—
1 cm above	No	—
1 cm above	No	No
1.5 cm above	No	No
1.5 cm above	Marked	Marked
1 cm above	No	No
0.2 cm above	No	No
At junction	No	No
None found	No	No
At junction	No	No
None found	No	No
0.5 cm above	No	No
None found	No	—
None found	No	—
1 cm above	No	No
At junction	No	No

Fig 1.—Photograph of distal esophageal mucosa made at operation upon patient 19, showing bulging varices. There is no gross evidence of esophagitis.

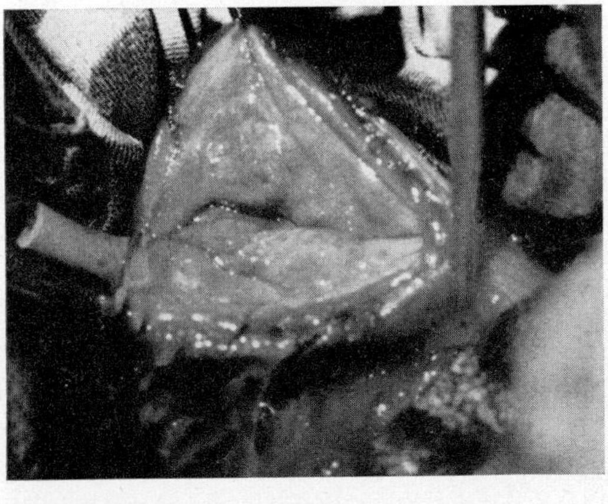

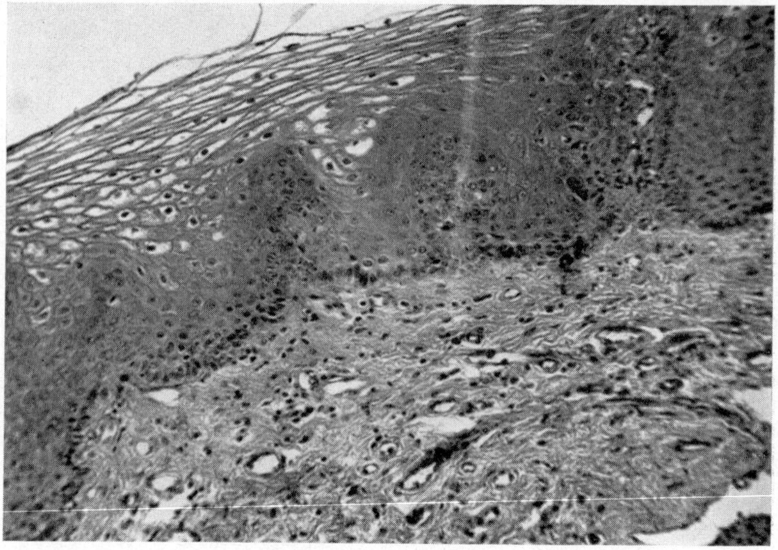

Fig 2.—Photomicrograph of distal esophagus of patient 10 showing numerous submucosal veins and absence of inflammatory infiltrate. There is no evidence of esophagitis despite the fact that the patient continued to ingest alcohol after the onset of bleeding. ×140.

ture of vessels or mucosal tears and is not believed indicative of inflammation.[4]

Comment

Evidence in Support of the Acid-Peptic Hypothesis.—In 1945, Baronofsky and Wangensteen [1] found in dogs and rabbits that obstruction of the portal vein, or of the venous drainage from the stomach, greatly enhanced the production by histamine of duodenal, gastric, and esophageal ulcers. Furthermore, they showed that resection of 90% of the stomach afforded marked, although not complete, protection against the development of histamine-induced ulcers. From these studies, the authors concluded that portal hypertension abets the ulcer diathesis and they postulated that varix bleeding in patients with portal hypertension was likely the result of erosion by acid-peptic juice. On the basis of their experimental work, Wangensteen and Baronofsky proposed the operation of near-total gastrectomy as the treatment for varix hemorrhage.[2,15] After a clinical trial of this operation with some successes and some failures, the authors emphasized that excision of gastric tissue in excess of that necessary to cure the conventional ulcer diathesis was necessary, and they proposed that total gastrectomy be done.[3,16]

Fig 3.—Photomicrograph of distal esophagus of patient 19, showing no evidence of inflammation. ×140.

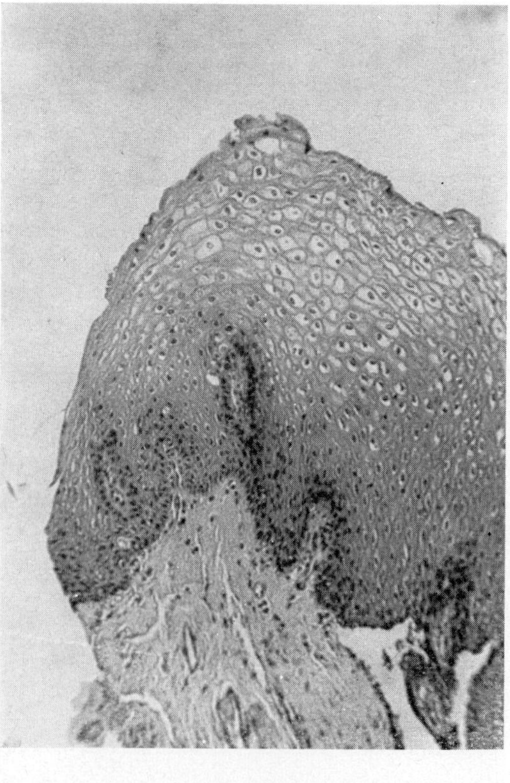

In 1953, Wagenknecht, Noble, and Baronofsky [14] conducted an autopsy study of the distal esophagus obtained from 44 patients who had bled massively from esophageal varices. In support of the acid-peptic hypothesis, they reported that 19, or 43.1% of the cases, showed ulcerative lesions with inflammatory infiltration of the esophageal mucosa overlying varices. Similar results of autopsy studies have been reported by Chiles and his associates [4] who found inflammatory erosions in 45 of 80 specimens, or 56%; by Ludington [7] who found esophagitis or erosions in 50% of 105 cases; and by Liebowitz [6] who observed esophagitis in 32 of 50 cases, or 64%.

In a recent study, Polish and Sullivan [13] performed esophagoscopy in 120 patients with esophageal varices, most of whom had cirrhosis, and found esophagitis in 33, or 27.5%. Forty-four of these patients underwent endoscopy within two weeks after bleeding, and in this group the incidence of esophagitis was 46%. None of the patients had had esophageal balloon tamponade within two weeks of the examination. In agreement with their findings, the authors cited the endoscopic study of Palmer [12] who observed esophageal varices in 14 of 100 patients with esophagitis and the comment of McGlone [8] who stated that in his experience 10% to 20% of patients with esophageal varices had esophagoscopic evidence of esophagitis.

The clear logic of the acid-peptic hypothesis, as well as the evidence accumulated to substantiate it, have made this explanation of varix rupture attractive to many experienced workers in the field of portal hypertension. Accordingly, a number of therapeutic measures in addition to total gastrectomy have been devised in part or wholly for the purpose of overcoming acid-peptic regurgitation. These include the operation of vagotomy, gastroenterostomy, and splenectomy combined with devascularization of the lower esophagus,[5] the interposition of a jejunal segment between the stomach and the esophagus,[9] and the use of local gastroesophageal hypothermia to control bleeding varices.[17]

Evidence Against the Acid-Peptic Hypothesis.—The major shortcoming of the autopsy and endoscopic studies showing esophagitis associated with bleeding varices is that none of them was performed at the time of onset of varix hemorrhage. This is more than a quibbling criticism, particularly as regards the autopsy investigations, since it is likely that before death, attempts were made over periods of time which are unknown, to stop the hemorrhage by the use of such devices as esophageal balloon tamponade and nasogastric tubes, all of which are capable of producing intense esophageal inflammation. No information is given on this score in any of the reports of autopsy studies. One has only to observe the esophagus at operation or autopsy after several days of treatment with an esophageal balloon tube or a simple nasogastric tube (which renders the sphincter mechanism incompetent and allows reflux of gastric juice) to be convinced of the validity of this criticism.

A number of cases have been reported in which varix hemorrhage has occurred in the absence of acid in the stomach or in spite of operations directed at eliminating acid or preventing reflux, such as total gastrectomy or the jejunal interposition procedure. These cases have been summarized by Liebowitz.[6] Although it is possible that acid-peptic erosion is only partially responsible for varix rupture, or is responsible in only some cases, these examples serve as circumstantial evidence against the acid-peptic hypothesis.

The interesting observations of Ostrow, Timmerman, and Gray [11] furnish another argument against the role of gastric acid in the pathogenesis of varix rupture. These authors studied all parameters of gastric secretion in 42 patients with cirrhosis and found *depression* of secretory activity in both "healthy" and decompensated cirrhotics and histamine anacidity in one third of the patients with decompensated liver disease.

The results of the present investigation indicate that reflux acid-peptic esophagitis is infrequently associated with varix rupture. In only 1 of the 20 patients, or 5%, examined at the time of bleeding was gross or microscopic evidence of esophagitis demonstrated. The finding of esophagitis in this patient was not surprising since he had been vomiting and ingesting large quantities of alcohol for several days when hemorrhage intervened. In fact, it is somewhat surprising that esophagitis was absent in several other patients who had been drinking up to the time of onset of bleeding and who entered the hospital with alcoholic intoxication. Since it is hardly likely that acid-peptic reflux would erode a varix without producing inflammation in the immediately adjacent tissue, these results provide strong evidence against the acid-peptic hypothesis of varix rupture.

This study does not prove that increased portal hydrostatic pressure is responsible for rupture of esophageal varices. It is not within the province of this report to review the pros and cons of this theory. Nevertheless, the hydrostatic pressure hypothesis remains the most logical and attractive explanation of why esophageal varices bleed.

Summary and Conclusions

Rupture of esophageal varices has been attributed to erosion by reflux acid-peptic esophagitis and to increased portal hydrostatic pressure. Support of the acid-peptic hypothesis has come from animal experiments which showed that portal hypertension abets the ulcer diathesis, and from autopsy and endoscopic studies which showed a significant incidence of esophagitis in patients who bled from esophageal varices. These studies all suffer from the justifiable criticism that they were not performed at the time of onset of varix hemorrhage.

In order to evaluate the importance of esophagitis in varix rupture, gross and microscopic examinations of the esophagus were conducted at the time of bleeding in 20 unselected cirrhotic patients with varix hemorrhage. These studies were obtained during the course of transesophageal varix ligations which were performed from 4¾ to 56 hours after the onset of hemorrhage, but within 16½ hours of the onset of bleeding in 18 of the patients.

In only 1 of the 20 cases (5%) was gross or microscopic evidence of esophagitis found. This patient had been vomiting and ingesting alcohol up to the time of bleeding. In the other 19 cases, the esophageal mucosa was free of inflammation and in 16 of these, the point of varix rupture was located and had the appearance of a clean tear. The results of this investigation indicate that esophagitis was infrequently associated with varix rupture and provide strong evidence against the acid-peptic hypothesis.

Marshall J. Orloff, MD, Harbor General Hospital, Torrance, Calif.

REFERENCES

1. Baronofsky, I. D., and Wangensteen, O. H.: Obstruction of Splenic Vein Increases Weight of Stomach and Predisposes to Erosion or Ulcer, Proc Soc Exp Biol Med 59:234-238, 1945.

2. Baronofsky, I. D.: Portal Hypertension, With Special Reference to the Acid-Peptic Factor in the Causation of Hemorrhage and Extensive Gastric Resection in Its Treatment, Surgery 25:135-168, 1949.

3. Baronofsky, I. D.: in discussion on Habif, D. V.: Treatment of Esophageal Varices by Partial Esophagogastrectomy and Interposed Jejunal Segment, Surgery 46:212-237, 1959.

4. Chiles, N. H.; Baggenstoss, A. H.; Butt, H. R.; and Olsen, A. M.: Nature of Bleeding in Esophageal Varices, Gastroenterology 25:565-573, 1953.

5. Gray, H. K., and Whitesell, F. B., Jr.: Hemorrhage from Esophageal Varices: Surgical Management, Ann Surg 132:798-810, 1950.

6. Liebowitz, H. R.: Pathogenesis of Esophageal Varix Rupture, JAMA 175:874-879, 1961.

7. Ludington, L. G.: A Study of 158 Cases of Esophageal Varices, Surg Gynec Obstet 106:519-526, 1958.

8. McGlone, F. B.: Panel Discussion: The Evaluation of Clinical Methods for Examining the Esophagus, Gastroenterology 35:92-103, 1958.

9. Merendino, K. A., and Dillard, D. H.: The Concept of Sphincter Substitution by an Interposed Jejunal Segment for Anatomic and Physiologic Abnormalities at the Esophagogastric Junction, Ann Surg 142:486-506, 1955.

10. Orloff, M. J.: A Comparative Study of Emergency Transesophageal Ligation and Nonsurgical Treatment of Bleeding Esophageal Varices in Unselected Patients With Cirrhosis, Surgery 52:103-116, 1962.

11. Ostrow, J. D.; Timmerman, R. J.; and Gray, S. J.: Gastric Secretion in Human Hepatic Cirrhosis, Gastroenterology 38:303-316, 1960.

12. Palmer, E. C.: Subacute Erosive (Peptic) Esophagitis, AMA Arch Intern Med 94:364-374, 1954.

13. Polish, E., and Sullivan, B. H., Jr.: Esophagitis Associated With Hemorrhage From Esophageal Varices, Ann Intern Med 54:908-911, 1961.

14. Wagenknecht, T. W.; Nobel, J. F.; and Baronofsky, I. D.: Nature of Bleeding in Esophageal Varices, Surgery 33:869-874, 1953.

15. Wangensteen, O. H.: The Ulcer Problem, Canad Med Ass J 53:309-331, 1945.

16. Wangensteen, O. H.: Surgical Lesions of the Esophagus, Rev Gastroenterol 19:525-549, 1952.

17. Wangensteen, O. H.; Salmon, P. A.; Griffen, W. O., Jr.; Paterson, J. R. S.; and Fattah, F.: Studies of Local Gastric Cooling as Related to Peptic Ulcer, Ann Surg 150:346-360, 1959.

"Directional" Flow Patterns in Portal Hypertension

Assessment by Spleen Pressure and Percutaneous Splenoportography

FRANCIS C. JACKSON, MD, PITTSBURGH

If a portacaval shunt is to be considered satisfactory treatment in the prevention of hemorrhage from gastroesophageal varices, it should be offered a cirrhotic patient with intrahepatic obstruction of portal blood flow and a functioning coronary vein visualized by splenoportography. The value of the prophylactic shunt would depend upon the significance of the coronary vein to bleeding varices.

The importance of such a consideration was suggested early in our experience. Studies on three cirrhotic patients indicated that a clinical significance may be attached to the first collateral channels, or branches of the splenic vein, filling with dye during these venographic studies, particularly, the prompt opacification of the coronary vein.

In one patient (Fig 1*A*) with frequent hemorrhages from varices, a large coronary vein represented the only venous channel providing a route for portosomatic blood flow. In a second instance (Fig 1*B*), the only vein so functioning was a large inferior mesenteric vein. This patient with portal hypertension never developed varices, clinically, and died one year later in hepatic coma. A third patient was admitted with recurrent anemia and all studies, including portal venography (Fig 2*A*), supported a diagnosis of thrombosis of the portal vein. The coronary vein was not visualized. Two years later, after repeated, massive hemorrhage, a second study showed the previously unfilled coronary vein to be opacified and associated with huge gastric varices (Fig 2*B*).

As the result of this experience, a study of all splenoportograms was undertaken. The patterns of collateral circulation in these studies were classified into five classes in accord with the filling of branches of the splenic vein. The term "Directional Flow" refers to the tendency of the injected opaque material to enter the collateral circulation via these initial or primary channels. Ninety-five per cent of all dye studies can be assigned to one of these classes.

Materials and Methods

The splenoportograms and clinical records of 260 studies performed since 1954 have been reviewed. The 223 patients selected had benign or malignant disease of the liver and pancreas and, clinically, were suspected of having portal hypertension. Twenty-seven patients received more than one examination (two to five). Tissue diagnoses were obtained in all but 12 patients. Those with serious clotting defects or in the terminal stages of their disease were excluded. Splenomegaly was not a requirement, and patients with ascites or jaundice were not excluded for these reasons alone.

Presented at the 20th Annual Meeting of the Central Surgical Association, Chicago, Feb 21-23, 1963.

From the Veterans Administration Hospital, Pittsburgh, and the Department of Surgery of the University of Pittsburgh School of Medicine.

A portion of this investigation was supported by a Cooperative Study of Gastroesophageal Varices being conducted by the Veterans Administration, departments of medicine and surgery.

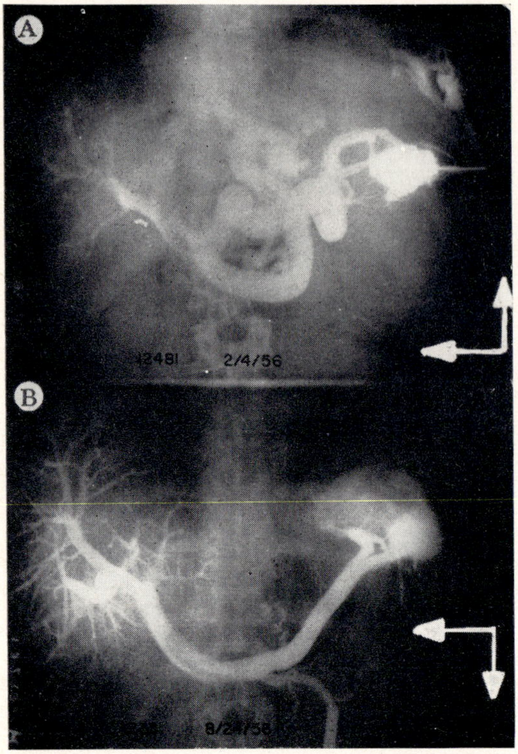

Fig 1.—*A,* the large coronary vein is the only collateral vessel in this patient with recurring hemorrhage from varices. *B,* Varices were not demonstrated on either esophagoscopy or portography in this patient with portal hypertension (spleen pressure 32.0 mm Hg) who died one year later in hepatic coma.

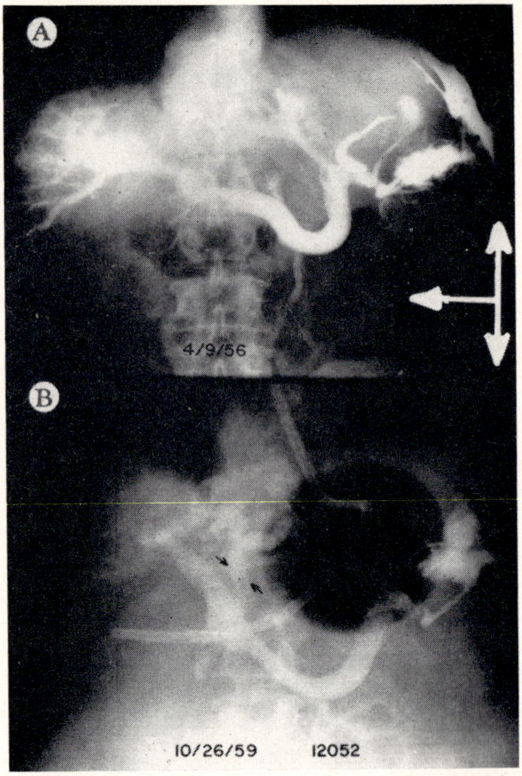

Fig 2.—*A,* this portogram confirms the clinical impression of thrombosis of the portal vein and gastroesophageal varices in a patient with anemia. *B,* three years later a massive hemorrhage occurred, and a restudy of the patient in Fig 2*A* demonstrated a recanalized portal vein, a coronary vein, and larger varices.

The technique used in the early period and reported[1] was similar to that described by others,[2,3] with the exception that fluoroscopy was not used as a control. A pressure transducer and recorder (Fig 3), instead of a fluid manometer, records the intrasplenic pressure, and a multiplane seriographic unit obtains both lateral and anterior-posterior films.

Local anesthesia, augmented by intravenous meperidine (Demerol) (200 ml in 500 ml of 5% glucose in distilled water), is used exclusively. The usual puncture site is 9.0 cm anterior to the spine (table) in the ninth intercostal space (mid- or posterior axillary line). The transducer (Fig 3) is 12.0 cm above the table or zero level, ie, the anterior border of the second lumbar vetebra,[3] and is connected to a recorder calibrated with a deflection sensitivity of 1.0 mm per 1.0 mm Hg and recording speed of 1.0 cm per second. The depth of the spleen is determined by intermittent aspiration via the No. 22-gauge needle during the injection of the local anesthetic.

With the patient apneic, a No. 18-gauge needle attached to a 10 ml syringe is placed into the spleen, approximately 2.0 cm deeper than the predetermined capsular depth. Upon introduction, the needle is flushed and a polyethylene tubing from the transducer is attached. The patient then breathes slowly. With a stable pressure and artefacts synchronous with respiration (Fig 4), a tracing is recorded for ten seconds. Forty milliliters of sodium diatrizoate (50% Hypaque) is then injected in seven to nine seconds. Fifteen serial films (four in the lateral projection) are exposed at one-second intervals beginning midway through the injection. An amount of 5 to 10 ml of a saline suspension of Gelfoam or Oxycel gauze is administered as the needle is withdrawn. The total elapsed time for the entire procedure is usually less than one minute, since a longer period may result in extensive injury to the spleen. Studies which failed to opacify the splenic or portal veins were discarded from review. In 40 instances (15%), the dye was improperly injected and did not enter the spleen.

A splenoportogram for classification in this study must have dye demonstrated within the splenic and portal veins sufficient for the caliber of these and

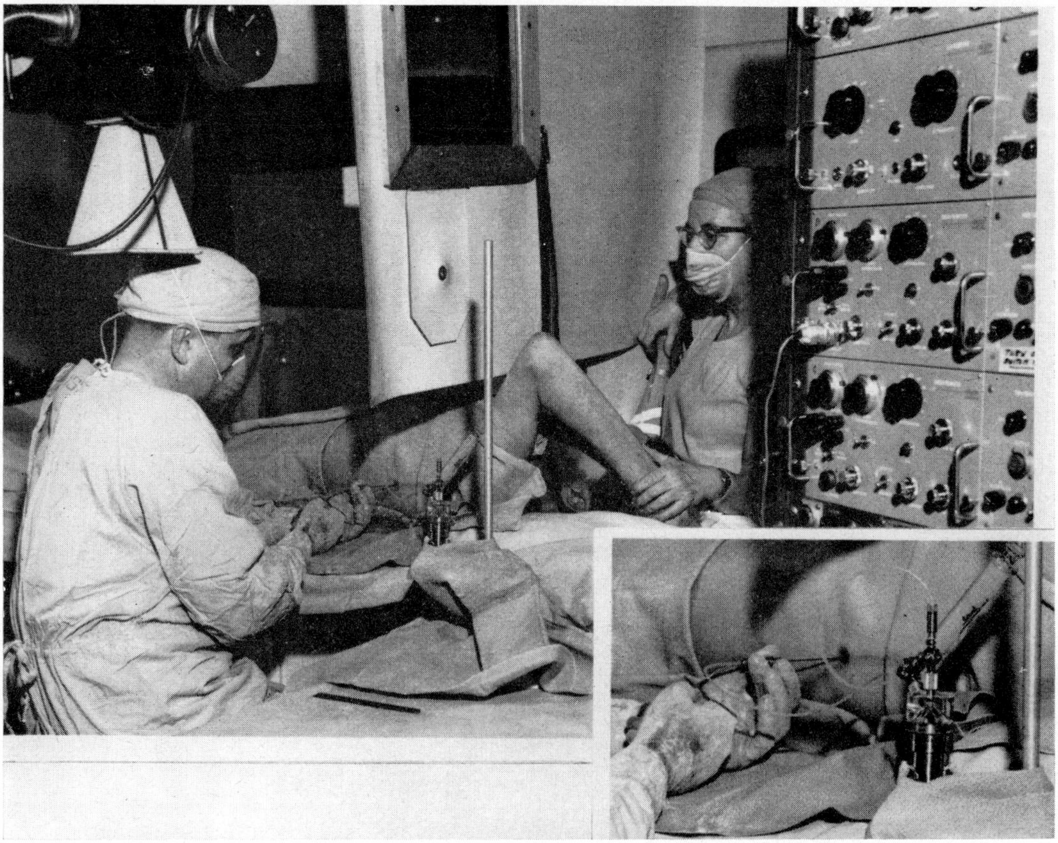

Fig 3—Spleen pressures are obtained with a pressure transducer (range 0 to 50 mm Hg) which is placed 12.0 cm above the x-ray table. This is the zero level or the anterior border of the body of the second lumbar vertebra.[3]

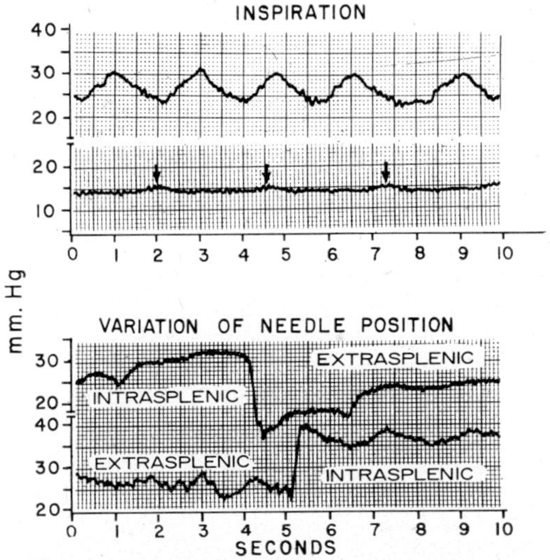

Fig 4.—A ten-second spleen pressure tracing is an adequate record and aids in reducing the time during which the needle is within the pulp. Deep and shallow respirations appear as artefacts. The mean pressure is taken from the extremes on the tracing. Changes in the position of the needle appear as abrupt alterations in tissue pressure.

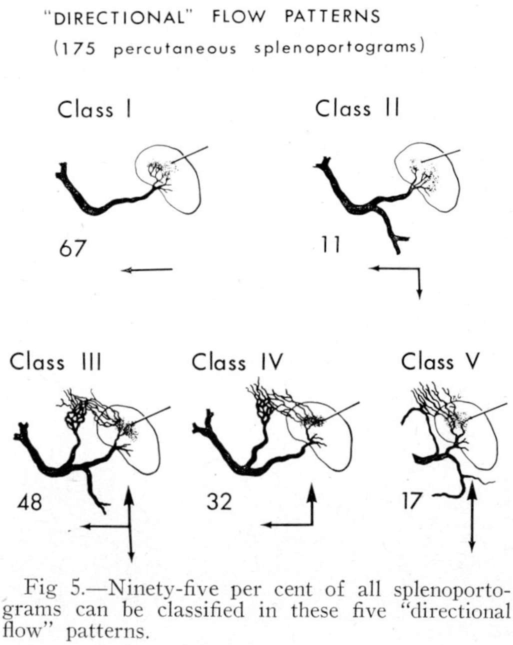

Fig 5.—Ninety-five per cent of all splenoportograms can be classified in these five "directional flow" patterns.

TABLE 1.—*Distribution of Flow Patterns by Classes in Splenoportograms*

Class	Total Studies	Studies in Cirrhotics	Studies in Noncirrhotics
I	67 (38) *	40	27
II	11 (6)	7	4
III	48 (28)	41	7
IV	32 (18)	29	3
V	17 (10)	7	10
Total	175 (100)	124 †	51

* Parentheses indicate %.

† Four are repeat studies with a different pattern in the same patient.

other principal vessels to be visualized on one or more films. An exception was made in partial or complete splenic and/or portal vein obstruction. Patients with appreciable extrahepatic block formed class V. Eliminated were those portograms where the umbilical veins were the only collateral vessels (four studies). Studies of the patency of portacaval shunts, the majority of repeat or serial portograms, and a number of other studies which were unsatisfactory for evaluation because of technical defects or insufficient clinical data were also discarded. The 175 remaining studies were classified into cirrhotic and noncirrhotic groups as follows (Fig 5 and Table 1).

Class I is the normal study of portal blood flow as demonstrated by venography. No collateral vessels are visible, and the dye promptly enters the sinusoidal system within the liver (Fig 8*A*).

Class II is seen when dye refluxes mainly through the inferior mesenteric vein and other caudal branches of the splenic vein. The portal vein is opacified. The collateral blood flow in this group is ultimately into the inferior vena cava (Fig 1*B*).

Class III shows dye filling branches of the splenic vein in both a cephalic as well as a caudal direction. The coronary, short gastric and the inferior mesenteric veins, along with many small and large collateral vessels associated with the pancreatic and mesenteric systems, may be visualized although all may not be opacified in an individual patient (Fig 2*A* and *B*, 8*B*, and 9*B*).

Class IV has the retrograde flow primarily identified with the coronary and short gastric veins. The portal vein and its intrahepatic branches are always visible. The important feature is the marked diversion of dye into the vessels identified with the development of gastroesophageal varices (Fig 1*A* and 9*A*).

Class V represents partial or complete occlusion of the splenic or portal veins, and extensive perisplenic collateral beds are visualized (Fig 10, *A* and *B*). However, the dye may enter the portal vein late in the study. Either the gastroepiploic, inferior mesenteric, or short gastric systems may be recognized. When a coronary vein fills, the dye enters the portal vein beyond the site of obstruction. In two instances, although the dye remained in the splenic system, the portal veins were patent at operation, indicating that this pattern is not always diagnostic for extrahepatic block.

The definition of cirrhosis in this study includes the following pathological descriptions: periportal fibrosis; fatty metamorphosis; and Laennec's,

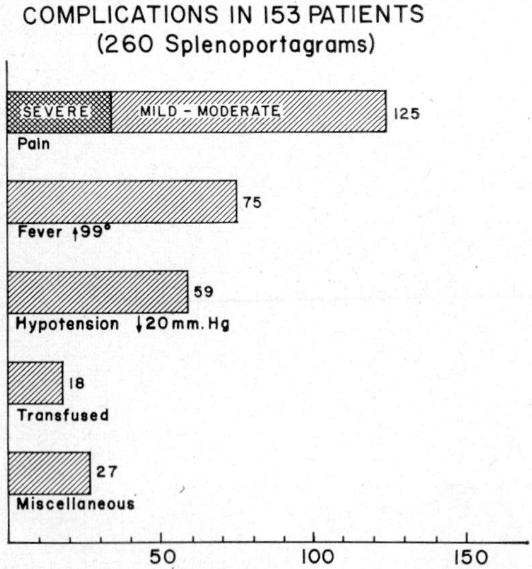

Fig 6.—The complication rate in terms of discomfort and morbidity following splenoportography is still high. Six of the patients received transfusions during a laparotomy which followed the percutaneous splenoportogram. Several techniques described in the text have reduced some of these hazards.

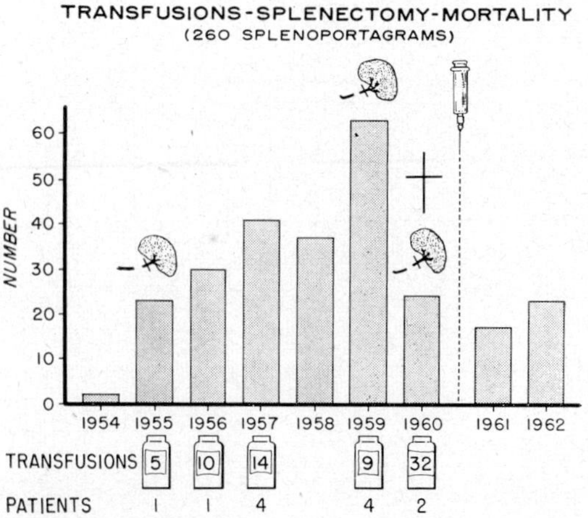

Fig 7.—Three splenectomies and one death have resulted from splenoportography in this series. The injection of a suspension of absorbable materials (Gelfoam or Oxycel) has apparently reduced this morbidity.

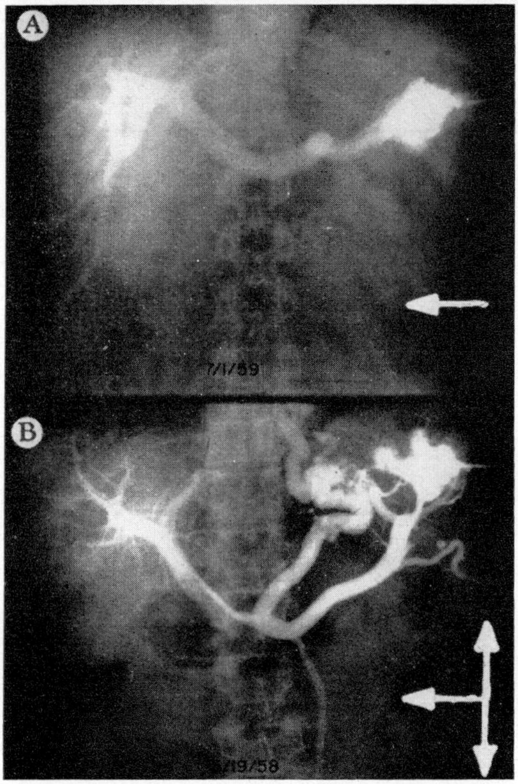

Fig 8.—*A,* this is a class I or normal flow pattern in a patient with cirrhosis and a high spleen pressure (35.0 mm Hg). *B,* the class III flow pattern is typical of that seen in patients clinically selected for portacaval shunts. The spleen pressure in this instance is 32.0 mm Hg. A large coronary vein is the primary collateral vessel.

biliary, or postnecrotic cirrhosis. The "noncirrhotic" refers to the patient with a liver biopsy which was either normal, contained a neoplasm, or the patient had a disease other than cirrhosis. Varices were identified at esophagoscopy, portography, or postmortem examination.

Spleen pressures were obtained on 165 patients. The spleen pressure represents the mean pressure on the respiratory artefact recorded to the nearest 0.5 mm Hg. The normal spleen pressure in this series is 13.0 ± 4.5 (SD) mm Hg.

For this report, the "directional flow" patterns are evaluated in terms of spleen pressure, the opacification of the coronary and other branches of the splenic vein, the demonstration of esophagogastric varices by both esophagoscopy and venography, hemorrhage from varices, and the death rate of the cirrhotic patients. The noncirrhotic patients served as controls.

Complications

The hazards of percutaneous splenoportography should not be underestimated.

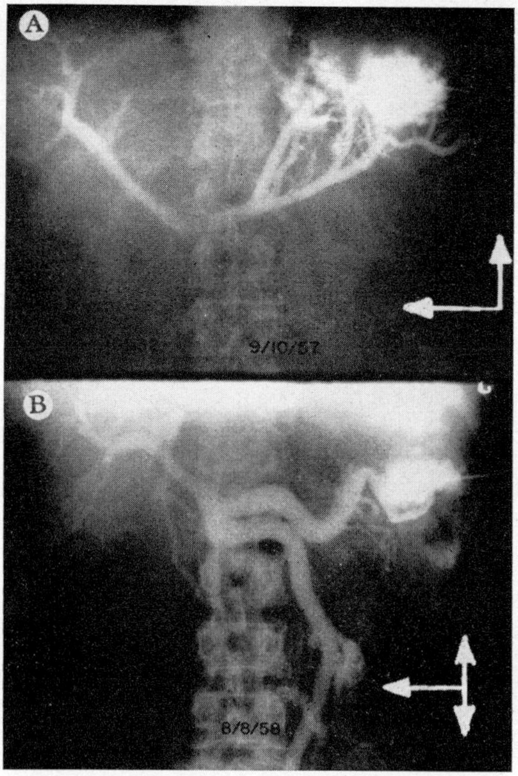

Fig 9.—*A,* this portogram was performed on a patient with a class IV flow pattern and a spleen pressure of 31.5 mm Hg. He died after exsanguination one month later. *B,* the large inferior mesenteric vein visualized on this study of a class III pattern was obtained in a patient with a spleen pressure of 26.5 mm Hg. He is alive 4½ years later without hemorrhage. Although varices and other cephalic collaterals are noted, the pattern is suggestive of class II.

The number of complications (153) (Fig 6) was considerably more than reported by others.[3] Earlier in the series, few limitations were placed upon splenoportography. The selection was dictated by the importance of the information to be elicited. Complications occurred despite careful selection and attention to technique.

Fifty-eight per cent of the patients complained of pain. It was the most common complication and is produced by dye or blood in the peritoneal cavity. Severe pain was more common when a 70% dye was used. Since the use of a 50% concentration, the frequency has been substantially reduced. Fever (an oral temperature over 99 F [37.2 C]) was frequent. It should not be

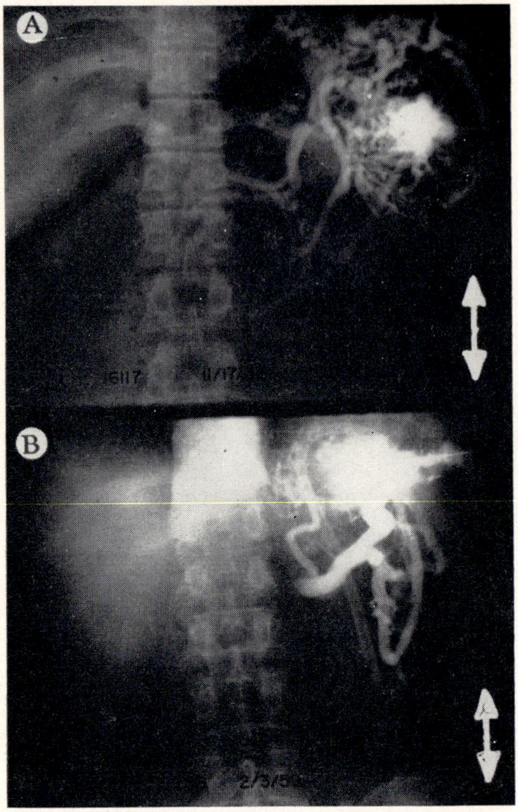

Fig 10—*A,* this class V pattern is from a cirrhotic patient with thrombosis of his splenic vein. He has never hemorrhaged, and his spleen pressure is 17.5 mm Hg. *B,* there is complete obstruction to the splenic vein in this instance of a class V pattern of a patient with carcinoma of the pancreas and a spleen pressure of 34.0 mm Hg. Death occurred from massive hemorrhage.

attributed to bacteremia [3] but to hemoperitoneum.

The hypotension (a drop of 20 mm Hg or more in systolic pressure), which occurred in 59 patients, is related not only to blood loss but to the intravenous meperidine. This usually occurs within the first six hours. Twelve patients received a plasma expander or blood (Fig 7); six additional patients received blood in the operating room. Splenectomy was necessary in three patients. The mean blood loss in twenty patients who had immediate laparotomy was 183 ml.

The single death occurred in a 41-year-old alcoholic patient admitted in precoma with hemorrhage, ascites, and jaundice. After three months of therapy, a splenoportogram was attempted but failed. The patient died nine days later after receiving 22 units of blood and when hemorrhage from varices had recurred. This type of patient is not considered to be a good selection for percutaneous splenoportography unless the procedure is to precede emergency or other surgery.

Three steps in the current technique seem to help control bleeding from splenic puncture. First, the period during which the needle is in the spleen is limited to 60 seconds, if possible. Secondly, the respiratory artefacts are identified on a stable pressure tracing, confirming the intrasplenic position of the needle (Fig 4). The dye is not injected unless the position is assured by this tracing. And, lastly, a suspension of Gelfoam or Oxycel gauze is injected as the needle is withdrawn. There have been few episodes of hypotension (only 4 in the past 41 studies) since the use of these substances. Dextran or blood transfusions have not been necessary in the past two years. Now, when immediate laparotomy is performed, little or no blood may be found in the peritoneal cavity. The value of this technique was originally demonstrated on a controlled series of normal and hypertensive dog spleens by noting a substantial decrease in bleeding from a needle puncture.[4] No adverse effects have been attributed to these materials.

Results

The distribution of the five classes of "directional flow" is shown in Table 1 and Fig 5. While a substantial number of patients with cirrhosis (40 of 120) demonstrate normal portal venograms, the majority (classes III and IV) reflect the high frequency of collateral circulation with portal hypertension. Since extrahepatic portal (splenic vein) block is more common in patients with pancreatic disease, the class V pattern is the most common abnormal flow pattern in the noncirrhotic group (10 of 24).

Splenic pressures were recorded in 165 of the 175 studies (Table 2). A significant difference ($P<0.01$) in pressure existed between the class I (normal) and classes III, IV, and V of the cirrhotic studies. There is

TABLE 2.—*Spleen Pressures by Classes of Splenoportograms*

	With Cirrhosis		Without Cirrhosis	
Class	No. of Observations	Spleen Pressure *	No. of Observations	Spleen Pressure *
I	40	20.5±7.5	24	14.6±6.0
II	7	19.0±5.5	4	17.0±5.0
III	35	28.0±7.5	9	22.5±7.0
IV	30	29.5±7.0	3	21.0±2.0
V	4	28.5±9.0	9	27.0±9.5
Total	116		49	

* Mean ± SD. The mean zero level is 12 cm anterior to the table or the anterior border of the first lumbar vertebra. The normal spleen pressure (9 observations) is 13.0 ± 4.5 mm Hg.

a similar pressure differential among the noncirrhotics of classes III, IV, and V, confirming the elevation of spleen pressures when collateral flow from any cause is demonstrated by the dye injection. There is no significant difference between the pressures of classes III, IV, and V as groups. However, there was a significant elevation of spleen pressure ($P<0.05$) among the patients who hemorrhaged with flow patterns of classes III, IV, and V when compared with the nonbleeders of these groups; 30.2±0.97 (SE) versus 26.3±1.6 (SE). From additional data, it is also predicted that with a mean pressure at or above 25.0 mm Hg, 76% of patients could be expected to hemorrhage, while less than 44% would bleed below this level ($P<0.01$).

The appearance of varices and the frequency of hemorrhage is summarized for the cirrhotic and the noncirrhotic groups of patients in Tables 3 and 4. Hemorrhage from gastroesophageal varices, as may be expected, occurs in classes III, IV, and V and is entirely absent when the portograms are normal or in class I (Fig 8*A*). The single exception to this was a patient who had a splenic vein thrombosis and had recanalized this vessel sufficiently so that the dye did not reflux into the branches of the splenic vein. When readmitted, bleeding, a repeat study indicated he had developed a class III flow pattern.

Gastroesophageal varices were not visualized on the portal venograms in classes I and II (Table 3), and varices reported by the esophagoscopist were usually small and frequently absent on restudy. This indicates a group of false positive reports or the low order and variability of portal hypertension in these classes. It may, also, indicate the current limitations of radiographic technique in defining small collateral vessels. The more frequent recognition of gastric and esophageal varices on the venograms in classes III, IV, and V can only be ascribed to the distinct limitations of esophagoscopy.

There is no statistical significance to the frequency of hemorrhage among classes III, IV, and V. However, when the *coronary vein* is visualized (Fig 8*B* and 9*A*, Table 4), there tends to be a significantly greater proportion of bleeders ($P<0.05$). An interesting observation is that the majority of the patients recommended clinically for portacaval shunts had coronary veins visualized by portography.

The sample of patients in class II is too small, at this time, to suggest that primary retrograde blood flow over the inferior mesenteric vein affords protection from

TABLE 3.—*Frequency of Varices and Hemorrhage Among Patients With Cirrhosis by Classes of Splenoportograms*

Class	Studies	Not Esophagoscoped	With Varices on Esophagoscopy	With Varices on Portography	With Hemorrhage From Varices
I	40	7	13	0	1
II	7	1	4	0	1
III	41	3	36	41	28
IV	29	4	18	29	23
V	7	1	5	7	3
Total	124	16	76	77	56

Varices are frequently reported by the esophagoscopist when collateral vessels are not demonstrated on the portal venograms. However, hemorrhage is more frequent when varices are noted on the films.

TABLE 4.—*The Visualization of the Coronary Vein and Its Relation to Hemorrhage From Varices Among Patients With Cirrhosis in Classes III and IV*

	Class III			Class IV		
Coronary Vein	Studies	With Hemorrhage	With Portacaval Shunt	Studies	With Hemorrhage	With Portacava Shunt
Filled with dye	31	23	12	20	17	12
Not filled with dye	10	5	2	9	6	2
Total	41	28	14	29	23	14

There is some significance ($p < 0.05$) to the opacification of the coronary vein on the portal venogram and hemorrhage from varices. This is also true when the spleen pressure is at or above 25.0 mm Hg ($p < 0.01$).

hemorrhaging varices. One patient in class III with a huge inferior mesenteric vein as the primary collateral vessel has not hemorrhaged in the four years after his portal venography despite a spleen pressure of 26.5 mm Hg (Fig 9*B*).

TABLE 5.—*Frequency of Varices and Hemorrhage From Varices Among Patients Without Cirrhosis*

Class	No. of Studies	With Varices (Portography Only)	With Hemorrhage
I	27	0	0
II	4	0	0
III	7	6	0
IV	3	3	1
V	10	10	3
Total	51	19	4

Hemorrhage from varices does occur in noncirrhotic patients; however, these patients usually die of a neoplasm rather than hemorrhage.

Noncirrhotic patients with well-developed collateral circulations also bled, but much less frequently (Table 5). The majority of these patients had carcinoma and no doubt died before hemorrhage from varices could occur (Fig 10*B*).

Death in the 120 cirrhotic patients occurred most frequently in classes III, IV and V. Seventy-five of these patients have survived (Table 6). Seventeen died during or after a portacaval shunt. Hemorrhage was the primary cause of the other deaths (12 of 28 patients). Nine of 11 patients in classes III and IV dying from bleeding had coronary veins visualized on the film studies. While hemorrhage from varices was a factor in the deaths of 4 noncirrhotic patients (Table 5), it was of limited significance in the presence of their tumors.

Comment

Percutaneous portal venography was first performed in 1951.[5] Subsequently, the measurement of splenic pulp pressure was demonstrated to be a reliable index of portal venous pressure.[6] These combined procedures for the first time permitted an assessment of the intact human portal circulation and, particularly, some understanding of the pathogenesis of portal hypertension.

The established concept that the elevation of spleen or portal pressure is related to the

TABLE 6.—*Death Among Patients With Cirrhosis by Classes of Splenoportograms*

			Cause of Death			
Class	Patients	Dead	Coma	Hemorrhage	Misc.	Died Post Shunt
I	39	5	1	0	4	0
II	7	3	2	0	1	0
III	39	18	1	9	3	5
IV	29	14	2	2	1	9
V	6	5	1	1	0	3
Total	120	45	7	12	9	17

Nine of the 11 patients in class III and IV who died of hemorrhage had a coronary vein demonstrated on the splenoportogram.

extent of the liver disease has been confirmed by others.[7] The degree of collateral circulation on portal venography also has a recognized relationship to hepatic failure and to portal pressure.[8] However, the appearance of gastroesophageal varices and the unpredictable onset of massive hemorrhage among individual cirrhotic patients with similar ranges of elevated portal pressure have not entirely been explained.

The major predisposing factor to bleeding is assumed to be the presence of the gastroesophageal varices themselves. These collateral channels are the result of a retrograde blood flow which has developed over the coronary and short gastric branches of the splenic (portal) vein. However, it is the experience of this study that varices may be identified in a number of patients in whom the coronary vein is not visualized in the portal venogram. Usually the varices in these patients are reported on esophagoscopy. Hemorrhage is less frequent in these instances, although it does occur when the varices are confirmed on portography (Table 3).

The early experience in this study of portal venography also suggested several questions. First, do individual cirrhotic patients develop a predominant collateral blood flow limited to certain branches of the portal system which may increase or decrease their chances of hemorrhage from varices? Secondly, if a classification of collateral vessels is demonstrated by venography and there is a significant frequency of hemorrhage in one or more of the classes, is the recommendation of a prophylactic portacaval shunt for such a patient justified?

A careful examination of a large number of splenoportograms has indicated that a classification of collateral blood flow could be devised (Fig 5). With the exception of extrahepatic portal obstruction (class V), the reasons for the directional flow patterns are not clear. Many anatomical, physiological, and technical factors may decide whether the opaque dye enters any one particular group of collateral veins as opposed to another. However, it does appear that a clinical significance can be attached to the tendency of the injected material to do one of two things: (1) enter the sinusoidal system of the liver without filling the branches of the splenic vein or (2) opacify the coronary vein. In this study, when the flow was normally through the liver, there was only 1 instance of hemorrhage among 40 cirrhotics.

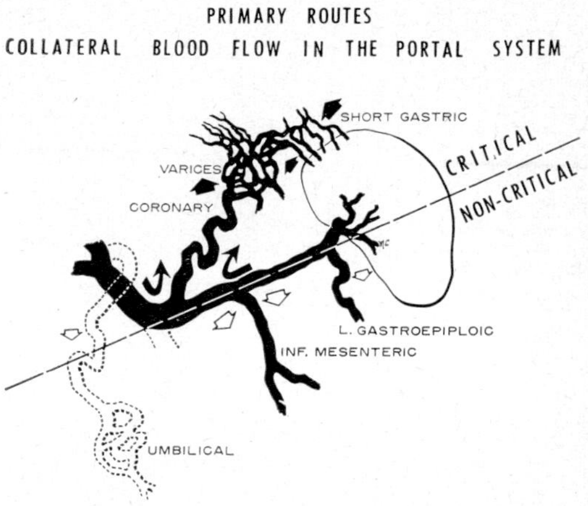

Fig 11.—While there are many factors predisposing to hemorrhage from varices, the demonstration of collateral blood flow over the coronary and short gastric veins may be considered the most critical feature of all classes in the five directional flow patterns.

The demonstration of the coronary vein in any one of the five classes of collateral blood flow is associated with hemorrhage from varices to a reasonable degree of significance ($P<0.05$). Therefore, a flow pattern which demonstrates large amounts of dye in a cephalic direction from the splenic vein may be called "critical" (Fig 11). This is a particularly serious collateral flow in terms of bleeding when the spleen pressure is 25.0 mm Hg or higher ($P<0.01$).

With the exception of the normal flow pattern (class I), there is still no evidence that natural portosomatic shunting, as in class II, is any more than a temporary safeguard against bleeding varices. There is insufficient material for evaluation.

Summary

Five classes of collateral or "directional" blood flow have been suggested by a review of 175 studies from among 260 percutaneous splenoportograms. The classification is based upon the selective appearance of the dye in branches of the splenic vein.

In terms of hemorrhage from esophageal varices, a clinically "critical" flow pattern is described which involves the coronary and short gastric veins.

When the coronary vein is visualized, there is some significant frequency of bleeding from varices ($P<0.05$). These bleeders, also, have higher spleen pressures ($P<0.05$), and a distinctly higher rate of hemorrhage occurs at pressures at or above 25.0 mm Hg ($P<0.01$).

It is suggested that if the prophylactic portacaval shunt is of value in the prevention of hemorrhage from varices, it should be considered when the coronary vein is a major collateral vessel.

A technique to reduce the number of complications from percutaneous splenoportography is also described.

Statistical data was provided by Edward B. Perrin, PhD, Department of Preventive Medicine, University of Washington School of Medicine, Seattle, Wash.

Francis C. Jackson, MD, Chief, Surgical Service, Veterans Administration Hospital, University Dr, Pittsburgh 40, Pa.

REFERENCES

1. Jackson, F. C.; Longabaugh, E. E.; Happel, J. L.; Kline, J. J.; and Croup, M. M.: A New Method for Evaluating Portal Hypertension, Scientific Exhibit, AMA Arch Surg 77:294, 1958.

2. Turner, M. D.; Sherlock, S.; and Steiner, R. E.: Splenic Venography and Intrasplenic Pressure Measurement in the Clinical Investigation of the Portal Venous System, Amer J Med 23:846, 1957.

3. Panke, W. F.; Bradley, E. G.; Moreno, A. H.; Ruzicka, F. F., Jr.; and Rousselot, L. M.: Technique, Hazards and Usefulness of Percutaneous Splenic Portography, JAMA 169:1032, 1959.

4. Davis, D. D., and Jackson, F. C.: Unpublished data.

5. Boulvin, R.; Chevalier, M.; Gallus, P.; and Nagel, M.: Contribution à l'étude du syndrome d'hypertension portale: Etude clinique et portographique, Acta Gastroent 14:795, 1951.

6. Atkinson, M., and Sherlock, S.: Intrasplenic Pressure as Index of Portal Venous Pressure, Lancet 1:1325, 1954.

7. Moreno, A. H.; Rousselot, L. M.; and Panke, W. F.: Studies on Portal Hypertension: II. Correlation Between Severity of Pathologic Involvement of the Portal System and Variations in Tension, Surg Clin N Amer 38:421, 1958.

8. Rousselot, L. M.; Moreno, A. H.; and Panke, W. F.: Studies on Portal Hypertension: IV. The Clinical and Physiopathologic Significance of Self Established (Nonsurgical) Portal Systemic Venous Shunts, Ann Surg 150:384, 1959.

DISCUSSION

On papers by Drs. Zuidema et al, Orloff and Thomas, and Jackson.

Dr. William J. Fry, Ann Arbor, Mich: Our experience with splenoportography has now reached somewhat over 200 patients. We have generally reserved this examination for patients who are candidates for shunt or who have questionable neoplasm of the pancreas. This is occasionally helpful in determining the operability of the patient who is considered for a pancreatoduodenectomy, in that it may rule out the invasion of the portal vein by tumor.

Complications in our hands have been relatively low. We have had to use a total of only seven transfusions in these 200 patients. One patient required three pints of blood in order to stabilize, and one pint each for an additional four patients, and in no instance have we had to carry out splenectomy.

We have not used any hemostatic agents such as Dr. Jackson has. We have paid a great deal of attention, however, to prothrombin time and the clotting time of these patients. We have discarded the use of pressures at the time of splenoportography because when we did use these we found a higher incidence of failure rate because of diffusion of the dye around the capsule of the spleen. The complication of bleeding occurred in these patients, and we felt it was too long a period of time to leave the needle in the spleen. If one desires a pressure, at least in our hands, we have elected to do this at a separate time.

We wonder if the patients with flow directed to the coronary vein with subsequent bleeding may not have represented a poor-risk group. This certainly would raise the mortality rate of shunting and perhaps make it prohibitive.

This technique may prove very useful in selecting some patients for prophylactic shunting procedures. It must be emphasized that evaluation of liver function is of prime importance.

There is one additional use that splenoportography may be used for. This photograph shows a patient who had intractable ascites and a very mild fill of the collateral. Another photograph of a postoperative portacaval shunt shows a very patent side-to-side shunt. An injection in the liver of the intrahepatic vein shows directional flow backward down into the side-to-side shunt and up the inferior vena cava. We have felt this might be helpful in other instances in determining the patency of a splenorenal shunt.

Dr. E. F. Bernstein, Minneapolis: Dr. Orloff's paper presents evidence which appears to conflict with the thesis that bleeding from esophageal varices is the result of acidpeptic activity.

In 1945, (*Canad Med Ass J* 53:309, 1945), Wangensteen first postulated the relationship of regurgitation of acid peptic juice to esophageal erosion. In subsequent papers Wangensteen and his associates developed the thesis of the extreme sensitivity of the esophageal mucosa to acid peptic digestion. These studies served as the basis for the treatment of bleeding esophageal varices due to extrahepatic portal obstruction with good liver function, by total gastrectomy or complete excision of the acid peptic secretory area of the stomach.

The difficult problem of treating extrahepatic portal obstruction in patients in whom splenorenal or mesenteric-portal shunt is impractical or has failed has been approached in three ways: gastric resection, esophageal resection, and, more recently, esophageal freezing. In Dr. Wangensteen's operative series there are three patients in whom either a total gastrectomy or an esophagoantrostomy was done, 17 or more years ago, who have continued well without recurrent hemorrhage. However, during this same interval of time there have been a number of failures. Dr. Richard Varco has five patients in whom he has resected the distal third of the esophagus, one to five years ago, re-establishing alimentary tract continuity with an interposed subcutaneous jejunal loop leading back to the stomach. Only one of these patients has had a single episode of bleeding since.

These two approaches have recently been supplemented by a third, involving esophageal freezing, which has been performed in two patients with multiple episodes of bleediing after a long list of operative procedures. One had undergone prior total gastrectomy and the other an extensive Billroth II procedure. Both patients were treated with three episodes of esophageal freezing in an attempt to provoke sufficient inflammatory reaction in the mucosa to establish a covering for the exposed varices, and in the hope that thrombosis of the varices themselves might follow in consequence of the freeze.

The balloon of Dr. S. L. Wangensteen was used, with a small globular distal end, a 250 cc capacity, and a long esophageal component. This segment of the balloon remains in the upper fundus of the stomach, and the narrower proximal reaches of the balloon extend up the distal two thirds of the esophagus.

In the dog's stomach and esophagus, frozen several times, both mucosa and submucosa become thickened. It is probably a reasonable thesis that if the varices were well covered by an intact mucosal layer, esophageal bleeding would be less likely. In other words, it is reasonable to assume a mucosal erosion is an accompaniment of bleeding from esophageal varices. While the follow-up on these patients is still quite short, neither has bled since the freezing.

In cirrhotic patients with varices, such as described by Dr. Orloff, the mortality after any operation procedure is prohibitively high. In these cases some nonoperative approach, such as multiple episodes of esophageal freezing, may have something to offer.

Dr. John J. Cranley, Cincinnati: I compliment Dr. Orloff for bringing out the mechanistic theory of bleeding of esophageal varices. I would like to make just one point.

The order of magnitude of venous pressure elevation in patients with portal hypertension is approximately the same as the abnormal pressure elevation in patients with venous insufficiency of the lower extremity. If we are correct in our assumption that this chronic abnormal elevation of venous pressure can cause deterioration of the subcutaneous tissue and erosion of the skin, then it seems equally reasonable to suppose that the same pressure could cause destruction of the esophageal mucosa.

Dr. Alfred M. Keirle, Cincinnati: Dr. Zuidema has described in his paper the abnormalities that we see in patients with cirrhosis and Eck fistula dogs, and especially in sodium, potassium, and ammonium ions. He also not only further demonstrates that the blood ammonia elevation causes the exogenous type of hepatic coma, but the paper alludes to the fact that an elevated blood ammonia actually may precipitate the endogenous coma by competing for and disturbing potassium metabolism.

In a study of the renal metabolism of ammonia we certainly see that there is a great competition between sodium, potassium, and ammonium for the transportation mechanisms across the cellular membranes. When one looks at the action of these resins they almost seem physiological indeed.

In Dr. Zuidema's paper the actual rise of the blood potassium over an eight-hour period was from 4.6 to 5.6 mg/cm. One would certainly have to be concerned, first of all, whether this rise is greater in the patient who is bleeding than in the patient being treated for hepatic coma without bleeding. Secondly, one would be interested in what the elevation of the blood potassium is as the treatment is prolonged over the course of a day or two. Certainly one must be most careful in renal failure.

It also would be very interesting to note whether the patients who do have an elevated blood potassium will stop or reduce the amount of absorption from the intestine of the potassium liberated from the resin.

I think this mechanism of treatment certainly allows a great possibility of individualizing the treatment of the patient. In the kidney you can give compounds that are not absorbed, that will alter the secretion or absorption of these various ions. It would be interesting if a resin could be devised in which an inert substance, or one that could not be absorbed from the intestine, could be used in an exchange for ammonia or potassium.

Dr. Jacob Berman, Indianapolis: I should like like to ask that we reorient ourselves concerning the problems of hepatic cirrhosis, and with this in mind I call your attention to some very fundamental clinical facts.

1. As you heard today, the cause of cirrhosis in general is unknown, with few exceptions, but at least in nutritional cirrhosis the process is not irreversible.

2. Cirrhotics do not all have esophageal varices, and if they do have varices this does not necessarily presage hemorrhage.

3. People without cirrhosis may have varices and they may bleed.

4. The studies that we have heard today have shown us that it is probably not possible completely to bypass the liver and have it function normally.

5. Dr. Jackson's observations confirm what many of us have called hepatopetal and hepatofugal flow, and this is important in assessing our patients.

6. I think we need to take a new look at the arterial side of this problem, for the following reasons: (*a*) we have had good postmortem injection studies of the hepatic arterial tree, and they are very revealing; (*b*) I have perfused dozens of cirrhotic livers, and I came to some definite conclusions with these perfusions, but these, again, were on cirrhotic livers that had been removed post mortem.

7. There is still cogent evidence that the cause of bleeding is not entirely venous, and I believe that many of these bleeders have arteriovenous (AV) communications and angiomatous transformations not only of the liver but of the spleen and the entire portal bed.

How do I come to this conclusion? Besides the many experimental evidences, we have the following clinical findings: (1) the cut vein at the time of operation has a pulsatile flow; (2) the blood is bright red; (3) the splanchnic veins often pulsate; (4) the AV oxygen difference between the hepatic arterial and the portal venous system is very, very low in the normal, it is 4-6 vol%; in the cirrhotic roughly 1.5 to 3 vol%; (5) these patients have a hypervolemia such as we see in AV fistula; (6) lastly, our experimental evidence supports the role of arteriovenous communications.

I do hope that Dr. Jackson and others interested in hepatic cirrhosis will make more accurate studies on the in vivo behavior of the hepatic arterial and the lymphatic systems of the normal and cirrhotic liver.

Dr. George D. Zuidema, Ann Arbor, Mich: In response to Dr. Keirle's question, we feel that hypokalemia may indeed be a serious problem in these patients. We have studied one patient who presented with a blood ammonia of 270$\mu g\%$ who was comatose. Her serum potassium was 2.5. We corrected the serum potassium, and within 12 hours the patient's blood ammonia was completely normal and she was responsive. She received no treatment other than this. This points up, to our minds at least, the importance that potassium plays in this whole picture.

In general, in our clinical experience we have used the sodium-cycle resin in patients with normal serum potassium levels or patients with poor renal function. To date we have used this in nine patients, two of whom developed temporary ammonia intoxication after portacaval anastomosis. Four were in terminal hepatic failure, and three patients had bleeding esophageal varices, depressed sensorium, and increased blood ammonias.

In the experience we have had with two patients with ammonia intoxication after portacaval anastomosis, blood ammonia levels were well over 300$\mu g\%$ after operation. Resin therapy was begun, and blood ammonia fell to normal levels. After the resin was stopped, ammonia levels remained low as long as the patient was kept on a 40 gm protein diet. When this was raised to 70 gm of protein, ammonia levels increased slightly until liver function improved. They then returned to normal. This was a patient with postnecrotic cirrhosis.

One patient, a 17-year-old boy from Michigan's Upper Peninsula, who had both postnecrotic cirrhosis and who was a chronic alcoholic had a prompt response to the resin given by gastric tube after his portacaval shunt. When this was stopped, the ammonia level promptly rose. He received some more by enema, and the ammonia subsided.

We are accumulating an experience with resin therapy now and feel that it has a real promise in patients with exogenous ammonia intoxication. In patients with endogenous ammonia intoxication and terminal hepatic failure, we are less optmistic. Although we have been able to lower their blood ammonia levels, we, as well as everyone else who has studied these patients, have been unable to see any improvement in their clinical condition.

Dr. E. F. Bernstein, Minneapolis: It troubles us considerably that some other investigators have been unable to duplicate our experimental findings, in which gastric freezing has been demonstrated to be quite safe in the experimental animal. Certainly our experience in man, which currently includes somewhat more than 300 patients treated without mortality either directly or indirectly related to the freezing, indicates that the procedure is safe. Moreover, it is effective in depressing gastric secretion long enough in most instances to permit ulcer craters to heal.

The hazards observed by Dr. Welch and cited by Dr. Eckert, I feel certain, are very real, but are due to minor but important differences in technique. These items involve the actual temperature of the perfusing alcohol, the systemic temperature of the perfused animal, the thickness and distention of the gastric balloon, and the duration of the freezing period. One must not skate too close to the brink of disaster in one's anxiety to secure secretory depression. Among 143 patients whose stomachs were frozen for either 45 or 50 minutes, not a single instance of postfreezing melena or gastric ulceration has been observed.

It would appear that a relatively narrow zone divides safe freezing, attended by secretory depression, and gastric necrosis accompanied by irrevocable complications. We are continuing to explore this border area to define more exactly safe and effective means of attaining our desired ends. If morbidity as well as mortality can be completely deleted, gastric freezing should come to play an important role in the control of some aspects of the peptic ulcer diathesis.

Dr. Marshall J. Orloff, Torrance, Calif: I will grant that every operation which has been done for portal hypertension has had some successes. It is only those procedures which provided a consistent degree of success that will have long-lasting value. The operation of total gastrectomy, as Dr. Bernstein has said, has had some successes. It has also had some failures, as had the procedures of distal esophagectomy and interposition. When these operations succeed I suspect that the reason for success is not the reduction of acid but is some interference with blood flow. Perhaps the same comment may be applied to the effect of gastroesophageal hypothermia, which, as the Minnesota group has shown us, not only reduces acid but perhaps more importantly reduces blood flow.

Our study did not prove that increased hydrostatic pressure is responsible for esophageal varix rupture, but I cannot resist the opportunity to express the opinion that this is the main cause, as Dr. Cranley stated in his discussion. Dr. Jackson's beautiful demonstrations of the huge coronary vein coming directly off of the portal vein, I think, in part account for the effect of increased hydrostatic pressure on the varices. The effect of pressure and flow is immediate, since the connection between the esophageal varices and the main stream of the portal vein is so direct.

Moreover, I believe the sucking action of the chest, with its negative pressure, has something to do with why esophageal varices bleed.

Finally, may I point out that the time when reflux of acid peptic juice is at its maximum is when the patient is in the horizontal position. Yet, few patients develop varix rupture while they are asleep. Rather rupture occurs commonly during an act which involves straining. I think Liebowitz has shown this, and in our studies we have often obtained a history of straining when specific inquiry was made. Straining and contraction of the abdominal muscles and descent of the diaphragm are capable of raising the portal pressure tremendously, and perhaps rupture of the varices is a consequence.

Dr. Francis C. Jackson, Pittsburgh: In answer to Dr. Fry's comment that the measurement of spleen pressure adds valuable time to the procedure, I would like to say that the combined technique which we are utilizing now, of spleen pressure and percutaneous splenoportgraphy, consumes exactly 60 seconds. The use of the manometer, we agree, adds a dangerous period of time to the period the needle is in the spleen. We also agree that the degree of liver disease is probably the prime factor in the pathogenesis of the associated portal hypertension and its complications. We would like to point, out, however, that if patients can be studied safely—and I emphasize this because we feel our technique is beginning to be safe (and it was not at first)—these patients can be studied earlier in their disease. This hemorrhagic pattern can then be defined, and they may be considered candidates for prophylactic portacaval shunt when they are otherwise good surgical risks.

We agree that the demonstration of the anatomical factor here, ie, demonstrable coronary vein, is only one of the many factors in the development of varices and the appearance of hemorrhage. However, we feel that this is one of the prime predisposing factors and not the precipitating factor of bleeding.

I agree with Dr. Berman that the very complex arteriovenous development which appears both in the liver and in the splanchic circulation does contribute, in a number of patients with portal hypertension, to the pathogenic process.

The patient demonstrated in our Fig 1*A* with a huge coronary vein, is shown after his portacaval shunt. Note the refilling of the coronary vein and the reappearance of his varices. You will, also, notice he has an intrahepatic obstruction to his inferior vena cava. This patient bled massively just before he died.

Significance of Post-Traumatic and Postoperative Oliguria

ROBERT W. HOPKINS, MD; GABRIEL SABGA, MD; POINCIANO BERNARDO, MD; ISRAEL PENN, MD; AND F. A. SIMEONE, MD, CLEVELAND

Hippocrates recognized the value of the urine as an aid in the prognosis of many disorders, and his references to the characteristics of the urine are numerous.[1,2] Homer Smith [3] quotes Constantine Africanus, writing in Salerno in the eleventh century, as stating that the "urine is better than the pulse to discover the disease from which the patient suffers."

Oliguria is a common finding following trauma, major surgery, hemorrhage, and sepsis. The oliguria may result from structural damage to renal tubules,[4-7] from impaired renal blood flow in the absence of structural damage to the kidney,[8,9] or from antidiuresis.[10,11]

This report presents the urinary findings of patients during or following severe hemorrhage and of patients who were in "septic shock." These are compared with the findings in the urine of patients who were oliguric during and after major elective surgery to see if fundamental differences exist with regard to causes for the diminished urinary flow.

Material

The urine has been studied from seven patients undergoing major elective surgery, from seven other patients during or after severe hemorrhage, and from three patients in "septic shock." Of the the seven patients undergoing elective surgery, six were oliguric with a urinary flow of less than 0.5 ml per minute. Two of the seven patients who had bled were oliguric (less than 0.5 ml per minute) for periods from 20 hours to 4 days, and two were totally anuric. Oliguria was observed in two of the three patients with "septic shock," while the third was totally anuric during the period of observation. The urinary findings of the ten patients with oliguria of less than 0.5 ml per minute form the basis for this report.

Three of the six patients with oliguria undergoing elective surgery had thoracic procedures, including one pneumonectomy, one resection of a pulmonary sequestration, and one hiatus herniorrhaphy. Abdominal procedures included one portacaval shunt, one splenorenal shunt (through a thoracoabdominal approach), and one elective subtotal gastrectomy. Four of the patients received no intravenous fluids prior to the induction of anesthesia, and two received 5% dextrose in distilled water at rates of 50 and 37 ml per hour throughout the preceding 12 hours. During the period of observation, 5% dextrose in distilled water was administered slowly (mean rate 39 ml per hour). Whole blood was administered to replace blood lost at surgery.

Of the two oliguric patients who had bled, one was a 31-year-old woman who developed severe intraperitoneal bleeding following vaginal hysterectomy. A laparotomy and ligation of the right ovarian artery, performed 6 hours before these observations were made, failed to control the bleeding. The patient had been oliguric since the conclusion of the hysterectomy 14 hours before the present observations were made. A total of 5,000 ml of whole blood and 1,000 ml of dextrose and distilled water were administered during this period. Oliguria and oligemia continued for an additional 8 hours, until a second laparotomy and ligation of the right internal iliac artery controlled the bleeding. An additional 2,500 ml of whole blood was given prior to surgery. The present observations were made during this 8-hour period of oliguria and during the subsequent period of recovery. After ligation of the external iliac artery, the patient made an uneventful recovery and was discharged from the hospital ten days later.

The second patient with hemorrhage was a 56-year-old man who was admitted six weeks before the time of this study because of cirrhosis of the liver with esophageal varices and ascites. Stools were guaiac-positive throughout his hospital stay. He developed massive gastrointestinal bleeding five days before these observations were made. He had received 1,300 ml of packed erythrocytes during this

Presented at the 20th Annual Meeting of the Central Surgical Association, Chicago, Feb 21-23, 1963.

From the Department of Surgery, Western Reserve University School of Medicine and the Cleveland Metropolitan General Hospital.

Supported by the Department of the Army contract number: DA-49-193-M.D. 2022.

time. An additional 1,000 ml of whole blood and 1,000 ml of 5% dextrose and water were administered during the eight hours prior to death. Four hours after the studies were begun, he suddenly vomited a large quantity of blood and died almost immediately. The patient was known to have renal disease while he was in the hospital, and the blood urea nitrogen had gradually climbed to 120 mg% by the time of death. Autopsy revealed the presence of severe chronic pyelonephritis with tubular atrophy and dilation. No evidence of recent acute damage to the kidney was noted. Findings included Laennec's cirrhosis with esophageal varices, and massive gastrointestinal hemorrhage. This patient is the only patient with known renal disease in the group studied and is therefore of particular interest for comparison.

Of the two patients with oliguria who were in septic shock, one was a 42-year-old woman with known cirrhosis who had previously been admitted for ascites and jaundice. On the day prior to the present admission, she had developed a high fever. Her arterial pressure was 120/82 on admission (5:30 am). It dropped to 108/40 at 2½ hours after admission, and she was placed on metaraminol. At 3 pm, while still receiving metaraminol intravenously, she vomited approximately 250 ml of dark blood. An additional 200 ml of dark blood was aspirated with a Levin tube, and 1,600 ml of coffee-ground material was aspirated from her stomach during the next 10 hours. No further bleeding was observed during her hospitalization. The total urinary output in the first 24 hours in the hospital was 350 ml. The present observations were begun 20 hours after admission after the patient had received 3,000 ml of whole blood and 1,750 ml of 5% dextrose in distilled water. Observations were continued for 10 hours during which time 500 ml of 5% dextrose and water was administered. The patient died 10 hours after these observations were completed. A culture of the blood drawn on admission grew *Escherichia coli.* At autopsy, the microscopic examination of the kidney showed occasional foci of tubular degeneration with vacuolar nephropathy, but most of the kidney appeared normal. The patient also had Laennec's cirrhosis and esophageal varices.

The second patient in septic shock was a 56-year-old man who underwent esophagectomy for carcinoma of the esophagus four days prior to the study. A segment of colon was interposed between the proximal esophagus and the stomach. The patient eventually died because of impairment to the venous return from the transposed colon with subsequent necrosis of this segment. The patient went into shock and became oliguric twenty hours before the present observations were started. The patient had been given 2,000 ml of 5% dextrose in water and 1,000 ml of 5% dextrose in saline prior to the study. Observations were continued until the patient's death 20 hours later. An additional 1,000 ml of 5% dextrose in water, 2,000 ml of whole blood, and 500 ml of macromolecular dextran were administered before death. At autopsy, the kidneys appeared normal both grossly and microscopically.

Methods

An indwelling catheter was placed in the bladder for collection of samples of urine at intervals of 15 to 60 minutes. Urine was collected by aspiration of the catheter without washout. Arterial blood was obtained for analysis from a cannula inserted into the brachial or radial artery. Arterial pressures were recorded with a Statham P23 strain gauge transducer attached to the arterial cannula. Central venous pressures were recorded from a catheter inserted via the basilic vein into the superior vena cava. Cardiac outputs were calculated from the dilution of indocyanine green dye according to the Hamilton-Stewart principle. The circulating blood volume was measured from the dilution of radioactive iodinated serum albumin with the Volemetron. The tables of Nadler, Hidalgo, and Bloch [12] were used to obtain values for estimated normal blood volumes where control data from the patient were not available. The osmolalities of the blood and urine were determined from the depression of the freezing point with a Fiske osmometer. The pH of the urine and blood was measured with a Cambridge glass electrode pH meter. The concentration of sodium and potassium in urine and blood was measured with a flame photometer using lithium as an internal standard.

The osmolar clearance (C_{osm}) was calculated from the urinary osmolality (U_{osm}), the osmolality of the plasma (P_{osm}), and the urinary volume (V) as described by Smith [13] according to the following formula:

$$C_{osm} = U_{osm} V / P_{osm}$$

The tubular reabsorption of free water (T_cH_2O) * was calculated according to the following formula:

$$T_cH_2O = C_{osm} - V$$

The T_cH_2O is an index of the concentrating activity of the kidney. A high T_cH_2O indicates concentration of the urine, a low T_cH_2O indicates a lack of concentration, and a negative T_cH_2O indicates dilution of the urine.

Results

Hemodynamic Factors.—The patients undergoing major operative procedures tolerated the procedures well and were at no

* The T_cH_2O is the net amount of free water reabsorbed to produce a urine more concentrated than the glomerular filtrate. It is the same as negative free water clearance (C_{H_2O}).

TABLE 1.—*Hemodynamic Observations*

	Arterial Pressure, Mm Hg	Blood Volume, Liters	Cardiac Index, Liters/Min/sq meter	Venous Pressure, Cm Saline	Durat of Oliguria, Hr
Elective surgery (6 patients)					
Preoperative	143/91	4.93	2.21	6.10	—
Oliguria	116/79	4.44	1.76	15.8	8.6
Shock (4 patients)					
Normal *	126/75	4.14	—	—	—
Oliguria	99/67	4.26	1.81	11.5	38
Hemorrhage (2 patients)					
Normal *	120/75	3.69	—	—	
Oliguria	104/78	2.85	1.37	9.8	22-96
Septic shock (2 patients)					
Normal *	131/75	4.56	—	—	27-31
Oliguria	94/59	5.67	2.25	13.2	

* Normal arterial pressures were obtained 1 to 60 days before shock.
The Tables of Nadler et al (reference 12) were used to estimate "normal" blood volumes.

time in clinical shock. Hemodynamic data are presented in Table 1. The mean arterial blood pressures for the group during the period of oliguria were lower than the control values but were not lower than the range of normal in four of the six patients. The arterial pressure dropped to 70/50 or 60/40 for periods of 15 to 20 minutes in two patients whose blood volumes were recorded as normal at the time of hypotension. The average blood volumes of the patients during the period of oliguria also were below control values. The cardiac index demonstrated a decrease from 2.21 preoperatively to 1.76 liters per minute per square meter during the period of oliguria.

The arterial pressures of the patients in shock were lower than those undergoing elective surgery (mean 99/67). The blood volumes of the patients in oligemic shock were low (mean 2.85 liters, 23%below expected normal), whereas they were normal or high in patients with septic shock. The cardiac index was very low (0.74 liters per minute per square meter) in one patient, who was actively bleeding, while it was within the range of normal for the other patient who had bled and those in septic shock, who were observed after fluid replacement.

Urinary Findings.—The findings in the patients undergoing elective surgery differed from those of the patients with bleeding or septic shock. The urine of the operative cases was characterized by an osmolality twice that of the plasma, a moderately low sodium, and a moderately high potassium, whereas the urine of the patients who had bled or were in septic shock was characterized by an osmolality close to that of the plasma, a low concentration of sodium, and a moderately high concentration of potassium (Table 2).

The mean rate of flow of the urine of the patients undergoing surgery was 0.36 ml per minute. The average urinary osmolality during oliguria ranged from 520 to 876 mOsm per kilogram of water with a mean for the group of 663 mOsm per kilogram. This compares with a mean of 420 mOsm per kilogram

TABLE 2.—*Urinary Findings of Patients*

Patients	Flow, Ml/Min	Osmolality, mOsm/Kg	Sodium, mEq/Liter	Potassium, mEq/Liter	pH	C_{osm}, Ml/Min	$T^c_{H_2O}$, Ml/Min	U:P Osmolality
Elective surgery (6 patients)								
Preoperative *	1.61	420	116	65	6.4	2.21	0.56	1.43
Oliguria	0.36	663	48.7	80	5.5	0.88	0.48	2.27
Shock (4 patients)	0.21	348	14.1	62	5.15	0.26	0.05	1.29
Hemorrhage (2 patients)	0.21	359	13.5	54	5.4	0.28	0.07	1.14
Septic shock (2 patients)	0.21	337	14.7	66	5.0	0.24	0.03	1.21

* Includes two patients who were hydrated and four patients who received no fluids for eight hours preoperatively.

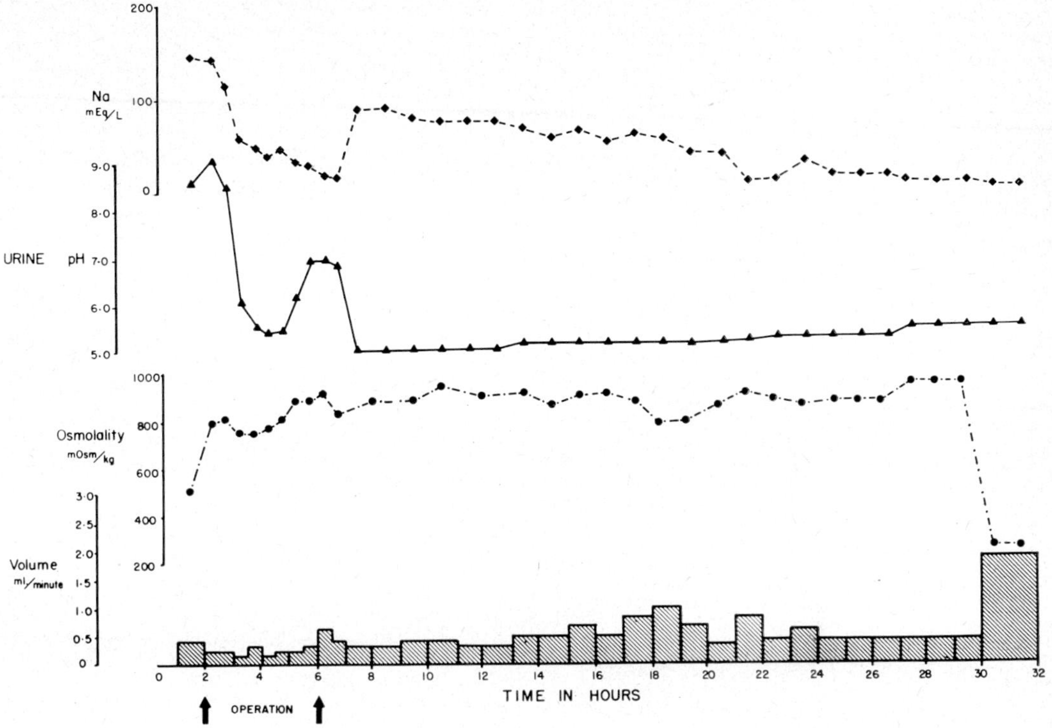

Fig. 1.—Data from a patient who was oliguric while undergoing a transthoracic repair of a hiatus hernia. The urinary osmolality was high until diuresis occurred 24 hours postoperatively.

preoperatively. The osmolar concentration of the urine during oliguria was approximately twice that of the plasma, with a mean U:P ratio for the group of 2.27 with a standard deviation of 0.48. The mean osmolar clearance was 0.88 ml per minute, and the mean T_cH_2O was 0.48 ml per minute. The average concentrations of sodium in the urine during oliguria ranged from 24 to 96 with a mean of 49 mEq per liter for the group. The lowest concentrations of sodium found in individual samples of urine from each patient ranged from 5 to 81 with a mean for the group of 25 mEq per liter. The mean concentration of potassium in the urine for the group was 80 mEq per liter. The patients excreted an acid urine throughout. No differences were apparent during oliguria between patients who had been hydrated preoperatively and those who were not. The findings from a patient undergoing a hiatus herniorrhaphy are demonstrated in Fig 1.

The urinary findings of the two patients with hemorrhage and oliguria and of the two in septic shock were similar and will be considered together as "patients in shock." The mean urinary volume for the group was 0.21 ml per minute. The average osmolalities of the urine of the individual patients in this group ranged from 303 to 370 with a mean for the group of 348 mOsm per kilogram. The ratio of the osmolalities of the urine to those in the plasma was low with a mean of 1.21 and a standard deviation of 0.11. The mean osmolar clearance was 0.26 ml per minute, and the mean T_cH_2O was only 0.05 ml per minute. The U:P osmolar ratio and the T_cH_2O of the group in shock were significantly lower than those of the patients undergoing elective surgery, indicating an inability of the patients in shock to form a concentrated urine. The urinary sodiums were low in the four patients in shock in the present study, with the average concentrations in the urine ranging from 9.9 to 19.4 mEq per liter (mean 14.1). The lowest values obtained from individual specimens from the four patients ranged from 1 mEq per liter to 16.6, with a mean of 8 for the four patients. An acid urine was excreted by the patients in

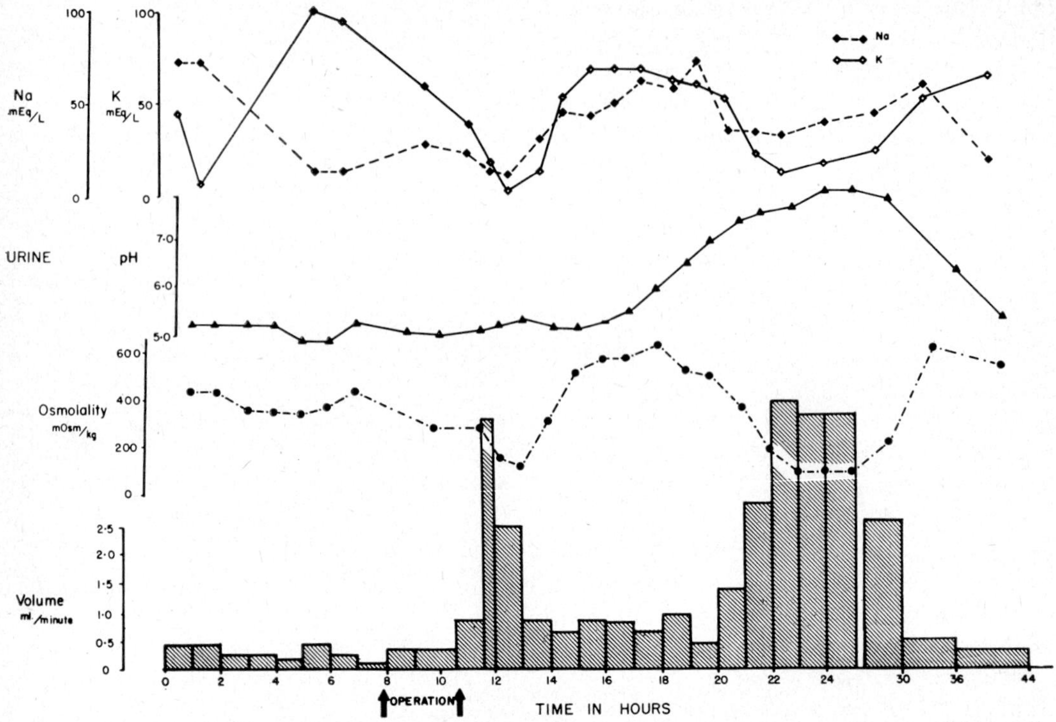

Fig. 2.—Data from a patient with intraperitoneal bleeding after vaginal hysterectomy. Prior to the final operation and control of the bleeding, she was oliguric with a urinary osmolality only slightly above that of the plasma. The urinary concentration of sodium dropped to low levels. After the hemorrhage was controlled, a higher urinary osmolality was found except during periods of diuresis.

shock. The mean of the urinary concentration of potassium was 62 mEq per liter. The findings in the patient with postoperative bleeding are presented in Fig 2.

Findings in the Plasma.—The values for osmolalities, concentrations of sodium and potassium, and pH in the plasma are given in Table 3. A moderate hyponatremia was observed in the patients in shock, but the difference in this small group of patients is not statistically significant. A transient hyperkalemia was observed in the patients undergoing elective surgery. Hyperkalemia was observed also in the patients in shock. A severe acidosis (average pH of the blood, 7.11) was observed in one of the patients in septic shock. The remainder of the oliguric patients with hemorrhage and septic shock and the patients undergoing elective surgery had a mean arterial pH during the period of oliguria of 7.35.

Comment

The urine of the patients in this study who were oliguric in hemorrhagic or septic shock demonstrated a failure of osmotic concentra-

Table 3.—*Osmolality, Electrolytes, and pH in Plasma*

	Osmolality, mOsm/Kg	Sodium, mEq/Liter	Potassium, mEq/Liter	pH
Elective surgery (6 patients)				
Preoperative	292	145	6.3	7.38
Oliguria	292	139	6.5	7.35
Shock (4 patients)	287	134	7.0	7.30
Hemorrhage (2 patients)	278	133	7.0	7.35
Septic shock (2 patients)	297	136	7.0	7.24

tion by the kidney. In contrast, a concentration of the urine to twice the osmolality of plasma was achieved by kidneys of the patients undergoing major elective surgery. This difference in concentrating ability of the kidney may help to differentiate the possible causes for the oliguria following trauma and hemorrhage, surgery, or serious sepsis.

Pringle et al,[14] in 1905, noted the oliguria which followed the induction of ether anesthesia and surgery and warned that the "inhibition of renal activity must exercise a most injurious effect on the general metabolism and the condition of the patient." The finding of oliguria after the induction of ether anesthesia with or without surgery has been confirmed by Dudley et al [10] and Aprahamian et al.[11] These authors demonstrated that the effects of anesthesia and surgery on the urine were similar to the effects observed after the administration of vasopressin. Hemorrhage is the most potent stimulus for the production of antidiuretic hormone. An increased level of antidiuretic hormone has been found in the jugular venous blood of animals after hemorrhage [15] or after a decrease in blood volume.[16] Changes in blood volume may, therefore, be followed by antidiuresis. Oliguria may be produced by a reduction of renal blood flow and arterial pressure, as demonstrated by Bounous et al,[9] although the response may be modified by autoregulation of the blood supply to the kidney.[17] Oliguria may also be the consequence of damage, either structural or functional, to the kidney itself. The clinical entity of post-traumatic renal insufficiency and similar forms of acute renal failure have been well recognized since the extensive studies emanating from World War II.[4-6]

The oliguria observed after surgery or in patients in shock could, therefore, result from antidiuresis, inadequate renal perfusion, or renal damage. Of help in differentiating these causes for oliguria is the osmotic concentration of the urine together with the concentration of sodium in the urine.

In the generally accepted countercurrent multiplier theory, concentration of the urine depends (*a*) upon the integrity of the function of the countercurrent loop in the renal medulla and (*b*) upon the presence of the antidiuretic hormone (ADH). The osmolality of the tissues in the renal papillae is normally four to five times that of the plasma. Urine in the descending limb of Henle's loop becomes hyperosmotic as it equilibrates with the progressively more concentrated interstitial fluid in the renal medulla. The hyperosmolality of the interstitial fluid is maintained primarily by active transfer of sodium from the urine in the ascending limb of Henle's loop to the interstitial fluid. The urine becomes hypo-osmotic with respect to plasma by the time it reaches the distal tubule. Although the mechanism and site of action of ADH are not entirely clear, the distal tubule and collecting ducts are thought to be relatively impermeable to water and solutes in the absence of ADH, and a dilute urine results. Under the influence of ADH, the permeability of the distal tubule and collecting ducts to water is increased to a greater extent than to solutes. As the urine descends in the collecting ducts through the hyperosmotic medulla, water leaves the urine in relatively greater amounts than solutes, and a concentrated urine is formed. Necessary to the formation of the concentrated urine, therefore, is the maintenance of the hyperosmolality of the renal papillae and the presence of the antidiuretic hormone.†

Oliguria with failure of concentration of the urine, as observed in the patients in shock in this study, indicates the presence of abnormal renal function. Impairment of the concentrating ability may result from functional damage to renal tubules and consequent inability to maintain the normal hyperosmolality of the renal medulla. In this instance, a urinary osmolality similar to that of the plasma would result, with oliguria resulting from obstruction to flow of urine in damaged tubules.

† Some increase in osmolality of the urine above that in the plasma has been demonstrated by Berliner and Davidson [18] in the absence of ADH in animals with a critical reduction of blood flow by partial occlusion of their renal artery. Osmolalities as high as 475 mOsm per kilogram have been obtained under these circumstances.

Decreased osmolality of the urine with oliguria may also result from marked reduction of glomerular filtration and a consequent decrease in the total amount of sodium delivered to the renal tubules. Kramer and co-workers [19,20] have demonstrated that blood in the capillary loop of the renal medulla flows at a rate close to that of urine in the countercurrent loops. When renal blood flow is reduced to a critical extent, the glomerular filtration and flow of urine in the countercurrent loops are reduced to a greater extent than capillary blood flow, and less sodium is available to the tubules. A "washout" of medullary hyperosmolality occurs, and failure of urinary concentration results. The ability of the tubules to function, however, may remain normal under these circumstances. Sodium is removed from the tubular fluid, and a low final concentration of sodium is observed. A continuing, but critically reduced glomerular filtration, may, therefore, result in oliguria with a urinary osmolality close to that of the plasma.

Although the urine of the patients in this study who were oliguric in hemorrhagic or septic shock demonstrated a failure of osmotic concentration of the urine, the concentrations of sodium in the urines were very low, ranging from lows of 1 to 16 mEq per liter. This indicates active removal of sodium by renal tubules. In acute tubular necrosis, the sodium levels in the urine are generally above 60 mEq per liter,[7,21] suggesting that while some tubules may continue to function normally, others are transmitting essentially unchanged glomerular filtrate. The low urinary sodiums in the patients in the present group, therefore, suggest that acute tubular necrosis has not developed in these patients and that failure of renal function occurs primarily from lack of an adequate glomerular filtration with poor perfusion of the kidney. The formation of an acid urine in these patients also indicates the absence of tubular damage. It is of particular interest to note that the patient who had severe chronic pyelonephritis at autopsy had urinary sodiums of 8 to 16 mEq per liter and a pH of 5.4, suggesting that the remaining tubules continued to function normally.

The urine of normally hydrated subjects to whom vasopressin is administered is characterized by high urinary osmolality and a low urinary volume. Crabbe [22] found urinary osmolalities averaging 940 mOsm per liter and urine flows of 0.86 ml per minute after the administration of vasopressin. This effect was augmented by the administration of aldosterone, although the oliguria and osmolal concentration of the urine were not as great as with dehydration alone.

The mean of the urinary flow rates of the patients undergoing elective surgery was 0.36 ml per minute with an osmolality of 663 mOsm per kilogram. These findings suggest the continued function of the concentrating mechanism in the renal medulla and an effect of the antidiuretic hormone as suggested by the studies of Dudley et al.[10] An effect of antidiuresis alone, however, does not appear to be sufficient to account entirely for oliguria of the extent observed. The rate of flow of urine was less than that observed by Crabbe [22] in dehydrated subjects or subjects to whom vasopressin had been administered, while the osmolality of the urine was also less. The operative patients in the present series were not "healthy young subjects," but they did not present known renal disease. Although the clinical conditions of these patients during surgery appeared to be satisfactory, some decreases in arterial pressure, cardiac index, and blood volume did occur. It is likely that these factors were associated with a decreased perfusion of the kidneys which was not sufficient to impair significantly the concentrating mechanism but which led to a reduction of urinary output beyond that which could be explained by an effect of antidiuresis alone.

Summary and Conclusions

The urinary findings were observed in two patients in hemorrhagic shock and two patients in "septic" shock who were oliguric. The observations were compared with findings in the urine of six patients who were oliguric during and following major surgery.

The urine of the patients in "shock" was characterized by an osmolality of the urine similar to that of plasma, a low concentration of sodium, a low pH, and a moderately high concentration of potassium. The urine of the patients undergoing elective surgery had significantly higher osmolalities, moderately low concentration of sodium, a low pH, and a high level of potassium.

The findings from the patients in shock suggest poor perfusion of the kidney with continued function of renal tubules. The findings from the patients undergoing elective surgery indicate an effect of antidiuresis.

Robert W. Hopkins, MD, Metropolitan General Hospital, 3395 Scranton Rd, Cleveland 9, Ohio.

REFERENCES

1. Adams, F.: The Genuine Works of Hippocrates: Translated From the Greek by Francis Adams, Baltimore: The Williams & Wilkins Company, 1939.

2. Major, R. H.: A History of Medicine: Volumes I and II, Springfield, Ill: Charles C Thomas, Publisher, 1954.

3. Smith, H. W.: De Urina, JAMA 155:899, 1954.

4. Mallory, T. B.: Hemoglobinuric Nephrosis in Traumatic Shock, Amer J Clin Path 17:427, 1947.

5. Burnett, C. H.; Shapiro, S. L.; Simeone, F. A.; Beecher, H. K.; Mallory, T. B.; and Sullivan, E. R.: Post-Traumatic Renal Insufficiency, Surgery 22:994, 1947.

6. Oliver, J.; MacDowell, M.; and Tracy, A.: The Pathogenesis of Acute Renal Failure Associated With Traumatic and Toxic Injury: Renal Ischemia, Nephrotoxic Damage and the Ischemuric Episode, J Clin Invest 30:1305, 1951.

7. Meroney, W. H., and Rubini, M. E.: Kidney Function During Acute Tubular Necrosis: Clinical Studies and a Theory, Metabolism 8:1, 1959.

8. Langston, J. B.; Guyton, A. C.; and Gillespie, W. J., Jr.: Acute Effect of Changes in Renal Arterial Pressure and Sympathetic Blockade on Kidney Function, Amer J Physiol 197:595, 1959.

9. Bounous, G.; Shumacker, H. B.; and King, H.: Studies in Renal Blood Flow, Ann Surg 151:47, 1960.

10. Dudley, H. F.; Boling, E. A.; LeQuesne, L. P.; and Moore, F. D.: Studies on Antidiuresis in Surgery: Effects of Anesthesia, Surgery and Posterior Pituitary Antidiuretic Hormone on Water Metabolism in Man, Ann Surg 140:354, 1954.

11. Aprahamian, H. A.; Vanderveen, J. L.; Bunker, J. P.; Murphy, A. J.; and Crawford, J. D.: The Influence of General Anesthetics on Water and Solute Excretion in Man, Ann Surg 150:122, 1959.

12. Nadler, S. B.; Hidalgo, J. U.; and Bloch, T.: Prediction of Blood Volume in Normal Human Adults, Surgery 51:224, 1962.

13. Smith, H. W.: Principles of Renal Physiology, New York: Oxford University Press, 1956.

14. Pringle, H.; Maunsell, R. C. B.; and Pringle, S.: Clinical Effects of Ether Anaesthesia on Renal Activity, Brit Med J 2:542, 1905.

15. Weinstein, H.; Berne, R. M.; and Sachs, H.: Vasopressin in Blood: Effect of Hemorrhage, Endocrinology 66:712, 1960.

16. Share, L.: Acute Reduction in Extracellular Fluid Volume and Concentration of Antidiuretic Hormone in Blood, Endocrinology 69:925, 1961.

17. Winton, F. R.: Present Concepts of the Renal Circulation, AMA Arch Intern Med 103:495, 1959.

18. Berliner, R. W., and Davidson, D. G.: Production of Hypertonic Urine in the Absence of Pituitary Antidiuretic Hormone, J Clin Invest 36:1416, 1957.

19. Kramer, K.; Thurau, K.; and Deetjen, P.: Hemodynamics of Kidney Medullary Substance: Part I. Capillary Passage Time, Blood Volume, Circulation, Tissue Hematocrit and Oxygen Consumption of Kidney Medullary Substance in Situ, Pflueger Arch Ges Physiol 270:251, 1960.

20. Thurau, K.; Deetjen, P.; and Kramer, K.: Hemodynamics of Kidney Medullary Substance: Part II. Interrelationships Between the Vascular and Tubular Counter-Flow System in Arterial Pressure Increases, Water Diuresis and Osmotic Diuresis, Pflueger Arch Ges Physiol 270:270, 1960.

21. Sporn, I. N.; Lancestremere, R. G.; and Papper, S.: Differential Diagnosis of Oliguria in Aged Patients, New Eng J Med 267:130, 1962.

22. Crabbe, J.: The Role of Aldosterone in the Renal Concentration Mechanism in Man, Clin Sci 23:39, 1962.

DISCUSSION

Dr. James M. Stokes, St. Louis: The topic discussed by Dr. Hopkins has been and continues to be of critical interest to surgeons. The difference between physiologic oliguria and pathological oliguria is of critical importance in assessing therapy after operation. Dr. Hopkins has indicated the various factors which may affect urine flow rates in the postoperative patient. In general, urine flow rates of 300 to 400 cc per 24 hours or about 0.33 cc per minute is the lowest which can be attained in the human under conditions of maximal concentrating ability of the kidney. Flow rates below this level are definitely pathological, whereas flow rates above this level either may be the result of physiologic antidiuresis or may also be the result of intrinsic renal disorders. There are only three primary renal factors which affect the urine output. These have been summarized in the slide. Assuming a constant solute load, that is, a load of urea or solute to be excreted, the two remaining factors which determine urine flow rates are the filtration rate and the tubular water reabsorption from the filtrate. Under ordinary circumstances only about 1% of the filtrate —which amounts to 180 liters—about 1% to 2% of this amount escapes as urine. The 99% is reabsorbed by the tubules. If the solute load is constant, then changes in either the filtration rate or the tubular water reabsorption and their relative relations to one another will determine the final urine output. This slide divided into four quadrants shows the combinations of filtration rate and tubular water removal which affect urine flow. Any physiologic or pathologic disorder ultimately affects one of these two processes. Under ordinary circumstances of glomerular and tubular balance the urine flow is about 1% of a filtration. If neither of these two are changed, urine flow rate remains the same. In quadrant 2 if the filtration rate remains the same or is increased by the plus sign and the tubular water reabsorption is decreased, the urine flow rate will remain the same or increase. Quadrants three and four demonstrate the only combinations of glomerular and tubular functions which can result in diminished urine output. These are decreased filtration rate and increased tubular removal of water or decreased filtration rate and decreased removal of water. Acute injuries to glomerular or tubular function, and these are rarely completely separable, will result in great diminution in urine flow.

The problem in the postoperative patient is to determine whether the oliguria is physiologic in the result of antidiuresis or is pathologically the result of renal injury. As Dr. Hopkins indicated, the urine plasma osmolality ratio, that is, the concentration of urine in excess of the plasma, will give some indication of renal concentrating ability and thus of renal reserve. However, as Berliner has shown, reductions in filtration rate up to 30% may also produce a concentrated urine independently of the antidiuretic stimulus, also misleading since this might be interpreted as evidence of good kidney function.

This may seem paradoxical since it takes away from the surgeon one of the recommended diagnostic tests for renal function. It is also possible to have high urine flow rates with very reduced renal function in the presence of solute diuresis. That is, if a concentrated solute is infused such as 10% glucose or urea, the urine output may be increased from 5 to 10 ml per minute even though renal function is quite low. We demonstrated this in the sodium-depleted animal, and it is also demonstrated in the kidney with high-grade arterial obstruction receiving hyperosmotic urea solution. Thus although urine flow is certainly a guidepost for renal function it may not be considered the essential factor of kidney function. A test for normal renal function quite easily obtained is the urine plasma creatine ratio. If the passage of creatine is elevated above 1.5 mg%, it is almost indicative of impairment of renal filtration rate and of renal function. If the urine plasma ratio of creatine is above 20 this would indicate reasonable concentrating ability of the kidney. Furthermore, as Dr. Hopkins indicated, if the urine plasma osmolality ratio is two or above, the kidney is certainly concentrating effectively. Since the plasma osmolality is about 300, any urine osmolality of 400-600 would indicate adequate renal concentrating ability if the plasma creatine were also within normal limits.

Dr. John Hager Wulsin, Cincinnati: The clinical study carried out by Dr. Hopkins and his associates brings out an extremely practical point, namely, that in shock or after trauma the quality of the urine is probably as important as the quantity.

There are a number of factors that influence renal function and flow after this type of stimulus or stress. Blood pressure is known to us all. The state of volume replacement is likewise important. I would like to call attention to the influence of catecholamines on urine flow after trauma or shock. It is recognized that circulating catecholamines are high after such stimuli, and furthermore, levarterenol is often given exogenously by doctors to raise pressure. Exogenous catecholamines can suppress urine flow, even though the normal blood pressure is present.

Let us focus our attention on endogenous catecholamines. Experimentally, if one bleeds a dog massively, the urine flow stops. If one blocks endogenous catecholamines with an antagonist such as guanethidine, we have observed on a number of occasions that the animals will produce urine despite very low pressures, which should prevent renal perfusion of a satisfactory level. Even without giving these blocked animals volume replacement, urine flow can be observed.

I would like to present a somewhat analogous clinical situation in which large amounts of endogenous norepinephrine are suddenly withdrawn from a patient.

This is a young woman with a pheochromocytoma, who was markedly hypertensive. Throughout the operation she put out relatively little urine. With removal of the tumor, as so often happens, the blood pressure dropped down below shock levels, and we started a drip of phenylephrine (Neo-Synephrine) rather than levarterenol. The pressure bounded right back up but then fell rather promptly within the next ten minutes, stabilizing at a very low level of 60/40 for another two hours.

Despite her low pressure (60/40), what was most striking was the very prompt diuresis, ranging between 0.5-2.0 cc/min, that started within four minutes after removal of the tumor and persisted for 1½ hours despite the low blood pressure. After two hours the blood pressure came back to normal, phenylephrine was discontinued, and the patient recovered uneventfully. Unfortunately we did not measure changes in osmolarity in the urine. The patient's diuresis was interpreted as resulting from sudden release of vasoconstriction in the renal arterioles after removal of the pheochromocytoma.

DR. FRASER N. GURD, Montreal, Canada: Dr. Michael Kaye of our Renal Service at The Montreal General Hospital has done studies of renal function on surgical cases during operations. Indwelling ureteral catheters add to the accuracy of measurement of urine production. To our astonishment Dr. Kaye has shown that there is often complete cessation of urine production for about 30 minutes during major operations.

When urine flow stops so completely it is difficult to determine the cause by clearance studies. However, from evidence at hand from several cases, Dr. Kaye has indicated that a drop in renal blood flow is the cause of the acute oliguria, rather than any effect of antidiuretic hormone. Nevertheless, we have found that mannitol is effective in preventing or reversing intraoperative oliguria. This action of mannitol is not completely clear.

There can be little doubt that the renal tubule in which urine has almost ceased to flow is exceptionally vulnerable to superimposed damage, such as shock or a transfusion reaction. I would like to ask Dr. Hopkins if he has any comment on the use of mannitol in the prophylaxis of renal failure.

Dr. Wulsin has raised the question of the use of adrenergic blocking agents in relation to improving renal blood flow. Although we are most interested in the subject and agree that some protection is afforded the kidney by the use of these drugs, we have not used them as primary treatment of acute oliguria. Our preference is to invoke volume replacement and all conventional measures first.

DR. ROBERT E. L. BERRY, Ann Arbor, Mich: Regardless of the complicated renal physiology involved, the interpretation of low urinary flow after operation or injury is of maximum practical importance.

Inadequate water intake is probably one of the most uncommon causes of inadequate urine flow following operation or injury and, excepting conditions of high environmental temperatures, low relative humidity, and high fever, it has been overemphasized as a cause of "oliguria." The obligatory oliguria, as stressed by Dr. Hopkins, is of considerable importance and I for one would like to thank him for his re-emphasis.

The wheel of time has inevitably brought us back to a new period when emphasis upon sodium salt replacement during operation and the early postoperative hours has again achieved some popularity. I should like to restate this problem as follows: the administration of isotonic solutions of sodium as a source of free water during operation and in the early postoperative hours is not without hazard and can be a triggering mechanism for complications. For the routine cholecystectomy, thyroidectomy, hernia, appendectomy, and amputation the administrations of isotonic sodium solutions has more to be said against than for it. In operations of considerable magnitude, however, it would appear good practice to administer isotonic sodium solutions to compensate for the edema of operative dissection and the resultant soft tissue injury. The amount to be given should be governed by the wisdom of experience, adequacy of circulation, rate of urine excretion, and urine specific gravity or osmolality.

And then there is the matter of oliguria due to renal tubular damage. Under these circumstances the renal concentrating ability is poor and the osmolality of urine is markedly decreased. The importance of this differential diagnosis cannot be overemphasized, because if accurate appraisal is not made very serious mistakes in treatment now result.

Another "gray zone" exists for those individuals who have undergone slow sodium depletion over a period of a few days. These patients often demonstrate low urine volumes with "middle range" specific gravity and urine osmolality. These individuals have difficulty in elaborating either a concentrated or dilute urine. Under these circumstances the administration of sodium-free water is a deadly form of treatment, as loads of water without sodium are poorly tolerated. The patient can easily be thrown into almost total anuria, and the symptoms of "water intoxication" become rapidly apparent.

Attention to the significance of a given urine volume is most essential if serious maltreatment is to be avoided. Diagnosis means almost everything.

DR. J. CUTHBERT OWENS, Denver: Last year at this meeting we reported our experiences with central venous pressure. This simple bedside technique is a valuable adjunct during oliguria and anuria to rule out the possibility of dehydration or hypovolemia as the cause for decreased urine output, and, if a true renal shutdown exists, to avoid overhydration. In evaluating these patients clinically, we have frequently been misled regarding the functioning blood volume.

One of our residents, Dr. Cerilli, has reported that suprarenal aortic occlusion up to eight hours in normally hydrated monkeys did not result in acute renal failure. However, dehydration increased the renal effects of suprarenal aortic occlusion. This needs to be considered in vascular surgery.

I should like to ask Dr. Hopkins if he checked central venous pressure in his patients.

DR. ROBERT W. HOPKINS, Cleveland: In response to Dr. Stokes' question about creatinine, we have only measured the blood creatinine. We have not done clearance studies on these patients, for two reasons: first, they presented very complicated problems, and second, they were severely oliguric. These observations were a part of a larger study made of the patients in shock.

I would like to comment briefly on Dr. Wulsin's observations. We, too, have been interested in the effect of catecholamines and blocking agents on the urinary output and renal blood flow. In the laboratory we are using a standardized preparation and are not able to demonstrate an improvement using either hydralazine or trimethaphan alone without blood replacement or fluid replacement in oligemic animals. We have tried trimethaphan in a few patients. We thought in one or two anuric patients, who subsequently died, that we did observe a small output of urine which might not otherwise have occurred, but we have no conclusive evidence with regard to this.

Dr. Gurd raised a very interesting question with respect to the use of mannitol in patients who are oliguric. We have had very little experience with it, but have thought a good deal about it and are planning to use it in the future to see what results we will obtain.

I do not think there is much doubt that mannitol can induce what I like to think of as a mechanical diuresis. It is an osmotic diuresis. I do not believe there is very good evidence to show that mannitol will increase glomerular filtration, but once the mannitol gets into the glomerular filtrate it will tend, by virtue of its osmotic effect, to keep urine in the tubule and flowing out from the kidney.

Whether this mechanical (osmotic) effect will be beneficial to the kidney in the long run, we do not know. I do not think there is good experimental evidence as yet to suggest that it does have a protective effect. There is no question but that it can increase urinary output. Whether this helps the organism as a whole, we have yet to see.

Dr. Berry emphasized the "gray zone," which is the one we were discussing today. Our patients with oliguria were betwixt and between. As he emphasized, we feel that the composition of the urine is of the greatest importance in determining what is going on in the patient and in the kidney. We emphasized particularly the importance of the osmolality of the urine. If this cannot be obtained, the specific gravity is second best. The determination of the sodium in the urine is also of great importance.

In answer to Dr. Owens' question, we did measure the central venous pressures in these patients. A number of the surgical patients studied during operation had thoracic procedures, and the central venous pressure in all of them was elevated during the period of time the chest was open. In the rest of the surgical patients it was generally normal. In patients in shock, throughout most of the period the venous pressure tended to be either low or within the normal range.

We measured blood volumes in these patients and in the patients in oligemic shock. In all the procedures their blood volumes tended to be low. Patients in septic shock had measured blood volumes that were high.

Myocardial Contractile Force in Experimental Hemorrhagic Shock

Some Observations

JACK C. COOLEY, MD, AND C. L. McINTOSH, MS, URBANA, ILL

The problem of managing hemorrhagic shock has always been a challenge to the physician. As early as the turn of the century this condition was recognized, and during each of the great wars signal advances were made in its treatment. Heretofore blood pressure and pulse rate have been the primary clinical parameters observed in patients with hemorrhagic shock. Ancillary observations have also been recorded on skin temperature, sweating, and skin color. Laboratory tests, including hemoglobin, red blood cell count, hematocrit, and blood volume have been helpful in judging blood replacement therapy. The state of irreversible shock has received much discussion in the

Presented at the 20th Annual Meeting of the Central Surgical Association, Chicago, Feb 21-23, 1963.

From the Section of Thoracic and Cardiovascular Surgery, Carle Memorial Hospital and Carle Clinic (Dr. Cooley); and from the Department of Physiology, University of Illinois (Mr. McIntosh).

This study was made possible by a grant from the United States Public Health Service.

literature and was attributed for many years primarily to failure of the peripheral circulation with capillary paralysis and pooling of peripheral blood.

Recently the heart has been strongly implicated as the organ which determines irreversibility in shock whether caused by hemorrhage of other etiologies. Unfortunately, even the experimental analysis of cardiac function following severe hemorrhage is difficult. Studies on coronary artery flow and myocardial muscle metabolism during hemorrhage have been accomplished but leave something to be desired as to accuracy and interpretation.

A third parameter is now available for the experimental evaluation of cardiac function under the stress of shock—the direct measurement of the contractile force of the heart muscle. This measurement is made by sewing a strain gauge to the myocardium and recording on a galvanometer the force of the isometric cardiac muscle contraction under the gauge. The results are accurate and reproducible and are important because they reflect a summation of all of the increments of pathologic myocardial physiology.

Using this parameter a group of experiments were conducted in animals in which the myocardial contractile force was recorded under conditions of varying degrees of severe hemorrhagic shock.

Materials and Methods

Twenty-one large mongrel dogs weighing from 13 to 22 kg were used. For anesthesia pentobarbital sodium was employed in the dose of 30 mg per kg. The right femoral artery and vein were isolated and cannulated with small polyethylene tubes. The systemic blood pressure was measured with a Statham pressure transducer (type P23 AC) and recorded with a Grass polygraph via the right femoral artery. Drug infusion and blood replacement were carried out via the right femoral vein. A large polyethylene cannula was introduced into the left femoral artery which was used for hemorrhaging the animals.

Each operation was carried out while employing an endotracheal tube and an automatic cyclic breathing apparatus. The pleural cavity was entered laterally in each animal through the left fifth intercostal space. The left lung was packed out of the field, exposing the left heart. The pericardium was opened and reflected with interrupted silk sutures. The Sutfin strain gauge was used in all animals to monitor contractile force and consists of two 350 ohm resistance gauges cemented on opposite sides of a 0.012 in. thick brass plate and insulated with Turtox imbedding plastic. Wires led from the gauge to a recording galvanometer. Fig 1 shows the dimensions of this gauge. The gauge was attached to the myocardium with two 00 silk sutures, 1.5 cm apart (Fig 2). For control purposes the left ventricular contractile force and systemic blood pressure values were recorded before closing the pericardium. The left lung was inflated and a routine closure of the chest wall carried out. The automatic cyclic breathing apparatus was discontinued and the animal allowed to recover until a constant contractile force and systemic blood pressure value were obtained in the closed chest preparation.

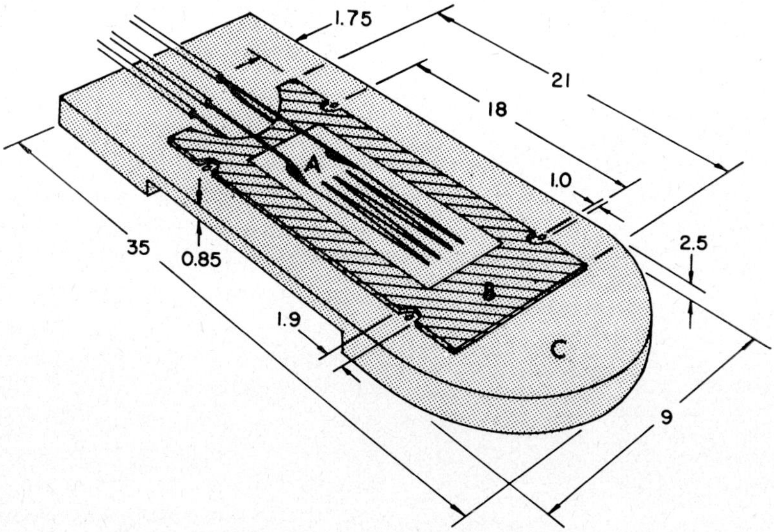

Fig 1.—The Sutfin strain gauge, showing dimensions in millimeters and the various parts: *A*, 350 ohm strain gauge; *B*, bronze plate 0.03 mm thick; *C*, embedding plastic.

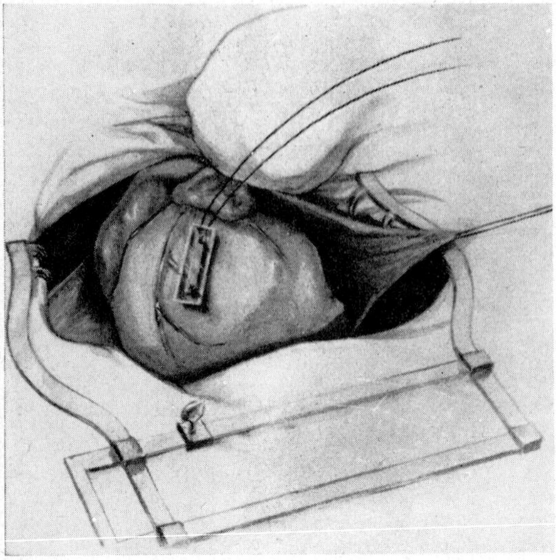

Fig 2.—A diagrammatic sketch of the Sutfin strain gauge attached to the left ventricular myocardium.

The percentage of total blood volume hemorrhaged was calculated on the basis of 92.5 ml of blood per kilogram of body weight.[1] Each animal was hemorrhaged via the left femoral artery to three levels of its estimated blood volume, 30% to 39%, 40% to 49%, and 50% to 60%. Each level of hemorrhage was reached in approximately 10 to 15 minutes, followed by a 10-minute control period. At each level of hemorrhage the animals were treated in one of four ways.

Group A was considered the control group and consisted of three animals. These animals were hemorrhaged to the various levels, and no treatment was administered. After each hemorrhage period the animals were allowed to recover for a period of ten minutes, during which time the left ventricular contractile force (LVCF) and femoral arterial blood pressure (FABP) were recorded continuously.

Group B consisted of seven animals treated with (L-) levarterenol (Levophed) after hemorrhage. The drug was administered on a weight basis, ranging from 1μg to 6μg of levarterenol per kilogram of body weight. A constant infusion apparatus was used enabling a relatively constant rate of infusion of the levarterenol over a ten-minute period. After the drug administration the animals were allowed a ten-minute control period prior to hemorrhaging to the next level.

The four animals in Group C were treated with 60% blood replacement after hemorrhage. Heparinized at the time of hemorrhage, the animal's own blood was used for transfusion. It was administered at the rate of about 10 cc per minute until 60% of the amount hemorrhaged had been replaced. The animals were allowed 30-minute control periods after blood replacement.

Seven animals comprised Group D. These were treated at each hemorrhage level with a combination of drug infusion (L-levarterenol) and 60% blood replacement. The drug and blood combined were administered to four of the seven animals in this group, while the other three received the two treatments separated by ten-minute control periods. A 30-minute control period followed the combined treatment prior to further hemorrhage.

After hemorrhaging to the 50% to 60% level, the surviving animals were allowed to establish control levels for 30 minutes, then were hemorrhaged to the point where myocardial contractile force could no longer be maintained, and they died.

Experimental Results

Group A—Control.—The three animals operated on in this group were intentionally progressively hemorrhaged without treatment until their death. The heart rate showed a gradual rise until just before death when it dropped precipitously. Blood pressure began to decline in most instances at the hemorrhage range of 30% to 40% of the estimated blood volume and declined seriously after 40% to 50% of the blood volume was depleted. In all three animals left ventricular contractile force continued with only slight decreases until just before death. Once a serious change took place in this parameter, cardiac standstill and death soon followed. Of interest was the fact that the left ventricular contractile force was so stable long after marked deterioration of the blood pressure. Fig 3 is a graph of a typical animal in the control group and illustrates some of the points mentioned. This animal was unique in the fact that an estimated 89% of the blood volume was withdrawn before serious changes occurred in the intensity of the myocardial contractile force. Average figures for percentage decrease in both blood pressure and contractile force at three levels of hemorrhage are shown in the Table.

Group B—Treatment With Levarterenol. Seven animals were progressively hemorrhaged to three predetermined levels. After reaching each level levarterenol was administered followed by ten-minute control periods. The Table gives the average percentage decrease from controls after hemorrhage and treatment at the various levels of

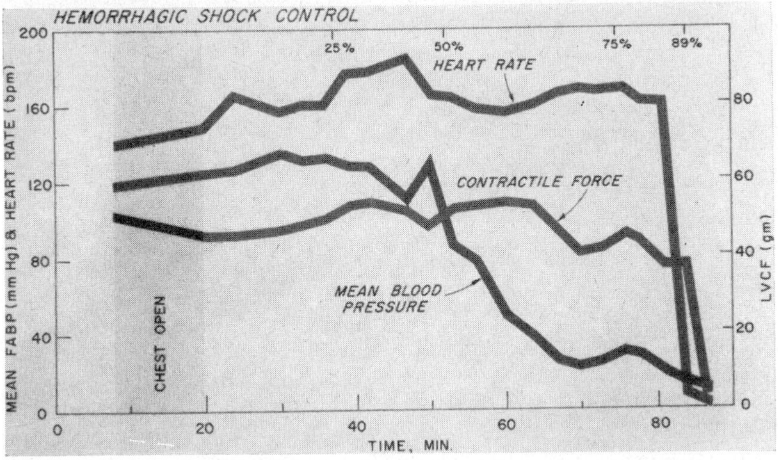

Fig 3.—Graph of a typical control animal. The percentages above refer to the amount of the animal's calculated blood volume hemorrhaged.

estimated blood volume depletion. In evaluating the effect of the drug it is interesting to note the very poor average response to the drug of both blood pressure and contractile force as indicated by a minimum return toward control figures. With levarterenol the contractile force shifted only 2% at the first level of hemorrhage, 6% at the second, and 12% at the third.

Fig 4 is a typical graph of an animal treated with levarterenol and indicates the relative stability of the contractile force as compared with the blood pressure. When contractile force severely decreased at the 69.5% hemorrhage level in this animal, however, a single injection of levarterenol of 5μg/kg had no effect on any of the three parameters, and death ensued rapidly.

Group C—Treatment With 60% Blood Replacement.—Sixty per cent blood replacement was used in treating the four animals that comprised this group. At each level of hemorrhage the animal's own blood was replaced to 60% of the amount previously lost. Anticipating a shift of a certain amount of extracellular fluid into the vascular system during the period required for hemorrhage, only 60% of the withdrawn blood was replaced rather than returning all of it. The Table indicates that a greater response occurred toward the control figures in both blood pressure and contractile force with this treatment than when levarterenol was used. Contractile force returned an average of 7% at the first level of hemorrhage, 24% at the second level, and 13% at the third level. Fig

Average Percentage Decrease in Blood Pressure and Contractile Force at Three Levels of Hemorrhage

	Effect of Hemorrhage % Decrease from Control		Effect of Treatment % Decrease from Control	
	Mean FABP	LVCF Syst.	Mean FABP	LVCF Syst.
Control (Group A-3 dogs)				
30%-39%	—26	—4	—	—
40%-49%	—42	+2	—	—
50%-60%	—59	—5	—	—
Treated with levarterenol (Group B-7 dogs)				
30%-39%	—30	—28	—20	—26
40%-49%	—55	—37	—45	—31
50%-60%	—82	—50	—70	—38
Treated with 60% blood replacement (Group C-4 dogs)				
30%-39%	—56	—11	—45	—4
40%-49%	—81	—47	—19	—23
50%-60%	—77	—52	—41	—39
Treated with drug and blood replacement (Group D-7 dogs)				
30%-39%	—30	—50	—10	—31
40%-49%	—66	—65	—10	—27
50%-60%	—72	—73	—12	—23

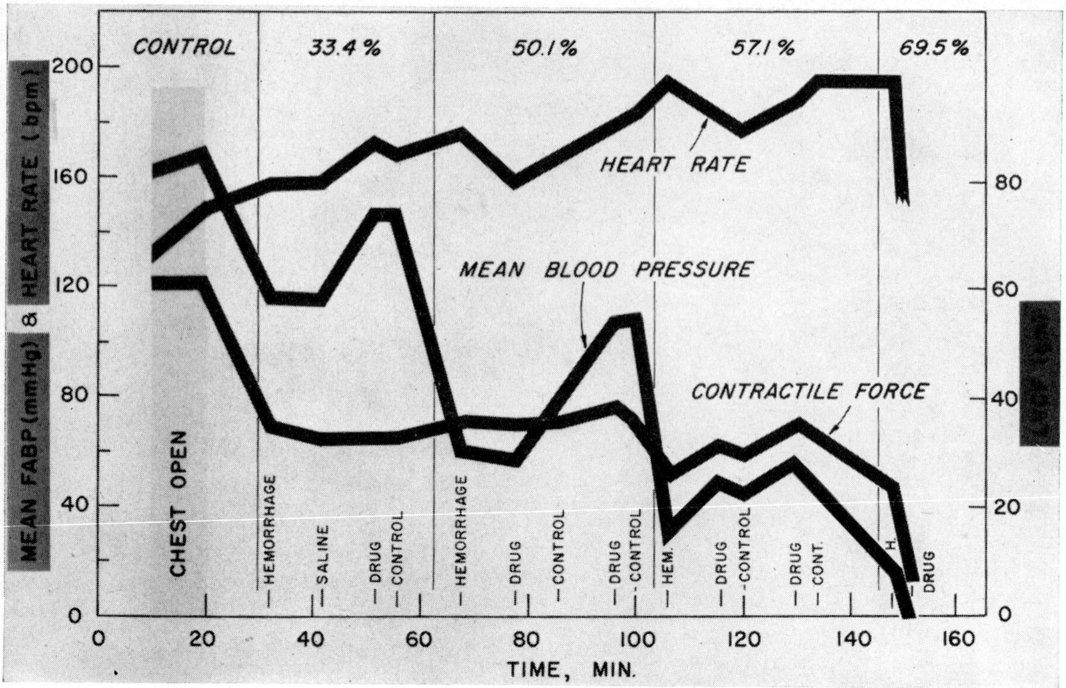

Fig 4.—Graph of an animal in which induced hemorrhagic shock was treated by levarterenol.

5 is a graph of a typical animal in the 60% blood replacement group and shows the lability of blood pressure in the earlier stages of hemorrhage and the relative stability of the contractile force in these same stages. At the 57% hemorrhage level severe decreases in contractile force are noted and rapid blood replacement no longer has any effect.

Group D—Treatment with both Levarterenol and 60% Blood Replacement.—A

Fig 5.—Graph of an animal in which induced hemorrhagic shock was treated with 60% blood replacement. Darkened vertical areas indicate time of blood replacement.

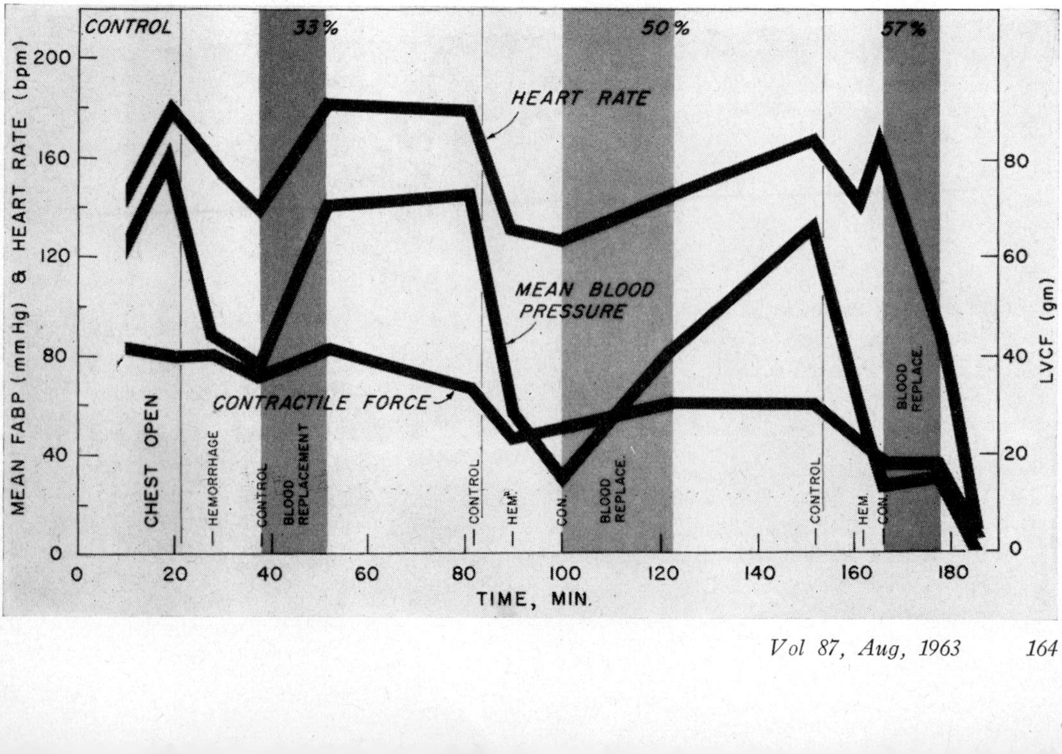

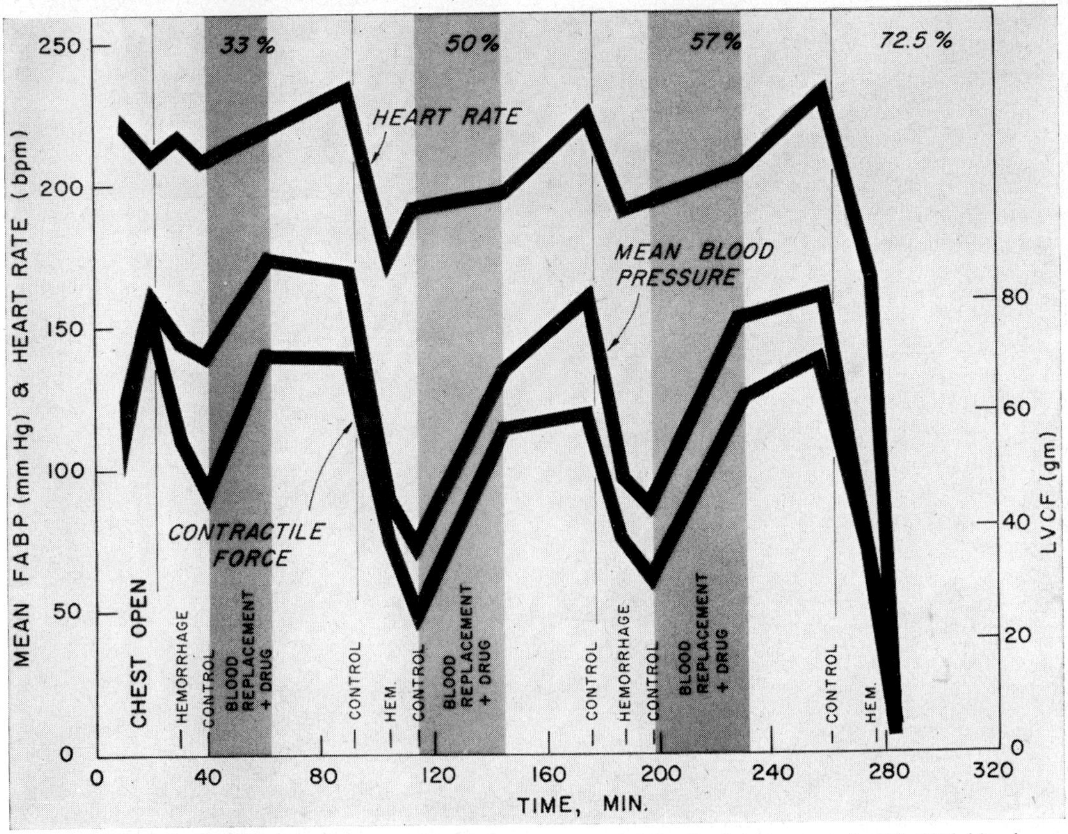

Fig 6.—Graph of an animal in which induced hemorrhagic shock was treated with 60% blood replacement combined with levarterenol.

combination of levarterenol and 60% blood replacement was used to treat the seven animals comprising this group. At this level of hemorrhage drug and blood were given, then followed by a control period for circulatory adjustment. The Table indicates that the contractile force shifted more toward control figures in this group than in either of the other two treated groups. At the first level of hemorrhage, a 19% average return occurred, with a 38% return at the second level and a 50% return at the third level. Fig 6 is a graph of a typical procedure in which both levarterenol and 60% blood replacement were used in treating hemorrhagic shock. More lability is noted in the contractile force, being almost as labile as the blood pressure. Both blood pressure and contractile force returned more nearly to the control level with each level of hemorrhage when treated with both drug and blood. When hemorrhage had progressed to the 72.5% level, irreversibility occurred with a sudden severe fall in contractile force and subsequent death despite rapid administration of both drug and blood.

Fig 7 is the graph of another animal treated with both blood and drug. In this instance after 50% of the estimated blood volume had been hemorrhaged almost no blood pressure was recorded for 20 minutes although the contractile force was still at almost 30 gm, or one half of control value. Before severe deterioration had occurred in contractile force, levarterenol was administered followed by 60% blood replacement. Both myocardial contractile force and blood pressure responded to this therapy, and the animal was allowed to survive. His postoperative convalescence was uneventful. In a number of similar experiments specific treatment was not given until after severe deterioration of the myocardial contractile force to one third or less of the control value, and

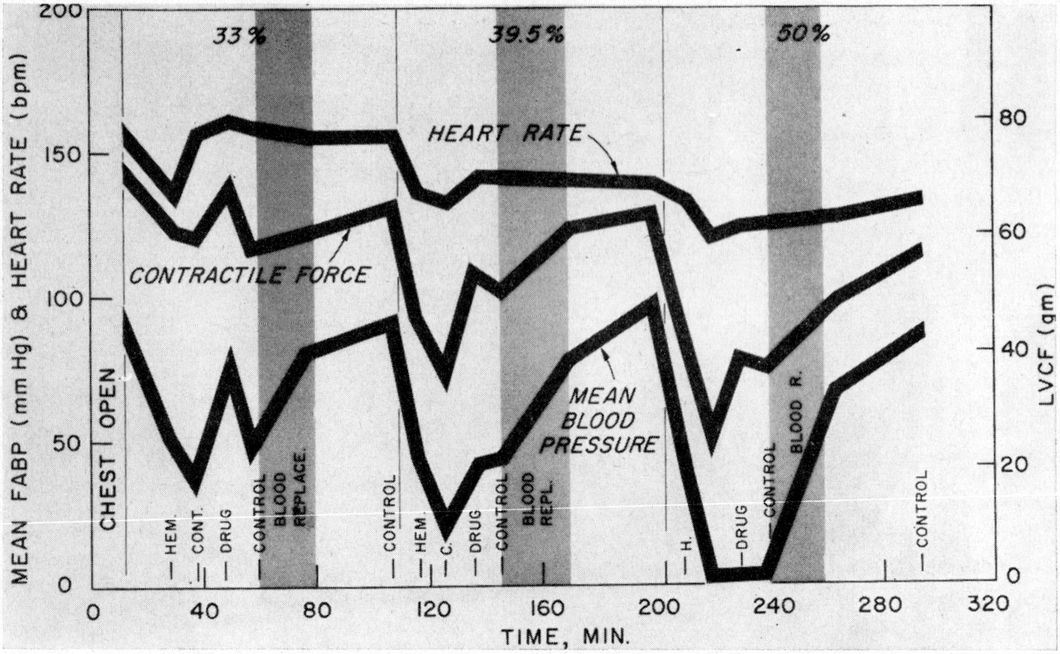

Fig 7.—Graph of an animal in which induced hemorrhagic shock was treated with 60% blood replacement and levarterenol. Treatment was given before irreversibility had occurred, and animal survived.

death occurred in each instance despite treatment.

Fig 8 presents a graphic analysis of the percentage of change from control levels in blood pressure and myocardial contractile force before and after treatment. Each graph illustrates a separate level of estimated depletion of the blood volume and is an average for all of the animals in a given therapy group. It is noteworthy that blood pressures responded best toward control readings at each level of hemorrhage after treatment with combined levarterenol and 60% blood replacement. A similar conclusion is reached concerning myocardial contractile force although the change is not as great. The remarkable response of myocardial contractile force to treatment with combined levarterenol and 60% blood replacement at the 50% to 60% hemorrhage level suggests the superiority of the combined treatment in this group of experiments.

Comment

Evidence continues to mount that the heart plays a leading role in the development of irreversible shock. Abnormalities in other organ systems of the body, however, may act as initiating factors in shock. Examples include burn shock, bacteremic shock, neurogenic shock, and traumatic shock. In these instances the heart probably enters the picture in the later phases. In hemorrhagic shock, however, evidence is accumulating that the heart becomes significantly affected early and may be the first part of the circulatory system to be damaged seriously. Wiggers and associates [2-4] have studied pressure and ventricular volume curves in the experimental animal and have demonstrated that both the force of contraction and the volume of blood ejected by the ventricles decrease as hemorrhagic shock progresses. They also noted an increase in right atrial pressure in late hemorrhagic shock if blood was reinfused.

Guyton and Crowell [5] have implicated the fatal role of the heart in hemorrhagic shock by conducting experiments in which they bled animals until the mean blood pressure was 30 mm of mercury and held them at that level by first withdrawing small amounts of

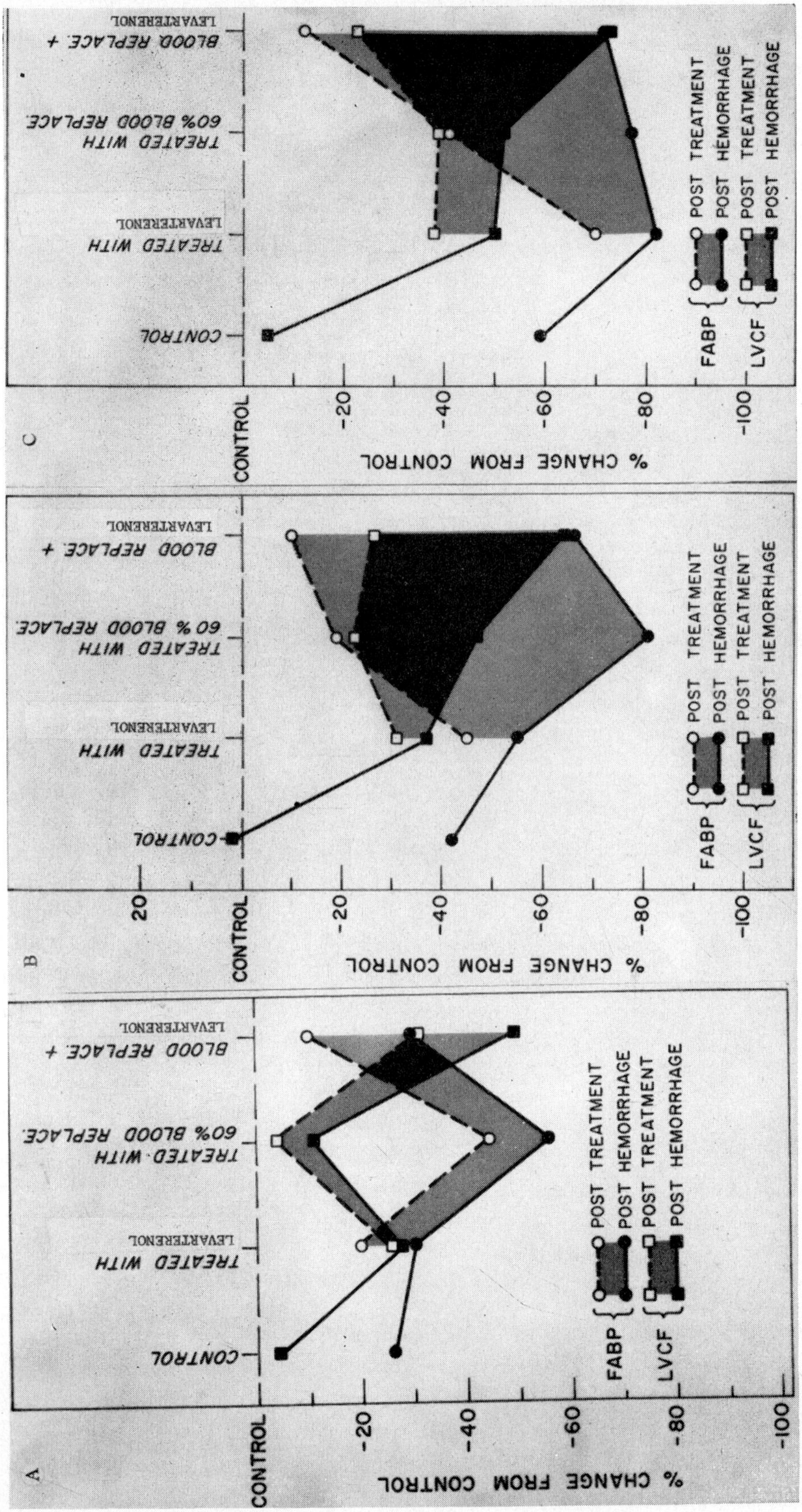

Fig 8.—Graphic analysis of the effect of the various treatments on femoral arterial blood pressure (FABP) and left ventricular contractile force (LVCF) at three different levels of hemorrhage: *A*, first level, 30%-39%; *B*, second level, 40%-49%; *C*, third level, 50%-60%. Dots represent an average of all animals in each treatment group.

blood and then gradually adding larger and larger amounts as the state of irreversibility was reached. In the terminal stages of these experiments large amounts of blood were infused, and the left atrial pressure rose steadily until it equalled the systemic pressure. They demonstrated that once the shock had become progressive, left atrial pressure rose while systemic pressure declined. In a normal heart, the systemic pressure would be expected to rise in the face of significant elevation of left atrial pressure. Guyton and Crowell also measured total peripheral resistance in animals in irreversible hemorrhagic shock and found it to be at a normal level. Thus venous congestion or pooling was not thought to be a cause of the animal's death, since much more blood was infused into the animal than could possibly have pooled in any area of the body. They concluded that the problem was not one of diminished venous return but rather the heart's inability to pump blood.

These same authors studied animals in hemorrhagic shock during the transition phase from reversible to irreversible shock. They were unable to pinpoint significant changes in cardiac output or oxygen consumption during the transition phase. The most significant change during this critical period was a gradual rise of the left atrial pressure. This rise continued until the animal died, suggesting that irreversible shock may be due to acute cardiac failure.

Opdyke and Foreman [6] recorded coronary artery flow in experimental hemorrhagic shock in the presence of hypotension. They found that during the hypotensive phase coronary artery flow diminished. In similar experiments Edwards, Siegel, and Bing [7] noted that coronary flow and myocardial oxygen consumption were below control levels during the normovolemic phase as well as during the oligemic phase of hemorrhagic shock, indicating that reinfusion of blood fails to correct the metabolic disturbance initiated during hemorrhage.

Michal [8] and co-workers, and Bing and Ramos [9] have stressed the importance of adequate oxygen supply to the myocardium. Since the heart muscle is primarily adapted to perform aerobically, a diminution in oxygen supply rapidly curtails normal myocardial working capacity. Significant changes noted in cardiac muscle metabolism occurring with anoxia included increased lactate and pyruvate production, increased glycogenolysis, rapid dephosphorylation of high-energy phosphate compounds with formation of inorganic phosphorus, and a decline of adenosine triphosphate. The summation of these profound metabolic changes is depressed myocardial function with resulting decreased cardiac output and stroke volume and further diminution of coronary flow and oxygen supply.

The observations made on myocardial contractile force reported here further implicate the heart as the organ responsible for irreversibility in hemorrhagic shock. The forceful contraction of the myocardium depends upon normal blood and oxygen supply as well as normal metabolism. Serious derangements in contractile force would be expected if proper nutrition of the heart muscle were not maintained, and this fact was demonstrated in our animals. The contractile force in the untreated or control animals changed little as compared to the blood pressure, and in all instances the blood pressure became severely depressed before serious depression occurred in the contractile force. In some instances in the control group a lag of 30 to 40 minutes occurred between severe hypotension and a definitive drop in contractile force. This undoubtedly signifies the period during which myocardial anoxia was present but had not yet seriously affected myocardial metabolism and function. When myocardial function became seriously impaired as evidenced by definitive decreases in myocardial contractile force, the death of the animal occurred soon thereafter. This same phenomenon of irreversibility after marked depression of contractile force was also noted in the treated groups. Once a severe drop in the contractile force had occurred, death could not be prevented by even large doses of either pressor amine, blood, or both combined. However, if treatment was initiated before a severe change had occurred in this parameter, the animal often could be salvaged.

Therapeutic methods for the management of severe hemorrhagic shock are suggested by the study of the myocardial contractile force. In this group of experiments, three different types of treatment were utilized as previously outlined. Levarterenol alone gave the least response of the three. Neither blood pressure nor cardiac contractile force showed significant recovery. These findings concur with those of Frank[10] and his associates who studied the effect of levarterenol on circulation of the dog in hemorrhagic shock and found that the fundamental defect leading to death was not corrected by this drug. Despite these findings they felt that pressor amine was beneficial until specific therapeutic measures could be instituted because of its ability to increase coronary, cerebral, and adrenal blood flow. The use of 60% blood replacement alone produced a satisfactory change in both blood pressure and cardiac contractile force toward control levels but would not prevent death once severe depression of the myocardial contractile force had occurred. The combination of 60% blood replacement and levarterenol gave the most consistently sustained changes toward control values of both parameters. For this reason the combination treatment seemed to be the most satisfactory. Partial replacement of blood volume associated with increased flow to coronary, cerebral, and adrenal vessels undoubtedly explains this advantage.

Germane to the discussion of these results in the experimental animal is the implication for the management of severe hemorrhagic shock in man. Although human organ systems and reflexes are more complex, many of the basic responses under conditions of hemorrhagic shock are similar to those of the experimental animal. Protection of myocardial function by early administration of pressor amine and blood replacement is suggested for the management of severe degrees of hemorrhagic shock in man.

Summary

The effect of severe hemorrhagic shock on myocardial contractile force has been studied in 21 experimental animals. Three types of therapy were used for the shock including levarterenol, 60% blood replacement, and a combination of these two. The following conclusions are suggested by these experiments:

1. Myocardial contractile force is a much more stable parameter than is the blood pressure in evaluating hemorrhagic shock.

2. When severe diminution occurs in myocardial contractile force secondary to hemorrhage, death of the animal is imminent, and treatment is ineffectual.

3. The combination treatment employing levarterenol and 60% blood replacement routinely gave the best response in myocardial contractile force and blood pressure at the more severe levels of hemorrhagic shock.

4. The important role of the heart in determining irreversibility in hemorrhagic shock is further substantiated.

Jack C. Cooley, MD, Section of Thoracic and Cardiovascuear Surgery, Carle Memorial Hospital, Urbana, Ill.

REFERENCES

1. Sjostrand, T.: in Handbook of Physiology, edited by W. F. Hamilton and P. Dow, Baltimore: The Williams & Wilkins Company, 1962, Sect 2. Circulation, vol 1, p 52.

2. Wiggers, C. J., and Werle, J. M.: Cardiac and Peripheral Resistance Factors as Determinants of Circulatory Failure in Hemorrhagic Shock, Amer J Physiol 136:421-432, 1942.

3. Wiggers, C. J., and Middleton, S.: Cardiac Output and Total Peripheral Resistance in Post-Hemorrhagic Hypotension and Shock, Amer J Physiol 140:677-687, 1944.

4. Wiggers, C. J.: Failure of Transfusions in Irreversible Hemorrhagic Shock: Study of Central Venous Pressures, Amer J Physiol 144:91-101, 1945.

5. Guyton, A. C., and Crowell, J. W.: Dynamics of the Heart in Shock, Fed Proc 20 (suppl 9):51-60, 1961.

6. Opdyke, D. F., and Foreman, R. C.: Study of Coronary Flow Under Conditions of Hemorrhagic Hypotension and Shock, Amer J Physiol 148:726-739, 1947.

7. Edwards, W. S.; Siegel, A.; and Bing, R. J.: Studies on Myocardial Metabolism: Coronary Blood Flow, Myocardial Oxygen Consumption, and Carbo-

hydrate Metabolism in Experimental Hemorrhagic Shock, J Clin Invest 33:1646-1661, 1954.

8. Michal, G.; Naegle, S.; Danforth, W. H.; Ballard, F. B.; and Bing, R. J.: Metabolic Changes in Heart Muscle During Anoxia, Amer J Physiol 197:1147-1151 1959.

9. Bing, R. J., and Ramos, H.: The Role of the Heart in Shock, JAMA 181:871-873 1962.

10. Frank, E. D.; Frank, H.; Jacob, S.; Weizel, H.; Korman, H.; and Fine, J.: Effect of Norepinephrine on Circulation of the Dog in Hemorrhagic Shock, Amer J Physiol 186:74-78, 1956.

Regional Blood Flow and Oxygen Consumption in Experimental Hemorrhagic Shock

GUSTAVO BOUNOUS, MD; LAWRENCE G. HAMPSON, MD; AND FRASER N. GURD, MD, MONTREAL

The fundamental element in the treatment of hemorrhagic shock is the correction of the deficit of blood volume before critical changes have occurred which render the shock irreversible. In the dog which has been subjected to severe hemorrhagic shock the reinfusion of shed blood almost invariably leads to a recovery of blood pressure and cardiac output. This recovery is short-lived in animals which have passed the point of reversibility, and it is a matter of the greatest difficulty to explain why one animal will go on to survive while another will die.

During the period of hypotension the perfusion of tissues and the consumption of oxygen are both greatly reduced. The degree of depression of oxygen consumption during shock has been shown by Guyton and Crowell to bear a relationship to recovery.[11] Immediately after reinfusion the oxygen consumption rises along with the blood pressure and cardiac output, but it has been shown in our laboratory that the degree of recovery of oxygen consumption is very closely related to the survival of the animal. In surviving animals the over-all oxygen consumption after reinfusion rises to above control or preshock levels, suggesting a capacity to resume normal aerobic metabolism and to restore the oxygen deficit. In animals which have reached the irreversible stage the total oxygen consumption does not recover to preshock levels.[22] These findings led us to question whether the failure to resume full preshock oxygen consumption which was observed in nonsurviving dogs was the result of an over-all tissue effect or was a limitation peculiar to one or more specific organs or systems. It occurred to us that, in view of the weight of evidence implicating the intestine and liver in the genesis of irreversible shock,[8,15,19] our studies should be extended to investigate blood flow and oxygen consumption in these organs throughout the course of hemorrhagic shock and reinfusion.

The circulation of blood to splanchnic organs during hemorrhagic shock has been studied extensively. However, the data obtained have been based as a rule upon the functional integrity of the organ being studied, the results being subject to errors when cellular function has been disturbed as a re-

Presented at the 20th Annual Meeting of the Central Surgical Association, Chicago, Feb 21-23, 1963.

Fellow of the Royal College of Surgeons of Canada and Fellow of the American College of Surgeons (Dr. Hampson, Dr. Gurd); Medical Research Council (Canada) Scholar (Dr. Bounous).

From the McGill University Surgical Clinic of the Montreal General Hospital.

Assisted by grants-in-aid from the Medical Research Council and the Defense Research Board of Canada.

sult of ischemia. On the other hand the data obtained using electromagnetic flow meters are difficult to evaluate. Some investigators have found a marked percentage reduction of mesenteric blood flow during shock,[1,13,10,16] some a significant redistribution of available blood flow in favour of abdominal viscera.[2] Others have shown no significant changes in the mesenteric circulation as compared with the systemic blood flow.[21,6,9,20] Recently, more direct attempts have been made by Selkurt [21] and others [17,3,12,23] to clarify not only the relationship between systemic and regional hemodynamics during a standard shock procedure but the more intricate problem of partition of oxygen utilization during shock.

The purpose of the present investigation was to study blood flow and oxygen consumption in a representative peripheral vascular bed (hind limb), in the mesenteric bed, and in the liver. Each area was to be analyzed as a fraction of total cardiac output and over-all oxygen consumption and in relation to survival and nonsurvival. Measurements were to be taken not only during the hypovolemic stage of shock but also after reinfusion of shed blood.

Materials and Methods

Dogs ranging in weight from 15 to 19 kg and anesthetized with pentobarbital sodium were used.

In group 1 blood flow and O_2 uptake of a limb were studied during hemorrhagic shock by the introduction of a large cannula into an external iliac vein through a small abdominal incision. The blood was drained per gravity into a graduated burette and returned to the animal by pump via the left jugular vein. Arterial and iliac venous blood samples were analyzed for O_2 content using the Van Slyke method.

In group 2 the mesenteric circulation alone was studied. The method entails division of the main extrahepatic portal vein with cannulation of each end of the vein with a 24 F plastic catheter (Pharmaseal). The portal flow is allowed to collect by gravity drainage into a graduated burette and is then returned into the proximal portal vein by a pump which is regulated so that the blood is returned at the same rate as it is being delivered from the distal portal vein. A pressure transducer is inserted in the pumping section of the extracorporeal apparatus. Mesenteric circulation is thus studied as if it were independent of the intrahepatic vascular

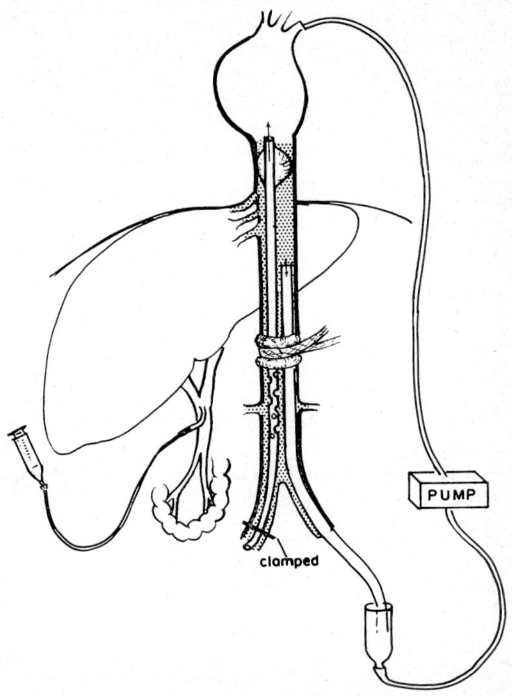

Fig 1.—Method used for measurement of hepatic venous outflow in the study of hepatic and gastrointestinal hemodynamics.

resistance. Arterial and portal venous blood samples were analyzed for O_2 content.

For experiments in Group 3, a new method was developed that allows direct measurement of both hepatic and gastrointestinal hemodynamics without interference with the integrity of the portal vein (Fig 1). The abdomen is entered through a midline incision extending about 10 cm below the xiphoid, and surgical manipulation can be accomplished without undue exposure of bowel or handling of the liver. A 24 F catheter is introduced through the left femoral vein and is passed into the inferior vena cava so that the end lies at the point of entry of the hepatic veins. Through this catheter hepatic venous outflow may drain freely into a burette and is then delivered by pump into the left jugular vein. In order to provide uninterrupted free drainage of blood from the infrahepatic vena cava, a second plastic catheter 18 F is introduced through the right femoral vein and passed into the vena cava so that its open end lies approximately 8 cm above the diaphragm. There are multiple holes in that part of this catheter lying caudad to the renal veins. A balloon is placed around the tip of the catheter for occlusion of the thoracic inferior vena cava above the hepatic veins. A heavy cloth tape is drawn taut over an encircling piece of compressed Ivalon sponge about the vena cava and the indwelling catheters; the tape is placed just above the renal veins and above the proximal level of the multiple holes described. With inflation of the balloon (8 cc of air) effective occlusion of the thoracic vena cava is accomplished without a thoractomy which would inevitably affect our O_2 studies, while the multiple holes guarantee the renal venous return without an outside shunt which would certainly affect the animal's temperature. By intermittent clamping of the hepatic artery the portal contribution to hepatic venous flow may be determined; for this purpose hepatic blood flow is measured after clamping of the hepatic artery for 30 seconds. A small polyethylene catheter is introduced into the portal vein through the pancreaticoduodenal vein for sampling of portal vein blood and measurement of portal blood pressure. In addition arterial, portal vein, and hepatic vein blood samples were taken during various stages of the experiments and analyzed for O_2 content; this, combined with flow measurements, furnished information concerning O_2 utilization of the intestine and the liver during shock.

The following procedures were common to all groups of experiments. The burette was kept approximately 10 cm below the level of the vena cava in order to ensure free drainage without collapse of the vena cava and tributary veins. The burette and the extracorporeal tubing were primed with fresh heparinized blood from a donor dog prior to each experiment. By stopping the pump and recording the time interval required for the accumulation of a given volume of blood in the burette, blood flows could be calculated. All animals were heparinized by the I.V. administration of 1 mg of heparin per kilogram just prior to the introduction of the venous cannulas.

The burette, during these experiments, was kept in warm water (40 C) to prevent cooling of the dog. Previous experience has shown that such water temperature is sufficient to prevent cooling in a normal dog during extracorporeal circulation. Hemorrhagic shock in itself caused a gradual temperature drop from an average control of 38 C to 34-35 C in most animals. No attempt was made to interfere with the hypothermic effect of hemorrhagic shock by increasing the temperature of the water bath.

The standardized shock procedure employed involved bleeding into an elevated reservoir bottle through a plastic catheter introduced into the femoral artery, until a level of 30-35 mm Hg arterial pressure was attained. This pressure was maintained for 30 minutes, the level of the bottle then being raised sufficiently to elevate systemic blood pressure to about 60 mm Hg for a further 30-minute period. The catheter to the reservoir was then clamped, and the animal's homeostatic mechanisms were not interfered with for another hour, during which time blood pressure tended to fall gradually. The reservoir blood was then rewarmed and retransfused during an interval of about ten minutes. Blood samples for measurement of O_2 content were usually drawn at the end of the 15-minute control period, during the 60 mm Hg period, at the end of the hour in which the catheter connecting the animal with the bottle had been clamped, and 15-20 minutes after retransfusion of blood. We were particularly concerned with drawing samples when a stable organ blood flow was observed; the relative stability of the organ blood flow, rather than a precise time, was the essential factor in determining the moment at which to draw blood samples. At least three flow determinations were made immediately before and after the sampling of blood.

In each dog a continuous measurement of total body O_2 consumption was made possible by a recording spirometer, and cardiac output was determined by the Fick principle, utilizing blood samples from the right ventricle and the aorta drawn simultaneously with the organ venous blood.

Results

The data relating to group 1 are reported in Table 1. The blood flow of the limb is on the average 4.9 cc/kg/min, or 3.5% of car-

TABLE 1.—*Group 1, Systemic and Hind*

	Regional							
	Control		60 MM/HG		Clamped		Transfused	
No. of Dog	Ext. Iliac Blood Flow	O_2 Consumption of Limb	Ext. Iliac Blood Flow	O_2 Consumption of Limb	Ext. Iliac Blood Flow	O_2 Consumption of Limb	Ext. Iliac Blood Flow	O_2 Consumption of Limb
1833	4.5	0.315	1.8	0.170	2.1	0.130	8.3	0.318
1729	3.1	0.178	1.25	0.169	1.25	0.155	6.6	0.180
1810	5.35	0.218	0.71	0.105	0.71	0.100	4.6	0.241
1865	8	0.380	1.2	0.158	1	0.121	6.2	0.372
1800	3.8	0.207	0.37	0.065	0.73	0.102	3.8	0.153
1896	4.8	0.260	0.95	0.142	1	0.159	5.3	0.201
Mean	4.9	0.259	1.0	0.134	1.1	0.127	6	0.244

* All measurements given in cubic centimeters per kilogram per minute.

diac output; O_2 consumption is 0.259 cc/kg/min, or 4.8% of the total O_2 consumption. During the hypovolemic stage the iliac blood flow decreases to 20% and 22% of control while cardiac output falls to 22% and 25% of control. The difference is minimal. After retransfusion of blood, iliac blood flow returns to 122% of control while cardiac output is 103%. The O_2 consumption of the limb during shock falls to 51% and 49%, the total O_2 consumption somewhat less (59% and 65% of control). After transfusion the O_2 consumption of the limb rises to 94%, while the total body consumption is 89% of control.

Mesenteric blood flows and O_2 studies in group 2 animals are shown in Table 2 in conjunction with systemic studies. The term "mesenteric" seems to us more appropriate in this particular instance, as the hemodynamic pattern of the portal system was here studied as it is determined solely by the mesenteric vascular resistance without the effect of the hepatic resistance. The control determinations show an average mesenteric blood flow of 17.9 cc/kg/min, or 13.2% of the cardiac output (135 cc/kg/min). The control gastrointestinal O_2 consumption is, on the average, 0.658 cc/kg/min, or 11% of the total O_2 consumption (6.1 cc/kg/min). After one hour of shock mesenteric blood flow falls to 36% of control while cardiac output falls to 28%; one hour later the corresponding values are 29% and 23%. The difference between the two means is below the margin of statistical significance. After transfusion mesenteric blood flow returns well above control, 153% of control, and has risen percentage-wise more than cardiac output (136%). During the hypovolemic period gastrointestinal and total O_2 consumption fell to 71% and 72%, and 65% and 61% of control, respectively. Here again, as for the blood flow, the mesenteric values are somewhat above the corresponding systemic value by approximately the same amount. The striking difference between regional and systemic values is shown after retransfusion of blood. The pattern here is reversed; gastrointestinal O_2 consumption is still only 72% of control, as it was during the terminal stage of shock, while total O_2 consumption has returned near control (92%). The pattern for O_2 consumption is therefore, at this stage, entirely the opposite of the blood flow relationship between the two areas. The significance of this particular feature in determining irreversibility will be further illustrated in group 3 in which this phenomenon is even more accentuated since the three survivors have been subtracted from the average. In group 3 the same parameters were measured with the different method allowing a normal portal circulation. Eight nonsurviving dogs were studied. The data are recorded in Table 3. The mean control figures compare nicely with group 1; mean portal blood flow 21.7 cc/kg/min and O_2 consumption 0.730 cc/kg/min. The percentage fall of portal blood flow during hypo-

Limb Blood Flow and O_2 Consumption *

Systemic							
Control		60 MM/HG		Clamped		Transfused	
Cardiac Output	Total O_2 Consumption	Cardiac Output	Total O_2 Consumption	Cardiac Output	Total O_2 Consumption	Cardiac Output	Total O_2 Consumption
197	5.13	45.5	30.6	43.6	2.9	81	3.7
120	6	42.5	4.5	50	5.25	275	5.7
107	4.76	14.8	1.9	17.7	2	70	3.5
290	11	60	6.1	63	6.5	319	9.3
150	4	19	2.9	25	3.05	152	4.6
123	6.5	44	3.8	54	4.7	123	6.3
141	5.34	32.3	3.18	36.2	3.5	146	4.7

173 *Bounous et al*

volemia is almost the same as that of cardiac output 25%, 21% and 24%, 25%, respectively. The blood flow ratio between the two areas observed in group 2 after retransfusion is again manifest in this group; although the total amount of increase is less, portal blood flow rises to 124% of control while cardiac output is 99% of control. Control total body O_2 consumption in this group is on the average 5.1 cc/kg/min (Table 4). Gastrointestinal O_2 consumption falls to 72% of control in the first hour; this figure is precisely the same as in group 2. Total O_2 consumption at the same time has fallen to 65% of control. In the second hour the two values are 56% and 60% of control, respectively. After retransfusion the gastrointestinal O_2 consumption continues to fall (40% of control), despite the marked increase in blood flow, while total O_2 consumption returns to 96% of the control level.

In Table 3 are reported the individual data in group 3 in which both hepatic and gastrointestinal circulations were studied in eight nonsurviving dogs. The control liver blood is on the average 31.2 cc/kg/min, or 29.2% of cardiac output, and hepatic O_2 consumption is 0.881 cc/kg/min, or 17.2% of the total O_2 consumption. From these values hepatic flow falls during shock to 25% and 20%, returning to 105% of control after transfusion; at the same time cardiac output falls to 24%, 25% and then returns to 99% of control. Hepatic circulation shows a pattern very similar to the systemic circulation during all stages of shock. The hepatic oxygen consumption, however, is more markedly reduced during the hypovolemic stage of shock (48%, 43% of control—total 64%, 60%) but returns above control following retransfusion (112%).

In Tables 5 and 6 are reported the data on the three dogs in group 3 which survived the shocking procedure. In these animals the control values were similar to the remainder of group 3. Hepatic blood flows fell with hypotension to 30% and 26% of controls, while cardiac output decreased to 23% and 18%; portal flow fell to 29% and 26% of control. The hepatic O_2 consumption did not differ significantly from the surviving dogs of group 3 during the hypovolemic stage of shock (46% and 49% of control). The striking difference between survivors and nonsurvivors is observed in the O_2 utilization of the gastrointestinal tract. In the surviving group this value fell to 77% of control at the end of the first hour but rose to 97% before transfusion, returning to 103% of control after retransfusion of blood. Those animals failing to survive showed a falling gastrointestinal O_2 consumption despite adequate return of mesenteric blood flow following blood replacement.

Comment

The data reported in the literature concerning measurements of hepatic and portal blood flow and O_2 consumption are at variance.

TABLE 2.—*Group 2, Systemic and Gastrointestinal Blood*

	Regional							
	Control		60 MM/HG		Clamped		Transfused	
No. of Dog	Portal Blood Flow	Gastrointestinal O_2 Consumption	Portal Blood Flow	Gastrointestinal O_2 Consumption	Portal Blood Flow	Gastrointestinal O_2 Consumption	Portal Blood Flow	Gastrointestinal O_2 Consumption
1904	19.6	0.441	9.25	0.210	7	0.350	31.3	0.284
1899	20	0.660	9.9	0.520	5		32.3	0.388
1914	18.3	0.683	6.7	0.620	5.3	0.507	25	0.442
1743	12	0.570	3.7	0.400	4.4		25	0.487
1776	13	0.710	5.2	0.360	4.7	0.420	16.6	0.540
1795	21	0.700	4.1	0.450	3.3	0.450	27	0.758
1940	21.3	0.841	7.2	0.745	6.3	0.655	35	0.420
Mean	17.9	0.658	6.58	0.472	5.2	0.476	27.5	0.474

* All measurements given in cubic centimeters per kilogram per minute.

The problems and difficulties related to the production of a reliable and standardized shock preparation are well known; individual variations in response to hemorrhage still represent the predominant source of error in computing results and averages. The efforts to determine more accurately the anatomical sites and physiological mechanisms concerned in the irreversibility of shock have created a second major problem for investigators. It is our opinion, as will be later shown, that particularly in the splanchnic area great effort and special care must be directed toward obtaining reliable control determinations. We shall, therefore, briefly review some of the principal reports found in the literature with regard to blood flow and O_2 data in the splanchnic area.

Blalock,[4] using a direct method, observed an average hepatic blood flow of 27 cc/kg/min; Hinshaw [13] obtained an average control hepatic blood flow of 13 cc/kg/min, while Ballinger,[3] using an indicator-dilution technique, obtained an average hepatic flow of 56 cc/kg/min; Werner [23] reported the hepatic flow to represent 32% of cardiac output, while Bradley [6] showed it to be 20%. In our observations the mean hepatic blood flow was 31.2 cc/kg/min, or 29.2% of the cardiac output, in one group and 31.2 cc/kg/min, or 30% of the cardiac output, in the other. Using a direct method, Selkurt observed portal blood flow to average 19 cc/kg/min; our portal flow measurements averaged 17.9 cc/kg/min in one group and 21.7 cc/kg/min in the other. Hinshaw,[13] using a flowmeter, observed the femoral blood flow to average 5 cc/kg/min; our average for the external iliac is 4.9 cc/kg/min.

The average arterial O_2 content was 15% in Ballinger's report,[3] 16% in Blalock's [4]; our arterial O_2 averages per group are 17.64%, 15.64%, 15.7%, 17.04%. Ballinger obtained a portal vein O_2 average of 12.6% with an arterioportal gradient of 3.3 cc%; our portal O_2 averaged 12.2% and 11.95%, with arterioportal gradient of 3.50 in one group and 3.43 in the other. The similarity of these figures is important to us, as Ballinger measured blood flow with an indirect method with little or no trauma in the preparation and yet the control O_2 data for the portal blood showed little difference from our data. The portal vein-hepatic vein gradient was 1.4 in the controls of Ballinger and 1.7 in ours.

Splanchnic O_2 consumption was calculated by Blalock [4] at 1.48 cc/kg/min of O_2, and by Selkurt [21] at 2.01 cc/kg/min; our corresponding figures are on the average 1.611 cc/kg/min in one group and 1.738 cc/kg/min in the other.

Differential Organ Flows.—Selkurt [21] observed that the hepatic artery normally contributes 36% of the hepatic blood flow and 70% of the liver oxygenation. Blalock [4] noted that the portal blood flow represents 80% of the total hepatic circulation. In our experiments it was found that the hepatic artery contributes 30% of liver flow and 58% of liver O_2 consumption, while the reverse figures are true for the portal vein.

Flow and O_2 Consumption: Divided Portal Vein *

Systemic							
Control		60 MM/HG		Clamped		Transfused	
Cardiac Output	Total O_2 Consumption	Cardiac Output	Total O_2 Consumption	Cardiac Output	Total O_2 Consumption	Cardiac Output	Total O_2 Consumption
165	7.3	56	4.16	58	3.9	130	5.3
194	6.7	51.5	3.6		2.57	265	5.5
100	6.2	43	4.8	36	4.5	151	5.1
65	5	30	3.25			245	5.5
106	5	20	3.8	21	3.8	93	4.9
204	5.9	28.7	3.7	23.6	3.4	200	5.4
110	6.6	35	4.6	40	4.8	204	7.26
135	6.1	37.8	4.0	32.3	3.73	184	5.57

175 Bounous et al

TABLE 3.—*Group 3, Splanchnic Blood Flow and O_2 Consumption (Nonsurvivors)* *

		Control		60 MM HG		Clamped		Transfused	
No. of Dog	Organ	Blood Flow	O_2 Consumption	Blood Flow	O_2 Consumption	Blood Flow	O_2 Consumption	Blood Flow	O_2 Consumption
2156	Liver								
	Hepatic	13	0.637	3.3	0.550	1.6	0.270	8.7	0.270
	Portal	21	0.318	3.4	0.065	2.9	0.056	25.3	0.652
	Total	34	0.955	6.7	0.615	4.5	0.326	34	0.920
	Gastrointestinal	21	0.720	3.4	0.444	2 9	0.430	25.3	0.116
	Splanchnic	34	1.675	6.7	1.059	4.5	0.756	34	1.036
2139	Liver								
	Hepatic	10.1	0.404	1	0.150	1	0.122	5	0.220
	Portal	21	0.287	2.4	0.094	2.2	0.124	18	0.385
	Total	31.1	0.691	3.4	0.240	3.2	0.246	23	0.605
	Gastrointestinal	21	0.563	2.4	0.260	2.2	0.146	18	0.407
	Splanchnic	31.1	1.253	3.4	0.500	3.2	0.392	23	1.012
2078	Liver								
	Hepatic	10	0.510	4.5	0.457	2.1	0.248	3.5	0.132
	Portal	30	0.367	8	0.129	6.8	0.273	44.5	1.520
	Total	40	0.877	12.5	0.586	8.9	0.521	48	1.652
	Gastrointestinal	30	1.200	8	0.681	6.8	0.501	44.5	0.200
	Splanchnic	40	2.077	12.5	1.267	8.9	1.022	48	1.852
2074	Liver								
	Hepatic	8.5	0.479	1.3	0.170	1.8	0.120	2.3	0.075
	Portal	20	0.258	5.5	0.141	4.7	0.122	26.2	0.530
	Total	28.5	0.737	6.8	0.311	6.5	0.242	28.5	0.605
	Gastrointestinal	20	0.807	5.5	0.578	4.7	0.190	26.2	0.336
	Splanchnic	28.5	1.544	6.8	0.889	6.5	0.432	28.5	0.941
2036	Liver								
	Hepatic	10.6	0.598	0.8	0.067				
	Portal	16	0.254	3.2	0.052	2.0	0.02		
	Total	26.6	0.852	4.0	0.119	2.0	0.02		
	Gastrointestinal	16	0.700	3.2	0.232	2.0	0.216		
	Splanchnic	26.6	1.552	4	0.351	2	0.236		
2171	Liver								
	Hepatic	8.6	0.446	3.9	0.420	3	0.380	8.4	0.320
	Portal	18.4	0.190	6.3	0.060	5	0.040	19.6	0.484
	Total	27	0.636	10.2	0.480	8	0.420	28	0.804
	Gastrointestinal	18.4	0.726	6.3	0.630	5	0.600	19.6	0.268
	Splanchnic	27	1.362	10.2	1.110	8	1.020	28	1.072
2196	Liver								
	Hepatic	8.5	0.550	1.4	0.215	1.6	0.220	8	0.380
	Portal	25.5	0.930	5.6	0.100	7.2	0.361	32	1.088
	Total	34	1.480	7	0.315	8.8	0.581	40	1.468
	Gastrointestinal	25.5	0.620	5.6	0.680	7.2	0.560	32	0.432
	Splanchnic	34	2.100	7	0.995	8.8	1.141	32	1.900
2233	Liver								
	Hepatic	7	0.420	2.7	0.320	2.2	0.271	5	0.200
	Portal	22	0.400	9.4	0.400	6	0.207	24	0.662
	Total	29	0.820	12.1	0.720	8.2	0.478	29	0.862
	Gastrointestinal	22	0.510	9.4	0.656	6	0.480	24	0.300
	Splanchnic	29	1.330	12.1	1.370	8.2	0.958	29	1.162
Mean	Liver								
	Hepatic	9.5	0.506	2.4	0.293	1.9	0.233	5.8	0.228
	Portal	21.7	0.375	5.5	0.130	4.6	0.148	27	0.760
	Total	31.2	0.881	7.9	0.423	6.5	0.381	32.8	0.988
	Gastrointestinal	21.7	0.730	5.5	0.520	4.6	0.415	27	0.295
	Splanchnic	31.2	1.611	7.9	0.943	6.5	0.796	32.8	1.283

* All measurements given in cubic centimeters per kilogram per minute.

It is interesting to note that this ratio is maintained during the hypovolemic stage of shock.

Fig 2 illustrates the findings during shock expressed as percentage changes from control. It is apparent from our figures that blood flow in the organ studied falls by almost the same amount as does the cardiac output. Our observations tend to support the concept that during hypovolemic shock there is no particular adjustment of vascular resistance in the areas studied. From the

TABLE 4.—*Group 3, Cardiac Output and Total O_2 Consumption (Nonsurvivors)**

No. of Dog	Control		60 MM HG		Clamped		Transfused	
	Cardiac Output	O_2 Consumption	Cardiac Output	O_2 Consumption	Cardiac Output	O_2 Consumption	Cardiac Output	O_2 Consumption
2156	110	4.9	19	3.2	20	3.2	108	4.2
2139	135	5.2	16	1.9	15.6	1.9	95	3.8
2078	135	6.2	47	5.4	48	5.5	137	6.1
2074	100	5.3	23	3.8	39	3.5	83	5.3
2036	70	3.8	22	2.2	12	1.2		
2171	90	5.4	26	3.5	21	3.5	123	5.2
2196	100	5	21	2.9	26	3.4	95	5.1
2233	115	5	40	3.6	37	3.5	100	4.4
Mean	107	5.1	26.7	3.3	27.3	3.1	106	4.9

* All measurements given in cubic centimeters per kilogram per minute.

data collected it would definitely appear that the local hemodynamics are adjusted to shock in a way that is comparable to the average changes in the whole body. The constancy of blood flow pattern is also observed in the hepatic artery-portal blood flow ratio within the liver which is maintained through the hypovolemic stage of shock, as shown in Fig 3. In the survivors of group 3 the hepatic and portal blood flows appear to be slightly increased (7%-8%) in relation to the cardiac output; the significance of these data is questionable because of the small number of observations and the minimal difference. After retransfusion of blood the portal blood flow is constantly above control and rises to a greater degree than the cardiac output.

Hepatic Resistance.—It has been suggested [7,9] that the muscular coat of the hepatic veins in dogs can contract, producing a sphincter-like mechanism which impedes portal flow. This feature has been assumed to be characteristic of the dog, making data on splanchnic hemodynamics in dogs diffi-

TABLE 5.—*Group 3, Splanchnic Blood Flow and O_2 Consumption (Survivors)**

No. of Dog	Organ	Control		60 MM HG		Clamped		Transfused	
		Blood Flow	O_2 Consumption	Blood Flow	O_2 Consumption	Blood Flow	O_2 Consumption	Blood Flow	O_2 Consumption
2053	Liver								
	Hepatic	3.2	0.210	2.4	0.213	1.8	0.251	1.5	0.079
	Portal	22	0.945	9.8	0.135	8.4	0.148	27.5	0.825
	Total	25.2	1.155	12.2	0.348	10.2	0.399	29	0.904
	GI								
	Splanchnic	22	0.740	9.8	0.750	8.4	1.034	27.5	0.728
		25.2	1.895	12.2	1.098	10.2	1.199	29	1.633
1111	Liver								
	Hepatic	9	0.450	3.4	0.470	3.6	0.610	3.5	0.120
	Portal	24.5	0.250	6.6	0.360	6.4	0.320	43	0.635
	Total	33.5	0.700	10.0	0.830	10.0	0.930	46.5	0.750
	GI	24	0.940	6.6	0.630	6.4	0.772	43	0.860
	Splanchnic	33.5	1.640	10.0	1.460	10	1.645	46.5	1.640
2211	Liver								
	Hepatic	12.5	0.600	2.4	0.215	1.2	0.156	6.5	0.180
	Portal	22.5	0.540	4.1	0.011	3.2	0.04	34	0.232
	Total	35	1.115	6.5	0.216	4.4	0.160	40.5	0.412
	GI	22.5	0.570	4.1	0.345	3.2	0.370	34	0.715
	Splanchnic	34.0	1.655		0.661	4.4	0.530	40.5	1.127
Mean	Liver								
	Hepatic	8.2	0.420	2.7	0.299	2.2	0.339	3.8	1.125
	Portal	23	0.578	6.8	0.165	6	0.157	34.8	0.564
	Total	31.2	0.998	9.5	0.464	8.2	0.496	38.6	0.689
	GI	23	0.740	6.8	0.575	6	0.728	34.8	0.768
	Splanchnic	31.2	1.738	9.5	1.039	8.2	1.221	38.6	1.457

* All measurements given in cubic centimeters per kilogram per minute.

TABLE 6.—*Group 3 Cardiac Output and Total O_2 Consumption (Survivors)* *

No. of Dog	Control		60 MM HG		Clamped		Transfused	
	Cardiac Output	O_2 Consumption	Cardiac Output	O_2 Consumption	Cardiac Output	O_2 Consumption	Cardiac Output	O_2 Consumption
2035	98	3.9	32	2.5			65	4.3
1111	100	5	23.5	3.4	20.3	3.4	157	5.3
2211	128	5.3	23	2.6	21	3.2	210	5.6
Mean	109	4.7	26.1	2.8	20.6	3.3	144	5

* All measurements given in cubic centimeters per kilogram per minute.

cult to assess in terms of the relationship to human physiology. After retransfusion of blood, portal pressure rises to twice control values. In our observation, as in Selkurt's, this value rises from 10 mm Hg control, and 8.8 mm Hg during hypovolemia, to 20 mm Hg after blood has been retransfused. It has been assumed that this rise was characteristic of the dog because of its particular hepatic sphincter-like mechanism opposing portal flow and causing intestinal pooling of blood by a back pressure effect.

We have demonstrated that the observed increase in portal pressure does not appear to interfere with mesenteric circulation. In group 2 the hepatic resistance is bypassed, while in group 3 the portal blood flows as usual against the hepatic resistance. The average portal and cardiac output post-transfusion values in percentage of control are, respectively, 153%, 136% (difference 17%) for group 2; 124%, 96% (difference 28%) for group 3 nonsurvivors; 151%, 132% (difference 19%) for group 3 survivors. Incidentally we might stress the necessity for simultaneous measurement of cardiac output; should this determination have been omitted, and the post-transfusion increment of portal flow be compared with control portal flow rather than with simultaneous cardiac output, the calculation would have shown only a 124% increase in group 3 nonsurvivors, significantly less than the 153% figure observed in group 2. Our observations would lead us to agree with Zanetti [24] that portal hypertension per se does not play a causative role in irreversible shock. Johnson [14] concluded from intestinal

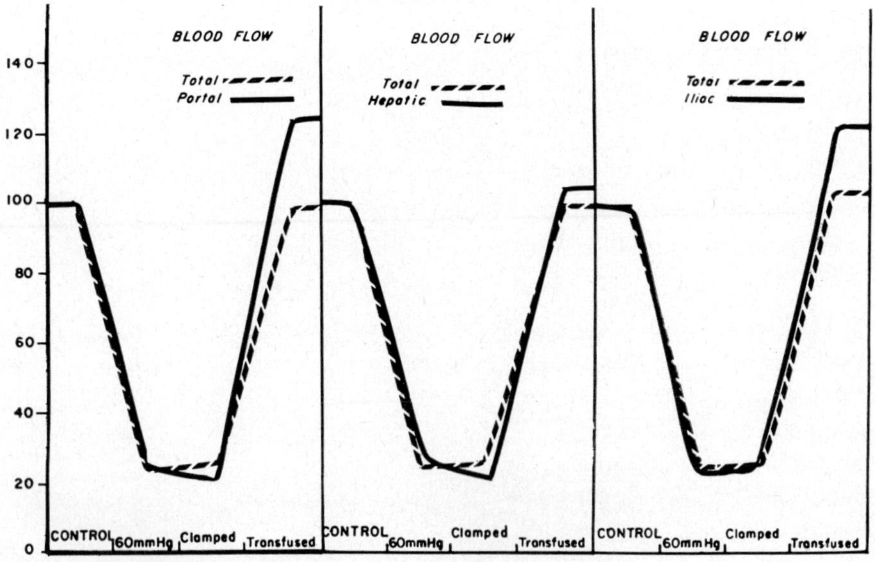

Fig 2.—Response of local blood flow to hemorrhagic shock: patterns of portal, hepatic, and iliac blood flows shown as percentages of control values. Simultaneous measurements of cardiac output are expressed as total blood flow.

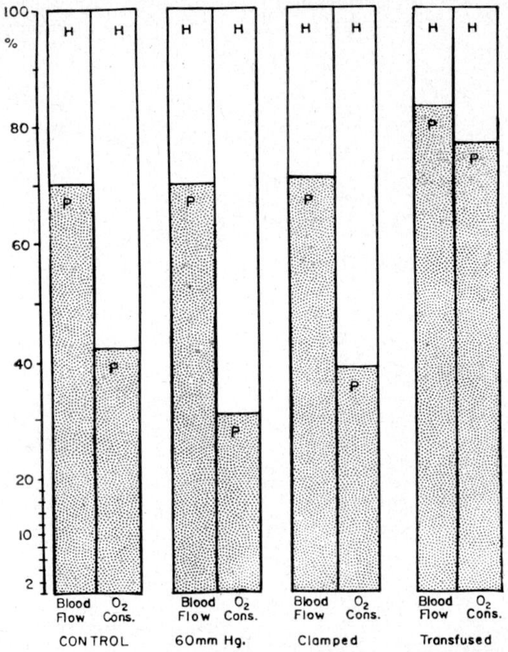

Fig 3.—Relative contributions (%) of hepatic artery (*H*) and portal vein (*P*) to total liver blood flow and oxygenation in the course of hemorrhagic shock and retransfusion.

weight measurements that intravascular pooling of blood in the intestine is not a necessary feature of hemorrhagic shock. Following transfusion we observed, as did Selkurt, a large increase in portal flow which accounts at this stage for 77% of the total hepatic circulation. At this phase of normovolemic shock most of the hepatic flow and oxygenation is contributed by the portal system (Fig 3).

Mesenteric Oxygen Consumption.—We have divided our hypovolemic period into two phases of hypotension, one controlled, the other uncontrolled. Initially the situation is presumably reversible but it gradually deteriorates to an irreversible state. If studies were continued only during hypovolemia the difference between survivors and nonsurvivors would be trivial, blood flow and O_2 consumption being reduced in both cases by approximately the same amount as the cardiac output and total O_2 consumption. Organ O_2 consumption shows a more differential and characteristic pattern in our studies; it is certainly a study of this parameter that allows us to comment as to the anatomical site and characteristics of irreversibility. We have sufficient evidence to show that the feature that most distinctly differentiates reversibility from irreversibility in shock is manifest following retransfusion of blood; it is neither blood flow nor blood pressure, but the O_2 consumption of the gastrointestinal tract. We have found constantly at this stage mesenteric blood flows well above control values, as are the cardiac output and the hepatic and the iliac blood flows. However, in irreversibly shocked animals, the difference in O_2 content between aortic and portal blood is so small (1.18 vol%) that the calculated O_2 consumption of the gastrointestinal tract is on the average less than half the control value. At this time the oxygen consumptions of the other organs studied are either at or above control values. In the three dogs that survived, however, intestinal O_2 consumption had returned to control values.

We feel that there can be two reasons why blood flows but O_2 is not extracted: either the capillary circuit is bypassed, or the tissue cells have become unable to carry out oxidative metabolism.

In group 2 this phenomenon is also evident though to a lesser degree. In these animals no attempt was made to check survival after shock, while in group 3 the three survivors were subtracted from the average making even more striking this characteristic feature of irreversible shock. In the terminal stage of shock the difference between survivors and nonsurvivors is striking in the gastrointestinal tract O_2 uptake. Group 2 containing both survivors and nonsurvivors shows no appreciable change, but the nonsurvivors of the third group show a significant fall from the value observed in the first stage of shock. In dogs that survived, however, gastrointestinal O_2 consumption has already returned near control values in the terminal stage of shock and continues to rise after transfusion (Fig 4).

It is our hypothesis that the reason for this significant difference in O_2 consumption between intestine, on the one hand, and liver and leg, on the other hand, is already present

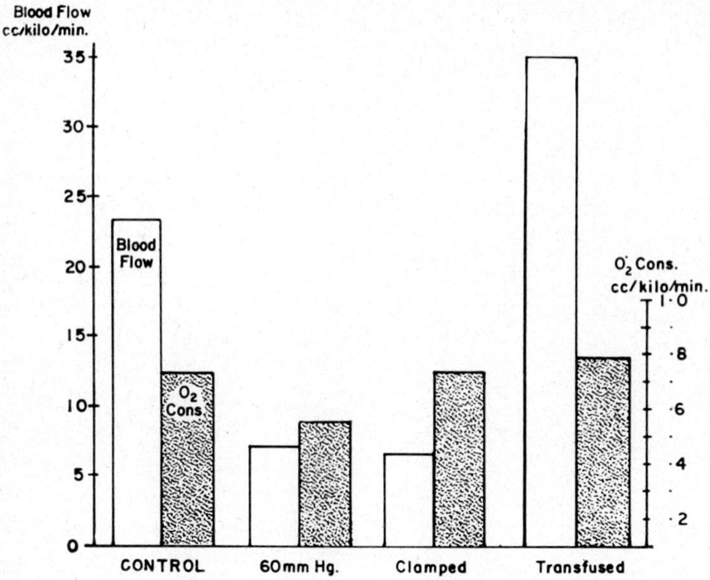

Fig 4.—Relation of mesenteric blood flow to O_2 consumption during hemorrhagic shock and following retransfusion in group 3 surviving animals. Adequate recovery of oxygen consumption is shown.

in the terminal stage of hypovolemic shock. At this stage, however, the blood flow in all areas is so greatly reduced, and the O_2 uptake of the organs consequently so small, that the changes in capacity for O_2 utilization that may have occurred as a consequence of direct ischemic or toxic damage cannot be seen. When the tissue cells are forced to a low level of metabolic activity by reduced cardiac output, as in the hypovolemic phase of shock, their different potentiality cannot be appreciated; however, when, after transfusion, blood flow is greatly increased in every organ, the basic difference between intestine and liver is manifest. The reason why intestinal O_2 consumption is resumed in some dogs while in others it progressively declines can be only a matter of speculation. In the former group mesenteric circulation did not fall below a critical level that we might estimate at around 6 cc/kg/min (or one third of control) for a period of about one hour. The intestinal O_2 consumption values of the post-transfusion phase in dogs

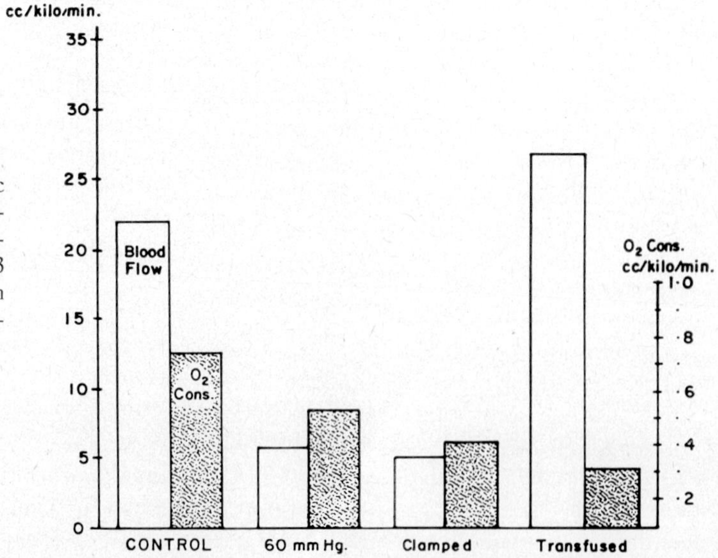

Fig 5.—Relation of mesenteric blood flow to O_2 consumption during hemorrhagic shock and following retransfusion in group 3 nonsurviving animals. Failure in adequate recovery of oxygen consumption is shown.

that died are, in our opinion, the result of a progressive decrease in capacity for O_2 utilization which originated at some stage of the hypovolemic phase of shock and that, once started, continues to decline totally unaffected by favorable changes in blood circulation (from control of 0.730 to 0.520, 0.475 and 0.295 cc/kg/min) (Fig 5). This phenomenon probably involves the intestinal mucosa which normally utilizes the greater portion of the arterial-portal O_2 difference.

With reference to the hypothesis regarding a possible critical level of mesenteric blood flow, it is of interest to comment on our previous experience with cross clamping of the thoracic aorta [5] and the similar observations of Pontius.[18] The mortality following one hour of clamping of the aorta above the diaphragm was found to be 80%, while all dogs in which the aorta was clamped below the subclavian artery survived. Blood flow distal to the clamp in the latter group was reduced to almost the critical point of one third of control, while in the former group it fell well below this value. Death in these dogs occurred within a few hours.

An interesting feature of spanchnic hemodynamics appears from our control studies. The blood flow through the portal vein represents 20% of the cardiac output while the O_2 consumption is only 15% of the total O_2 consumption; at the same time the blood flow through the liver is 29.2% of the cardiac output and the O_2 consumption is only 17.2% of the total body O_2 consumption. This data correlates very well with a peculiar characteristic of the gastrointestinal hepatic circulation. Obviously these two areas of the splanchnic system are perfused by a circulation of blood in excess of their tissue needs for oxygen. The blood that flows and oxygenates the intestine must still perfuse the liver and provide it with over 40% of its oxygen supply. When, however, both organs are considered together our control studies show that gastrointestinal and hepatic blood flow is 30% of the cardiac output, while at the same time O_2 consumption of the gastrointestinal tract and liver is 31% of the total body O_2 consumption. The similarity of these two figures is important in supporting the validity of our determinations.

Hepatic Oxygen Consumption.—The characteristic relationship between intestinal and hepatic O_2 uptake is shown in our hypovolemic studies and particularly in the post-transfusion determinations. During the terminal stage of hypovolemic shock the hepatic vein O_2 in our dogs was decreased to 3.12 vol%. Selkurt obtained an average hepatic vein O_2 content of 3.22% and 2.06% in the terminal stage of a protracted period of hypovolemic shock. Presumably when O_2 saturation in the portal blood reaches a critical level (perhaps below 6 vol%) the liver will receive blood in which the level of O_2 saturation is so low that there is little margin left for further O_2 extraction. It is our hypothesis that this is why the liver O_2 consumption was always found to fall slightly more than the total body O_2 consumption in group 3 both during the 60 mm Hg period and after one hour of clamping. After transfusion the hepatic circulation is almost entirely portal in origin. At this stage the dependence of the liver upon the availability of portal oxygen is obvious. In dogs that died (group 3) the intestine did not extract a great amount of O_2, the portal blood was highly oxygenated (15.96 vol%), and the portal-hepatic vein gradient 2.69 vol%. In these dogs the liver was offered a more favorable O_2 gradient and the extraction of O_2 was good; in this series therefore the hepatic O_2 consumption returned above control levels (Fig 6). In the dogs that lived (group 3) the intestine utilized a reasonable amount of oxygen, the portal blood oxygen was 14.10 vol%, and the portal-hepatic vein gradient only 1.58 vol%. In these dogs the liver was offered less oxygen and the hepatic O_2 consumption was, therefore, well below control, the blood flow patterns not being greatly different in the two groups. This serves to illustrate our contention that the pattern of intestinal O_2 consumption, rather than the hepatic O_2 consumption, was the determinant cause of early death following retransfusion of blood.

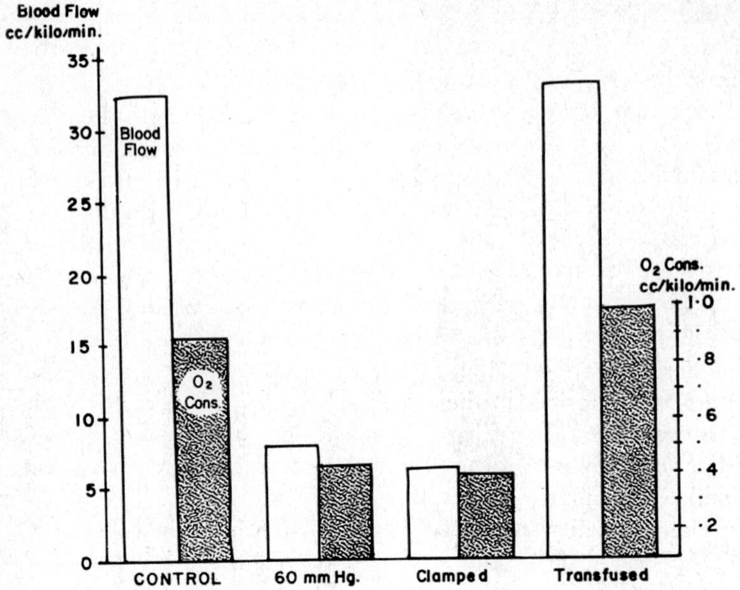

Fig 6.—Relation of hepatic blood flow to O_2 consumption during hemorrhagic shock and following retransfusion in group 3 nonsurviving animals. Adequate recovery of hepatic O_2 consumption is evident.

Significance of Results

The medical literature concerning visceral O_2 consumption during hemorrhagic shock is scarce indeed. In 1952 Werner [23] measured splanchnic O_2 consumption and estimated hepatic blood flow with the sulfobromophthalein (Bromsulphalein) method. He found that the fraction of cardiac output passing through the splanchnic bed remained the same during hypovolemic shock; similar observations were made regarding splanchnic O_2 consumption. Hamrick [12] observed a 60% reduction in hepatic blood flow during mild hemorrhagic shock with no change in splanchnic O_2 consumption thanks to an increase in mean arteriovenous difference. However, in sustained shock with mean blood pressure down to 35 mm/kg a 69% reduction in hepatic blood flow was observed with simultaneous decrease in splanchnic O_2 consumption. The splanchnic O_2 consumption to total O_2 consumption ratio did not show a consistent change in severe shock. In 1956 Selkurt [21] published a very interesting and complete analysis of hepatic and mesenteric hemodynamics during a standard hemorrhagic shock. He noted that O_2 utilization was diminished in both the intestinal tissue and the liver in approximately equal proportions. He stated that the possible significance of reduced O_2 utilization by the intestine was still obscure. Selkurt [21] observed that after transfusion intestinal O_2 utilization remained reduced at about 74% of control despite a good blood flow. In his commendable effort for accuracy in statistical analysis, Selkurt calculated this 74% reduction to be below the mathematical margin of statistical significance, and no attempt was made to investigate further or interpret this phenomenon. Selkurt did not divide his series of nine dogs into survivors and nonsurvivors. The constancy of this finding in dogs that died compared with adequate return of O_2 consumption in survivors has led to our deductions concerning its predominant role in the genesis of irreversible shock. It is of interest to observe that the 74% reduction figure for intestinal O_2 uptake in Selkurt's series is comparable to the 72% for the corresponding value in our group 2. In this group we did not differentiate between survivors and nonsurvivors. This average represents, in our opinion, a value standing somewhere between the two extremes represented by survivors and nonsurvivors in group 3, the former containing only nonsurvivors (reduction to 40% of control), and the latter the survivors (return to 103% of control).

The statistical analysis of the control and post-transfusion difference in our group 2 shows $P=46.3$ with a difference between the two means of 184; this difference is more than three times the P (138.9), and it should therefore be considered statistically significant. In group 3 (nonsurvivors), however, the difference between the two means (control and post-transfusion) is 435, well above three times the corresponding P ($P=80.3$). The difference between the two main groups in group 3 is overwhelmingly significant, while in group 2 it is barely above the statistical requirements of significance.

The maintenance of an adequate mesenteric blood flow has been shown to protect animals subjected to hemorrhagic shock.[15] It would seem that the intestinal changes observed in experimental shock studies are a result of ischemia and/or anoxia of the intestine during hypotension. While lack of oxygenation of tissues during shock may be due initially to inadequate blood flow, the inability of the tissue cells to extract oxygen with the resumption of adequate flow after reinfusion may be due either to arteriovenous shunting with bypassing of capillary beds or to irreversible cellular changes which preclude resumption of oxidative metabolism. Studies are in progress in our laboratory to evaluate metabolic changes at the level of the intestinal mucosal cell during shock and after reinfusion. The possible influence of drug therapy in improving O_2 delivery to the intestine during the critical stage of late shock is also under investigation.

Summary

A new technique has been devised which allows direct measurement of hepatic blood flow using a small abdominal incision and with internal shunting of infrahepatic blood.

The circulation of blood in the limb, in the mesenteric, and in the hepatic vascular beds has been shown to be greatly reduced during the hypovolemic stage of shock. Simultaneous measurements of cardiac output have revealed, however, that the percentage contribution of each of these territories to the total circulation remains approximately the same during hypovolemia. It would appear that local hemodynamics are adjusted to hemorrhagic shock in a way that reflects closely the average changes of the whole body.

The most striking observation concerned the O_2 consumption of the gastrointestinal tract in the post-transfusion period of dogs that died. Immediately after reinfusion the mesenteric circulation returned to well above control values, but the oxygen consumption of the gastrointestinal tract was reduced to 40% of control. Conversely, after reinfusion O_2 consumption returned to control or slightly above in the gastrointestinal tract of the dogs that survived.

In dogs that died, hepatic O_2 consumption was returned to control or above in the post-transfusion stage, while in the three surviving animals this value was well below control. It would, therefore, appear that the intensity of oxidative metabolism of the liver as reflected by the O_2 uptake of this organ is not directly related to survival in hemorrhagic shock. It would seem that the hepatic O_2 consumption is a reflection of O_2 offered to the liver after retransfusion. Inadequate oxygen utilization of the intestine results in high portal vein O_2 content with a resultant increase in hepatic O_2 consumption.

After transfusion of blood the portal blood pressure rises to nearly twice the control level. This factor, however, does not reflect a decreased mesenteric circulation by back-pressure effect. When the hepatic resistance is bypassed by division of the portal vein, the percentage increase in portal blood flow in relation to cardiac output is almost the same as in dogs with portal vein intact.

Conclusion

Irreversible hemorrhagic shock in the dog would appear to be related to a failure of intestinal tissues to take up oxygen after the expiration of a critical period of time at a critically low level of blood flow. Beyond this point in time the resumption of an adequate flow of oxygenated blood is ineffective in raising oxygen utilization in the intestine.

Gustavo Bounous, MD, McGill University Surgical Clinic, Montreal General Hospital, Montreal, Canada.

REFERENCES

1. Abel, F. L., and Murphy, Q. R.: Mesenteric, Renal, and Iliac Vascular Resistance in Dogs After Hemorrhage, Amer J Physiol 202:978, 1962.

2. Andersen, M. N.; Hambraeus, G.; Alfano, G. A.; and Schenk, W. G., Jr.: Distribution of Splanchnic and Peripheral Blood Flow During Acute Reduction in Circulatory Rate, Ann Surg 153:477, 1961.

3. Ballinger, W. F., II, and Vollenweider, H.: The Effect of Acute Hemorrhage Upon Hepatic Blood Flow and Splanchnic Oxygen Consumption in Dogs, Surgery 48:758, 1960.

4. Blalock, A., and Mason, M. F.: Observations on the Blood Flow and Gaseous Metabolism of the Liver of Unanesthetized Dogs, Amer J Physiol 117: 328, 1936.

5. Bounous, G., and King, H.: Cross Clamping of the Descending Thoracic Aorta, AMA Arch Surg 78:519, 1959.

6. Bradley, S. E.; Marks, P. A.; Reynell, P. C.; and Meltzer, J.: The Circulating Splanchnic Blood Volume in Dog and Man, Trans Ass Amer Physicians 66:294, 1953.

7. Cull, T. E.; Scibetta, M. P.; and Selkurt, E. E.: Arterial Inflow Into Mesenteric and Hepatic Vascular Circuits During Hemorrhagic Shock, Amer J Physiol 185:365, 1956.

8. Frank, E. D.; Frank, H. A.; Jacob, S. W.; Fine, J.: Hepatic Blood Flow in Experimental Hemorrhagic Shock, Amer J Physiol 202:7, 1962.

9. Friedman, J. J.: Mesenteric Circulation in Hemorrhagic Shock, Circ Res 9:561, 1961.

10. Gregg, D. E.: in Shock: Pathogenesis and Therapy; An International Symposium, edited by K. D. Bock, Berlin: Springer-Verlag, 1962.

11. Guyton, A. C., and Crowell, Z. W.: Dynamics of the Heart in Shock, Fed Proc 20:51, 1961.

12. Hamrick, L. W., Jr., and Myers, J. D.: Effect of Hemorrhage on Hepatic Blood Flow and Splanchnic Oxygen Consumption of Dog, Circ Res 3:65, 1955.

13. Hinshaw, D. B.; Peterson, M.; Huse, W. M.; Stafford, C. E.; and Joergenson, E. J.: Regional Blood Flow in Hemorrhagic Shock, Amer J Surg 102:224, 1961.

14. Johnson, P. C., and Selkurt, E. E.: Intestinal Weight Changes in Hemorrhagic Shock, Amer J Physiol 193:135, 1958.

15. Lillehei, R. C.: The Intestinal Factor in Irreversible Hemorrhagic Shock, Surgery 42:1043, 1957.

16. Longerbeam, J. K.; Lillehei, R. C.; and Scott, W. R.: The Nature of Irreversible Shock: A Hemodynamic Study, Surg Forum 13:1, 1962.

17. Osten, W.: Behavior of the Splanchnic Area and of the Total Organism in Hemorrhagic Shock in Animal Experiment, Z Ges Exp Med 131:30, 1959.

18. Pontius, R. G.; Brockman, H.; Hardy, E. G.; Cooley, D. A.; and DeBakey, M. F.: The Use of Hypothermia in the Prevention of Paraplegia Following Temporary Aortic Occlusion: Experimental Observations, Surgery 36:33, 1954.

19. Powers, L. H., and Schloerb, P. R.: Intestinal Factor in Irreversible Hemorrhagic Shock, Surg Forum 9:40, 1958.

20. Reynell, P. C.; Marks, P. A.; Chidsey, C.; and Bradley, S. E.: Changes in Splanchnic Blood Volume and Splanchnic Blood Flow in Dogs After Haemorrhage, Clin Sci 14:407, 1955.

21. Selkurt, E. E., and Brecher, G. A.: Splanchnic Hemodynamics and Oxygen Utilization During Hemorrhagic Shock in the Dog, Circ Res 4:693, 1956.

22. Thompson, B. G.; Hampson, L. G.; and Gurd, F. N.: The Relationship of Oxygen Consumption, Oxygen Debt, and Cardiac Output to Survival of Dogs in Hemorrhagic Shock, in preparation.

23. Werner, A. Y.; MacCanon, D. M.; and Horvath, S. M.: Fractional Distribution of Total Blood Flow to and Oxygen Consumption of the Liver as Influenced by Mild Hemorrhage, Amer J Physiol 170:624, 1952.

24. Zanetti, M. E.: Significance of Elevated Portal Vein Pressure in Etiology of Hemorrhagic Shock, Amer J Physiol 171:538, 1952.

Studies on Viscosity Alterations in Shock

I. Effect of High and Low Viscosity Dextrans Upon Plasma and Red Cell Volumes

WILLIAM C. SHOEMAKER, MD, CHICAGO

Viscosity alterations have been invoked to explain certain phenomena associated with shock and other disturbed circulatory states. Unfortunately, methods for the measurement of the viscosity of blood in vivo are not yet available. However, in vitro measurements of the relative viscosity may be obtained by measuring the shear stress at various shear rates in samples of blood or plasma withdrawn from the patient or experimental animal. Alternatively, the effects of viscosity alterations may be studied by physiologic measurements before and after addition of highly viscous materials to a biological preparation. Sucrose is polymerized to dextrans of various molecular weights and viscosities by the bacteria, *Leuconostoc mesenteroides* [1]; these dextrans may be fractionated to provide material of relatively uniform viscosity and molecular weight for clinical and experimental studies.[2] The physiologic effects of viscosity alterations produced by the administration of high or low viscosity dextran then may be observed and studied in vivo.

The intravenous administration of high molecular weight, high viscosity dextran to dogs and rabbits will produce the classic signs of shock, and the use of low molecular weight, low viscosity dextrans will alleviate these effects. Gelin [3] has shown that the high molecular weight dextran produces intravascular aggregation, which is directly observable in the sclera of rabbits. Studies from this laboratory [4] have demonstrated intravascular cellular aggregation in the hepatic sinusoids of the intact rabbit produced by high viscosity dextran and restoration of relatively normal flow after administration of low viscosity dextran. Moreover, an increased hepatic resistance, which has been shown to occur in hemorrhagic shock,[5] was demonstrated after administration of high viscosity dextran in the perfused canine liver. Increased hepatic resistance, demonstrated by decreased flow with constant perfusion pressure or increased pressure with constant flow, was alleviated by the administration of low viscosity dextran, provided the changes in hepatic physiology had not proceeded to an irreversible point.[4]

The present studies were undertaken to determine if the addition of high viscosity dextran would reproduce the delayed equilibration of labeled red cells previously observed in hemorrhagic shock.[6] Second, the influence of low viscosity dextran on these red cell alterations was investigated.

Methods

Mongrel dogs weighing between 11 and 20 kg were splenectomized under standard aseptic technique. After recovery from this procedure, polyethylene catheters (PE 240) were placed in a femoral artery and vein. On the day of the experiment, 50 ml of the dogs' own blood was withdrawn into a sterile plastic bag, and the cells were washed with saline and labeled with Cr^{51} by Read's modification [7] of the method of Sterling

---

Presented at the 20th Annual Meeting of the Central Surgical Association, Chicago, Feb 21-23, 1963.

From the Department of Surgical Research, Hektoen Institute, Cook County Hospital, and the Department of Surgical Research, Michael Reese Hospital and Medical Center.

Supported in part by grants from the United States Public Health Service and by the Charles H. and Rachel M. Schwab Memorial Foundation.

Dextrans supplied by A. B. Pharmacia, Uppsula, Sweden.

and Gray.[8] Methods for measuring the equilibration patterns of T-1824 (Evans blue dye) and the injected, labeled red cells as well as the techniques for sampling and calculation of plasma and red cell volumes have been previously described.[6]

High molecular weight (mean mol wt 1,200,000) highly viscous (viscosity, η=0.67) dextran, 1 gm/kg body weight, was administered intravenously in 250 ml of isotonic saline usually over a 20- to 30-minute period. Low molecular weight (mean mol wt 40,500), low viscosity (η=0.17) dextran was given intravenously as a 6% solution in isotonic saline at 2 gm/kg body weight. The dogs were studied in an unanesthetized state.

Labeled red cells, T-1824, and the dextrans were injected into the femoral vein catheter. Four- to five-milliliter blood samples were withdrawn at ten-minute intervals from the femoral artery catheter. The blood was centrifuged and the plasma separated from the cells. Aliquots of the packed cells were assayed for Cr^{51} using a NaI well-type scintillation counter and pulse height analyzer; counting time was extended to give counting errors of ± 1% to 2%. The plasma samples were analyzed colorimetrically for T-1824 in a Coleman or Beckman spectrophotometer at a wave length of 620 mμ. Plasma volumes in the control and experimental conditions were calculated from samples taken at ten-minute intervals over a period of one hour or more.[9] The volumes of the rapidly circulating, slowly circulating, and total circulating red cells were calculated using compartmental analysis of the delayed equilibration curve as previously described.[6] Noncirculating red cell volume was calculated from the difference between the control red cell volume and the total circulating red cell volume after dextran.

Microhematocrit measurements were made at frequent intervals on samples of arterial blood (Art H). The total body hematocrit (TBH), representing the percentage of red cells in the blood volume, was obtained as the total circulating red cell volume divided by the total circulating red cell volume plus the plasma volume. Finally, the ratio of the total body hematocrit to the arterial hematocrit, TBH/Art H, was calculated.

Results

Arterial hypotension and tachycardia were produced with rapid, intravenous administration of high viscosity dextran, 1 gm/kg body weight; profound hypotension and, on occasion, death followed 2 gm/kg body weight doses.

The mean control plasma volume of this series of dogs was 555±29 (SE) ml. There was an increase in plasma volume to 813±63 (SE) ml after intravenous administration of high viscosity dextran, 1 gm/kg body weight ($P<0.01$).

In the normal control period, mixing of injected, labeled red cells within the intravascular space occurred within ten minutes

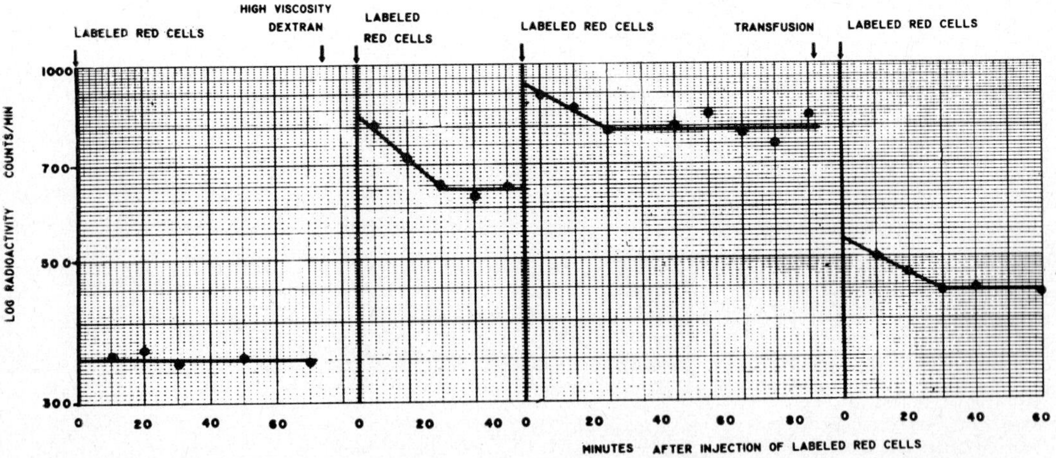

Fig 1.—Labeled red cell equilibration curves before and after high viscosity dextran in a representative experiment. Labeled red cells were first injected in the normal, control period indicated by arrow and vertical line at left. The radioactivity of red cells was relatively constant after this first injection, as indicated by the horizontal line. High viscosity dextran was then injected, and one-half hour later labeled red cells were again injected at the time indicated by the second vertical line and arrow. There was a sharp decrease in red cell radioactivity for a short period of time as the injected labeled red cells mixed in a larger and larger red cell volume. This was followed by a leveling off to constant values. Similar equilibration patterns were shown on two subsequent injections of labeled red cells at the vertical lines. A transfusion was given between the third and fourth injection.

as in previously reported series.[6] However, the intravenous administration of high viscosity dextran produced a delayed equilibration of the labeled red cells but not of the plasma indicator. Fig 1 illustrates a representative experiment. Calculation of red cell volumes was based on the equilibration curves, using compartmental analysis. After high viscosity dextran was injected, there was a decreased rapidly circulating red cell volume, a decreased total circulating volume, and the appearance of slowly circulating and noncirculating red cell volumes. The mean control total circulating red cell volume was 370 ml. After injection of high viscosity dextran, the average total circulating red cell volume was 335 ml. Of the latter, 252 ml was calculated to be rapidly circulating; 83 ml was slowly circulating. These equilibration characteristics and red cell volume changes were comparable to those observed in hemorrhagic shock.[6]

The arterial hematocrit decreased from a mean control of 32% to 24% after administration of high viscosity dextran. The TBH fell from a mean of 31% to 27%; the ratio, TBH/Art H, increased. This increased ratio suggests that at any one time there is a greater volume of red cells in the microcirculation than in the large vessels.

Direct observation of the transilluminated liver in vivo gives qualitative evidence of a microcirculatory defect described by Knisely [10] as "sludging," or intravascular, cellular aggregation. Measurement of the equilibration characteristics of injected, labeled red cells provides a quantitative estimation of the rapidity of the red cell circulation. The hypothesis is made that the results of these two independent approaches are essentially reflections of the same underlying phenomenon; that is, sludging, which can be observed directly but not quantified, and red cell equilibration, which can be measured but not seen, are microscopic and macroscopic aspects of the same pathophysiologic process. A number of predictions based on this hypothesis were framed and tested experimentally.

The development of intravascular cellular aggregation in response to the intravenous administration of high viscosity dextran takes a definite period of time depending on the dose given and other experimental conditions. Usually 20 to 30 minutes are required to produce this lesion in a moderately severe

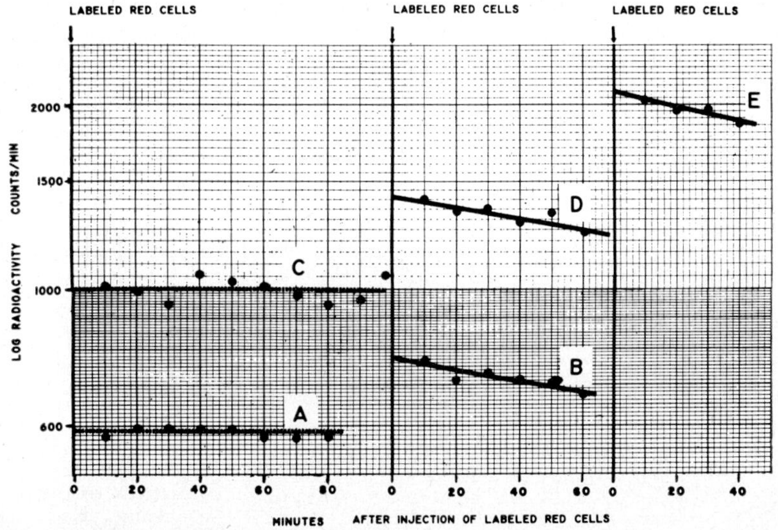

Fig 2.—Equilibration of labeled red cells: effect of the time between injection of high viscosity dextran and labeled red cells. High viscosity dextran was given during a 3-minute period, and 12 minutes later labeled red cells were injected as shown by the left vertical line and arrow. Radioactivity of the animal's circulating red cells was relatively constant (shown by dotted line, curve *A*). Two hours and ten minutes later a second injection of labeled red cells was given at center vertical line. There was a progressive decrease of red cell radioactivity at this time as shown by solid line of curve *B*. After the completion of curve *B* the sequence was repeated. A second rapid injection of high viscosity dextran was given, and 13 minutes after this, labeled red cells were injected; curve C again demonstrated a relatively horizontal, but erratic line. Another labeled red cell injection, 2½ hours later, demonstrated delayed mixing (curve *D*). Finally, 14 hours later delayed mixing was still demonstrable (curve *E*). Thus, delayed red cell mixing was not observed 12 to 13 minutes after high viscosity dextran but was observed two hours or more after this dextran.

form. On the basis of time taken to develop intravascular, cellular aggregation after high viscosity dextran, it may be predicted that injection of the Cr^{51}-labeled red cells within a few minutes after intravenous administration of the high viscosity dextran would not reproduce the two-compartment curve. If the mixing of the labeled red cells in the total red cell volume occurred before the aggregation of a sizeable proportion of the unlabeled cells, the progressive aggregation of red cells after the dextran injection would include both labeled and unlabeled cells without distinction. This was confirmed experimentally and is illustrated in Fig 2.

Direct observations of the hepatic sinusoids in the very late stages of shock produced by either high viscosity dextran or hemorrhage indicate that there are engorged, swollen sinusoids in which the aggregated cells do not appear to move over periods of several hours. At this stage it also would be anticipated that the two-compartment curve would not be found; but a relatively horizontal curve, primarily indicating a decreased total circulatory red cell volume, would be expected. The aggregated red cells caught in the microcirculation would not be expected to equilibrate with the injected, labeled red cells within the active circulation. Again, the delayed equilibration curve was observed infrequently in the terminal and preterminal states.

We have observed the time course of the delayed equilibration curves, and the volume changes derived from them, both clinically and experimentally. A slowly moving red cell volume appears; this volume progressively increases in size; subsequently it is replaced by noncirculating red cells before death. This pattern is entirely consistent with the development of the microcirculatory lesion, where there is a progressive slowing of cells in the microcirculation leading eventually to completely motionless cell aggregates.

Administration of low viscosity dextran during the course of the 90 or 120 minutes allowed for sampling during the high viscosity dextran equilibration curve would not be expected to change the equilibration pattern appreciably. The "disaggregation" or reversal of cellular aggregation also requires a finite period of time. In addition to the time factors there must be a measurable difference between the radioactivity of the slowly moving or noncirculating red cells and the rapidly moving cells before changes between these pools can be detected by the techniques described. For example, if low viscosity dextran were administered during the second or horizontal portion of a two-compartment curve, no change would be demonstrable, since equilibration of the injected labeled red cells in the total circulating red cell volume would be complete at this time. Under these circumstances the amount of radioactivity in the rapidly and slowly circulating red cells would be the same, and a return of slowly circulating cells into the active circulation would not be detectable. If low viscosity dextran were injected during the period of decreasing radioactivity in the labeled red cell equilibration curve, there would be only an earlier leveling off to constant levels of red cell radioactivity. Further, the addition of low viscosity dextran shortly after high viscosity dextran would not give clearly defined results, since the use of a two-pool or two-compartment analysis presumes at least a relatively steady state. Measurements under rapidly changing physiologic conditions produce curves which are uninterpretable.

The effect of low viscosity dextran was observed in the following manner. During the normal, control period, the animal's circulating cells were allowed to mix with a large dose of labeled red cells. High viscosity dextran was given, and several hours were allowed for aggregation of the circulating cells. A large volume of unlabeled, washed red cells from a donor animal then was given to reduce the radioactivity of the rapidly circulating red cells. Cells which had become noncirculating or "sequestered" then would have a higher radioactivity than that of the rapidly circulating cells, since the latter were diluted with transfused, unlabeled donor cells. Low viscosity dextran then was infused rapidly and red cell radioactivity

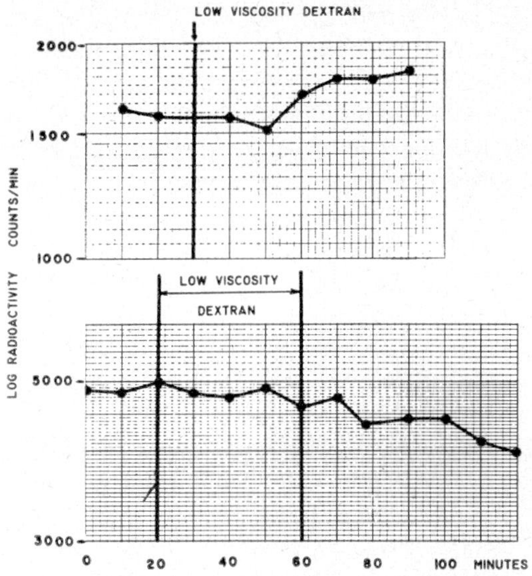

Fig 3.—Effect of low viscosity dextran on red cell movements. Upper section: A large injection of labeled red cells was given and after this an injection of high viscosity dextran. After a period of 2½ hours a tranfusion of unlabeled red cells was given to reduce the radioactivity of the rapidly circulating red cells leaving the noncirculating cells more radioactive. Then low viscosity dextran was rapidly injected, shown by the arrow and vertical line. This resulted in increasing levels of circulating red cell radioactivity suggesting re-entry of the more radioactive noncirculating red cells. Lower section: High viscosity dextran first was given, and 24 hours later labeled red cells were injected so that the actively circulating red cells had higher radioactivity. Then an infusion of 50 gm of low viscosity dextran was given, as shown by the arrow in the figure above. There was a decrease of red cell radioactivity suggesting a dilution of the circulating red cells by relatively unlabeled, previously noncirculating cells.

measured before and after this infusion. There was a significant increase in the red cell radioactivity in samples withdrawn after low viscosity dextran administration (Fig 3). This increased radioactivity could only come from the re-entrance of the more highly labeled, previously noncirculating cells into the active circulation.

Disaggregation of red cells also was observed in conditions where the actively circulating cells had higher radioactivity than the noncirculating red cells. A large dose of chromium-tagged red cells was injected into an animal which previously had been given high viscosity dextran. Under these circumstances, the noncirculating red cells had lower radioactivity. Then 50 gm of low viscosity dextran was infused intravenously. A decrease in the radioactivity of the circulating red cells was observed, suggesting re-entrance of less highly labeled, previously noncirculating cells into the circulating red cell volume (Fig 3).

Comment

The data of the present study indicate that the administration of high viscosity dextran to the intact unanesthetized dog produced arterial hypotension, tachycardia, delayed mixing of labeled red cells, and the appearance of a slowly circulating and a noncirculating red cell volume. Incident to these red cell volume changes there was an increase in plasma volume after administration of high viscosity dextran. The blood volume, calculated on the basis of total circulating red cell volume plus plasma volume, increased after high viscosity dextran. Shock, in these circumstances, was normo- or hypervolemic. The delayed red cell mixing occurred although the whole blood volume was normal or increased.

The effects of shock induced by administration of high viscosity dextran were qualitatively and quantitatively similar to alterations observed in hemorrhagic shock [6] and thermal injury [11]; namely, the loss of rapidly circulating red cell volume and the concomitant appearance of a slowly circulating, then noncirculating red cell volume. Thus, the red cell equilibration defect of shock is reproducible by administration of a high viscosity dextran and is reversed in part by low viscosity dextran. This suggests the possibility that increased plasma viscosity incident to decreased velocity may be one of the mechanisms operative in the production of shock.

The appearance of slowly circulating and noncirculating red cells is consistent with the cellular aggregation in hepatic sinusoids and postcapillary venules observed by direct microscopy. The similar time course of these two phenomena also suggests an interrelationship. Moreover, predictions based upon observations of the microcirculatory alterations were borne out experimentally in the labeled red cell equilibration studies.

The studies reported herein provide direct evidence for the so-called phenomenon of "sequestration." Sequestration, which has been a frequently invoked explanation for many physiologic effects of shock, is an ill-defined concept which implies that there is a volume of blood hidden somewhere and in some obscure fashion. Although there is considerable indirect evidence suggesting that sequestration does occur in shock, direct evidence of sequestered cells has not been available. Appearance of increased radioactivity in the circulating red cells after low viscosity dextran administration when the noncirculating red cells had higher radioactivity indicates mobilization of the noncirculating cells. If delayed red cell mixing bears a direct relationship to cellular aggregation, then these experiments also provide evidence for disaggregation of previously aggregated red cells.

Summary

Dextrans of high and low viscosity were found to be useful tools for investigation of the effects of viscosity alterations in the intact animal.

High molecular weight, high viscosity dextran produced arterial hypotension, tachycardia, increased plasma volume, and delayed equilibration of injected labeled red cells. Calculations of red cell volumes based upon these equilibration curves indicate the appearance of a slowly circulating red cell volume as well as a decrease in the rapidly circulating and total circulating red cell volumes.

High viscosity dextran decreased the arterial hematocrit markedly and the total body hematocrit moderately. The ratio, TBH/Art H, increased; this suggested a redistribution of red cells within the vascular compartment so that there were proportionately more cells in the microcirculation than in the large vessels.

A relationship between the previously observed intravascular, red cell aggregation and the failure of labeled red cells to equilibrate normally was explored. The hypothesis was proposed that delayed red cell equilibration may be a reflection of cellular aggregation (sludging). If so, calculations of red cell volumes based upon the delayed equilibration curve may, under specified conditions, reflect a quantitative estimation of the extent of the cellular aggregation.

Administration of low molecular weight, low viscosity dextran increased the plasma volume. It also produced an increase in the radioactivity of the circulating red cells, when the noncirculating red cells had greater radioactivity than those circulating, and a decrease in radioactivity of the circulating red cells when the noncirculating red cells had less radioactivity. This suggested a re-entrance of noncirculating red cells into the active circulation and may represent disaggregation of previously aggregated or sludged cells.

William C. Shoemaker, MD, Director, Department of Surgical Research, Hektoen Institute for Medical Research, Cook County Hospital, 1835 W Harrison, Chicago, Ill.

REFERENCES

1. Grönwall, A., and Ingelman, B.: Untersuchungen über Dextran und sein Verhalten bei parenteraler Zufuhr, Acta Physiol Scand 7:97, 1944.

2. Thorsén, G.: The Use of Dextrans as Infusion Fluids, Surg Gynec Obstet 109:43, 1959.

3. Gelin, L. E.: Studies in Anemia of Injury, Acta Chir Scand suppl 210:1-30, 1956.

4. Gelin, L. E., and Shoemaker, W. C.: Hepatic Blood Flow and Microcirculatory Alterations Induced by Dextran of High and Low Viscosity, Surgery 49:713, 1961.

5. Shoemaker, W. C.; Walker, W. F.; and Turk, L. N., III: The Role of the Liver in the Development of Hemorrhagic Shock, Surg Gynec Obstet 112:327, 1961.

6. Shoemaker, W. C., and Iida, F.: Studies on the Equilibration of Labeled Red Cells and T-1824 in Hemorrhagic Shock, Surg Gynec Obstet 114:539, 1962.

7. Read, R. C.: Studies of Red-Cell Volume and Turnover Using Radiochromium, New Eng J Med 250:1021, 1954.

8. Sterling, G., and Gray, S. J.: Determination of Circulating Red Cell Volume in Man by Radioactive Chromium, J Clin Invest 29:1614, 1950.

9. Noble, R. P., and Gregersen, M. I.: Blood Volume in Clinical Shock, J Clin Invest 25:158 and 172, 1946.

10. Knisely, M. H.; Block, E. H.; and Warner, L.: Selective Phagocytosis, Kongelige Danske Videnskabernes Selskab Biol. Skrift. 4:1, 1948.

11. Iida, F.; Richter, H. M., Jr.; and Shoemaker, W. C.: Measurement of Rapidly and Slowly Circulating Red Cell Volumes in Thermal Injury, Surg Gynec Obstet 114:701, 1962.

DISCUSSION

ON PAPERS BY DRS. COOLEY AND MCINTOSH, HAMPTON ET AL, AND SHOEMAKER

DR. WILLIAM DRUCKER, Cleveland: I should not like to confine my remarks to the paper by Dr. Gurd and his associates because the other papers, particularly the one by Dr. Cooley, raise a problem in semantics which has bothered many of us.

We all know that the treatment of shock is very simple: one merely replaces the lost blood volume. If this is done promptly with adequate amounts of blood, there is no problem. But if we delay treatment, more and more blood is required and frequently other forms of therapy must be employed to maintain a satisfactory circulatory state. Is this the human counterpart of experimental irreversible shock? We do know that in clinical medicine the phenomenon or irreversible shock is rarely, if ever, seen. But irreversible shock has a very clear meaning to the investigator. A very good understanding of this can be derived by reviewing Dr. Carl Wigger's book, in which he discusses the problem of interpreting death from hemorrhage.

In the laboratory death from hypovolemia can occur in two ways. Death can occur because the animal has been bled out and remains bled out until death (hypovolemic death): this is a different form of death from that which occurs sometimes after transfusion of all blood that was removed (normovolemic death).

In Dr. Cooley's very interesting studies I think it would be important to determine what is irreversibility. It seems to me that in his study, even though occasional transfusions were given, he might be studying the death that occurs from serious and untreated hemorrhage. It would be important to know what percentage of his untreated animals died after transfusion, if one is to compare this as irreversible shock with what is conventionally designated in the laboratory as irreversible shock.

There are two different mechanisms that lead to death. During the period of hemorrhage there are many compensatory mechanisms that come into play. In time these fail and the animal or human will die. This is not irreversible shock; this is the loss of physiological adjustment to hypovolemia.

An animal eventually will die after transfusion even though we employ other therapeutic measures.

Many investigators have been interested for some time in the effect of hypovolemia on the intestinal mucosa. This was initially observed by Dr. George Whipple in the first part of the century. More recently the work of Drs. Lillehi, Vischer, and co-workers in Minnesota has indicated that we must look closely at the intestine to interpret irreversible shock. Is it a circulatory maladjustment? In view of the work by Dr. Hampson, Dr. Bounous, and Dr. Gurd, we must ask, is it a metabolic maladjustment? Their work suggests that hypovolemia produces an irreversible metabolic change in a specific anatomic area—the intestine. This is reflected by the failure of the intestine to take up oxygen after transfusion. A similar failure to resume a normal uptake of oxygen after transfusion did not occur in the other tissues they studied, namely liver and muscle.

Why does this occur? Does it perhaps reflect the technique they employed? Is this a reproducible technique? I understand in talking with Dr. Hampson that it is reproducible with minimal variation. Do these results occur because they have studied only certain phases in the dynamic sequence of events that occur during shock? If they were to study other phases would they find similar differences? Are the intestinal cells still alive but incapable of resuming oxidative metabolism?

Strictly from a philosophical standpoint, this work opens for all of us broad new vistas for investigation. Why not remove the intestine and study its metabolism as an isolated tissue as we have done with the diaphragm from hypovolemic rats? With regard to epinephrine we do know (and I think it is very important in reference to Dr. Cooley's work) that if either epinephrine or levarterenol is given in large quantities (ie, more than 2.5μg/kg/min over four hours) it will cause death in the experimental normovolemic animal with all of the metabolic changes characteristic of hemorrhagic shock plus extensive necrosis of the intestine. The effect of epinephrine therefore is pertinent in consideration of the pathogenesis of irreversible shock. Although epinephrine may not be deterimental as an acute infusion when an animal (or man) is dying from exsanguination, we should be very cautious in the use of levarterenol or epinephrine as a prolonged infusion for either normovolemic or hypovolemic shock.

Now the question must be asked on the basis of the work reported by Dr. Hampson and his colleagues—what effect do catecholamines, adrenal steroids, endotoxin, and various pharmacological agents (ie, dibenzyl-β-chlorethylamine [Dibenamine]) have on the ability of the intestine to take up oxygen in normovolemic and hypovolemic animals?

DR. THEODORE DRAPANAS, Buffalo: I arise to emphasize the significance of the techniques of study that Dr. Shoemaker has just presented to us. As he has pointed out, it is a well-known phenomenon that blood volume studies in patients in shock are unreliable unless you allow for a much prolonged equilibration time, especially if you use Cr^{51}-labeled red cells.

Dr. Shoemaker has nicely shown that the mixing pattern is similar to that which may occur in a two-compartment system—that is, first you get immediate mixing followed by a rather slow mixing, and by extrapolation you can actually determine what size this slow-mixing compartment is.

I would suggest to you that these techniques now offer an experimental model whereby one can actually measure the sequestration of red cells in many experimental and clinical conditions. The obvious implications in this study are that sequestration of red cells may be related to sludging of the microcirculation in oligemic shock and that the infused tagged red cells were not being rapidly mixed into the altered microcirculation.

Here, then, is a method by which we can now not only determine the actual sequestered volume but also determine the effects of some pharmacologic agents on the microcirculation. Dr. Shoemaker has shown us very nicely what happens, for example, with low viscosity dextran.

I would like to ask Dr. Shoemaker if he has extended his studies and what results he has obtained, if any, with the use of some of the other agents commonly used in the therapy of oligemic shock—vasopressors or perhaps some of the ganglionic blocking agents or phenoxybenzamine (Dibenzyline).

Dr. Fiorindo A. Simeone, Cleveland: I was especially interested in Dr. Cooley's presentation in regard to the role of the heart in "irreversibility." It is interesting that despite the different kinds of model that we have used in our own laboratories, the data are somewhat similar, particularly the data that Dr. Cooley showed in his first slide.

Of interest is the fact that, while the data are similar, the interpretations are somewhat different. In this problem of "irreversibility," of course, we feel that the central point is the capillary loop where the business of the circulation is done. Various things happen when this circulation is disturbed, including "irreversibility" and death.

For keeping conditions normal around this capillary loop, a number of physiologic mechanisms are available. The heart is a unit of the homeostatic mechanism responsible for maintaining capillary circulation and tissue perfusion. It functions, of course, as a pump.

Our data have led us to believe that the heart is not the trigger mechanism or the leading point which drags after it a breakdown in a number of other mechanisms concerned with this capillary circulation which is the central point in the problem of shock, and the reasons we think so are these:

We have used a somewhat different strain gauge from the one that Dr. Cooley has described, but the results are comparable. We have found that, when an animal is bled to a level which leads to "irreversibility," at first there is a preliminary increase in the mechanical tension that the heart is able to develop. Others, too, have seen this. During the period of hypotension and oligemia the myocardial force with each contraction is low; with reinfusion of the reservoir blood the force comes up again, often to normal levels and sometimes above normal.

Here is the important point: our animals, in a state of "irreversibility" after reinfusion show all of the signs of going downhill and on to death long before the myocardial strain gauge shows a diminution in its ability to exert contractile force. Dr. Cooley's first slide showed the same thing, and actually Dr. Cooley mentioned that this may be due to the cardiotonic actions of catecholamines and the sympathetics. Regardless of what it is due to, the fact remains that the heart is able to exert tension at that point, yet the animal is dying. Its blood pressure continues downward and it goes on to death. This was the first observation that made us believe that the heart was not the key functional unit that dragged everything else down after it.

The second thing is that the central venous pressure—that is, the right atrial and even the left atrial pressures—do not rise as the animal is deteriorating and is about to die, until it is actually dying. The venous pressures stay normal or actually are below normal in the normovolemic, hypotensive animal. Besides that, we have transfused our normovolemic, hypotensive animals with donor blood equivalent to their calculated blood volumes. Their blood pressure will go up and remain up as long as transfusion is continued, cardiac function will improve, and the venous pressures will not rise above normal range until the animals are just about to die.

For these two reasons especially, we do not think the heart is the leading point that goes on to a breakdown of all homeostatic mechanisms leading to death of the animal.

Dr. Paul R. Schloerb, Kansas City, Kan: Dr. Hampson's paper really gets very much to the crux of the matter, that is, actual measurement of tissue perfusion.

I would like to ask whether or not he has investigated the effect of adrenergic blocking agents upon tissue oxygen uptake.

Secondly, regarding Dr. Shoemaker's paper, I wonder if he would speculate a little more about the anatomy of this physiologic abnormality which he has so beautifully elucidated. The phenomenon of splanchnic sequestration in the dog, apparently due to a developed hepatic vein sphincter valve mechanism, seems pretty well agreed upon, although it is not at all established that this is true in the human.

I wonder if splanchnic sequestration does account for any part of this, and whether Dr. Shoemaker has attempted to quantify it.

Dr. Jack C. Cooley, Urbana, Ill: Dr. Drucker, I can only agree with your comments that we do have to do further studies on animals that are hemorrhaged to the point of irreversibility and that are allowed to survive and later die. There is certainly a group that will do this; you think the animal is going to survive, and later the animal does not survive. Contractile force studies must be done on this group.

Whether this has something to do with irreversible changes in the metabolic abilities of the cardiac muscle or, as Dr. Hampson has brought into the discussion, the intestinal factor with irreversible changes in the mucosa of the intestine with formation of endotoxins or other substances that later cause the death of these animals, we do not understand.

I was very grateful to Dr. Simeone for his discussion. Several years ago he was the chairman of a large discussion group of physiologists, surgeons and others interested in this problem, in Washington, D. C., in a conference on shock, and I greatly respect his opinions. Our interpretations, as illustrated by my paper and his findings, are somewhat different, but I think in the main the contractile force assumptions that we have made are pretty much the same.

I would like to mention the work of Guyton and Crowell, referred to by Dr. Hampson originally, in regard to some of the points Dr. Simeone made. I think this work was a monumental study. They hemorrhaged animals until the mean blood pressure came down to 30 mm Hg. They kept on hemorrhaging these animals to keep their pressure at 30 mm Hg. In other words, they would not allow the mean pressure to get above 30 mm Hg. They would stop if it started to go below. Finally, when irreversibility had been reached and there was evidence that the systemic pressure was going down, they would transfuse the animal with large amounts. Once irreversibility occurred, the blood pressure tended to go down and down, and they had to transfuse more and more. Extremely large volumes had to be used to keep the systemic pressure at 30 mm Hg. They monitored left atrial pressure and found that the left atrial pressure gradually rose. Finally it came to as high a figure—in other words, 30 mm Hg—as the systemic pressure. Their conclusion was that this was evidence that heart failure was an important factor in producing irreversibility in hemorrhagic shock.

I mention this work because it does introduce another study that perhaps has some effect on this over-all picture.

Dr. Fraser N. Gurd, Montreal, Canada: One of our preparations represents a new method which Dr. Bounous has developed for the simultaneous direct evaluation of both mesenteric and hepatic blood flow in the dog. The other technique, which Dr. Hampson omitted from his presentation for lack of time, gives a direct measurement of mesenteric flow alone. The portal vein is divided and blood is drained into a burette and pumped back into the proximal portal vein. This not only measures portal flow directly but also removes the influence of hepatic resistance. In answer to one of Dr. Schloerb's questions, the phenomenon of an ultimate failure of oxygen uptake in the intestine occurred also in the group from which hepatic resistance had been excluded in this way.

Dr. Schloerb also asked about adrenergic blocking agents. So far our data show an improvement in mesenteric flow in the late hypotensive period when a blocking agent is introduced.

Personally, I am of the opinion that success in the treatment of shock consists in the maintenance or restoration of visceral flow, and of venous return to the heart, during the stage of shock in which irreversible damage might occur. What the treatment is does not matter provided that it is well calculated to accomplish these ends. Transfusion may be good treatment, or an expander, or saline; or a drug designed to improve tissue perfusion by adjusting vascular resistance. As usual, treatment depends upon the genuine underlying diagnosis.

We feel that, despite our conventional preoccupation with hemodynamics, a certain moment arrives when blood flow becomes irrelevant to the survival of the animal and when proferred oxygen is no longer accepted by cells. We are hoping to be able to add support to this hypothesis within the next few months.

Dr. William C. Shoemaker, Chicago: Although we have not observed the effects of vasopressors or blocking agents on red cell equilibration, we have measured the hemodynamic and physiologic effects of vasopressors, such as epinephrine, levartenol, and serotonin on hepatic hemodynamics and metabolism. A marked increased hepatic resistance, as well as profound metabolic changes, occur after epinephrine and levarterenol in the unanesthetized dog. The reason we have not gotten around to measuring the effects of vasodilators or blocking agents in either type of experimental preparation is that we are more interested, at least as the first step, in investigating the underlying hemodynamic and physiologic mechanisms involved in the development of the shock syndrome. We would first like to know what is happening in shock; then we will try to understand how these vasodilators or other agents affect the outcome.

I have been asked to speculate a little about what happens to all this noncirculated blood volume and how it relates to the defect of shock, whatever that may be! The defect of shock, of course, is exceedingly elusive; we are all talking about something that is exceedingly difficult to define precisely. To my mind, there are at least four or five different types of circulatory nonuniformity involved in the development of underlying lesion of shock.

First, there is a redistribution of cardiac output. Initially, there is an increase in percentage of cardiac output to the central organs—the brain, lungs, liver, and coronary circulations—and concomitantly, less blood flow to the periphery. There is probably also a redistribution of flow within organs, that is, the medulla as opposed to the cortex of the kidney and the longer versus the shorter arcs in the liver. There is a redistribution of blood volume, the so-called sequestration of blood presumably in the splanchnic area. In my mind, this is induced by increased hepatic venous resistance changes at the level of the outlet sinusoidal sphincter rather than the vena cava-hepatic vein junction, which is the site of the so-called throttle valves. Our measurements of the pressure gradients across the sinusoids are increased after hemorrhagic shock.

Fourth, and more importantly, there is a redistribution of blood volume along the course of the vascular tree—that is, as the blood transverses from artery to capillary to postcapillary venule to vein. Cellular aggregation, or "sludging," occurs in the postcapillary venule in the peripheral circulation, and in the sinusoids of the liver. Finally, there is an alteration we have only recently begun to study; namely, changes in the velocity of the red cell flow independent of the velocity of the plasma flow.

If allowed a final observation, I should like to say that we, and others, have presented studies having to do with the effects of one or more agents on a particular experimental situation. Perhaps it is time we forget about measuring "effects" and turn our attention to the underlying mechanisms of the disease process.

Editorials

How Cardiac Surgery Transformed Surgery

Broadly speaking, a cardiac surgeon is a general surgeon who, of necessity, has had to explore in some detail and even to expand upon pertinent aspects of the sciences basic to general surgery. He has become the prototype of an operating surgeon, basing clinical action on clinically oriented research. Although seeking information to help him solve specific problems within his own special interests, the cardiac surgeon inevitably made multiple practical contributions to the management of similar problems in general surgery. He has stimulated surgical investigation and teaching, and, as a by-product of his therapeutic achievements, he has been a challenge to the diagnostic ability of a variety of medical practitioners. His ability to operate successfully for a broad spectrum of cardiovascular diseases placed squarely before them new diagnostic and therapeutic obligations.

A vital need on the part of the cardiac surgeon has been a truer practical understanding of basic physiopathologic processes governing survival following major trauma. Careful, and yet aggressive, pre- and postoperative care for his type of patients had critical bearing on their survival. This hard-won basic knowledge is now being adopted by the general surgeon, resulting in lower morbidity and mortality following all forms of major surgery and trauma.

Therapeutic advances in general surgery which occurred primarily because of the interests of the cardiac surgeon are multiple. A few examples would include: recognition and management of the metabolic acidosis of hypoxia with its profound effect upon cardiac output and the general circulation (all patients with shock); better and more precise control of blood volume maintenance and blood loss replacement (using continuous venous pressure monitoring and frequent blood volume determinations); attention to the importance of adequate respiration while simultaneously minimizing the energy expenditure of achieving ventilation (tracheotomy and supported respiration are as applicable to the emphysematous "cardiac" who has had resection of his gastric carcinoma as to the postoperative tetralogy of Fallot patient). In general, we conclude that the development of cardiac surgery has given solid example of the need for a better understanding of basic body physiology in good patient care. Science was made respectable, and "milliequivalent" was no longer a dirty word. Now one hears general surgeons talking of low-output heart failure, of metabolic acidosis, of water loading, and of low-sodium lethargy in a fashion that was unheard of 15 years ago.

Although patients had been suffering from sudden death in the operating rooms of our hospitals for many, many years, the management of acute cardiac arrest and the techniques of resuscitation were perfected because of cardiac surgery. Continuous monitoring devices were developed for use with all anesthesias, and electrical defibrillators (with staff knowledge of how to use them) have become a part of every hospital. Cardiac resuscitation is as pertinent to the patient undergoing tonsillectomy or gastrectomy as to one having repair of ventricular septal defect. There can be no doubt of the fact that hundreds of patients having general surgical procedures have been saved because the cardiac surgeon has taught general surgeons the techniques of treating cardiac arrest.

Remember the dread that doctors had of considering any form of surgery in a patient with heart disease? Remember the many extensive, learned, and futile discussions about what a patient with a cardiac condition could "stand" in the way of surgery, when they had, for example, intestinal obstruction or carcinoma of the rectum? Such discussions were manifestations of both the ignorance and the prejudice which had existed in this sphere for so long. Then the cardiac surgeon began performing major procedures on very sick hearts with low mortality rates. The "cardiac" patient obviously could tolerate a cardiac operation of the first magnitude with very slight risk. Equally obviously, such a patient with a general surgical problem could also be operated upon whenever the procedure was clearly indicated and the surgeon involved had the type of knowledge necessary to nurse a patient with a sick heart through major surgery. The general surgeon is learning to do this.

Postoperative care of the really sick patient needs special equipment and specially trained personnel. The cardiac surgeon insisted on such practices, and now recovery rooms and intensive therapy units have become widely established in modern hospitals.

Two very important techniques of broad application were first developed for cardiac surgery:

1. General body hypothermia now is used in many forms of surgery, particularly in patients with vascular lesions, cerebral disease, cirrhosis, pancreatitis, and thyrotoxicosis. Above all, hypothermia has critical potential in the future of the transplantation of tissue and organs.

2. Total (or partial) body perfusion has become a stimulating experimental tool in the study of general physiology, a technique for the treatment of the failing circulation in circulatory collapse, and a method for regional perfusion in cancer therapy. The methodology originated as a means to achieve open-heart operative procedures.

A by-product of devising new operations has been the development of new instruments and prosthetic devices, based on a broad study of plastic and other implantable prosthetic materials. Thus an extensive armamentarium of instruments including nontraumatic clamps, special sutures, hemostatic agents, and recording monitors were developed. Many of these have subsequently been widely adopted in general surgical use.

The problems associated with massive transfusion came under close scrutiny as total cardiopulmonary bypass became a more frequent procedure. Since, for a period, all perfusions were in essence an experiment in massive transfusion, a great stimulus was given to a critical evaluation of current techniques for the storage of blood, to the development of new coagulants and anticoagulants, and to a better understanding of the clotting mechanism and its disturbances. This knowledge is as applicable to an exenteration of the pelvis as it is to repair of coarctation of the aorta; and blood banking procedures have been extensively modified because of this newer information.

Perhaps the most important contribution of the cardiac and vascular surgeon to the growth of general surgery has been a demonstration of the need for surgical experimental laboratories. No previous branch of surgery had so clearly shown the importance of developing in the laboratory the techniques and instrumentation necessary to solve the challenge of operation on new and difficult anatomic problems. Gastric surgery, biliary surgery, and pulmonary surgery evolved mainly through human experiment, and in the early days of these developments the mortality and morbidity was staggering (ie, gastrectomy 60%; pneumonectomy 40%). Interestingly enough, cardiac surgery emerged almost full-fledged from the laboratory before its first application to the patient, and even the very earliest series of patients with surgical repair of patent ductus arteriosus, coarctation of the aorta, and pulmonary valvular stenosis, for example, was performed at operative mortality rates less than those still existing in gastric resection or cholecystectomy (ie, less than 2%).

The creation of these laboratories, in turn, had a profound effect upon surgical training, upon basic concepts in general surgery, and upon the development of many other fields within general surgery. Thus gynecologists have used vascular-anastomotic techniques to correct sterile fallopian tubes. Urologists have stopped occasionally taking out the wrong kidney for renal hypertension and have learned arterial bypass procedures. Orthopedists have learned to recognize and treat vascular injuries. Vascular injection diagnostic procedures have become widespread in all specialties. General surgeons treating major trauma have begun to repair lacerated arteries rather than to ligate them; and kidney transplants depend on vascular-anastomotic techniques.

In these research laboratories (created largely because of the interest of the cardiac surgeon) there worked an increasing number of young surgeons in training. Here they have encountered a renewed emphasis on surgical techniques—asepsis, hemostasis, and the gentle handling of tissue (the atraumatic surgery so essential to repair of the cardiovascular system). Thus, the surgical experimental laboratory has become a prime site for graduate surgical training—a tool to discipline the mind in research and to mold sound surgical technique. If it had done nothing else, the establishment by cardiac surgery of the surgical experimental laboratory would symbolize the breadth and depth of its contributions to general surgery.

Finally, the rapid growth of cardiac surgery in the last three decades has been an extensive challenge to the entire medical profession. For the first time in history, since the possibility of complete cure was now possible, the cardiologist had to face up to the fact that he was unable to make a completely accurate diagnosis of the particular type of cardiac disease from which his patients suffered. He realized that he did not really understand these diseases intimately. His response to this challenge was dramatic. There soon emerged a more accurate knowledge of the pathogenesis, pathology, physiopathology, and life history of various congenital and acquired forms of heart disease, a better understanding of signs and symptoms, and, thus, a markedly sharpened diagnostic acumen. Ancillary techniques such as cardiac catheterization and angiocardiography were devised. By careful analysis, the cardiologist finally began really to understand the electrocardiogram. He dramatically showed to the world that physicians can rise magnificently to new challenges for better patient care. No stimulus to the better understanding of heart disease in general and of all aspects of normal and abnormal circulation has ever been so successful in accelerating the pace of human understanding. Anesthesiologists, radiologists, internists, and pediatricians have all made tremendous strides in the conquest of these problems. It is obvious to all that the value of this newer knowledge has also benefited the general surgical patient as much as anyone. This is an era which demands precise preoperative diagnosis and deeper basic understanding of normal and abnormal physiology, bacteriology, and biochemistry for adequate care of the sick or traumatized patient. Cardiac surgery has had repercussions reaching from experimental biologic science to advanced therapeutics.

The cardiac surgeon *is* a specialist, yes, but he is a general surgeon in his training and, in fact, in his thinking. He regards the patient as a psychobiologic entity and his heart as a specific problem. His contributions to the practice of surgery have left a mark on the art which has changed its entire aspect. He need feel no shame for being one of "those cardiac surgeons"; and he can draw comfort from the fact that the surgeon who scoffs, though sarcastic, is using his contributions in every facet of his daily practice.

Henry Swan, MD
303 Josephine St
Denver

Intrathoracic Pheochromocytoma

A Case Report

RONALDO LUNA, MD
IRVING KATZ, MD
AND
RICHARD W. ERNST, MD
DALLAS, TEX

Intrathoracic pheochromocytoma is an entity which is seldom diagnosed prior to surgery. Only five cases out of 14 described in the literature, including our own, were diagnosed prior to surgery. This is predominantly due to the bizarre symptomatology in the presence of an intrathoracic pheochromocytoma, as well as to the fact that one suspects such a tumor in the mediastinum only if the patient has the full-blown symptomatology.

Submitted for publication Nov 2, 1962.

Senior Resident in Cardiothoracic Surgery (Dr. Luna); Resident in Surgery (Dr. Katz); Acting Chairman, Division of Cardiothoracic Surgery (Dr. Ernst).

Division of Cardiothoracic Surgery, Department of Surgery, The University of Texas, Southwestern Medical School.

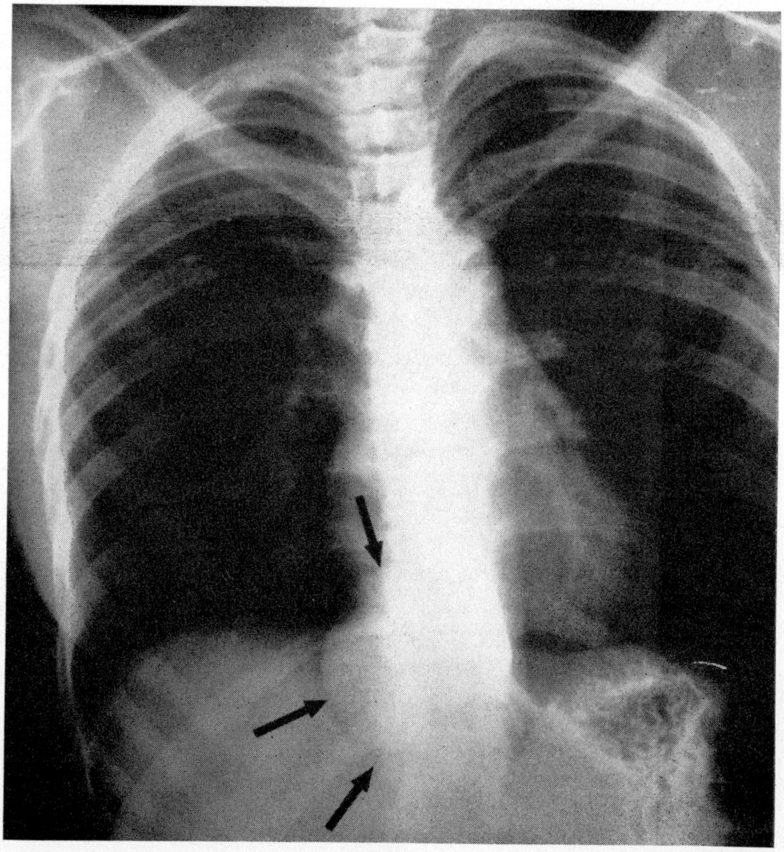

Fig 1.—Posterior-anterior view. Arrow indicates position of neoplasm.

Report of a Case

This 26-year-old Negro female was seen in the emergency room of Parkland Memorial Hospital on various occasions for the last four years. Every time she was seen her blood pressure and pulse were normal. For the last two years prior to admission she complained of intermittent right lateral chest pain, which on occasion was also present over the sternum. On one occasion the pain was very severe and was accompanied by shortness of breath. She was diagnosed to have anxiety each time. Other admissions to the emergency room were because of abdominal complaints due to pelvic inflammatory disease. On one of her last visits to the emergency room a routine chest x-ray revealed the presence of a homogeneous mass located just above the diaphragm in the right posterior gutter. It measured approximately 6 cm in transverse diameter (Figs 1 and 2). The patient was referred to the chest surgery service but did not keep her appointment. She returned to the emergency room again one year later complaining of palpitation, dizziness, and soreness in the vertex of her head and was again referred to the chest surgery service.

Physical examination on admission revealed the blood pressure to be 130/80, pulse 90, and the remainder of the physical examination was essentially normal. An electrocardiogram taken on this admission was normal. Repeat chest x-ray (Figs 1 and 2) again revealed the mass as previously described. The patient was prepared for surgery. The preoperative fasting blood sugar was 124 (normal in this laboratory 120 mg%). CBC, urinalysis, BUN, and electrolyte studies were all within normal limits.

On Aug 17, 1961, the patient underwent a right thoracotomy using endotracheal anesthesia consisting of nitrous oxide and halothane (Fluothane). Upon palpation of the tumor the blood pressure rose to 180/140, and it was at this time that a pheochromocytoma was suspected. Attempts were then made at completely ligating the vascular channels to the tumor. However, this was technically not feasible, because the tumor was extremely vascular. Upon removal of the tumor the blood pressure fell to 70/40. Metaraminol (Aramine) and phenylephrine (Neosynephrine) were started with the return of a normal blood pressure. The postoperative course was characterized by occasional hypotensive epi-

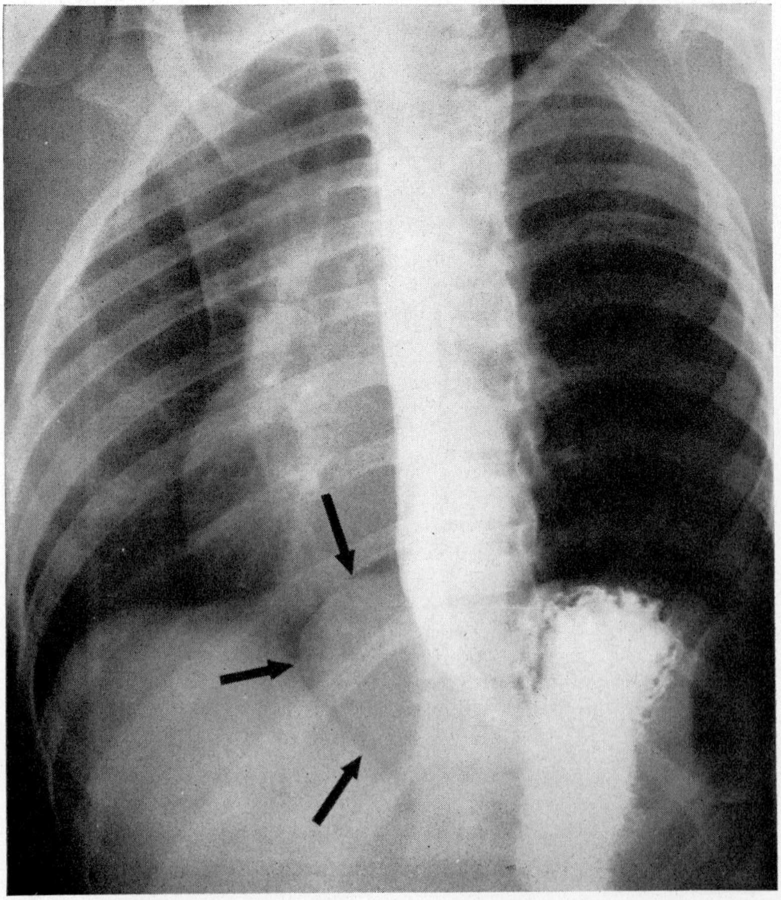

Fig 2.—Left anterior oblique view. Arrows indicate postion of neoplasm in low right posterior mediastinum.

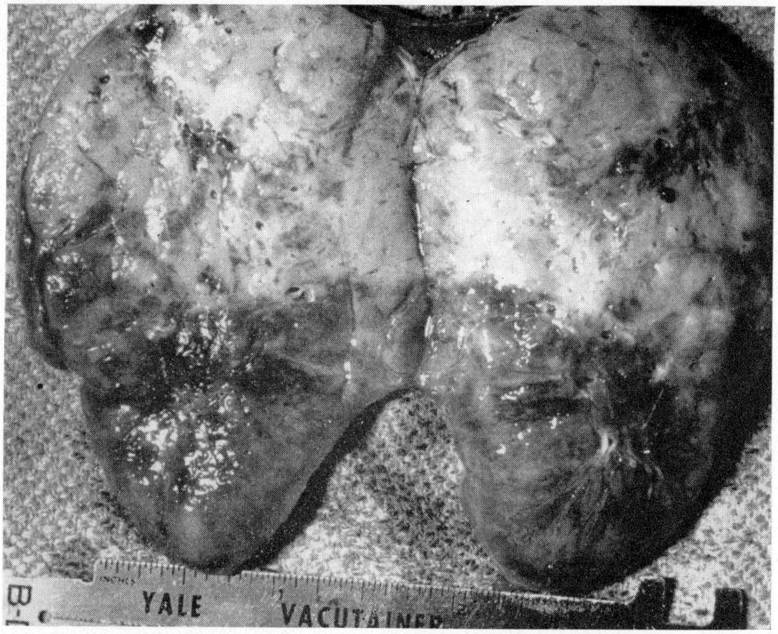

Fig 3.—Gross appearance; cross section of tumor.

sodes which were readily controlled by intravenous metaraminol. From the fourth postoperative day on the patient had a stable and normal blood pressure. The patient was discharged on the tenth postoperative day and has been asymptomatic since then.

Gross and Microscopic Description of Tumor.—The specimen consisted of a tumor mass measuring 8 × 6 × 3 cm and weighed 80 gm. The tumor was well encapsulated, soft, and tan, with multiple small yellow flecks and multiple small hemorrhagic flecks. The microscopic examination revealed numerous packets of cells with the packets varying markedly in size. The stroma separating these packets consisted of a very delicate fibrous tissue framework containing numerous capillaries. The cells within these packets consisted primarily of a cell with a very regular hyperchromatic round nucleus and with abundant vesiculated cytoplasm. In small areas the cytoplasm was somewhat more scanty and less vesicular, but the nuclei varied only slightly in overall size and staining characteristics. The pathological diagnosis was pheochromocytoma (Figs 3, 4, and 5).

The tissue assay of the tumor revealed 2.296 mg per gram of tissue of levarterenol bitartrate

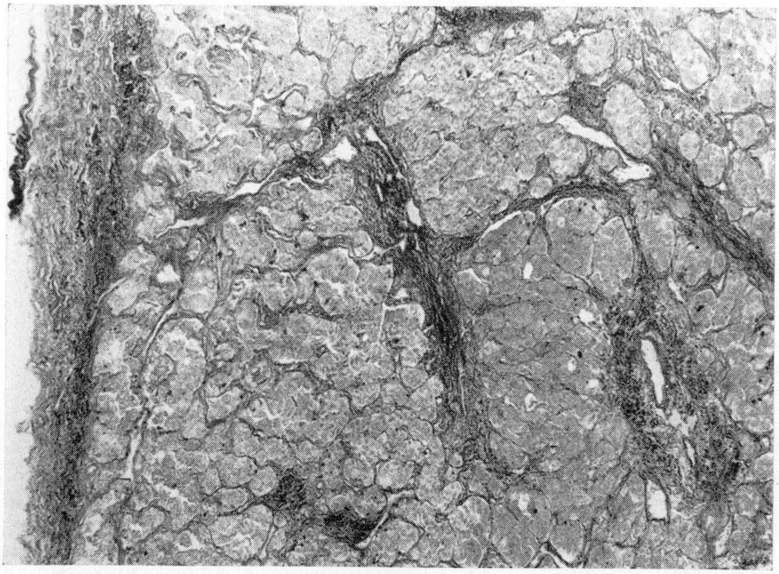

Fig 4.—Microscopic appearance. Note the well-developed capsule. Reduced about 34% from mag × 120.

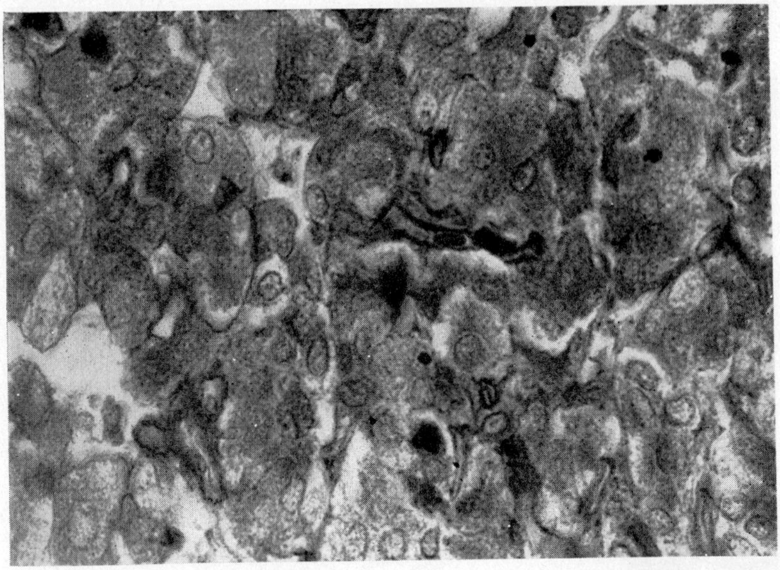

Fig 5.—Microscopic section revealing cellular detail. Reduced about 34% from mag × 800.

(norepinephrine) and 0.26 mg per gram of tissue of epinephrine.

Comment

Reviewing the cases presented in the literature [1-11] and adding our own it is noted that the symptomatology can vary significantly. Fifty per cent of the patients complained of intermittent headaches; 50% complained of profuse perspiration; 25% complained of chest pain; 50% complained of palpitation, and only 50% had changes in blood pressure. This probably explains the fact that only five of these cases were diagnosed preoperatively. If one suspects a pheochromocytoma preoperatively, the usual tests [12,13] with the detection of the neoplasm should be carried out in order to be prepared for the rather dramatic pressure changes which do occur on the operating table. The average age of all patients is 31 years. This is a small group and, therefore, the sex distribution may not be significant. However, in the group there were eight males and six females.

There are a few points which can aid in a correct preoperative diagnosis, however. A patient with a mass in the mediastinum, especially when this patient falls into the younger age group and complains of intermittent headache, profuse perspiration, and palpitations accompanied occasionally by dizzy spells, should be suspected to have a pheochromocytoma. If we can also observe a change in the blood pressure, this will add significantly to the completeness of the picture.

Even when the diagnosis is not made preoperatively, it is essential that the surgeon realizes the possibility of a pheochromocytoma once he has opened the chest. Here, important information consists of the appearance of the tumor, which usually is a very vascular one deriving its blood supply from many sources. In addition, it is often noted that the blood pressure may rise significantly during manipulation of the tumor. This is almost always followed by a severe drop of the pressure to shock level. It is essential at this time that the patient be treated with a vasoconstrictive drug such as metaraminol and/or phenylephrine. When this is done immediately, the patient should not suffer any ill effects from this marked drop in blood pressure and should be controllable without too much difficulty postoperatively until the blood pressure becomes stabilized. Although we have not had this experience, we propose that if the blood pressure cannot be stabilized by the conventional means postoperatively it is quite likely that the patient has multiple pheochromocytomata rather than just one,[7-10] which demonstrates that pheochromocytomata can occur anywhere along the sympathetic chain in the abdomen, chest, or neck. Cahill[13] classifies the symptoms of a pheochromocytoma into the silent, the paroxysmal, and the continuous hypertensive. The silent type occurs in an individual who may have a pheochromocytoma without experiencing any of the effects of its presence. This type is usually discovered at x-ray, operative exploration, or at autopsy. It is in this type of unsuspected neoplasm that a dreaded anesthetic mortality or pressure change may occur. Those that experienced paroxysmal hypertension were frequently difficult to differentiate from hyperthyroidism or psychoneurosis prior to the advent of specific diagnostic tests. Of known tumor cases, 30% to 40% experience the paroxysmal form of hypertension. Questioning of these patients will usually reveal a history of acute attacks of palpitations, headaches, anxiety, restlessness, sweating, and a feeling of exhaustion.

Summary

The fourteenth case in the world's literature of an intrathoracic pheochromocytoma is presented. A review of the cases presented is made in an attempt to find means by which the tumor can be diagnosed preoperatively and treated in the most prudent manner. The major symptoms preoperatively are compiled. The symptomatology on the operating table as well as the tumor appearance is discussed. The postoperative management is mentioned.

We are indebted to Vernie A. Stembridge, MD, Professor of Pathology, University of Texas, Southwestern Medical School for his able assistance in the interpretation of the histologic sections.

Richard W. Ernst, MD, Acting Chairman, Division of Thoracic and Cardiac Surgery, The University of Texas, Southwestern Medical School, 5323 Harry Hines Blvd, Dallas 35.

REFERENCES

1. Miller, J. W.: Ein Paraganglion des Brustsympathicus, Zbl Allg Path 35:85-94, 1924-1925.

2. Phillips, B.: Intrathoracic Pheochromocytoma, Arch Path 30:916-921, 1940.

3. Maier, H. C.: Intrathoracic Pheochromocytoma with Hypertension, Ann Surg 130:1059-1065, 1949.

4. Nissen, R.: Chirurgische Moglichkeiten in der Behandlung der Hypertonie, Mschr Psychiat Neurol 117:316-337, 1949.

5. Overholt, R. H.; Ramsay, B. H., and Meissner, W. A.: Intrathoracic Pheochromocytoma: Report of a Case, Dis Chest 17:55-62, 1950.

6. McLeish, G. R., and Adler, D.: A Case of Intrathoracic Pheochromocytoma with Hypertension, Acta Med Scand 152 (Supp 306):135-144, 1955.

7. Cone, T. E., Jr.,; Allen, M. S., and Pearson, H. A.: Pheochromocytoma in Children, Pediatrics 19:44-56, 1957.

8. Euler, U. S., and Von Strom, G.: Present Status of Diagnosis and Treatment of Pheochromocytoma, Circulation 15:5-13, 1957.

9. Pampari, D., and Lacerenza, C.: Intrathoracic Pheochromocytoma, J Thorac Cardiov Surg 36:174-181, 1958.

10. Maier, H. C., and Humphreys, G. H.: Intrathoracic Pheochromocytoma, J Thorac Cardiov Surg 36:625-641, 1958.

11. Green, W. O., and Bassett, F. H.: Intrathoracic Pheochromocytoma: Report of a Case, Amer J Clin Path 35:142-146, 1961.

12. Roth, G. M.; Flock, E. V.; Kvale, W. F.; Waugh, J. M., and Ogg, J.: Pharmacologic and Chemical Tests as an Aid in the Diagnosis of Pheochromocytoma, Circulation 21:769-778, 1960.

13. Cahill, G. F.: Pheochromocytoma, Bull NY Acad Med 29:749-764, 1953.

Intestinal Hemorrhage in von Recklinghausen's Disease

N. PERRYMAN COLLINS, MD
BALTIMORE

Neurogenic Tumors as Cause

Patients with multiple neurofibromatosis are prone to develop neurogenic tumors within the peritoneal and retroperitoneal spaces, but such a tumor arising in the wall of the bowel is extremely unusual. In a collected review of 1,399 patients with a benign small intestinal tumor only 90 had a neurogenic tumor, and in only 14 were there cutaneous manifestations of von Recklinghausen's disease.[1] Intestinal bleeding produced by such a tumor has occasionally been observed,[2-5] and in some instances hemorrhage has been massive.[2-4] Perforation [6] as well as intestinal obstruction [7] from these tumors has been reported. During a period of seven years there have been two patients with von Recklinghausen's disease who have undergone surgery at The Johns Hopkins Hospital for bleeding neurogenic tumor of the intestinal tract. Because of the rarity of intestinal bleeding from a neurogenic tumor in patients with multiple neurofibromatosis and the difficulty in establishing a correct diagnosis for the cause of bleeding, the clinical records of these patients are presented.

Report of Cases

CASE 1.—A 39-year-old Negro female elevator operator at this hospital was admitted for the ninth time to the hospital on April 15, 1955, because of rectal bleeding. She had been known to have von Recklinghausen's disease for many years, and five years previously had undergone removal of a 16 × 9 cm neurofibroma of the right thigh because of difficulty in bending her knee. For at least four years prior to the current admission she had been known to have a chronic anemia of blood loss type which was thought probably to be a result of menorrhagia which had been present for about a year. Consequently, she underwent total abdominal hysterectomy but the anemia persisted. One year later, for the first time, she was found to have occult blood in her feces. Her hematocrit on admission to the hospital at that time was 23%. All diagnostic procedures, including gastrointestinal x-rays and a barium enema, were negative for a source of bleeding. Sigmoidoscopy was unremarkable except for demonstrating the presence of severe internal and external hemorrhoids. She was given 1,500 ml of whole blood, and hemorrhoidectomy was done. She was well for a short time after discharge from the hospital but was subsequently found to be anemic again and was treated with iron medication without response. One month prior to the current admission she was hospitalized again with a hematocrit of 20%, and again repeat x-ray studies were normal, although her feces remained consistently positive for occult blood. She was given 2,500 ml of whole blood which raised her hematocrit to 40%. She was discharged and remained well without evident bleeding until the day prior to admission, when she passed approximately an ounce of bright red blood after a normal bowel movement. She came to the hospital and was admitted. At this time she appeared thin and deformed, having a dorsal scoliosis and innumerable neurofibromata and café au lait spots of varying sizes on her skin. The rest of the physical examination was unremarkable except for her nail beds and mucous membranes which were pale. Her hematocrit was 27%, and the remainder of the laboratory examinations were essentially normal. A long intestinal tube was passed, and the intestinal content was aspirated at various

Submitted for publication Dec 26, 1962.

Resident in Surgery, The Johns Hopkins Hospital.

From the Department of Surgery, The Johns Hopkins University School of Medicine and Hospital.

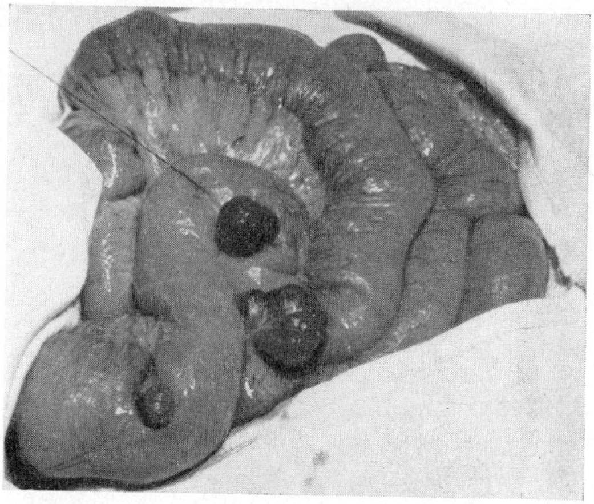

Fig 1 (case 1).—Three of the six tumors in the segment of jejunum at the time of operation.

levels and examined for occult blood. Guaiac-positive aspirate was first obtained after the tube had passed a distance of 7½ ft. It was felt that she probably had a neurogenic tumor in her small intestine causing the bleeding, and consequently she was transfused and operated upon. The proximal 2 ft of jejunum had six yellowish-red tumors, all of which were pedunculated, arising from the antemesenteric border of the intestine and varying in size from 1 to 4 cm in diameter (Fig 1). Approximately two feet distal to these was a single tumor of similar nature, and several much smaller (2-3 mm) ones were on the duodenum and stomach. No other tumor or abnormalities were found. The proximal 2 ft of jejunum containing the six tumors was resected, and an end-to-end anastomosis was done. Examination of the resected bowel showed that these tumors arose in the wall of the bowel and one had ulcerated through the mucosa. Each of these tumors on histologic examination was found to be typical of a neurilemmoma (Fig 2). The patient's postoperative course was uneventful, and she was discharged on the tenth postoperative day. She had no further gross bleeding, her stools remained negative for occult blood, and the anemia did not recur. She did well for six years thereafter but died suddenly from a massive cerebral vascular accident.

Case 2.—A 47-year-old white housewife was admitted for the third time to this hospital on Nov 5, 1962, passing gross blood per rectum. She was known to have had von Recklinghausen's disease since early childhood but had otherwise been in good health until three years previously when she was admitted to the medical service of the hospital for the first time with dyspnea and ankle edema and complaining of having passed tarry and grossly bloody stools for several days' duration. She was found to be severely anemic with a hematocrit of 14%. Gastrointestinal and small intestinal x-ray examinations were normal. A barium enema, however, demonstrated an area of questionable extrinsic pressure on the sigmoid colon. She was given 4,000 ml of whole blood during this hospitalization, resulting in a satisfactory rise in hematocrit to a normal level. The source of the bleeding was never determined, and she was subsequently discharged. She was followed in the clinic where she was found to have persistent occult blood in the feces but otherwise was felt to be in good health. One year later she again passed tarry stools over a three-day

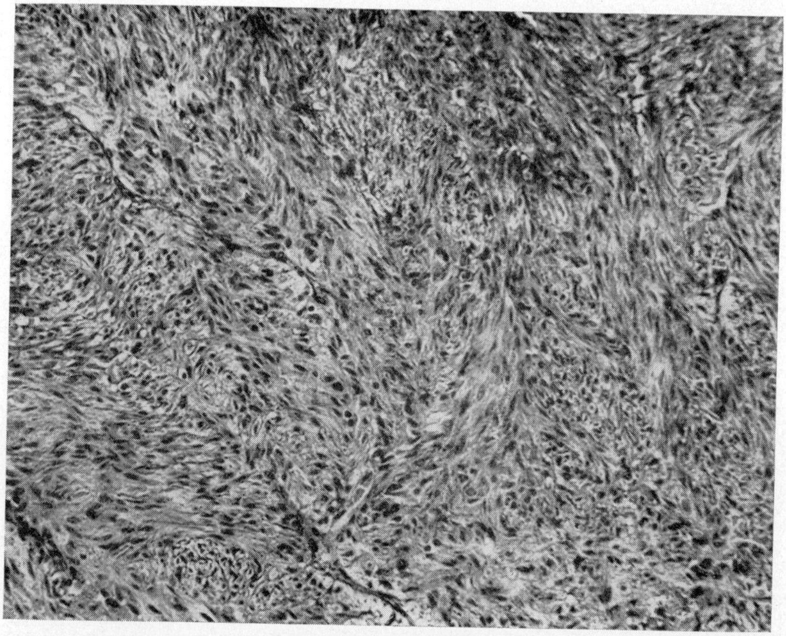

Fig 2.—Histologic pattern of neurilemmoma. All of the resected tumors showed the same pattern. Hematoxylin and eosin; reduced 11% from mag × 200.

period, became weak, and was readmitted to the hospital again on the medical service. At this time she was in mild shock, and it was found that her hematocrit had fallen from a previously normal level to 23%. Repeat gastrointestinal x-ray examination again was normal. The barium enema this time was normal, but the small intestinal x-rays showed questionable pressure from an extrinsic mass in the pelvis. She was given 5,500 ml of whole blood during this hospital stay and was discharged again without a definitive diagnosis. She did well after discharge for ten months and then began passing bloody bowel movements. She came to the hospital and again was admitted on the medical service. Physical examination was unremarkable except for

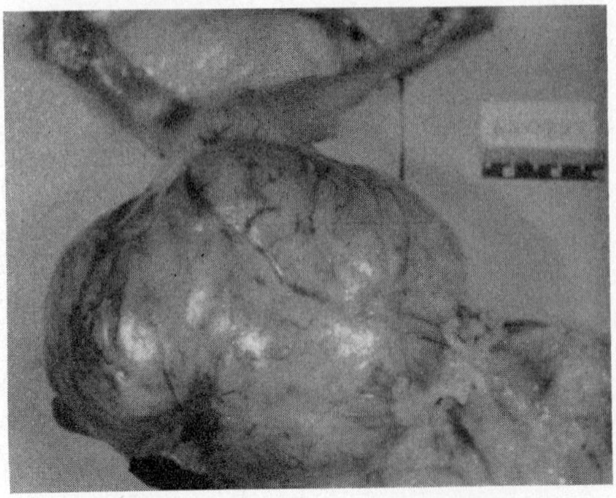

Fig 4 (case 2).—Intestinal neurilemmoma. The resected portion of bowel and mesentery is at the top of picture and the tumor with attached omentum at the bottom.

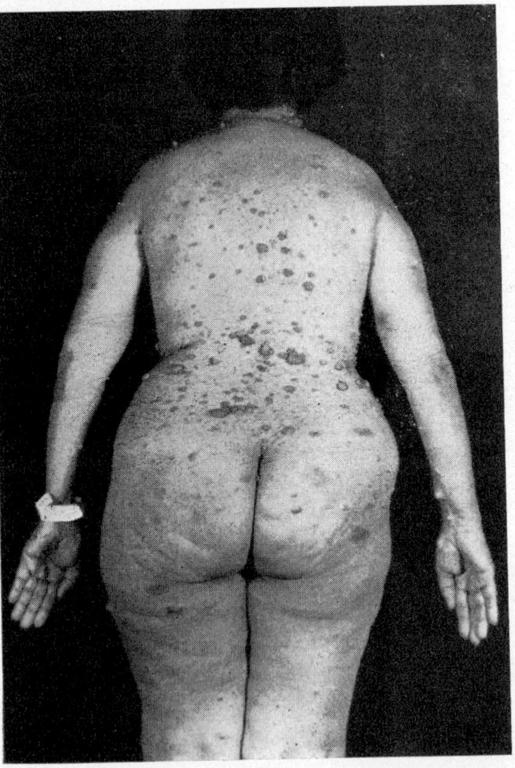

Fig 3 (case 2).—Patient showing typical skin tumors and café au lait spots of von Recklinghausen's disease.

multiple neurofibromata, café au lait spots of the skin (Fig 3), and evidence of anemia. Repeat gastrointestinal x-rays and barium enema were normal. Shortly after admission she began bleeding profusely, passing large quantities of blood per rectum. She required 4,000 ml of whole blood in a period of eight hours to maintain a normal pulse and blood pressure. She was operated on as an emergency procedure at which time, through a midline abdominal incision, a 9 × 11 cm round tumor arising from the antemesenteric border of a loop of ileum was found (Fig 4). This mass was in the ileum about two to three feet proximal to the ileocecal valve and was firmly attached to the pelvic peritoneum by a dense adhesion thereby pulling this loop of ileum into the pelvis. A portion of the greater omentum was also attached. The intestine in this region and distally was distended with blood in the lumen. By differential occlusion of the intestinal lumen the source of bleeding was localized to the segment of ileum containing the tumor. A 14 cm length of ileum containing the tumor was resected along with the attached segment of mesentery, greater omentum, and adhesive band. The intestinal continuity was re-established by an end-to-end ileoileostomy. Two smaller (1-2 cm) similar tumors were found on the antemesenteric border of the ileum near the ileocecal valve. These were excised. Further exploration of the abdominal cavity revealed no other tumor or abnormalities. Examination of the specimen revealed that a large area of ileal mucosa overlying the tumor had been ulcerated (Fig 5 and 6). The histologic pattern of the major tumor and the two smaller ones was that of a neurilemmoma (Fig 7), and it was clearly

Fig 5.—Segment of ileum opened to show large area of ulceration of mucosa produced by the tumor.

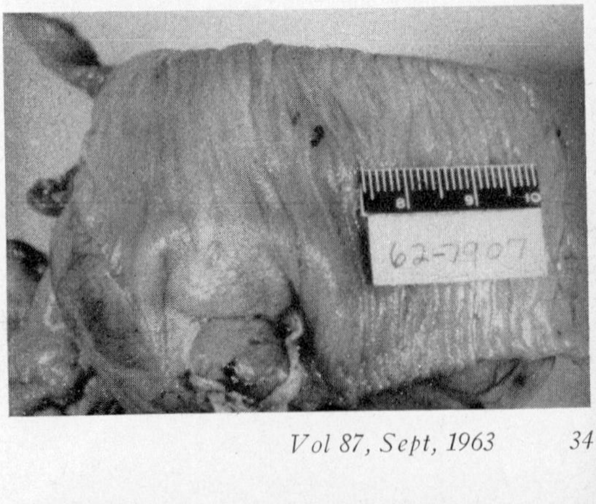

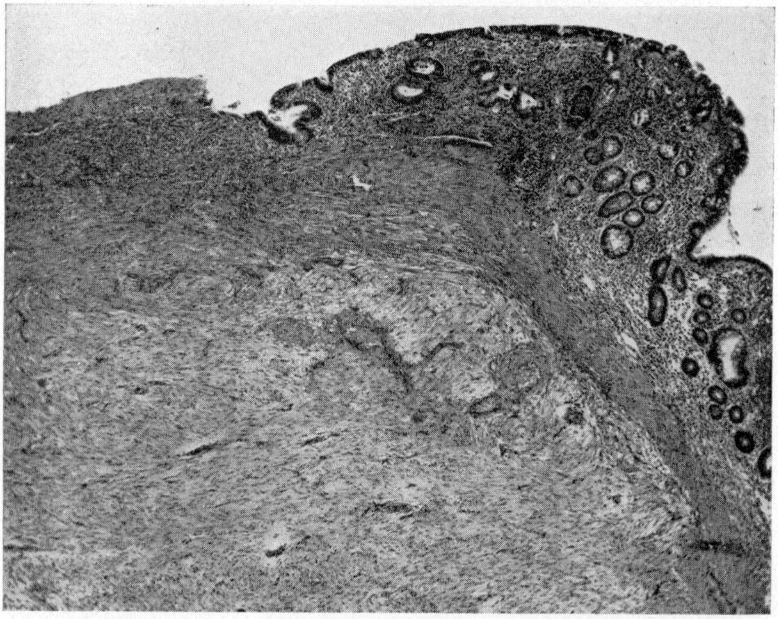

Fig 6.—Histologic appearance of tumor with area of ulceration. The tumor is in the submucosa stretching and thinning the overlying muscularis mucosa. Hematoxylin and eosin; reduced 11% from mag × 50.

demonstrated that the tumors arose in the wall of the intestine. She did well after surgery, having no further bleeding, was discharged on the tenth postoperative day, and has continued to remain well.

Comment

The presence of a small bowel tumor is difficult to detect and is most often discovered at the time a patient is operated on for intestinal obstruction, the obstruction most frequently being due to intussusception but occasionally to volvulus or to blockage of the lumen by the tumor itself. Less commonly, intestinal bleeding may occur and in one large series was present in 30% of patients with small bowel tumors.[1] In a third of these patients the bleeding was massive. In the group of patients that had only occult bleeding and anemia, a surprisingly large number of them were followed for many years without a correct diagnosis of the

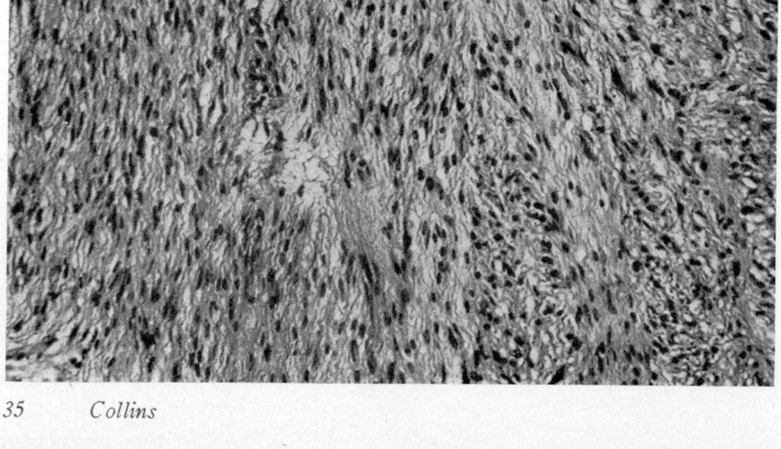

Fig 7 (case 2).—Histologic pattern of neurilemmoma. Hematoxylin and eosin; reduced 10% from mag × 200.

cause of bleeding being made. This usually resulted in the patient being hospitalized on many occasions and requiring numerous transfusions. The bleeding in patients with intestinal neurogenic tumors is usually chronic, leading to symptoms of weakness, fatigue, and exertional dyspnea, but occasionally massive hemorrhage will occur.

Both of the patients in this report had evidence of occult bleeding and anemia for several years, and in addition the second patient had experienced three episodes of massive hemorrhage superimposed on the occult bleeding. The first patient had been admitted on three previous occasions over a two-year period for anemia and had received a total of 4,500 ml of whole blood before surgery was undertaken. The second patient had been admitted to the hospital three times in three years with rather severe intestinal bleeding and had received 13,500 ml of whole blood prior to undergoing operation which had to be done as an emergency procedure. It would have been more desirable had surgery been undertaken in each of these patients earlier and particularly so in the second patient. Although intestinal neurogenic tumors are unusual in patients with von Recklinghausen's disease, the presence of this type tumor should be strongly considered in such a patient in whom intestinal hemorrhage occurs, whether occult or gross. Since a preoperative diagnosis may be very difficult to establish with any certainty, abdominal exploration should be done when there is evidence of intestinal bleeding. Neurogenic tumors in patients with von Recklinghausen's disease are likely to undergo sarcomatous changes, but in these two patients as well as in others reported the tumors were benign, and it has been possible to remove the tumor or tumors by resecting a minimal amount of bowel, since these tumors tended to be more or less localized to a short segment of intestine. After removal of the segment of bowel containing the tumor these patients have had no further bleeding, thereby eliminating the necessity for numerous hospitalizations and multiple blood transfusions as well as minimizing the hazard of a possible exsanguinating hemorrhage.

N. Perryman Collins, MD, Resident in Surgery, The Johns Hopkins Hospital, Baltimore, Md.

REFERENCES

1. River, L.; Silverstein, J.; and Tope, J. W.: Benign Neoplasms of the Small Intestine: A Critical Comprehensive Review with Reports of 20 New Cases, Int Abstr Surg 102:1, 1956.

2. Farrar, T., and Chappell, F. W.: Severe Gastrointestinal Hemorrhage Resulting From Recklinghausen's Disease, AMA Arch Surg 79:106, 1959.

3. Shaiken, J.: Tumors of the Small Bowel, Amer Pract 3:388, 1952.

4. Shaw, R. C.: Von Recklinghausen's Disease of the Small Intestine Associated With Skin Lesions, Amer J Surg 80:360, 1950.

5. Wilson, J. S., and Anderson, A. A.: Cutaneous and Intestinal Neurofibromatosis, Amer J Surg 100: 761, 1960.

6. Warshauer, F. B., and Nelson, R E.: Neurofibroma of Jejunum with Perforation: A Case Report, Amer Surg 19:467, 1953.

7. Collins, J. D.: Neurofibroma of the Small Intestine, Ann Surg 119:362, 1944.

Annular Pancreas and Duodenal Obstruction in the Neonate

A Review

JOHN M. JACKSON, MD
FAIRFIELD, ALA

Annular pancreas is a condition in which pancreatic tissue forms a partial or complete ring encircling the descending duodenum. The condition may manifest itself in infancy, childhood, or adult life. It is an unusual cause of duodenal obstruction in the neonatal period. A recent patient with annular pancreas presenting as duodenal obstruction in a newborn infant has prompted this review of neonatal operative cases.

Tiedemann [1] is frequently given credit for the first description of annular pancreas. However, Ravitch and Woods,[2] after reviewing Tiedemann's original article, have credited Ecker with the first description of the anomaly in humans.

Pathology-Embryology [3-4]

The pancreas develops as dorsal and ventral out-pouchings from the entodermal lining of the foregut at the 3-4 mm stage. The dorsal anlage, growing more rapidly than the ventral bud, forms the body, tail, and part of the head of the pancreas. The ventral anlage is carried away from the duodenum by the lengthening common bile duct to which it is attached. At approximately the seventh week, in normal gut rotation, the ventral bud lies in contact with the right caudal border of the dorsal bud, and fusion occurs (Fig 1). The main pancreatic duct of Wirsung is derived from the duct of the ventral anlage and the distal portion of the dorsal anlage. The accessory pancreatic duct of Santorini, when present, is derived from the proximal portion of the duct of the dorsal anlage. Most authors feel that the initial abnormality in the development of annular pancreas is a fixation of the free end of the ventral pancreatic anlage. With subsequent rotation of the duodenum, the ventral pancreatic anlage is drawn out and encircles the descending duodenum (Fig 2). As fusion of the tip of the ventral anlage and the anterior aspect of the dorsal anlage occurs, encirclement of the duodenum becomes complete.

Clinical Picture

Annular pancreas may be clinically manifested by either acute or chronic progressive low-grade duodenal obstruction. Occasionally it is seen as an incidental finding at autopsy.

Acute duodenal obstruction with vomiting, dehydration, and weight loss is seen more often in infants. Abdominal distention is usually absent because of the high obstruction. The vomitus may or may not contain bile, depending on the exact site and degree of obstruction. If the obstruction is incomplete, the symptoms may be less acute, and the infant may be admitted as a feeding problem with weight loss.

Confirmatory abdominal x-rays, with or without opaque media, usually reveal the "double bubble" sign with air fluid levels in the stomach and proximal duodenum. With

Submitted for publication Dec 3, 1962.

From the Department of Surgery, Lloyd Noland Hospital.

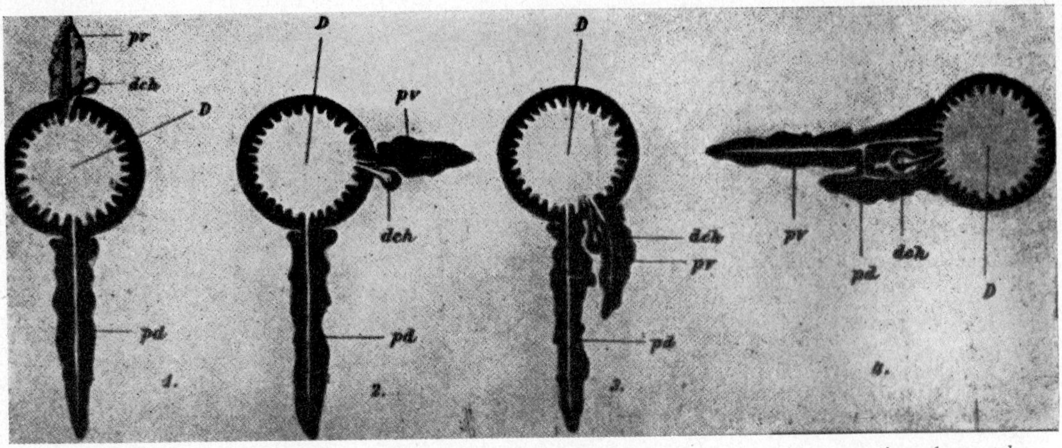

Fig 1.—The ventral pancreatic anlage, *pv,* migrates toward the dorsal pancreatic anlage, *pd,* to fuse and enclose between them the ductus choledochus, *dch.* The ducts of the ventral and dorsal anlagen anastomose as can be seen in the last figure. Duodenum, *D.* (After Lecco[27]) (Reproduced with permission of *Surgery, Gynecology and Obstetrics,* 54 E Erie St, Chicago, Illinois 60611.)

complete obstruction, no air will be seen distal to the duodenum.

Treatment

Numerous surgical procedures have been described for the treatment of annular pancreas. These include various bypass procedures and direct attack on the obstructing annular lesion.

Division of the ring of pancreatic tissue is fraught with numerous complications and physiologically fails to take into consideration the basic pathological condition. Even if the ring could be safely divided, the minute caliber of the duodenum, which has been encircled by pancreatic tissue since the seventh week of gestation, would still require some type of bypass procedure.

Retrocolic side-to-side duodenojejunostomy is the simplest and most effective operation for correction of the obstructing

Fig 2.—Development of annular pancreas is demonstrated. The ventral pancreatic anlage (*pv*) becomes fixed at its free end, during its subsequent migration with the rotation of the duodenum (*D*) the ventral anlage is drawn out, and, with the fusion of the two anlagen, the pancreas comes to surround the duodenum. Dorsal pancreatic anlage (*pd*), ductus choledochus (*dch*). (After Lecco[27]) (Reproduced with permission of *Surgery, Gynecology and Obstetrics,* 54 E Erie St, Chicago, Illinois 60611.)

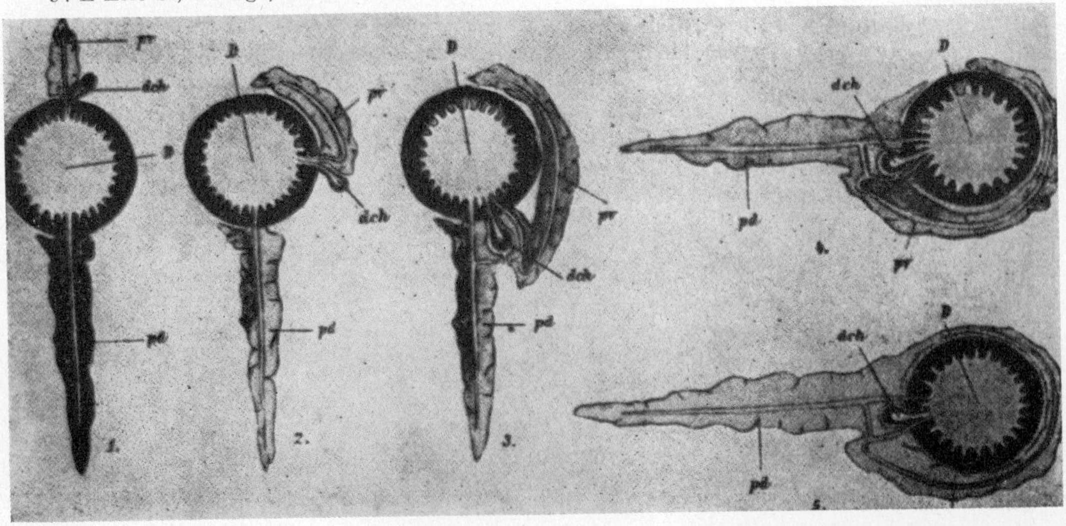

Fifty-Five Previously Reported Cases

Author *	Date	Age, Sex	Operation	Results	Coexisting Anomalies
Vidal (5)	1905	3 days, M	Posterior gastroenterostomy	Died	Duodenal stenosis
Gross & Chisholm (7)	1944	3 days, F	Duodenojejunostomy	Cure	Malrotation
Burger & Alrich (8)	1949	4 days, F	Duodenoduodenostomy	Died	Duodenal stenosis
Glover & Barry (9)	1949	2 days, F	Division of ring Duodenojejunostomy	Died	Duodenal stenosis
Ravitch & Woods (2)	1950	3 days, F	Anticolic duodenojejunostomy	Cure	Duodenal stenosis
Ravitch & Woods	1950	8 days, M	Gastroduodenostomy	Cure	Duodenal atresia, malrotation, portal vein over duodenum
Shapiro, Dzurik, & Gerrish (10)	1952	4 days, F	Gastroduodenostomy	Cure	Duodenal atreasia
Shapiro, Dzurik, & Gerrish	1952	6 days, F	Duodenoduodenostomy	Died	Mongolism, duodenal stenosis
Shapiro, Dzurik, & Gerrish	1952	17 days, M	Duodenoduodenostomy	Cure	Mongolism, duodenal stenosis
Shapiro, Dzurik, & Gerrish	1952	8 days, F	Duodenoduodenostomy	Cure	Duodenal atresia
Wilson & Bushart (11)	1952	4 wk, M	Posterior gastrojejunostomy	Cure	None
Wilson & Bushart	1952	9 days, M	Posterior duodenojejunostomy	Died	None
Gross (12)	1953	2 days, F	Duodenojejunostomy	Died	Malrotation
Gross	1953	1 day, F	Duodenojejunostomy	Cure	Meckel's diverticulum
Gross	1953	5 days, F	Duodenojejunostomy	Cure	None
Gross	1953	5 days, F	Duodenojejunostomy	Cure	Possible mongolism
Gross	1953	1 day, M	Duodenojejunostomy	Died	Congenital heart disease, esophageal atresia
Gross	1953	5 days, M	Duodenojejunostomy	Cure	Malrotation
Gross	1953	1 day, M	Duodenojejunostomy	Died	Esophageal atresia, imperforate anus, congenital heart disease
Gross	1953	2 days, M	Duodenojejunostomy	Cure	Possible mongolism
Kiesewetter & Koop (13)	1954	18 days, M	Division of ring (secondary gastrojejunostomy)	Died	Duodenal stenosis, mongolism
Kiesewetter & Koop	1954	4 days, M	Duodenojejunostomy (secondary gastrojejunostomy)	Died	Duodenal stenosis
Kiesewetter & Koop	1954	6 days, F	Gastrojejunostomy and gastrostomy	Died	Esophageal atresia, tracheo-esophageal fistula, duodenal atresia
Kiesewetter & Koop	1954	5 days, M	Duodenojejunostomy	Cure	Duodenal atresia, malrotation, accessory spleens
Kiesewetter & Koop	1954	3 days, F	Duodenojejunostomy	Cure	None
Small & Berman (14)	1954	3 days, M	Posterior duodenojejunostomy	Cure	None
Hope & Gibbons (15)	1954	14 days, M	Resection of ring (secondary anterior gastrojejunostomy)	Died	Mongolism, duodenal stenosis
Hope & Gibbons	1954	5 days, M	Duodenojejunostomy (secondary gastrojejunostomy)	Died	Duodenal stenosis
Hope & Gibbons	1954	6 days, F	Posterior gastroenterostomy and gastrostomy	Died	Tracheo-esophageal fistula, duodenal atresia
Hope & Gibbons	1954	5 days, M	Gastrojejunostomy	Died	Malrotation, duodenal atresia
Hope & Gibbons	1954	7 days, F	Section of band crossing the 4th portion of duodenum and freeing of ligament of Treitz (secondary duodenoduodenostomy)	Cure	Duodenal fibrosis, 4th portion, malrotation, agenesis of right lung, Sprengel's deformity, deformity of spine
Rickham (16)	1954	2 days, M	Duodenojejunostomy	Cure	Tricuspid atresia
Rickham	1954	8 days, M	Duodenojejunostomy	Died	Duodenal atresia
Rickham	1954	4 days, F	Duodenoduodenostomy	Cure	None
Cohen & Potter (17)	1954	3 wk, F	Duodenojejunostomy	Died	Tetralogy of Fallot, ductus arteriosus, patent foramen ovale, duodenal stenosis
Carroll (18)	1955	3 wk, F	Lysis of adhesion (secondary duodenojejunostomy)	Died	Malrotation
Carroll	1955	4 wk, M	Posterior gastrojejunostomy	Cure	None
Carroll	1955	8 days, M	Duodenojejunostomy	Died	None
Carroll	1955	2 wk, F	Duodenojejunostomy	Cure	None
Farringer (19)	1955	19 days, F	Posterior duodenojejunostomy	Cure	None
Frucht (20)	1956	3½ wk, F	Duodenojejunostomy	Cure	Malrotation, mongolism
Wilkinson & Simms (21)	1957	2 days, F	Duodenojejunostomy	Cure	None
Large (22)	1957	4 days, M	Posterior gastroenterostomy	Died	None
Weatherill, Forgrave, & Carpenter (23)	1958	9 days, M	Retrocolic duodenojejunostomy	Died	None
Weatherill, Forgrave, & Carpenter	1958	3 days, M	Retrocolic duodenojejunostomy	Cure	None

Fifty-Five Previously Reported Cases—Continued

Author *	Date	Age, Sex	Operation	Results	Coexisting Anomalies
Gilroy & Adams (24)	1960	2 days, F	Posterior gastrojejunostomy	Died	Duodenal stenosis
Hays, Greaney, & Hill (25)	1961	3 days, F	Retrocolic duodenojejunostomy	Cure	Peritoneal bands across duodenum
Hays, Greaney, & Hill	1961	3 days, F	Retrocolic duodenojejunostomy	Cure	None
Hays, Greaney, & Hill	1961	2 days, M	Retrocolic duodenojejunostomy	Cure	Mongolism
Hays, Greaney, & Hill	1961	6 days, M	Retrocolic duodenojejunostomy	Cure	None
Hays, Greaney, & Hill	1961	2 days, M	Gastrostomy, colostomy	Died	Tracheo-esophageal fistula, imperforate anus and cryptorchid
Hays, Greaney, & Hill	1961	2 days, M	Retrocolic duodenojejunostomy	Died	Tracheo-esophageal fistula
Hays, Greaney, & Hill	1961	5 days, M	Retrocolic duodenojejunostomy	Died	Mongolism, malrotation, duodenal stenosis, Meckel's diverticulum
Kie, Wittebol, & Lunding (26)	1961	7 days, M	Mobilization of duodenum, Secondary duodenojejunostomy	Died	Mongolism
Kie, Wittebol, & Lunding	1961	2 wk, F	Duodenojejunostomy	Cure	None

* Parentheses indicate reference numbers.

lesion. This procedure was utilized in our recent patient with an excellent result.

Review of Neonatal Operative Case Reports

The first successful operative procedure for annular pancreas was performed by Vidal in 1905.[5] Fifty-four additional case reports recorded in the English literature have had surgery during the neonatal period. Twenty-five of these 55 patients died, a mortality rate of 45% (see Table).

The operative procedure in four cases included division of the ring of pancreatic tissue with primary or secondary bypass procedures. All of these patients died.

Fourteen infants had gastroenterostomy, gastroduodenostomy, or duodenoduodenostomy. Six, or 43%, died.

Duodenojejunostomy was performed in 33 cases with 12 deaths, a mortality rate of 36%.

Three patients had lysis of adhesions or mobilization of the duodenum. All three had secondary bypass procedures. Two of these infants died postoperatively. Gastrostomy and colostomy were performed on a single patient who died.

Coexisting congenital anomalies were a major factor in the high mortality reported in these cases. Thirty-nine, or 70% of the reported cases, had at least one associated anomaly. Duodenal stenosis or atresia was the most frequently reported anomaly associated with annular pancreas. It was described in 22 of the 54 patients, or 40%. It is this condition in the neonatal period which negates simple division of the pancreatic ring. In all four of the patients who had division of the ring there was some degree of duodenal stenosis. Whelan and Hamilton[6] feel that this frequent association of the two anomalies may be more than coincidental. They point out that evolution of the gut from the solid stage occurs at the same time as normal gut rotation, and any temporary arrest in development at this stage might explain the association of the two defects.

Other associated anomalies include stigmata of mongolism in 18%, malrotation of the gut in 18%, tracheo-esophageal fistula or esophageal atresia in 9%, and congenital heart lesions in 7%.

Imperforate anus, cryptorchism, Meckel's diverticulum, portal vein over duodenum, Sprengel's deformity, deformity of the spine, and agenesis of the lung have been occasionally reported to coexist with annular pancreas.

There were no associated anomalies in our recent patient.

Summary

An additional case of annular pancreas causing duodenal obstruction in the newborn is added to the growing number of cases reported.

A discussion of annular pancreas as a cause of duodenal obstruction in the neonatal period is presented.

The fifty-five previously reported cases requiring surgery for duodenal obstruction in the neonatal period are reviewed.

Retrocolic duodenojejunostomy is recommended as the surgical procedure of choice for this condition.

John M. Jackson, MD, Chief Resident, Department of Surgery, Lloyd Noland Hospital, Fairfield, Ala.

REFERENCES

1. Tiedemann, F.: Deutsch Arch Physiol 4:403, 1818, cited by Van Der Horst, L. F.: Annular Pancreas, Arch Surg 83:249, 1961.
2. Ravitch, M. M., and Woods, A. C., Jr.: Annular Pancreas, Ann Surg 132:1116, 1950.
3. Arey, L. B.: Developmental Anatomy, 5th ed, Philadelphia: W. B. Saunders Company, 1947.
4. Howard, N. J.: Annular Pancreas, Surg Gynec Obstet 50:533, 1930.
5. Vidal, E.: "Quelques cas de chirurgie pancréatique," in Proceedings of the XVIII Congress of Surgery, Paris, 1905, p 739, cited by Howard, N. J.[4]
6. Whelan, T. J., Jr., and Hamilton, G. B.: Annular Pancreas, Ann Surg 146:252, 1957.
7. Gross, R. E., and Chisholm, T. C.: Annular Pancreas Producing Duodenal Obstruction, Ann Surg 119:759, 1944.
8. Burger, R. E., and Alrich, E. M.: Annular Pancreas, Report of a Case, Southern Surgeon 15: 83, 1949.
9. Glover, D. M., and Barry, F. M.: Intestinal Obstruction in the Newborn, Ann Surg 130:480, 1949.
10. Shapiro, D. J.; Dzurik, F. J.; and Gerrish, E. W.: Obstruction of Duodenum in the Newborn Infant Due to Annular Pancreas, Pediatrics 9:764, 1952.
11. Wilson, H., and Bushart, J. H.: Annular Pancreas Producing Duodenal Obstruction, Ann Surg 137:818, 1953.
12. Gross, R. E.: The Surgery of Infancy of Childhood: Its Principles and Techniques, Philadelphia: W. B. Saunders Company, 1953.
13. Kiesewetter, W. B., and Koop, C. E.: Annular Pancreas in Infancy, Surgery 36:146, 1954.
14. Small, W. T., and Berman, C. Z.: Annular Pancreas Producing Duodenal Obstruction in Infancy, New Eng J Med 251:191, 1954.
15. Hope, J. W., and Gibbons, J. F.: Duodenal Obstruction Due to Annular Pancreas With Differential Diagnosis of Other Congenital Lesions Producing Duodenal Obstruction, Radiology 63: 473, 1954.
16. Rickham, P. P.: Annular Pancreas in the Newborn, AMA Amer J Child 29:80, 1954.
17. Cohen, G. J., and Potter, J.: Annular Pancreas in a Premature With Other Congenital Anomalies, Clin Proc Child Hosp (Wash) 10: 192, 1954.
18. Carroll, D. S.: Annular Pancreas, Southern Med J 48:1270, 1955.
19. Farringer, J. L., Jr.: Annular Pancreas in Infants and Children, Surgery 37:638, 1955.
20. Frucht, D. A.: Annular Pancreas in Infancy, AMA J Dis Child 92:182, 1956.
21. Wilkinson, L. H., and Simms, A. G., II: Annular Pancreas, Amer Surg 23:317, 1957.
22. Large, P. G.: Annular Pancreas, S Afr J Lab Clin Med 3:281, 1951.
23. Weatherill, D.; Forgrave, E. G.; and Carpenter, W. S.: Annular Pancreas Producing Duodenal Obstruction in the Newborn, AMA J Dis Child 95:202, 1958.
24. Gilroy, J. A., and Adams, A. B.: Annular Pancreas, Radiology 75:568, 1960.
25. Hays, D. M.; Greaney, E. M., Jr.; and Hill, J. T.: Annular Pancreas as a Cause of Acute Neonatal Duodenal Obstruction, Ann Surg 153: 103, 1961.
26. Kie, A. T.; Wittebol, P.; and Lunding, J.: Annular Pancreas, Acta Paediat 50:72, 1961.
27. Lecco, T. M.: Zur Morphologie des Pancreas annulare, cited by Howard, N. J.[4]

Segmental Distribution of Peripheral Atherosclerosis

ADOLF SINGER, MD
BROOKLYN, NY

Atherosclerosis is a generalized disease of the arterial system. The localization of atherosclerotic lesions is of importance to the surgeon, as it determines the site and mode of direct surgical attack. It is also of significance in the natural history and prognosis of this disease.

The distribution of atherosclerotic lesions in the arterial tree is also of theoretical interest. A predilection for certain sites would suggest that local factors are relevant to the more general problem of the pathogenesis of atherosclerosis.

This study was undertaken to investigate the localization of atheromatous deposits in certain parts of the arterial system. Definite, frequently recurring patterns of atherosclerosis were found in the arteries to the lower limbs, and the clinical implications are noted. Some conclusions are drawn concerning mechanical factors in atheroma production, and these will be discussed subsequently.

Material and Methods

An analysis of 205 arteriograms of patients with varying degrees of lower limb ischemia due to atherosclerosis has been made. The arteriograms were from patients who attended St. Mary's Hospital, London, between 1953 and 1957. Their clinical condition has been reported elsewhere (Singer and Rob, 1960). Commencing with the abdominal aorta from just below the origin of the renal arteries, each named artery, except the common femoral, was divided into three equal segments. The width of the vessel was assessed by direct measurement of the width of the column of radiopaque contrast material present in the lumen. Measurements were made at three equidistant points within each segment, the final figure for that segment being the mean of these three separate determinations. Each individual measurement was made with calipers, the width being read against a millimeter scale. At each point on a vessel chosen for measurement, three separate estimations were carried out, and the average of these was accepted as the width of the lumen at this point.

The amount of narrowing of any given segment of a vessel due to atherosclerosis was determined by comparing its width with a figure obtained from a similar study of eight normal adult arteriograms. Where the width of the dye column was normal but its density reduced owing to a posterior plaque, this was noted as an equivalent degree of narrowing.

Three degrees of disease were recognized. First degree narrowing ("a") is a reduction of the lumen up to one third of its diameter. Second degree narrowing ("b") is a reduction of the lumen up to two thirds of its diameter. Third degree ("T") means complete occlusion of the vessel (Table 1).

Results

There were 120 femoral arteriograms and 85 lumbar aortograms. The results are presented graphically in Fig 1 and 2. Table 2 expresses the severity of atherosclerosis, in each arterial segment, as a percentage.

Comment

In the aorta below the origin of the renal arteries, the upper third was normal in 70% of arteriograms, and the lower third in only 28%. Conversely all degrees of disease were

Submitted for publication Dec 18, 1962.

Associate Chief of Surgery, The Mount Sinai Hospital Greenpoint Services Unit, Brooklyn, and Assistant Attending Surgeon, The Mount Sinai Hospital, New York.

TABLE 1.—*Degree of Arterial Narrowing*

Condition of Vessel	Aorta	Common Iliac Artery	External Iliac Artery	Common Femoral Artery	Superficial Femoral Artery	Popliteal Artery
Normal "N" midpoint of vessel	15.5 mm	8.5 mm	7.5 mm	6.5 mm	5.75 mm	4.5 mm
First degree narrowing "a"	Lumen of vessel narrowed to 2/3 of normal					
Second degree narrowing "b"	Lumen cf vessel narrowed to 1/3 of normal					
Thrombosis "T"	Lumen of vessel completely occluded					

All measurements are the mean of three separate estimations. Irregular vessels (internal iliac and profunda femoris arteries) and calf vessels were assessed by measurements and general extent and pattern of radiological filling of each vessel.

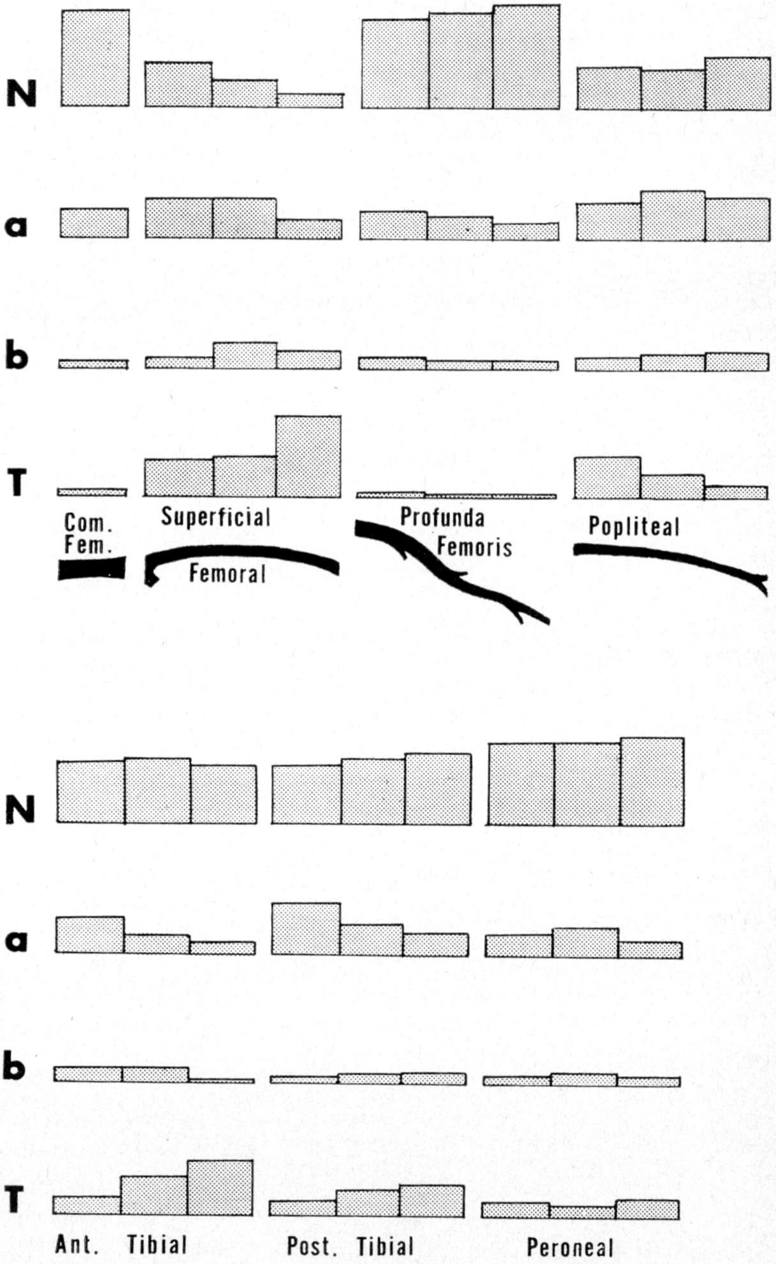

Fig 1.—Graphic representation of the distribution and severity of atheromatous narrowing and occlusion in 120 patients presenting with femoropopliteal atherosclerosis (see Tables 1 and 2).

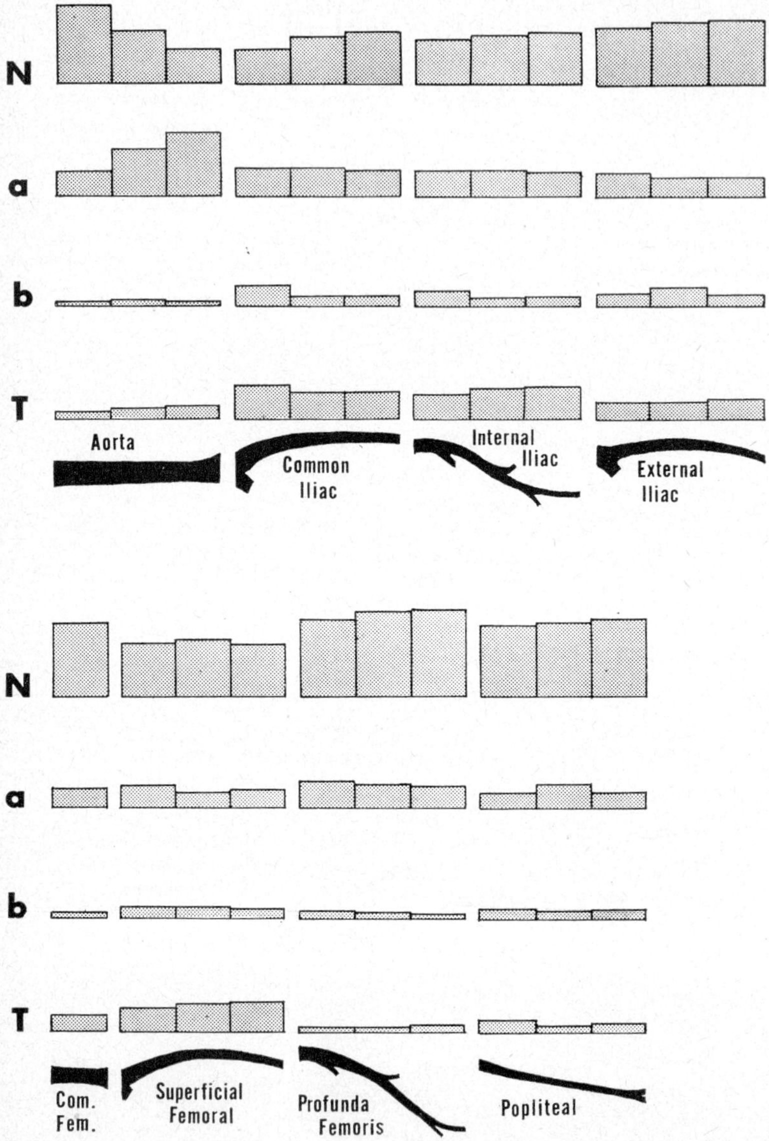

Fig 2.—Graphic representation of the distribution and severity of atheromatous narrowing and occlusion in 85 patients presenting with aortoiliac atherosclerosis (see Tables 1 and 2).

most marked in the lower third, this being most evident for first degree narrowing ("a") which occurred in 57% in the lower portion, and in only 21% in the upper portion of the vessel. The common iliac arteries show the opposite pattern, but to a less extent. Complete occlusion is only slightly more common in the proximal (30%) than in the distal (25%) segment. The finding of a normal lumen is distinctly more frequent in the distal segment (44%) than in the proximal segment (28%). This confirms the frequency of atherosclerosis in the region of the aortic bifurcation (Fig 3). Because disease at this site is often relatively localized, it is particularly suitable for treatment by thromboendarterectomy.

The superficial femoral artery shows the highest incidence of severity stenosis and thrombosis. In only 34% was the upper third considered normal, and the lower third in only 8% (Fig 4).

The relative freedom from disease of the common femoral artery (68% normal) and of the lower third of the popliteal artery (55% normal) makes these the obvious sites for anastomosis of bypass grafts, with the best chance of prolonged patency (Fig 5 and

TABLE 2.—*Percentage Severity of Atherosclerosis*

Group 1. Femoropopliteal Atherosclerosis

	N1	N2	N3	a1	a2	a3	b1	b2	b3	T1	T2	T3
Common femoral	71			22			5			2		
Superf. femoral	34	20	8	30	30	14	7	19	14	29	31	64
Profunda femoris	69	73	78	21	18	13	8	8	8	2	1	1
Popliteal	32	31	42	28	38	34	9	13	14	31	18	10
Ant. tibial	47	49	45	28	13	11	10	10	3	15	28	41
Post. tibial	45	50	53	37	24	21	6	6	5	12	20	21
Peroneal	63	63	67	20	21	14	7	9	6	10	7	13

Group 2. Aortoiliac Atherosclerosis

	N1	N2	N3	a1	a2	a3	b1	b2	b3	T1	T2	T3
Aorta	70	47	28	21	41	57	4	5	4	5	7	11
Common iliac	28	42	44	25	25	23	17	8	8	30	25	25
Internal iliac	40	43	44	23	23	22	13	8	7	24	26	27
External iliac	50	55	56	21	17	17	12	11	9	17	17	18
Common femoral	65			17			4			14		
Superf. femoral	50	51	48	19	14	17	11	11	10	20	24	25
Profunda femoris	67	71	72	23	22	21	7	4	3	3	3	4
Popliteal	63	66	70	16	22	16	9	8	9	12	4	5

Figures express percentage of each segment of a named vessel with a particular degree of narrowing (see Table 1). The suffix (1,2,3) refers to the first, second, or third segment of each vessel (eg, common iliac a2=25 means that 25% of common iliac arteries showed first-degree narrowing in their middle third).

6). The sparing of the profunda femoris artery (essentially normal in 72%) is of significance in the conservative treatment of patients with lower limb atheroma, as it forms the basis of the collateral circulation which will often maintain nutrition to an ischemic limb (Fig 7).

Fig 3.—Atherosclerosis of aortic bifurcation and of the common iliac arteries.

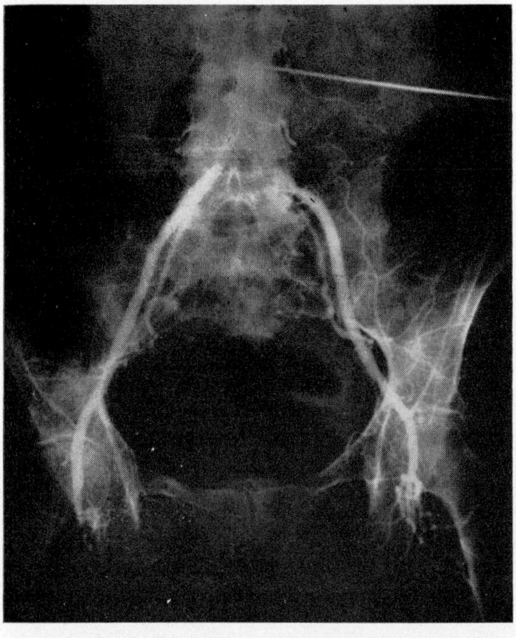

The theoretical implications of this study are also worthy of attention. Arterial thrombosis in these patients is almost certainly the end result of progressive narrowing due to atherosclerosis, irregularity of the vessel wall, and increasing slowing of the local circulation. The lower third of the superficial femoral artery is the most severely affected segment of the vessel in this survey, a finding previously reported by other authors (Lindbom, 1950; Mavor, 1956). But the results show a marked difference in incidence of occlusion of this segment of artery between patients having primarily femoral artery disease (64% thrombosed) and those who have significant narrowing or occlusion above the inguinal ligament (25% thrombosed). A similar lesser incidence of thrombosis of the upper third of the popliteal artery is noted in those patients with significant disease of the aorta and iliac arteries (12%) when compared with the figure (31%) for patients with femoral artery disease. These observations suggest that the reduced blood pressure and

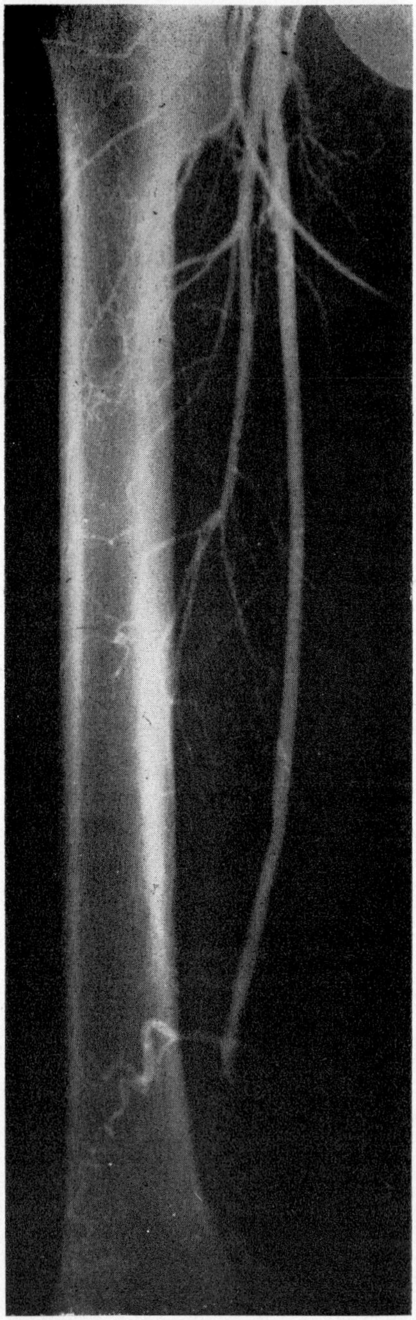

Fig 4.—Classical segmental occlusion of superficial femoral artery in lower Hunter's canal.

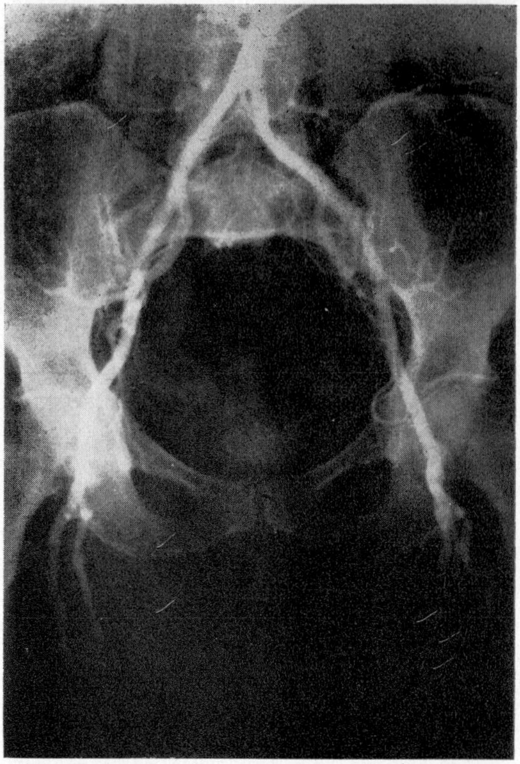

Fig 5.—Severe atheroma of superficial and profunda femoris arteries at their origin, with virtually normal external iliac and common femoral arteries.

flow distal to a stenosis or complete obstruction result in a diminished production of atherosclerosis in that segment of the artery. The earlier development of narrowing or occlusion in the proximal part of a vessel seems to exert a protective effect on its more distal parts.

This phenomenon is readily explicable in terms of the presently established major theories of the pathogenesis of atherosclerosis. Page (1954) suggests that the lateral filtration pressure acting on the arterial wall is the important local factor in the production of atheromatous lesions. Duguid (1946, 1948) maintains that intimal damage caused by the passing blood stream leads to deposition of thrombi which by way of fatty degeneration later become atheromatous lesions. With both these mechanisms reduction of blood pressure will reduce atheroma production.

Winternitz (1937) holds the view that subintimal hemorrhages undergo fatty degeneration to produce atheromatous deposits. Reduced blood pressure would diminish their occurrence where they arise from within the lumen of the vessel but would be less significant if caused by hemorrhages from the vasa vasorum.

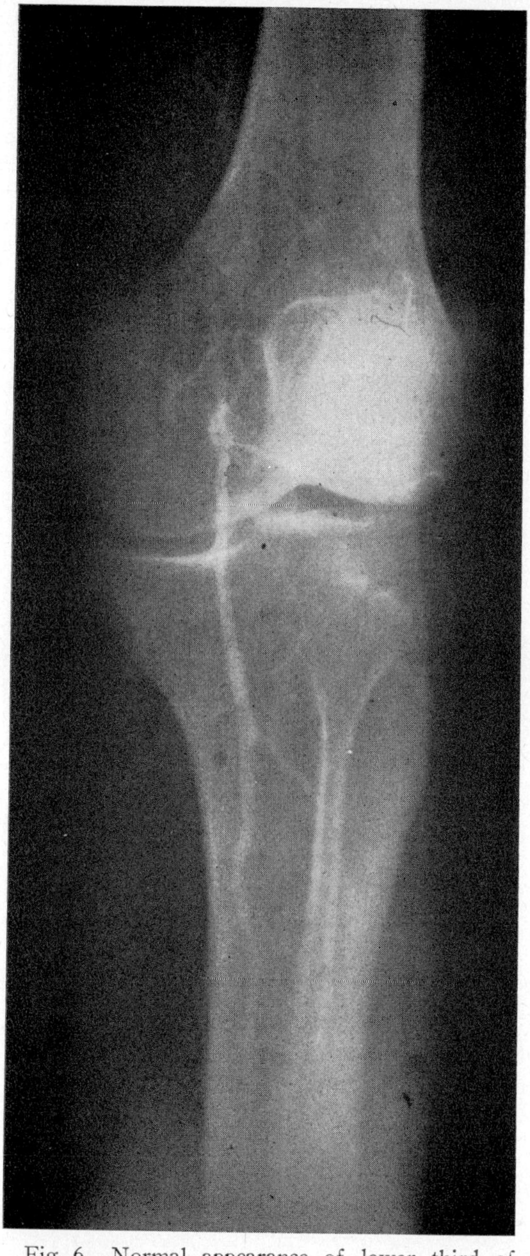

Fig 6.—Normal appearance of lower third of popliteal artery, with moderately severe disease above and below.

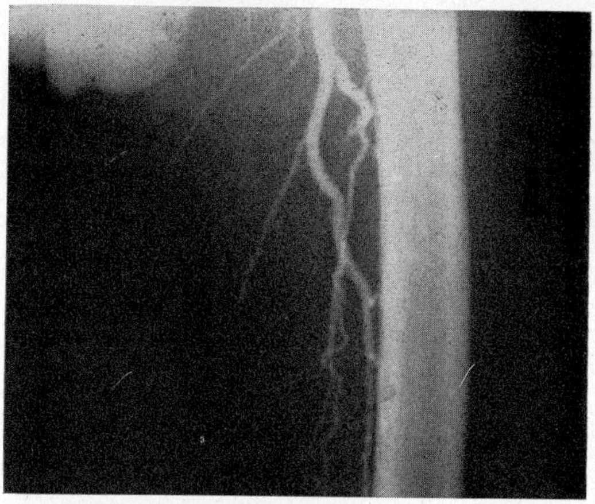

Fig 7.—The superficial femoral artery is completely occluded. The profunda femoris artery appears normal and supplies collaterals almost down to the knee.

General support for the hypothesis of protective stenosis on the basis of reduced blood pressure is also derived from the converse finding of the frequent association of hypertension and atherosclerosis in man. In analyzing groups of patients presenting with peripheral atherosclerosis, significant hypertension was present in 25% of 105 patients (Massarelli and Estes, 1957); 35% of 280 patients (Hines and Barker, 1940); 60% of 359 patients (Singer and Rob, 1960). Comparable figures are also quoted by other authors in this field (McDonald, 1953; Starer and Sutton, 1958). In the experimental animal, it has similarly been found that raised blood pressure increases the incidence of atheroma deposition to a significant degree (Bronte-Stewart and Heptinstall, 1954; Moss et al, 1951). Experiments being carried out by me at the present time further confirm the protective effect of proximal stenosis in reducing the deposition of experimental atheroma in animals.

The theory recently developed by Texon (1957, 1960) proposed the opposite view, that areas of artery wall subjected to reduced blood pressure are more susceptible to atheroma deposition. There is no obvious way of reconciling this opinion with the observations in this study.

No satisfactory explanation can be offered for the frequent sparing of the profunda femoris artery, a finding also noted by previous authors (Lindbom, 1950; Dible, 1956). This vessel is unusual in that its course leads it through the large muscle masses of the adductors of the thigh, where it is exposed to frequent compression. Although this may reduce blood flow and pressure, it may equally cause local damage, a mechanism which is often held responsible for the high incidence of atherosclerosis in the superficial femoral artery where it passes through the adductor hiatus. At the same time, acute angulation of the profunda femoris is probably prevented by its proximity to the femur, thus tending to protect against local artery wall damage. The rapid reduction in diameter of this vessel during its course may be a further factor contributing to its relative lack of atheroma deposits. This finding was recently emphasized by Young et al (1960) in a study assessing the atheroma distribution in the coronary arteries of man, where similar circumstances are present.

Summary

A survey of 205 arteriograms of patients with lower limb atherosclerosis is presented with an analysis of segmental deposition of atheroma. The various patterns of pathology are described, and their significance in reconstructive vascular surgery and in the evaluation of the natural history of the disease is commented on.

The concept of the protective effect of proximal arterial stenosis and thrombosis is supported by these findings, and its significance is stressed in relation to theories of the pathogenesis of atherosclerosis.

Adolf Singer, MD, Department of Surgery, The Mount Sinai Hospital Greenpoint Services Unit, Brooklyn, NY.

REFERENCES

1. Bronte-Stewart, B., and Heptinstall, R. H.: Relationship Between Experimental Hypertension and Cholesterol-Induced Atheroma in Rabbits, J Path Bact 68:407 (Oct) 1954.

2. Dible, J. H., in Peripheral Vascular Disorders, by P. Martin, R. B. Lynn, J. H. Dible, and I. Aird, Baltimore: The Williams & Wilkins Company, 1956.

3. Duguid, J. B.: Thrombosis as Factor in Pathogenesis of Aortic Atherosclerosis, J Path Bact 60: 57-61 (Jan) 1948.

4. Duguid, J. B.: Thrombosis as Factor in Pathogenesis of Coronary Atherosclerosis, J Path Bact 58:207-212 (April) 1946.

5. Hines, E. A., Jr., and Barker, N. W.: Arteriosclerosis Obliterans: Clinical and Pathologic Study, Amer J Med Sci 200:717-730 (Dec) 1940.

6. Lindbom, A.: Arteriosclerosis and Arterial Thrombosis in Lower Limb Roentgenological Study, Acta Radiol (Stockholm) supp 80:1-80, 1950.

7. McDonald, L.: Ischaemic Heart Disease and Peripheral Occlusive Arterial Disease, Brit Heart J 15:101-107 (Jan) 1953.

8. Massarelli, J. J., Jr., and Estes, J. E.: Atherosclerotic Occlusion of the Abdominal Aorta and Iliac Arteries: A Study of 105 Patients, Ann Intern Med 47:1125 (Dec) 1957.

9. Mavor, G. E.: Pattern of Occlusion in Atheroma of Lower Limb Arteries: Correlation of Clinical and Arteriographic Findings, Brit J Surg 43: 352-364 (Jan) 1956.

10. Moss, W. G.; Kiely, J. P.; Neville, J. B.; Bourque, J. E.; and Wakerlin, G. E.: Effect of Experimental Renal Hypertension on Experimental Cholesterol Atherosclerosis, Fed Proc 10:94, 1951.

11. Page, I. H.: Atherosclerosis, National Academy of Sciences Publication No. 338, Washington, DC: the Academy, 1955, p 5.

12. Singer, A., and Rob, C. G.: The Fate of the Claudicator, Brit Med J 2:633 (Aug 27) 1960.

13. Starer, F., and Sutton, D.: Aortic Thrombosis, Brit Med J 1:1255, 1958.

14. Texon, M.: A Hemodynamic Concept of Atherosclerosis, With Particular Reference to Coronary Occlusion, AMA Arch Intern Med 99: 418-427 (March) 1957.

15. Texon, M.; Imparato, A. M.; and Lord, J. W.: The Hemodynamic Concept of Atherosclerosis, AMA Arch Surg 80:47 (Jan) 1960.

16. Winternitz, M. C.; Thomas, R. M.; and LeCompte, P. M.: Studies in the Pathology of Vascular Disease, Amer Heart J 14:399, 1937.

17. Young, W.; Gofman, J. W.; Tandy, R.; Malamud, N.; and Waters, E. S. G.: The Quantitation of Atherosclerosis: II. Quantitative Aspects of the Relationship of Blood Pressure and Atherosclerosis, Amer J Cardiol 6:294-299 (Aug) 1960.

Are Benign Gastric Ulcers Really Benign?

P. A. DUHAMEL, MD
M. A. BLOCK, MD
AND
W. S. HAUBRICH, MD
DETROIT

In a practice involving large numbers of unselected gastric ulcer patients, the problem of medical intractability and recurrence of benign peptic ulcers in the stomach has posed, for us, a greater difficulty than the initial differentiation from gastric cancer. Rigid adherence to a policy of thorough diagnostic study and, in appropriate cases, reliance on a strictly interpreted therapeutic trial have permitted an accuracy of differentiation approaching 99%. Nevertheless, in the satisfaction of being able to discern the benign from the malignant gastric ulcer, one can easily lose sight of the eventual gravity of benign ulcer disease. To confirm our suspicions of this gravity, we have reviewed the later courses of our patients with apparently benign gastric ulcer disease.

Submitted for publication Dec. 18, 1962.

From the Divisions of General Surgery and Gastroenterology, Henry Ford Hospital.

Patients Comprising the Study

At Henry Ford Hospital from Jan. 1, 1945, through Dec. 31, 1955, the diagnosis of benign gastric ulcer was initially recorded for 474 patients. It is emphasized that this group does *not* include patients first presenting with ulcerated tumors of the stomach.

There were 353 males and 121 females. Their ages ranged from 10 to 83 years, with 81% in the fifth, sixth, and seventh decades (Table 1).

By far the commonest presenting complaint was epigastric distress (Table 2) which for at least half of these patients had been noted for more than a year. A few patients presented with acute and massive hemorrhage which necessitated immediate

TABLE 1.—*Age Distribution of 474 Patients with Gastric Ulcer*

Age Yr.	No. Patients	Total %
10-19	1	0.2
20-29	16	3.4
30-39	51	10.8
40-49	117	24.6
50-59	168	35.5
60-69	100	21.1
70-83	21	4.4
	474	100.0

TABLE 2.—*Frequencies of Presenting Complaints Among 474 Patients with Gastric Ulcer. Some Patients Had Several Complaints, so Percentages Total More than 100*

Complaint	% of 474 Cases
Epigastric distress	86
Hemorrhage	18
Nausea, vomiting	19
Weight loss (over 20 lb.)	7
Acute free perforation	2.5

surgical intervention. Occasionally, a gastric ulcer was detected only in the investigation of anemia in the absence of gastrointestinal complaints.

Radiographic studies were accomplished in all except nine patients whose hemorrhage required immediate operation. In the radiographs of 16 patients, gastric ulcer craters were not apparent and were found only at gastroscopy, laparotomy, or necropsy. Significantly, in 96.6% of cases the site and extent of gastric ulcers were accurately demonstrated by x-ray (Fig. 1). None of 18 ulcers situated along the greater curve of the stomach proved to be malignant. It is remarkable that evidence of duodenal ulcer or cap deformity was noted in nearly half of the cases.

Fractional gastric analysis, employing in almost all instances a modified Ewald meal, was recorded in about three-fourths of the cases. The peak "free HCl" exceeded 50 mEq. per liter in 44%. Only three patients had an apparent histamine achlorhydria, and one of these proved to have a gastric carcinoma.

Gastroscopy was undertaken in 241 patients. About 70% of examinations disclosed apparently benign gastric ulcers, 10% were erroneously described as revealing malignant lesions, and 20% provided inadequate views of the stomach.

An insignificant number of exfoliative cystology examinations were done at this hospital prior to 1955.

Thirteen (2.7%) of the 474 gastric ulcers, considered at the first impression as probably benign, later proved to be malignant.

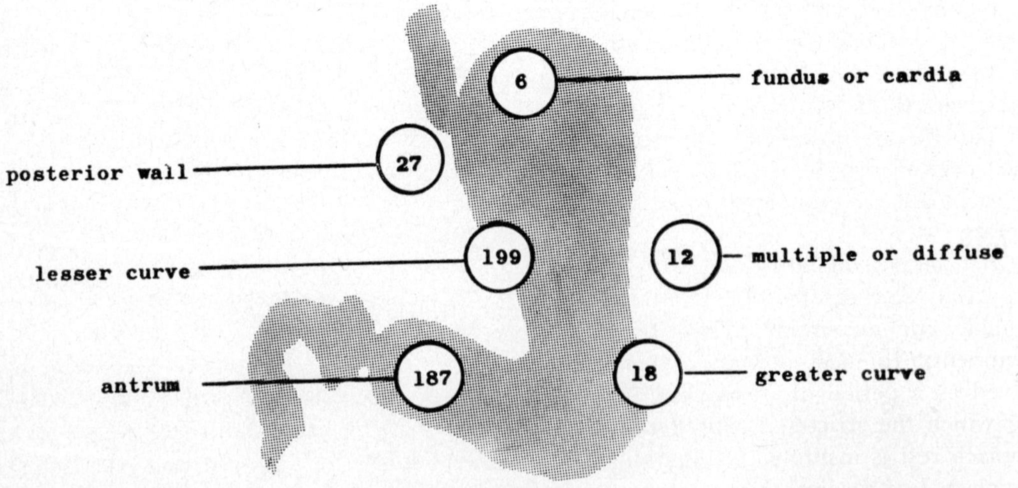

Fig. 1.—Sites of 449 gastric ulcers as demonstrated by x-ray. Remarkably, there was concomitant deformity of the duodenal cap in 214 of these cases.

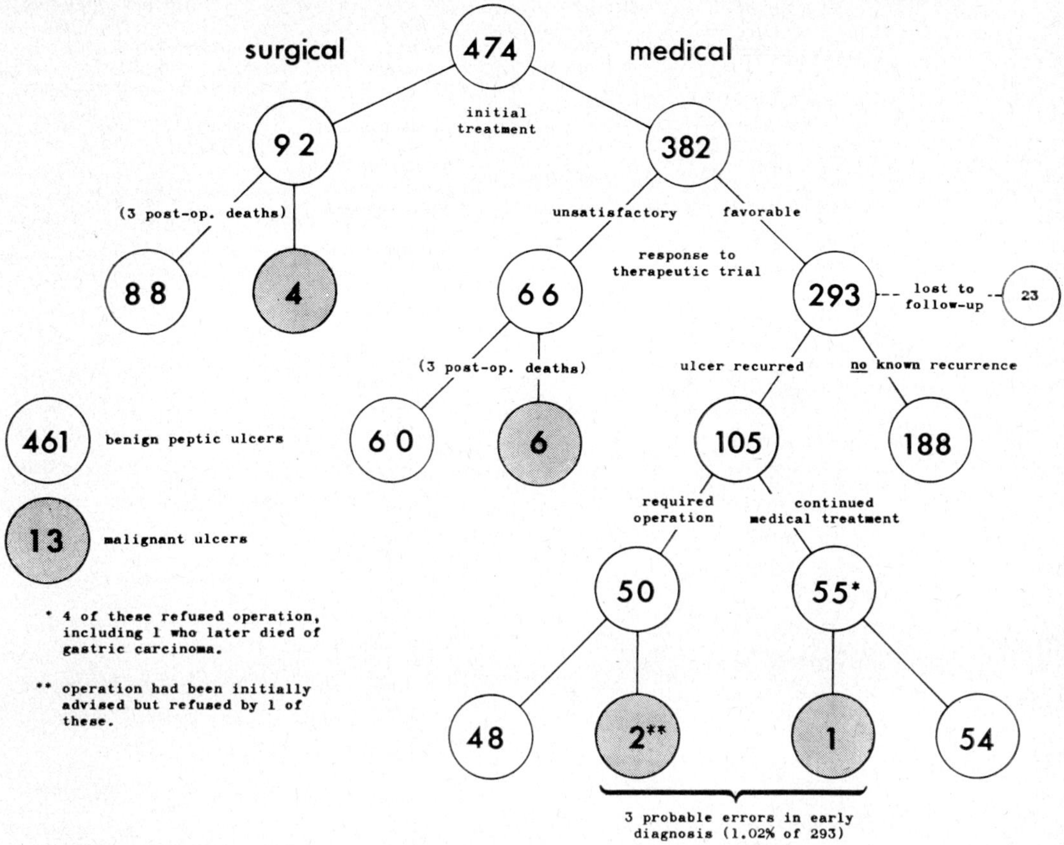

Fig. 2.—Chart depicting the immediate and ultimate courses of 474 patients seen because of ulcers in the stomach wall (see text). Patients with ulcerated gastric tumors have been deliberately excluded.

Results of Treatment

The initial and subsequent management of the 474 gastric ulcer patients is charted in Figure 2. Customarily, at Henry Ford Hospital, medical and surgical methods of treatment are not considered as competing remedies. Rather, a majority of gastric ulcer patients are observed jointly by medical and surgical consultants who seek to apply, in each case, a mutually agreed choice of therapy.

Medical Treatment.—Following the first appraisal, 382 cases (81%) were deemed suitable for an initial course of medical treatment. In most instances, this is conceived as a period of therapeutic trial during which the strictest form of physiologic stomach rest is instituted. Embarking on an initial trial of medical therapy never is construed as an irrevocable course and always requires a second decision at the completion of the trial period.

Sixty-six patients, at first considered worthy of a medical therapeutic trial, failed to fulfill the criteria of initial healing (complete relief of symptoms, reduction in the size of crater by at least one-half, and no persistent or superimposed filling defect) in radiographic studies after two or three weeks of strict stomach rest. For these patients, a surgical remedy was then invoked. In 60 cases, the ulcers were benign although often complicated by confined perforation. Malignant ulcers were found in six patients, none of whom survived five years.

In this series, 293 patients were considered to have responded favorably to the therapeutic trial. Of these, 188 (64.5%) have had no known recurrence of gastric ulcer (over two-thirds were subsequently observed from 5 to 16 years). The remaining 105 patients, although initially responding satisfactorily, were found later to have recurrent gastric ulcers. As many as four recurrences occurred following intervals of 5 months to 19 years. Thirteen sustained grave complications of which four died. Surgical intervention was required eventually by 50 of these patients (Fig. 1). Of the 55 patients requiring continued medical treatment, operation was advised but refused by four, and one of these died of gastric carcinoma.

Surgical Treatment.—For 92 patients, the diagnosis of gastric ulcer being provisionally established, surgery was considered as the primary treatment of choice. In 12, immediate operations were necessitated by emergency (eight for acute free perforation, four for hemorrhage). Of the eight patients whose perforated gastric ulcers were closed, three later required partial gastrectomy. There were three postoperative deaths, one after closure and two following gastric resections. Cancer was found in four of the 92 patients, but in one the carcinoma originated in the pancreas and eroded the stomach wall resulting in a mucosal ulceration. One of these four has survived his operation by 12 years; the remaining three have died of their disease.

The necessity of surgery after a brief medical trial and because of later recurrence has been discussed above and is depicted in Figure 2. It is to be noted that a total of 208 patients, or 44%, ultimately required surgery. The operative mortality rate was 4%.

Comment

It is believed that the patients comprising this study are typical of gastric ulcer problems encountered in a large, unselected practice. The chief problems in evaluating the need for surgical intervention are (*a*) to distinguish benign and malignant ulcers, and (*b*) to assure a remedy for benign ulcer disease which is intractable to medical therapy. While not denying the importance of the former, our impression is that the problem of recurrence and intractability of benign gastric ulcers is often underestimated.

Frequency of Malignancy.—Little difficulty is encountered in distinguishing, from a careful interpretation of the initial radiographic study, ulcerated gastric tumor defects from ulcers appearing within the stomach wall. Patients with ulcerated tumor defects, as previously stated, have been purposely excluded from this study. Among 474 ulcers apparently within the stomach wall, 13 (2.7%) were found to have a malignant base. Four of these occurred in patients whose ulcers were considered to be complicated and, from the first, unsuited to medical therapy. Six were detected by their failure to meet the criteria of a brief, strict, therapeutic trial. Therefore, only three malignant ulcers (1.02%) remained to represent errors in differential diagnosis. This compares favorably with the results reported by Paustian and his associates [3] who employed a similar program. A record of almost 99% accuracy, achieved by currently available diagnostic methods diligently applied, indicates to us that the problem of distinguishing benign from malignant ulcers approaches resolution.

Recurrence of Benign Gastric Ulcers.—The indication for invoking a surgical remedy for gastric ulcer disease, in our experience, is more often the failure of medical therapy to induce a lasting remission. Unquestionably, some ulcers in the stomach wall are acute lesions, the nature of which is to heal promptly and to not recur. It is presumed that many of the 188 cases with no known recurrence (Fig. 1) were in this category. Nevertheless, of 293 patients responding favorably to initial medical treatment, 105 (35.5%) were known to have recurred. Because these are only the known cases, we must assume this is a minimum figure. Fifty of these patients later required definitive surgical treatment of their ulcer disease, 11 undergoing emergency surgery for a life-endangering complication. The recurrence rate, determined in our patients, of 35.5% compares with that of 24.6% reported by Larson et al.,[1,2] 27% by Paustian et al.,[3] and 33% by Smith et al.[4] Swynnerton and Tanner[5] found 75% of medically treated gastric ulcers recurred.

Adding the 66 cases failing the initial therapeutic test, we find that the gastric ulcers in 171, or 44.5%, of 382 patients first chosen for medical treatment proved to be refractory or recurrent. Some of these patients were meanwhile exposed to the risk of complication in their disease which, in fact, did occur in a small but appreciable fraction.

This, then, provides a basis on which benefit to be derived from the surgical treatment of gastric ulcers must be judged. Our experience suggests that even one recognized recurrence in benign gastric ulcer activity usually denotes chronicity. Benign peptic ulcers can and do recur despite assiduous medical attention. Our opinion is that unless there are concomitant circumstances contraindicating operation, the patient with a chronic, recurring gastric ulcer is best served by a surgical remedy of his disease.

Summary and Conclusions

A review of 474 gastric ulcer patients emphasizes two problems: (*a*) discerning benign and malignant lesions, and (*b*) a recurrence rate in benign gastric ulcers of at least 35%.

Using generally available diagnostic methods and adhering strictly to criteria by which a brief therapeutic trial is interpreted, accuracy in discerning benign and malignant lesions approached 99%. Inadvertent neglect of a malignant gastric ulcer is almost always avoidable.

The likelihood of malignancy in a gastric ulcer which heals satisfactorily during a brief trial period of closely supervised medical therapy is less than the risk of gastric resection.

Almost half of 359 patients initially selected for a therapeutic trial eventually required a surgical remedy because of failure to heal or recurrence of their gastric ulcers.

The problem of recurrence and subsequent complication in benign gastric ulcer disease, in our experience, more often weighs in favor of invoking a surgical remedy than does fear of overlooking an occult malignancy.

Melvin A. Block, M.D., Associate Surgeon, Division of General Surgery, Henry Ford Hospital, Detroit 2.

REFERENCES

1. Larson, N. E.; Cain, J. C., and Bartholomew, L. G.: Prognosis of the Medically Treated Small Gastric Ulcer: I. Comparison of Follow-Up Data in 2 Series, New Engl. J. Med. 264:119 (Jan. 19) 1961.

2. Larson, N. E.; Cain, J. C., and Bartholomew, L. G.: Prognosis of the Medically Treated Small Gastric Ulcer: II. Ten Year to 19 Year Follow-Up Study of 391 Patients, New Engl. J. Med. 264:330 (Feb. 16) 1961.

3. Paustian, F. F.; Stein, G. N.; Young, J. F.; Roth, J. L. A., and Bockus, H. L.: The Importance of a Brief Trial of Rigid Medical Management in the Diagnosis of Benign Versus Malignant Gastric Ulcer, Gastroenterology 38:155, 1960.

4. Smith, F. H.; Boles, R. S., Jr., and Jordan, S. M.: Problem of Gastric Ulcer Reviewed, J.A.M.A. 153:1505, 1953.

5. Swynnerton, B. F., and Tanner, N. C.: Chronic Gastric Ulcer: Comparison Between a Gastroscopically Controlled Series Treated Medically and a Series Treated by Surgery, Brit. Med. J. 2:841, 1953.

Johannes Scultetus (1595-1645)

E. LEE STROHL, MD, CHICAGO

In my daily rounds at the hospital, I invariably encounter Johannes Scultetus—in his binder which is used each day on several of my patients.

In asking the medical students or members of the house staff to apply a Scultetus binder, the name Scultetus is hardly known, nor is the term "many-tailed binder."

Who was this surgeon who designed the Scultetus, or many-tailed, binder?

Johannes Scultetus (1595-1645) was one of the outstanding surgeons of the 17th century. He was born at Ulm, Germany, and later in his life became the City Physician.

It was the custom for scientists of that era, in their writings, to use the Latin form of their name. The reason was that the writings were in Latin. Johannes Scultetus is the Latin translation for his German name, Johann Schulte.

He attended the University of Padua, Italy, where he received his MD degree from that institution at the age of twenty-six, in 1621.[1]

After graduation, he was a military surgeon in the German Army during part of the Thirty Year Wars, in the period 1618 to 1648. Undoubtedly, his military experience influenced this young surgeon in his bold and daring surgical attack on patients. He was always ready to intervene, surgically, on the slightest provocation. It has been recorded that he was one of the most enterprising and venturesome surgeons of his era.

While the 17th century medical men were disputing about many far-fetched ideas, which could not be proved, surgeons of that time, feeling that they were dealing with facts, were willing to leave the theorizing to others. Surgeons, therefore, began the improvement of their instruments, tools, and operative technique. The attempt to standardize these areas of surgery was undertaken by Johannes Scultetus, although Dallas Groce had carried on similar work about a century before. Scultetus' observations and innovations were published at a later date.[2]

Scultetus possessed great mechanical ingenuity, and incorporated his own ideas in the design of instruments, creation of bandages, and description of operative procedures.

The instruments, bandages, and operative procedures were illustrated in his own hand, and each one was carefully described. He is especially remembered for the large number of bandages that he introduced to surgery, each being adapted to its specific purpose.

On Scultetus' death, at the age of fifty, he was considered one of the outstanding surgeons of the world.

Had the ingenuity of Scultetus emphasized simplicity rather than complexity, his contributions would have been more outstanding and his reputation even greater.

Armamentarium Chirurgicum, his only contribution to the literature, was published at Ulm, in 1655, ten years after his death.[3] The following year it was published at The Hague.[4] This work, a Latin text, which includes one hundred of Scultetus' observations, is a veritable picture book of 17th century surgery, and went through many editions. The innovations and complex devices that Scultetus developed, or modified, are demonstrated. In addition, surgical techniques used in the reduction of fractures and dislocations, amputation of limbs, breasts, and other surgical procedures are shown.

Modern surgery is indebted to this great German surgeon. It is not only remarkable,

Submitted for publication Dec 26, 1962.

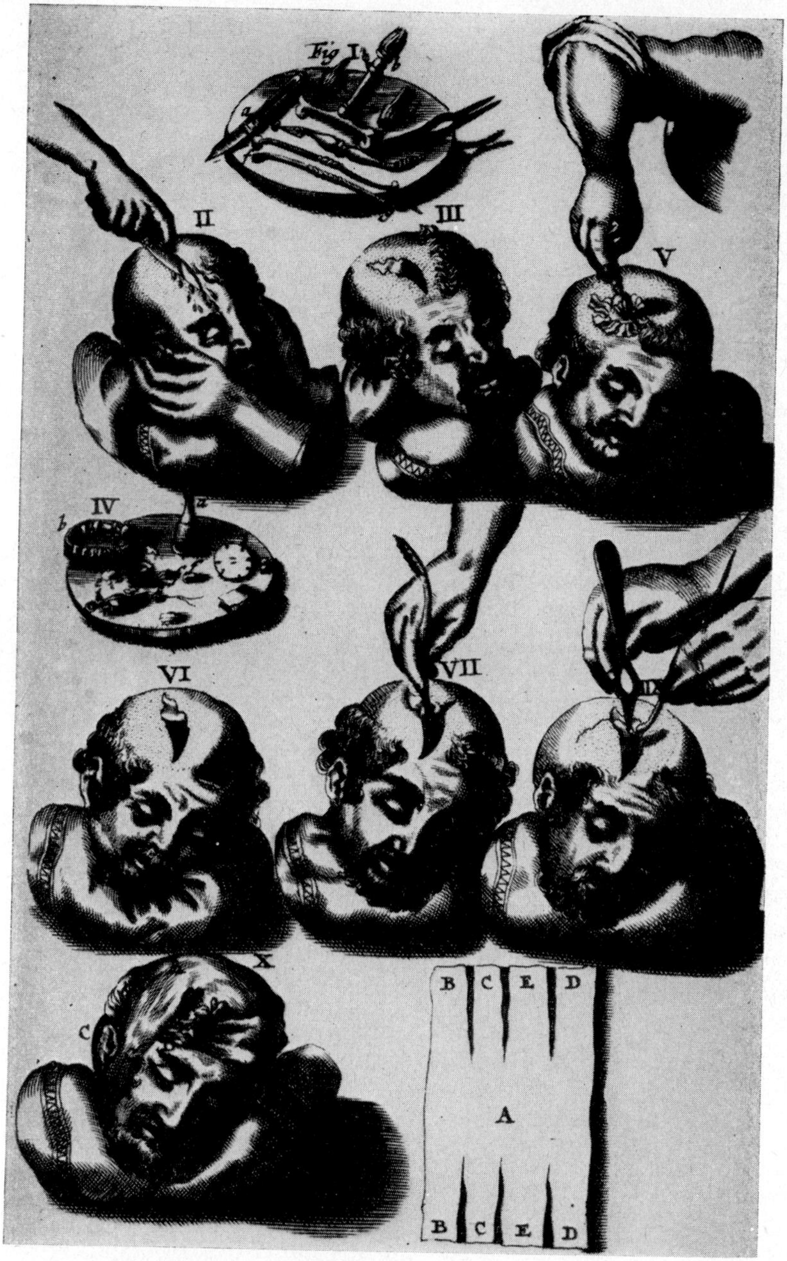

Table XXXI from page 96 of *Armamentarium Chirurgicum,* 1656, by Johannes Scultetus. Note the many-tailed binder (Scultetus binder) lower right.

but almost phenomenal, that in this modern scientific era, with all of the advances that have been made, we are still using one of Scultetus' contributions—the many-tailed binder.

E. Lee Strohl, MD, 122 S Michigan Ave, Chicago 3, Ill.

REFERENCES

1. Leonardo, R. A.: Lives of Master Surgeons, New York, Froben Press, Inc., 1948, pp 387 and 388.

2. Brown, A.: Old Masterpieces in Surgery, Surg Gynec Obstet 47:131 (July) 1928.

3. Scultetus, J.: Armamentarium Chirurgicum, Ulm, Germany, Balthasar Kuhnen, 1655, pp 131.

4. Scultetus, J.: Armamentarium Chirurgicum, The Hague, Adrian Vlacq, 1656, pp 318. (This book is in the rare book collection of the American College of Surgeons as a gift from the late H. Winnett Orr, MD, FACS.)

Post-Traumatic Temporal Artery Aneurysm

A Recurrent Surgical Curiosity

RUBEN F. GITTES, MD
AND
MARK M. KARTCHNER, MD
BOSTON

Three cases of post-traumatic temporal artery aneurysms were encountered in our hospital during the past two years. This entity was new in our experience and found to be ignored in present-day textbooks. We have undertaken here the presentation of these cases and a review of the literature on this relatively benign but curious surgical entity.

Report of Cases

CASE 1.—A 26-year-old truck driver was seen complaining of a "cyst" on his left forehead. A 2.5×1.5 cm. soft tissue mass was noted over the left eyebrow and presumed to be a dermoid cyst. At exploration under local anesthesia the mass was found to be a saccular aneurysm of the anterior branch of the temporal artery with weak pulsations which was easily resected. The cavity of the aneurysm was almost filled with organizing thrombus. The patient then recalled having been kicked in the forehead while inebriated three weeks earlier. No laceration had occurred, and the progressively enlarging mass had developed subsequently.

CASE 2.—A 32-year-old technician entered with a pulsatile mass on the left forehead. Five weeks earlier he had fallen while inebriated and required suture of a laceration on the right side of his scalp. While no injury was noted on the left side at the time, the pulsatile mass had appeared overlying the temporal ridge of the frontal bone and progressively enlarged. Pressure on the temporal artery proximally abolished the pulsations. Skull films and other routine studies were negative. A 0.7 cm. saccular aneurysm of the anterior branch of the temporal artery was easily resected under local anesthesia.

Submitted for publication Dec. 26, 1962.

Department of Surgery, Massachusetts General Hospital and Harvard Medical School.

CASE 3.—A 15-year-old schoolboy was initially seen because of poor vision which he attributed to a blow from a hockey stick to the left temporal region four weeks previously. The blow had felled him to the ice but did not lacerate the skin nor render him unconscious. Ophthalmologic examination confirmed preexisting myopia, and in addition the patient was found to have a 1.5 cm. pulsatile mass 2 cm. above the lateral aspect of the left eyebrow; pulsations could be stopped by proximal pressure. After negative skull x-rays, the mass, a saccular aneurysm of the left temporal artery with clearly defined vessels proximally and distally, was resected under local anesthesia. The sac was filled with layered organizing thrombus (Fig. 1, *A* and *B*).

Comment

These small aneurysms characteristically develop in the temple over the easily palpated lateral ridge of the frontal bone, the temporal line (Fig. 2). The artery compressed against the ridge by a blow to the side of the head is locally crushed to varying degrees, either extravasating blood and resolving slowly to a false aneurysm or weakening its wall by partial transection which slowly develops a saccular aneurysmal dilatation. Antonio Scarpa, the Italian surgeon, commented[1] on their formation in 1808:

> Therefore, with regards to the aneurysms of the external arteries of the body of a smaller size, the rupture of the temporal artery, in consequence of a blow, is not at all a rare case, the integuments covering it remaining uninjured, under which the effused blood collecting itself forms a circumscribed swelling with pulsation, and all the characters which were said to be proper of the *true* aneurysm. . . . I have twice had occasion to observe and cure the

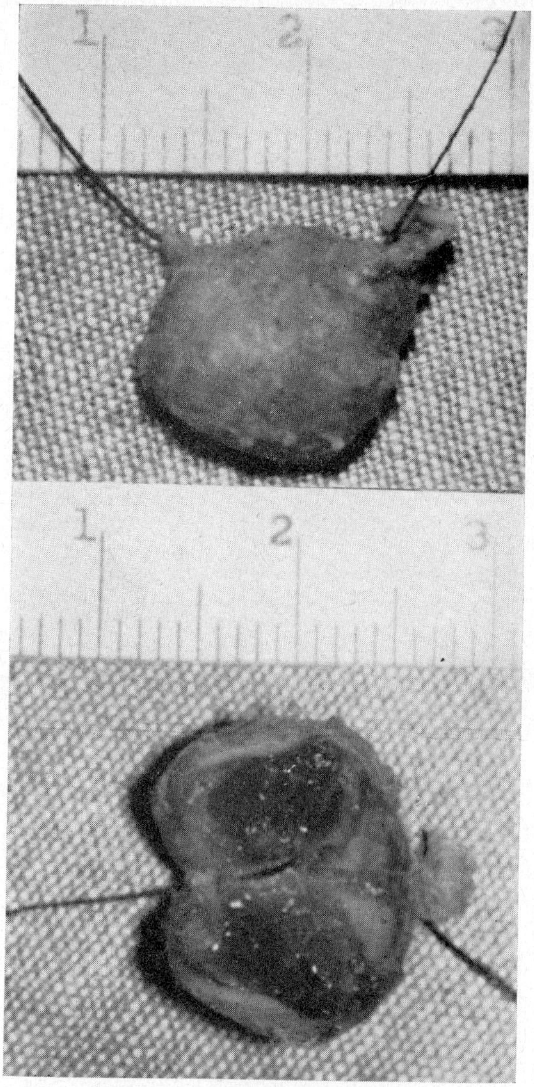

Fig. 1 (Case 3).—*A*, excised aneurysm with characteristic saccular shape showing a silk thread in lumen of entry and exit. *B*, opened specimen showing the thickened wall and organizing thrombus.

aneurysm of the temporal artery. . . . On opening the tumor I found the artery ruptured and I accomplished the cure by means of compression.

Diagnosis should present no problem, but the slow development of the lesion after relatively minor trauma and the dampening of pulsations by accumulating thrombus has led to preliminary diagnosis of dermoid cyst as in our Case 1. Spontaneously arising aneurysms of the temporal artery are rarely encountered, usually cirsoid [2] or arteriosclerotic.[3] A continuous bruit may suggest post-traumatic arteriovenous fistula, which has been reported.[4] Treatment can still be carried out as outlined in 1771 by Donald Munro,[5] rival of John Hunter as anatomy and surgery lecturer in London:

. . . to make an incision and lay bare the artery in the middle of the forepart; to open the cyst, and evacuate its contents; to tie the artery above and likewise below where it is dilated to prevent bleeding from any anastomotic branches that may open into this artery. This operation can almost only be done in the extremities and in the branches of the temporal artery.

The early literature is dotted with references to temporal artery aneurysms resulting from blood-letting procedures. Lorenz Heister's textbook of surgery in 1750 included a chapter entitled "Of Arteriotomy in the Temples" in which he stated that "this operation is not so often performed at present with us, as it was formerly among the ancient surgeons, for fear of the profuse bleeding or an aneurysm, which may be occasioned by wounding this vessel. . . ." [6] By 1861, the *Lancet* mentioned that "as usually seen, aneurysms of the temporal artery originate in wounds produced by cupping" while reporting [7] a case in a medical student, struck on the temple by a stone, who brought about consolidation and resorption of the lesion by keeping steady digital pressure on it while studying. Sword dueling among university students was reported [8] as a common cause of temporal aneurysms in Germany at one time. By 1935 Winslow and Edwards [4] were able to collect from the literature 79 cases of post-traumatic temporal aneurysm while reporting one case of their own. Since that exhaustive review there have been five more cases in the world literature.[9-13]

Review of our hospital's records for the past 25 years failed to turn up any cases in addition to the three here reported. With more refined means of blood-letting now in use and the protection of today's university gladiators with football helmets, post-traumatic temporal artery aneurysm may continue to be found only rarely, a recurrent surgical curiosity.

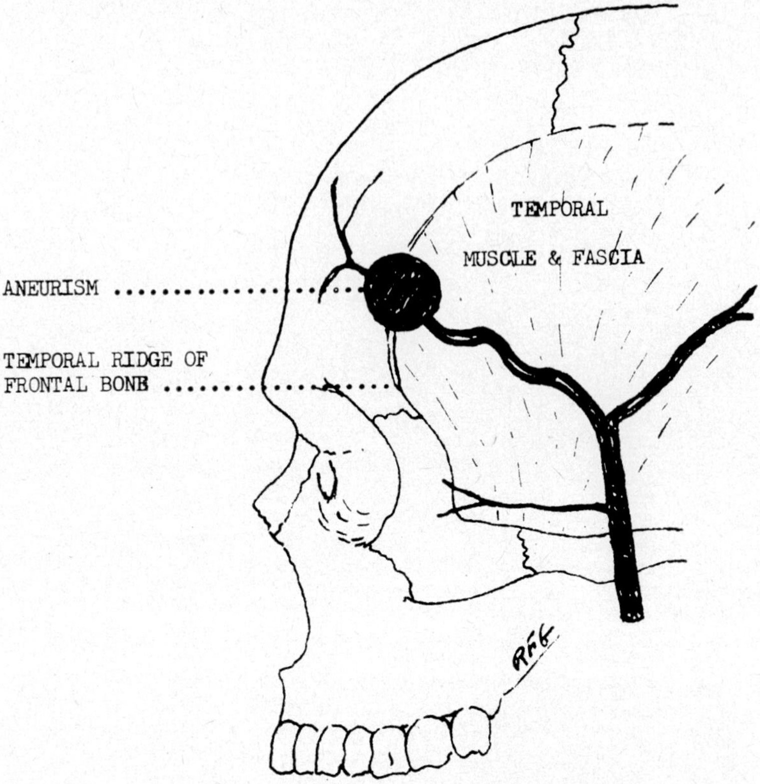

Fig. 2.—Characteristic location of traumatic temporal aneurysms, overlying the temporal ridge just beyond the cushioning of subjacent muscle.

Summary

Three cases of post-traumatic temporal aneurysm are described. This lesion, once common in days of blood-letting from the temples and of clashing sword duels, is now an unusual but easily recognized and remedied surgical curiosity.

Ruben F. Gittes, M.D., Department of Surgery, Massachusetts General Hospital, Boston 14, Mass.

REFERENCES

1. Scarpa, A.: Treatise on the Anatomy, Pathology, and Surgical Treatment of Aneurism, translated by J. H. Wishart, Edinburgh, 1808, pp. 184-185.

2. Brown, R. K., and Mehnert, R. H.: Aneurysm of the Temporal Artery: A Spontaneous Case Cured by Operation, Surgery 12:711-715, 1942.

3. Martin, W. L., and Shoemaker, W. C.: Temporal Artery Aneurysm, Amer. J. Surg. 89:700-702, 1955.

4. Winslow, N., and Edwards, M.: Temporal Aneurism: Analysis of Cases Reported in the Literature to June 1, 1934, and Report of a Case of Traumatic Origin, Amer. J. Surg. 28:696-702, 1935.

5. Munro, D.: Observations on Aneurysms, in Essays and Observations, Physical and Literary, Vol. iii, Edinburgh, 1771, p. 147.

6. Heister, L.: General System of Surgery, London, 1750, p. 353.

7. Aneurism of the Temporal Artery: Cure by Compression, Lancet 2:135, 1861.

8. Erb, K. H., and Hahn, E.: Aneurysmen der Arteria temporalis als Folge von Mensurverletzungen, Zbl. Chir. 58:2610-2613, 1931.

9. Judica, G.: Intorno ad un caso di aneurisma traumatico della arteria temporale, Gazz. Int. Med. Chir. 45:327-328, 1935.

10. Feurer, M.: Aneurysma der Arteria temporalis, Schweiz. Med. Wschr. 68:822-823, 1938.

11. Lopez Mansilla, R., and Aguilar, A.: Aneurisma traumatico de la arteria temporal superficial, Sem. Med. (B. Air.) 1:157-158, 1938.

12. Favero, F., and Veiga de Carvalho, H.: Aneurisma traumatico da arteria temporal superficial esquerda, Brasil Med. 55:577-578, 1941.

13. Smith, F.: Case of Traumatic Aneurism of the Right Superficial Temporal Artery, Brit. J. Surg. 37:241-242, 1949.

Intravenous Protein Hydrolysates

Favorable Influence on Postoperative Nitrogen Balance

JOSEPH C. PEDEN, JR., MD
ALEXANDRE OHIN, MD
PAUL T. WILLIAMS, MD
AND
HENRY WEATHERS, MD
ST. LOUIS

The efficacy of parenteral protein alimentation in the postoperative patient remains in dispute in spite of many pertinent studies reported in the medical literature. Information which is available strongly points to significant nitrogen sparing attributable to the use of intravenous protein digests, but rigidly controlled balance studies in postoperative patients have not been described. The present investigation is directed toward this purpose.

We have made a comparison of parenteral protein feedings with isocaloric oral protein feedings as well as with protein-free parenteral feedings by means of nitrogen balance measurements. The results of this study indicate that parenteral protein feeding is almost equivalent to an identical oral protein feeding in nitrogen sparing. Both oral and parenteral protein feedings cause marked increases in nitrogen balance when compared to isocaloric, protein-free parenteral feedings. While nitrogen sparing may not be of obvious benefit for short periods, prolonged nitrogen losses or the excessive nitrogen losses said to follow major operative procedures may be detrimental.

In the course of the present study, ancillary observations on the catabolic effect of operative trauma have been made. In the uncomplicated operative procedure the change in nitrogen balance attributable to the operation alone has been small.

Methods

Part 1.—Two feeding programs were selected which were equivalent in all respects except for their caloric and carbohydrate proportions. The first diet provided 900 calories; 76 gm. of protein (12 gm. of nitrogen) and 60 mEq. of both sodium and potassium each day. This diet was given parenterally by means of 2,000 ml. of a 5% hydrolyzed protein and 5% glucose * plus 1,000 ml. of 5% glucose in water; 30 mEq. of potassium were

Submitted for publication Dec. 26, 1962.

From the Metabolic Service, Homer G. Phillips Hospital, and the Department of Surgery, Washington University School of Medicine, St. Louis, Mo.

* Amigen supplied by Baxter Laboratories, Inc., Morton Grove, Ill.

TABLE 1.—*The Mean of Nitrogen, Sodium, and Potassium Oral Nutrition of Patients Operated On and Those*

			No Operation				
	Intake * Col.		No. Patients	Parent.	Oral	Parent.	No. Patients
Nitrogen Balance (Gm)	900	Mean	10	−2.5	+0.9	−0.6	10
		S D		4.98	4.02	3.37	
		S E		1.66	1.34	1.29	
	1,960	Mean	6	+1.9	+4.3	+2.2	10
		S D		2.84	2.20	3.37	
		S E		1.27	0.99	1.38	
Sodium Balance (mEq)	900	Mean	10	−1.2	+7.4	+7.6	10
		S D		26.2	17.0	27.4	
		S E		8.7	5.7	9.1	
	1,960	Mean	6	+12.2	+24.6	+18.1	10
		S D		18.4	16.9	25.8	
		S E		8.2	7.6	11.5	
Potassium Balance (mEq)	900	Mean	10	+0.7	+7.8	+4.9	10
		S D		17.2	17.1	22.1	
		S E		5.7	5.7	7.4	
	1,960	Mean	6	+18.8	+30.6	+24.2	10
		S D		21.6	13.3	13.9	
		S E		9.7	5.9	6.2	

* Each daily feeding provided 76 gm. of protein (12.0 gm. of nitrogen) and 60 mEq. of both sodium and potassium. Nonprotein supplements account for the different caloric equivalents of the 2 feedings.

added to the hydrolyzed protein which then provided a total daily intake of 60 mEq. of both potassium and sodium. The oral intake was made up of a properly proportioned mixture of dextrimaltose and milk-protein solids † with added sodium to provide a similar daily intake.

The second diet contained additional carbohydrate so that its energy equivalent equalled 1,960 calories per day; otherwise it was similar to the first diet. The parenteral feeding consisted of 2,000 ml. of a 5% protein hydrolysate with 12.5% fructose and 2.4% ethyl alcohol ‡ plus 1,000 ml. of 10% glucose in water. The oral mixture was similar to that of the 900 calorie diet with sufficient dextrimaltose added to provide an additional 1,060 calories per day.

Postoperative patients and others not operated on were fed alternately in three day periods, parenterally, orally, and parenterally, beginning with the first postoperative day in patients who had undergone cholecystectomy, hysterectomy, or colectomy. During parenteral feeding periods only water or noncaloric drinks were permitted by mouth. Twenty-four hour urinary collections were made, and measurements of total nitrogen, sodium, and potassium losses were made, from which balance computations were derived. Fecal losses were not determined, nor were the insignificant gastric tube suction losses of nitrogen measured in the patients in whom short periods of suction were used.

† Protenum, provided by Mead, Johnson and Co., Evansville, Ind.

‡ Amigen, high calorie solution, supplied by Baxter Laboratories, Inc., Morton Grove, Ill.

Ten unoperated and ten postoperative patients were studied on each diet except for those not operated on who received the 1,960 calorie diet when only six patients were studied.

Part 2.—In this study we made observations on the effect of operation alone on nitrogen, sodium, and potassium balances as well as the effect of isocaloric protein-containing and protein-free feedings during the postoperative period. Three types of feedings were given to each patient, all of them providing 900 calories and 60 mEq. of both sodium and potassium each day. One feeding was protein-free and consisted of parenteral glucose; the other two contained 76 gm. of protein or protein hydrolysate (12 gm. of nitrogen) given orally and parenterally respectively. Each patient was given either glucose or protein hydrolysate parenterally for three days preoperatively, and the same feeding was continued for the first three postoperative days. The alternate parenteral diet was then given for the next three days and the oral diet the final three days, or this order was reversed. Four patients were started with the protein-free feeding preoperatively and three with the parenteral protein hydrolysate.

Results

Part 1.—The means of balance studies of nitrogen, sodium, and potassium are tabulated in Table 1, and an analysis of the statistical significance of the differences of the means is presented in Table 2.

Balances During Parenteral and Not Operated On

Postoperative		
Parent.	Oral	Parent.
−1.9	+1.7	−0.9
3.15	3.18	4.81
1.05	1.06	1.70
−2.7	+1.4	−1.5
3.42	3.46	3.86
1.14	1.15	1.29
+21.5	+37.5	+32.4
7.2	9.1	9.4
2.4	3.0	3.3
−2.9	+20.7	−12.3
27.6	13.7	28.1
9.2	4.6	9.4
+8.2	+23.7	+12.0
17.7	9.7	22.3
5.9	3.2	7.9
+12.7	+31.7	+8.3
25.0	13.0	20.4
8.3	4.3	6.8

Mean nitrogen balance during oral alimentation in the postoperative period and in patients not operated on is greater than that during parenteral feeding, but the differences are not of statistical significance. While postoperative nitrogen balance during oral alimentation is significantly greater than that of a previous period of parenteral feeding, a subsequent three day period of parenteral feeding is not significantly less in nitrogen balance than that during the oral feeding. Consequently, the apparent differences are probably due to the relative proximity of the period of study to the operative period rather than due to the method of feeding. The effect of operation on nitrogen balance is also demonstrated by significant differences of the means of nitrogen balance during the periods of parenteral feeding found in patients receiving 1,960 calories not operated on and operated on. However, no significant differences were found with a 900 calorie intake.

In patients not operated on, the nitrogen balance during parenteral feeding is not found to be significantly different than that recorded during oral alimentation. Further, the provision of an additional 1,060 calories by means of added carbohydrate over and above that present in the 900 calorie diet does not significantly influence the nitrogen balance of patients operated on or not operated on. In short, the nitrogen balance of patients both operated on and not operated on has not been shown to be significantly influenced by the method of feeding nor by the caloric intake within the range of 900 to 1,960 calories per day.

Examination of the data presented in Tables 1 and 2 in regard to sodium balance indicates that sodium retention found in

TABLE 2.—*A Statistical Analysis of the Means of Nitrogen, Sodium, and Potassium Balances*

Calories		900 No Op.	900 Postop.	1,960 No Op.	1,960 Postop.
Nitrogen Balance	P_1:0 *	0	+	0	+
	P_2:0	0	0	0	0
	P_1:P_2	0	0	0	0
Sodium Balance	P_1:0	0	++	0	+
	P_2:0	0	0	0	++
	P_1:P_2	0	++	0	0
Potassium Balance	P_1:0	0	+	0	+
	P_2:0	0	0	0	++
	P_1:P_2	0	0	0	0

	Nitrogen			Sodium			Potassium		
	P_1	0	P_2	P_1	0	P_2	P_1	0	P_2
900 Cal., no op:op.	0	0	0	+	++	++	0	+	0
1,960 Cal., no op:op.	++	0	+	0	0	+	0	0	0
No op., 900:1,960	+	+	0	0	0	0	0	++	+
Op., 900:1,960	0	0	0	+	++	++	0	0	0

* P_1, first parenteral feeding period; 0, oral feeding period; P_2, second parenteral feeding period; +, significant difference of means at 5% probability level; ++, significant difference of means at 1% probability level.

postoperative patients is greater in those fed orally; retention is significantly greater regardless of the method of feeding during 900 caloric intakes compared to 1,960 caloric intakes. These phenomena are not present in patients not operated on.

The results of the study of potassium balance are interesting in that mean balance was positive during each three day period regardless of route of administration, operative status, or caloric intake. Potassium retention is usually greater during oral than during parenteral alimentation; the influence of operation on potassium balance appears to be variable and of uncertain significance.

Part 2.—In this study, during three day periods, patients received three different isocaloric feedings; one was protein-free, and the other two contained 76 gm. of protein administered either orally or parenterally. A three day preoperative feeding was always given parenterally, and the same feeding was given during the first three postoperative days. The data of seven patients studied do not warrant statistical analysis. However, it is clear that: (1) Nitrogen balance during parenteral protein feeding is similar to that produced by oral feeding; (2) both oral and parenteral protein feedings greatly reduce nitrogen deficits compared to those observed with isocaloric protein-free feedings; (3) a major opera-

TABLE 3.—*A Comparison of Nitrogen, Sodium and Potassium Balance Preoperatively and Postoperatively in Patients Receiving Isocaloric Intakes Containing 76 Gm. of Protein Given Parenterally and Orally, and Protein-Free Infusions*

(A)

Balance (Mean)	Days Intake *	Preoperative 3-1 CHO Infus.	Postoperative 1-3 CHO Infus.	4-6 Parent. Protein	7-9 Oral Intake	Remarks
N gm.	1	—5.8	—3.5	+2.7	+3.3	Left colectomy
	2	—6.1	—8.6	—1.9	—	Cholecystectomy
Na mEq.	1	—60.4	+34.0	+12.0	+49.4	(154 mEq Sodium)
	2	+71.9	+117.0	+54.6		(3 days pre- and postop.)
K mEq.	1	+11.2	+31.0	—48.7	+9.1	(only 30 mEq potassium intake)
	2	—14.6	+5.3	+43.0		(3 days pre- and postop.)

(B)

Balance (Mean)	Intake	CHO Infus.	CHO Infus.	Oral Intake	Parent. Protein	Remarks
N gm.	1	—5.3	—6.3	—2.4	—1.9	Vagotomy & antrectomy
	2	—7.0	—7.8	+5.9	+3.1	Gastrojejunostomy; ca. stomach, malnourished
Na mEq.	1	+19.3	+20.8	+30.6	+22.6	
	2	—57.3	+31.0	+52.8	+51.6	
K mEq.	1	—7.2	—27.8	—51.9	—38.8	
	2	—73.4	—45.5	+10.3	+12.9	

(C)

Balance (Mean)		Parent. Protein	Parent. Protein	CHO Infus.	Oral Intake	Remarks
Nitrogen Gm.	1	+6.1	+4.2	—10.3	+8.2	Sigmoid resection for diverticulitis
	2	+2.4	+3.0	—12.6	+4.8	Cholecystectomy
	3	+8.0	+7.0	—10.5	+5.0	Cholecystectomy
Sodium mEq.	1	+37.6	+25.4	+21.5	+41.6	
	2	—1.2	+23.2	+8.9	+34.3	
	3	+50.4	+45.9	+38.2	+50.0	
Potassium mEq.	1	+37.3	+5.2	+28.6	+43.0	
	2	+11.4	+10.9	+15.1	+10.8	
	3	+40.8	+11.4	+35.7	+24.9	

* All daily intakes isocaloric (900Cal) with 60 mEq of sodium and potassium unless indicated otherwise in Remarks. Parenteral protein and oral diets provided 76 gm of protein (12.0 gm of nitrogen) a day.

tion itself usually affects nitrogen balance little (Table 3—A, B, and C).

In four of seven patients there was a considerable increment in sodium retention during the immediate postoperative period when compared to preoperative sodium balance, and in three of these four patients preoperative sodium balance was negative on a 60 mEq. intake. Sodium retention in all cases persisted during the nine day postoperative period regardless of changes apparently produced by operation.

Potassium balance is not consistently influenced by the protein character of the feedings, the route of feeding, or the effect of operation in these cases.

Comment

In the evolution of parenteral therapy, initial efforts were concerned with the administration of medicinal agents rather than alimentation.[1] Elman [2] substantially developed the concept of parenteral protein alimentation first, in 1937. His investigation led to the refinement and proved usefulness of a complete amino acid mixture produced through the enzymatic digestion of casein. Acid hydrolysates of casein are incomplete in essential amino acids and require the addition of tryptophane or cystine (or choline or methionine) for efficient utilization.[3-5] In multiple clinical observations, Elman [6-8] demonstrated the positive effect of intravenous casein hydrolysates on nitrogen balance and serum albumin in patients not operated on. Brunschwig, Clark, and Corbin [9] reported a sustained positive nitrogen balance for ten days in a 36-year-old female with intestinal obstruction due to pelvic inflammation, using 3,000 ml. of 5% glucose and 5% protein hydrolysate per day as the sole nutriment; positive nitrogen balance was maintained for 12 days in a patient given 3,000 ml. of 10% glucose and 5% protein hydrolysate per day and nothing by mouth. Shohl, Butler, Blackfan, and MacLachlan [10] reported that intravenous alimentation with amino acids in infants maintained nitrogen balance as well as did the same amount of protein by mouth. Hartmann [11] substantiated these observations in older children. Allen [12] showed that intravenous plasma as the sole source of protein intake is as effective as oral alimentation in the growth rate and nitrogen balance of puppies up to 99 days. A similar study of intravenous amino acids as the sole protein source was unsatisfactory and permitted no conclusions.

Thus, the usefulness of intravenous protein alimentation in unoperated patients has been repeatedly confirmed and, while similar results are expected and have been assumed in the postoperative period, observations available are somewhat incomplete and without controlled studies. In view of the reports of large losses of nitrogen in the urine in the postoperative period, up to 20-35 gm. a day,[13] the need for parenteral protein alimentation is clear. Elman [13] perhaps best summarized the role of simple starvation in the pattern of postoperative nitrogen deficits, and Holden et al.[14] have more recently emphasized this concept. Wilkinson [15] observed no appreciable alteration on postoperative nitrogen balance through the use of intravenous casein hydrolysates. This point of view is not the more common, however, and Brunschwig [16] observed a reduction or even a complete correction of nitrogen deficits in patients undergoing cholecystectomy and treated with intravenous glucose and protein hydrolysate. In this uncontrolled study, it was also noted that intravenous protein feeding was just as effective as oral protein on nitrogen balance. Elman [6] reported a negative nitrogen balance of 12 to 16 gm. a day in the first six days after closure of a perforated peptic ulcer when 4,000 ml. of 10% glucose in water per day was given; for the next 11 days, 80 gm. of nitrogen given parenterally changed the nitrogen balance to −4 to +2 gm. per day, and when parenteral protein was discontinued, nitrogen balance ranged from −8 to −10 gm. per day.

Holden et al.[14] have reported convincing evidence of the efficacy of parenteral protein alimentation on nitrogen balance in postoperative patients. After hemigastrectomy and vagotomy in one patient, urinary losses of nitrogen averaged 6.0 gm. per day for five days on parenteral carbohydrate feeding. Positive nitrogen balance was accomplished thereafter through the use of 3,000 ml. of 10% fructose and 5% protein hydrolysate per day. In a second patient, mean daily nitrogen losses of 10 gm. per day on an intake of 3,000 ml. of 5% glucose after closure of a perforated gastric ulcer were reduced to 2.0 gm. per day when the patient received 2,000 ml. of 5% glucose and 5% protein hydrolysate, and 1,000 ml. of 10% glucose per day. In 14 men after subtotal gastrectomy who received an average of 20 cal. per kg. of body weight through the use of parenteral carbohydrate, nitrogen deficits averaged 10-12 gm. per day. Seven other men subjected to subtotal gastrectomy received 25 cal. per kilogram of body weight including 9 gm. of nitrogen parenterally per day with a mean nitrogen deficit of 8 gm. per day.

Thus the evidence of these and other observations [17-20] reported in the literature suggests that parenterally administered protein feeding can effect nitrogen balance postoperatively. Yet this evidence has not been acceptable to many, probably in part due to data inadequately controlled. It was this situation which prompted our experiment. We were predominately interested in postoperative patients who had undergone major surgical procedures; patients not operated on were included as controls and for comparison with the observations of earlier studies. Data in Table 1 indicate that while the mean of nitrogen balance during oral alimentation is greater than that of parenteral alimentation, the difference of the means is not greater than that attributable to random sampling errors, and this is true in patients operated on and not operated on. The reasons for a significant difference between the means of oral feeding and parenteral feeding during the first three postoperative days but not during the third three postoperative days are not apparent. With the 1,960 calorie feeding, postoperative nitrogen losses appear to be greater than in patients not operated on. Apparently small increments in nitrogen balance found in unoperated patients who receive 1,060 additional calories are present in only insignificant proportions in postoperative patients. Striking improvement in nitrogen balance is observed in Part 2 of the experiment when oral and parenteral protein alimentation is compared to protein-free feeding in postoperative patients. This study also substantiates the observations and conclusions of Elman and Holden who emphasized that protein starvation during the postoperative period is the main cause of the large negative nitrogen balance regularly recorded postoperatively and that the so-called stress response is a very minor factor. In brief, we have observed only insignificant differences in the nitrogen balance of the postoperative and preoperative periods. Both oral and parenteral protein feedings greatly reduce the postoperative negative nitrogen balance when compared to nonprotein feedings. Certainly, short-term negative nitrogen balance may be well tolerated as far as we can observe. However, in long-term parenteral therapy, following operation or not, and in patients in whom protein destruction is increased, the use of parenteral protein feeding is indicated and can serve as an efficient substitute for oral feeding.

The observations on sodium balance confirm those of many investigators. The daily administration of 60 mEq. of sodium is followed by slight sodium retention postoperatively, and this retention is greater when the sodium is given orally than when given intravenously. The greatest retention of sodium was observed in patients who received the subcaloric (900 calorie) intake. However, postoperative sodium retention in the patients studied here and in other observations has appeared to be quite variable, and in some patients it is completely absent when 60 mEq. were given daily. Thus, while the general rule pertains, there are many variations, and in the sick postoperative patient in whom the most careful control is indicated the measurement of urinary sodium losses is urgently required.

Potassium balance appears to be little influenced by operative procedures; somewhat greater balance is attendant upon oral as opposed to parenteral feeding; and 60 mEq. of potassium per day are adequate to supply potassium losses in patients not operated on and in those operated on who do not have unusual losses.

Joseph C. Peden, Jr., M.D., 100 N. Euclid Ave., St. Louis 8.

REFERENCES

1. Elman, R.: Parenteral Alimentation in Surgery, Chapt. 1, New York, Paul B. Hoeber, Inc., Medical Book Dept. of Harper & Bros. 1948.

2. Elman, R.: Intravenous Injection of Amino Acids in Regeneration of Serum Protein Following Severe Experimental Hemorrhage, Proc. Soc. Exper. Biol. Med. 36:867, 1937.

3. Elman, R.: Urinary Output of Nitrogen as Influenced by Intravenous Injection of a Mixture of Amino Acids, Proc. Soc. Exper. Biol. Med. 37: 610, 1938.

4. Elman, R., and Weiner, D. O.: Intravenous Alimentation with Special Reference to Protein (Amino Acid) Metabolism, J.A.M.A. 112:796, 1939.

5. Elman, R.: Time Factor in Retention of Nitrogen after Intravenous Injection of a Mixture of Amino Acids, Proc. Soc. Exper. Biol. Med. 40:484, 1939.

6. Elman, R.: Parenteral Replacement of Protein with the Amino Acids of Hydrolyzed Casein, Ann. Surg. 112:594, 1940.

7. Elman, R.: Maintenance of Nitrogen Balance by the Intravenous Administration of Plasma Proteins and Protein Hydrolysates, Physiol. Rev. 24: 372, 1944.

8. Elman, R.: Time Factors in the Utilization of a Mixture of Amino Acids (Protein Hydrolysate) and Dextrose Given Intravenously, J. Clin. Nutr. 1: 287, 1953.

9. Brunschwig, A.; Clark, D. E., and Corbin, N.: Postoperative Nitrogen Loss and Studies on Parenteral Nitrogen Nutrition by Means of Casein Digest, Ann. Surg. 115:1091, 1942.

10. Shohl, A. T.; Butler, A. M.; Blackfan, K. D., and MacLachlan, E.: Nitrogen Metabolism During the Oral and Parenteral Administration of the Amino Acids of Hydrolyzed Casein, J. Pediat. 15: 469, 1939.

11. Hartmann, A. F.; Meeker, C. S.; Perley, A. M., and McGinnis, H. G.: Studies of Amino Acid Administration, J. Pediat. 20:308, 1942.

12. Allen, J. G.; Stemmer, E., and Head, L. R.: Similar Growth Rates of Litter Mate Puppies Maintained on Oral Protein with Those on the Same Quantity of Protein as Daily Intravenous Plasma for 99 Days as Only Protein Source, Ann. Surg. 144:349, 1956.

13. Elman, R.: Acute Starvation Following Operation or Injury with Special Reference to Calorie and Protein Needs, Ann. Surg. 120:350, 1944.

14. Holden, W. D.; Grieger, H.; Levey, S., and Abbott, W. E.: The Effect of Nutrition on Nitrogen Metabolism in the Surgical Patient, Ann. Surg. 146:563, 1957.

15. Wilkinson, A. W.; Billing, B. H.; Nagy, G., and Stewart, C. P.: Nitrogen Metabolism After Surgical Operations, Lancet 1:533, 1950.

16. Brunschwig, A., and Corbin, N.: Clinical Study of Relative Efficiency for Nitrogen Metabolism of Casein Digest Administered Intravenously and Protein Ingested by Mouth, J. Surg. 14:898, 1943.

17. Messinger, W. J.: Nitrogen Equilibrium and Degeneration of Serum Protein Following Intravenous Use of Amino Acids, Arch. Intern. Med. 72: 91, 1941.

18. Gardner, C. E., Jr., and Trent, J. C.: Intravenous Amino Acid Administration in Surgical Patients Using an Enzymatic Casein Digest, Surg. Gynec. Obstet. 75:657, 1942.

19. Riegel, C.; Koop, C. E.; Dres, J.; Stevens, L. W., and Rhoads, T. E.: The Nutritional Requirements for Nitrogen Balance in Surgical Patients During the Early Postoperative Period, J. Clin. Invest. 26:18, 1947.

20. Peters, J. P.: Effect of Injury and Disease on Nitrogen Metabolism, Amer. J. Med. 5:100, 1948.

Experimental Venous Thrombosis and Thrombectomy

A. G. ROSS SHEIL, MB, BS, BA
AND
DAVID C. SABISTON, JR., MD
OXFORD, ENGLAND

Venous thrombosis continues to represent a troublesome and even fatal complication of a variety of medical and surgical disorders. Numerous methods of treatment have been employed in both the prevention and the management of this condition, but it is generally agreed that much yet remains to be done in the satisfactory solution of this difficult problem.

In the recent past direct thrombectomy has been advocated for acute and chronic venous occlusion. This has been employed in the femoral and iliac vessels particularly, and encouraging results have been reported by several observers.[1,2] In the present study an attempt has been made to devise a reliable method for the production of experimental thrombosis in large veins and to follow the natural history of such lesions with an investigation of the results following thrombectomy.

Submitted for publication Dec. 26, 1962.

From the Nuffield Department of Surgery, The University of Oxford, and The Radcliffe Infirmary, Oxford, England.

Methods

Twelve mongrel dogs (10-20 Kg.) were employed. Following premedication with morphine (1.25 mg. per kilogram) and chlorpromazine hydrochloride (Largactil) 1 mg. per kilogram, anesthesia was induced with veterinary pentobarbital (Nembutal) 0.4 ml. per kilogram. A long midline incision was made in the abdomen, and the inferior vena cava was exposed from the renal veins to the bifurcation. This technique has been described in detail elsewhere.[5] Briefly, the lumbar branches in this segment were isolated, ligated, and divided, and a small polythene catheter was introduced through one and passed into the inferior vena cava. A segment of vena cava between the renal and iliac veins was isolated by vascular clamps, and 2 ml. of concentrated (90%) phenol were injected through the catheter and allowed to remain for one minute. The phenol was then aspirated and the segment of vena cava irrigated several times with heparinized saline. The vascular clamps were then removed, and the venous circulation reestablished. The incision was closed, and the animal observed for a varying period. Subsequently the animal was killed or underwent reoperation. Venograms of the inferior vena cava were obtained by the insertion of a small nylon catheter into the femoral vein with injection of radio-opaque contrast medium. The catheters were left in place and filled with heparinized saline if

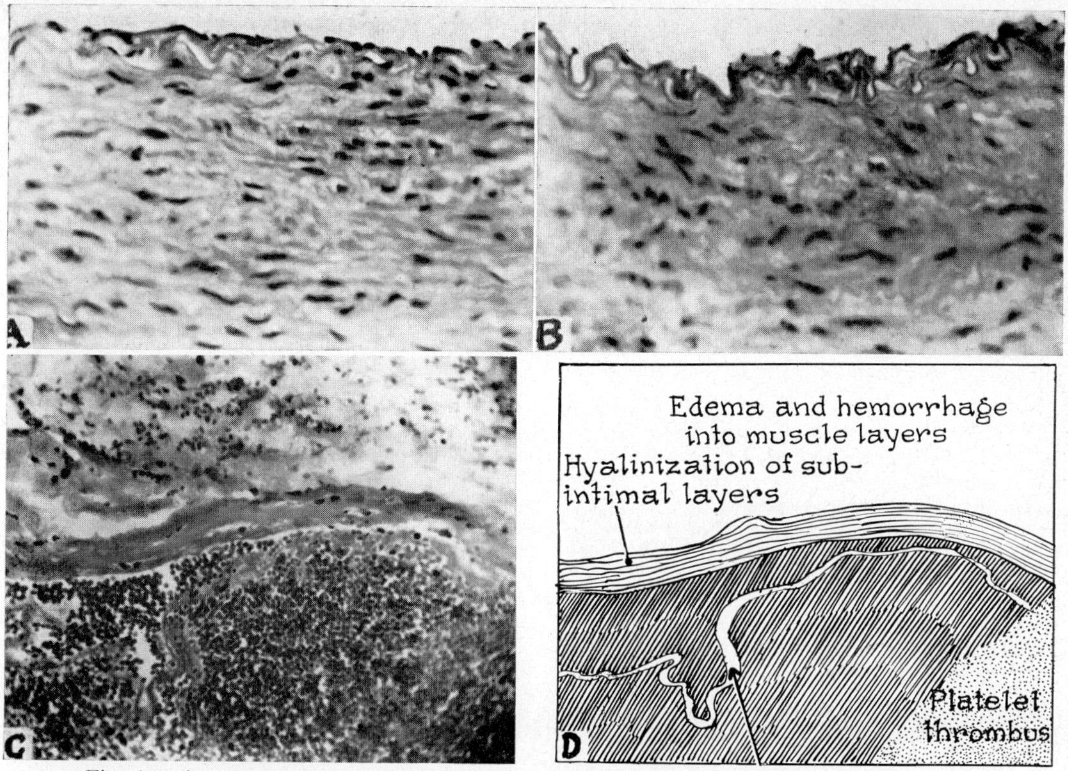

Fig. 1.—*A*, cross-section of the wall of a normal inferior vena cava of the dog. Reduced about 29% from mag. × 270. *B*, section of portion of the wall of the inferior vena cava immediately after exposure to concentrated phenol for one minute. Although the tissue becomes grossly opaque and white the microscopic changes are minimal. Reduced about 29% from mag. × 270. *C*, section of part of the wall of the inferior vena cava three days after exposure to phenol. The intima has separated completely, and there is hyalinization of the subintimal layers. Edema and hemorrhage of the muscle layer are present. *D*, diagrammatic illustration of Figure 1*C*. Arrow indicates separation of intima.

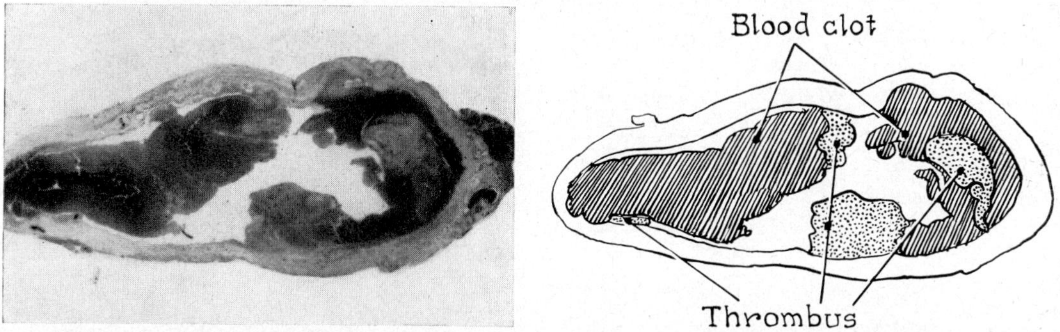

Fig. 2.—Section of inferior vena cava of dog three days after application of phenol. A thrombus composed of fibrin, platelets, leukocytes, and erythrocytes has formed in part of the lumen, and the remainder is blood clot.

further venograms were to be obtained on subsequent days.

Five animals were observed from three days to three weeks and then killed. In each instance thrombosis was complete after the fourth day (Figs. 1 and

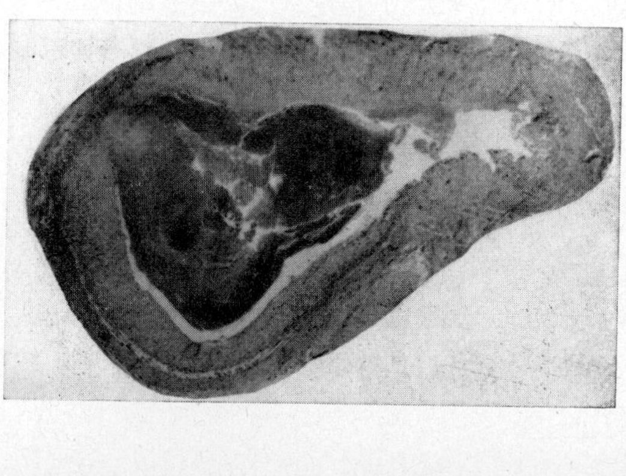

Fig. 3.—Section of inferior vena cava of the dog three weeks after exposure to phenol. Organization of the thrombus is proceeding. The apparent lumen is an artefact due to shrinkage of the thrombus from the vessel wall. At operation no blood flowed through the inferior vena cava, and venograms obtained at three weeks showed complete occlusion. × 10.

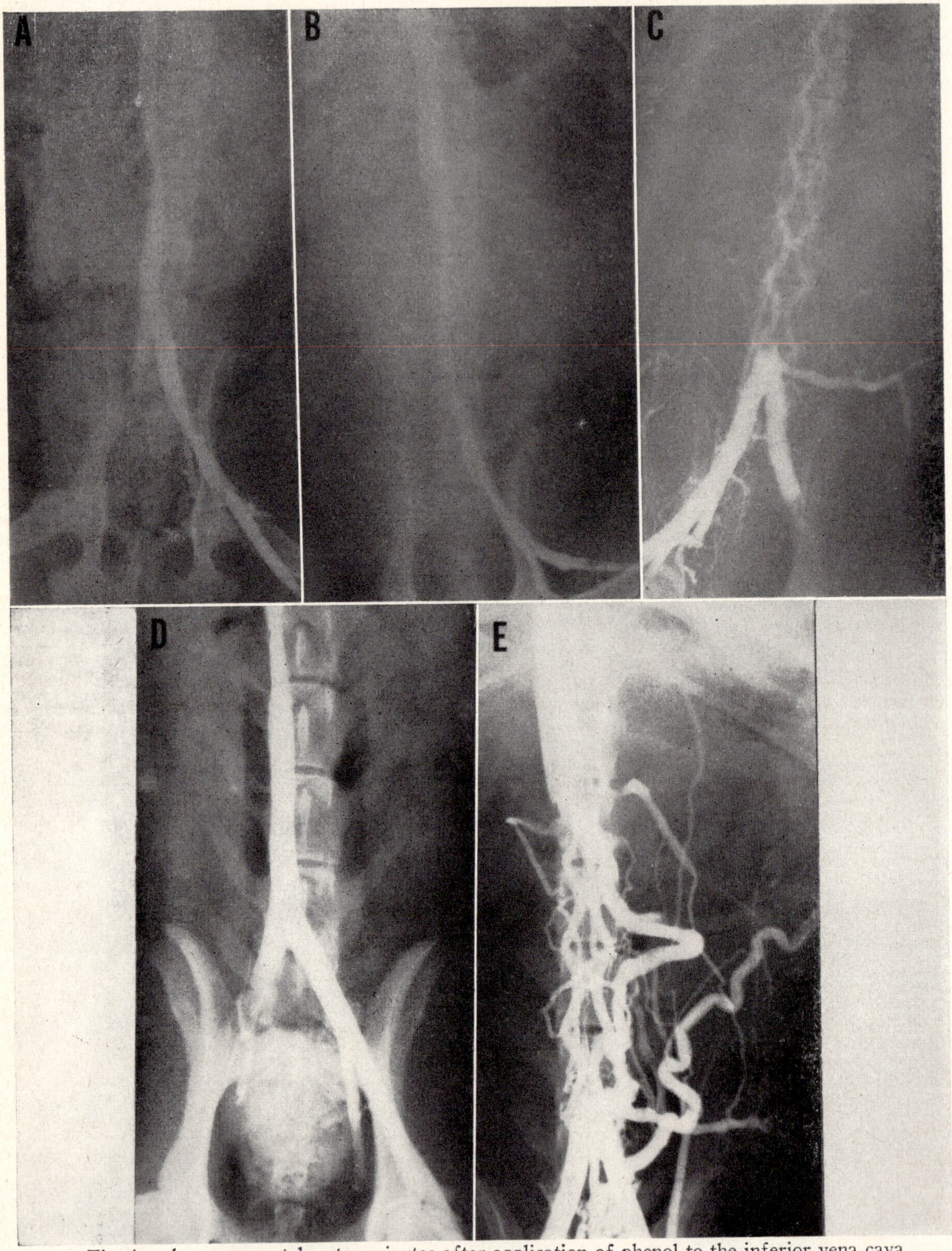

Fig. 4.—*A,* venogram taken ten minutes after application of phenol to the inferior vena cava. A constriction of the inferior vena cava just below the entrance of the renal veins is demonstrated. *B,* venogram taken three days after exposure to phenol with injection of contrast medium into the left femoral vein. A narrow channel is present. No collaterals are demonstrable at this time. *C,* venogram taken five days after exposure to phenol. There is now complete occlusion of the inferior vena cava, and collateral circulation is well developed. *D,* venogram taken after removal of the thrombus from the inferior vena cava. The lumen remains smooth, but the constriction below the level of the entry of the renal veins remains. *E,* venogram obtained three days after removal of thrombus from inferior vena cava. Complete occlusion is present with massive collateral circulation.

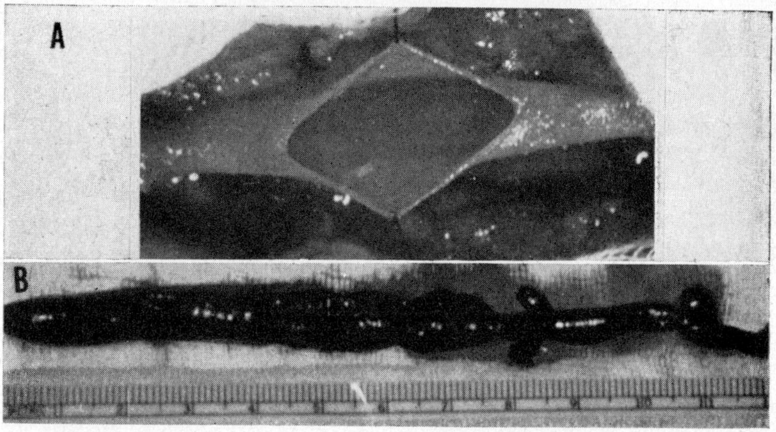

Fig. 5.—*A,* the internal surface of the inferior vena cava after thrombectomy. *B,* the thrombus after removal from the inferior vena cava.

2), and at three weeks the vena cava had become greatly contracted and contained organized thrombus (Fig. 3). Venograms demonstrated progressive narrowing of the lumen of the inferior vena cava with complete occlusion by the fourth day (Fig. 4). In seven animals ***thrombectomy*** was performed on the fourth to the seventh day. The previous midline incision was reopened, and the vena cava was incised longitudinally for about 3 cm. with careful removal of the thrombus and closure with No. 6-0 silk (Fig. 5). The results showed that the thrombus could be totally removed; the residual internal surface of the vena cava appeared smooth, but rethrombosis occurred in each instance within 3 days (Table).

Comment

Experimental venous thrombosis has been produced previously by a variety of means including mechanical trauma, obstruction, foreign bodies, chemical injury, and by electric current.[3-7] In our experience the introduction of a small amount of concentrated phenol into the venous lumen for a short period has produced thrombosis consistently. The method has been used previously to evaluate experimental pulmonary embolism and has proved quite satisfactory.[5]

In the present studies an attempt has been made to evaluate the course of complete venous thrombosis and of the response to *thrombectomy.* The results show that total occlusion of the inferior vena cava occurs by the fourth day after phenol injury and that both true thrombus and blood clot are initially present. With the passage of time the thrombus becomes organized, and the vein wall contracts. Concomitant with this process is the development of a massive venous collateral circulation.

Thrombectomy.—This procedure may be easily performed in these preparations with return of normal blood flow through the inferior vena cava. Serial venograms demon-

Results of Application of Phenol to Isolated Segment of Inferior Vena Cava

Expt. No.	Procedure	Result
1 2 3	Venogram at 3 wk.; immediate killing of animal	Total occlusion of inferior vena cava with development of collateral circulation; grossly, cava appeared as fibrous cord; microscopic examination showed organized thrombus in lumen
4	Daily venograms & killing at 4 days	Gradual occlusion; complete thrombosis after 4 days
12	Killed at 3 days	Thrombus, incomplete occlus. of vena cava
5 6 7 9	Thrombectomy after 7 days; venograms 3 days later	Complete occlus. by thrombus, 7 days; complete reocclusion 3 days after thrombect. demonstrated by venograms; extensive collat. circulation demonstrated
10	*Thrombectomy* at 6 days; venogram, day following	Complete occlus. at 6 days & complete reocclus. after thrombect.; extensive collat. circulation
11	Daily venograms & *thrombectomy* after 6 days foll. by venograms	Gradual occlus.; complete thrombosis after 5 days; gradual reocclus. with complete thrombosis foll. thrombectomy within 2 days
13	*Thrombectomy* after 5 days; killing, day foll.	Complete thrombotic occlus. & incomplete reocclus., foll. day

strate that reocclusion characteristically occurs by the second or third day. Extensive collateral circulation persists if it has already developed, or it appears if the thrombectomy is performed a short time after appearance of a complete thrombotic occlusion. It should be emphasized that this method for the production of experimental thrombosis is one which produces a *thrombus* similar to that occurring in human venous thrombosis, although the mechanism of production differs from that found in the clinical condition. This factor may be of considerable importance in the secondary thrombosis consistently observed following thrombectomy.

Summary

A method producing chemical intimal injury is described which consistently produces large venous thrombi similar in microscopic appearance to those occurring in humans. Total thrombotic occlusion of the inferior vena cava below the renal veins is followed by the development of a massive collateral circulation. Subsequent thrombectomy may be easily performed with restoration of blood flow in the vena cava, but rethrombosis regularly develops within several days.

David C. Sabiston, Jr., M.D., Associate Professor of Surgery, The Johns Hopkins Hospital, Baltimore 5.

REFERENCES

1. Haller, J. A.: Thrombectomy for Acute Ileofemoral Venous Thrombosis, Arch. Surg. 83:448, 1961.

2. Mahorner, H.; Castleberry, J. W., and Coleman, W. A.: Attempts to Restore Function in Major Veins which are the Site of Massive Thrombosis, Ann. Surg. 146:510, 1957.

3. Marin, H. M., and Stefanini, M.: Experimental Production of Phlebothrombosis, Surg. Gynec. Obstet. 110:263, 1960.

4. Robertson, H. R.; Perrett, T. S.; Colbeck, J. C., and Moyes, P. D.: Reaction of Wall of Vein to Intraluminal Blood Clot, Surg. Gynec. Obstet. 98: 705, 1954.

5. Sabiston, D. C.; Marshall, R.; Dunnill, M. S., and Allison, P. R.: Experimental Pulmonary Embolism: Description of a Method Utilizing Large Venous Thrombi, Surgery 52:9, 1962.

6. Wessler, S.: Experimentally Produced Phlebothrombosis in the Study of Thrombo-Embolism, J. Clin. Invest. 32:610, 1953.

7. Williams, R. D., and Carey, L. C.: Studies in the Production of "Standard" Venous Thrombosis, Ann. Surg. 149:381, 1959.

Pyloric Atresia

JERROLD M. BECKER, MD; KEITH M. SCHNEIDER, MD; AND ALFRED E. FISCHER, MD, NEW YORK

Atresia of the pylorus has been reported in 16 newborn infants. Eleven of these have survived.

Two of the patients were under 5 lb (2,267 gm) in weight at birth. Seven were female, eight were males, and in one case the sex of the patient was not indicated.

This case is reported to describe a method of surgical treatment which we feel is useful in all cases of gastric, duodenal, and high jejunal obstruction in the newborn.

Report of a Case

The patient was born on Oct 16, 1961, weighing 5 lb 4 oz (2,381.36 gm). Because of polyhydramnios, a tube was passed into the infant's stomach to rule out esophageal atresia. Six cc of clear gastric fluid was obtained.

The baby was given feedings of 5% glucose-water starting at 12 hr of age. Some spitting up of feedings was noted. The vomitus was not bile stained.

At 24 hr of age, a plain film and upright of the abdomen were obtained. Gas could be seen to fill the stomach, but no gas was noted distally.

On Oct 18, 1961, the infant was taken to the operating room with an infusion via a "cut down." An 8F nasogastric tube was used to decompress the stomach. Under satisfactory cyclopropane anesthesia the abdomen was opened through a transverse incision, one finger-breadth above the umbilicus. The incision extended from the midline out into the right flank.

The stomach was larger than normal and hypertrophied. The small bowel was collapsed. Ten cc of saline were injected into the duodenum through a 24-gauge needle. The saline was traced down the small bowel and around the colon. The saline did not pass retrograde into the stomach, and air could not be milked into the duodenum from the stomach. The site of obstruction appeared to be the proximal pylorus.

A 2 cm longitudinal incision was made across the pylorus from the gastric to the duodenal end. A membranous web 2 mm in thickness was found completely occluding the lumen. The web was excised, and the posterior mucosa approximated with interrupted 50 chromic sutures.

A Stamm gastrostomy was then performed, using two purse-string sutures of No. 4-0 atraumatic chromic catgut. An 8F polyethylene catheter and a 14F Foley catheter were brought through a stab wound in the center of the left rectus muscle and led through the gastrostomy opening into the stomach. The polyethylene catheter was advanced through the pylorus and duodenum, and threaded approximately 15 cm into the jejunum. The Foley balloon was inflated with 3 cc of saline and pulled up against the anterior wall of the stomach as the purse-string sutures were tied. The outer purse string was sutured to the peritoneum with the stomach pulled up against the anterior wall.

The longitudinal incision through the pylorus was then closed transversely with interrupted No 50 Atraumatic silk. The peritoneum and fascia were approximated with vertical figure-of-eight sutures

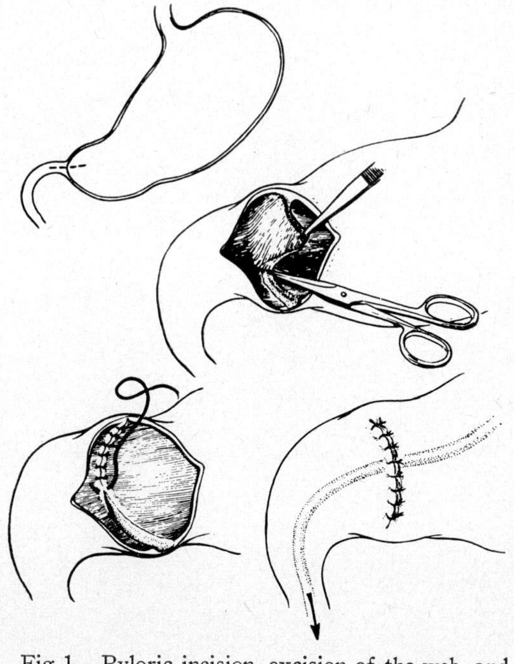

Fig 1.—Pyloric incision, excision of the web, and type of closure with indwelling feeding tube.

Submitted for publication Jan 16, 1963.

Departments of Surgery and Pediatrics, The Mount Sinai Hospital.

of No 32 wire. Skin edges were approximated with interrupted No 4-0 silk (Fig 1).

The infant was given penicillin and tetracycline for eight days after the operation.

Postoperatively, the gastrostomy tube was placed on gravity drainage, and the jejunostomy tube was occluded. After 24 hours, the patient's gastric drainage was instilled into the jejunostomy tube. After 48 hours, glucose and dilute electrolyte solution was instilled into the jejunostomy tube. On the third postoperative day, formula was given through the jejunostomy tube.

Intravenous fluids were discontinued on the third postoperative day. On the eighth postoperative day, skin sutures were removed.

On the ninth postoperative day, the baby pulled out both the gastrostomy tube (the balloon was deflated) and the jejunostomy tube.

On the tenth postoperative day, oral feedings were started and were well tolerated. The baby was kept on Nutramigen during the hospital stay.

On the 14th hospital day, the gastrostomy incision was noted to be closed.

The baby was discharged on the 22nd hospital day weighing 4 lb 13 oz (2,183 gm).

At 6 mo of age the baby weighs 14 lb (6,350 gm) and is on a normal diet.

Comment

Despite the rarity of this condition, the diagnosis of pyloric atresia should not be difficult. The mothers are frequently noted to have polyhydramnios (over 2,000 cc of amniotic fluid). In nine cases of pyloric atresia, this finding has been described (Table). In fetuses with high intestinal obstruction, swallowed amniotic fluid cannot reach the small intestinal mucosa to be absorbed, and therefore it accumulates. Clatworthy[1]

Findings in 16 Cases of Pyloric Atresia

Author	Yr.	Birth Weight Lb.	Polyhydramnios	Operation (Day)	Pathology	Type Operation	Result	Sex
Bennett	1937	7^{3}	+	4th	Web	Atresia overlooked; Ramstedt procedure	D	F
Metz	1940	8^{3}		3rd	6 cm. apart double web	Radial incision of webs & nasogastric tube into duodenum	L	M
Touroff	1940	6	+	5th	Web	Radial incision of web & pyloroplasty	L	F
Holladay	1946	5^{5}		7th	2 cm. defect	Gastrojejunostomy	D	M
Burnett	1947		+	2nd	1 cm. defect	Atresia overlooked; closure of perforation of stomach	D	M
Benson	1951	6	+	6th	Web	Excision of web	L	F
				13th		Edema found		
				27th		Gastrojejunostomy		
Fell	1951			12th	Web	Gastrojejunostomy	D	Not listed
Lemak	1951	Not recorded	+	7th	Web	Excision of web	L	F
				12th		Opening probed		
				19th		Gastrojejunostomy		
Brown	1959	$3^{5\ 1/2}$		10th	Internal cord 0.6 cm.	Excision of cord & pyloroplasty; gastroduodenal tube	L	F
Brown	1959	$3^{8\ 1/2}$		7th	Web	Incision of web; nasogastric tube into duodenum	L	M
Lauste	1959	6^{8}	+	5th	Antrum cord	Gastrojejunostomy	L	M
Salzberg	1960	5^{5}	+	1st	Web	Gastrojejunostomy	D	F
				9th		Ileostomy		
Davis	1961	$5^{3\ 1/2}$	+	6th	Web	Incision of web & pyloroplasty	L	M
				12th		Duodenal intubation via gastrostomy		
Wurtemberger	1961	5^{8}		6th	Web	Ramstedt procedure	L	F
				9th		Perforation of web		
				23rd		Gastrojejunostomy		
Becker	1961	5^{4}	+	2nd	Web	Excision of web & pyloroplasty; jejunal intubation via gastrostomy	L	F
Kornfeld	1962	8^{1}		3rd	2 mm. defect	Gastroduodenostomy	L	M
Kornfeld	1962	Not recorded		3rd	Web	Excision of web; gastroduodenojejunostomy & gastrostomy	L	M

reports polyhydramnios in 45% of mothers whose infants had duodenal or jejunal obstruction.

The babies vomit within the first 24 hours of life and cannot retain feedings. The vomitus is not bile stained. The upper abdomen is frequently distended.

X-rays reveal a dilated stomach with no gas beyond the pylorus (Fig 2). It is not necessary to use contrast material to make or confirm the diagnosis.

The operative findings, techniques, and results of the cases reported in this literature are listed in the Table. Fourteen patients had membranous atresia. Three patients presented with a loss of continuity of the bowel, in the pyloric region, for 2 mm and 1 and 2 cm. One patient had double pyloric web.

Two patients had, obviously, inadequate surgery, with performance of a Ramstedt procedure in one,[2] and simple closure of a gastric perforation in the other.[3] Both of these patients died.

Fig 2.—X-ray of the abdomen revealing the absence of any air in the gastrointestinal tract beyond the pylorus.

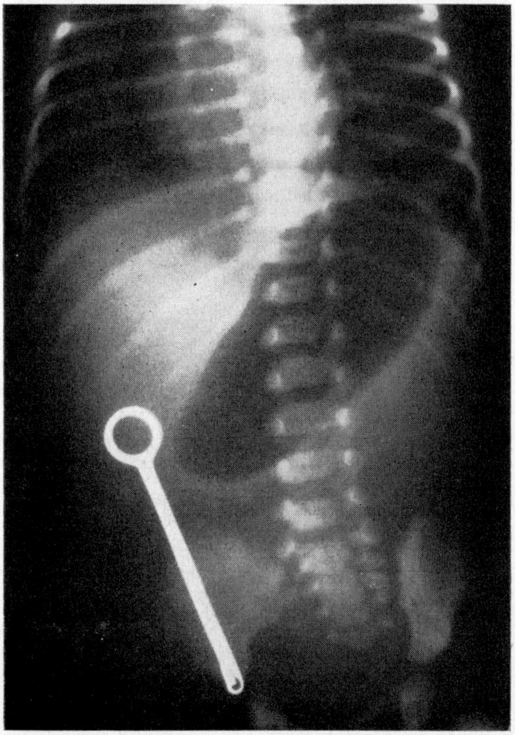

There are 12 patients who survived after surgery for pyloric atresia.

One of the survivors required two operative procedures, and three required a third procedure.

Davis' patient [4] had an incision of the web and pyloroplasty at 6 days of age. At 12 days of age a duodenal intubation was performed via a gastrostomy.

Benson's [5] patient had an excision of the pyloric diaphragm at 6 days of age, and at 13 days of age he was reexplored and found to have stomal edema. The baby required a third procedure, a gastrojejunostomy, at 27 days of age. A gastrointestinal series at 2 mo of age revealed that the gastrojejunostomy had closed as the pyloric edema subsided.

Wurtemberger's [6] patient had a pyloromyotomy performed on the sixth day of life. On the ninth day, the pyloric web was perforated and dilated, and a tube passed via a gastrostomy opening into the duodenum. Two weeks after the operation a gastrointestinal series showed opaque medium passing through the pylorus along the tube. A short time later the child began to vomit again, and a gastrojejunostomy was performed.

Lemak's [7] patient was operated on at seven days of age. The membrane was incised and "sutured so that patency was present." A gastrointestinal series five days later revealed a high degree of obstruction after 6 hr. At surgery, there was edema at the pylorus. Seven days after the second operation, the baby began to vomit, and a gastrojejunostomy was performed.

Of four [8-11] patients treated by gastrojejunostomy alone, three died. Even if this procedure resulted in an acceptable mortality, the probable high incidence of marginal ulcer would make this operation inadvisable.

Kornfeld,[12] who reported two cases of pyloric atresia successfully treated, suggested the use of a side-to-side gastroduodenostomy.

All four [13,14] patients who were treated by incision or excision of the web, and the addition of a feeding tube passed distal to the site of surgery, survived with a single operation.

The technique used in this case has been used successfully by us, for duodenal atresia and stenosis and high jejunal obstruction, for the past four years. It was previously described by Glover in 1949.

The gastrostomy tube affords excellent decompression of the stomach without the need of an irritating tube running through the pharynx. There is no need for elaborate formulas for replacement of gastric drainage, since this fluid is reintroduced into the intestinal tract via the jejunal tube. This tube also affords a method of supplying an adequate caloric intake. Another advantage of placing the jejunal tube in through the gastrostomy opening is that there can be no narrowing of the already minute small bowel lumen such as would occur through an independent enterostomy. It is well known that gastrostomy tubes can be well tolerated for months or even years. However, some authors have hesitated to use a tube across a suture line. We have found, however, that a Size 5 F polyethylene tube has been tolerated for 2-3 weeks.

Summary

A case of pyloric atresia in the newborn period is reported. The patient is the 12th survivor of the 17 newborns with pyloric atresia recorded in the literature.

The usual cause of obstruction is a web completely occluding the lumen. Surgical therapy has consisted of incision or excision of the web and/or a bypass procedure (gastrojejunostomy).

The authors suggest a technique of excision of the web, gastrostomy, and passage of a feeding tube into the jejunum via the gastrostomy opening through the anterior abdominal and gastric walls.

The major advantages of this method include good decompression of the stomach and early alimentation through the jejunal tube.

This method has successfully been used in all varieties of high intestinal obstructions in the newborn.

Jerrold M. Becker, MD, Klingenstein Pavilion, The Mount Sinai Hospital, 1176 Fifth Ave, New York 29.

REFERENCES

1. Lloyd, J. R.; Clatworthy, H. W., Jr.: Hydramnios as an Aid to the Early Diagnosis of Congenital Obstruction of the Alimentary Tract: A Study of the Maternal and Fetal Factors, Pediatrics 21:903-909, 1958.

2. Bennett, R. J., Jr.: Atresia of the Pylorus, Amer J Dig Dis 4:44, 1937.

3. Burnett, H. A., and Halpert, B.: Perforation of the Stomach of a Newborn Infant with Pyloric Atresia, Arch Path 44:318-320, 1947.

4. Davis, D. A., and Douglas, K. R.: Congenital Pyloric Atresia, A Rare Anomaly: Report of a Successful Case, Ann Surg 153:418-422, 1961.

5. Benson, C. D., and Coury, J. J.: Congenital Intrinsic Obstruction of the Stomach and Duodenum in the Newborn, AMA Arch Surg 62:856-866, 1951.

6. Wurtemberger, H.: Gastrict Atresia, Arch Dis Child 36:161-163, 1961.

7. Lemak, L. L.: Roentgenological Manifestations of Gastroduodenal Ulceration in the Newborn, Amer J Roentgenol 66:191-199, 1951.

8. Holladay, L. J.: Case Report of Congenital Aplasia of the Pylorus, J Indiana Med Ass 39:350-351, 1946.

9. Fell, E. H.: In discussion of Benson and Coury, 1951.

10. Lauste, L. W., and Mestit, W.: Atresia of the Pyloric Antrum, Proc Roy Soc Med 52:1027-1028, 1959.

11. Salzberg, A. M., and Collins, R. E.: Congenital Pyloric Atresia, AMA Arch Surg 80:501-505, 1960.

12. Kornfeld, H. J.: Pyloric Atresia and Its Repair, Surgery 51:569-573, 1962.

13. Metz, A. R.; Householder, R., and LePree, J. F.: Obstruction of the Stomach Due to Congenital Double Septum with Cyst Formation, Trans West Surg Ass 50:242-251, 1940.

14. Brown, R. P., and Hertzler, J. H.: Congenital Prepyloric Gastric Atresia: A Report of 2 Cases, AMA J Dis Child 97:857-862, 1959.

15. Glover, D. M., and Barry, F.: Intestinal Obstruction in the Newborn, Ann Surg 130:480-511, 1949.

16. Touroff, A. S. W., and Sussman, R. M.: Congenital Prepyloric Membranous Obstruction in a Premature Infant, Surgery 8:739-755, 1940.

Practical Methods of Short-Term Storage of Homografts

LCDR RICHARD B. GRESHAM, MC, USN
LT VERNON P. PERRY, MSC, USN
AND
CDR VERA K. THOMPSON, MC, USN

Introduction

A practical concept of tissue banking must evolve from clinical demand and economic feasibility. It is the purpose of this paper to present methods of tissue procurement and processing which are satisfactory for limited storage periods and are within the economic capabilities of the average community hospital.

The ready availability of tissues from the recently deceased should enable surgeons to meet their requirements for all homografts which are currently practical for human transplantation. Studies based upon tissue culture of postmortem tissues indicate that viability is retained by most of these tissues for at least 24 hours after clinical death.[1] The practice of removing tissues for human transplantation within this 24 hour period has been substantiated by the clinical results obtained from the use of this material in a large number of patients.[2] It is therefore possible for the physician to use cadavers as a source of satisfactory homografts within a convenient 24 hour period provided the body has been stored in a morgue at +4 C from the time of death until graft excision.

Submitted for publication Jan 9, 1963.

Tissue Bank Department, US Naval Medical School, National Naval Medical Center, Bethesda 14, Md.

The opinions and views expressed are those of the authors and are not to be construed as official or necessarily reflecting those of the Medical Department of the United States Navy or the Naval Service at large.

Experience has shown that permission is easily obtained from the next-of-kin for excision of specific tissues for human transplantation. A simple form signed by the legal next-of-kin and witnessed by the requesting physician is all that is legally required in most states[3] (Fig 1).

If the tissues are not to be sterilized prior to storage, formal surgical preparation of the cadaver must precede their removal under aseptic conditions. This must include shaving and cleansing with a surgical soap followed by preparation of the skin with an antiseptic and surgical draping. If the skin is to be stored, strong antiseptics should not be used as this may alter cell viability. Multiple preparations with a surgical detergent followed by rinsing with sterile saline is more feasible for the preparation of this tissue. Because of the state of the physiology of these tissues and their loss of normal mechanisms to combat local bacterial contamination, this procedure must be extremely meticulous. If the tissues are to be sterilized, excision may be performed under less than operating room conditions but should include cleansing of the skin to avoid gross contamination with foreign materials.

Tissues which are currently of practical value for human transplantation include skin, bone, fascia, dura, and cartilage.[4] Although a variety of methods are available for processing each of these tissues, only those which have been found to be relatively simple and have withstood clinical trial are presented.

Standard Form 523B
Promulgated by
Bureau of the Budget
Circular A-32 Revised

U. S. GOVERNMENT PRINTING OFFICE · 1958—O-482714

CLINICAL RECORD | **AUTHORIZATION FOR TISSUE DONATION**

In the event authorization for tissue donation is obtained by letter, telegram, or mechanically recorded telephone call, paragraphs 1 and 2 shall be completed by hospital authorities and the letter, telegram, or memorandum confirming telephone call of authorization attached to this form for permanent file.

NAME AND LOCATION OF HOSPITAL
1.

DATE

2. You are hereby authorized to remove the following-named tissue from the remains of

.... (Name of deceased) .... for donation to the Tissue

Bank of .... (Name of hospital)

.... (Specify: tissue, eg. bone, artery, cartilage, skin, fascia, dura, nerve, tendon, etc.)

Authority is also granted to use the tissue in grafts upon living persons, or to dispose of the tissue in a suitable manner.

Signature of witness ....

Signature .... (Person authorized to consent)

Address ....

Address ....

Authority to consent ....

PATIENT'S IDENTIFICATION (*For typed or written entries give: Name—last, first, middle; grade; date; hospital or medical facility*)

REGISTER NO. WARD NO.

AUTHORIZATION FOR TISSUE DONATION
Standard Form 523B

Fig 1.—Form used at the US Navy Tissue Bank to obtain permission for excision of grafts.

Simple Refrigeration

Fresh skin homografts may be maintained in a viable condition in excess of two weeks by simple refrigeration storage.[5] The skin grafts may be removed with an electric dermatome. Usually split thickness grafts measuring 0.010 to 0.015 in. are most desirable. If large quantities of skin are to be removed from a single cadaver, excision of the grafts should not involve areas which might be exposed on burial. In general it is best to limit donor sites to areas below the nipple line, avoiding the upper extremities, hands, and neck.

After aseptic removal, the skin is wrapped in gauze sponges soaked in a saline solution of antibiotics and stored in sterile bottles in an ordinary refrigerator. This method is particularly suitable for procurement of tissues from a single cadaver for use within a few days on a severely burned patient.

Nutrient Media

Viable storage of many tissues may be accomplished using various types of nutrient solutions. Experiences of the US Navy Tissue Bank are based upon the storage of skin in media containing Earle's balanced salt solution [6] and 10% pooled human serum maintained at normal refrigerator temperatures of +3 to +5 C.

Human split-thickness skin stored in this media in tightly sealed glass units will survive for six to eight weeks.[7] This will permit the collection of skin from several sources to be stored in anticipation of a future grafting procedure. Human skin autografts stored by this method have resulted in permanent clinical takes similar to fresh autografts,[8] permitting storage of excess grafts for use at a later date on the same patient. Other tissues such as fascia and dura may also be temporarily stored in nutrient media.

Storage in nutrient media provides for cell maintenance at the depressed level of metabolic activity accomplished by lowered temperatures. In addition, the buffering capacity of the media compensates for accumulating cell acid catabolites while the cell oxygen demands are significantly decreased by the lowered temperature.

Earle's balanced salt solution complete with $NaHCO_3$ and phenol red indicator may be purchased commercially in sterile bottles.* To this solution is added pooled human serum 10% by volume, 200 units of penicillin, and 0.1 mg of streptomycin per ml. The serum may also be obtained commercially or procured from the local blood bank and processed by the following method: Raw serum is obtained from whole blood drawn into 600 ml sterile blood-collection bottles free of anticoagulants. The blood is refrigerated for a minimum of one hour to assure maximum clot retraction. The clotted blood is then centrifuged in a refrigerated centrifuge at a temperature of +5 C at approximately 2,300 rpm (1,370 g) for 30 minutes. After centrifugation the serum is aspirated with a sterile 50 cc syringe and a long needle into storage flasks. The flasks should not be filled more than half full. If more than one unit of blood is obtained, the serum should not be pooled at this time but stored in separate flasks in a freezer. The serum is pooled immediately before media preparation after it has been determined that the Kahn is negative. Pooled serum is desirable in that antigens or toxins from a single donor are diluted by pooling and thus more favorable to cell survival.

If these procedures are carried out under sterile conditions and cultured for bacterial contaminants, further sterilization is not necessary. However, if sterilization is required this can be accomplished after mixing the serum with the salt solution followed by closed filtration sterilization through a Selas filter according to methods described by Perry and Kindred.[9] The final solution should be sealed in sterile glass containers and maintained in a refrigerator at +3 to +5 C until ready for use. Under these conditions the solution may be stored for three to six months.

Using a 200 cc jar,† approximately 75 sq cm of skin are rolled in perforated cellophane,‡ lightly tied with a silk suture, and placed in 180 cc of the nutrient media. This results in a ratio of about 2.4 cc of media for each square centimeter of skin, and allows a 20 cc air space between the surface of the media and the lid of the container. A small sheet of sterile Teflon (0.003″ thick)§ is used between the screw lid and the jar to assure a tight seal and to prevent the media from coming in contact with the metal lid. The 200 cc bottle is placed in a larger jar to protect the sterility (Fig 2).

The phenol red index of acid catabolite accumulation as evidenced by a change i[illegible] color from a cherry red to an orange-yell[illegible] indicates the need for a change in nut[illegible]nt media solution. One half of this s[illegible]on should be changed under sterile c[illegible]ons with bacterial cultures being tak[illegible] the time of the change. Tissues m[illegible]a[illegible]fely stored by this method for a[illegible] six weeks.

Thimero[illegible]

Nonviable tissues m[illegible] by a variety of methods for l[illegible]f time. The use of thimerosal [illegible] to preserve

* Sources: Microbiological Associates, Inc., Bethesda, Md; Flow Laboratories, Inc., Arlington, Va; Cappel Laboratories, West Chester, Pa; Difco Laboratories, Detroit, Mich.

† Source: Owen[illegible] Company, Alton, Ill.

‡ Source: M[illegible]ociates, Inc., Bethesda, Md.

§ Source[illegible], Washington, D.C.

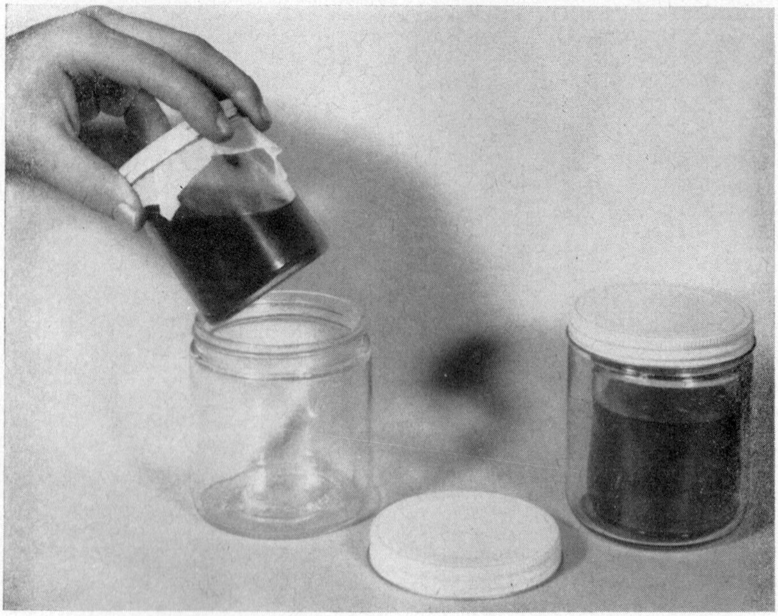

Fig 2.—Double bottle unit used for tissue storage.

cartilage and bone has been well documented in the literature.[10,11] This method has been used by the US Navy Tissue Bank for the storage of cartilage homografts.

Under sterile conditions the cartilage is removed from the costal cartilages of the ribs and cleaned of soft tissues, cut into desired lengths, cultured, and placed in sterile glass jars containing 1:1,000 solution of aqueous thimerosal.|| Containers similar to those used for nutrient media storage are satisfactory for this purpose. The grafts re temporarily stored in this solution at 4 C for 14 days, after which they are re- r ed from the thimerosal, recultured, and th sited in a fresh 1:1,000 solution of re sal. The tissue is then stored in a evi tor where it is observed weekly for clou f clouding of the solution. If ture curs, the tissue should be recul- shoul deposited. If contaminated it planta rded. Prior to surgical im- saline. ssue is washed in sterile stored homografts have been years. od for as long as seven

|| Source Company, Indianapolis, Ind.

Freezing

Modern freezing techniques have made possible the viable storage of many tissues.[12] However, the techniques and storage systems are too complex for the average hospital. If viability is not the prime object, then less refined methods may be utilized to store nonviable tissues for limited periods of time. The frozen storage of bone homografts is currently practiced by many hospitals utilizing material taken from surgical procedures such as rib resections in thoracotomies. Clinical results reported by Wilson indicate a reasonable degree of success.[13] The bone may be removed at the time of surgery or from a cadaver under sterile conditions. It is cut into proper size, gently washed in saline to remove excess blood and fat, and placed in a sterile bottle with a screw top lid as previously described. This bottle may be placed in a second sterile container to assure the sterility of the first. The doubly bottled tissue may then be placed in a household deep freezer where storage is considered to be safe for about three months. Although longer periods of storage have been used, gross changes in color and bone texture have been noted on prolonged frozen storage. The effects of these changes on the clinical application of the graft are not known.

Sterilization Methods

Nonviable tissues procured under less than sterile conditions require some type of sterilization prior to storage. Over the past years the US Navy Tissue Bank has used both ethylene oxide and β-propiolactone as sterilizing agents for potential human homografts. Both of these agents have given satisfactory results. This approach has been more recently applied to the processing of dura which is removed in the morgue under unsterile conditions, and sterilized in 1% β-propiolactone prior to freeze-drying.

The concentrated β-propiolactone ¶ is first diluted to a 10% concentration by the addition of distilled water. Further dilution to 1% is accomplished by the addition of a bicarbonate saline solution. The bicarbonate saline is made by adding 16.8 gm of sodium bicarbonate to 1,000 ml of normal saline.

The tissue to be sterilized is covered with the 1% β-propiolactone and incubated at 37 C for three hours. It is then washed in a phosphate buffer solution which is prepared as follows: disodium hydrogen phosphate, 7.755 gm; potassium dihydrogen phosphate, 1.6557 gm; distilled water, 1,000 ml. The buffered phosphate solution is autoclaved prior to use. Once the tissue has been processed, bacterial cultures are taken to confirm sterility. The tissue may then be frozen or stored in nutrient media.

Summary

A variety of methods are currently available for the storage of human homografts. However, many of these are not practical for use where equipment and personnel are limited. Techniques of storage and sterilization of human homografts have been presented in sufficient detail to enable the surgeon to process and store these tissues in limited quantity for a limited period of time. It is with this practical approach that every hospital can have within its capabilities a functional tissue bank.

¶ Source: Testagar & Co., Inc., Detroit.

R. B. Gresham, Lieutenant Commander, Medical Corps, US Navy, US Naval Medical School, Bethesda 14, Md.

REFERENCES

1. Perry, V. P.; Pappas, A. M.; Zink, G. A.; and Stevenson, R. E.: Tissue Culture Studies of Tissues Removed at Post-Mortem Procedures, to be published.

2. Gresham, R. B.; Perry, V. P.; and Wheeler, T. E.: US Navy Tissue Bank: Report on Current Methods and Experimental Approaches to the Future, JAMA 183:13 (Jan 5) 1963.

3. Medical-Legal Source Material for Tissue Procurement, staff publication, Virology Research Resources Branch, National Cancer Institute, National Institutes of Health, 1961.

4. Hyatt, G. W.: The Tissue Bank: Present and Future, Milit Med 125:523-531 (Aug) 1960.

5. Brown, J. B., and Fryer, M. P.: Postmortem Homografts, Springfield, Ill: Charles C Thomas, Publishers, 1960, p 31.

6. Earle, W. R.: Production of Malignancy in Vitro: IV. The Mouse Fibroblast Cultures and Changes Seen in Living Cells, J Nat Cancer Inst 4:165 (Oct) 1943.

7. Young, J. M., and Hyatt, G. W.: Stored Skin Homografts in Extensively Burned Patients, AMA Arch Surg 80:208-213 (Feb) 1960.

8. Connelly, J. R.: Aggression in the Treatment of Burns, Southern Med J, to be published.

9. Perry, V. P., and Kindred, R. G.: A Closed System of Filtration for Sterilization, US Armed Forces Med J Med Tech Bull 7:36-40 (Jan-Feb) 1956.

10. O'Connor, G. B.: Merthiolate: A Tissue Preservative and Antiseptic, Amer J Surg 45:563 (Sept) 1939.

11. Reynolds, F. C.; Oliver, D. R.; and Ramsey, R. H.: Clinical Evaluation of the Merthiolate Bone Bank and Homogenous Bone Grafts, J Bone Joint Surg (Amer) 33A:873-883 (Oct) 1951.

12. Perry, V. P.: Techniques of Viable Tissue Storage, Fed Proc 22:102 (Jan-Feb) 1963.

13. Wilson, P. D.: Experience With Use of Refrigerated Homogenous Bone, J Bone Joint Surg 33B:301-315 (Aug) 1951.

Acute Intestinal Obstruction Caused by Food

A Case Report

MAURICE A. CLAMAN, MD
GALESBURG, ILL

Although acute intestinal obstruction is a relatively common surgical disease, it is not widely recognized that the ingestion of foodstuffs can produce the disease. The extensive review of Ward-McQuaid in 1950 called more attention to the clinical entity, and since then other authors have added their experiences.[6]

It has become apparent that while most foodstuff obstructions occur in grossly normal gastrointestinal tracts, a disproportionate number occur in patients who have previously had partial gastrectomies.[1-5] Evidently the food bolus, passing rapidly into the intestine through the surgically altered stomach, arrives at the ileum poorly digested with its fibrous components intact and, becoming impacted there, causes the obstruction.

It is reasonable to assume that even in the absence of rapid intestinal transit such an obstruction might occur if poorly digested food becomes lodged in an area of preexisting intestinal stenosis. The following case illustrates this phenomenon.

Submitted for publication Jan. 4, 1963.

Report of a Case

On March 18, 1961, a 49-year-old white male transient was admitted to St. Mary's Hospital, Galesburg, Ill., complaining of severe cramping abdominal pain and vomiting. The symptoms began about 12 hours previously and became progressively worse. There had been accompanying moderate abdominal distention. No flatus had been passed since the onset of the pain. On the previous night, the patient had eaten fresh coconut for the first time in his life. He attributed his present illness to "bad coconut," although the person who had shared the coconut with him had assured him at the time, that it tasted like all coconuts. The patient's past history was noncontributory except for an appendectomy which had been performed many years previously.

Physical examination revealed a moderately distended abdomen. There were high-pitched bowel sounds appearing in rushes. These rushes were accompanied by severe cramping abdominal pain. X-ray examination of the abdomen revealed dilated small bowel loops in the upper abdomen, and these contained fluid levels.

An exploratory laparotomy was performed. The small bowel, as far as proximal ileum, was dilated. Beyond this point the small bowel was collapsed. At the point of obstruction was a symmetrical circumferential fibrotic narrowing of the small intestine with no surrounding adhesions. This narrowing reduces the lumen of the intestine to roughly one-third of its normal cross-sectional diameter. For 10 cm. proximal to this area of narrowing the intestine was filled with densely packed, poorly masticated particles of coconut, each measuring 2 to 3 cm. in its greatest diameter. None of these had passed the narrowed area. An enteroplasty was performed through the stricture, opening the bowel in the longitudinal direction and closing it transversely. The coconut was removed through the enterotomy. The abdomen was closed. The patient had an uneventful postoperative course and was discharged from the hospital on the eighth postoperative day.

Comment

Certain fibrous foods can, under proper circumstances, cause acute intestinal obstruction. Oranges are the most common offenders, but the list includes numerous substances from the prosaic peach to such esoteric items as turtle eggs and grasshoppers. Most such episodes occur in otherwise-normal gastrointestinal tracts. There is, however, an increased likelihood of obstruction by food in the presence of inadequate gastric digestion, as might occur after partial gastrectomy, or when there is a preexisting intestinal stenosis. The reported case illustrates the latter situation.

Summary

The author has reported a case of intestinal obstruction caused by coconut meat impacted in an area of congenital ileal narrowing.

Maurice A. Claman, M.D., Medical Arts Clinic, Galesburg, Ill.

REFERENCES

1. Bowen, F. H.: Obstruction of the Small Bowel Due to Boli of Ingested Coconut: A Report of 2 Cases, Amer. Surg. 22:1076, 1956.

2. Davies, D. G. L., and Lewis, R. H.: Food Obstruction of the Small Instestine, Brit. Med. J. 2:545, 1959.

3. Davies, S. I.: Intestinal Obstruction by Food, Lancet 2:998, 1956.

4. Norberg, P. B.: Intestinal Obstruction Due to Food, Surg. Gynec. Obstet. 113:149, 1961.

5. Spurzem, R. R., and Desser, P. L.: Intestinal Obstruction Due to Phytobezoar Following Gastric Resection, Surgery 42:493, 1957.

6. Ward-McQuaid, J. N.: Intestinal Obstruction Due to Food, Brit. Med. J. 1:1106, 1950.

Effect of Endocardial Incisions on Myocardial Blood Flow

BANNING G. LARY, MD
MIAMI

Surgical attempts to correct coronary insufficiency by increasing the blood flow to the myocardium have been directed toward supply from extracardiac sources or reconstruction of the coronary arteries.[1] That a rich plexus of intramyocardial blood vessel anastomoses between the branches of the coronary arteries and the myocardial cavities exist is known.[2,3] Cases have been reported where obstruction of both coronary arteries has apparently been compatible with life,[4] and it is speculated that part or all of the myocardial nourishment was supplied by intramyocardial vessels communicating with the heart cavities. It is known that these communications are the source of myocardial blood supply in certain lower animals. Experiments were devised in an attempt to increase the blood flow to the myocardium directly from the left ventricular cavity.

Submitted for publication Jan 9, 1963.

Department of Surgery, University of Miami, School of Medicine.

Supported in part by grants from the United States Public Health Service (H-3651), and the Heart Association of Greater Miami.

Method

Twenty-six mongrel dogs weighing between 8 and 15 kg were anesthetized with 25 mg/kg pentobarbital sodium (Nembutal) intravenously, and the lungs were mechanically ventilated with room air through a cuffed intratracheal tube with aseptic technique. The chest was entered through the left fourth intercostal space, and the pericardium incised anterior to the phrenic nerve. In two animals initial attempts to create small communications by multiple perforations with a cutting skin needle resulted in fatal ventricular fibrillation (Fig 1). The remaining 24 animals were divided into two groups of 12 each.

In group 1 the anterior descending coronary artery was transected between two 00 cotton ligatures just distal to the septal branch, and in one animal an accessory branch also was transected. Four to eight endocardial incisions were immediately made with a Freer mucosa knife inserted through the apex that had been injected with 1% lidocaine hydrochloride (Xylocaine) (Fig 2).

In group 2, four to eight endocardial incisions were made in eight animals, and one deep endocardial incision directly under the anterior decending coronary artery was made in four animals. The pericardium was approximated loosely with 000 chromic, excepting in one animal where there was congenital absence of the pericardium. The chest was closed while the lungs were expanded with

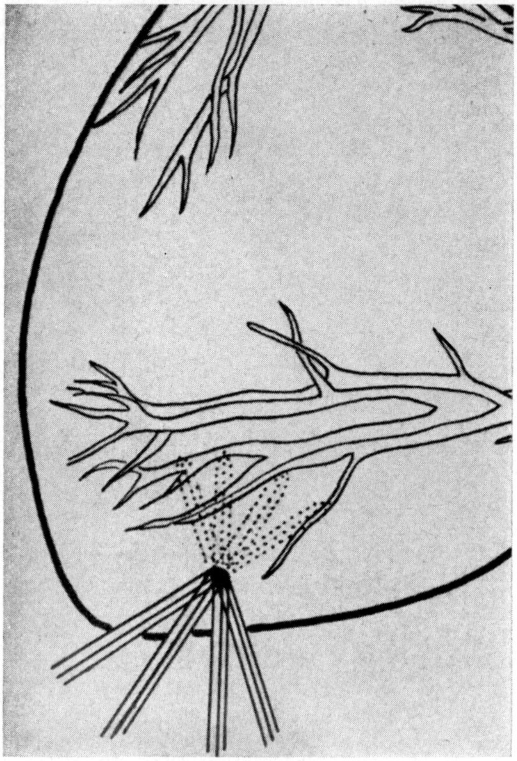

Fig 1.—Multiple needle punctures radiating from a single epicardial entrance which resulted in ventricular fibrillation in two animals.

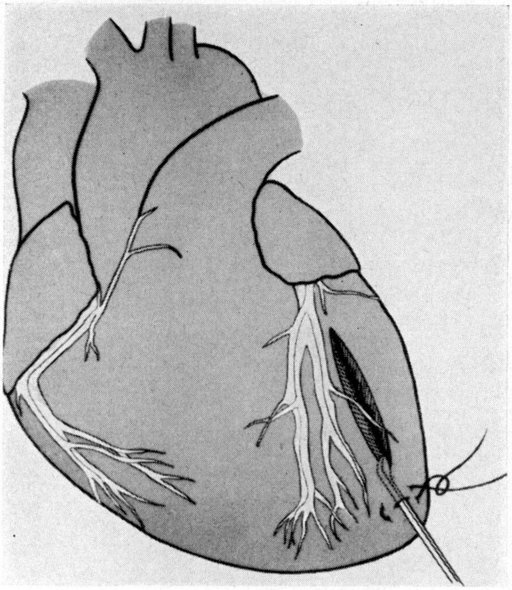

Fig 2.—Method of making endocardial incisions with a Freer mucosal knife.

running 00 chromic on the muscles and subcuticular fascia. One animal died from pneumonia in group 1 and one each from chest wall hemorrhage and mechanical failure of the respirator in group 2. Surviving animals in group two were subjected to ligation and transection of the anterior descending coronary between 251 and 255 days later. The influence of any extracoronary myocardial communications that may have formed by attachment of the pericardium to the myocardium was obviated by cutting all adhesions. Animals which survived this procedure were sacrificed after two and three months. These hearts were immediately flushed with saline, and, while still warm, the anterior descending coronary artery distal to the site of transection was injected at 140 mm Hg with vinyl acetate as described by Day.[5] The myocardium was removed by gentle water jet after maceration in 10% potassium hydroxide for three days.

Results

In group 1, four animals lived more and seven lived less than one month. All but two of the seven died the day of surgery.

In group 2 one animal was lost, and only one animal lived less than one month. Three of these remaining eight animals failed to survive ligation and transection of the anterior descending coronary. However, two of these died from hemorrhage or infection. (The Table summarizes these results.)

Comment

While some have reported a mortality of 10%-48% [6-9] following ligation of the ante-

Summary of Experimental Results

Group 1	
Animals with 4-8 endocardial incisions and concomitant anterior descending coronary artery ligation and transection	
Lived >1 mo	4
Lived <1 mo	7
Total: 11	
Group 2	
Animals with 4-8 endocardial incisions only	
Lived >1 mo	4
Lived <1 mo	1, and 1 lost
Total: 6	
Animals with 1 deep endocardial incision	
Lived >1 mo	4
Lived <1 mo	0
Total: 10	
8 survivors subjected to anterior coronary ligation and transection	
3 lived less than one month (of which 2 died from infection and hemorrhage)	
5 lived more than one month (all subjected to coronary artery injection study)	

rior descending coronary artery, most[10-16] agree that with careful attention to preservation of the septal branch and ligation of accessory branches the mortality is in the neighborhood of 70%-90%. Double ligation and transection were employed to assure complete interruption of proximal blood source and to remove the objection of simple ligation.

A mortality of 64% in group 1 would correspond to the latter figures and would also indicate that multiple endocardial incisions are well tolerated even with immediate prior ligation of the anterior decending coronary artery. In some animals the incisions actually appeared to decrease the area of cyanosis and improve the heart beat. However, since the mortality is the same expected from ligation of the anterior decending coronary artery alone, no proof exists that protection could be afforded from acute ligation by ventricular blood entering the myocardial blood vessel plexus.

The high survival rate (9 of 10) in group 2 would collaborate the findings that dogs tolerate both multiple shallow or one deep endocardial incision well. When two of the eight animals in group two are excluded because of hemorrhage and infection at the second operation, it is seen that five of six animals which had endocardial incisions survived ligation of the anterior decending coronary.

Autopsy on the animals that expired frequently revealed blood clots on the endocardium in the early postoperative period but none in long-term survivors. In many animals there was no gross evidence where the endocardial incisions had been made. Study of the ventricular endocardium at the time of injection and the casts failed to reveal the formation of vessels of arteriolar size or larger. In all cases, however, the vessel remained patent distal to the site of ligation and transection.

Sabiston[17] has discussed the "throttling" effect of ventricular contraction on coronary artery blood flow, and Menno[18] has shown that the normal systolic to diastolic flow ratio is approximately one to six in major coronary vessels. Myocardial flow directly from the ventricle has not been measured; however, one could reason myocardial-ventricular anastomosis might fill during diastole or systole. It is conceivable that with the relaxation in diastole a partial vacuum would draw blood from the ventricle into the myocardium, or, conversely, the increased pressure during systole might force blood directly into the myocardium.

Goldman[19] attempted to bring ventricular blood directly to the myocardium by transmyocardial "U" shaped and straight arterial grafts and straight polyethylene grafts. In these experiments, there were extensive epicardial to pericardial adhesions which were not separated when challenged by anterior coronary artery ligation. Massimo and Boffi[20] used a "T-tube" of polyethylene inserted in the "spongy layer" of the myocardium with one end projecting into the ventricular lumen. Both of these methods offer a limited area of myocardium to ventricular blood.

The present study tremendously increases the communicating surfaces, particularly when multiple incisions were employed.

Conclusions

Dogs tolerate well one deep and four to eight shallow endocardial incisions.

1. Endocardial incisions do not appear to protect animals from anterior coronary artery ligation and transection done immediately prior to the incisions.

2. Endocardial incisions made months previous may protect the animal from acute ligation of the anterior descending coronary artery.

Banning G. Lary, MD, 1550 NW 10th Ave, Miami 36, Fla.

REFERENCES

1. Crafoord, C.: Some Aspects of Surgery for Coronary Disease, Surgery 49:215-222, 1961.

2. Schlesinger, M. J.: An Injection Plus Dissection Study of Coronary Artery Occlusions and Anastomoses, Amer Heart J 15:528-568, 1938.

3. Gregg, D. E., and Sabiston, D. C., Jr.: Current Research and Problems of the Coronary Circulation, Circulation 13:916-927, 1956.

4. Leary, T., and Wearn, J. T.: Two Cases of Complete Occlusion of Both Coronary Orifices, Amer Heart 5:412-423, 1930.

5. Day, S. B.: The Utilization of Vinylite Plastic Casts to Demonstrate Coronary and Intercoronary Anastomotic Vessels, Surgery 41:220-226, 1957.

6. Manning, G. W.; McEachern, C. G.; and Hall, G. E.: Reflex Coronary Artery Spasm Following Sudden Occlusion of Other Coronary Branches, Arch Intern Med 64:661-674, 1939.

7. Chardack, W. M.; Bolgan, F. J.; Olson, K. C.; Gage, A. A.; and Farnsworth, W. E.: Mortality Following Ligation of the Anterior Descending Branch of the Left Coronary Artery in Dogs, Ann Surg 141:443-450, 1955.

8. Marcus, E.; Hasbrouck, E. E.; and Wong, S. N.: Myocardial Revascularization, AMA Arch Surg 74:225-231, 1957.

9. Carter, B. N.; Gall, E. A.; and Wadsworth, C. L.: An Experimental Study of Collateral Coronary Circulation Produced by Cardiopneumonopexy, Surgery 25:489-509, 1949.

10. Bakst, A. A.; Costas-Durieux, J.; Goldberg, H.; and Bailey, C. P.: Protection of the Heart by Arterialization of the Coronary Sinus, J Thorac Surg 27:433-441, 1954.

11. Beck, C. S.; Stanton, E.; Batiuchok, W.; and Leiter, E.: Revascularization of the Heart by Graft of Systemic Artery Into Coronary Sinus, JAMA 137:436-442, 1948.

12. Glover, R. P.; Davila, J. C.; Kyle, R. H.; Beard, J. C., Jr.; Trout, R. G.; and Kitchell, J. R.: Ligation of the Internal Mammary Arteries as a Means of Increasing Blood Supply to the Myocardium, J Thorac Surg 34:661-678, 1957.

13. Stanton, E. J.; Schildt, P.; and Beck, C. S.: The Effect of Abrasion of the Surface of the Heart Upon Intercoronary Communications, Amer Heart J 22:529-538, 1941.

14. Vineberg, A. M., and Niloff, P. H.: Value of Surgical Treatment of Coronary Artery Occlusion by Implantation of Internal Mammary Artery Into Ventricular Myocardium, Surg Gynec Obstet 91:551-561, 1950.

15. Sabiston, D. C., Jr., and Blalock, A.: Physiologic and Anatomic Determinants of Coronary Blood Flow and Their Relationship to Myocardial Revascularization, Surgery 44:406-423, 1958.

16. Vansant, J. H.: Technique of Experimental Ligation of the Anterior Descending Coronary Artery, Surgery 49:387-391, 1961.

17. Sabiston, D. C., Jr., and Gregg, D. E.: Effect of Cardiac Contraction on Coronary Blood Flow, Circulation 15:14-20, 1957.

18. Menno, A. D., and Schenk, W. G., Jr.: Dynamics of Coronary Arterial Flow: Flow Alterations Resulting From Certain Surgical Procedures and Drugs of Surgical Importance, Surgery 50:82-90, 1961.

19. Goldman, A.; Greenstone, S. M.; Pruess, F. S.; Strauss, S. H.; and Chang, E. S.: Experimental Methods for Producing a Collateral Circulation to the Heart Directly From the Left Ventricle, Thorac Surg 31:364-374, 1956.

20. Massimo, C., and Boffi, L.: Myocardial Revascularization By a New Method of Carrying Blood Directly From the Left Ventricular Cavity into the Coronary Circulation, Thorac Surg 34:257-264, 1957.

Congenital Atresia and Stenosis of the Colon

DONALD A. PECK, MD
HUGH B. LYNN, MD
AND
LLOYD E. HARRIS, MD
ROCHESTER, MINN

Atresia or stenosis of the colon is a rare congenital anomaly. In 1673, Binninger reported the first case of colonic atresia, and Gaub reported the first survival with this anomaly in 1922. In recent years the number of survivals has increased. A better understanding of etiology as well as the marked increase in successfully treated patients reported on in the world literature has prompted this present review.

Definitions and Classification

Definitions.—In this review we shall consider only congenital atresia and stenosis of the colon and shall not include malformations of the anus and rectum (particularly Type 4 imperforate anus,[16] which might be considered a form of atresia of the pelvic colon, but will not be discussed since it is traditionally classified as a form of imperforate anus). The term "atresia" refers to complete occlusion of the lumen of the bowel, while stenosis refers to partial occlusion. Although occasional cases of colonic stenosis in children and adults have been reported, we have excluded these and are concerned only with the stenosis that precipitates clinical findings in the newborn similar to those in atresia of the colon. The use of the term "congenital microcolon" has added confusion by suggesting a distinct pathologic entity, rather than the undilated colon to which it properly refers.

Classification.—We shall use the classification of Louw[27] for the clinical types of atresia and stenosis.

Stenosis: This refers to a narrowing of the intestinal lumen and may vary from a slight reduction in diameter to an almost complete occlusion. The mesentery is intact.

Atresia, Type I: This refers to a diaphragmatic occlusion of the lumen. The mesentery is intact.

Atresia, Type II: The proximal and distal blind ends are joined by a cordlike remnant

Submitted for publication Jan. 11, 1963.

Fellow in Surgery, Mayo Foundation (Dr. Peck); Section of Pediatric Surgery (Dr. Lynn); and Section of Pediatrics (Dr. Harris).

Mayo Clinic and Mayo Foundation.

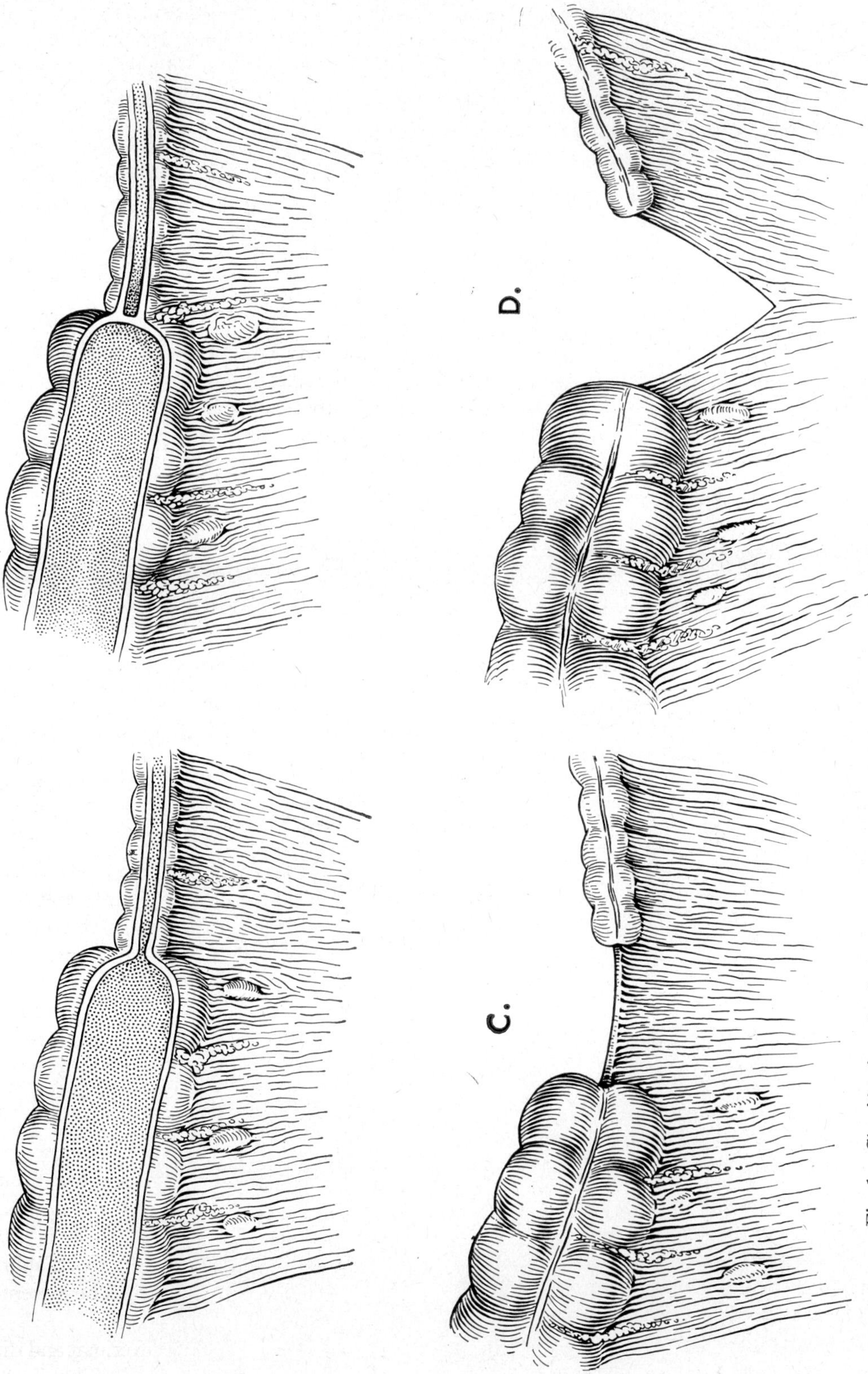

Fig. 1.—Classification of colonic stenosis or atresia. *A*, stenosis; *B*, atresia, Type I; *C*, atresia, Type II; *D*, atresia, Type III.

of the bowel. The mesentery may be either intact or absent as it relates to this intestinal remnant.

Atresia, Type III: There is no remnant connecting the proximal and distal segments of bowel. There is a wedge-shaped defect in the mesentery.

These four categories are illustrated diagrammatically in Figure 1. In the case of multiple occlusions, more than one type may occur in the same patient.

Incidence

Atresia and stenosis of the colon are most commonly considered an incidental part of the larger problem of congenital intestinal obstruction. Accurate evaluation of the incidence of intestinal atresia and stenosis is difficult. Evans, in his extensive review of 1,498 cases, estimated the incidence to be one in 1,500 births. Colonic atresia constituted 10% of his series. Others have considered the incidence of intestinal atresia to be as low as one in 20,000 births. Atresias and stenoses of the colon were present in 4% to 15% of several large series reported by Lynn and Espinas. In the period 1950 through 1959, Larson and co-workers found only one case of colonic atresia among 16 patients with intestinal atresia or stenosis treated at the Mayo Clinic.

Etiology

Many theories have been advanced to explain the genesis of intestinal atresia. Any proposed theory must account for the observed clinical types of atresia, as well as for the presence of bile, squamous epithelial cells, and lanugo hair that have been found distal to the point of occlusion. The major theories may be grouped as they relate to early or to late intrauterine life.

Early Intrauterine Life.—Two theories relate to the period of organogenesis of the intestinal tract. The first is the concept of agenesis, or complete failure of development, which was used in the past to explain Type III atresias. The second theory is based on the observations of Tandler. An arrest is thought to occur during the solid stage of intestinal development, and is termed "failure of recanalization." Proponents of this concept attribute Type I atresia to a small persistent area of complete occlusion, while Type II occurs following the persistence of a larger occluded segment. Stenosis is thought to be the result of persistent partial occlusion. Support for the theory of failure of recanalization is twofold: (1) the association between the high clinical frequency of duodenal atresia and the high incidence of duodenal occlusion in embryos studied from this viewpoint, and (2) the association of other congenital defects with intestinal atresia, each thought to occur during the same period of fetal development. The association between clinical and embryologic duodenal occlusion suggests, but does not prove, the validity of this theory. Multiple congenital anomalies may be the result of a single embryologic insult, but multiple intrauterine accidents may occur at different periods of fetal development.

Tandler's original observations were limited to the duodenums of 11 human embryos. More recently, Lynn and Espinas studied 89 human embryos of five to eleven weeks' gestation. They observed vacuolation or complete epithelial occlusion of the intestinal lumen in only 27 specimens, and concluded that complete or partial occlusion was a frequent, although not a constant, phase in the normal development of the alimentary tract. Some degree of epithelial proliferation was observed in all specimens of five to seven weeks' gestation, while this was not observed in fetuses eight to eleven weeks old. Of the 27 specimens with either complete or partial occlusion, in 20 the occlusion was in the duodenum, while in only two was it in the colon —in the region of the rectum or rectosigmoid. Patten noted that the most common sites of plugging were in the upper part of the small intestine and in the rectum. Occlusion of the lumen of the colon has not been observed in the 5 to 11-week-old embryo except in the rectal region. However, occlusions in other parts of the colon occasionally may occur.

The observations of Santulli and Blanc make it difficult to accept any theory associated with early intrauterine life. They studied 52 cases of intestinal atresia and found bile droplets, squamous epithelial cells, or lanugo hair distal to the atresia or between segments of multiple atresias in 43 cases. Bile is not formed before the eleventh week, and squamous epithelial cells are not found until after the twelfth week of gestation. Lanugo hair does not become conspicuous until the sixth to seventh month of intrauterine life, although hair follicles may be demonstrated microscopically as early as the third month. Since squamous epithelial cells and lanugo hair are swallowed in utero, and bile enters the intestinal lumen in the duodenum, these components of meconium must pass the point of atresia prior to epithelial occlusion. Since failure of recanalization must occur before bile, squamous cells or lanugo hair are formed, we cannot accept either the concept of agenesis or the theory of recanalization as a satisfactory explanation for the majority of intestinal atresias.

Late Intrauterine Life.—The theories included in this category assume that the development of a normal intestine is followed by a subsequent intrauterine accident such as volvulus, kinking, intussusception, or vascular occlusion due to sclerosis or thrombosis.

The experimental studies of Barnard and Louw have clarified many aspects of the pathogenesis of intestinal atresia. They ligated one or more mesenteric vessels, or created a strangulated volvulus, in dog fetuses of 45 to 55 days' gestation. Eighty per cent of these fetuses were born alive, and all had either intestinal stenosis or atresia. All clinical types were represented. Incomplete obstruction of the vascular supply appeared to precipitate stenosis, and creation of a strangulated volvulus was followed by a membranous or diaphragmatic occlusion. Ligation of mesenteric vessels close to their origin produced atresias resembling clinical Types II or III, including the mesenteric defect. The devascularized segments had disintegrated and were absorbed completely in some, while a fibrous remnant remained in others. Earlier studies by Laufman and associates concerning obstruction of the small intestine by strangulation demonstrated no deleterious effect on the host when autolysis of the devascularized, sterile intestinal segment was allowed to proceed intraperitoneally. Thus the formation of an atretic intestinal segment may occur without fetal morbidity or mortality.

Although the concept of vascular occlusion appears to account for a majority of cases of either single or multiple atresias, the specific factors leading to vascular occlusion in utero remain obscure. Also this concept does not adequately explain the high frequency of other associated congenital anomalies. These defects may occur in the alimentary tract as well as in other systems. As an example, the occurrence of duodenal occlusion and mongolism is often observed.

At present there is no single pathogenetic theory able to account for all observed intestinal stenoses and atresias. The observations of Lynn and Espinas have established epithelial occlusion and recanalization as a frequent phase of intestinal development. However, there are no experimental data available to suggest that an arrest of development prior to recanalization results in intestinal atresia as it is clinically observed.

There is much to be learned concerning the etiology of intestinal atresia. Current concepts permit us to consider an arrest of development during recanalization or an intestinal vascular accident during the period of organogenesis as etiologic for those atresias found in association with other congenital anomalies. When atresia of the small intestine or colon is the only congenital defect, and if bile, squamous epithelial cells, or lanugo hair are observed distal to the atresia, then this type of atresia may be the result of an intestinal accident during late intrauterine life.

Review of Cases

Cases of colonic stenosis or atresia in which treatment has been successful are rare. We have reviewed the literature and found 36 reported cases in which patients lived be-

TABLE 1.—*Successfully Treated Colonic Atresia and Stenosis Proximal to the Splenic Flexure*

Author	Age	Sex	Type of Atresia	Site in Colon	Other Anomalies	Operations: No.	Operations: Basic Procedure *
Potts	33 hr.	M	III	Transverse	No	1	Colocolostomy (s-s)
Lemon & Walker	1 hr.	M	II	Cecum through splenic flexure	Yes	1	Ileodescending colostomy (s-s)
Lee & MacMillan	2½ da.	M	II	Transverse	No	4	Closure of cecal perforation; resection and colocolostomy; reresection & colocolostomy
Jemson	3 da.	F	?	Ascending	No	1	Colocolostomy (s-s)
Wilson & co-workers	36 hr.	F	I (both)	Cecum, transverse (2 atresias)	Yes	1	Resection of distal ⅔ of ileum; rt. hemicolectomy &i leosigmoidostomy
Suidmak & Regan	3 da.	M	II	Ascending	No	3	Resection, ileocolostomy (extraperitoneal & intraperitoneal)
Chester & Robinson	48 hr.	F	II	Transverse	No	2	Colostomy, ileocolostomy (e-s)
Rang	1½ hr.	M	II	Right half	Yes	1	Resection, ileocolostomy (e-s)
Hardin & Friesen	1 da.	F	III	Transverse	No	2	Colostomy; resection; ileocolostomy
Rang	2 da.	?	III	Right half (3 remnants of left colon present)	Yes	1	Ileostomy (lived 3 mo.)
Hecker	3 da.	M	III	Hepatic flexure	No	1	Colocolostomy (e-s)
Coryllos & Simpson	18 hr.	F	III	Transverse	Yes	2	Colocolostomy, wound dehiscence & anastomotic leak closed

* s-s, side-to-side; e-s, end-to-side.

yond the postoperative period. In addition, treatment was successful in two cases encountered at the Mayo Clinic, and these will be reported.

Tables 1 and 2 are a synopsis of those cases in which the patient survived after the treatment of atresia or stenosis of the colon. The cases included are only those in which

TABLE 2.—*Successfully Treated Colonic Atresia and Stenosis Distal to the Splenic Flexure*

Author	Age	Sex	Type of Atresia	Site in Colon	Other Anomalies	Operations: No.	Operations: Basic Procedure *
Gaub	33 hr.	M	II	Sigmoid	No	1	Colostomy
Gann & Hoffman	62 hr.	F	I	Sigmoid	No	1	Colocolostomy (s-s)
Feggetter	3 da.	M	I	Pelvic	Yes	5	Colostomy; colocolostomy; colostomy closure
Gerrish	1 da.	F	?	Sigmoid	No	2	Tube cecostomy, colocolostomy
Fox & Dvonch	26 hr.	M	I	Sigmoid	No	1	Colocolostomy (s-s)
Armitage & Armitage	52 hr.	M	III	Sigmoid	No	2	Colostomy; colocolostomy; colostomy closure
Hardin & Friesen	4 da.	F	I	Descending	No	3	Colostomy; colocolostomy; colostomy closure
Santulli & Blanc	?	?	Stenosis	Sigmoid	?	1	Colostomy (further operation contemplated)
Lasserre	7 da.	F	I	Sigmoid	No	2	Colostomy; resection; anast. of distal trans. colon to rectum (Swenson's method with rectum everted)
Beau & co-workers	3 da.	M	III	Transverse to sigmoid	No	1	Resection, ileosigmoidostomy (e-e)
Melenteev	50 hr.	M	III	Transverse to sigmoid	No	1	Colostomy
Cohn	36 hr.	M	II	Sigmoid	No	3	Colostomy; Mikulicz's spur with colostomy, & colocolostomy
Dalton	48 hr.	F	III	Transverse to sigmoid	No	1	Colostomy
Soave	50 hr.	M	II	Transverse to descending	No	3	Colostomy; colocolostomy (s-s); colostomy closure
Coryllos & Simpson	4 da.	F	II	Transverse to descending	No	4	Colostomy; resection & colocolostomy (e-s)

* s-s, side-to-side; e-e, end-to-end.

sufficient data (location, type, surgical procedure, and result) were available.

Nine cases of colonic stenosis or atresia reported in the literature are not included in the tables. Gross noted two survivors in his series of 140 cases of intestinal atresia. Santulli and Santulli and Blanc reported on two successfully treated patients with colonic atresia. One of these underwent colocolostomy but subsequently required colostomy because of anastomotic malfunction; reanastomosis was later performed successfully. No information other than survival was available in the second case. Coryllos and Simpson described two patients with stenosis of the sigmoid. One patient underwent a side-to-side anastomosis and is well; the other died at age three years following an attempt to close his colonic stoma. Three surviving cases of colonic atresia were reported by Pollock and Bergin. Treatment in two patients was resection and primary anastomosis, while a colonic stoma in the third patient was closed at a second operation. All three atresias were located proximal to the splenic flexure.

Analysis of the 27 cases summarized in Tables 1 and 2 and the two new cases presented herein reveals that approximately half of the defects involved the colon proximal to the splenic flexure and half involved it distal to this flexure. There were 14 lesions on the right side, and three of these involved the entire colon proximal to the splenic flexure. The transverse colon was the most common site of atresia, being involved in eight cases, in one of which the cecum was the site of a coexisting atresia. The ascending colon alone accounted for two cases. Lesions of the left side of the colon involved the sigmoid alone in eight cases, the descending colon alone in one, pelvic colon alone in one, the portion from the distal transverse colon to the sigmoid colon inclusive in three, and the distal transverse colon to the descending colon inclusive in two. In Heckel and Apfelbach's series of 29 patients, seven had the defect in the sigmoid, five in the ascending, three in the transverse, and two each in the ileocecal, splenic flexure, and descending colon. Eight patients had multiple lesions. It would appear that those portions of the colon with a free mesentery are the more common sites for atresia. Perhaps this is due to increased susceptibility to volvulus, or kinking with subsequent vascular occlusion.

Type II and Type III atresias appear to occur more commonly on the right, while Type I is most frequently encountered distal to the splenic flexure. Although the series reviewed here is small, the apparent association between clinical type of atresia and location suggests an etiologic relationship. Atresias of the right side may result most commonly from vascular occlusion close to the origin of the mesenteric vessels, while atresias of the left side may result from strangulated volvulus of the sigmoid.

Six patients in this review had other anomalies associated with colonic atresia. Two were operated on within two hours after birth for an abdominal-wall defect, and the atresia was found during exploration. Volvulus occurred in three cases. Other anomalies included incomplete rotation, failure of mesenteric fixation, and universal mesentery. One patient had erythroblastosis and a mild calcaneovalgus deformity of the right foot.

Report of Cases

CASE 1.—In July, 1956, a 1-day-old Caucasian boy, birth weight 3.0 kg., was referred here following his failure to pass meconium. Several episodes of bile-stained emesis had been observed prior to admission. At examination, the abdomen was found moderately distended, and minimal peristaltic sounds were audible. Roentgenograms of the abdomen, taken in the inverted position with a rectal thermometer in place, were interpreted as consistent with the presumptive diagnosis of imperforate anus. There were no other abnormalities noted.

The abdomen was explored through a left upper transverse incision. The distended blind end of the proximal part of the transverse colon presented in the operative field. Limited exploration failed to reveal any remnant of the colon distal to this Type III atresia. A single-barrel colonic stoma was fashioned, and the abdomen was closed. Postoperatively, the infant did well and was dismissed after 22 days of hospitalization.

In April, 1957, the patient was returned for a contemplated colorectal anastomosis. His weight had increased to 10.7 kg. He was given neomycin orally before operation.

On complete exploration, via a left rectus-retracting incision, the left portion of the colon was found to be present commencing just proximal to the splenic flexure. Patency of the distal part was established by irrigation and the passage of a rectal tube. The colonic stoma was taken down and the terminal 8 cm. of the proximal atretic colon resected. An end-to-oblique colocolic anastomosis in two layers reestablished continuity of the large bowel.

Postoperatively, nasogastric suction was instituted and antibiotics were given. Stool was passed on the third day. The patient did well except for a minor wound infection and was dismissed on the sixteenth postoperative day.

CASE 2.—A Causasian-Hawaiian-Chinese girl was admitted in December, 1961, at age 3 days. She had a history of failure to pass meconium since birth, increasing abdominal distention, and bile-stained emesis. She was the product of a full-term, uncomplicated pregnancy. There had been no history of hydramnios.

Examination revealed a moderately dehydrated, alert infant with marked abdominal distention. Weight was 3.15 kg. During the examination, a bile-stained emesis was noted. The abdomen was tympanitic, with minimal peristaltic activity. Rectal examination revealed an apparently normal rectum that was tight to the examining finger. A small quantity of opalescent mucoid material was passed following examination. No other anomalies were noted. Roentgenograms of the abdomen demonstrated marked distention of multiple loops of intestine with air-fluid levels. A presumptive diagnosis of atresia in the lower part of the intestine was made, and the patient was prepared for operation. Intravenous administration of fluids, antibiotic therapy, administration of vitamins K and C, and nasogastric suction were started preoperatively.

The abdomen was explored through a primary right lower transverse incision. A Type III atresia of the transverse colon was found. The proximal segment of the colon ended at the hepatic flexure, and the distal segment at the level of the splenic flexure was only a few millimeters in diameter. Patency and dilatation of the distal portion of the colon were confirmed by saline irrigation. The dilated proximal colonic segment and distal part of the ileum were decompressed, and the proximal colonic segment was resected. An end-to-side two-

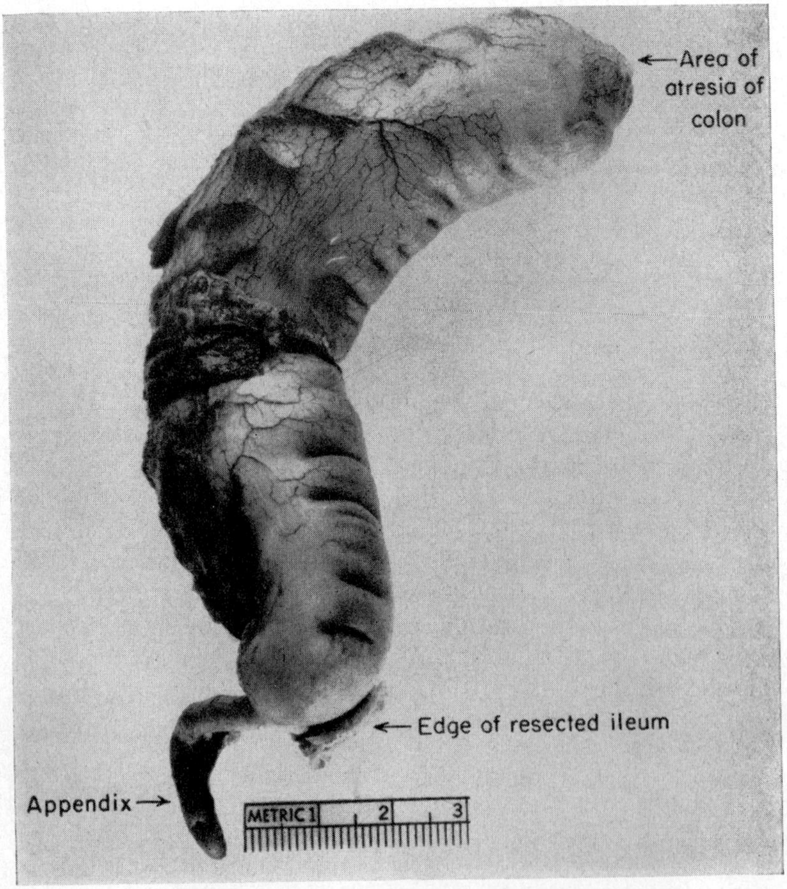

Fig. 2.—Excised segment of colon showing appendix and edge of ileum.

layer ileocolostomy was performed, and the abdomen was closed. Examination of the resected segment by the pathologist showed complete atresia of the colon 10 cm. above the cecum (Fig. 2). The ileocecal valve was competent.

Postoperatively, the patient did quite well, and stool was passed three days after operation. Oral feedings of a low-residue formula were started on the third day. The patient was dismissed on the ninth postoperative day. At three months of age she was well, gaining weight, and having two to three normal stools per day.

Diagnosis

Colonic atresia is similar clinically to atresia of the distal part of the ileum. Symptoms may develop during the first day of life or may not be apparent for several days. Failure to pass meconium, or the passage of atypical, unusual, or small amounts of meconium, should immediately alert the clinician to the possibility of intestinal obstruction. The development of progressive abdominal distention and the occurrence of vomiting, particularly when the vomitus is bile-stained, should be considered indicative of intestinal obstruction secondary to an anomaly until proved otherwise.[15] Nixon emphasized the abnormal character of bile-stained vomitus and its importance in the diagnosis of intestinal obstruction in the newborn. The emesis occurring with colonic and ileal atresia becomes progressively more fecal with the passage of time.

Fever and dehydration are later findings in neonatal intestinal obstruction. Perforation of the distended proximal segment may occur. The presence of a competent ileocecal valve in colonic atresia may lead to cecal perforation; this was the experience of Lee and MacMillan. Without surgical intervention peritonitis, shock, and death will follow.

Examination of meconium for the presence of cornified epithelial cells (Farber's test) was not used in either of the cases reported herein. The frequent occurrence of squamous epithelium distal to the site of atresia, as described by Santulli and Blanc, would make the results of the examination of meconium for squamous cells inconclusive.

The most valuable diagnostic aid in a suspected case of atresia of the distal part of the intestine is roentgenographic examination of the abdomen. Routine and upright roentgenograms of the abdomen showing the presence of distended loops of bowel with air-fluid levels confirm the impression of obstruction. Use of a barium enema has been suggested in the evaluation of a suspected colonic atresia; however, it has not been helpful in our experience. Hecker observed perforation of the blind end of the distal colon without an increase in intraluminal pressure during barium-enema examination. In addition to the danger of perforation, a plug of inspissated meconium may obstruct the retrograde flow of barium and provide erroneous information concerning the lowermost level of colonic patency. The condition of the distal colonic segment may be readily evaluated during operation. If clinical findings are inconclusive in an early suspected case, diagnosis may be established by roentgenographic study of the distal colon using aqueous radiopaque media. Perforation is the chief hazard of a contrast study, and if perforation occurs, immediate surgical intervention is mandatory.

The diagnosis of obstruction low in the intestine must occasionally be differentiated from (1) meconium ileus, or (2) cerebral injury that may suggest intestinal obstruction. Meconium ileus may be differentiated by the palpation of firm masses within the distended intestinal loops. The granular appearance of inspissated meconium on roentgenograms may be helpful. Gross points out that surgical intervention is necessary in the majority of cases. At operation the diagnosis is apparent, and appropriate treatment for either atresia or meconium ileus may be undertaken. Cerebral injury may occasionally mimic intestinal obstruction, with nausea and vomiting as prominent features. However, a history of birth injury, positive neurologic findings, and the passage of normal meconium should rule out intestinal atresia.

Other causes of intestinal obstruction in the newborn include anorectal malformations, incomplete rotation, and Hirschsprung's disease. All require surgical intervention for relief of symptoms.

Treatment

Adequate treatment of atresia or stenosis of the colon includes restoration of intestinal continuity as well as appropriate preoperative and postoperative management of these seriously ill patients.

Preoperative Care.—Surgical intervention is mandatory following the presumptive diagnosis of atresia. However, several hours employed in adequate preoperative preparation may mean the difference between a successful and an unsuccessful result. Dehydration may be partially corrected during this period; cut-down on a vein is preferable, and a cannula of sufficient size to permit blood replacement during operation should be used. Antibiotic therapy as well as supplemental treatment with vitamins K and C should be started, and blood should be cross-matched. Decompression of the distended abdomen may be started using intermittent nasogastric suction. An Isolette incubator is desirable, in the preoperative and early postoperative periods, for the administration of humidified oxygen and for better control of the infant's body temperature.

Operative Procedures.—The prime objective of surgical intervention in colonic atresia is the relief of intestinal obstruction, and secondarily the restoration of intestinal continuity. Ideally, relief of obstruction and restoration of continuity should be accomplished as a single procedure. However, the seriously ill, high-risk patient may tolerate only colostomy, and the restoration of continuity of the large bowel must be postponed.

The choice of anesthetic agent is best left to the experienced pediatric anesthesiologist. Similarly the type of incision employed will depend on the experience of the surgeon. However, adequate exposure is essential for exploration of the colon and the entire abdominal contents, considering always the possibility of multiple intestinal atresias or other associated intra-abdominal anomalies. After complete exploration, the proximal distended portion of the bowel is decompressed by aspiration, and patency of the distal portion may be established by injection of isotonic saline. If no obstructions are present, the saline will be observed to pass freely out of the anus. In addition to establishing patency of the distal segment, saline injection serves to dilate it.

In recent years both clinical and experimental evidence has been presented which strongly favors resection of the proximal dilated, hypertrophied segment of bowel. Louw[26] found necrotic changes, believed secondary to poor vascularity, in the proximal blind end of the jejunoileal atresias in nearly 50% of cases studied, while in 20% this end was frankly gangrenous. Nixon studied the motility of the proximal segment, and he concluded that the hypertrophied gut had adjusted to abnormal obstructive conditions and was inefficient in propulsive force when the normal intestinal pressure gradient was restored. In Nixon's clinical series, mortality associated with jejunoileal atresia was reduced by one-third when resection with anastomosis was substituted for primary anastomosis without resection. There have been six cases of colonic atresia in which primary anastomosis without resection was successful. In one of these,[20] abdominal distention persisted for one week postoperatively, suggesting propulsive atonicity of the proximal segment. In a second case, a leak in the colocolic anastomosis was associated with wound dehiscence six days after operation, despite decompression by means of tube cecostomy for the first three days. This patient was studied three months later, and the dilated ascending colon did not appear to be functioning normally. Gross advocated the use of an exteriorization operation, citing markedly improved results when compared with those from primary anastomosis. The exteriorization operation allows time for the distended proximal segment to recover its normal propulsive ability prior to the reestablishment of intestinal continuity. Resection of the distended proximal segment obviates the need for an exteriorization operation, avoids the hazards of atonicity and poor blood supply, and makes anastomosis technically simpler by reducing the discrepancy in size between proximal and distal colonic segments.

The surgical management of colonic atresia depends to a large degree on the location and extent of the defect. Of the 12 cases summarized in Table 1 and the two cases reported herein, colostomy was used successfully as an initial procedure in three cases, in all three of which the defect was in the transverse colon. Of the patients treated by primary anastomosis, approximately equal numbers were treated by primary anastomosis with resection of the proximal segment and by anastomosis without resection. Ileostomy was used in one case [34] with survival for three months, the patient dying ultimately from inanition. Ileostomy, with its associated depletion of body fluid and electrolytes, is usually poorly tolerated for any prolonged period in an infant. A colonic stoma proximal to the hepatic flexure functions much like a stoma in the terminal part of the ileum. If ileostomy or proximal colostomy must be considered as a first stage in atresia in the right colon, intestinal continuity should be restored within one or two weeks, and meticulous fluid and electrolyte replacement is essential during the interval. Colostomy was the primary procedure in 11 of the 15 cases listed in Table 2. Colostomy on the left side is well tolerated by the growing infant and allows considerable latitude for selecting the appropriate time for the restoration of intestinal continuity.

When the infant's condition is precarious during operation, or when there is doubt concerning the patency of the distal colonic segment, colostomy or ileostomy should be the procedure of choice. However, if the patient's condition permits, resection and primary anastomosis should be performed. The anastomotic type (end-to-end, side-to-side, or other combinations) is best left to the judgment of the surgeon in the individual case. The excised segment should include all of the markedly distended bowel, which is usually the remaining proximal colon when the defect is on the right side. Ten or more centimeters of left colon should be excised in order to ensure normal postoperative colonic motility. The creation of long blind loops proximal to the anastomosis should be avoided. In several cases, side-to-side colocolostomy performed in Type I atresia of the sigmoid, bypassing the atretic site, permitted restoration of continuity without impairment of colonic function.

Postoperative Care.—After surgical intervention, nasogastric suction should be maintained until active peristalsis has returned. In both cases reported herein, this occurred within 48 to 72 hours postoperatively. Intravenous administration of fluid and electrolytes is essential for the correction of residual dehydration and for daily maintenance until oral intake is sufficient for the infant's needs. Antibiotic therapy should be continued postoperatively for three to five days. For several weeks postoperatively, a diet which results in a minimal curd should be fed. Frequent digital rectal examinations have been helpful in stimulating bowel movements.

The functional potential of the distal colon has been of concern to many clinicians. However, we have not observed delayed or impaired motility following anastomosis. There is a period of reduced capacity, but the capacity increases during the postoperative period and corresponds to the period required for dilatation to normal caliber. Dilatation does not require enemas, but is effectively produced by the passage of normal intestinal content.

Comment

A striking feature of this series is the almost complete absence of nonabdominal congenital anomalies. In two cases a coexistent defect of the abdominal wall led to early diagnosis of the atresia, and may have contributed to the successful outcome. There have been no reports of successfully treated patients with associated cardiac, renal, or neurogenic anomalies. We may infer that the patients most amenable to successful treatment are those who have colonic occlusion as the only defect. The coexistence of volvulus, incomplete rotation, or failure of mesenteric fixation results in a more complex surgical problem, which has been successfully treated despite the presence of these other anomalies.

Untreated colonic atresia is incompatible with survival. Immediate corrective operation is mandatory. Surgical management should include resection of the proximal distended colonic segment. Although primary anastomosis without resection has been successful in some instances, it has been unsuccessful in many others because leakage of the anastomosis or persistent ileus have contributed to the infant's death. Primary anastomosis with resection appears to subject the infant to less risk than does anastomosis without resection.

Summary

Thirty-six cases of successfully treated congenital atresia or stenosis of the colon in the newborn are reported in the world literature. These cases have been reviewed, and two additional cases are reported. Etiology of this condition may relate to circumstances occurring in early or late intrauterine life.

Surgical treatment should include complete abdominal exploration, determination of patency of the distal colonic segment, resection of the distended proximal segment of colon, and primary anastomosis. Temporary colostomy or ileostomy should be avoided when the defect is in the right colon.

Mayo Clinic, Rochester, Minn.

REFERENCES

1. Armitage, G. L., and Armitage, H. V.: Congenital Atresia of the Sigmoid Colon, Amer. J. Surg. 96:580-583 (Oct.) 1958.

2. Barnard, C. N., and Louw, J. H.: The Genesis of Intestinal Atresia, Minnesota Med. 39:745; 753 (Nov.) 1956.

3. Beau, A.; Préyot, J., and Masse, P.: Atrésie colique congénitale: Rapport d'un cas de guérison, Mém. Acad. Chir. 86:741-746, 1960.

4. Binninger: Quoted by Evans, C. H.[9]

5. Chester, S. T., and Robinson, W. T.: Congenital Atresia of the Transverse Colon: A Case Report and a Review of the Literature, Ann. Surg. 146:824-829 (Nov.) 1957.

6. Cohn, B. D.: Congenital Atresia of the Colon, Amer. J. Surg. 104:861-865 (Dec.) 1962.

7. Coryllos, E., and Simpson, J.: Congenital Atresia of the Colon: Review of Literature and Report of 2 Cases, Dis. Colon Rectum 5:37-50 (Jan.-Feb.) 1962.

8. Dalton, G. R.: Atresia of the Colon, Clin. Proc. Child. Hosp. (Wash.) 14:70-75 (Mar.) 1958.

9. Evans, C. H.: Collective Review: Atresias of the Gastrointestinal Tract, Surg. Gynec. Obstet. 92:1-8 (Jan.) 1951.

10. Feggetter, S.: Congenital Intestinal Atresia, Brit. J. Surg. 42:378-388 (Jan.) 1955.

11. Fox, P. F., and Dvonch, L. A.: Congenital Atresia of the Sigmoid Colon, A.M.A. Arch Surg. 77:1008-1010 (Dec.) 1958.

12. Gann, M. E., and Hoffman, E.: Congenital Atresia of the Sigmoid, Amer. J. Surg. 83:605-609 (Apr.) 1952.

13. Gaub, O. C.: Congenital Stenosis and Atresia of the Intestinal Tract Above the Rectum: With a Report of an Operated Case of Atresia of the Sigmoid in an Infant, Trans. Amer. S.A. 40:582-638, 1922.

14. Gerrish, E. W.: Operative Management of Congenital Intestinal Atresia, Ann. Surg. 142:469-475 (Sept.) 1955.

15. Glover, D. M., and Barry, F. M.: Intestinal Obstruction in the Newborn, Ann. Surg. 130:480-509 (Sept.) 1949.

16. Gross, R. E.: The Surgery of Infancy and Childhood: Its Principles and Techniques, Philadelphia, W. B. Saunders Company, 1953.

17. Hardin, C. A., and Friesen, S. R.: Congenital Atresia of the Colon: Report of 2 Cases, A.M.A. Arch. Surg. 80:616-619 (Apr.) 1960.

18. Heckel, N. J., and Apfelbach, C. W.: Congenital Atresia of the Colon, Amer. J. Dis. Child. 34:1050-1055 (Dec.) 1927.

19. Hecker, W. C.: Kongenitale Colonatresie, ein klinischer Beitrag zum Ileus in der Neugeborenenperiode, Chirurg. 31:405-407 (Sept.) 1960.

20. Jemson, J.: Atresia of the Ascending Colon, Lancet 2:61-62 (July 14) 1951.

21. Larson, R. E.; Harris, L. E., and Lynn, H. B.: Intestinal Obstruction in the Newborn Infant, Proc. Mayo Clin. 36:516-524 (Sept. 27) 1961.

22. Lasserre, M. J.: Atrésie congénitale du Côlon gauche, Bordeaux Chir. 1:44-47 (Jan.) 1961.

23. Laufman, H.; Martin, W. B.; Method, H.; Tuell, S. W., and Harding, H.: Observations in Strangulation Obstruction: II. The Fate of Sterile Devascularized Intestine in the Peritoneal Cavity, Arch. Surg. 59:550-564 (Sept.) 1949.

24. Lee, C. M., Jr., and MacMillan, G .B.: Rupture of the Bowel in the Newborn Infant: Includ-

ing Case Report of Rupture in Large Intestine With Recovery, Surgery 28:48-66 (July) 1950.

25. Lemon, R. G., and Walker, J. N.: Congenital Evisceration with Atresia of the Colon, Texas J. Med. 44:449-454 (Oct.) 1948.

26. Louw, J. H.: Congenital Intestinal Atresia and Severe Stenosis in the Newborn: A Report on 79 Consecutive Cases, S. Afr. J. Clin. Sci. 3:109-129 (Sept.) 1952.

27. Louw, J. H.: Congenital Intestinal Atresia and Stenosis in the Newborn: Observations on Its Pathogenesis and Treatment, Ann. Roy. Coll. Surg. Engl. 25:209-234 (Nov.) 1959.

28. Lynn, H. B., and Espinas, E. E.: Intestinal Atresia: An Attempt to Relate Location to Embryologic Processes, A.M.A. Arch. Surg. 79:357-361 (Sept.) 1959.

29. Melenteev, M. G.: Surgery in Atresia of the Large Intestine, Vestn. Khir. Grekov. 87:100-101 (Aug.) 1961.

30. Nixon, H. H.: Intestinal Obstruction in the Newborn, Arch. Dis. Child. 30:13-22 (Feb.) 1955.

31. Patten, B. M.: Textbook of Human Embryology, Philadelphia, Blakiston Co., Division of McGraw-Hill Book Co., Inc., 1946.

32. Pollock, W. F., and Bergin, W. F.: Management of Intestinal Atresia at the Los Angeles Children's Hospital, Amer. J. Surg. 102:202-216 (Aug.) 1961.

33. Potts, W. J.: Congenital Atresia of Intestine and Colon, Surg. Gynec. Obstet. 85:14-19 (July) 1947.

34. Rang, R. H.: Congenital Atresia of the Colon, Indiana Med. Ass. J. 52:2160-2164 (Dec.) 1959.

35. Santulli, T. V.: Intestinal Obstruction in Newborn Infant, J. Pediat. 44:317-377 (Mar.) 1954.

36. Santulli, T. V., and Blanc, W. A.: Congenital Atresia of the Intestine: Pathogenesis and Treatment, Ann. Surg. 154:939-948 (Dec.) 1961.

37. Soave, F.: Su di un rarissimo caso di atresia dell'angolo splenico del colon (trattamento chirurgico—Guarigione), Minerva Pediat. 10:100-104 (Feb. 4) 1958.

38. Suidmak, J. J., and Regan, P.: Congenital Atresia of the Colon, Ann. Surg. 148:840-844 (Nov.) 1958.

39. Tandler: Quoted by Louw, J. H.[27]

40. Wilson, B. J.; Nelson, A., and Harshbarger, M.: Congenital Atresia of the Colon, Surg. Gynec. Obstet. 99:34-41 (July) 1954.

Portal Hypertension From Postbulbar Duodenal Ulcer

D. E. STRANDNESS, JR., MD, AND J. W. BELL, MD, SEATTLE

Introduction

Postbulbar duodenal ulcers comprise about 5% to 10% of all duodenal ulcers.[1-6] These lesions have a greater tendency to bleed massively, often are deeply penetrating, and frequently require surgical therapy. More uncommon complications of this ulcer are duodenal obstruction and obstruction of the common bile duct. Because of their location in the second portion of the duodenum, visualization on upper gastrointestinal series is often difficult. We have recently had the opportunity to observe two patients who had extrahepatic portal vein obstruction and portal hypertension resulting from this disease. The portal vein was occluded by massive periduodenal scarring and inflammation. Although many causes for extrahepatic vein obstruction have been noted, postbulbar duodenal ulcer has not been reported even as a cause.[7] Because of the problems encountered in differential diagnosis, these cases will be reported in detail.

Case 1.—This 68-year-old white male was admitted Jan 12, 1959, with a three-week history of epigastric pain relieved by antacids. The patient had a temperature of 100 F (37.8 C) and was found to have an epigastric mass which was exquisitely tender.

Laboratory Data: Hematocrit 33%, WBC 34,000/cu mm, alkaline phosphatase 20.5 units/100 ml, bilirubin 1.0 mg%. An upper gastrointestinal series revealed displacement of the lesser curvature of the stomach by a mass, but no esophageal varices or duodenal ulcer was visualized. The patient was treated conservatively with rapid resolution of the mass and decrease in temperature to a normal range. The alkaline phosphatase dropped to 10.5 units/100 ml prior to discharge.

During the intervening two years the patient felt well. One month prior to his second admission the dull epigastric pain returned. Two days before admission he passed the first tarry stool and vomited bright red blood. The patient's abdomen was normal. The hematocrit was 14%, direct bilirubin 0.4 mg%, alkaline phosphatase 4.3 units/100 ml, and thymol turbidity 9 cc.

An upper gastrointestinal series revealed extensive esophageal varices and question of a duodenal diverticulum. At esophagoscopy, varices were seen first at 30 cm and extended through the cardia. A percutaneous liver biopsy was normal.

Hospital Course: The anemia was corrected by six units of whole blood. The patient was carefully questioned and denied the use of alcohol. There was no past history of hepatitis. A splenoportogram revealed extrahepatic portal vein obstruction.

At laparotomy (Nov 7, 1961) the portal pressure was found to be 45 cm of H_2O. The portal vein was enmeshed in very dense fibrous tissue immediately adjacent to a large postbulbar ulcer which had penetrated completely through the wall of the second portion of the duodenum. It was our impression that the bleeding was secondary to the ulcer, and a 75% gastric resection with a gastrojejunal anastomosis was performed. A portacaval shunt would have been technically impossible because of the amount of scarring and inflammation. The left kidney had been removed years before for trauma; hence, a splenorenal shunt was out of the question. A subsequent upper gastrointestinal series 14 months later revealed persistence of the varices.

Case 2.—This 65-year-old white male was admitted on June 21, 1961, with a history of hematemesis and melena of one day's duration. The patient was asymptomatic prior to this episode but had been hospitalized elsewhere for one year before admission with bleeding from a "peptic ulcer." The patient allegedly drank rather heavily in the past but denied any drinking for the past year.

The patient arrived at the hospital in shock but responded well to whole blood. Laboratory: Hematocrit 34%, alkaline phosphatase 5.4 units/100 ml, bilirubin 2.1 mg%, total protein 6.8 gm, albumin 4.1 gm, prothrombin time 88% of normal, sulfo-

Submitted for publication Jan 9, 1963.

Clinical Investigator, Veterans Administration Hospital; Instructor in Surgery, University of Washington School of Medicine (Dr. Strandness). Chief, Surgical Service, Veterans Administration Hospital; Associate Professor of Surgery, University of Washington School of Medicine (Dr. Bell).

From the Surgical Service, Veterans Administration Hospital and Department of Surgery, University of Washington School of Medicine.

bromophthalein 14% (drawn while bleeding). An upper gastrointestinal series revealed esophageal varices and a postbulbar duodenal ulcer.

Hospital Course: On July 6, 1961, a laparotomy was performed, and a large, active penetrating ulcer was found 5 cm distal to the pylorus. The area of induration was adjacent to the common bile duct and related structures. The liver was grossly normal, and this was verified by biopsy. The spleen was normal in size. A 70% resection, vagotomy, and gastrojejunal anastomosis was carried out. The patient had an excellent convalescence.

A follow-up upper gastrointestinal series 14 months later revealed a normal esophagus without evidence of esophageal varices.

Comment

Case 1 posed a very difficult problem in diagnosis and management. In reviewing the history the sequence of events can be reconstructed as follows: (1) In 1959 he undoubtedly perforated the ulcer, with the resultant abscess in the lesser omental bursa; (2) regression of the mass with resultant scarring and portal vein obstruction occurred; (3) by the time of his second admission two years later, esophageal varices had developed which were very large and seen both by x-ray and esophagoscopy.

Failure to visualize the ulcer on upper gastrointestinal series further complicated the problem from a diagnostic standpoint. In retrospect, the duodenal diverticulum seen was a false one formed secondary to the ulcer. The normal liver biopsy ruled out intrahepatic causes of the portal hypertension. The splenoportogram was technically poor but did reveal extrahepatic obstruction of the portal vein. At the time of operation, the ulcer had completely destroyed the posterosuperior wall of the second portion of the duodenum. A very dense mass of scar tissue surrounded the ulcer and portal vein. The common bile duct was not visualized but was probably adjacent to and involved as well. We felt quite certain the bleeding was secondary to the ulcer and not the varices. It is of interest that the varices have persisted. The patient continues to have occult blood in his stools. Transfusions have not been required, and his anemia has responded to parenteral iron therapy. If massive bleeding should occur from the varices, the only alternative remaining would be to create a shunt between the superior mesenteric vein and inferior vena cava, or to resect the distal esophagus.

Case 2 was not as carefully documented but showed many of the same features. This patient was seen only a few months after the first patient, and we were alerted to the possible diagnosis by the finding of the postbulbar ulcer and lack of history or physical findings to suggest intrahepatic causes of the portal hypertension. In addition to the portal vein obstruction, this patient had a slight elevation of the serum bilirubin. It is of interest that with healing of the ulcer the portal obstruction was relieved and the esophageal varices regressed, as evidenced by the normal upper gastrointestinal series 14 months after operation.

Summary

Two unusual cases of portal hypertension secondary to postbulbar duodenal ulcer are presented. The scarring secondary to the ulceration was sufficient to obstruct the portal vein, resulting in esophageal varices. The diagnostic problems and therapy of these patients are discussed.

D. E. Strandness, Jr., MD, Department of Surgery, Veterans Administration Hospital, 4435 Beacon Ave, S, Seattle 8, Wash.

REFERENCES

1. Rauch, R. F.: Postbulbar Peptic Ulceration of the Duodenum, Ann Surg 144:57, 1956.

2. Cooke, L., and Hutton, C. F.: Postbulbar Duodenal Ulceration, Lancet 1:754-757, 1958.

3. Paterson, D. E., and Hancock, D. M.: Duodenal Stenosis Due to Post-Bulbar Ulcer, Brit J Radiol 31:660-665, 1958.

4. Swartz, J. M., and Rice, M. L., Jr.: Post-Bulbar Duodenal Ulcer With Particular Reference to its Hemorrhagic Tendency, Gastroenterology 26: 251, 1954.

5. Lonergan, W. M., and Kahn, A., Jr.: Post-Bulbar Duodenal Ulceration, Gastroenterology 17: 494, 1951.

6. Cunningham, W. L., Jr.; Del Junco, T.; and Wilk, S. P.: Postbulbar Duodenal Ulcer, Western J Surg 69:26 (Jan-Feb) 1961.

7. Hunt, A. H.: Contribution to the Study of Portal Hypertension, Edinburgh: E. & S. Livingstone, Ltd., 1957, pp 10-26.

Liver Photoscanning in Evaluation of Cancer Chemotherapy

DANIEL J. HANSON, JR., MD
A. BRADLEY SOULE, MD
O. S. PETERSON, JR., MD
CARLTON R. HAINES, MD
AND
CLINTON D. JANNEY, PhD
BURLINGTON, VT

The liver has always been a difficult organ to evaluate. Physical examination is often inaccurate. Laboratory procedures are available to determine various parameters of liver function, but these often are not sensitive enough to appreciate other than gross changes. Plain roentgenograms of the liver also are only of value when gross changes are present, and special radiographic techniques are frequently complicated procedures.

Submitted for publication Jan 28, 1963.

Formerly Research Associate in Radiology, University of Vermont College of Medicine and Affiliated Hospitals, presently Instructor, Department of Radiology, University of Kentucky College of Medicine (Dr. Hanson); Professor and Chairman, Department of Radiology (Dr. Soule), Associate Professor of Radiology (Dr. Peterson), Assistant Professor of Surgery (Dr. Haines), Associate Professor, Department of Radiation Physics (Dr. Janney), University of Vermont College of Medicine and Affiliated Hospitals.

From the Departments of Radiology and Surgery, University of Vermont College of Medicine and Affiliated Hospitals (Mary Fletcher Hospital and DeGoesbriand Memorial Hospital).

This study was supported by grant 1960-1961 No. 5 from the Vermont Division, American Cancer Society.

With the advent of effective chemotherapeutic agents, and more frequent use of radiation therapy to the liver, it is advantageous to have some relatively simple method of recording their effect on primary and metastatic neoplastic disease involving the liver. Photoscanning, using a suitable recording instrument and a radioactive compound, seems to meet these requirements. In the course of a study of diagnostic techniques in neoplastic disease of the liver, we have had the opportunity to do repeat examinations on patients receiving chemotherapy. Following are representative case reports in which liver scanning was valuable in evaluating therapy and selecting further courses of treatment.

Report of Cases

Case 1.—This 55-year-old white female was first admitted in May 1960 for investigation of a watery vaginal discharge of six week's duration. A hysterosalpingogram demonstrated trapping of contrast

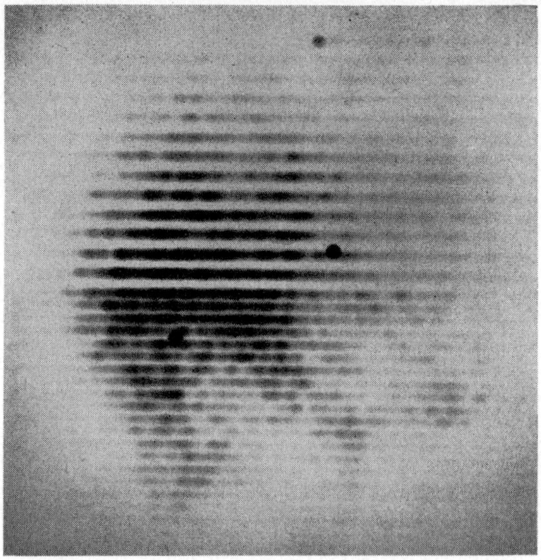

Fig 1 (case 1).—Liver scan in June 1961, demonstrating marked liver enlargement. (The three large black dots mark the midline of the right and left costal margins and the xiphoid process.)

media in the right fallopian tube, suggesting cavitation within a neoplastic process. At operation, a mass lesion was found in the right adnexa which histologically was poorly differentiated adenocarcinoma of the ovary. Abdominal hysterectomy and bilateral salpingo-oophorectomy were done. The patient was then given a course of external pelvic radiation to a calculated midtumor dose of 5,400 rad.

She was readmitted in June 1961 for investigation of crampy abdominal pain. On physical examination

Fig 3 (case 1).—March 1962, recurrence of liver enlargement and apparent complete replacement of the left lobe of the liver.

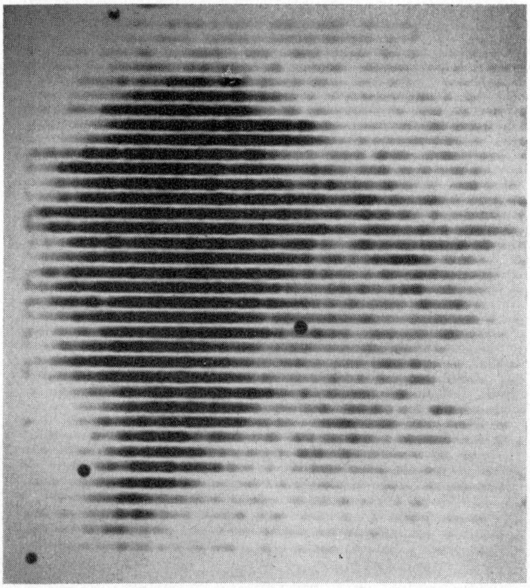

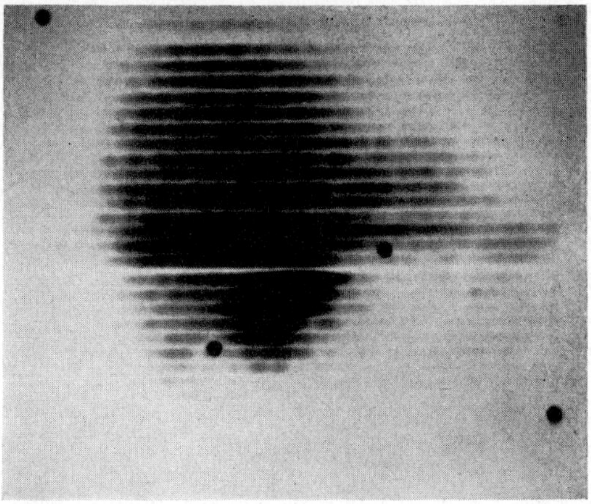

Fig 2 (case 1).—Scan in October 1961, in which the liver is of normal size and shape.

the liver margin was palpated 8 cm below the right costal margin. A chest film showed large rounded nodules in both lung fields consistent with metastatic disease. An I^{131}-labeled rose bengal liver scan (Fig 1) demonstrated marked enlargement of the liver, indicating metastatic disease. She was given 60 mg of thio-tepa intravenously over a three-day period and discharged subjectively improved. This was followed by an additional 60 mg, for a total of 120 mg in 30 days.

Chest films and a repeat liver scan were obtained in October 1961. These showed marked regression of the pulmonary metastases, and at this time the liver scan (Fig 2) was normal with no demonstrable metastatic nodules. Clinically the patient was feeling very well.

The patient was readmitted in March 1962 with swelling of the abdomen and legs. A repeat chest radiograph showed no recurrence of the chest

Fig 4 (case 2).—Initial scan, with evidence of multiple metastatic nodules.

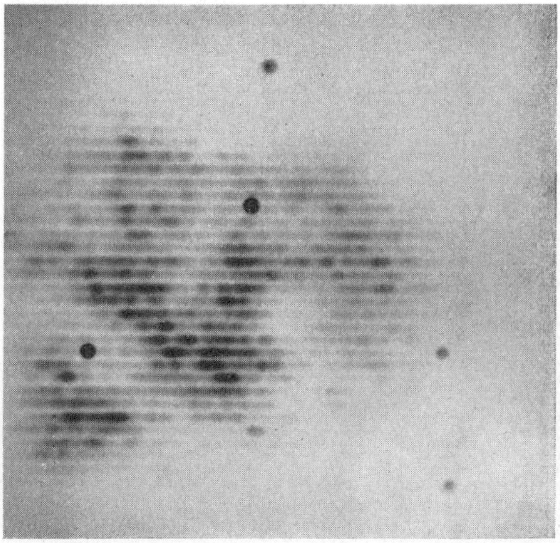

lesions, but a repeat liver scan (Fig 3) indicated that marked enlargement was again present with what appeared to be complete replacement of the left lobe of the liver by metastatic disease and with evidence of metastatic nodules in the right lobe of the liver. The patient failed to improve on further intravenous thio-tepa and died in May 1962.

CASE 2.—This 50-year-old white female was admitted in March 1962 with complaints of increasing weakness and fatigue following a small amount of rectal bleeding which occurred one month prior to admission. On physical examination the liver was readily palpable. Barium enema demonstrated a polypoid tumor within the ascending colon. A liver scan (Fig 4) showed evidence of multiple metastatic nodules throughout the liver.

The patient was explored, and, with identification of the tumor in the ascending colon, an ileo-transverse colostomy with resection of the terminal ileum, ascending colon, and a portion of the transverse colon, was done. Metastatic disease was visible in the liver, and a polyvinyl catheter was inserted through the gastroduodenal artery into the hepatic artery for infusion of 5-fluorouracil. A total of 5 gm was administered over a five day period. A course of external radiation to the liver was then given, with the patient receiving an estimated midlane tumor dose of 4,000 rad in a 30-day period.

She was readmitted in June 1962, when a repeat liver photoscan was done. This (Fig 5) demonstrated some reduction in size of the multiple nodules. A second course of 5-fluorouracil was administered, and the patient was discharged to continue to be followed.

CASE 3.—This 40-year-old white female was first admitted in November 1960 for therapy of recurrent malignant melanoma of the right lower extremity. She first noticed a black shiny "mole" on the medial aspect of the right knee in September 1959. This was resected completely in another hospital; when microscopic examination revealed a malignant melanoma, a right groin dissection was performed in October 1959. None of the removed nodes showed evidence of tumor.

On physical examination, there were multiple pigmented nodules scattered over the lower extremity. Since no other lesions could be found, isolation-perfusion of the right lower extremity was carried out using thio-tepa.

She was followed closely, and the lesions regressed well. In April 1961, a liver scan was done which was within normal limits. The patient continued to do well until February 1962 when a subcutaneous mass appeared in the right thigh. Hospitalization was advised for re-evaluation.

Physical examination and radiographs failed to demonstrate evidence of other disease. A repeat liver scan seemed unchanged from the initial examination. On the basis of these findings, amputation was recommended, but the patient refused. The right lower extremity was again perfused with thio-tepa, with simultaneous resection of the recurrent tumor mass. The patient was discharged to continue to be followed.

Fig 5 (case 3).—Scan after therapy, showing apparent reduction in the size and number of nodules.

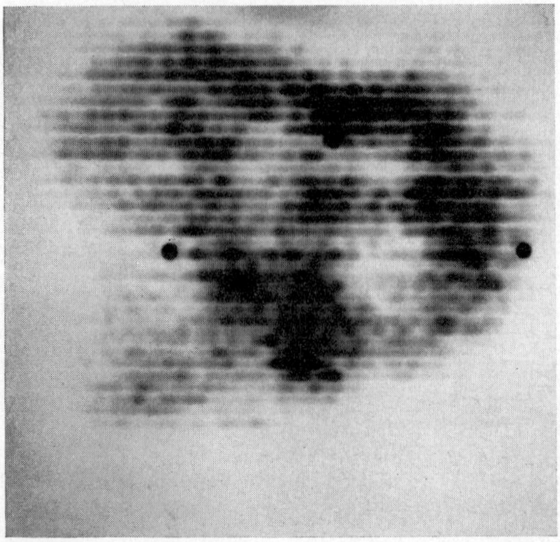

Technical Details

The medium used for liver scanning is rose bengal labeled with I^{131}. No special preparation of the patient is required. A dose of $3\mu c$ of the radioactive compound per kilogram of body weight is added to 5 cc of plain rose bengal utilized as a carrier. This is injected intravenously, and the patient is positioned beneath the scanner. Scanning is started 20 minutes after injection and is usually completed in a total elapsed time of one hour after injection. No reactions or side effects have been noted during or after the procedure.

A commercial photoscanner (Picker Magnascanner), utilizing a 3 in $\times$ 2 in sodium iodide scintillation probe fitted with a coarse focus 19-hole collimator, is used as the recording instrument. Both dot scans on paper and continuous tone scans on photographic films are obtained. The dot scans on paper are of most value in visualization of the outline of the organ, whereas the photographic patterns are helpful in appreciating abrupt changes in count rates in selected areas.

Comment

The value of liver photoscanning as a diagnostic method has been well established.[1,2,4-6,8-10] It has proved to be a valuable aid in clinical problems involving mass lesions of the right upper quadrant and has provided a simple, relatively rapid means of visualizing the size, shape, and position of an organ which had previously been difficult to examine. In addition, the amount of radiation exposure of the patient has been relatively low.[6,7]

Scintigrams of the liver have been especially helpful in cases in which primary or metastatic malignant neoplastic disease has been clinically suspected. With the advent of chemotherapeutic agents and development of new surgical techniques devised to deliver these agents to the liver, they have become of even greater value. There is obtained not only a permanent record of the initial amount of involvement, but an easily reproducible technique is at hand to evaluate response.

In addition, recently announced technical innovations have improved the diagnostic quality of liver scintigraphy. Use of a closed circuit television system [5] to view the scans allows variance of the contrast enhancement so that previously unappreciated small changes in film density can now be seen readily. Experimental and clinical work with I^{125}-labeled rose bengal by Endlich et al [3] indicates that scans with this isotope provide improved resolution and contrast. It also has the advantages of reduction of radiation dose to patients and longer shelf life, which will help to eliminate delay in performing the examinations.

Summary

Representative cases have been presented to demonstrate the feasibility of liver photoscanning as a method of evaluating the effect of chemotherapy and as a guide to further therapy in malignant neoplastic disease.

Daniel J. Hanson, MD, Department of Radiology, University of Kentucky, College of Medicine, Lexington, Ky.

REFERENCES

1. Bonte, F. J.; Bryan, H. L.; Krohmer, J. S.; and Mize, H. L.: Scintillation Scanning of the Liver, Southern Med J 53:754-763, 1960.

2. Doehner, G. A.; Powers, J. C.; and Ruzicka, F. F., Jr.: Scintigraphy and Portography: Their Value in the Diagnosis of Liver Disease, Radiology 74:912-927, 1960.

3. Endlich, H. E.; Harper, P.; Beck, R.; Siemens, W.; and Lathrop, K.: The Use of I-125 to Increase Isotope Scanning Resolution, Amer J Roentgen 87:148-155, 1962.

4. Fee, D. A., and Fedoruk, S. O.: Clinical Value of Liver Photoscanning, New Eng J Med 262:123-125, 1960.

5. Fleming, W. H.; McIlraith, J. D.; and King, E. R.: Medical Scintillation Scanning Utilizing Closed Circuit TV Contrast Enhancement, Amer J Roentgen 87:128-140, 1962.

6. Friedell, H. L.; MacIntyre, W. J.; and Rejali, A. M.: A Method for the Visualization of the Configuration and Structure of the Liver: A. Preliminary Clinical Investigations, Amer J Roentgen 77:455-470, 1957.

7. Holodny, E.; Lechtman, H.; and Laughlin, J. S.: Bone-Marrow Dose Produced by Radioactive Isotopes, Radiology 77:1-11, 1961.

8. Wagner, H. N., Jr.; McAfee, J. G.; and Mozley, J. M.: Diagnosis of Liver Disease by Radioisotope Scanning, Arch Intern Med 107:324-334, 1961.

Siliconized Dacron as a Pericardial Patch

MOHAMAD K. MAZUJI, MD, AND JAMES C. LETT, MD, HARLAN, KY

The clinical application of silicone rubber is based on a high degree of tolerance by the body and the lack of foreign-body reaction. This material has been used in plastic correction of facial bony defects and nasal deformities, soft tissue augmentation, tubes and valves for the relief of hydrocephalus, heart valve prostheses, and in repair of meningoceles and defects of the dura mater. Silicone rubber has been considered an ideal substitute for soft tissues.[1] It appears to be inert and nonirritating, to cause minimal fibrous tissue formation, and no foreign-body reaction. In this experiment Dacron, calendered with Silastic of 0.007 in. thickness—a fine, nonporous, resistant fabric—was studied, first to observe its fate as a partial pericardial prosthesis, and second to show the resultant neighboring tissue reaction in surgically produced pericardial defects. In a previous experiment,[2] the lack of peritoneal adhesion to a tubular drain and the occasional migration of the drain suggested that perhaps silicone is not an ideal soft tissue substitute. In referring to the statement given by Schofield in 1955,[3] an ideal prosthesis should have the following criteria:

1. It must unite with the surrounding tissue.
2. It should be chemically and biologically inert.
3. It should be as workable, pliable, and strong as the tissue it replaces.

In considering the above criteria, it is of interest to describe some difficulties and results encountered in this experiment.

Submitted for publication Jan 28, 1963.

Harlan Memorial Hospital.

This work was supported by a research grant from the Miners Memorial Hospital Association, Washington, DC.

Method of Investigation

Employing ten mongrel dogs, under general anesthesia, with a balloon-cuff endotracheal tube connected to an automatic respirator, through an incision in the left sixth interspace, a square defect in the pericardium from 25 to 64 sq cm in size was made. The defect was covered with a Silastic-Dacron patch using 00000 noncapillary braided silk for sutures in running fashion in seven dogs and 000 interrupted braided silk in three. The periphery of the prosthesis was plicated to maintain the curvature of the pericardial anatomy (Fig 1, *A* and *B*). No postoperative pleural drainage tube was inserted. The dogs recovered rapidly, except for one im-

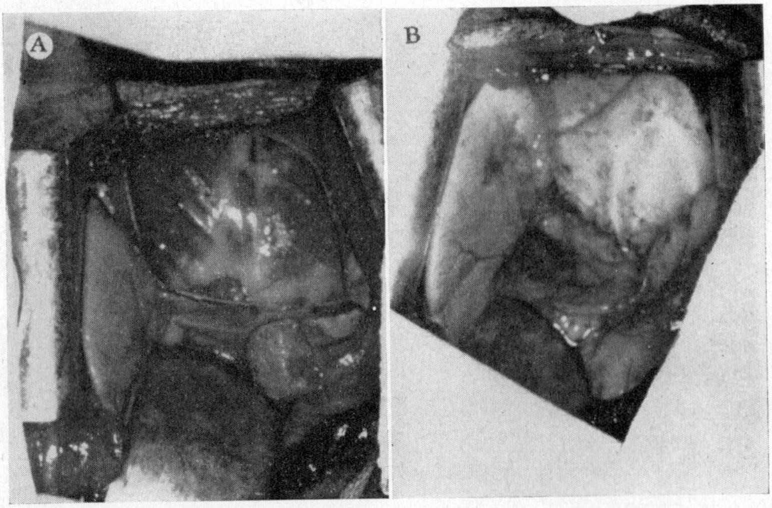

Fig 1.—*A*, pericardial defect. *B*, prosthetic patch in place.

Tabulation of Data

Dog No.	Weight, Lb	Date of Operation	Length of Observation, Mo	Size of Graft Sq Cm	Silk Suture Used	Fate of Graft
1	35	7/20/61	10	36	Running 00000	Migrated
2	36	7/27/61	5	37	"	"
3	31	8/ 5/61	4	42	"	"
4	37	9/10/61	3	52	"	"
5	25	9/15/61	3½	41	"	"
6	41	9/17/61	2	64	"	"
7	55	10/27/61	3	60	"	"
8	55	12/10/61	5	25	Interrup. 000	Partly attached
9	30	7/10/62	2	36	"	"
10	27	7/12/62	2	25	"	Held in place

mediate postoperative death which is not included in the series. The dogs were sacrificed after two to ten months for gross and microscopic examination.

Results

In seven dogs the grafts were found to have migrated to the most dependent portion of the left hemithorax. In two there was partial attachment of the prosthesis by the sutures to the anterior lower corner of the pericardial suture line, and in one the prosthesis was intact. In the last three animals interrupted 000 braided silk had been used (Table).

Dense fibrosis of the pleura and pericardium was noted around the migrated grafts with an increase in thickness from 0.33-0.5 mm to 5-10 mm (Fig 2). No adhesions were noted between the prosthetic material and the surrounding tissue, consisting of pericardium, pleura, and newly formed fibrous tissue, but fine to dense fibrous formation was present around the silk sutures.

Fig 2.—Macroscopic view: fibrous tissue formation around the graft.

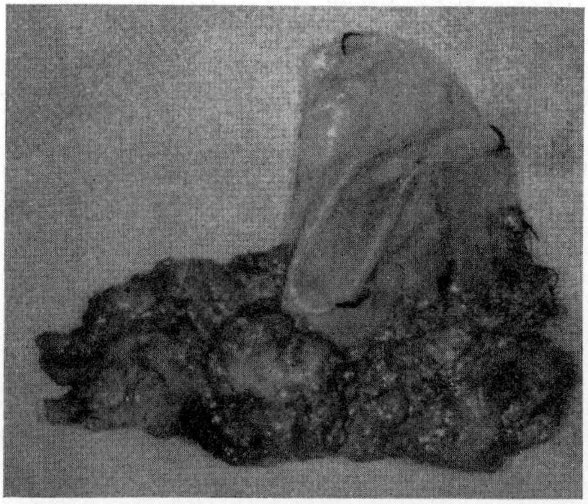

In all subjects the epicardium was thickened on the exposed surface with granulation, hyalinization, and fibrous tissue formation. There was no fibrous invasion into the myocardium under the thickened epicardium (Fig 3, *A* and *B*).

Microscopic study of the prosthesis-pericardial junction in the well-preserved suture lines showed no direct union of the prosthesis to the pericardium nor to the newly formed fibrous tissue. Mature collagenous tissue containing no giant cell foreign-body reaction was noted around the graft (Fig 4).

Dog No. 10.—The graft was found to be in place after two months, supported by dense fibrosis, more marked around the silk sutures. The edges of the graft between the sutures were sharp and free of adhesions. The outer surface of the graft was covered with thick fibrous tissue but was separated from it by a dead space. The contraction of this fibrous covering had caused folding of the graft.

Comment

In this experimental application of siliconized Dacron in a nonporous form as a partial pericardial replacement in ten dogs, the lack of union between the prosthesis and the surrounding tissue was noted in all subjects. This failure of union supports the contention that silicone does not become adherent when used in vivo. Considering the above fact, silicone as used in this experiment does not fulfill Schofield's first crite-

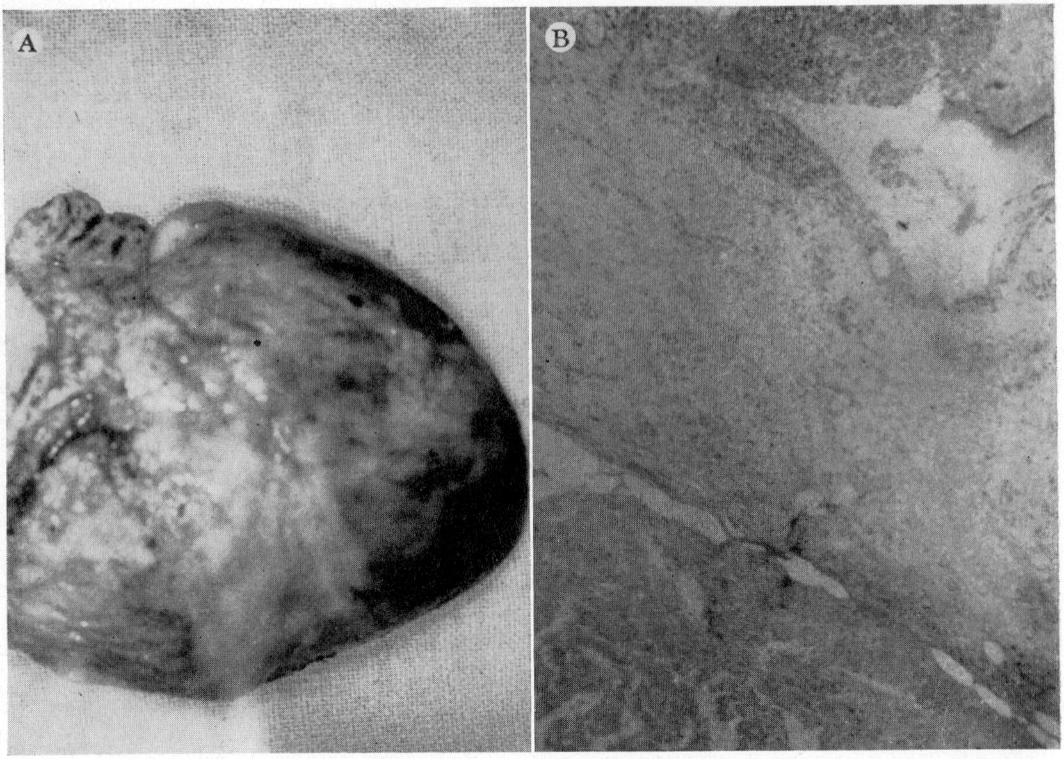

Fig 3.—*A,* macroscopic view: epicardial fibrous reaction. *B,* microscopic view: expicardial fibrous reaction. Reduced 38% from mag × 550.

rion for an ideal tissue substitute. It is thought that the continuous cardiopulmonary motion within the chest cavity was partly responsible for most of the sutures cutting through the pericardial margin.

The fibrous formation around the graft, together with the epicardial reaction of granulation progressing to mature fibrosis, is thought to be related to the mechanical irritation of the prosthesis.

Conclusions

1. This experiment suggests that a siliconized Dacron sheet, when used as a pericardial patch, is prone to migrate.

2. The restoration of the large defect in the pericardium, under these conditions, was uncertain because the sutures cut through the pericardial margins.

3. The epicardial reaction of granulation, hyalinization, and fibrous tissue formation in contact with the prosthesis may be related to the purely mechanical irritation of the graft (replacing friction of mesothelium on mesothelium by mesothelium on prosthesis).

4. The migration of the grafts is thought to be related to: a) the continuous motion of the heart, breaking some sutures and tearing other pericardial suture lines; and b) the lack of adherence of the pericardium to the prosthesis with failure of union at the suture line.

Summary

An experiment using siliconized sheets of Dacron for pericardial patches has been outlined.

The sheets did not unite with the surrounding tissue and did not form adhesions.

The prosthesis migrated to the most dependent portion of the hemithorax in seven dogs and became partially detached in two. It remained in place in one dog two months after the operation.

Fibrosis was found around the prosthesis and on a portion of the epicardium in contact with the prosthesis.

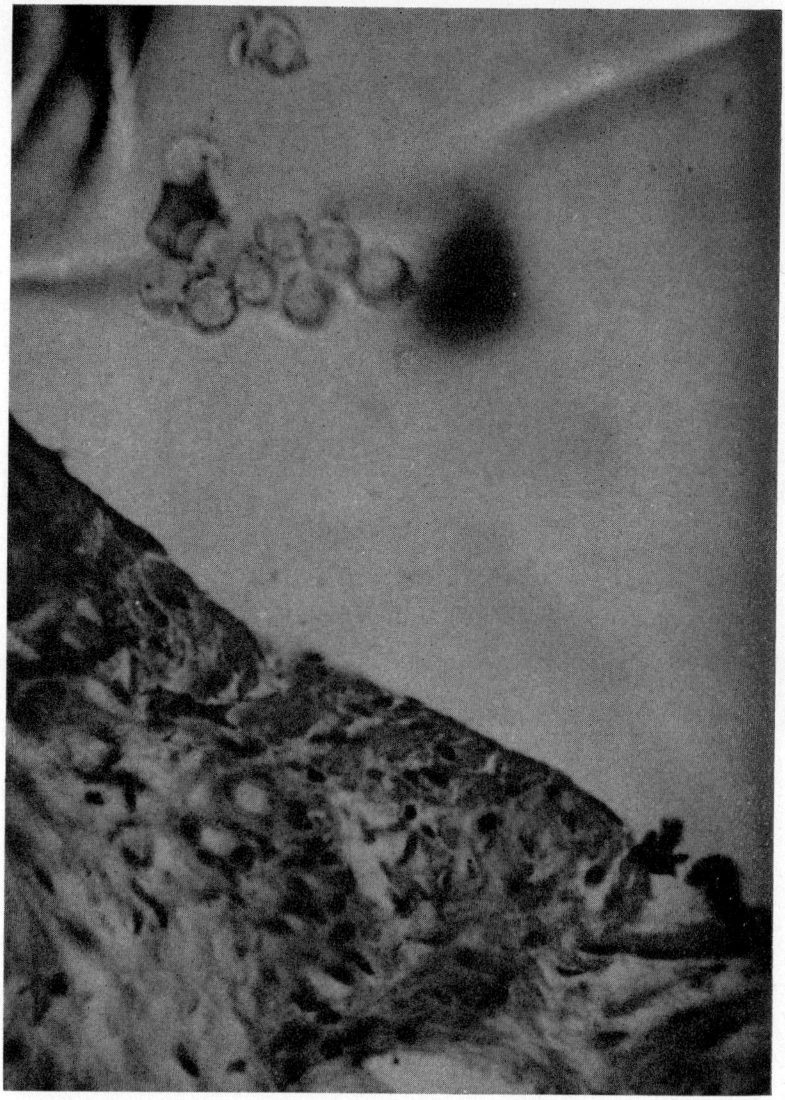

Fig 4.—Microscopic view: fibrous tissue reaction around the graft with a sharp line of demarcation and no foreign-body giant cell reaction. Reduced 14% from mag ×550.

This experiment suggests that under these conditions the closure of large pericardial defects cannot be successfully accomplished with siliconized sheets of Dacron.

Harlan Memorial Hospital, Harlan, Ky.

REFERENCES

1. Marzoni, F. A.; Upchurch, S. E.; and Lambert, C. J.: An Experimental Study of Silicone as A Soft Tissue Substitute, Plast Reconstr Surg 24: 600 (Dec) 1959.

2. Santos, O. A.; Hastings, F. W.; and Mazuji, M. K.: Effectiveness of Silicone as an Abdominal Drain, Arch Surg 84:643-645 (June) 1962.

3. Schofield, T. L.: Polyvinyl Alcohol Sponge: An Inert Plastic Material for Use as a Prosthesis in the Repair of Large Hernias, Brit J Surg 42: 176, 1955.

Quantitative Barrier of Synovium to Penicillin

HARRY C. MORGAN, MD
RONALD C. HERTEL, MD
AND
WARREN G. STAMP, MD
ST. LOUIS

Introduction

As a preliminary study of the microbiological effectiveness of parenterally administered penicillin in suppurative arthritis, the need for adapting quantitative methods of bio-assay to joint fluids became apparent. Recently, Jocson [4] has shown in humans that penicillin will cross synovial tissue. The distribution of electrolytes between plasma and joint fluids is in dynamic equilibrium obeying the laws of Donnan's equilibrium. The larger molecules, such as albumin, globulin, and mucin, behave differently.

It is the purpose of this paper to report a statistically reproducible quantitative method of measuring penicillin in the knee joint fluid of normal rabbits. The relationship of joint fluid concentration to circulating blood serum levels has been studied.

Submitted for publication Jan 22, 1963.

From the Orthopedic Surgery Division, Department of Surgery, School of Medicine, Washington University.

Supported by United States Public Health Service grant No. E-3522.

Methods

The potassium salt of crystalline penicillin G (benzylpenicillin) with a molecular weight of 372.48 and a theoretical potency of 1,595 units per milligram was chosen because of its widespread clinical usage. Penicillin concentrations were determined by an adaptation of the cylinder plate method of Grove and Randall.[3] The diameter of zones of inhibition of growth are compared to standard curves of known concentrations using *Sarcina lutea* as test organisms. Upon a base layer of 10 ml of Bacto antibiotic medium 1 is placed a seed layer of 4 ml of antibiotic medium 4 containing a 5% suspension of *S lutea*. The media are incubated 16 to 18 hours at 26 to 27 C with the solutions held in a 6 by 10 open-end cylinder planted on the media.

Using 3 to 5 kg New Zealand anesthetized male rabbits, simultaneous samples are obtained from each knee joint and the left auricle before and at 30 minutes after a single injection of 50,000 units per kilogram of crystalline potassium penicillin G into the paraspinus musculature. The joint samples are obtained by inserting a 15-gauge needle into the suprapatellar pouch of each knee joint. Into one knee 2 ml of Ringer's lactate is injected. Two minutes later all fluid recoverable is aspirated, yielding 0.8 to 2.0 ml. Into the opposite knee, 2 ml of pooled rabbit sera is injected and recovered in a similar manner. One milliliter aliquot is then used to make

Penicillin Levels in Serum and Knee Joints of Normal Rabbits Given 50,000 Units/Kg Benzylpenicillin

Time, Hr, After Injection, Hr	Blood Serum Units/Ml, Mean±SE	Joint Ringer's Lactate, Units/Ml, Mean±SE	Joint Pooled Serum, Units/Ml, Mean±SE
0	0	0	0
½	14.95±2.02 (27) *	1.58±0.22 (35)	1.74±0.23 (15)
1	10.35±1.53 (27)	1.21±0.19 (36)	2.02±0.46 (15)
1½	6.28±1.25 (28)	0.87±0.10 (36)	1.38±0.39 (15)
2	5.47±1.18 (27)	0.71±0.10 (39)	0.86±0.14 (14)
2½	3.56±0.50 (26)	0.47±0.09 (41)	0.53±0.12 (15)
3	3.06±0.93 (25)	0.32±0.04 (40)	0.38±0.11 (12)
3½	3.57±1.13 (20)	0.25±0.04 (37)	0.34±0.12 (9)
4	2.40±0.69 (26)	0.24±0.04 (42)	0.25±0.06 (15)
4½	1.11±0.20 (25)	0.13±0.03 (36)	0.21±0.06 (12)
5	1.42±0.39 (22)	0.13±0.03 (34)	0.16±0.07 (9)

* Number of determinations is shown in parentheses after each number.

three determinations of antibiotic concentration. If less than 1 ml is recovered two determinations are made.

Simultaneous blood samples of 2 ml are obtained by intracardiac aspiration using a 21 gauge needle. After centrifugation aliquots of 0.2 ml of serum are diluted with 0.8 ml of pooled rabbit sera. From this sample three determinations are made. Samples are taken at 30 minute intervals up to five hours. After the five hour reading, the joints are opened and the intra-articular placement of the needle is confirmed. Synovial tissue sections were then fixed in formalin and stained with hematoxylin and eosin. No difference in inflammatory response was noted between synovium exposed to Ringer's lactate and pooled rabbit sera.

Results

Maximum joint fluid concentrations are usually reached within the first 30 minutes after intramuscular injection of penicillin G which corresponds to the maximal circulating blood levels (Table). Thereafter the decrease in joint fluid concentration is dependent upon the decreasing blood level. Three to 3½ hours after injection, the blood level remains almost constant for a brief period and then declines further (Fig 1). This has occurred in almost every animal tested, and no explanation is available. This change has little effect in the joint concentration. Although the joint fluid concentrations using pooled sera as a diluent are significantly higher at one hour following injection, the rate of decline is comparable to the use of Ringer's lactate as the diluent. Variation is greater with sera than with Ringer's lactate. Although fewer observations were made with sera, there is evidence to suggest variation in protein concentration and pH may affect the biological activity of penicillin G (Fig 2). For this reason it is imperative that a well standardized and executed method of bio-assay is necessary to accurately reflect changing concentrations.

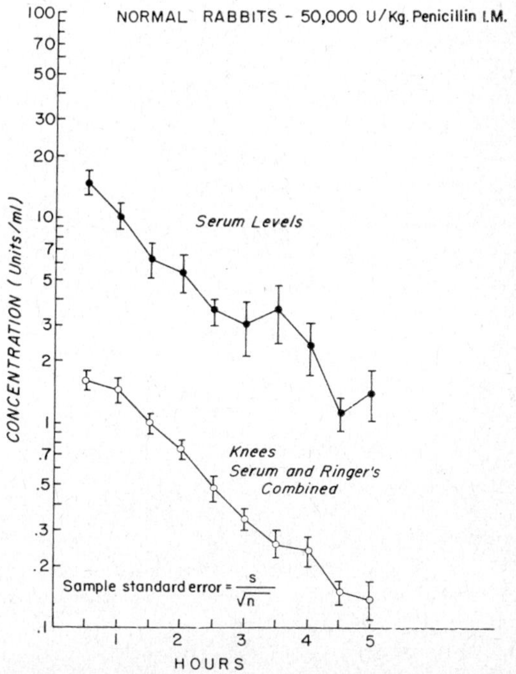

Fig 1.—Correlation of the circulating serum level with the simultaneous joint concentration is shown. The sample standard error of the mean is shown for each group of observations. Slope b (serum) = —0.29; slope b (joint) = —0.26; correlation coefficient (r) = +0.969.

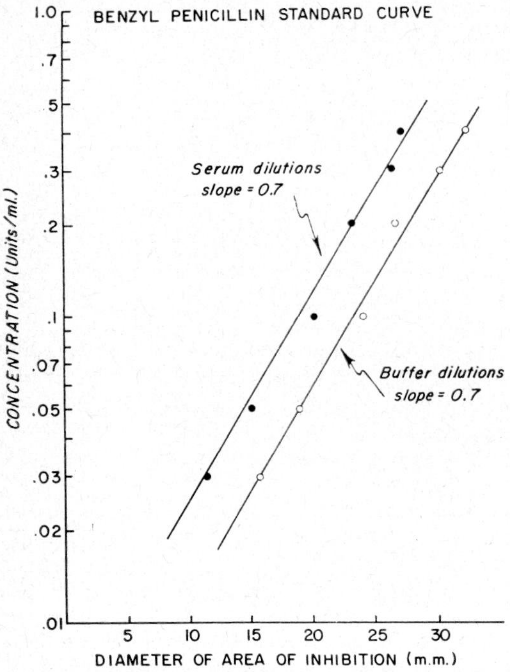

Fig 2.—Standard curves show similar slopes using two different diluents.

Penicillin molecules when injected intramuscularly cross the synovium in significant quantities at a predictable rate.

Summary

A reliable method of quantitative bioassay of potassium penicillin G has been adapted to measure penicillin concentrations in knee joint fluid of small animals using Ringer's lactate as a diluent.

Penicillin crosses normal synovial tissue in significant quantities.

The rate of change in penicillin concentration in knee joints of rabbits is a function of the circulating blood level.

There is a significant barrier to penicillin G molecules with molecular weight of 373 to cross normal synovium. Joint concentrations approximate 10% of circulating serum concentration.

Harry C. Morgan, MD, Assistant Professor of Orthopedic Surgery, Washington University School of Medicine, 600 S Kingshighway, St. Louis 10, Mo.

REFERENCES

1. Bunn, P. A.; Knight, R.; and Amberg, J.: Relative Merits of Serial Dilution and Cup-Plate Assays for Determination of Blood Levels of Penicillin in the Use of Different Diluents in Both Methods, Antimicrob Agents Ann 1960:231-239.

2. Edlund, T.: Studies on Absorption of Colloids and Fluids from Rabbit Knee Joints, Acta Physiol Scand, 18 (Suppl 62):1-108, 1949.

3. Grove, D. C., and Randall, W. A.: Assay Methods of Antibiotics, New York: Medical Encyclopedia, Inc., chap 2, 1955.

4. Jocson, C. T.: The Diffusion of Antibiotics Through the Synovial Membrane, J Bone Joint Surg (Amer) 37:107-114, 1955.

Adenocarcinoma of the Appendix

A Report of Four Cases

MAJID A. QURESHI, MD; WILLIAM T. FOLEY, MD; AND CHARLES D. HAFNER, MD, MS, CINCINNATI

Although adenocarcinoma of the vermiform appendix is a rare disease, it merits periodic consideration. In 1951 Hughes [1] accepted only 19 of the cases which he studied from the literature as true primary lesions of the appendix. Earlier reports were misleading, inasmuch as carcinoids were often recorded as grade 1 adenocarcinomas. Collins [2] discovered an incidence of 0.082% after studying 50,000 specimens, while McGregor [3] reported an incidence of only 1 in 30,000. Brown and Husni [4] reviewed the literature from 1900 to 1957 and found 52 cases. Since their report, the total was extended to 66 by Tarasidis,[5] and more recently to 83 by Wilson's composite study from several hospitals in Vancouver, Canada.

This neoplasm in the early stages remains asymptomatic. However, as the condition progresses, it can manifest itself in a variety of ways. For instance, Niceberg [7] reported a case presenting as an abdominal fistula associated with a polypoid lesion at the base of the appendix. One of the cases in our series presented as a large fungating mass with multiple mucus-draining sinuses. To our knowledge, no such case has been reported previously in the literature.

Clinical Material

During the 11-year period from 1952 through 1962, four cases of adenocarcinoma of the appendix have been treated at our hospitals.

Case 1.—A 73-year-old white male was admitted to the hospital on Dec 10, 1957, with a history of severe lower abdominal pain of two week's duration. This was described as intermittent and throbbing in character. There was no associated nausea, vomiting, or change in bowel habits. Physical examination revealed evidence of generalized arteriosclerosis. In the right lower quadrant of the abdomen a tender, firm, nonmobile, 3×4 cm mass was palpable.

Laboratory studies were: hemoglobin 13.5 gm, hematocrit 44%, and white blood cell count 10,300 with a normal differential. A barium enema demonstrated only diverticula of the descending and sigmoid colon.

After complete evaluation, the patient was taken to the operating room on Dec 16, 1957, where a granulomatous-appearing lesion (Fig 1) was found, suggesting that only an appendectomy be performed. However, when microscopic examination revealed an adenocarcinoma of the appendix (Fig 2), the patient was prepared for a right colectomy. At the time of the second procedure, the cecum was entirely free, but there were metastases to the regional lymph glands. A progress examination in December of 1958 revealed a large abdominal mass, and the patient died three months later.

Case 2.—A 66-year-old white male was admitted to the hospital on Feb 13, 1957, with a history of severe pain in the right lower quadrant for two days. During the two weeks prior to admission, however, he had experienced a milder pain which was aggravated by exertion. Physical examination revealed evidence of arteriosclerotic heart disease with auricular fibrillation. A 6 cm mass was palpable in the right lower quadrant of the abdomen.

Laboratory studies on admission were: hemoglobin 14 gm, hematocrit 45%, and white blood cell count 16,000 with 76 polymorphonuclears.

A standard McBurney's incision was made, and an abscess secondary to a perforated appendix was

Fig 1.—Gross specimen of adenocarcinoma of appendix.

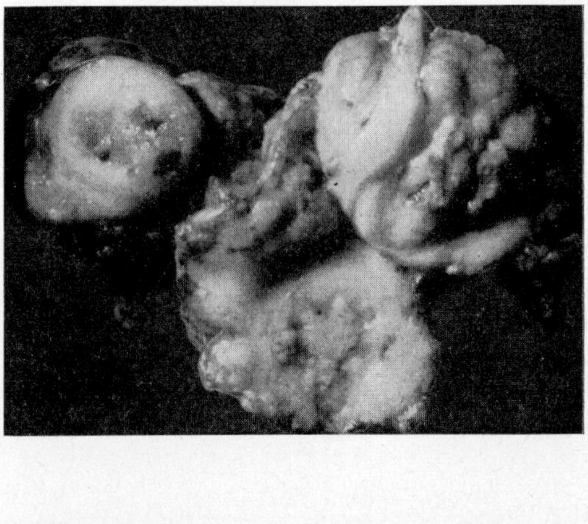

Submitted for publication Jan 28, 1963.

From the Departments of Surgery, Good Samaritan and St. Mary's Hospitals.

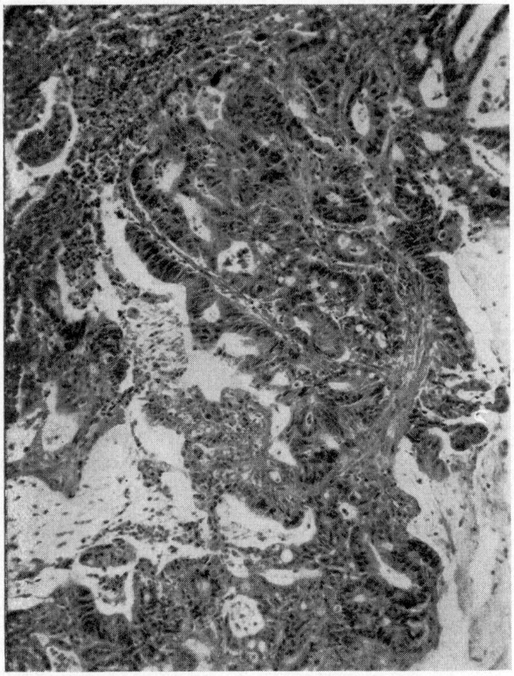

Fig 2.—Microscopic appearance of adenocarcinoma of appendix, showing glandular epithelium with anaplasia and mitosis.

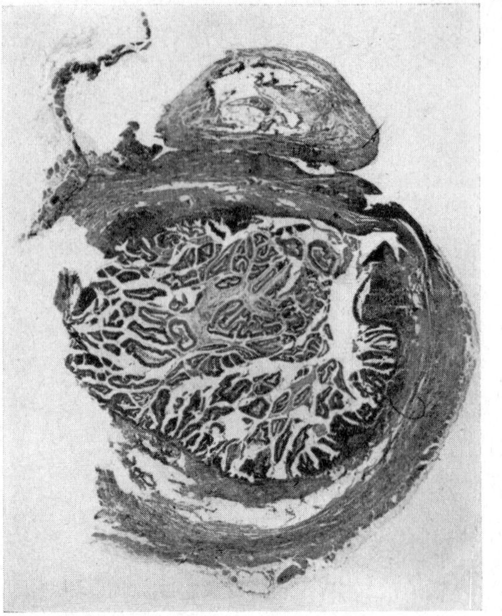

Fig 3.—Low-grade, mucinous-producing adenocarcinoma, limited to the lumen of the appendix.

found. It was possible to remove the appendix in addition to draining the abscess. Microscopic examination revealed a well-differentiated adenocarcinoma of the appendix. However, because of the patient's extremely poor cardiac status, a definitive procedure was delayed. Nevertheless, the patient was readmitted to the hospital on Sept 15, 1957, at which time laboratory studies including liver function tests and barium enema were normal. At the time of the second operation, extension of the lesion was found in the anterior abdominal wall and metastases were present throughout the peritoneal cavity. In two months, pulmonary involvement was demonstrated by roentgenography, and the patient died a few days later.

Case 3.—A 47-year-old white female was admitted to the hospital on June 25, 1959, with pain in the right lower abdomen, associated with nausea and vomiting 12 hours in duration. Physical examination revealed tenderness and guarding in the right lower quadrant highly suggestive of acute appendicitis. There was no palpable mass.

Laboratory studies were: hemoglobin 12.1 gm, hematocrit 43%, and white blood cell count 11,900 with 72 polymorphonuclears and 28 lymphocytes.

An emergency appendectomy was performed. Although the microscopic examination revealed acute appendicitis as suggested by the clinical picture, a low-grade, mucinous adenocarcinoma of the appendix was also discovered (Fig 3). The patient was re-explored 25 days later, at which time extensive adhesions were present between the terminal ileum and the uterus. A frozen section revealed no evidence of malignancy. Nevertheless, a hysterectomy, bilateral salpingo-oophorectomy, and right colectomy were performed. Pathological examination revealed no residual tumor in the cecum or regional lymph nodes. The patient is alive and well 3½ years later, with no evidence of recurrence.

Case 4.—An 80-year-old white female was admitted to the hospital on July 2, 1962, with a fractured left femoral shaft and an ulcerating mass in the right lower quadrant of the abdomen. This mass was 10 cm in diameter and contained multiple fistulous openings which discharged mucoid material onto the skin. There was no history of fecal drainage or disturbance in bowel habits. The patient experienced intermittent episodes of localized discomfort which were relieved by expressing accumulated mucoid material from the openings. Biopsy revealed a colloid adenocarcinoma.

Laboratory studies revealed: hemoglobin 8.5 gm, and normal white blood cell count. A barium enema roentgenogram demonstrated an extra-luminal mass displacing the cecum and ascending colon, but not involving the mucosa (Fig 4).

After the patient was prepared with blood transfusions, an intramedullary nail was inserted to stabilize the femoral shaft fracture. On July 30, 1962, an en bloc resection of the abdominal wall mass and right colectomy was performed. The defect in the anterior abdominal wall was repaired by fascia lata and sartorius muscle. Microscopic examination confirmed a colloid adenocarcinoma in the area of the appendix, no remnant of which

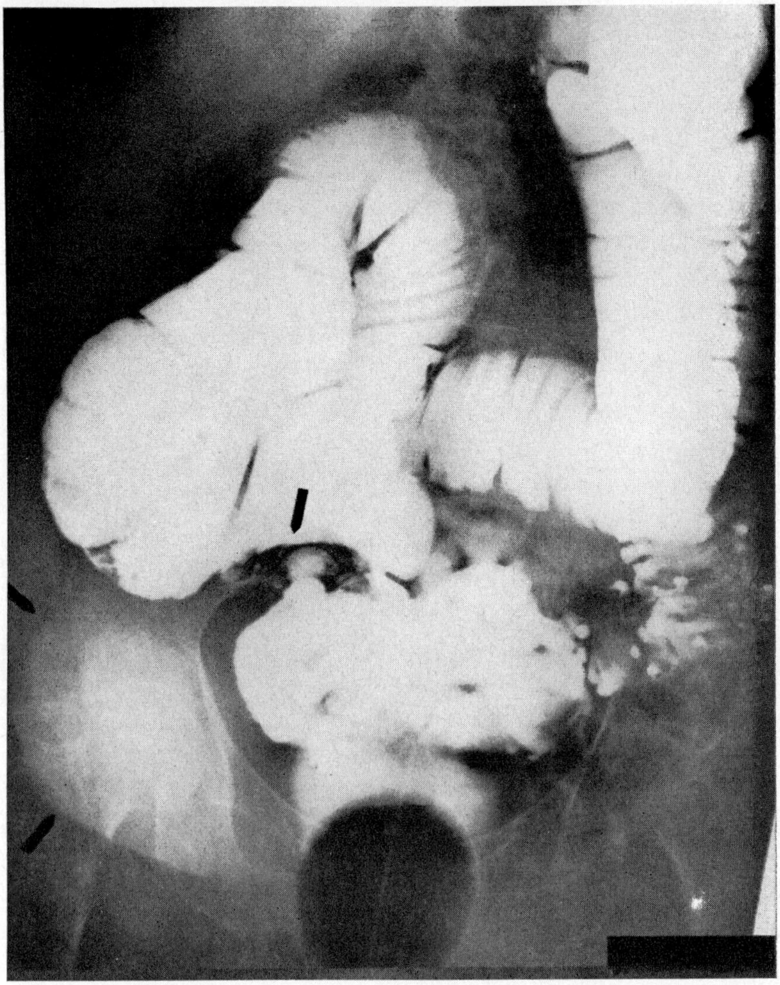

Fig 4.—Roentgenogram showing large, extraluminal mass displacing cecum and ascending colon superiorly.

could be identified. However, the cecum and lymph nodes were free of tumor. The patient is alive and well, without evidence of recurrence six months later.

Comment

In the very early stage of adenocarcinoma of the appendix it may be found coincidentally as the patient is treated for acute appendicitis or one of its complications, such as rupture and abscess formation. Certainly the neoplasm itself is asymptomatic at this time, and it is the acute inflammatory picture that focuses surgical attention on the appendix. Nevertheless, as the tumor itself enlarges, it may cause vague discomfort in the right lower quadrant, and a mass eventually becomes palpable in this area. As the neoplastic disease progresses, it may appear as a large, ulcerating, fungating mass with multiple mucous drainage sinuses. The different modes of presentation of all 87 cases from the literature, including the four in our series, are presented in the Table. In the advanced stages, it is frequently difficult to differentiate a large mass in this location as arising from the appendix or from some neighboring structure such as the cecum. For example, in case 4 careful gross and microscopic examinations were required to establish that the large ulcerating lesion was a direct extension of the primary adenocarcinoma of the appendix. To our knowledge, no such case has been reported to date, although Crile[8] reported one case with a mucous sinus subsequent to peritoneal drainage for a ruptured appendix. Case 2 demonstrates the poor prognosis and course of this neoplasm when it is associated with a perforated appendicitis. This patient survived less than two years after the initial appendectomy. In contrast to this, the patient whose early adenocarcinoma is found coexisting with an uncomplicated appendicitis should enjoy the best prognosis. In the latter circumstance, however, it is almost impossible to establish this diagnosis at the time of the initial appendectomy because of the associated inflammatory reaction. Consequently, a more definitive procedure seems indicated once the microscopic sections reveal the true identity of the lesion. A radical right colectomy with resection of the regional lymphatics appears to be the operation of choice. This should be performed as soon as possible when the patient is over the initial surgical procedure and an adequate bowel preparation has been accomplished. Simple appendectomy is probably sufficient for preinvasive adenocarcinomas.

Although a barium enema is usually of little aid in the diagnosis of this condition, Nardell[9] reported one case of his own and cited another from the Mayo Clinic series where the preoperative diagnosis was made by roentgenography. In these two cases, there was a filling defect in the cecum and the appendix could not be visualized. Similarly, roentgenograms were helpful in the diagnosis of one case in our series (Fig 4).

Modes of Presentation of Carcinoma of Appendix: 87 Cases

Symptoms	No. of Cases	%
Appendicitis	50	57.5
Rt. lower quadrant pain	7	8
Rt. lower quadrant mass	11	12.6
Incidental finding at surgery	12	13.8
Miscellaneous:	7	8
Pelvic mass		
Carcinoma of cecum		
Abdominal distention		
Perforated viscus	(One case each)	
Generalized carcinomatosis		
Abscess right flank		
Mucous-draining sinuses		
Total	87	100

Summary

Adenocarcinoma of the appendix is a relatively rare pathological entity. The limited literature concerning this condition has been reviewed. The four patients in our series are reported bringing the total number of recorded cases to 87. This tumor may present in a protean manner as indicated. Case 4 in our series appears to have a unique mode of presentation which has not been previously reported. It would appear, however, that the majority of these simulate acute appendicitis or one of its complications. The presence of perforation and abscess formation would seem to alter the prognosis considerably. The more favorable situation exists in those patients in whom an early, asymptomatic adenocarcinoma is found coincidentally with an uncomplicated acute appendicitis, or at the time of an incidental appendectomy. In these patients a radical right colectomy, in our opinion, should be performed as soon as possible after the diagnosis is established.

Majid A. Qureshi, MD, Peripheral Vascular Laboratory, Good Samaritan Hospital, Cincinnati 20, Ohio.

REFERENCES

1. Hughes, J. H.: Adenocarcinoma of the Appendix, Brit J Surg 39:282, 1951.

2. Collins, D. C.: A Study of 50,000 Specimens of the Human Vermiform Appendix, Surg Gynec Obstet 101:437, 1955.

3. McGregor, J. K., and McGregor, D. D.: Adenocarcinoma of the Appendix, Surgery 48:925, 1960.

4. Brown, H. W., and Husni, A. H.: Ruptured Adenocarcinoma of the Appendix: Review of the Literature and Case Presentation, Surgery 42:953, 1957.

5. Tarasidis, G. C.; Goodall, H. M.; and Farringer, J. L., Jr.: Adenocarcinoma of the Vermiform Appendix, Surg Gynec Obstet 115:287, 1962.

6. Wilson, R.: Primary Carcinoma of the Appendix, Amer J Surg 104:238, 1962.

7. Niceberg, D. M.; Feldman, S.; and Mandelberg, A.: Adenocarcinoma of the Vermiform Appendix, Surgery 40:560, 1956.

8. Crile, G., Jr., and Glen, C. G.: Primary Adenocarcinoma of the Appendix With Development of a Mucous Fistula, US Nav Med Bull 47:328, 1947.

9. Nardell, S. G.: Adenocarcinoma of the Appendix, Brit J Surg 41:136, 1953.

Fibrocystic Disease and Carcinoma of the Breast

MARTIN SWERDLOW, MD
AND
L. J. HUMPHREY, MD
CHICAGO

The objective of this project is the study of the relationship between fibrocystic disease and carcinoma of the breast. We divided our study into three parts: a microscopic study of fibrocystic disease preceding the development of carcinoma; of fibrocystic disease that did not eventuate as carcinoma in a minimal period of ten years, and the microscopic changes in breast tissue adjacent to carcinoma of the breast. The last group will be reported separately.

Our purpose is not the discovery of any possible statistical relationship but rather the micropathological characterization of the fibrocystic disease. It is our feeling that "fibrocystic disease" is too broad a concept or diagnosis for purposes of uncovering a possible relationship to carcinoma. Our goal is to observe the differences, if any, in the microscopic character of the fibrocystic disease that did or did not precede the development of carcinoma, and later to compare these with changes in carcinomatous breasts.

The relationship of fibrocystic disease to carcinoma has been studied and reported using either clinical statistics or correlating microscopic changes. In 1940, Warren reported carcinoma developing from three to four times more frequently in breasts with chronic cystic mastitis than in normal breasts. Lewison reported carcinoma developing in 1.8% of 385 patients operated upon for benign breast disease, while Pessagno found carcinoma developed in 12% of 108 patients with a previous biopsy for cystic disease of the breast.

Foote and Stewart in an extensive study reported on the incidence of histologic changes in cancerous and noncancerous breasts. They concluded there were no significant differences in any specific histologic changes between cancerous and noncancerous breasts, although cancerous breasts had five times more atypical papillomatosis. From a study of 76 cases of benign breast disease, Cole and Rossiter, in 1944, concluded that ductal hyperplasia was the most likely microscopic change. Tellem et al recently reported atypical hyperplasia six to seven times more frequent in cancerous versus benign breast lesions. Marcuse found that fibrocystic disease variants characterized by pronounced epithelial proliferation were almost twice as frequent in patients requiring multiple excisions than in those who had had only one operation, and that this association between the degree of epithelial hyperplasia and the tendency toward continued activity was independent of the patient's age.

Methods and Material

Clinical.—The microscopic slides of 630 breast biopsies and mastectomy specimens were reviewed. These specimens were from female patients seen at Research and Educa-

Submitted for publication Jan 24, 1963.

Clinical Associate Professor of Pathology (Dr. Swerdlow); Instructor in Surgery and Clinical Fellow American Cancer Society (Dr. Humphrey).

From the Departments of Pathology and Surgery, University of Illinois at the Medical Center.

TABLE 1.—*Criteria for Microscopic Changes*

	Slight 1	Moderate 2	Severe 3	Severe 4
Small ducts (interlobular); and large ducts	Slight proliferation, no cellular atypia, normal organization	Slight proliferation of cells, crowding, lumen and organization persist; no atypia	Marked cellular proliferation, lumen narnarrow, some atypia	Solid, no lumen; cellular atypia; loss of polarity with disorganization
Lobules: alveolar, terminal, intralobular ducts	Slight increase in lobular size and/or slight proliferation of ductal cells	Slight increase in lobule size and/or moderate proliferation of ductal cells; lumens persist	Increase in lobular size and/or marked proliferation of ductal cells, some atypia, lumens persist	Lobules increased in size, marked proliferation of ductal cells, cellular atypia, loss of polarity
Fibrosis	Slight increase with separation of lobules	Increase, separation lobules, compression lobules and ducts, some extension into lobules	Marked increase, compression or extension into lobules	Severe with complete disruption of lobules, compression of ducts, obliteration periductal and perilobular loose stroma
Sclerosing adenosis	Present			
Papilloma(s)	Single	Multiple	Single or multiple with atypia	
Apocrine epithelial changes	Present			
Cyst(s)	Single	Multiple		

tion Hospitals of the University of Illinois during the period of 1946 to 1955. Thirteen patients each had a biopsy diagnosed as fibrocystic disease and later a second biopsy interpreted as carcinoma. Sixty patients each had a biopsy diagnosed as fibrocystic disease and did not develop carcinoma in a minimal period of ten years. These patients are reported in this paper.

In one patient the carcinoma developed in the opposite breast; all the others developed carcinoma on the same side. The patients developing carcinoma ranged in age from 24 to 62 years with an average of 47 years. The average difference in years between the fibrocystic disease biopsy and the carcinoma biopsy was 5.4 years with a range from 1.3 to 13 years. Six of these patients were multipara.

The average age of the 60 patients with fibrocystic disease that did not eventuate in carcinoma was 43.5 years with a range from 17 to 84 years. The number of children, size of the lesion, and duration of the lesion were comparable to the fibrocystic disease-carcinoma group. The size of the benign lesions was also comparable.

A nipple discharge was present in 10% of the 60 patients not developing carcinoma compared to 39% of the fibrocystic disease-carcinoma group. Pain occurred in 37% of those not developing carcinoma and in 23% of those eventually developing carcinoma. The location of the benign tumors was also comparable in both groups.

Those patients who did not develop carcinoma had gynecological pathology in 20% of the cases and thyroid disease in 15%, com-

TABLE 2.—*Fibrocystic Disease Preceding Carcinoma*

	No Change 0	Slight & Moderate 1	Slight & Moderate 2	Slight & Moderate (1+2)	Severe 3	Severe 4	Severe (3+4)	Total Cases
Small interlobular ducts	3	3	4	7	1	2	3	13
Large ducts	1	2	3	5	3	4	7	13
Lobules: alveolar, terminal, intralobular ducts	4	1	6	7	1	1	2	13
Fibrosis	0	0	5	5	1	7	8	13
Sclerosing adenosis	7	6						13
Papillomatosis	6	7						13
Apocrine changes	7	6						13
Cysts			13					13

TABLE 3.—*Fibrocystic Disease Not Complicated by Carcinoma*

	No Change	Slight & Moderate			Severe			Total
	0	1	2	(1+2)	3	4	(3+4)	Cases
Small interlobular ducts	4	6	15	21	21	14	35	60
Large ducts	16	19	13	32	3	6	9	57 *
Lobules: alveolar, terminal, intralobular ducts	4	5	6	11	21	22	43	58 *
Fibrosis	0	0	5	5	29	26	55	60
Sclerosing adenosis	43	17						60
Papillomatosis	47	8	4					60
Apocrine changes	30	30						60
Cysts	19	1	40					60

* Material inadequate to evaluate in all cases.

pared to 39% and 23% of those patients that subsequently did develop carcinoma.

Pathological.—Microscopic sections stained with hematoxylin and eosin were examined. Changes in the smaller interlobular ducts, larger ducts, lobules (alveolar, terminal, intralobular ducts), and fibrous tissue were recorded and graded from 1 to 4. Also noted was the presence or absence of sclerosing adenosis, papilloma(s), apocrine epithelial changes, and cyst(s). Table 1 lists the criteria for the various grades of changes.

Results

The changes are presented in Tables 2 and 3.

Comment

Although it is difficult to generalize from these observations, it seems apparent from the tables that fibrocystic disease occurring in the biopsies that preceded the development of carcinoma was characterized by:

1. Slight to moderate hyperplasia of the epithelial cells lining the smaller ducts
2. A moderate to severe hyperplasia of the epithelial cells lining the larger ducts
3. A slight to moderate hyperplasia of the lobules and intralobular ducts
4. Moderate to severe fibrosis in all cases
5. An almost equal likelihood of the presence or absence of sclerosing adenosis, apocrine epithelial changes, and papilloma(s)
6. The presence in all cases of cyst(s)

The fibrocystic disease in those patients whose disease was not complicated by carcinoma in a minimal period of ten years was characterized by:

1. A moderate to severe hyperplasia of the epithelial cells lining the smaller ducts of most cases
2. Either no changes, or slight to moderate hyperplasia of the epithelial cells lining the larger ducts of most cases
3. A severe hyperplasia of the lobules and intralobular ducts
4. A severe degree of fibrosis in most cases
5. The absence of sclerosing adenosis in most cases
6. The absence of papillomas in most cases
7. Apocrine changes in half of the cases
8. Multiple cysts in most, but not all, cases

Fig 1.—Small interlobular ducts with slight hyperplasia. Hematoxylin and eosin; reduced 27% from mag × 125.

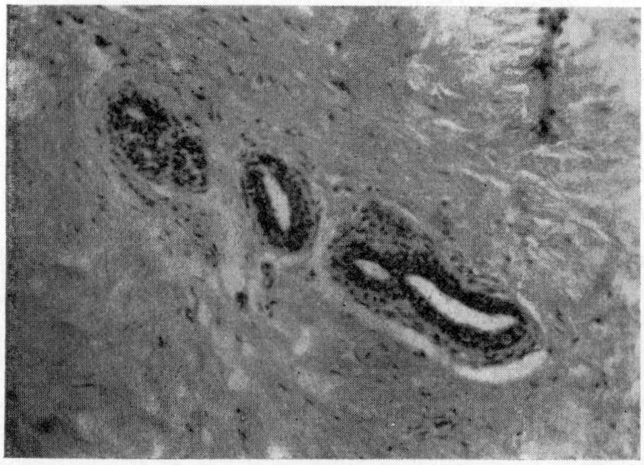

Fig 2.—Small interlobular duct with severe hyperplasia. Although the lumen persists, there is hyperplasia of lining cells with crowding, loss of polarity, and "atypical" cells. Hematoxylin and eosin; reduced 27% from mag × 440.

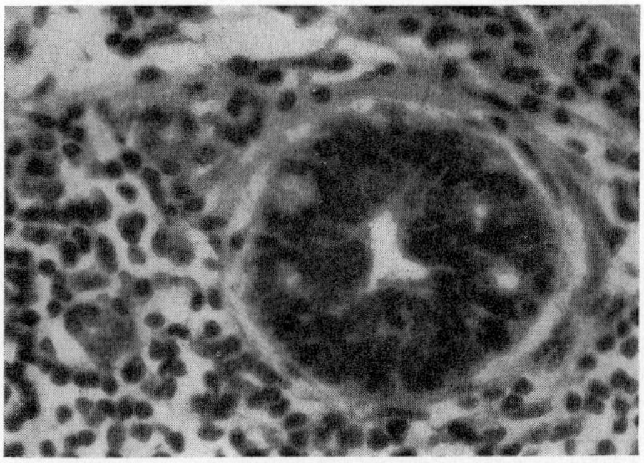

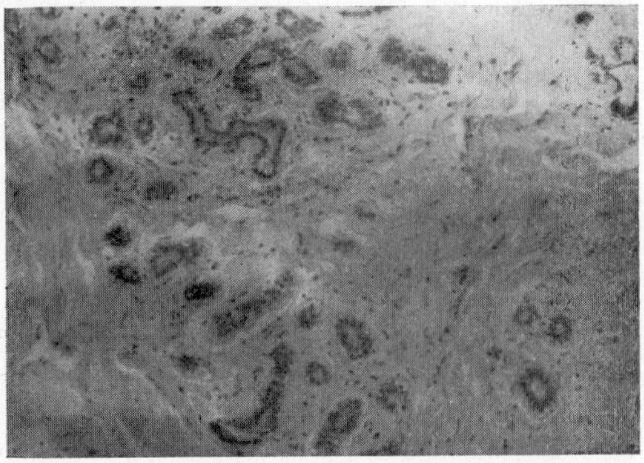

Fig 3.—Lobule with grade 3 fibrosis. Hematoxylin and eosin; reduced 27% from mag × 125.

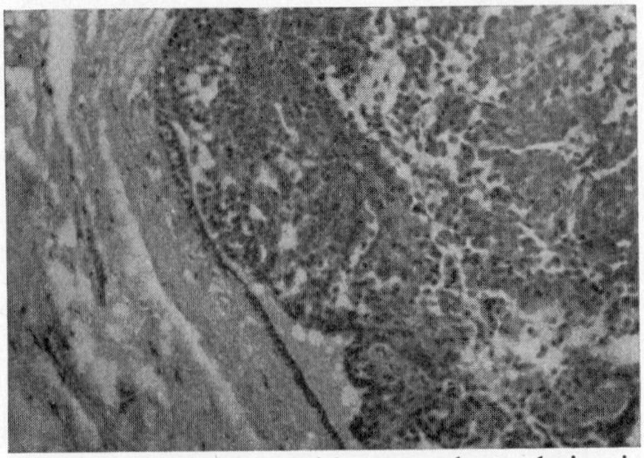

Fig 4.—Large duct with severe hyperplasia: in our study a significant change in fibrocystic disease preceding carcinoma of the breast. Hematoxylin and eosin; reduced 27% from mag × 125.

A comparison of these changes is difficult primarily because the series are not comparable in number. There does, however, appear to be a different emphasis of pathological changes.

The lesions that did not eventuate as carcinoma in the period of this study generally showed a more pronounced florid hyperplasia of all components of the breast tissue.

The lesions complicated by carcinoma showed a moderate to severe hyperplasia of the epithelial cells of the larger ducts, while the noncancerous group of lesions showed either no changes or slight to moderate changes.

The carcinomatous group showed a slight to moderate hyperplasia of the lobules, while the noncarcinoma group showed a severe hyperplasia.

Both groups showed a moderate to severe fibrosis in most cases.

The carcinoma group showed sclerosing adenosis in about half of the cases, while the noncarcinoma group contained areas of sclerosing adenosis in about one third of the cases.

The carcinoma group showed papillomas in about half of the cases, while papillomas were absent in most cases of the noncarcinoma group.

Both groups of breast lesions had apocrine changes in about half of the cases; the carcinoma group revealed cysts in all cases and the noncarcinoma group in most cases.

Summary

Breast biopsies of 13 patients with fibrocystic disease complicated by carcinoma and breast biopsies of 60 patients with fibrocystic disease not complicated by carcinoma in a ten-year period were reviewed. These sections stained with hematoxylin and eosin were microscopically characterized and compared. The outstanding microscopic differences in the two groups of patients were the moderate to severe epithelial hyperplasia in the larger ducts of the breast in those cases complicated by carcinoma and the more marked hyperplasia in the lobules and smaller ducts in the uncomplicated cases.

Martin Swerdlow, MD, Associate Professor, Department of Pathology, University of Illinois College of Medicine, 1853 W Polk St, Chicago 12, Ill.

REFERENCES

1. Cole, W. H., and Rossiter, L. J.: Chronic Cystic Mastitis: With Particular Reference to Classification, Ann Surg 119:573, 1944.

2. Foote, F. W., and Stewart, F. W.: Comparative Studies of Cancerous Versus Noncancerous Breasts, Ann Surg 121:6 and 197, 1945.

3. Lewison, E. F., and Lyons, J. G., Jr.: Relationship Between Benign Breast Disease and Cancer, AMA Arch Surg 66:94, 1953.

4. Marcuse, P. M.: Fibrocystic Disease of the Breast, Amer J Surg 103:428, 1962.

5. Pessagno, D. J.: Cystic Disease of the Breast, Amer Surg 23:65, 1957.

6. Tellem, M.; Prive, L.; and Meranze, D. R.: Four-Quadrant Study of Breasts Removed for Carcinoma, Cancer 15:10, 1962.

7. Warren, S.: The Relation of "Chronic Mastitis" to Carcinoma of the Breast, Surg Gynec Obstet 71:257, 1940.

Lumbar Sympathectomy

Effects on Vascular Responses in the Lower Extremity of Patients With Arteriosclerosis Obliterans

DAVID A. TICE, MD
GEORGE E. REED, MD
EDWARD J. MESSINA, BS
EMMETT CLEMENTE, MS
AND
WALTER REDISCH, MD
NEW YORK

Introduction

Reports on the clinical results of lumbar sympathectomy have varied from great satisfaction to the denial of any essential benefit.[1,2] Clinical evaluation of therapeutic results in chronic disease is notoriously difficult.[3] On the other hand, it must be admitted that a rationale established on purely experimental basis may not necessarily always be borne out by clinical experience. Nevertheless, if reliable methods to ascertain the physiologic effects of a procedure are available, it is preferable to establish such on an objective basis rather than to rely on clinical impressions.

With this in mind the effects of lumbar sympathectomy upon blood flow to skin and muscles of the lower extremity in patients with arteriosclerosis obliterans were measured plethysmographically.

Methods and Material

Presympathectomy measurements of blood flow were made on 12 limbs in eight patients with nongangrenous obliterative atherosclerosis. In six, unilateral sympathectomy was performed and postsympathectomy data (two to four weeks after the operation) are available. The nonsympathectomized contralateral extremity was studied in three. All patients were male, their ages ranging from 54 to 72, with an average of 63 years. None had any evidence of cardiac or renal decompensation.

Percutaneous femoral arteriography or translumbar aortography was performed in all patients using 50% or 70% diazotrate (Hypage) to determine the extent and location of the peripheral arterial disease prior to the initial studies of blood flow. Patients selected for study and sympathectomy all demonstrated arteriosclerosis obliterans in the iliofemoral-popliteal system not amenable to direct arterial reconstruction or graft. Patients with gangrene, loss of tissue, or ulcerations were not included in this study.

Submitted for publication Jan 16, 1963.

From the Cardiovascular Unit of The New York University Medical Center, Departments of Surgery and Medicine of New York University School of Medicine, and the New York University Research Service, Goldwater Memorial Hospital.

This work was supported in part by the United States Public Health Service under grant No. HE-03097-06 and in part by the Health Research Council of The City of New York under contract No. U-1089.

Lumbar sympathectomy was performed through an anterolateral, extraperitoneal approach. The lumbar sympathetic chain was exposed, the preganglionic and postganglionic fibers divided, and the chain including the ganglia L-1 through L-4 excised. Pathological confirmation of specimen was obtained in each case.

Blood flow was measured with an air transmission venous occlusion two-channel plethysmograph. Skin and muscle flow were calculated using a previously described method.[4,5] This method permitted simultaneous measurements of segmental blood flow to one calf and to the other foot, respectively. By reversing the procedure in control experiments reliable checking of results was facilitated. Only changes of 0.5 ml/100 ml of tissue or more were considered significant.

The constant-environment laboratory was kept at 55% humidity in all experiments. Resting flows were measured at 20 C and 25 C environmental temperature. Blood flow responses to a physiologic "dilator" stimulus (Gibbon-Landis procedure) were tested at 20 C (mild vasoconstrictor stimulus) in six subjects.[6] Responses to regional exercise[7] were tested in four of the eight patients at 20 C; in three extremities this could not be done because of severe intermittent claudication; there was no change in this after sympathectomy. Responses to a levarterenol (Noradrenaline) infusion were tested in six subjects at 25 C (mild vasodilator stimulus). From 0.48-0.8 mg of levarterenol in 200 ml of 5% glucose was infused within 30-45 minutes (80-100 drops/minute), after blood flow measurements had been ascertained to remain constant during an infusion of physiological saline at the same rate for 10-15 minutes.

Table 1.—*Resting Perfusion Values in Three Limbs Before and After Sympathectomy, ML/100 CC of Tissue/Minute at 20 C and 25 C: New Method*

	Before		After	
	Average	Range	Average	Range
	Resting Skin Perfusion			
At 20 C	2.1	1.5-3.1	4.0	3.2-4.7
At 25 C	2.6	1.8-3.6	3.2	2.5-4.7
	Resting Muscle Perfusion			
At 20 C	1.6	1.4-1.7	1.4	1.0-1.7
At 25 C	2.0	1.6-2.4	1.9	1.3-3.0

Comment

Skin perfusion at 20 C was significantly higher after sympathectomy, but the increase was below the level of significance at 20 C. Muscle perfusion was essentially unchanged by the operation (Table 1).

Table 2.—*Average Responses to Gibbon-Landis Procedure in Six Limbs Before and After Sympathectomy*

Change in Skin Perfusion		Change in Muscle Perfusion	
Before	After	Before	After
+60%	−32%	None	−14%

+ indicates increase, — indicates decrease in per cent of resting perfusion at 20 C.

Before sympathectomy, skin perfusion increased during the Gibbon-Landis procedure by 60%, while muscle perfusion showed no change. After sympathectomy, skin perfusion decreased by 30% and there was a slight decrease in muscle perfusion in response to the Gibbon-Landis test (Table 2). Systemic arterial pressure (measured at the brachial artery) remained unaltered throughout all experiments. Thus the alteration in responses cannot be explained by a borrowing-lending phenomenon within the limb. It is realized that bone flow is not accounted for in the methods used.

In response to regional exercise, there were slight increases in skin before sympathectomy but slight decreases after sympathectomy; in contrast there were increases in muscle flow of about 100% elicited before sympathectomy, but these were somewhat smaller (about 80%) after the operation (Table 3).

It appears, therefore, that the only objective benefit derived from the procedure within two to four weeks after operation is an increase in perfusion of the resting skin. No change was recorded in the subjective complaints of six patients after sympathec-

Table 3.—*Average Responses to Regional Exercise in Four Limbs Before And After Sympathectomy*

Change in Skin Perfusion		Change in Muscle Perfusion	
Before	After	Before	After
+14%	−14%	+111%	+80%

+ indicates increase, — indicates decrease in per cent of resting perfusion at 20 C.

Table 4.—*Average Responses to Levarterenol Infusion in Six Limbs Before and After Sympathectomy*

Change in Skin Perfusion		Change in Muscle Perfusion	
Before	After	Before	After
—51%	—72%	—26%	—39%

+ indicates increase, — indicates decrease in per cent of resting perfusion at 25 C.

Table 5.—*Average Responses to Levarterenol Infusion in Three Nonsympathectomized Limbs Before and After Sympathectomy of Contralateral Limbs*

Change in Skin Perfusion		Change in Muscle Perfusion	
Before	After	Before	After
—50%	—50%	—44%	—44%

+ indicates increase, — indicates decrease in per cent of resting perfusion at 25 C.

tomy; one 72-year-old patient felt that his leg was warmer than before the operation.

There was a significant decrease in both skin and muscle perfusion in response to levarterenol under all experimental conditions. The decreases were somewhat more marked in the skin. After sympathectomy, these responses were invariably enhanced. An interesting observation was that in the skin the flow decrease in response to levarterenol was only 30%-50% in some subjects but 60%-90% in others; in muscle it was always between 20% and 50%. After sympathectomy, originally lesser skin responses were increased to high response level (Table 4).

Since levarterenol is, to our present-day knowledge, the most important physiologic vasoconstrictor in the internal milieu, the above represents an undesirable result of sympathectomy.

Responses in the limb not operated on appeared uninfluenced by sympathectomy performed on the contralateral side. There was no significant change in any of the parameters. Table 5 indicates the responses to levarterenol. This makes a "borrowing-lending" phenomenon from one extremity to the other most unlikely.

Summary

All early effects of lumbar sympathectomy upon blood flow to the lower extremity appear undesirable except for an increase in perfusion of the resting skin.

Blood flow responses in the extremity not operated on are not altered by sympathectomy on the contralateral side.

David A. Tice, MD, Department of Surgery, New York University School of Medicine, 550 First Ave, New York 16, NY.

REFERENCES

1. DeTakats, B.: Place of Sympathectomy in the Treatment of Occlusive Arterial Disease, AMA Arch Surg 77:655, 1958.

2. Warren, R.: The Diagnosis and Treatment of Chronic Obliterative Arterial Disease of the Extremities, Practitioner 175:248, 1955.

3. Steele, J. M., and Redisch, W.: Use of Drugs in the Treatment of Peripheral Vascular Disease, J Chronic Dis 4:327, 1956.

4. Redisch, W.; Wertheimer, L.; Delisle, C.; and Steele, J. M.: Comparison of Various Vascular Beds in Man: Their Responses to a Simple Vasodilator Stimulus, Circulation 9:63, 1954.

5. Redisch, W.; Besseghini, I.; and Steele, J. M.: Distribution of Blood Flow to the Human Extremity in Response to Physiologic and Pharmacologic Stimuli, Fed Proc 19:90, 1960.

6. Gibbon, J. H., and Landis, E. M.: Vasodilatation in the Lower Extremities in Response to Immersing Forearms in Warm Water, J Clin Invest 11:1019, 1932.

7. Redisch, W.; Antonio, A.; Bogdanovich, A.; and Steele, J. M.: Vasomotor Responses to Exercise in the Extremities of Subjects With Vascular Disease, Circulation 19:583, 1959.

Effects of Hypothermia on Myocardial Contractile Force

HARVEY W. BENDER, MD
W. GERALD AUSTEN, MD
TAKEO TSUNEKAWA, MD
AND
PAUL A. EBERT, MD
BETHESDA, MD

It is well known that general body hypothermia results in a decrease in heart rate and an associated increase in ventricular contractile force. Previous studies of this temperature effect on myocardial activity have been restricted to isolated heart preparations or intact animals in which the entire body was cooled.[1-4] The present studies were designed to investigate the site of action of hypothermia on myocardial contraction in intact animals utilizing separate cardiopulmonary and systemic perfusion systems.

Materials and Methods

Adult fasting mongrel dogs weighing 16 to 22 kg were used. After induction of anesthesia with intravenous thiopental (20 mg/kg) a cuffed endotracheal tube was inserted and ventilation was maintained by a positive pressure respirator supplying room air. A bilateral anterior thoracotomy was performed through the fourth intercostal spaces and the sternum transected. Heparin was administered intravenously.

Cardiopulmonary bypass was then effected by draining venous blood from the venae cavae to a Kay-Cross rotating disc oxygenator and returning it through a Brown-Harrison heat exchanger into the femoral artery. A separate perfusion system was established by draining blood from the ascending aorta into a reservoir and pumping it through a second heat exchanger into the pulmonary artery (Fig 1). A clamp was then placed across the ascending aorta just proximal to the brachiocephalic artery, thus separating the two perfusion systems. The systemic arterial pressure, ascending aortic pressure, and the signal from a Walton-Brodie strain gauge arch attached to the left ventricle were recorded on a multichannel oscillograph. The flows in both circuits were adjusted so that the pressures proximal and distal to the aortic clamp were equal. A telethermometer probe in the esophagus and a thermistor in the left ventricular myocardium enabled continuous recording of the systemic and myocardial temperatures.

Submitted for publication Feb 20, 1963.
From the Clinic of Surgery, National Heart Institute.

In nine dogs these two perfusion systems were utilized to cool the systemic circulatory bed to an esophageal temperature of 15 C while the heart temperature was maintained in the normal range. The animals were then rewarmed to normal levels. In four of these dogs the temperatures of the heat exchangers were then reversed so that the systemic circuit remained normothermic while the heart and lungs were cooled. In the remaining five dogs the aortic clamp was removed and the entire animal was then cooled.

In three additional animals the cardiopulmonary circuit was modified so the heart and lungs could be perfused separately (Fig 2). In these dogs the aorta was not cross clamped and the heart was included in the systemic perfusion system. The second circuit perfused only the lungs; pulmonary venous blood was collected through a large left atrial cannula and was pumped through a heat exchanger into the pulmonary artery. In these dogs the lungs were cooled to 15 C while the heart and systemic temperatures were maintained at normothermic levels.

Results

Systemic Cooling With Heart and Lungs Normothermic.—In the nine animals cooled to an esophageal temperature of 15 C, the average heart temperature was maintained at 35 C. During cooling or rewarming there was no significant change in left ventricular contractile force and only a very slight decrease in heart rate (Fig 3 and 4).

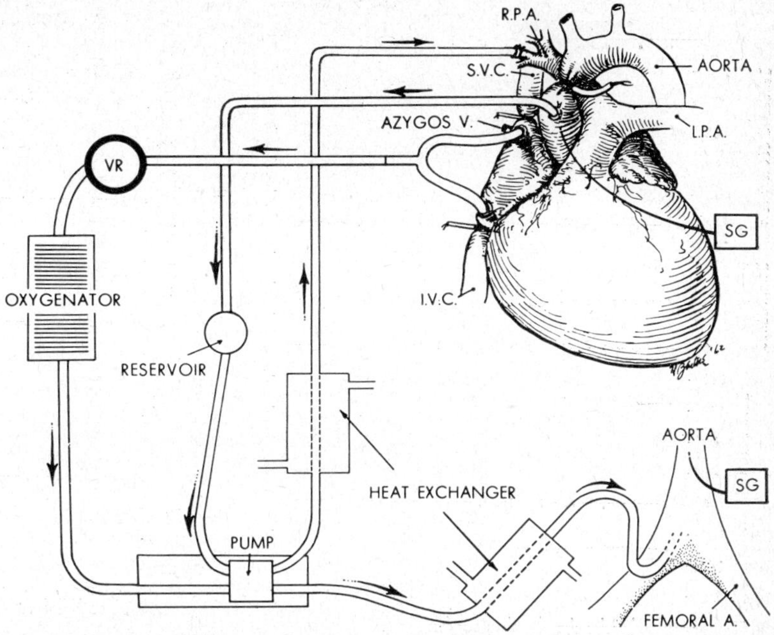

Fig 1.—Schematic representation of the cannulations and extracorporeal circuits employed to separate the cardiopulmonary and systemic circulations.

Cardiopulmonary Cooling With or Without Systemic Cooling.—When the heart and lungs were cooled with or without systemic cooling, significant changes in heart rate and contractile force occurred (Fig 3 and 4). At a myocardial temperature of 25 C a decrease in heart rate of approximately 67%, to an average rate of 40 beats per minute, occurred in both groups. An associated increase in contractile force of approximately 40% also occurred.

Pulmonary Cooling With Heart and Systemic System Normothermic.—With isolated pulmonary cooling to 15 C there was no significant change in contractile force or heart rate (Fig 5).

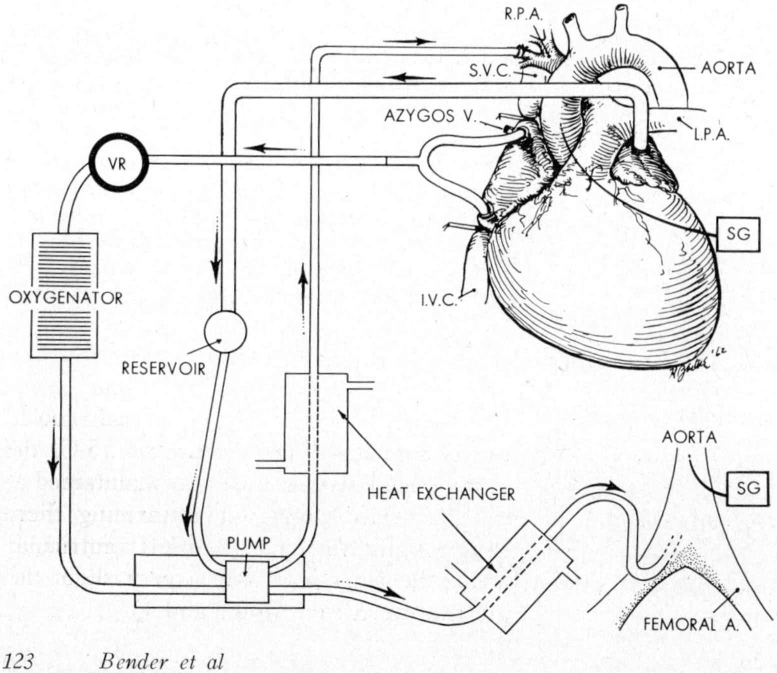

Fig 2.—Schematic representation of the cannulation and extracorporeal circuits employed to isolate the pulmonary circulation.

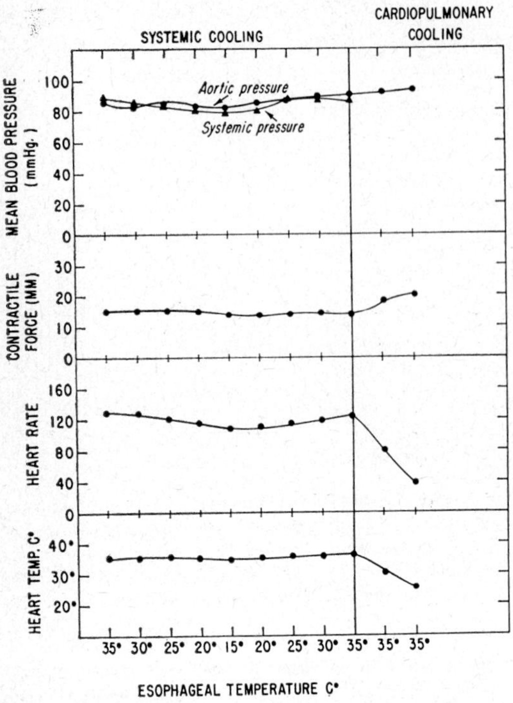

Fig 3.—Average change in blood pressure, contractile force, heart rate, and heart temperature associated with changes in esophageal temperature. To the left of the solid line only systemic cooling was produced; to the right of the line only cardiopulmonary cooling was accomplished.

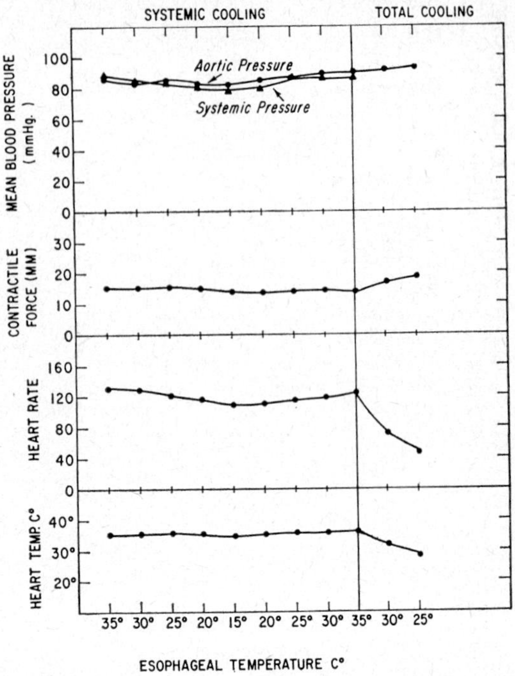

Fig 4.—Average changes in blood pressure, contractile force, heart rate, and heart temperature associated with changes in esophageal temperature. To the left of the solid line only systemic cooling was produced; to the right of this line total body cooling occurred.

Comment

The changes in heart rate which have previously been observed during moderate hypothermia (29-32 C) have been presumed to be the direct effect of low temperature on the heart. At these temperatures neurogenic reflexes are still active and, at least in part, could be responsible for the bradycardia observed during moderate hypothermia.

In the present experiments, no change in heart rate or contractile force occurred when the entire body was cooled while the heart and lungs were kept normothermic. In addition, isolated pulmonary cooling failed to produce any alteration in cardiac action. One might postulate that the above findings are due to the fact that neural pathways are not responsive when the body temperature is 15 C, but if this is so, some change in rate would have been observed at higher temperatures since these animals were gradually cooled and rewarmed. Furthermore, investigation in this laboratory has shown that the normothermic dog heart will respond to electrical stimulation of the vagus nerves and the stellate ganglia at temperatures as low as 15 C. Thus, these studies demonstrate that no central or peripheral receptors relating to cardiac action are activated by decreasing temperatures and that the change in heart rate observed during hypothermia is entirely a direct effect of cold on the heart.

The effect that temperature has on myocardial contractile force could not be accurately evaluated from this study since the heart rate became so slow at low temperature. The signal from the Walton-Brodie strain gauge arch increased in amplitude at low temperatures, but the upstroke recorded from the arch was much slower when the rate decreased. Thus, the observed increase in amplitude may not represent a true increase in the strength of contraction since the first derivative would probably be much

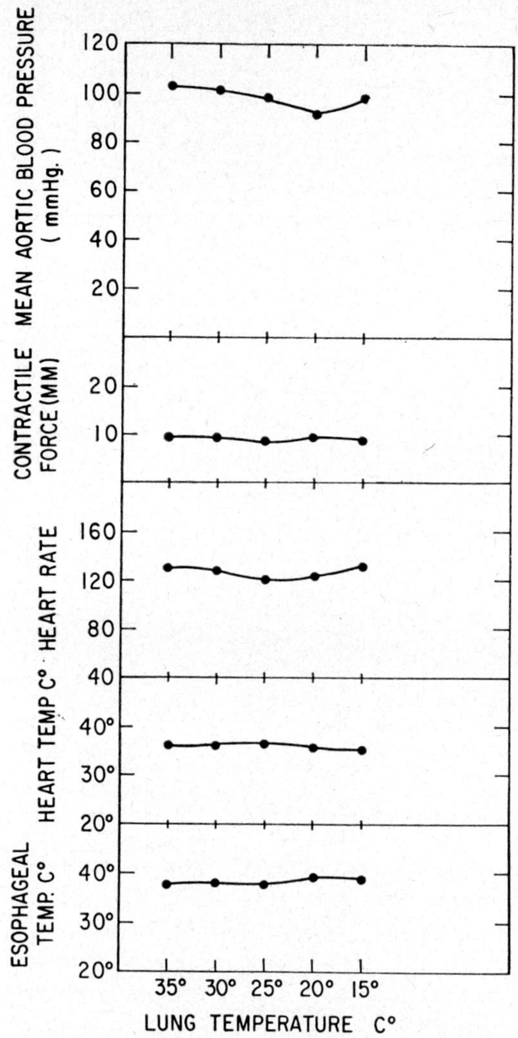

Fig 5.—Average changes in blood pressure, contractile force, heart rate, heart temperature, and esophageal temperature associated with changes in lung temperature.

lower during hypothermia. The reduction in cardiac output and peripheral pressure observed in hypothermic animals with intact circulatory systems may result, at least in part, from the inability of the heart to maintain a normal rate at these temperatures.

Summary

Employing separate perfusion circuits, the temperatures of the heart, lungs, and systemic system were independently altered to determine the site of cardiac action of hypothermia in the dog. There was no significant change in either heart rate or contractile force with systemic cooling alone. During cardiopulmonary cooling, with or without systemic hypothermia, marked alterations in heart rate and contractile force occurred, but no changes were noted with isolated pulmonary cooling. These observations lead to the conclusion that the site of cardiac action of decreased body temperature is the heart itself.

Harvey W. Bender, MD, c/o Andrew G. Morrow, MD, Chief, Clinic of Surgery, National Heart Institute, Department of Health, Education & Welfare, Bethesda 14, Md.

REFERENCES

1. Garb, S., and Chenoweth, M. B.: Electrogram of Isolated Papillary Muscle of the Cat Heart, Amer J Physiol 156:27, 1949.

2. Trede, M.; Foote, A. V.; and Maloney, J. V., Jr.: Pathophysiologic Aspects of Profound Hypothermia With Extracorporeal Circulation, Ann Surg 154:210 (Aug) 1961.

3. Goldberg, L. I.: Effects of Hypothermia on Contractility of the Intact Dog Heart, Amer J Physiol 194:92, 1958.

4. Brown, T. G., Jr., and Cotten, M. D.: Evaluation of Factors Enhancing Cardiac Force During Hypothermia, Fed Proc 15:405, 1956.

"Spontaneous Rupture" of the Spleen: One Mechanism

Routine Splenectomy Challenged

JAMES D. HARDY, MD
AND
RICHARD L. YELVERTON, MD
JACKSON, MISS

The surgeon is frequently surprised and dismayed when in the course of upper abdominal surgery the spleen is found to be denuded of a portion of its capsule. This most frequently occurs "spontaneously" at the point where the various tissues or ligaments attach to the spleen at the cephalad or caudad extremes of the hilum. The defect may have been caused by traction on the splenic attachments, and, of course, actual instrumental trauma may have been inflicted upon any portion of the spleen.

When bleeding from a denuded portion of the spleen results in detection of the capsular tear, the surgeon commonly concludes that splenectomy is indicated to prevent possible further hemorrhage in the postoperative period. That is, the diagnosis of splenic injury has often been considered an indication for immediate splenectomy.

Submitted for publication Feb 26, 1963.

Department of Surgery, University of Mississippi Medical Center.

Aided by USPHS Grant No. A-5122(cl).

In the course of transabdominal repair of an esophageal hiatal hernia, we observed a phenomenon which to us shed light upon at least one mechanism of "spontaneous rupture" of the spleen during operation in the absence of direct trauma. This case caused us to revise our thinking regarding the inevitability of splenectomy where mere loss of capsular surface has occurred.

Report of Case

A 64-year-old white woman was operated upon for the repair of a severely symptomatic sliding esophageal hiatal hernia. Despite the fact that she was obese, the transabdominal approach was elected, since complete abdominal exploration was desired. There was considerable inflammatory reaction in the region of the esophageal hiatus, and exposure was tedious and difficult even with the left lobe of the liver retracted to the right after division of the triangular ligament. Great care was taken to avoid injury to the spleen. This organ was noted to be small (Figure, *A*), and packs were then placed carefully to exclude it from the operative field. Scattered adhesions were present throughout the abdomen, doubtless secondary to cholecystectomy performed previously. In due course the hiatal

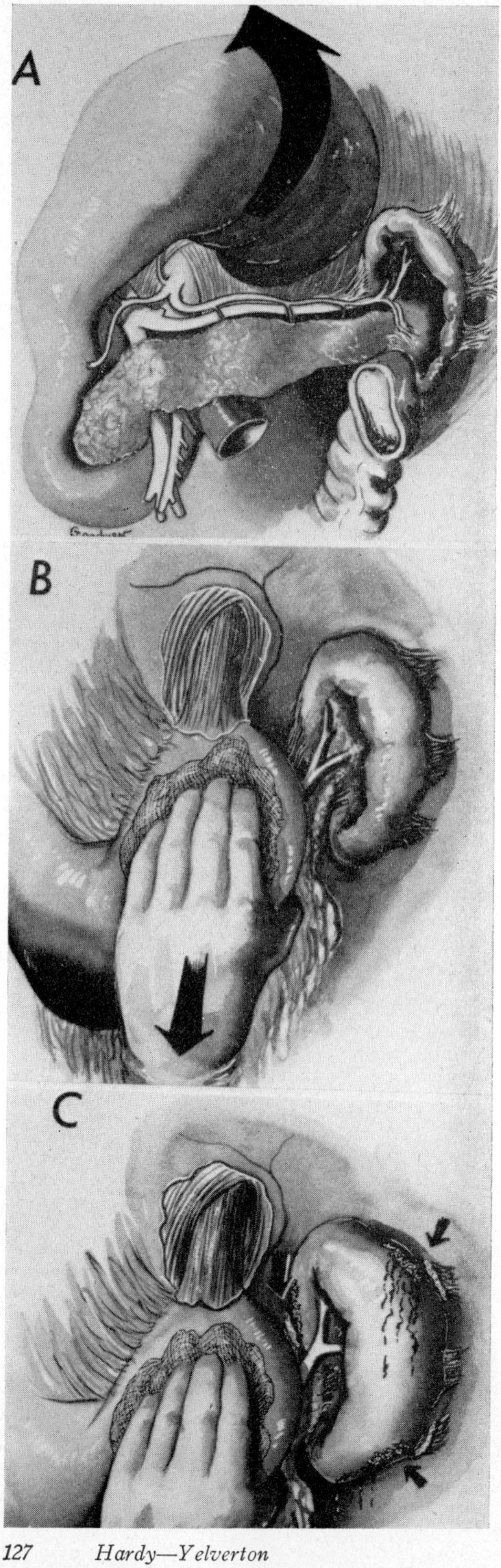

hernia was exposed, the hiatal opening was satisfactorily reduced in size with appropriately placed silk sutures, and the cardioesophageal junction with the remnants of the phrenoesophageal ligament were joined with interrupted sutures to the newly established diaphragmatic aperture. Several additional sutures were used to tack the fundus of the stomach to the undersurface of the left hemidiaphragm.

Meanwhile, it had been observed that the downward retraction of the stomach, with pressure also exerted posteriorly (Figure, *B*), had resulted in considerable distention and enlargement of the splenic vein. Traction on the tail of the pancreas and the splenic pedicle had been carefully avoided.

Presently blood was observed flowing from behind the sponges which had been placed to protect the spleen from trauma. These were carefully removed, to reveal marked splenic enlargement to a size at least four or five times the volume that had existed when this organ had been first visualized prior to repair of the hiatal hernia. On more careful inspection it was apparent that adhesions on the posterior surface of the spleen had been put under stretch and had torn free, a portion of the splenic capsule being avulsed at each site (Figure, *C*). A similar mechanism was considered possibly operative in producing a small denuded area in the cephalad portion of the splenic hilum.

The pressure upon the retroperitoneal pancreas and splenic vein having been released, the splenic vein and the spleen both diminished in size. Meanwhile, the bleeding from the denuded areas slowed markedly, and after perhaps ten minutes of observation this bleeding ceased. And inasmuch as no deep or pulp injury had been inflicted, it was elected not to remove the spleen, and the abdomen was closed.

The patient made an uneventful recovery.

Comment

In 1958 Orloff and Peskin [1] reviewed all previously reported cases of spontaneous rupture of the normal spleen. The mechanism herein described was not mentioned, though we would admit that this case represented a most unusual circumstance. The spleen was fixed to the undersurface of the anterior chest wall and left hemidiaphragm by a number of short and dense fibrous ad-

A, the usual anatomic relationships are demonstrated, with the exception of the splenic adhesions. The spleen was normal in size when first exposed. *B*, posterior pressure exerted upon stomach, compressing pancreas and splenic vein, causing spleen to enlarge. *C*, avulsion of areas of splenic capsule by dense adhesions as spleen rapidly enlarged to a size at least four times that which existed at the beginning of the operation.

hesions. As the organ was caused by splenic vein compression to enlarge rapidly to a size several times that which existed at the beginning of the operation, certain of these unyielding adhesions were put under tension and they pulled away from the spleen, taking with them a portion of the delicate capsule. However, since the damage to the spleen was superficial, clotting occurred once the high splenic pulp pressure had been lowered by removing the pressure previously exerted upon the splenic vein.

Failure to Perform Splenectomy.—There has been an increasing awareness that splenectomy is not always an innocuous procedure and that the indications for splenectomy might well be re-examined. The present case again emphasized that loss of splenic capsular integrity need not represent a categorical indication for splenectomy, provided that bleeding ceases either spontaneously or after application of some material such as Gelfoam.

Summary and Conclusions

A case is reported in which multiple sites of avulsion of the splenic capsule occurred during splenic enlargement, in the course of difficult abdominal exposure of an esophageal hiatal hernia.

The capsular avulsions were produced not by direct trauma but by tension on scattered short dense fibrous adhesions as the spleen enlarged rapidly due to splenic vein compression.

When pressure on the splenic vein caused by downward retraction of the stomach was released, a reduction in the sizes of the distended splenic vein and spleen occurred. Bleeding from the denuded surfaces then ceased, and splenectomy was not performed. No previous report of a similar clinical observation has been found.

1. It is suggested that rapid enlargement of the spleen, placing tension upon hilar attachments or adhesions elsewhere, may represent one mechanism of spontaneous rupture of the spleen.

2. Splenectomy is not routinely indicated in the management of minor capsular avulsions.

James D. Hardy, MD, Professor & Chairman, Department of Surgery, The University of Mississippi Medical Center, 2500 N State St, Jackson 6, Miss.

ADDENDUM

Since the manuscript was submitted, three similar cases have come to our attention. In each instance a small tear in the splenic capsule was successfully treated without splenectomy.

REFERENCE

1. Orloff, M. J., and Peskin, G. W.: Spontaneous Rupture of the Normal Spleen: A Surgical Enigma, Int Abstr Surg 106:1, 1958.

Internal Cooling for General Hypothermia

MARSH H. HOLT, MD
AND
F. JOHN LEWIS, MD
CHICAGO

Introduction

In previous publications on this subject,[2,3] we have reported the use of intragastric cooling as an adjunct to external blanket refrigeration in the induction of general hypothermia as used at the Northwestern University Medical Center and, more recently, at the West Virginia University Medical Center. The purpose of this paper is to report the continued successful use of an internal means of temperature control as well as to describe a refinement of our original cooling device.

Subjects

Thirty-six surgical patients were cooled and rewarmed in this study. A summary of pertinent data is given in Table 1. Twenty-six craniotomies were performed for meningiomas, intracranial aneurysms, subdural hematomas, an arteriovenous fistula, a pituitary tumor, and a fibrosarcoma. The seven surgical heart lesions included: aortic stenosis, atrial septal defect, and ventricular septal defect. A carotid endarterectomy, renal endarterectomy, and a thoracic aneurysm were the three vascular disorders operated upon.

Method

The intragastric apparatus contains a closed system circuit and is composed of a balloon attached to a double lumened tube * and a heat exchange unit (Figure) with attachments to a Therm-O-Rite † refrigerating unit. As in external cooling procedures, a rectal thermometer is inserted, and the patient is encased in a moist sheet, protectively padded at the sacrum, knees, heels, and toes. A Therm-O-Rite blanket is then wrapped around the patient.

The gastric heat exchange unit consists of a hollow cylinder through which cooling fluid from the Therm-O-Rite unit is circulated. In the center of the cylinder is an 18 ft coil of ¼ inch stainless steel tubing. Water is circulated through the coil by a centrifugal pump,‡ which requires submersion

Submitted for publication Feb 4, 1963.

Department of Surgery, Northwestern University Medical School, Chicago, and West Virginia Medical Center, Morgantown.

Supported in part by United States Public Health Service grant H-2879.

* Manufactured by Davol Rubber Company, Providence, RI.

† Therm-O-Rite Production Company, Buffalo.

‡ Little Giant Vaporizer Co, Oklahoma City.

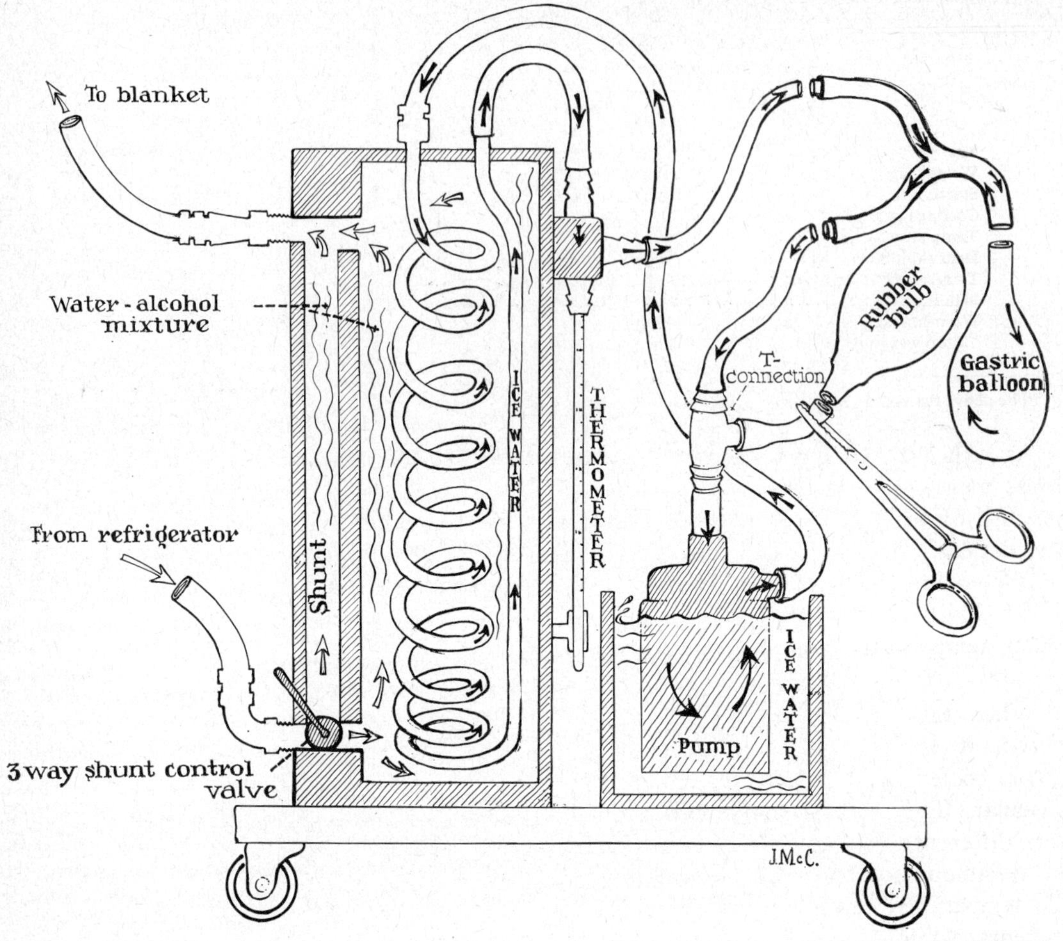

Schematic drawing of heat exchange unit in intragastric cooling circuit. See text for explanation.

during operation (Figure). From the metal coil, water passes through the intragastric balloon via a double lumen esophageal tube and back to the pump. A monitoring thermometer is inserted in the circuit distal to the heat exchange coil.

In preparation for use, the tubing and balloon are connected and filled with water by way of a T-connector as is seen in the Figure. Prior to insertion, the balloon is collapsed by withdrawing fluid from the closed system and, after endotracheal intubation, is passed into the stomach by way of the mouth. The balloon is then expanded with approximately 100 cc of water by its introduction into the closed system through the T-connector. Its location in the stomach is checked by exerting a light traction on the esophageal tubing. If the balloon is above the cardia it is easily withdrawn by this maneuver. After the balloon's position is determined to be within the stomach, an additional 400 cc of water is introduced into the cooling system. Circulation through the balloon is begun, and the heat exchange unit is connected to the Therm-O-Rite tubing in series with the blanket(s).

During cooling, the Therm-O-Rite temperature is maintained at approximately O C (32 F) and that of the intragastric fluid at 8 C (46.4 F). Circulation through the balloon is two liters per minute.

While rewarming, the blanket temperature is no higher than 46 C (114.8 F) and the balloon 41 C (105.8 F). The balloon temperature is controlled by adjustment of a shunt control valve (Figure) which diverts the warming fluid pumped from the Therm-O-Rite away from the gastric heat exchange unit.

Results

A tabulation of the patients' temperature responses to cooling and warming is given in Table 1. The data are presented according to type of surgery and sex of the individual.

TABLE 1.—*Summary of Data of 36 Surgical Patients* *

	Group 1 Neurosurgery		Group 2 Cardiovascular Surgery	
	M, 16	F, 10	M, 7	F, 3
Age, yr	42 (27-69)	38 (17-64)	47 (18-65)	35 (18-44)
Weight, kg	78.6 (66-95)	56.4 (48.3-64.5)	71.4 (59.1-88.2)	51.4 (48.2-56.8)
Starting temp, C	36.5 (35.1-38.2)	36.4 (36.0-37.0)	36.7 (35.2-38.0)	37.1 (36.4-38.0)
Cooling rate, min/C/kg	0.29 (0.25-0.35)	0.34 (0.29-0.42)	0.35 (0.19-0.59)	0.38 (0.27-0.52)
Temp stop cooling, C	32.2 (30.8-34.6)	32.1 (31.2-32.7)	32.6 (32.0-33.8)	31.3 (30.0-32.2)
Drift rate, min/C/kg	0.30 (0.26-0.36)	0.46 (0.32-0.76)	0.48 (0.21-0.88)	0.51 (0.41-0.61)
Temp start warming, C	30.3 (28.2-32.8)	29.0 (28.1-30.2)	29.8 (29.5-30.7)	29.4 (28.8-29.0)
Minimum temp, C	29.5 (27.8-31.6)	28.7 (27.7-30.2)	30.0 (27.1-31.2)	28.9 (28.8-29.0)
Warming rate, min/C/kg	0.35 (0.26-0.41)	0.51 (0.35-0.56)	0.38 (0.36-0.39)	0.67 (0.51-0.77)
Stop warming, C	33.8 (32-35)	33.2 (32-35)	34.0 (32-35)	33.7 (32-35)

* The above figures are means with ranges given in parentheses.

As expected, cooling was found to progress more rapidly than warming, probably because of the 30-35 C differential between the patients' normal temperatures and that of the cooling fluid, while there was only a 15-17 C difference between the cooled patients' temperatures and that of the warming fluid.

When the two major groups are compared, it is clear that the neurosurgery group cooled more rapidly than the cardiovascular. The most obvious explanation for this difference is that there was no change in the amount of body surface area utilized for temperature control in the neurosurgical patients, while the latter group was cooled for a short initial period, and then the chest or abdomen was exposed for surgery.

The drift rate following cessation of active cooling was most rapid in the male neurosurgical patient group. There was no significant difference in the rate of temperature change in this group during the active cooling phase and the drift period. In the other three groups, the drift rate was from 0.12 to 0.13 min/C/kg slower than during active cooling. No clear explanation was found for this apparent discrepancy. One possible factor might, again, be the higher average fat content of the female's subcutaneous tissues. This insulation might explain the sex difference in the neurosurgical group but apparently is not as significant in the second group wherein periods of extensive body surface exposure are required for surgery.

When Group 1 was evaluated according to sex and age, as seen in Table 2, it was found that the younger members of each sex responded to cooling and warming more rapidly than the other members.

An evaluation of the same group according to total weight by sex showed that the heavier members of both sexes cooled slightly more rapidly than did the lighter ones. The warming rate was not consistently affected by total body weight.

As seen in Table 1, the rate of temperature change during either cooling or warming was more rapid in males than in females in both surgical groups. In explaining this difference we believe that the higher amount of adipose tissue usually found in females acts as an insulation against either direction of temperature change. Baker [1] clearly demon-

TABLE 2.—*Neurosurgery Patients (Group 1)*

No.	Yr	Cooling *	Warming *
According To Age			
16 M	<42	0.27	0.34
	>42	0.34	0.37
10 F	<36	0.31	0.38
	>36	0.35	0.48
According To Weight			
No.	Kg	Cooling *	Warming *
16 M	>78.6	0.31	0.35
	<78.6	0.29	0.35
10 F	>56.4	0.37	0.45
	<56.4	0.34	0.47

* Average rates given in min/C/kg.

strated this in 1956 while working with men of varying degrees of obesity.

No controlled study was made concerning the effects of various preoperative medication and anesthetic agents on temperature response. Casual observations, however, did not result in support of chlorpromazine or promethazine (Phenergan) as aids in increasing the rate of temperature change in either direction. An accurate appraisal was not possible because of the many variables encountered. No occurrences of burns or frostbite were noted at the temperatures used. There were no clinical changes in gastric function in any patient nor in HCl and pepsinogen determinations in several patients, and no functional or histological derangement was noted in experimental studies in dogs.

As previously discussed [2,3] the advantages of the addition of intragastric heat exchange in general hypothermia are a more rapid temperature change and accuracy in control with minimal risk and technical involvement. The unit used for the accomplishment of this end has been herein described. Its usefulness lies in the convenience of completing the usual hypothermia case during a morning's operating time without the problems and dangers of extracorporeal heat exchange methods.

Summary

A further presentation is offered on the advantageous use of intragastric temperature control as an adjunct in general hypothermia. A device is described which accomplishes this end with no encountered deleterious side effects, minimal technical involvement, and minor expense. Observations are recorded on rates of temperature change according to sex, weight, and type of surgery performed.

Dr. Nichols Wetzel and Dr. Byron M. Bloor helped in the collection of data for this paper.

F. John Lewis, MD, Department of Surgery, Northwestern University Medical School, 303 E Chicago Ave, Chicago 11, Ill.

REFERENCES

1. Baker, P. T., and Daniels, F., Jr.: Relationship Between Skinfold Thickness and Body Cooling for Two Hours at 15 C, J Appl Physiol 8:409-416, 1956.

2. Holt, M. H.; Benvenuto, R.; and Lewis, F. J.: General Hypothermia With Intragastric Cooling, Surg Gynec Obstet 107:251-254, 1958.

3. Holt, M. H.; Benvenuto, R.; and Lewis, F. J.: General Hypothermia With Intragastric Cooling: A Further Study, Surg Forum 9:287-291, 1958.

Intrahepatic Cholangiography

FRANK G. MOODY, MD; THANE ASCH, MD; AND FRANK GLENN, MD, NEW YORK

A detailed knowledge of intrahepatic cholangiographic anatomy is essential for the recognition and management of pathology within the proximal biliary tree. The following postmortem study was designed to focus on the details of human intrahepatic anatomy. An associated clinical study was directed toward assessing the value of our present cholangiographic methods in demonstrating the proximal biliary tree.

Norman[6] was one of the first to stress the importance of good proximal cholangiography in the management of stones within the substance of the liver. Fainsinger[1] demonstrated the value of the correlative study of postmortem casts and cholangiograms of the human liver. We have combined a clinical and postmortem approach in order to assess ways in which we might improve the quality of our visualization of the proximal biliary tree and our ability to interpret variations and pathology within it.

Postmortem Study

Injection-corrosion preparations of 20 fresh human cadaver livers were compared with their respective postmortem cholangiograms. The cholangiograms were performed in air with propyliodone, the liver molded over sponge to conform to its in vivo contour. The bile ducts, portal vein, and hepatic artery were injected with 15% vinyl acetate. Digestion of the hepatic parenchyma was carried out with 20% potassium hydroxide. A sturdy replica of the intrahepatic vasculature and biliary tree was obtained in this manner. Twelve of the 20 specimens were grossly normal and had been obtained from subjects who were clinically free of hepatic or biliary tract disease. The remaining eight specimens were grossly abnormal. There were two cases of advanced Laennec's cirrhosis, two with metastatic carcinoma, and one each of chronic passive congestion, massive fatty infiltration, obstruction of the distal bile duct, and retained cystic duct stump post cholecystectomy. All of the specimens were studied to determine their intrahepatic biliary architecture.

Submitted for publication April 6, 1963.

From The Departments of Surgery and Radiology, The New York Hospital-Cornell Medical Center.

Intrahepatic Anatomy

The bilaterality of the liver was confirmed by McIndoe and Counseller in 1927.[5] Hjortsjö recognized the segmental pattern of the intrahepatic architecture in 1949.[3] Healey and Schroy,[2] in 1953, described the normal intrahepatic anatomy as encountered in their study of 100 injection-corrosion preparations of human postmortem livers. Their nomenclature and description are complete and clearly stated. They will be applied throughout the following text.

The human liver is divided into right and left lobes by a major or lobar fissure. This division can be identified on the visceral hepatic surface by a line which transects the gallbladder bed and the fossa for the inferior vena cava. This fissure has no external landmarks on the anterior or superior surface of the liver. In vivo, it lies in a sagittal plane. The middle hepatic vein courses throughout its length, but it is free of biliary radicles or branches of the portal venous or hepatic arterial systems.

The right lobe of the liver is divided into anterior and posterior segments by the right segmental fissure. This fissure lies in a coronal plane, and has no surface landmarks. The right hepatic vein courses within this space.

The left lobe is divided into a medial (quadrate lobe) and lateral segment by the

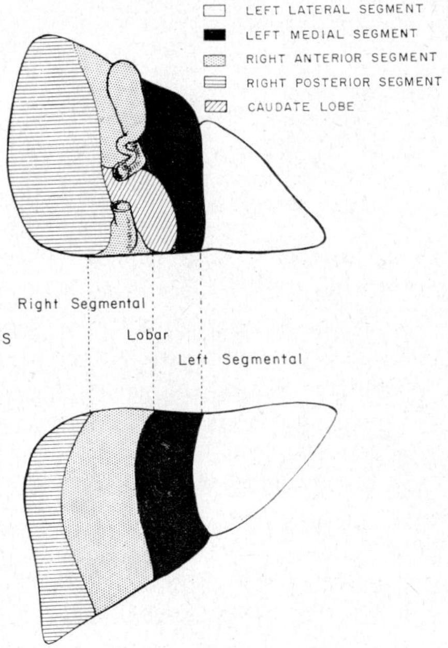

Fig 1.—Diagram of the major segments of the human liver. The dorsal surface is above, ventral below. The major lobar and segmental fissures are identified.

left segmental fissure. This can readily be identified on the surface of the liver as the umbilical fossa or area of attachment of the falciform ligament. This fissure lies in a sagittal plane and is occupied by the left hepatic vein.

The caudate lobe is most conveniently considered a separate mass of hepatic parenchyma which arises from the posterior superior segment of the right lobe. It extends to the left where its bulk lies behind the medial segment of the left lobe.

The segments of each lobe divide in turn into superior and inferior areas. The major divisions of the liver and their respective fissures are portrayed diagrammatically in Fig 1.

Intrahepatic biliary drainage is segmental in distribution and forms an anatomic unit with the respective segmental hepatic artery and portal vein. Fig 2 is a composite sketch of the most common pattern of biliary drainage. The hepatic venous system is intersegmental, occupying the space of the major fissures and interdigitating with branches of the portal vein within the hepatic parenchyma. Each area is drained by a third order duct. The segmental ducts are second order, and the major lobar ducts are the primary biliary radicles.

The most common pattern is a bifurcation of the right and left hepatic ducts within the hilum of the liver. The right hepatic duct in turn divides at a variable distance within the substance of the liver to form the anterior and posterior segmental ducts. These then divide into inferior and superior area ducts. Fig 3 and 4 are a cast and cholangiogram of a grossly normal postmortem liver which demonstrates this common pattern.

The left hepatic duct assumes a gentle, anterior superior course to the left and divides at a variable distance from its origin into the medial and lateral segmental ducts. The

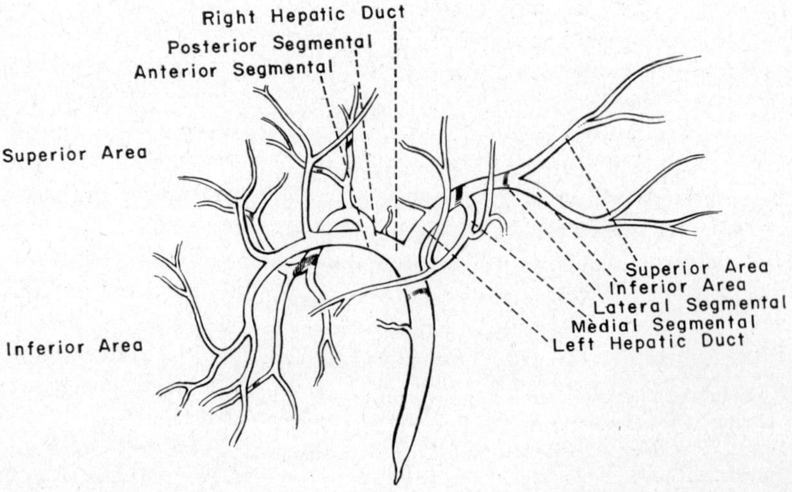

Fig 2.—Composite sketch of the human biliary tree. It has been extended to the fifth order of branching.

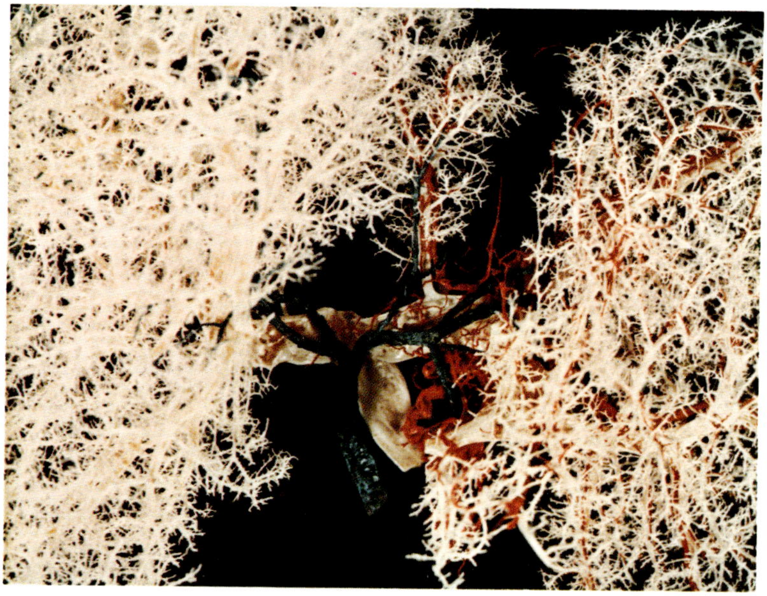

Fig 3. — Vinyl acetate cast of a normal postmortem liver demonstrating the most common branching of the segmental ducts.

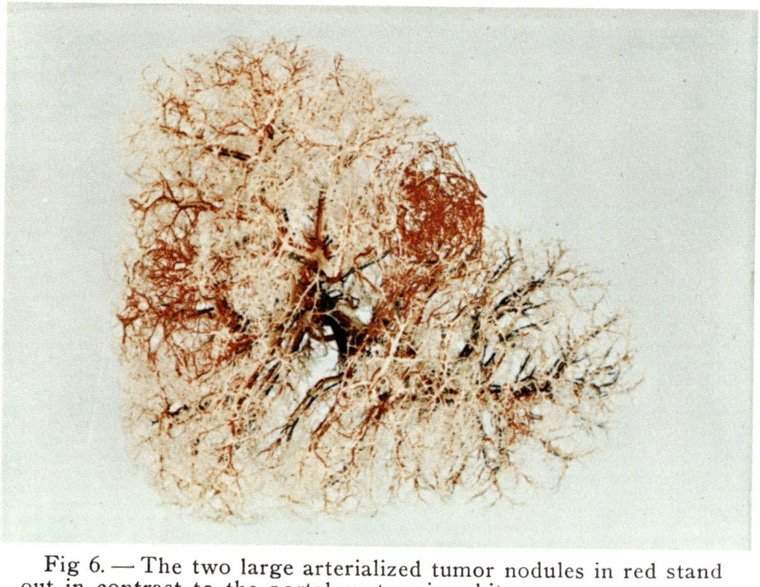

Fig 6. — The two large arterialized tumor nodules in red stand out in contrast to the portal system in white.

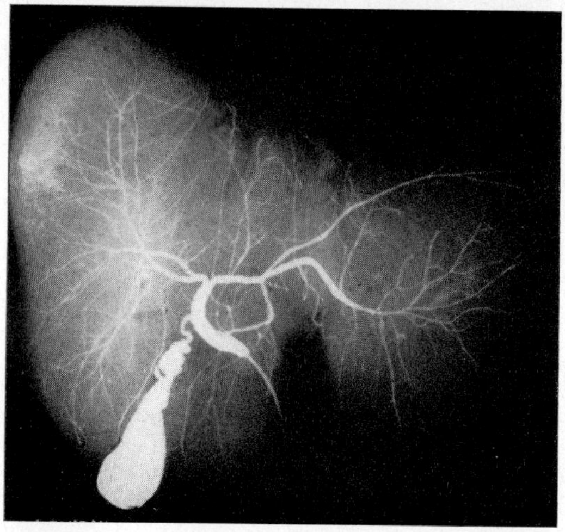

Fig 4.—Postmortem cholangiogram of the cast in Fig 3. Comparing cast with cholangiogram facilitates identification of the anterior and posterior segmental ducts.

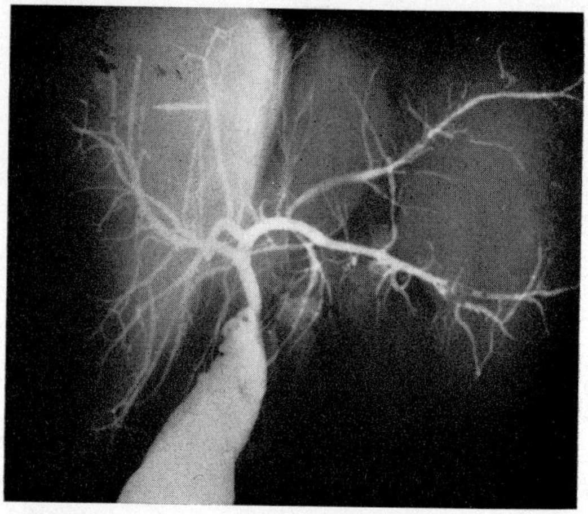

Fig 5.—Postmortem cholangiogram in which the right posterior segmental duct drains into the left primary hepatic duct.

former arises at an acute angle just proximal to the umbilical fossa, courses anteriorly, and branches to drain the various areas of this segment. The lateral segmental duct divides at the umbilical fossa to form the superior and inferior area ducts. The caudate lobe drains into both the right and the left ductal systems.

There are numerous variations to this pattern. The most common involve the right ductal system and are related to the level at which the segmental ducts join to form the right hepatic duct. The two segmental ducts may arise from the common hepatic duct at the same or different levels, or commonly, one may drain into the left hepatic duct. The latter variation occurred in 28% of the cases studied by Healey and Schroy.[2] Fig 5 is a postmortem cholangiogram which demonstrates this pattern.

The most common variations of the left ductal system involve the origin of the ducts which drain the medial segment. They may arise from a single trunk or in a number of combinations. Occasionally they arise from the common hepatic duct directly. This was encountered twice in the present study. The medial segment may in addition drain into an area duct of the lateral segment. It is important to recognize this variation when removal of only the left lateral segment of the liver is contemplated.

Distortions of the intrahepatic ductal system from biliary tract or intrinsic hepatic disease are not common. There was no discernible effect on the proximal biliary tree in the two cases of Laennec's cirrhosis even though there was marked disruption of the surface architecture from fibrous scarring and hepatic regeneration. Chronic passive congestion and fatty infiltration also had no grossly evident effect on the cast or cholangiogram.

Fig 6 and 7 are the cast and cholangiogram of a liver which contained several large metastatic tumor nodules from a carcinoma in the head of the pancreas. The nodules filled with red plastic via injection of the hepatic artery stand out in contrast to the white background of the portal venous system. There were no bile ducts or branches of the portal vein within these nodules. The arrow on the cholangiogram identifies displacement of a duct draining the superior area of the anterior segment of the right lobe. A second liver studded with multiple small nodules from a chorioepithelioma revealed no distortion of the intrahepatic biliary tree.

Fig 8 and 9 are an anterior-posterior (AP) and lateral cholangiogram, respectively, of the biliary tree which contained a cystic duct remnant. There were no appar-

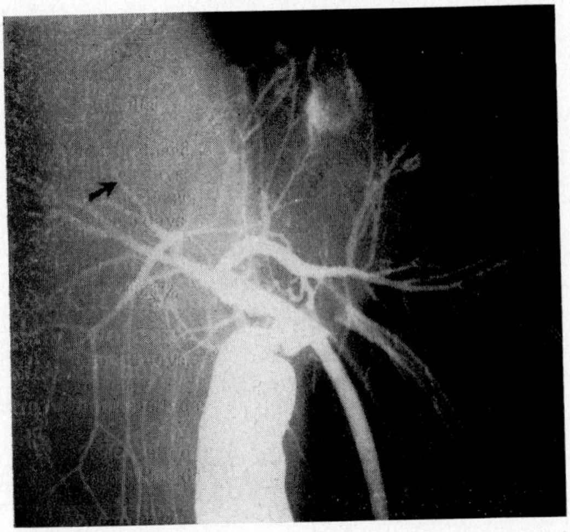

Fig 7.—This is a postmortem cholangiogram of the cast in Fig 6. The arrow identifies the superior area duct of the posterior segment which is bowed laterally by the tumor nodule.

ent changes within the proximal biliary tree. The cholangiograms however are a good example of the value of the lateral view in demonstrating the distribution of the right ductal system. It is in fact essential for positive identification of the anterior from the posterior segmental ducts.

Clinical Study

One hundred and fifty cases in which an operative and/or postoperative tube cholangiogram was obtained were reviewed to assess the value of our present cholangiographic methods. Our attention was focused on the visualization of the proximal biliary tree. Sixty-eight of the operative studies were considered to be inadequate for accurate interpretation; thirty-two of the postoperative studies were in this category. The Table is a list of the factors which contributed to the unsatisfactory nature of these cholangiograms.

Fig 8.—Postmortem cholangiogram demonstrating a postcholecystectomy biliary tree with a large cystic duct remnant. This conventional AP cholangiogram does not demonstrate the spatial relationship of the segmental ductal systems of the right lobe. The radiopaque area in the lower portion of the right lobe is extravasation of dye at a biopsy site.

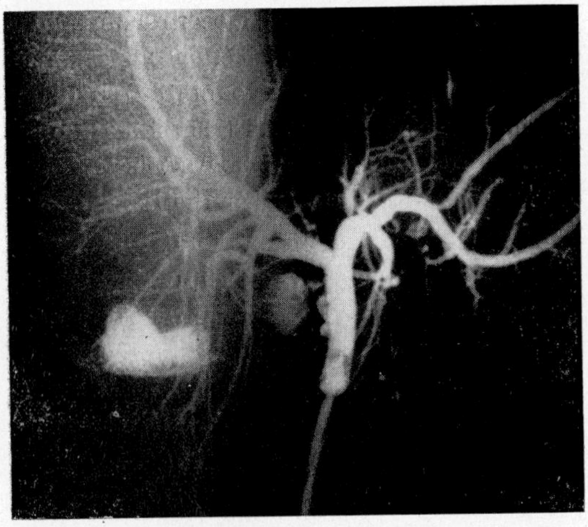

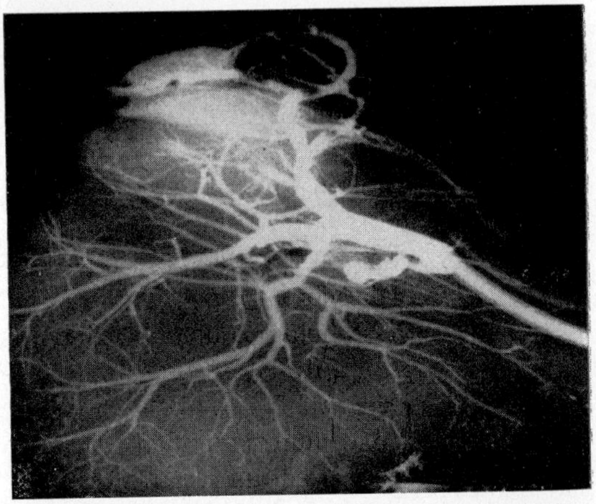

Fig 9.—This lateral cholangiogram of Fig 8 demonstrates the value of this view in studying the right ductal system. The left ductal system is above, the right anterior segmental in the middle, and the right posterior segmental below.

Poor radiographic technique accounted for the greatest number of unsatisfactory operative cholangiograms. The reasons for this are multiple and are related in part to the fact that these studies are performed in the operating room with the patient covered with sterile drapes. Positioning, tube distance, and proper timing are difficult under these circumstances. Portable equipment is employed, and the facilities for developing films are not as ideal as those within the

Major Deficit in 100 Unsatisfactory Cholangiograms

	Operative	Postoperative
Poor technique	39	8
Poor filling	15	22
Superimposition	10	2
Poor position	4	0
Total	68	32

x-ray department. The relatively few inadequate studies obtained for technical reasons in the postoperative group attest to the validity of these factors.

Poor filling of the intrahepatic biliary tree accounted for the largest number of inadequate studies in the postoperative group. The majority of cases were due to poor filling of the left hepatic duct (17 cases). There were only two cases in the operative group where the left hepatic duct failed to fill. The remaining cases of poor filling were related to inadequate instillation of contrast material into a markedly dilated ductal system. The high incidence of inability to fill the left ductal system in the postoperative studies bears explanation. It may be related in part to the anterior course of this duct in the supine position. The fact that most of these studies were performed by gravity filling was probably of equal importance in this inability to fill the left ductal system. The relative ease with which contrast material passes through the sphincter of Oddi in the postoperative studies may also play a role.

Superimposition of the bile ducts was a relatively frequent occurrence in the cholangiograms taken at the operating table. This is compounded by the fact that the patient cannot be rotated to gain an optimal view of the ductal system. It is further complicated by the presence of a dilated biliary tree which is frequently present during operative studies.

Comment

Our technique for performing operative and postoperative cholangiograms has been outlined in a previous publication.[4] There are several additional factors which may contribute to improved visualization of the proximal biliary tree.

Positioning of the patient on the cassette prior to operation is an important initial step toward insuring a good cholangiogram. The cassette should extend from the anterior superior spine of the iliac crest to the level of the third dorsal vertebral spine. An accurate measurement of the patient's anterior-posterior depth should then be made, since this is essential in determining the correct radiographic exposure.

The performance of an operative cholangiogram requires the cooperation of the surgeon, x-ray technician, and anesthesiologist. The surgeon is responsible for the adequate filling of the biliary tree with a contrast agent. The volume of material required to fill a dilated ductal system can be estimated by the instillation and aspiration of a measured amount of saline. It is important to use a dilute water-soluble contrast agent in order to avoid obscuring small stones within a heavy radiopaque column.

The instillation of opaque material should be carried out by gravity. Its forceful introduction may lead to a chemical cholangitis or pancreatitis. Proximal filling can be aided by placing the patient in a moderate head-down position. Digital compression of the distal common duct is of value at the operating table when free flow of contrast agent into the duodenum is encountered. This is an important maneuver when the distal end of a T-tube is passed through the sphincter of Oddi.

Once adequate filling of the entire biliary tree is obtained, then the x-ray tube should be properly positioned to insure that the roentgenogram is centered on the midaspect of the common duct. This in our experience gives sharp focus to the full extent of the biliary tree. Respiratory motion should be controlled by the anesthesiologist to prevent blurring of the finer details of the smaller biliary radicles.

Adequate postoperative cholangiograms are much easier to obtain. Proximal filling of the left ductal system is the single most difficult feature of this type of study. This can sometimes be facilitated by placing the patient in the prone position. Postoperative cholangiography however has many advantages over similar studies performed in the operating room. Proper positioning to overcome superimposition can be easily accomplished under fluoroscopic control. Oblique and lateral views can be obtained to gain an optimum view of the intrahepatic biliary radicles. It should be pointed out however that a lateral cholangiogram can be taken in the operating room by holding a cassette encased in a sterile wrap against the patient's right side, and this should be done when intrahepatic pathology is suspected.

This cholangiographic review was undertaken primarily to assess the quality of the intrahepatic portion of the operative and postoperative cholangiograms performed in this hospital. Several interesting radiographic findings deserve comment. Twenty-one major anatomical variations were encountered. There were nine studies in which the right posterior segmental duct joined the left hepatic duct above the branching of the primary radicles. In eight cases, a segment of the right ductal system joined the common duct below the level of primary branching. In one case, this junction was at the level of the cystic duct. The left medial segmental duct arose from the inferior area duct of the lateral segment of the left lobe in one study and from the common hepatic duct in two others.

There were seven cases in which the intrahepatic radicles were filamentous in character. This was present in one of the postmortem livers studied and represents an extreme variation in the caliber of the normal biliary tree.

Numerous cases of dilatation of the proximal biliary tree were studied. In obstruction of short duration, the intrahepatic radicles were normal in caliber, while the extrahepatic ducts were relatively much larger in size. This delay in intrahepatic dilatation is probably related to the parenchymatous support afforded to the ducts within the substance of the liver. When obstruction is complete and prolonged, however, the proximal biliary tree then becomes progressively dilated, and the smaller radicles lose their taper and become cylindrical in shape. In extreme cases, portions of the intrahepatic ductal system may become saccular in appearance.

Three cases of intrahepatic calculi were reviewed. In each study there was a radiolucent defect within an opaque filled biliary radicle. Absence of filling of an area of the biliary tree was sought for as a possible clue of ductal obstruction from tumor or stone. We did not encounter such a case, and concluded from this search that excellent visualization of the finer biliary radicles would be required to make this a reliable and practical sign.

We were disappointed in the general quality of the proximal portions of the tube cholangiograms. There are numerous technical limitations to the adequate visualization of the proximal biliary tree, many of which can be improved upon as discussed above. The correlative study of postmortem cholangiograms and their representative plastic casts was invaluable in gaining a three-dimensional concept of the intrahepatic biliary architecture. When high-quality proximal cholangiograms are obtained at the time of the primary operation, then an accurate knowledge of the normal intrahepatic biliary architecture affords an opportunity to recognize and treat intrahepatic pathology.

Frank Glenn, MD, Department of Surgery, The New York Hospital, 525 E 68th St, New York 21, NY.

REFERENCES

1. Fainsinger, M. H.: The Radiology of the Intrahepatic Biliary Tree, S Afr J Med Sci 15:51-66, 1950.

2. Healey, J. E., Jr., and Schroy, P. C.: Anatomy of the Biliary Ducts Within the Human Liver, AMA Arch Surg 66:599-616, 1953.

3. Hjortsjö, C. H.: The Topography of the Intrahepatic Duct Systems, Acta Anat (Basel) 11:599-615, 1951.

4. Kantor, H. G.; Evans, J. A.; and Glenn, F.: Cholangiography: A Critical Analysis, AMA Arch Surg 70:237-252, 1955.

5. McIndoe, A. H., and Counseller, V. S.: The Bilaterality of the Liver, Arch Surg 15:589-612, 1927.

6. Norman, O.: Studies on the Hepatic Ducts in Cholangiography, Acta Radiol (Stockholm) suppl 84:1-81, 1951.

Peritoneal Fluid pH After Perforation of Peptic Ulcers

The Myth of "Acid-Peritonitis"

JOHN M. HOWARD, MD
AND
LOKENDRA M. SINGH, MD
PHILADELPHIA

The board-like abdomen, characteristic of a perforation of a peptic ulcer, has always been described by the surgeon as being secondary to an "acid-peritonitis." Seemingly, this statement found its place in medical literature many years ago and, like many other statements, does not appear to have a basis in factual observation.

Methods and Materials

The current study consists of measurement of the pH of the peritoneal fluid in 59 patients who were found to have had an acute perforation of a peptic ulcer. The fluid was taken at laparotomy as soon as the peritoneum was incised, and the pH was measured using Nitrazine paper or a Beckman pH meter.

Each of the patients studied gave a history indicative of free perforation within 24 hours of the time of operation. Almost all of the patients had board-like rigidity immediately prior to operation. In several instances the ulcer had sealed spontaneously, but, in the majority, the ulcer crater was still patent. Forty-six of the ulcers appeared to be duodenal, six were gastric, and in seven instances, the surgeon was uncertain as to whether the site was duodenal or pyloric.

Results

The pH of the peritoneal fluids is demonstrated in the Figure. In all but one instance the fluid was alkaline, although the pH was often below the normal pH of the blood. The single exception revealed no unusual clinical findings; it occurred in a patient several hours after perforation of a duodenal ulcer which was immediately distal to the pylorus.

Comment

Although peritoneal fluid has been examined cytologically by many workers, no mention of pH of the fluid has been made by them. The current studies confirm our earlier observations [3] and the original studies of Moretz and Erickson [1,2] who found the peritoneal fluid alkaline in 16 of 20 patients

Submitted for publication Feb 26, 1963.

From the Department of Surgery Hahnemann Medical College.

Supported by grant AM-02723 from the National Institute of Arthritis and Metabolic Diseases.

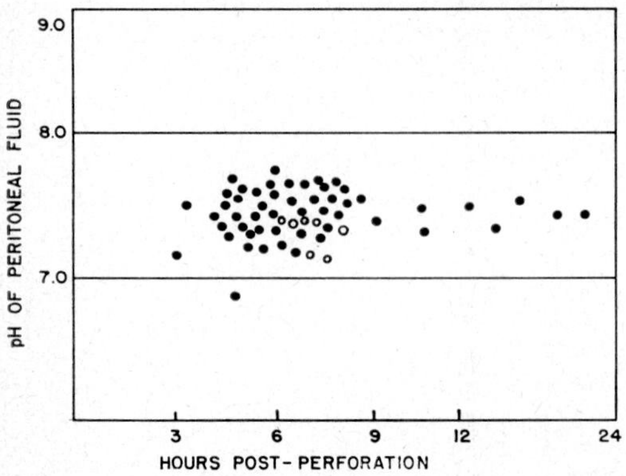

The pH of peritoneal fluid following perforation of a peptic ulcer. The black dots record the reaction to Nitrazine paper, the open circles the pH as measured on a Beckman pH meter.

after perforation of an ulcer. They extended the studies in dogs to show that dilute hydrochloric acid (0.05 N), when instilled intraperitoneally in amounts of 50 ml per kilogram of body weight, was neutralized within 35 minutes (neutral reaction to nitrazine paper) and became alkaline within one hour.

The current studies do not demonstrate the pH of the fluid at the moment of perforation. On several occasions Allen [4] has examined at the time of operation both the peritoneal fluid and the gastric juice. Neither fluid was acid. This observation suggested to him the possibility that the initial insult of perforation stopped the secretion of acid by the stomach. Doubtlessly, the fluid is often initially acid, and possibly the low pH has an influence in initiating the board-like rigidity, but *at the time of laparotomy* the board-like rigidity is not due to an acid peritoneal fluid. Furthermore, the determination of the pH on fluid obtained by paracentesis in patients with an acute abdomen may have little diagnostic value.

Summary

Studies of peritoneal fluid collected at the time of laparotomy from 59 patients with perforation of a peptic ulcer revealed that in 58 the fluid was alkaline.

John M. Howard, MD, Department of Surgery, Hahnemann Medical College & Hospital, 230 N Broad St, Philadelphia 2, Pa.

REFERENCES

1. Moretz, W. H., and Erickson, W. G.: Peritoneal Tap as an Aid in Diagnosis of Acute Abdominal Disease, Amer Surg 20:363, 1954.

2. Moretz, W. H., and Erickson, W. G.: Neutralization of Hydrochloric Acid in the Peritoneal Cavity, AMA Arch Surg 75:834, 1957.

3. Amerson, J. R.; Howard, J. M.; and Vowles, K. D. J.: Amylase Concentration in Serum and Peritoneal Fluid Following Acute Perforation of Gastroduodenal Ulcers, Ann Surg 147:245, 1958.

4. Allen, J. G.: Personal communication to the authors.

Effect of Hypoxia on Pulmonary Vasculature of the Dog

JOSEPH R. LANCASTER, MD
PAUL B. STEWART, MD
JAMES LENNERTZ, MD
JAMES COVELL, MD
AND
PETER V. MOULDER, MD
CHICAGO

There are conflicting reports and conflicting concepts in the literature as to the effect of hypoxia on the pulmonary circulation. An array of studies has been done in perfused lungs, anesthetized animals, and unanesthetized humans which indicate a rise in pulmonary vascular resistance in response to hypoxia.[1-8] Other studies, which show elevation in pulmonary artery pressure with concomitant rise in cardiac output, indicate vasodilatation and no increased resistance. There are also studies which indicate an irregularity in resistance response.[12,13] Boake et al [14] produced increased pulmonary vascular resistance in animals breathing 8% oxygen and partially reversed the effect with perfusion of some oxygenated blood into the pulmonary artery. Lanari-Zubiaur and Hamilton [15] found "nonsignificant" resistance changes in their anoxia studies and raised the teleological question: "It is doubtful that a vigorous pulmonary constrictive response to anoxic breathing could long survive in evolutionary development."

All observers agree that there are pulmonary circulatory changes of moderate to profound intensity following hypoxia. This is the conceptual problem: usually there is a marked increase in pressure; in some experimental instances flow is preset though fixed; in others output has increased. In fixed flow experiments this indicates increased vascular resistance; interpretation in the second has been decreased, unchanged, or increased resistance depending upon the extent of the increase in cardiac output at the time of measurement!

In this basic area each group studying the pulmonary circulation should present its findings and interpretation to help in resolution of this problem.

Submitted for publication Feb 25, 1963.

American Cancer Society Fellow (Dr. Lancaster); work performed during tenure as National Research Council Student Fellows (Dr. Lennertz, Dr. Covell).

From the Department of Surgery, University of Chicago.

Supported by grants-in-aid from the John A. Hartford Foundation and the Chicago Heart Association.

Methods

This series was performed on ten healthy mongrel dogs weighing between 17 and 23 kg, anesthetized with morphine sulfate and chloralose, and intubated with a large, cuffed, endotracheal catheter. All dogs autoventilated throughout the experiment, with room air during control studies, and with varying percentages of nitrogen and oxygen via an intervening nonrebreathing valve [16] for attainment of the hypoxic state.

Pulmonary artery pressure was obtained via a No. 7 Cournand type catheter passed from an external jugular vein, left atrial pressure via a 17 T Ross transseptal needle introduced through the same vein. Central aortic pressure was obtained via a polyethylene catheter passed through the femoral artery. Statham P 23 d strain gauges and a Grass polygraph were used for transducer and recorder, respectively. Separate catheters were passed into the inferior vena cava and thoracic aorta for performing dye dilution curves. Indocyanine green (Fox) dye was injected into the former and blood was drawn from the latter through a Colson densitometer at a rate of 50 ml/min, and the dye curve was inscribed on a Texas rectilinear recorder. Cardiac output was calculated from the dye dilution curves by the forward triangle method with occasional validation by the classical Stewart-Hamilton area method.[17]

Arterial oxygen saturation was determined by the method of Van Slyke and Neill.[18]

The pulmonary vascular resistance was calculated with the formula:

$$TPR = \frac{PAm - LAm}{CO} \times 1332$$

TPR indicates total pulmonary resistance (dynes sec cm^{-5}); *PAm*, mean pulmonary artery pressure (mm Hg); *LAm*, mean left atrial pressure (mm Hg); *CO*, cardiac output (liters/min). Studies were performed after 2 min stabilization at the desired level. Two sets of readings were made at each level.

Results

The results are summarized in the Table and depicted graphically in the Figure. The mean value for mean pulmonary artery pressures with the dogs autoventilating room air was 10.4 mm Hg (SD *±1.14). When the respiratory gas mixture was 92% N_2 and 8% O_2, the mean value obtained for the mean pulmonary artery pressures was 10.0 mm Hg (SD±1.85); and with 95% N_2 and 5% O_2 mixture, the mean value of the mean pulmonary artery pressures was 12.5 mm Hg (SD±0.88).

The left atrial pressures during the control periods had a mean value of 4.5 mm Hg (SD±1.82). During the hypoxic periods obtained with 92% N_2 and 8% O_2, the mean value for the mean left atrial pressures was 4.2 mm Hg (SD±1.82). In the hypoxic period obtained with 95% N_2 and 5% O_2, the value was 3.5 mm Hg (SD±1.32).

The mean value for the cardiac outputs taken during the control periods was 1.82 liters/min (SD±0.45). Values during the hypoxic periods were 2.58±0.94 liters/min for 92% N_2-8% O_2 and 2.78±0.62 liters/min for 95% N_2-5% O_2.

The mean value for calculated total pulmonary vascular resistance during the control periods was 259 dynes sec cm^{-5}, during the hypoxia produced with 92% N_2-8% O_2, 179 dynes sec cm^{-5}, and during the hypoxia of 95% N_2-5% O_2, 259 dynes sec cm^{-5}.

The degree of hypoxia obtained was indicated by arterial oxygen saturations with average values at 30 minutes of 47% for the 92% N_2-8% O_2 and 20% for the 95% N_2-5% O_2.

All animals developed a slight rise in the mean aortic pressure of 10-15 mm Hg during the periods of hypoxia with moderate hyperventilation and slight increase in cardiac rate.

*SD indicates standard deviation.

Effect of Hypoxia: Summary

Inspired Oxygen, %	Arterial Oxygen Saturation, %	Pulmonary Artery Mean Pressure, Mm Hg	L. Atrial Mean Pressure, Mm Hg	*PAm—LAm*, Mm Hg	Cardiac Output Liters/Min	Vascular Resistance, Dynes Sec Cm^{-5}
21 (air)		10.4	4.5	5.9	1.82	259
8	47	10.0	4.2	5.8	2.58	179
5	20	12.5	3.5	9.0	2.78	259

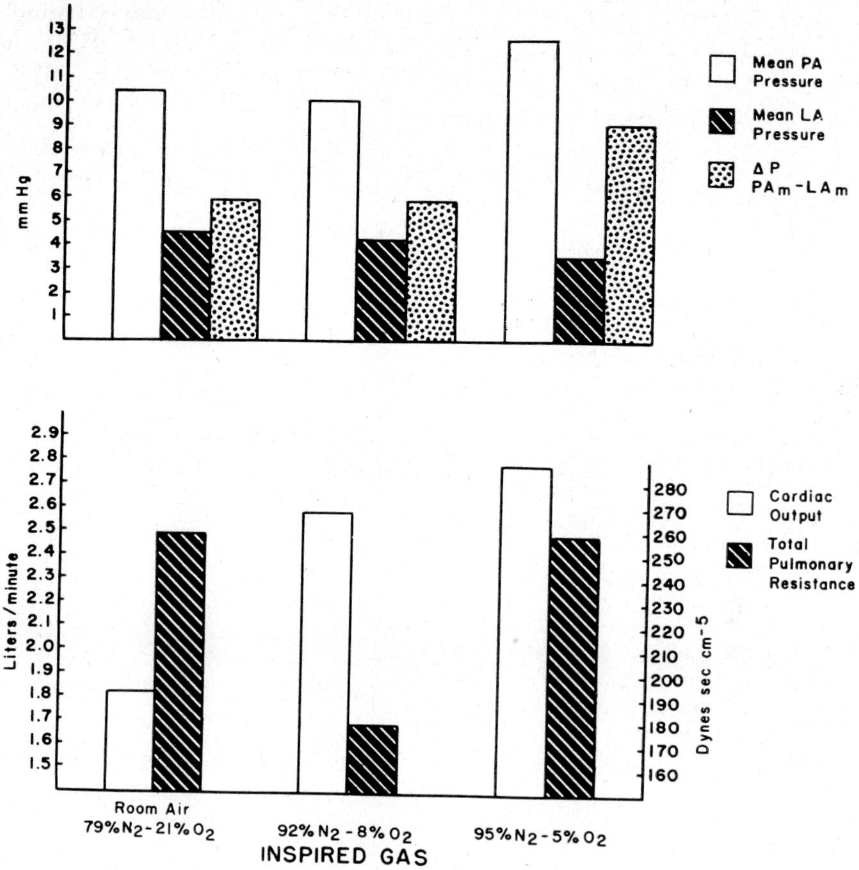

The effect of hypoxia on pulmonary circulatory parameters .

Comment

The disagreement in the literature regarding the effect of hypoxia on the pulmonary vasculature is in part a difference in interpretation of data. An increase out of proportion to a rise in mean pressure can occur in systolic pressure in the pulmonary artery in response to hypoxia, and this is important as a pulsatile phenomenon but does not indicate in itself any over-all vascular change. Furthermore, there are striking visible reactions indicated by tachycardia, increased stroke volume, and so forth. That these changes are or are not associated with an increased pulmonary vascular resistance seems to be the important point of controversy. These data show a variation in response and *striking hemodynamic changes,* but no evidence for increased pulmonary vascular resistance. Hypoxia created by breathing 8% oxygen caused no increase in the mean left atrial pressure, whereas the hypoxia brought about by the inhalation of 5% oxygen produced a slight rise in the mean pulmonary artery pressure. In both instances there was an increase in the cardiac output and this indicated little change in vascular resistance; however, the usual response to increased blood flow in the normal lung is a fall in resistance and stability of pressure, and *in this sense the response is abnormal.*

It would seem that the intense concern over pulmonary vascular resistance phenomena in this and other studies is unfortunately preventing a look at the entire cardiovascular reaction to hypoxia in which moment to moment, even systolic-diastolic pressure flow relationships need to be determined and related to local and central nervous stimuli and response.

There has been important concern for knowledge in this area, since the patient with pulmonary hypertension undergoing cardiac surgery is sensitive, often lethally so, to hypoventilation. Present studies are concerned with the effect of hypoxia in the pulmonary hypertensive preparation[19] and correlation with changes in pCO_2 and pH.

Conclusions

In the closed-chest, normal dog under morphine-chloralose anesthesia hypoxia produced by breathing gas of reduced oxygen tension produces complex and intense cardiohemodynamic changes:

Cardiac output increased from a normal of 1.82 liters/min to 2.58 liters/min with 8% oxygen, and to 2.78 liters/min with 5% oxygen.

Mean pulmonary artery pressure increased with inhalation of 5% O_2, but not with 8% O_2.

No significant change occurred in mean left atrial pressure.

No increase in calculated total pulmonary vascular resistance occurred.

Peter V. Moulder, MD, Department of Surgery, The University of Chicago, 950 E 59th St, Chicago 37.

REFERENCES

1. von Euler, U.S., and Liljestrand, G.: Observations on the Pulmonary Arterial Blood Pressure in the Cat, Acta Physiol Scand 12:301, 1946.

2. Motley, H. L.; Cournand, A.; Werkö, L.; Himmelstein, A.; and Dresdale, D.: The Influence of Short Periods of Induced Acute Anoxia Upon Pulmonary Artery Pressures in Man, Amer J Physiol 150:315, 1947.

3. Nissel, O. I.: The Action of Oxygen and Carbon Dioxide on the Bronchioles and Vessels of the Isolated Perfused Lungs, Acta Physiol Scand 21 (suppl 73):5, 1950.

4. Duke, H. N.: Pulmonary Vasomotor Responses of Isolated Perfused Cat Lungs to Anoxia and Hypercapnia, Quart J Exp Physiol 36:75, 1951.

5. Fishman, A. P.; McClement, J.; Himmelstein, A.; and Cournand, A.: Effects of Acute Anoxia on the Circulation and Respiration in Patients With Chronic Pulmonary Disease Studied During the "Steady State," J Clin Invest 31:770, 1952.

6. Lewis, B. M., and Gorlin, R.: Effects of Hypoxia on the Pulmonary Circulation of the Dog, Amer J Physiol 170:574, 1952.

7. Siebens, A. A.; Smith, R. E.; and Storey, C. F.: Effect of Hypoxia on Pulmonary Vessels in Man, Amer J Physiol 180:428, 1955.

8. Duke, H. N.: The Site of Action of Anoxia on the Pulmonary Blood Vessels of the Cat, J Physiol 125:373, 1954.

9. Beyne, J.: Influence de l'anoxémie sur la grande circulation et sur la circulation pulmonaire, CR Soc Biol 136:399, 1942.

10. Nahas, G. G.; Visscher, M. B.; Mather, G. W.; Haddy, F. J.; and Warner, H. R.: Influence of Hypoxia on the Pulmonary Circulation on Non-narcotized Dogs, J Appl Physiol 6:467, 1954.

11. Rodbard, S., and Harasawa, M.: The Passivity of the Pulmonary Vasculature in Hypoxia, Amer Heart J 57:232, 1959.

12. Aviado, D. M., Jr.; Ling, J. S.; and Schmidt, C. F.: Effects of Anoxia on Pulmonary Circulation: Reflex Pulmonary Vasoconstriction, Amer J Physiol 189:253, 1957.

13. Nissel, O. I.: The Influence of the Blood Gases on the Pulmonary Vessels of the Cat, Acta Physiol Scand 23:85, 1951.

14. Boake, W. C.; Daley, R.; and McMillan, I. K.: Observations on Hypoxic Pulmonary Hypertension, Brit Heart J 21:31, 1959.

15. Lanari-Zubiaur, F. J., and Hamilton, W. F.: Effect of Unilateral Anoxia on Pulmonary Circulation, Circ Res 6:289, 1958.

16. Rattenborg, C.: Anestesiventil: Ventil til cirkelsystem og kunstig ventilation uden genandining [Anesthetic valve; valve to the circulatory system and artificial ventilation without re-respiration], Ugeskr Laeger 118:1168, 1956.

17. Hamilton, W. F.; Moore, J. W.; Kinsman, J. M.; and Spurling, R. G.: Studies on the Circulation: Further Analyses of the Injection Method, and of Changes in Hemodynamics Under Physiological and Pathological Conditions, Amer J Physiol 99:534, 1932.

18. Peters, J. P., and Van Slyke, D. D.: Quantitative Clinical Chemistry (Methods), Baltimore: The Williams & Wilkins Company, 1931 vol 2.

19. Evans, R. H.; Bresler, H. L.; Lennertz, J. A.; Harrison, R. W.; and Moulder, P. V.: Increased Shunt Tolerance Provided by Experimental Production of Biventricular Hypertrophy, Circulation 24:930, 1961.

Perforation of the Gallbladder

Analysis of Twenty-One Cases

C. G. McEACHERN, MD
AND
R. E. SULLIVAN, MD
FORT WAYNE, IND

Although perforation of the acute gallbladder is not a common occurrence, a significant number of cases of acute cholecystitis will progress to perforation under conservative management.

In 1949 Diffenbaugh et al [1] collected from the literature 630 cases of perforation of the gallbladder among 5,272 cases of acute cholecystitis. This series summarized the experiences of 27 different surgeons and indicated an average incidence of 11.9% of perforations in acute cholecystitis. The incidence varied in different series from 2.5% to 25%.

In 1934, Niemeier [2] classified perforations of the gallbladder into three groups, namely: (1) acute perforation into the free peritoneal cavity, (2) subacute perforation with formation of a localized pericholecystic abscess, (3) chronic perforation with formation of an internal biliary fistula. The localized type of perforation is by far the most frequent. The other types of perforation are much less frequent.

Submitted for publication Feb 4, 1963.

This paper presents a study of 21 cases of acute perforation of the gallbladder which fall into types 1 and 2 of Niemeier's classification; ie, perforation into the free abdominal cavity and perforation with formation of a pericholecystic abscess. Cases of Niemeier's type 3, ie, perforation with formation of an internal biliary fistula, are not included in this study.

This series of 21 patients with acute perforations of the gallbladder were operated on either by us or under our supervision during the 12 year period of Jan 1, 1948, to Dec 31, 1959. During this time, 218 patients underwent surgery for acute cholecystitis. According to these figures, the incidence of perforation of the gallbladder in acute cholecystitis in this series is 10.4% (Table 1).

Classification

In 12 cases, or 57.1%, the perforations were of the Niemeier type 1, or acute free perforations (Table 1). In nine cases or 42.8%, the perforations were of the Niemeier type 2, or perforation with formation of a pericholecystic abscess.

Sex

Ten or 47.5% were women, and 11 or 52.5% were men (Table 2). Fourteen patients or 66.6% were 60 years of age and over. Eight of these were women, and six were men.

Age

The age incidence by decades is depicted in Table 3. The youngest patient was a man

TABLE 1.—*Incidence and Types of Perforation*

	No. of Cases	%
Acute cholecystitis	218	
Perforations	21	
Incidence of perforations		10.4
Niemeier type 1	12	57.1
Niemeier type 2	9	42.8

TABLE 2.—*Sex Incidence*

	No. of Cases	%
Female	10	47.5
Male	11	52.5
Over 60 Yr (66.6%)		
Female	8	38.1
Male	6	28.5

TABLE 3.—*Age Incidence*

Age	No. of Cases	%	
40-49	1	4.5	28.5 (40-59)
50-59	5	24.0	
60-69	5	24.0	71.5 (60-89)
70-79	8	38.0	
80-89	2	9.5	

aged 48; the oldest was a woman aged 89. The average age of the ten women was 68 years, and of the 11 men the average was 66 years. The average age of the total group was 67 years. Six or 28.5% were under 60 years of age; 15 or 71.5% were 60 years or over.

TABLE 4.—*Symptoms*

	No. of Cases	%
RUQ pain	21	100.0
Vomiting	14	66.6
Nausea	17	81.0
Gen. abdom. pain	6	28.6
Chills & fever	6	28.6

Symptoms

Pain in the right upper quadrant was present in all 21 cases (Table 4). Nausea was present in 17 cases. Vomiting was present in 14 cases. Generalized abdominal pain was present in six cases. Chills and fever occurred in six cases.

Incidence of Jaundice

Four cases or 19% were jaundiced as evidenced clinically and by elevation of the serum bilirubin (Table 5).

History of Previous Attacks

Sixteen or 76.2% gave a history of more than one previous attack (Table 6). Three patients or 14.3% gave no history of previous disease of the gallbladder. Two patients or 9.5% gave a history of one previous cholecystic attack.

TABLE 6.—*History of Previous Attacks*

	No. of Cases	%
None	3	14.3
One previous	2	9.5
More than one	16	76.2

Duration of Present Illness

Three cases of acute cholecystitis perforated on the second day (Table 7). Four cases perforated on the third day. Five cases perforated on the fourth day. Three cases perforated on each of the fifth and sixth days. One case perforated on each of the seventh, ninth, and tenth days. Thus 57.1% perforated in four days; 85.7% perforated in six days. All perforated within ten days.

TABLE 5.—*Incidence of Jaundice*

	No. of Cases	%
Jaundice	4	19.0
No jaundice	17	81.0

Diagnosis

In eight cases, a preoperative diagnosis of perforated cholecystitis was made (Table 8). In six cases, the diagnosis was acute chole-

TABLE 7.—*Perforation in Relation to Duration of Disease*

	No. of Cases	%	Total %
1st day	0	0	0
2nd day	3	14.2	14.2
3rd day	4	19.1	33.3
4th day	5	23.8	57.1
5th day	3	14.2	71.4
6th day	3	14.2	85.7
7th day	1	4.8	90.2
9th day	1	4.8	95.2
10th day	1	4.8	100.0
Total	21		

TABLE 8.—*Pre-Operative Diagnosis*

		No. of Cases
Perforation of the gallbladder		8
Acute cholecystitis		6
Acute cholecystitis with jaundice		2
Peritonitis		3
Perforated viscus	1	
Etiology?	2	
Small bowel obstruction		1
Abdominal abscess		1

cystitis. In two cases, the diagnosis was acute cholecystitis with jaundice. A preoperative diagnosis of peritonitis was made in three cases. In one of these, the peritonitis was presumed to be due to a perforated viscus. In two cases, the etiology of the peritonitis was not ventured. A diagnosis of small bowel obstruction was made in one case, while a diagnosis of abdominal abscess was made in another.

Types of Operation

In 12 cases, cholecystectomy was performed (Table 9). Four of these cases did not survive. In two cases, cholecystectomy and exploration of the common duct was carried out. In six cases, cholecystostomy was performed. One case in this latter group did not survive. In one seriously ill patient, only drainage of the abdominal cavity was carried out. This patient survived and subsequently underwent a cholecystectomy and exploration of the common duct.

Causes of Death

Five deaths occurred in this series giving a mortality of 23.7% (Table 10). Three patients died of peritonitis, one died of pulmonary embolus, and one with uremia.

TABLE 9.—*Type of Operation*

	No. of Cases	%
Cholecystectomy	12	57.1
Cholecystectomy and common duct exploration	2	9.5
Cholecystostomy	6	28.6
Drainage	1	4.8

Comment

Perforation of the gallbladder, although rather infrequent, is attended by a significant mortality. The mortality rate of 23.8% in this series, which is consistent with the average mortality reported in the literature, attests to the seriousness of the condition.

The signs and symptoms of perforation of the gallbladder are not distinct, and, consequently, delay in diagnosis and subsequent delay in operative intervention are factors contributing to the high mortality rate. The most frequent diagnoses are acute cholecystitis and peritonitis. The diagnosis of impending perforations as evidenced by increasing pain, increasing pulse rate, progressive elevation of the temperature, and increasing leukocytosis has little foundation in fact.

TABLE 10.—*Causes of Death*

	No. of Cases	%
Peritonitis	3	14.3
Uremia	1	4.7
Pulmonary embolus	1	4.7
Total	5	23.7

It is significant that perforation is more common over the age of 60 years. In this series, 66.6% were 60 years of age or over. This is consistent with the increased incidence of acute cholecystitis in this age group.

The time of perforation is significant. One third of the cases perforated on the second and third day. Twelve cases or 57.1% perforated in the first four days. Eighteen cases or 85.1% perforated in six days. All had perforated within ten days. These figures would indicate that the conservative treatment of acute cholecystitis can be hazardous and supports the premise that early surgery is the treatment of choice in acute cholecystitis.

The treatment of perforative cholecystitis is surgical. Usually the choice of operation lies between cholecystostomy and cholecystectomy. Cholecystostomy is frequently the operation of choice in these seriously ill patients. However, if, in the opinion of the surgeon, cholecystectomy can be easily executed, it may be employed. Exploration of the common duct may occasionally be performed without materially increasing the risk. Rarely, simple drainage of the abdominal cavity in a desperately ill patient may be a lifesaving procedure and permit definitive surgery at a later date.

Since the majority of patients with perforation of the gallbladder give an antecedent history of one or more attacks of pain, it becomes evident that cholecystectomy performed at the time of the first attack would do much to lower the mortality in acute perforation. Better still, cholecystectomy performed when gallstones are first detected, even though symptomless, would further tend to decrease the ultimate mortality.

Peritonitis is the commonest cause of death. The other causes are those encountered in the postoperative phase of surgery, namely pulmonary embolus and uremia.

Summary

A series of 21 cases of perforation of the gallbladder treated in the 12 year period, Jan 1, 1948, to Dec 31, 1959, is presented.

In this group, 12 cases were of the Niemeier type 1; nine cases were of the Niemeier type 2.

There was no significant difference in the sex incidence; 71.5% of the patients were 60 years of age or over.

A history of more than one previous attacks was obtained in 76.2% of the cases.

Within four days 51.1% perforated; 85.7% perforated within six days. All perforated within ten days.

The diagnosis is difficult. Acute cholecystitis was the most frequent diagnosis. Peritonitis was the second most frequent diagnosis.

The diagnosis of impending perforation is very difficult.

The treatment of perforative cholecystitis is surgical. The operation must be selected to suit the particular case.

Five deaths occurred in this series; a mortality of 23.7%. The commonest cause of death was peritonitis.

C. G. McEachern, MD, 2424 Fairfield Ave, Fort Wayne, Ind.

REFERENCES

1. Diffenbaugh, W. G., et al: Gangrenous Perforation of the Gallbladder, Arch Surg 59:742, 1949.

2. Niemeier, O. W.: Acute Free Perforation of the Gall-Bladder, Ann Surg 99:922, 1934.

Inguinal and Femoral Hernias

WILLIAM B. RYDELL, JR., MD
HANOVER, NH

Surgical repair of an inguinal hernia is a frequently performed operation. Ideally, a hernia should be permanently cured by one operation and its repair attended by minimum morbidity.

But there is much to go wrong after a hernia repair; the atrophied testicle, the recurrent hernia, and other problems are seen all too often. This study evaluates our experience with the repair of inguinal and femoral hernias, tabulates the complications encountered in groin surgery, and considers the causes of recurrent hernias.

Clinical Material

The records of all patients undergoing inguinal or femoral hernioplasty at Mary Hitchcock Memorial Hospital between Jan 1, 1950, and Dec 31, 1959, were reviewed. During this period 1,162 patients underwent 1,286 operations in which 1,416 different hernias were repaired by the permanent and resident staff of this hospital. Approximately 40% of the patients had adequate long-term follow-up data in their records which, in this institution, include the outpatient records of the Hitchcock Clinic. All other patients were sent a questionnaire, and replies were received from 71%. We were thus able to follow 83% of the adults and 80% of the children for over two years.

The age distribution by decades is shown in the Figure. Approximately one third (123) of the children were under one year of age, and another 157 were between one and five years of age. After this initial childhood peak, there was a great drop in the second and third decades followed by a steady rise to a second peak incidence in the sixth and seventh decades. For purpose of analysis we arbitrarily divided the patients into two groups; those 14 years of age or over were classified as adults and those 13 years of age or under as children.

There was nothing unusual about the types of hernia encountered (Table 1). Over-all, 88.7% of the hernias occurred in males. The usual preponderance of right-sided hernias existed: 65% of the children and 56% of the adult hernias were on the right.

There were 22 irreducible hernias (6%) in children. Two were in females and presented no particular problem. Two males had a strangulated loop of bowel in the hernia sac. Four other patients (all under six months of age) had a strangulated testicle secondary to the incarcerated hernia. Orchiectomy was necessary in three of these infants; the

Submitted for publication Feb 20, 1963.

Resident in Surgery, Dartmouth Affiliated Hospitals, Dartmouth Medical School.

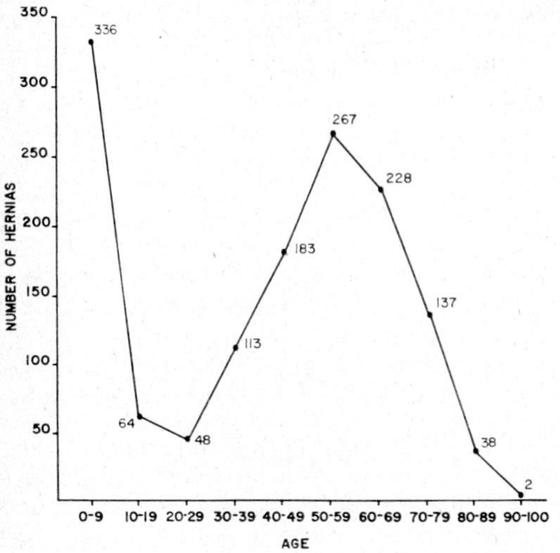

Age distribution of inguinal and femoral hernias.

other testicle was saved by incising the tunica albuginea for decompression. This testicle was normal to palpation seven years later. As emphasized by Hill et al[4] this complication seems limited to the very young. A strangulated testicle occurs frequently enough (20%) in irreducible infant hernias to make the prompt reduction of the hernia essential. If a strangulated testicle is found at surgery, decompression incisions in the tunica albuginia seem to offer a reasonable chance of saving the testicle.

In adults there were 99 irreducible hernias, an incidence of 9.3%. A third (35) of these hernias had strangulated contents, and resection was required in 16 patients. Omentum was resected in 12 patients and small bowel in 4 patients. Femoral hernias were most likely to be irreducible; 43 of 78 femoral hernias were irreducible at the time of surgery.

Sliding hernias were found in 45 adults. The sigmoid colon was the sliding viscus in 34 cases, and the cecum was present in the other 11 patients. Two female infants had a sliding hernia involving a tube and ovary.

TABLE 1.—*Types of Hernia Encountered in 307 Children and 855 Adults*

	Children		Adults		
	M	F	M	F	Totals
Indirect	328	32	578	62	1,000
Direct	1	—	164	8	173
Femoral	—	—	23	55	78
Ind.-dir.-fem.	—	—	1	—	1
Pantaloon	—	—	60	2	62
Recurrent	2	—	98	2	102
Totals	331	32	924	129	1,416

Appendectomy was done at the time of hernioplasty in 24 patients. We had no complications following this limited experience. Recent reports[1,6] have demonstrated the safety of appendectomy performed at the time of right inguinal herniorrhaphy.

Hydrocelectomy was done in 59 (18%) of the male children and in 36 (4%) of the adults.

Undescended testes were present in 23 children and 5 adults. Because of atrophy, six testes were removed. The remaining 22 patients (20 children and 2 adults) had an orchidopexy performed.

Orchiectomy was performed 32 times to facilitate the repair of difficult or recurrent hernias. Removal of the testis and cord does not guarantee favorable results as illustrated by the three recurrent hernias subsequently noted in this group of patients.

Mortality and Morbidity

Children.—There were no deaths following the 325 operations performed on children. Two patients developed systemic complications, a rate of 0.6%. Both children had pneumonia and both recovered uneventfully.

No wound complications occurred in females, but significant local complications were seen in 13 males (Table 2). In addition to the one major wound infection, eight patients developed silk sinuses.

Marked scrotal swelling was present in five patients. All of these testes were normal to palpation at the follow-up examination. The two boys with retracted testes underwent successful orchidopexy to replace the testis in the scrotum.

All four of the patients with recognized transections of the vas deferens were under five months of age. While two of these were repaired immediately, it is doubtful that patency was re-established in these tiny structures.

One child had an atrophied testis.

TABLE 2.—*Local Complications in Male Children Following 331 Inguinal Hernioplasties*

	No.	%
Major wound infection	1	0.3
Scrotal swelling (severe)	5	1.5
Cut vas deferens	4	1.2
Retracted testes	2	0.6
Testicular atrophy	1	0.3
Totals	13	3.9

TABLE 3.—*Mortality Following 961 Hernioplasties*

Age, Sex	Operation	Cause of Death	Clinical Course
50, M	McVay repair of recurrent pantaloon	Bronchopneumonia	Discharged well on 7th PO day; returned 1 week later, died on 16th PO day
69, M	Halsted & tantalum mesh repair of indirect	Pneumonia, liver necrosis, cirrhosis	Shock on 1st day; Staph. wound infection; bilateral bronchopneumonia; died on 3rd PO day
74, M	A. Halsted repair of incarcerated indirect hernia B. Left lumbar sympathectomy	Coronary occlusion	Died suddenly on 3rd PO day

Adults.—Three patients died in the postoperative period, a mortality rate of 0.31%. Causes of death, all verified by autopsy, are shown in Table 3.

Systemic complications occurred after 6.9% of the operations (Table 4). Cardiovascular and pulmonary complications occurred in 4%, causing two of the deaths and contributing to the other fatality. Thrombophlebitis was diagnosed in 13 patients and 5 of these patients suffered nonfatal pulmonary emboli.

A total of 70 patients required bladder catheterization postoperatively. Prostatic resection was required in 10 of these patients. Urinary tract infection secondary to the catheterization developed in 5 other patients.

Miscellaneous complications included five patients with acute gout and single occurrences of acute cholecystitis, intestinal obstruction, gastrointestinal hemorrhage, renal calculus, herpes zoster, liver necrosis, and acute psychosis.

Wound complications were present in 21 patients. There were 14 major infections and 7 hematomas (Table 5). An additional 55 male patients (6%) developed complications of the scrotum or cord.

The distressing appearance of a grossly swollen hemiscrotum occurred 24 times. Ten of these patients had hematomas of the scrotum and in 14 the swelling was due to swelling of the testicle itself. Atrophy of the testis developed in 7 of these patients.

Testicular atrophy, without antecedent swelling, was demonstrated in nine patients, giving a total of 16 atrophied testes.

A hydrocele developed in the late postoperative period in five patients. None of these patients had had a hydrocele before the hernioplasty.

Significant pain in the distribution of the ilioinguinal nerve was reported by 14 patients. Four of these patients were treated by a series of nerve blocks and relief was obtained by two patients.

Results

Children.—There are no recurrences among the 291 cases followed from 2 to 12 years. Of the total number of cases, 42%,

TABLE 4.—*Systemic Complications in Adults Following Inguinal Hernia Repair: 961 Operations*

	No.		%	
Cardiovascular—pulmonary	39		4.1	
Atelectasis, pneumonitis		24		2.5
Thrombophlebitis		13		1.4
Coronary occlusion		2		0.2
Urinary retention (req. T.U.R.)	10		1.0	
Urinary infection	5		0.5	
Miscellaneous	12		1.3	
Totals	66		6.9	

TABLE 5.—*Local Complications in Adults Following Repair of 1,053 Hernias*

	No.		%	
Wound	21		2.0	
Major infection		14		1.3
Hematoma		7		0.7
Scrotal & cord (924 male hernias)	62		6.7	
Marked swelling		24		2.6
Testicular atrophy		16		1.8
Postop hydrocele		5		0.5
Ilioinguinal neuritis		14		1.5
Cut vas deferens		3		0.3
Totals	83		8.7	

or 153 were followed for over 5 years. The majority of the repairs (83%) consisted of high ligation of the sac, with or without a few sutures to tighten the abdominal ring. A more extensive repair was used in the other patients, usually of the Ferguson type, but occasionally a Halsted or Cooper's ligament repair was utilized.

Bilateral hernias were found in 61 (20%) of the children. Half of these hernias were not clinically evident when the patient was first seen; 7 were discovered during "blind" contralateral exploration (a total of 10 blind explorations were done) and 23 became apparent at various intervals (1 month to 12 years) following unilateral herniorrhaphy.

The appearance of a contralateral hernia after a unilateral repair in children is a problem which has received much attention recently.[15] Whether a surgeon should routinely explore the opposite side when doing a unilateral hernioplasty has not been definitely determined, but we now believe that bilateral exploration should be done in females under six years of age and in any male under six years of age where the slightest suspicion of a contralateral hernia exists.

Adults.—We followed 871 (83%) patients for more than two years, and 567 (54%) were followed from five to twelve years. There are 65 known recurrences, a rate of 7.5%. The recurrences appeared as follows: 16 (24%) within six months, 39 (60%) within two years, 54 (82%) within five years, and the other 11 (18%) were discovered between five and ten years after hernioplasty.

Our results are tabulated by the method of repair and by the type of hernia (Table 6). Four types of repairs were used: Halsted I,[13] Bassini,[13] transversalis,[10] and Cooper's ligament.[10] A Halsted transplantation of the spermatic cord was added to several Cooper's ligament repairs. These are classified separately in Table 6.

Pantaloon hernias are listed as direct or indirect hernias depending upon the major component of the hernia. All recurrent hernias that were repaired during the period of study are included in Table 6.

When these recurrent hernias are excluded, the recurrence rates are 7.1% for indirect hernias, 4.6% for direct hernias, and 7.8% for femoral hernias, giving an over-all 6.6% recurrence rate for primary inguinal and femoral hernias. Repair of recurrent hernias failed 13 times, a rate of 16% for the 80 patients followed for more than two years. Recurrent direct hernias were the most difficult hernias to repair; 20% of these hernias recurred.

Recurrence rates reported by others are shown in Table 7. Those series that include children are indicated by an asterisk. If children were included in our figures, the recurrence rate for indirect hernias would be 5.1%, and our over-all recurrence rate would be reduced to 5.6%.

The first three series represent the personal series of men long interested in hernias. Their superior results are clearly evident from Table 7.

Comment

The mortality, systemic complication, and recurrence rates in children are acceptable

TABLE 6.—*Recurrence Rate by Method of Repair and by Type of Hernia*

Method of Repair	Indirect		Direct		Femoral		Totals	
Halsted I	31/344	9.0 *	11/109	10.0 *	—	—	42/453	9.3 *
Bassini	2/46	4.3	0/6	0.0	3/24	12.5 *	5/76	6.6
Transversalis	7/151	4.6	1/13	7.7	—	—	8/164	4.8
Cooper's ligament (McVay)	2/34	5.7	1/33	3.3	2/39	5.1	5/106	4.7
Cooper's ligament-Halsted	3/17	17.6	2/50	4.0	0/5	0.0	5/72	7.0
Totals	45/592	7.6	15/211	7.1	5/68	7.3	65/871	7.5

* Numerator of fraction indicates number of recurrences; denominator indicates number of cases.
† Columns marked with asterisk are %.

TABLE 7.—*Recurrence Rates (%) of Inguinal and Femoral Hernias*

Author	No. Cases Followed	Years Followed	Indirect	Direct	Femoral	Recurrent	Total
Estes (2) *	363	5-15	0.9	1.8	—	5.0	1.4
Koontz (7) †	386	1-22	—	—	—	2.0	0.8
McVay (12) †	580	2-11	3.2	1.0	0	0	2.2
Hagan (3) †	766	2-5	4.1	5.0	2.9	21.0	5.5
Levy (8)	490	1-3	4.8	10.5	—	12.3	6.7
Marsden (9)	1,602	3	5.2	7.4	—	19.0	6.8
Telle (16)	1,124	5-10	6.7	7.6	22.0	14.0	10.8
Present study	871	2-12	7.1	4.6	7.8	16.0	7.5

* Parentheses indicate references.
† Series that include children.
—Not stated in article.

and comparable to those reported by others. However, the development of local complications in nearly 4% of the patients is disconcerting. At least seven patients (the last three groups in Table 2) lost the use of a normal testicle after their hernioplasty, an incidence of 2.1%.

The mortality rate of 0.3% in adults is acceptable. An infection rate of 1.3% for "clean" surgery, while higher than one would like, is not unacceptable. But we had 62 other patients, over 6%, with local complications, all of which might have been prevented. Over 5% of the men lost the use of a normal testicle because of its removal or its atrophy following hernioplasty.

Analysis of our figures revealed that no individual surgeon or method of repair was responsible for an undue number of these complications. Careful dissection, meticulous hemostasis, and gentle handling of tissue are necessary if we are to reduce the frequency of these distressing complications.

We had an unsatisfactory recurrence rate for indirect hernias (Table 6). The original Halsted repair was used to repair more than half of these hernias, resulted in a 9.0% recurrence rate, and was chiefly responsible for the poor results. This repair has been shown to be inferior to other hernioplasties both clinically [3,14,16] and anatomically.[11] We are unable to show an overwhelmingly superior method to repair these common hernias, but feel that the transversalis repair, with its correct closure of the abdominal ring,[11] is preferable to those repairs using the inguinal ligament.

We feel that in the large indirect hernias a Cooper's ligament repair, as described by McVay,[10] should be used. However, in our hands, the recurrence rate has been disturbingly high with these large hernias.

We had a recurrence rate of 7.1% for direct hernias. The superiority of the Cooper's ligament repair for these hernias is illustrated in Table 6. McVay and Anson [11] and Isaac [5] have convincingly demonstrated the anatomy of this region and the importance of Cooper's ligament in the repair of these hernias. A Cooper's ligament repair resulted in a 3.6% recurrence rate for direct hernias, while other methods gave a combined 9.4% recurrence rate. This difference is due to the failure of the Halsted repair (even when buttressed with tantalum mesh as was done 12 times) to cure these more difficult hernias.

The Cooper's ligament repair was superior to other methods of repair in the treatment of femoral hernias. Its use resulted in a 4.5% recurrence rate as compared to a 12.5% recurrence rate for other methods of repair. Closing the femoral ring through a femoral approach or by utilizing the inguinal ligament represents a compromise with the anatomy of this region and should be expected to result in more frequent recurrences.

All recurrent hernias were reviewed critically in an effort to discover why the surgery failed. Of the 65 recurrences, a reasonable cause for the recurrence could be assigned to 43 cases on the basis of findings at reoperation or at physical examination (Table 8).

TABLE 8.—*Causes of Recurrence in 65 Recurrent Inguinal and Femoral Hernias*

	Inadequate Closure of Internal Ring	Missed Femoral or Indirect	Excess Tension	Direct Recurrence	Infection	Undetermined
Halsted I						
Indirect	13	6	2	2	1	7
Direct	2	2	—	3	—	4
Bassini						
Indirect	—	—	1	—	—	1
Femoral	—	2	—	—	—	1
Transversalis						
Indirect	1	—	1	1	—	4
Direct	—	—	1	—	—	—
Cooper's ligament						
Indirect	1	—	1	—	—	3
Direct	2	—	1	—	—	—
Femoral	—	—	—	—	—	2
Totals	19	10	7	6	1	22

The greatest number of recurrences occurred at or just lateral to the internal ring as indirect hernias. This occurred more frequently when the abdominal ring was not closed properly (and it is not correctly done by sewing the conjoined tendon to the inguinal ligament). It is important that the defect in the transversalis fascia be closed carefully, both medial and lateral to the cord, as is done in the transversalis repair. We found three indirect recurrences lateral to the cord after Halsted repairs.

A "missed" femoral hernia appeared eight times after a Halsted repair. In addition, two indirect hernias were overlooked when a femoral hernia was repaired via the femoral approach. Six of these ten hernias appeared within six months of the original surgery; two of them presented as strangulated hernias. Though some might argue that these do not represent recurrent hernias at all, we cannot agree with them. Any future herniation in the groin following repair of an inguinal or femoral hernia should be classified as a recurrence.

This type of recurrence is preventable. Careful finger exploration of the femoral ring via the indirect sac is an essential part of every indirect hernioplasty. The use of the Cooper's ligament repair in direct hernias would not only allow careful inspection of the femoral canal for unrecognized or incipient femoral hernias but would also repair the area so that future femoral herniation would be a negligible risk.

Because of the increased dissection and operating time needed with an inguinal approach, many surgeons utilize the femoral route to repair reducible femoral hernias in elderly or poor-risk patients. However, the femoral approach does not allow the surgeon an opportunity to discover and repair coexisting inguinal hernias and provides for an inferior repair of the femoral hernia. Its use is not recommended.

Excessive tension caused seven recurrent hernias. Two of these recurrences occurred because the suture line to the inguinal ligament broke down, one on the first postoperative day.

Four recurrent hernias were limited to a small area near the pubic tubercle and at reoperation were shown to be due to protrusions through the suture line in this area. We feel that it is important to carry the suture line down to the pubic tubercle in order to prevent this type of recurrence.

A large direct recurrence, when found at reoperation, was often the result of an inadequate repair of the floor of the inguinal canal. We did not see this type of recurrence after a Cooper's ligament repair.

We were impressed by the manner of recurrence of the hernias. We left behind 10 unrecognized hernias, sewed under excessive tension in 7 cases, and inadequately closed the abdominal inguinal ring in 19 other patients. Thus over half of the recurrent hernias could probably have been prevented.

A thorough search for a coexisting hernia, an accurate and anatomical closure of the abdominal inguinal ring, and careful suturing without excessive tension should substantially reduce a surgeon's incidence of recurrent hernias.

Summary and Conclusions

A clinical study of 1,416 inguinal and femoral hernioplasties is presented. Particular attention is given to postoperative complications and to the recurrence of the hernia. Our recurrence rate, based on a minimum two-year follow-up period, is 7.5%.

Many of the distressing complications occurring in the scrotum and wound are preventable. Gentle handling of tissue and careful hemostasis should reduce a surgeon's incidence of these complications.

We obtained unsatisfactory results with the Halsted I repair in both indirect and direct hernias.

A careful anatomical closure of the defect in the transversalis fascia produced by an indirect hernia is necessary for its successful repair.

The Cooper's ligament repair gives superior results when used to repair direct and femoral hernias. This method of repair should be used for the vast majority of these hernias.

William T. Mosenthal, MD, reviewed this paper critically.

William B. Rydell, Jr., MD, Huntley Road, Norwich, Vt.

REFERENCES

1. Eiseman, B.; Robinson, R. M.; and Brown, J. H.: Simultaneous Appendectomy and Herniorrhaphy Without Prophylactic Antibiotic Therapy, Surgery 51:578, 1962.

2. Estes, W. L., Jr.: Five Year End Results in the Treatment of Inguinal Hernia, Amer Surg 22:948, 1956.

3. Hagan, W. H., and Rhoads, J. H.: Inguinal and Femoral Hernias, Surg Gynec Obstet 96:226, 1953.

4. Hill, M. R., Jr.; Pollock, W. F.; and Sprong, D. H., Jr.: Testicular Infarction and Incarcerated Inguinal Herniae, Arch Surg 85:351, 1962.

5. Isaac, R. E.: Inguinal Hernia and the Iliopectineal Line, Brit J Surg 49:204, 1961.

6. Keeley, J. L., and Schairer, A. E.: Incidental Appendectomy During Repair of Groin Hernias, Surgery 52:421, 1962.

7. Koontz, A. R.: Personal Technique and Results in Inguinal Hernia Repair, JAMA 164:29, 1957.

8. Levy, A. H.; Wren, R. S.; and Friedman, M. N.: Complications and Recurrences Following Inguinal Hernia Repair, Ann Surg 133:533, 1951.

9. Marsden, A. J.: Inguinal Hernia: A Three-Year Review of 2,000 Cases, Brit J Surg 49:384, 1962.

10. McVay, C. B.: Hernia, Springfield, Ill: Charles C Thomas, Publisher, 1954.

11. McVay, C. B., and Anson, B. J.: A Fundamental Error in Current Methods of Inguinal Herniorrhaphy, Surg Gynec Obstet 74:746, 1942.

12. McVay, C. B., and Chapp, J. D.: Inguinal and Femoral Hernioplasty: The Evaluation of a Basic Concept, Ann Surg 148:499, 1958.

13. Ravich, M. M., and Hitzrot, J. M., II: Operations for Inguinal Hernia: Part I; Part II, Surgery 48:439 and 615, 1960.

14. Ryan, E. A.: Recurrent Hernias: An Analysis of 369 Consecutive Cases of Recurrent Inguinal and Femoral Hernias, Surg Gynec Obstet 96:343, 1953.

15. Sparkman, R. S.: Bilateral Exploration in Inguinal Hernia in Juvenile Patients, Surgery 51:393, 1962.

16. Telle, L. D.: Inguinal and Femoral Hernia: A Review of 1,694 Cases, Amer J Surg 93:433, 1957.

Portacaval Transposition in Experimental Hypertension

JOHN M. PALMER, MD, PALO ALTO, CALIF

Effect on Blood Pressure

Experimentally produced renal hypertension is usually attributed to the release into the blood stream of a humoral substance (renin) elaborated by the ischemic kidney. Renin is a proteolytic enzyme which acts upon a protein substrate synthetized in the liver [1] to form angiotensin I, an inactive decapeptide. From this decapeptide histadylleucine is hydrolyzed, leaving an octapeptide known as angiotensin II,[2] the active vasoconstrictor substance whose pressor activity is said to be ten times that of norepinephrine.[3] The actual time sequence of this reaction in vivo is unknown. The elevation in mean arterial pressure following constriction of the renal artery may occur within hours, but usually a period of two to three weeks transpires before significant elevation is seen. If the reaction described above is other than instantaneous, then an opportunity is presented for metabolic attack on the development of experimental hypertension.

Cerqua and Samaan [4] in 1939 reported a reduction in blood pressure in hypertensive dogs following omentorenopexy. The following year, Weeks et al [5] reported the same result from splenorenopexy. These authors concluded that the development of extensive collateral circulation to the ischemic kidney occasioned by these operations implemented the fall in blood pressure. However, the liver is well known for its ability to metabolize endogenous substances, and their results might be interpreted to suggest a metabolic alteration of renin due to inclusion of the ischemic kidney into the portal circulation. If this is true, then direct shunting of the renal venous blood through the portal circulation could lead to hepatic inactivation of the enzyme renin before it reaches the systemic circulation and therefore interrupt the sequence leading to development of hypertension. Such a result would be further evidence for the humoral basis of experimental renal hypertension.

The purpose of this study was to examine this thesis by transposition of the portal vein and the inferior vena cava in Goldblatt hypertensive dogs.

Materials and Methods

A. *Materials.*—Male and female mongrel dogs weighing from 16 to 24 kg made up the experimental groups. Hematocrit readings and serum creatinine determinations were serially performed throughout the experimental period. Blood pressures were measured by direct femoral artery puncture on the unanesthetized animal using a No. 20 gauge needle connected with vinyl plastic tubing * to a Statham pressure transducer and a Brush Mark II direct writing recorder. Arterial pressures were recorded once or twice weekly by the same persons throughout all periods.

B. *Methods.*—Experimental Animals: After a seven- to ten-week control period, five of six animals were subjected to a right nephrectomy, and one week later a Goldblatt clamp was applied to the left renal artery. The sixth animal underwent both procedures at one operation. These operations were performed through flank incisions and under pentobarbital sodium (Nembutal) anesthesia. After the development of hypertension (in five to nine weeks), these animals were subjected to transposition of the inferior vena cava and the portal vein after the method of Child et al.[6] All animals were fasted one day prior to surgery and received atropine 0.4 mg on the operative day. Under pentobarbital sodium anesthesia a midline abdomi-

Submitted for publication Feb 19, 1963.

* United States Catheter and Instrument Corporation, Glens Falls, NY.

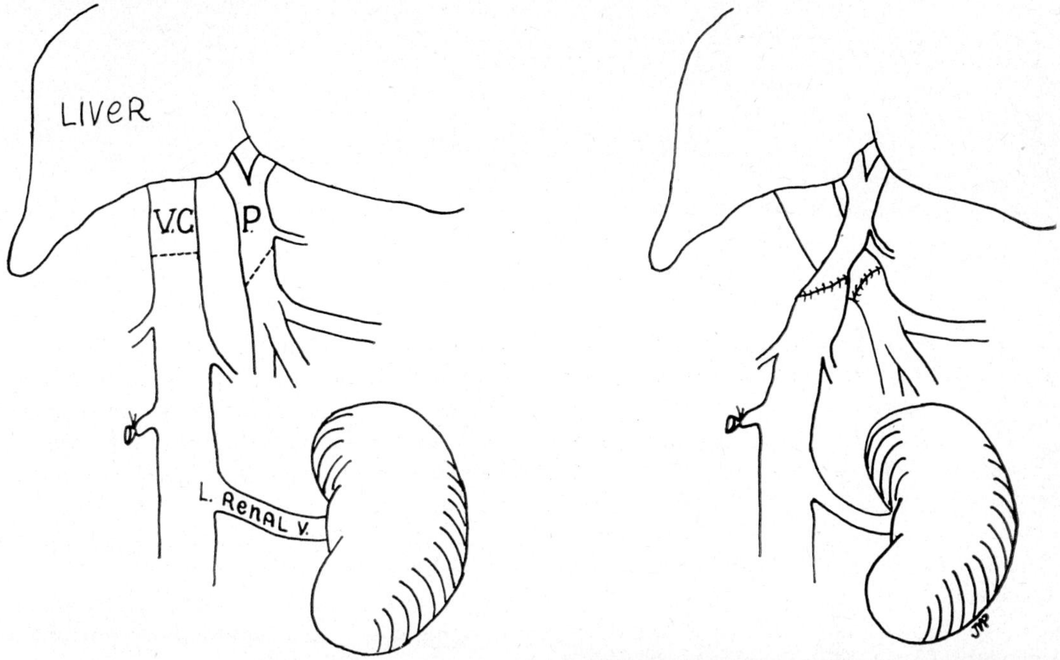

Fig 1.—Line drawing diagram of vascular anastomoses in portacaval transposition in the dog.

nal incision was made, and the portal vein, inferior vena cava, and superior mesenteric artery were identified and dissected free. The inferior vena cava was divided transversely, the superior mesenteric artery clamped, and, after a moment or two to allow for venous drainage, the portal vein was clamped and incised obliquely. The distal portal vein was immediately anastomosed to the proximal vena cava and the superior mesenteric clamp released. After this, the distal vena cava was anastomosed to the proximal portal vein (Fig 1).

Control Animals: After nine- and ten-week control periods, the animals were subjected to portacaval transposition, followed in one week by right nephrectomy. Arterial blood pressures were measured up to 17 weeks after the shunt. After all surgical procedures, the animals received penicillin 600,000 units a day for four days.

Portacaval transposition was demonstrated to be patent in all dogs by portal venography via the inferior vena cava. A representative roentgenogram of a functioning cavoportal anastomosis is shown in Fig 2. The anastomoses were patent at autopsy.

In four animals retrograde femoral aortography (methylglucamine diatrizoate [Renografin], 1 ml/kg) was performed to ascertain the extent of arterial collateral circulation to the remaining ischemic kidney.

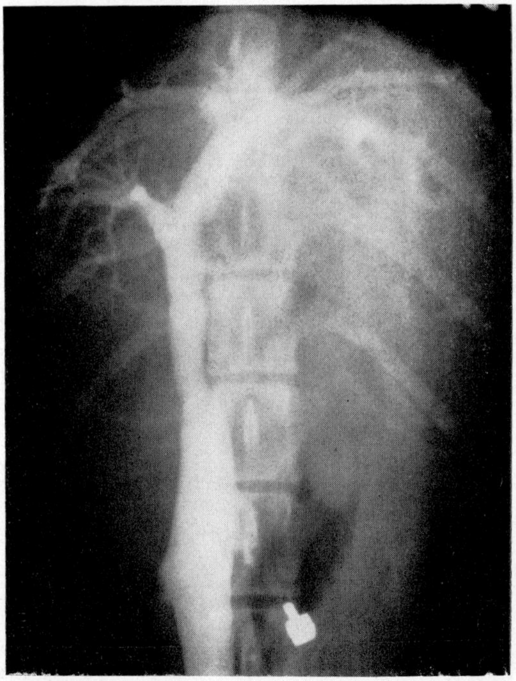

Fig 2.—Roentgenogram of patent anastomosis between distal vena cava and proximal portal vein in vivo in the dog. Catheter inserted via femoral vein into inferior vena cava. Contrast media fills the vena cava, portal vein, and hepatic portal system. Experimental dog No. 2.

Results

Blood pressure data for each experimental period are presented in Table 1. A remarkable individual variation in mean arterial pressure was observed in normal dogs. Of

TABLE 1.—*Mean Arterial Blood Pressure Recordings on Six Experimental and*

	Control Period				Goldblatt Period			
		Range				Range		
Dog No.	No. of Observ.	Systolic	Diastolic	Average	No. of Observ.	Systolic	Diastolic	Average
					Experimental Animals			
1	16 (14) *	154-220	88-129	195/104	11 (6) *	200-268	196-152	237/124
2	10 (9)	136-184	70-98	163/86	12 (8)	186-254	96-140	225/123
3	9 (5)	190-250	98-124	218/111	8 (6)	210-310	110-168	249/132
4	8 (5)	188-218	104-132	208/119	6 (4)	216-236	128-142	229/135
5	12 (7)	252-296	138-176	274/155	13 (8)	244-364	156-204	314/178
6	12 (9)	226-284	114-138	251/126	12 (9)	260-320	122-156	295/139
					Control Animals			
7	11 (11)	184-232	96-120	207/107				
8	10 (10)	194-244	108-140	223/127				

* Parentheses indicate duration of period of observation in weeks.

In this experimental group, a ries of 13 to 37 mm of Hg in mean diastolic pressure occured after application of the Goldblatt clamp. During the period following portacaval transposition, the mean diastolic pressure continued to rise in dogs No. 1, 2, and 4.In dog No. 3, no change occurred in mean diastolic pressure, and in dogs No. 5 and 6, the diastolic pressures were noted to fall after portacaval transposition. No significant change was noted in mean diastolic blood pressure in control animals after portacaval transposition.

the eight experimental animals, the lowest mean pressure during the control period was 163/86 (average of 10 observations), while the highest mean pressure was found to be 274/155 (average of 12 observations).

The experimental animals showed a rise in mean diastolic pressure of 13 to 37 mm Hg after application of the Goldblatt clamp. Three of these animals (No. 1, 2, and 4) showed a further mean elevation of 16, 9, and 8 mm Hg, respectively, in diastolic pressure in the period following portacaval transposition. Dog No. 3 showed essentially no change in blood pressure after portacaval transposition. Dogs No. 5 and 6 showed a fall in mean arterial pressure to the control level in the period following portacaval transposition. The two animals of the control group (dogs 7 and 8) showed no significant variation in blood pressure between the control and the transposition periods.

Results of creatinine determinations during the three periods are reported in Table 2. All dogs had slight to moderate elevations during the period of renal ischemia, but later returned to control readings in most cases. Hematocrit readings were never significantly altered from the preliminary control levels.

Comment

The marked variation in mean arterial blood pressure obtained in these animals during the control period points out the fallacy in assuming a "normal" blood pressure in the dog. These pressures are graphed in Fig 3A, 3B, and 4 and demonstrate the repeatability of pressures in the different periods. However, the inherent error of assuming a control blood pressure after only two or three determinations in one animal is apparent, and the necessity for individualization of each dog is obvious.

All animals thrived as long-term survivors and showed no untoward sequelae attributable to portacaval transposition. These findings were not unexpected since Child et al have demonstrated remarkable regenerative capacity of the liver in dogs following transposition[6] and hepatic function studies in these animals compare favorably with pretransposition measurements.[7]

Four dogs of the experimental group had no fall in arterial pressure following portacaval transposition. In fact, three of these dogs had a rise in pressure after the shunt. This result may represent the natural history of experimental hypertension for these dogs, ie, progressive scar formation in

Two Control Animals

No. of Observ.	Transposition Period Range Systolic	Diastolic	Average
14 (17) *	228-318	120-160	268/140
11 (7)	220-260	120-148	242/132
18 (15)	200-288	100-160	242/131
10 (12)	222-254	136-150	239/143
11 (11)	246-328	124-200	280/156
10 (6)	232-296	112-140	264/128
12 (11)	164-224	84-124	192/101
14 (14)	182-260	100-142	239/127

and around the renal artery leading to increasing renal ischemia. Two dogs had a fall in mean arterial pressure following transposition. The drop in pressure was striking in dog No. 6 but gradually declined in dog No. 5, the decline in the latter actually beginning in the mid-Goldblatt period (Fig 3B).

Aortograms were performed on dogs No. 1, 3, 5, and 6 to evaluate the extent of collateral circulation to the ischemic kidney. Dogs No. 3 and 5 developed extensive collateral vessels to the remaining kidney, and, as seen in Fig 5 (dog No. 5), the main renal artery was completely occluded by the clamp. Dogs No. 1 and 6 did not develop important collateral vessels and demonstrated excellent flow through the clamped renal artery (Fig 6, dog No. 6). Dogs No. 3 and 5 developed a sudden and permanent transverse myelitis following aortogram. It is of considerable interest that these dogs developed lumbar collateral circulation.

From these studies the possibility exists in dog No. 5 that increased blood flow to the kidney occurred secondary to development of collateral circulation from surrounding tissue. Dog No. 6 had a sudden fall in blood pressure coincident with portacaval transposition. While this is suggestive of a cause and effect relationship, it must be noted that dog No. 6 had the least hypertensive response of all to application of the Goldblatt clamp. No fall in blood pressure following portacaval transposition occurred in the other animals.

TABLE 2.—*Results of Serum Creatinine Determinations in the Experimental and Control Group*

Dog No.	Creatinine Reading, Mg % Control (Highest Reading)	Goldblatt (Highest Reading)	Transposition (Last Reading)
Experimental Animals			
1	1.72	1.10	1.31
2	1.48	3.20	1.62
3	1.24	1.64	1.12
4	1.00	1.46	0.90
5	1.06	2.00	0.92
6	1.15	1.30	0.92
Control Animals			
7	0.80		1.64
8	0.84		0.93

Slight elevation occurred after application of the Goldblatt clamp in two experimental dogs with subsequent return to values consistent with those during control period. Some elevation was noted in one of the control animals after portacaval transposition.

Fig 6.—Transfemoral aortogram in dog No. 6 demonstrating excellent arterial flow through the Goldblatt clamp and no renal collateral circulation.

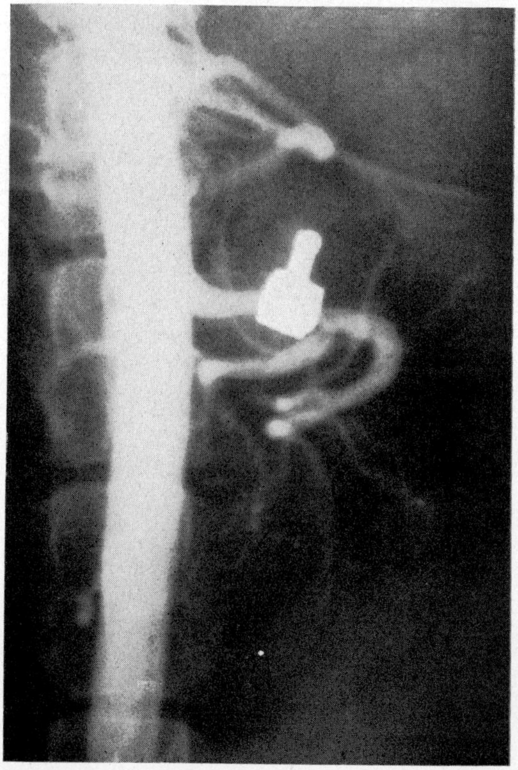

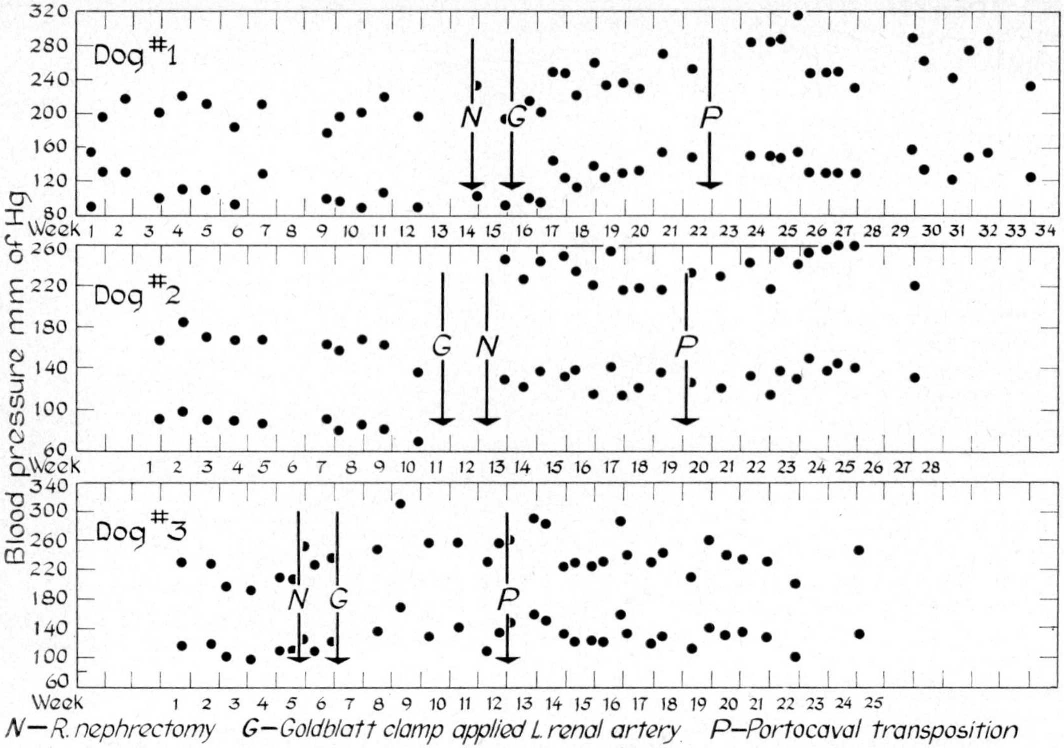

Fig 3A.—Graphic representation of serial arterial blood pressure recordings presented in Table 1, for three of the experimental dogs. Note the marked variations found in individual readings for each animal during the three periods. These figures point out the error in interpreting a single blood pressure recording as representative for the particular animal. The variation in individual canine blood pressures is also demonstrated (see text).

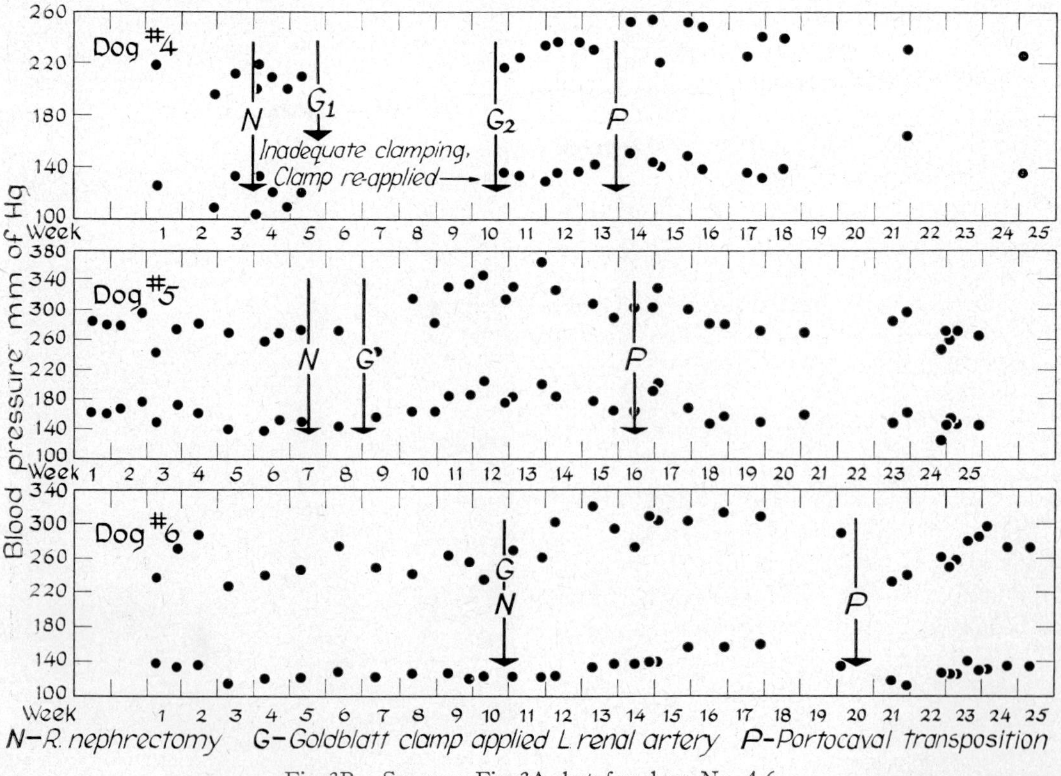

Fig 3B.—Same as Fig 3A, but for dogs No. 4-6.

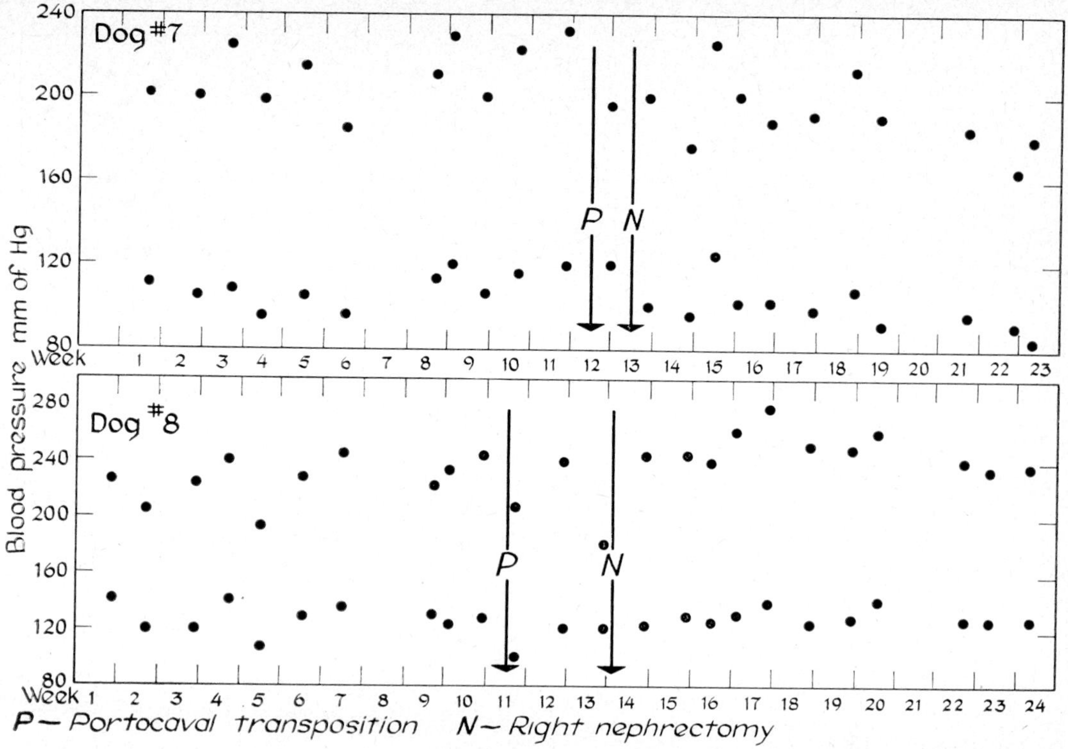

Fig 4.—Graphic representation of serial arterial blood pressure recordings in two control animals undergoing nephrectomy and portacaval transposition.

Fig 5.—*A,* transfemoral aortogram in dog No. 5 five months following application of Goldblatt clamp. Complete occlusion of left renal artery has occurred. The stump of right renal artery can be faintly seen. *B,* transfemoral aortogram in dog No. 5 demonstrating extensive renal collateral circulation which was sufficient to maintain life in this animal.

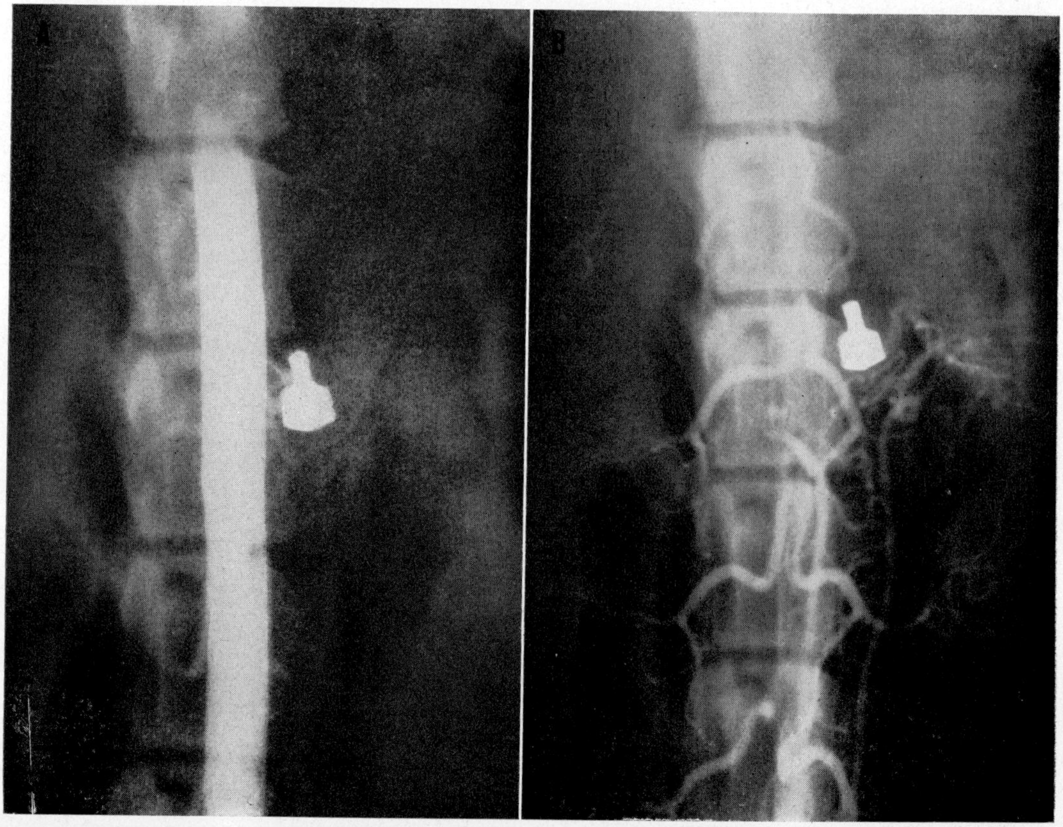

While shunting of the renal venous blood through the portal circulation in experimental hypertension is not a new idea, the limitations of earlier experiments encouraged further study. Child and Glenn[8] in a similar experiment were unable to alter the blood pressure in two hypertensive dogs subjected to reverse Eck fistula. A related study was performed in short-term experiments by Levy and Blalock[9] who failed to prevent the development of hypertension in four Goldblatt dogs previously subjected to anastomosis of the distal renal vein to the proximal splenic vein. Portacaval transposition has two advantages over these earlier methods: first, the crucial problem of patency of the distal caval to proximal portal vein anastomosis was verified in vivo by angiography in our experiments, and, second, the possibility of retrograde flow in the distal vena cava secondary to hepatic engorgement was ruled out in all animals at fluoroscopy.

In these experiments, we have been unable to demonstrate a fall in blood pressure in experimental hypertension following transposition of the portal vein and vena cava. Our results suggest at least three possibilities: (*a*) the assumption can be made that the liver has no control over the enzyme renin when it is elaborated from the ischemic kidney; (*b*) the possibility exists that the conversion of renin-substrate to angiotensin II is an instantaneous reaction occurring as soon as renin contacts renal venous blood; and (*c*) since the liver is thought to be the source of renin-substrate, shunting of the renal venous blood through the portal circulation may simply accelerate the rate of conversion of this globulin to angiotensin II.

Conclusion

The effect of portacaval transposition on Goldblatt-induced hypertension was studied in dogs. The experiments reported and the documented results lend no support to the hypothesis that diversion of renal venous blood into the portal circulation may reduce blood pressure in Goldblatt hypertension.

The development of permanent transverse myelitis in two hypertensive dogs subjected to transfemoral aortography with methylglucamine diatrizoate (Renograffin) is reported.

John M. Palmer, MD, Department of Surgery, Stanford Medical Center, 300 Pasteur Dr, Palo Alto, Calif.

REFERENCES

1. Page, I. H.: Influence of the Liver on Vascular Reactivity, Amer J Physiol 160:421, 1950.

2. Dustan, H. P.; Page, I. H.; and Poutasse, E. F.: Renal Hypertension, New Eng J Med 261:647, 1959.

3. Mendlowitz, M.; Wolf, R. L.; Gitlow, S. E.; and Naftchi, N. E.: "Angiotensin Studies in Hypertension," in Symposium on Angiotensin, American Heart Association Monograph No. 3, New York: American Heart Association, 1962.

4. Cerqua, S., and Samaan, A.: Cure of Experimental Renal Hypertension, Clin Sci 4:113, 1939.

5. Weeks, D. M.; Steiner, A.; Mansfield, J. S.; and Victor, J.: The Depressor Effect of Spleno-Reno-Pexy on Hypertension Due to Renal Ischemia, J Exp Med 72:345, 1940.

6. Child, C. G.; Barr, D. P.; Holswade, G. R.; and Harrison, C. S.: Liver Regeneration Following Portacaval Transposition in Dogs, Ann Surg 138:600, 1953.

7. Heer, F. W.; Silvius, D. E.; and Harper, H. A.: The Relation Between Hepatic Blood Flow and Function in Normal Dogs and Dogs With Cirrhosis After Portacaval Shunt or Transposition, Surg Forum 11:282, 1960.

8. Child, C. G., and Glenn, F.: Effect of Passing Renal Blood Through the Liver in Dogs With Experimental Hypertension, Arch Surg 36:376, 1938.

9. Levy, S. E., and Blalock, A.: Experimental Attempts to Prevent or Abolish the Hypertension That Is Associated With Renal Ischemia, Surgery 3:899, 1938.

Sodium Oxacillin in Surgical Infections

Clinical Evaluation

WILLIAM SCHUMER, MD
CHICAGO

Doyle and Nayler [1] in 1961 chemically coupled the diacetylization of 6-aminopenicillanic acid to 5-methyl-3-phenyl-4-isoxazolecarboxylic acid and produced a colorless, crystalline compound known as sodium oxacillin,* or MPI, or P-12. Its molecular weight is 441.43, and it is extremely stable in its dry state. It is freely soluble in water and in the state of solution may be stable for 24 hours at room temperature. Its most important attribute is that it is acid resistant. This allows it to be used as an oral preparation. It is penicillinase resistant and apparently ten times more active than methicillin against *Staphylococcus aureus,* coagulase positive. Reports reveal that *Staph aureus* is inhibited by MPI penicillin in concentrations of 1 mEq or less per milliliter. Its bactericidal end point lies between 2.5 and 5 mg/cc.[2] Numerous clinical studies have been carried out which reveal a marked antistaphylococcal activity.[3,4] MPI penicillin was a more active bacteriostatic and bactericidal agent against penicillinase-producing *Staphylococcus* and β-hemolytic *Streptococcus* than either benzathine penicillin G or methicillin.[5-9] There is also a reported effectiveness against pneumococci.

There have also been some rewarding reports concerning the use of oxacillin in severe staphylococcal infections such as osteomyelitis, cellulitis, pyelonephritis, and other tissue infections.

In view of the excellent reports on the drug and the ability to use it orally, it was decided to try MPI penicillin on staphylococcal and streptococcal surgical infections.

Submitted for publication Feb 4, 1963.

Assistant Professor Surgery, The Chicago Medical School; Associate, Mount Sinai Hospital; Attending, Hines Veterans Administration Hospital.

* The trade name of E. R. Squibb & Sons for sodium oxacillin is Resistopen.

Method and Materials

Fifty-two consecutive, surgical, staphylococcal and streptococcal infections were studied. All exudates and discharges of the infections were serially cultured, and sensitivities were performed. Oxacillin was given in dosages of 1 gm q. 6 h. for a total of

Method and Results of Study

Infection	Cultured Organism	Duration of Therapy, Days	Results	Untoward Reactions
		Soft Tissue		
Carbuncles:				
1	*Staph aureus* coag +	14	Resolution	0
2	*Staph aureus* coag +	10	Resolution	Nausea 1st 2 days
3	*Staph aureus* coag + β-hemolytic *Strep*	16	Resolution	0
4	*Staph aureus* coag +	21	Nonresolution	Diarrhea after 18 days
5	*Staph aureus* coag +	9	Resolution	0
6	*Staph aureus* β-hemolytic *Strep*	10	Resolution	Maculopapular rash
7	*Staph aureus* coag +	14	Resolution	0
8	*Staph aureus* coag +	12	Resolution	0
9	β-hemolytic *Strep*	10	Resolution	0
Total: 9		Average: 12.9	Resolution: 89%	Reactions: 33.3%
Abscesses:				
10	*Staph aureus* coag +	7	Localization	0
11	*Staph aureus* coag +	4	Incision & drainage, 7 day resolution	0
12	*Staph aureus* coag +	6	Resolution	Nausea
13	*Staph aureus* coag +	5	Resolution	0
14	*Staph aureus* coag +	5	Localization 5 days with incision and drainage	0
15	*Staph aureus* coag +	6	Resolution	0
Total: 6		Average: 5.5	Resolution: 100%	Reactions: 20%
Cellulitis:				
16	*Staph aureus* coag + β-hemolytic *Strep*	10	Resolution	0
17	*Strep* β-hemolytic	14	No effect	Nausea
18	*Strep* β-hemolytic	18	No effect	Diarrhea
19	*Staph aureus* coag +	16	Resolution	0
20	*Staph aureus*	9	Resolution	0
21	β-hemolytic *Strep*	8	No effect	Maculopapular rash
22	β-hemolytic *Strep* *Staph aureus*	10	Resolution	0
23	β-hemolytic *Strep*	14	Resolution	0
Total: 8		Average: 12.4	Resolution: 62%	Reactions: 38%
Total Soft Tissue: 23		Average Duration of Therapy: 11	Resolution: 83%	Untoward Reactions: 30%
		Wound Infection		
Cellulitis:				
24, hernia	*Staph aureus* coag +	7	Resolution	0
25, hernia	*Staph aureus* β-hemolytic *Strep*	5	Resolution	Nausea
26, appendectomy	*Staph aureus*	8	Drug discontinued due to rash	Maculopapular rash
27, cholecystectomy	*Staph aureus* β-hemolytic *Strep*	6	Resolution, culture neg	0
28, hernia	*Staph aureus* coag +	5	Resolution, culture neg	0
29, appendectomy	*Staph aureus* & *Staph albus*	8	Resolution, culture neg	0
30, cholecystectomy	*Staph aureus* coag + β-hemolytic *Strep*	10	Resolution, culture neg	0
31, hernia	*Staph aureus* coag +	9	Resolution, culture neg	Diarrhea
32, hernia	*Staph aureus*	11	Resolution, culture neg	Nausea
33, hernia	*Staph aureus*	6	Resolution	0
34, appendectomy	*Staph aureus* β-hemolytic *Strep*	8	Resolution	0
35, burn grafts	*Staph aureus*	7	Resolution, culture neg	Maculopapular rash
Total: 12		Average: 7.5	Resolution: 92%	Reactions: 42%
Abscesses:				
36, hernia	*Staph aureus* coag +	7	Incision & drainage, resolution 7 days	0
37, appendectomy	*Staph aureus*	6	Incision & drainage, resolution 6 days	0

Method and Results of Study—(Continued)

Infection	Cultured Organism	Duration of Therapy, Days	Results	Untoward Reactions
38, colon resection	*Staph aureus* coag + β-hemolytic *Strep*	4	Incision & drainage, resolution 5 days	0
39, gastric resection	*Staph aureus* coag +	5	Incision & drainage, resolution 5 days	0
40, hernia	*Staph aureus* coag +	8	No effect	0
41, hernia	*Staph aureus*	9	No effect	0
Total: 6		Average: 6.5	Resolution: 66.6 %	Reactions: None
Fistulae:				
42, colon resection	*Staph aureus* coag + *Paracolobactrum*	21	Resolution 16 days, culture neg	Nausea on 18th day
43, colon resection	*Ecoli Proteus mirabilis Staph aureus* coag +	18	Neg culture, 15th day	Nausea, rash
44, small bowel resection	*Staph aureus* coag +	24	Neg culture, 10th day	Nausea, diarrhea 21st day
45, colon resection	*Staph aureus* coag + β-hemolytic *Strep*	20	Neg culture, 16th day	Nausea 18th day
Total: 4		Average: 21	Resolution: 100 %	Untoward Reactions: 100 %
Total Wound Infections: 22	Average Duration of Therapy: 9.6		Resolution: 86 %	Reactions: 41 %
Septicemia:				
46, abdominal peritoneal resection	*Staph aureus* coag +	25	Neg culture, 18th day	No discernible effect
47, colon resection	*Staph aureus* coag +	30	Neg culture, 22nd day	No discernible effect
48, colostomy	*Staph aureus* coag +	24	Neg culture, 18th day	No discernible effect
49, colon resection	*Staph aureus* coag +	21	No effect, death	0
Total: 4		Average: 28	Resolution: 75 %	Reactions: None
Peritonitis:				
50, gastric resection	(Paracentesis) *staph aureus* enterococci	16	Resolution with hypothermia	0
51, ruptured gallbladder	(Paracentesis) *Staph aureus* enterococci	12	Resolution with hypothermia	Nausea, vomiting
52, ruptured diverticulitis	(Paracentesis) *Staph aureus* enterococci	18	Death with hypothermia	Nausea, vomiting
Total: 3		Average: 15	Resolution: 66.6 %	Reactions: 66.6 %
		All Cases		
Total Patients: 52	Average Duration of Therapy: 11.7		Resolution: 83 %	Untoward Reactions: 29 %

4 gm per day. The Table illustrates the method and results of the study.

Results of Therapy

The over-all result was 83% resolution in soft tissue infections. Twenty-three patients with soft tissue infections were studied. Of these nine had carbuncles, six had abscesses, and eight had cellulitis. All carbuncles except one had a positive *Staph aureus*. This exception revealed β-hemolytic *Streptococcus*. There were two cases with combinations of *Staphylococcus* and β-hemolytic *Streptococcus*. The one patient who did not respond to oxacillin was a 65-year-old female who had a carbuncle of the back. The lesion was treated for 21 days, but the patient after 18 days developed a severe diarrhea. During these 21 days the lesion changed very little. After the drug was discontinued the lesion extended itself with a production of sinus formation. Subsequent cultures revealed *Pseudomonas aeruginosa* which was sensitive to chloramphenicol (Chloromycetin).

Six patients with abscesses were included in this study. All revealed *Staph aureus;* four were coagulase positive, and the other two were negative. These patients responded well with localization after one week of therapy. Four of the six abscesses resolved spontaneously, and two of them necessitated incision and drainage. Eight patients with cellulitis were considered in this group. The cultures of the cellulitis revealed combinations of β-hemolytic *Streptococcus* and *Staph aureus,* coagulase positive. Two of the cellulitis cases had a pure culture of β-hemolytic *Streptococcus.* The largest number of failures in soft tissue infections was noted in the group of cellulitis. Of the eight cases, three revealed no effect. There was no correlative type of culture combinations which would set any pattern as to the failure. Of the 23 patients with soft tissue infections who were treated with sodium oxacillin, 17% did not react to the drug. Thirty per cent had untoward reactions, which included nausea, diarrhea, and maculopapular rash. The average duration of therapy was 12.9 days for the carbuncles, 5.5 days for the abscesses, and 12.4 days for the cellulitis; an over-all average of 11 days.

The study also included a group of 22 wound infections. There were 12 patients in this group who had cellulitis of the wound, four of which had combinations of β-hemolytic *Streptococcus* with *Staphylococcus.* One patient did not resolve his infection on the drug. This individual had to have the drug discontinued because of a severe skin manifestation (maculopapular rash). The average duration of therapy was 7.5 days. The over-all result yielded an 8% failure rate. Untoward reactions were very high, and five out of the 12 patients had some form of complication, including nausea, cutaneous reactions, and diarrhea.

Wound abscesses responded with resolution of the abscesses in four out of six patients. The over-all duration of therapy was 6.5 days.

The treatment of enteric fistula was attempted in four patients who had *Staph aureus* coagulase-positive cultures; however, there were two combinations with coliform bacteria and *Streptococcus pyogenes.* The over-all duration of therapy was 21 days. All of these patients had some form of gastrointestinal or cutaneous complication with the drug. All patients revealed a negative culture for *Staph aureus* during their therapy. It was found, however, that when the drug was discontinued the *Staph aureus* reoccurred, and the conclusion was drawn that surgery is still a necessary adjunct in the treatment of these particular complications.

Four patients with *Staph aureus* coagulase-positive septicemias, secondary to wound infections, were treated. Three out of the four septicemias revealed negative cultures from the 18th to the 22nd day. The average duration of therapy was 28 days. In these four patients there were no discernible untoward reactions.

Three patients with peritonitis secondary to dehiscence of gastrointestinal anastomosis were studied. Cultures were done by smearing and culturing paracentesis fluid. All were found to have *Staph aureus,* enterococci, and some coliform bacteria. Two out of these three cases resolved with localization of abscesses. Further paracentesis on these cases revealed a negative culture for *Staph aureus.* One of the patients died on the 18th day. The over-all duration of therapy was 15 days. Nausea and vomiting were noted in the therapy of two of these patients. All patients had adjunctive therapy which included hypothermia and adequate fluid replacement.

Comment

Sodium oxacillin has been thoroughly investigated in the treatment of staphylococcal infections. Numerous articles have shown that it is between 75% and 85% effective against *Staph aureus,* coagulase positive. Streptococcal disease does respond to the drug. In our study there has been an over-all good-to-excellent result in 83% of the cases. Of the nine cases that did not show any effect to the MPI penicillin, one had to be discontinued because of the cutaneous reaction; two were almost moribund, and both died soon after the drug was discontinued. It appeared in both of these latter cases that the drug had controlled the extent of the infection, but the patients continued to show a positive blood culture and a positive paracentesis. In the other six patients, three of whom had *Str pyogenes,* no reason could be found for the negative response to the drug.

Untoward reactions were usually found in the gastrointestinal tract or on the skin. The symptoms of the gastrointestinal tract were nausea, anorexia, vomiting, and diarrhea. Skin reactions were a maculopapular rash or a fine papular rash. Of the total patient load, 29% exhibited complications. Only in one case were the complications so severe that the drug had to be discontinued.

The average duration of therapy was approximately 11.7 days, but it was found that the drug could be continued for as long as 30 days without any signs of severe toxicity or untoward reactions.

Conclusions

1. In view of our studies it can be concluded that sodium oxacillin is a valuable drug in the control of surgical infections complicated with *Staphylococcus aureus,* coagulase positive.

2. β-hemolytic *Streptococcus* and enterococci are moderately sensitive to oxacillin.

William Schumer, MD, Mount Sinai Hospital, 2755 W 15th St, Chicago 8, Ill.

REFERENCES

1. Gourevitch, A.; Hunt, G. A.; Pursiano, T. A.; Carmack, C. C.; Moses, A. J.; and Lein, J.: Microbiological Evaluation of 5-Methyl-3-Phenyl-4-Isoxazolyl Penicillin, Antibiot Chemother NY 11: 780-789 (Dec) 1961.

2. Geraci, J. E.; Hoffmeister, R. T.; Nicols, D. R.; and Needham, G. M.: Preliminary Clinical and Laboratory Experiences With a New Oral Penicillin: 5-Methyl-3-Phenyl-4-Isoxazolyl Penicillin, Proc Mayo Clin 37:137-150 (Feb 28) 1962.

3. Simon, H. J., and Rantz, L. A.: The Newer Penicillins: I. Bacteriological and Clinical Pharmacological Investigations With Methicillin and Oxacillin, Ann Intern Med 57:335-343 (Sept) 1962.

4. Simon, H. J., and Rantz, L. A.: The Newer Penicillins: II. Clinical Experiences With Methicillin and Oxacillin, Ann Intern Med 57:344-362 (Sept) 1962.

5. White, A. C., and Smith, J.: Antistaphylococcal Activity of Penicillin P-12 (5-Methyl-3-Phenyl-4-Isoxazolyl Penicillin), Amer J Med Sci 243:202-208 (Feb) 1962.

6. Rutenberg, A. M.; Greenberg, H. L.; Levenson, S. S.; and Schweinburg, F. B.: Clinical Evaluation of 5-Methyl-3-Phenyl-4-Isoxazolyl Penicillin in Staphylococcal Infections, New Eng J Med 266: 755-759 (April 12) 1962.

7. Branch, A.; Rodger, K. C.; Tonning, H. O.; Lee, R. W.; and Power, E. E.: Laboratory and Clinical Experiences With a New Oral Synthetic Penicillin, 5-Methyl-3-Phenyl-4-Isoxazolyl Penicillin, Canad Med Ass J 86:97-101 (Jan 20) 1962.

8. Kallings, L. O.: The Susceptibility of Staphylococcal Hospital Strains to Methyl-Phenyl-Isoxazolyl Penicillin, Acta Path Microbiol Scand 54: 127-128, 1962.

9. Leduc, A., and Fontaine, J.: Etudes in vitro et in vivo d'une nouvelle pénicilline de synthèse: La 5-méthyl-3-phényl-4-isoxazolyl pénicilline, Canad Med Ass J 86:101-105 (Jan 20) 1962.

Significance of Meissner's Plexus in the Gastrin Mechanism

E. R. WOODWARD, MD
C. L. PARK, JR., MD
H. SCHAPIRO, MS
AND
L. R. DRAGSTEDT, MD
GAINESVILLE, FLA

The gastric phase of gastric secretion is mediated by the hormone *gastrin* which is elaborated by the antrum of the stomach. The exact cell of origin of this powerful hormone has not been determined; there are, however, many indications that intramural neural tissue plays an important role. Zeljong and Savich, working in Pavlov's laboratory, demonstrated that cocaine applied to the antral mucosa inhibited this hormonal mechanism.[1] This finding has been confirmed,[2] and other topical anesthetic agents without the vasoconstrictor properties of cocaine have a similar effect.[3] In addition topically applied atropine inhibits,[2] while topical acetylcholine potentiates, the gastrin mechanism.[4]

Baugh and co-workers stripped the seromuscular layer from the antrum, substituting the seromuscular coat of the colon.[5] This "hybrid antrum" responded normally to chemical stimuli, although the threshold for stimulation was increased. Since this dissection plane leaves the submucosa and submucous autonomic plexus of Meissner with the mucosa, it is clear that gastrin comes from one of these layers. Nyhus and his associates have dissected the antral mucosa from the muscularis through the submucous plane deep to the muscularis mucosae.[6,7] The mucosa remains in situ as a pedicle graft, receiving blood supply from the body of the stomach proximally and the duodenum distally. This procedure effectively obliterates the gastrin mechanism, indicating the possibility that the surgically destroyed submucosa has been important in the genesis of gastrin.

Both the above experiments have the disadvantage that they interfere seriously with the blood supply to the submucosa and mucosa of the antrum. Deloyers et al have studied the selective destruction of the myenteric plexus using 5% phenol.[8] This drug

Submitted for publication Feb 18, 1963.
The Department of Surgery, University of Florida, College of Medicine.
This work has been supported by National Institutes of Health Research Grants No. A 2372 and A 4178.

has been shown to be a specific destructive agent for all nervous tissue and in the above concentration causes minimal fibrosis and no necrosis. It was the purpose of the present experiment to determine if the submucous plexus of Meissner could be destroyed with 5% phenol without interference with the viability of the mucosa and the remainder of the submucosa.

Method

Seven dogs were prepared with Heidenhain pouches. After recovery from the surgical procedure, the animals were maintained on the standard laboratory diet with sodium chloride supplements to maintain electrolyte balance. The gastric juice secreted by the Heidenhain pouches was collected each 24 hours for 21 consecutive days. Volume, acid concentration, and daily HCl output were determined.

The animals were then reoperated upon, and the pyloric antrum was opened by an anterior wall gastrotomy. Thirty cubic centimeters of 5% phenol solution was injected into the submucosa with a fine hypodermic needle at four sites. The solution was diffused through the submucosa by digital massage. The gastrotomy was closed in layers.

One week later another 21-day collection period was repeated in each animal under identical conditions. Gastric juice collections were continued for a second three-week period in six of seven animals, for a third 21-day period in four, and for a total of five 21-day periods in two animals. The animals were sacrificed at the end of the experiment and histological examinations of the phenolized antrums made.

Results

Infiltration of the submucosa of the gastric antrum with 5% phenol produced an immediate blanching of the mucosa and to a lesser extent of the serosa, as observed at the operating table. However, all animals recovered and there was no indication of necrosis. The animals demonstrated a normal appetite and maintained a normal state of nutrition throughout the experiment, thus indicating that motor function was not seriously impaired.

The effect of chemical antroneurolysis on Heidenhain pouch secretion is summarized in the Table. The reduction in the first period varied from 38% to 90% in the seven animals. In one animal, No. 3, there was a progressive increase in periods 2 and 3 reaching a level only slightly below the control. In animal No. 5, secretion seemed to return in period 2 but was again markedly depressed in period 3. In the remaining four animals Heidenhain pouch secretion remained at low levels for long periods, up to 105 days in two studies.

The Effect of Chemical Antroneurolysis on Heidenhain Pouch Secretion

	Period *					
Dog No.	Control	I	II	III	IV	V
1	21	11	14			
2	52	15	20	16	19	16
3	39	24	29	33		
4	52	17				
5	26	7	21	10		
6	16	2	4	4	2	2
7	43	4	4			

* Each period 21 consecutive days. Average daily HCl output in mEq.

Necropsy revealed in each dog a stomach which appeared grossly normal in size, shape, and color, with no evidence of gastric retention. The mucosa of the pyloric antrum appeared grossly normal, but was somewhat less pliable and more adherent to the muscular coat. Histologic preparations from the antrum disclosed similar microscopic findings in all animals (Figure, *A*). In each there was complete absence of autonomic ganglia in the submucosa with only a few well-preserved nerve bundles remaining. There was moderate fibrosis in the submucosa with numerous, thin-walled ectatic blood vessels. There were minimal inflammatory reaction, and a moderate atrophy of the antral mucosa as indicated by some intestinal metaplasia in the pits of the gastric glands. The myenteric plexus was completely intact in all animals. Normal submucosa of the canine antrum is shown in the Figure, *B*.

Comment

Infiltration of the submucosa of the pyloric antrum with dilute phenol solution produced a striking reduction in gastric secretion in Heidenhain-pouch dogs. In four of the seven dogs studied, this reduction was

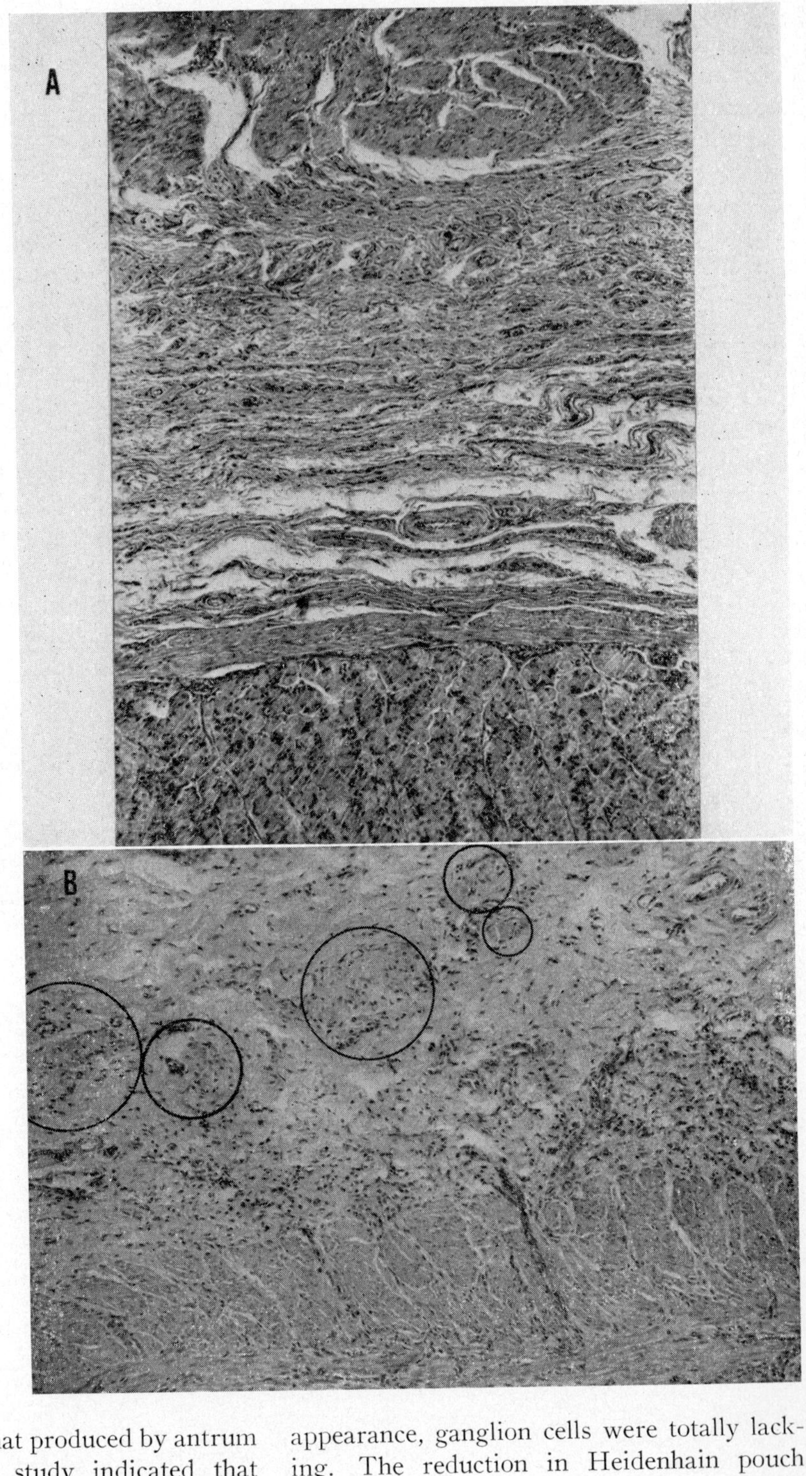

A, phrenolized submucosa of antrum, showing complete absence of ganglion cells composing Meissner's plexus.

B, submucosa of normal dog antrum, showing (circled) ganglia of Meissner's plexus.

in the same range as that produced by antrum resection. Histologic study indicated that relatively selective destruction of the ganglion cells in Meissner's submucous plexus had been achieved. Although nerve trunks were diminished in number and abnormal in appearance, ganglion cells were totally lacking. The reduction in Heidenhain pouch secretion was immediate and was sustained at a constant level for as long as 3½ months, indicating that the pathologic process was a static one. There was definite injury to other tissues as indicated by fibrosis and vascular ectasia in the submucosa and some atrophy in the mucosa. However blood supply had clearly been maintained in all cases.

Local anesthetics and anticholinergics [1-3] inhibit, and cholinergics [4] stimulate, gastrin release. The antrum still produces gastrin when its seromuscular coat is replaced by that of the colon.[5] Surgical destruction of the submucosa ablates the gastrin mechanism.[6,7] When one adds to these observations the data of the present experiment, it seems apparent that not only is Meissner's plexus intimately associated with the formation of gastrin but that, in all probability, the ganglion cells are the cells of origin of the hormone.

Summary and Conclusions

In seven Heidenhain pouch dogs, the submucosa of the pyloric antrum was infiltrated with 5% phenol solution. A drastic and sustained reduction in Heidenhain pouch secretion ensued. Histologic study indicated selective destruction of the ganglia constituting Meissner's submucous plexus.

It is probable that the ganglion cell of Meissner's plexus is the cell of origin of the hormone gastrin.

C. Ian Hood, MD, Department of Pathology, University of Florida, interpreted the histologic preparations.

E. R. Woodward, MD, Professor and Chairman, The Department of Surgery, College of Medicine, University of Florida, Gainesville, Fla.

REFERENCES

1. Zeljong, G. P., and Savich, V. V.: Concerning the Mechanism of Gastric Secretion, in Proceedings of Society of Russian Physicians (Jan-May) 1911-1912, quoted by Babkin, B. P.: Secretory Mechanism of the Digestive Glands, ed 2, New York: Paul B. Hoeber, Inc., Medical Book Department of Harper & Brothers, 1950, pp 470-471.

2. Woodward, E. R.; Lyon, E. S.; Landor, J.; and Dragstedt, L. R.: The Physiology of the Gastric Antrum, Gastroenterology 27:766, 1954.

3. Woodward, E. R., and Schapiro, H.: Effect of Local Anesthetics on the Isolated Antrum of the Stomach in Dogs, Amer J Physiol 192:479, 1958.

4. Robertson, C. R.; Langlois, K.; Martin, C. G.; Slezak, G.; and Grossman, M. I.: Release of Gastrin in Response to Bathing the Pyloric Mucosa with Acetylcholine, Amer J Physiol 163:27, 1950.

5. Baugh, C. M.; Bravo, J. L.; Barcena, J.; and Dragstedt, L. R.: Studies on the Site and Mechanism of Gastrin Release, AMA Arch Surg 76: 441, 1958.

6. Jones, T. W.; DeVito, R. V.; Nyhus, L. M.; and Harkins, H. N.: The Effect of Antroneurolysis Upon Antral Function of the Stomach, Surg Gynec Obstet 105:687, 1957.

7. Nyhus, L. M.; Chapman, N. D.; DeVito, R. V.; and Harkins, H. N.: The Control of Gastrin Release: An Experimental Study Illustrating a New Concept, Gastroenterology 39:582, 1960.

8. Deloyers, L.; Cordier, R.; and Duprez, M. A.: A New Approach to the Physiology of So-Called Cardiospasm: Experimental Production of Cardiospasm in Cats After Destruction of Auerbach's Plexus, Ann Surg 146:167, 1957.

Carcinoma of Tongue, Buccal Mucosa, and Mandible

Results From Surgical Treatment

RALPH F. BOWERS, MD
AND
WALTER H. HENLEY, MD
MEMPHIS

Selection of type of therapy for oral cancer is difficult to establish accurately and involves the use of x-ray therapy, combination of x-ray and surgery, surgery alone, and, if surgery, how extensive the procedure should be and whether the excision should be continuous with a lymphatic extirpation, interrupted lymphatic extirpation, or delayed lymphatic resection and advantage of the so-called commando procedure. Obviously, any attempt at solving these problems must include a survey of long-term results. One must realize that there is no consistency in the surgical attack by different surgeons.

A review of the literature reveals a five-year cure rate of 22% and 46% following radiation therapy alone.[1-3] Combinations of x-ray to source followed by radical neck dissection for carcinoma of the tongue yielded 25% in 1940 [4] and later 34.3% in 1951 [5] at Memorial Hospital in New York. All reports indicate better results in buccal mucosa carcinoma and alveolar ridge carcinoma than in the tongue.

Surgically, Slaughter [6] achieved 32% cure rate in intraoral cancer and Ward [7] reported an over-all rate of 40% and 35% for the tongue. In 1960, Slaughter [8] again reported 35% and 32% using different techniques. Kremen and Arhelger [9] in a recent publication report 68% five-year survival rate for tongue carcinoma treated surgically.

One recognizes immediately that there is no uniformity in the surgical series permitting accurate comparison, and lack of uniformity pervades the radiation reports also.

Enthusiasm for surgery has increased after the encouraging results of Kremen, Slaughter, and Ward.[6-11] More radical extirpations in continuity were attempted and seemed hopeful, particularly when the commando procedure began to better the results. This led surgeons to attack the lesions in the

Submitted for publication Feb 1, 1963.

From the Surgical Service, Veterans Administration Medical Teaching Group Hospital, and the Department of Surgery of the University of Tennessee College of Medicine.

hypopharynx and extensive posterior tongue lesions with involvement of the soft palate and peritonsillar area. The surgical gymnastics were mastered, but one must review the gain by experience. X-ray seemed nonvirile when lymph node metastases occurred. Perhaps the pendulum has swung too far toward surgery.

The area defies stereotyped procedures, and therefore any study is handicapped because of the different surgeons' abilities and philosophies. Also, it must be borne in mind that any individual operator over a period of years will from experience, new surgical modalities, fortifying medications, and other advantages change his surgical maneuvering in order to capitalize on these gain-producing matters. In other words, all follow-up studies in these lesions will lack consistency and therefore meaningful accuracy. However, if a single surgeon or a group of similarly trained surgeons report, as much consistency as possible will be attained.

In this study, it has proved to be advantageous to classify these lesions into four groups: carcinoma of the tongue, carcinoma of the buccal mucosa, carcinoma of the alveolar ridge, and carcinoma of the hypopharynx. Only one case of carcinoma of the hypopharynx has been handled in this series. Three patients with adamantinoma are included although most workers do not regard this as a malignant lesion.[12] However, the tendency to recurrence, if the lesion is not eradicated with the proper margin, is noted, and extension to the base of the skull has been occasionally seen. Metastases must indeed be rare.

There are 59 patients in the series, averaging 60 years of age, and 26 of the patients had carcinoma in the buccal mucosa, 22 in the tongue, seven in the alveolar ridge, one in the hypopharynx, and the three adamantinoma patients. All but one patient were male.

Mortality

There were five immediate postoperative deaths (mortality rate: 8.5%). Four occurred in extensive carcinoma of the tongue with involvement of the soft palate and hypopharynx and one in a hopeless extensive buccal mucosa lesion. Three patients were actually inoperable, and two died of *Staphylococcus* septicemia following aspiration pneumonia in spite of tracheotomy. One patient died because tracheotomy was not performed when aspiration difficulties arose after glossectomy and neck dissection. Postoperative plans provided use of tracheotomy immediately if any respiration difficulties arose. At night, a surgeon, unfamiliar with this plan, unfortunately delayed tracheotomy, which resulted in hypoxia, anoxia, cardiac arrest, and death. This death was the result of an error in technical judgment. Tracheotomy should have been done at time of operation or certainly promptly when difficulty arose. One patient died from infection of tracheotomy, carotid artery thrombosis, and aspiration pneumonia following radical neck dissection for metastatic cervical lymph node disease three years after the original extirpation operation. Another tongue patient died after glossectomy when the internal carotid artery was removed during radical neck dissection because it was invaded by tumor before the days of routine arterial grafting. Early good results and encouraging reports in the literature created enough enthusiasm to attempt these poorly selected procedures.[1-3,13-15] When one studies these deaths, it is obvious that the good results from radiation therapy, cobalt, million-volt machines, or interstitial radiation by radon seeds or radium were unfortunately ignored. It would be helpful if it is borne in mind that in each location, patients received either surgery alone, surgery plus radiation, or radiation followed by surgery.

Buccal Mucosa

These 26 cases include carcinoma of the floor of the mouth as well as that of the cheek (Table 1).

There were four *local excisions* with no postoperative deaths. Three are alive at two years, one year, and four months, respectively. One patient died of a heart attack 9½ years postoperatively with no evidence of cancer.

TABLE 1.—*Buccal Mucosa*

Operation	Total	Surgery Alone	Surgery + Radiation	Radiation + Surgery	Survivals: Plus 5 Yr	Survivals: Minus 5 Yr
Local excision	4	2	2		1	3
Local excision + mandibulectomy	2	1		1		2
Local excision + radical neck dissection	5	2		3	3	2
Local excision + mandibulectomy + radical neck dissection	15	9	3	3	6	9 (1) *
Total	26	14	5	7	10	16

* Immediate postoperative death.

There were two *local excisions plus mandibulectomy.* One patient died of carcinoma at one year and the other has been lost to follow-up.

Five patients had *local excision plus radical neck dissection.* Four of these patients have survived five years, eight years, nine years, and 11 years, respectively, without evidence of disease. One patient died of cancer 13 months after surgery.

Local excision plus mandibulectomy plus radical neck dissection numbered 15 patients with one postoperative death due to aspiration pneumonia and *Staphylococcus* septicemia. Of these, two died during the first year—one of cancer at seven months and the other patient died of acute pneumonitis at eight months. Three patients died during the second year—one from heart disease (no cancer at autopsy) and the other two patients died from cancer. Another patient died at 6½ years of generalized arteriosclerosis, cardiovascular disease, pneumonia, and pyelonephritis—no cancer was found at autopsy. One patient is alive one year; two are alive at more than two years; two are alive at more than five years; one patient is alive more than ten years with recurrence and has been treated with x-ray; and two other patients are alive more than 11 years without disease.

Of the 26 patients, 15 are still alive, 1 is lost to follow-up, and 10 have died. Sixteen of these patients could eat and talk satisfactorily.

Tongue

Twenty-two patients received operation (Table 2).

One patient had *local excision* and died at two years of bronchogenic carcinoma.

One patient who had *local excision plus mandibulectomy* is alive at one year and three months.

There were 12 patients with *local excision plus radical neck dissection* with three postoperative deaths. Three died during the first year of cancer; one patient from accident at three years (no cancer at postmortem examination); another patient died after six years of heart failure (no cancer at autopsy); two others died after seven years—one from

TABLE 2.—*Tongue*

Operation	Total	Surgery Alone	Surgery + Radiation	Radiation + Surgery	Survivals: Plus 5 Yr	Survivals: Minus 5 Yr
Local excision	1	1				1
Local excision + mandibulectomy	1	1				1
Local excision + radical neck dissection	12	5	3	4	4	8 (3) *
Local excision + mandibulectomy + radical neck dissection	8	6	2		2	6 (1) *
Total	22	13	5	4	6	16

* Immediate postoperative deaths.

TABLE 3.—*Alveolar Ridge*

Operation	Total	Surgery Alone	Surgery + Radiation	Radiation + Surgery	Minus 5 Yr Survivals
Local excision	2	2			2
Local excision + mandibulectomy	1	1			1
Local excision + radical neck dissection	1		1		1
Local excision + mandibulectomy + radical neck dissection	3	2		1	3
Total	7	5	1	1	7

aortic thrombosis and the other in an accident—and no tumor was found in either at necropsy; and one patient is still alive at seven years. One patient is lost to follow-up.

Eight patients underwent *local excision plus mandibulectomy plus radical neck dissection* with one postoperative death. Three died during the first year, two from cancer and one from unknown cause. One patient died after six years from carcinoma; three patients are still alive at four months, two years, and nine years, respectively. Twelve patients could eat and talk satisfactorily but with handicap.

Of the 22 patients in this group, five are alive without cancer at nine years, seven years, two years, one year, and four months, respectively. Seven died of cancer: one at six years, two at one year, two at eight months, one at seven months, and one at two months. Four died of other causes: two at seven years, one at six years, and one at three years in whom no cancer was found at autopsy. One patient died of unknown cause at 11 months. One patient is lost to follow-up and has probably died of cancer.

Alveolar Ridge

Seven patients were operated on (Table 3). Two patients had *local excision* with bone removal and are alive at two years and four years, respectively.

Local excision plus mandibulectomy: one patient is alive at one year.

Local excision plus radical neck dissection: one patient with rapidly growing carcinoma died at two months with recurrence in the mouth.

Local excision plus mandibulectomy plus radical neck dissection: one patient died at 2½ years of carcinoma. One patient is alive at two years, and another was alive with no disease at 4½ years when lost to follow-up.

All patients could eat and talk satisfactorily. Of the seven patients, four are still alive without disease—one at four years, two at two years, and one at one year. One other patient was alive with no disease at 4½ years and has been lost to follow-up. Two patients died of tumor—one at 2½ years and the other at two months. Patients operated on have not been followed long enough to establish five-year survival rate.

Commando

The commando procedure requires extirpation of at least the anterior half of the tongue, anterior floor of the mouth and mandible at the chin, combined with a suprahyoid neck dissection or radical neck dissection. Seven patients received this operation. Four patients (57%) are living but eat and talk with considerable difficulty. These lesions had their origin in the buccal mucosa which in our series has proved to be more satisfactorily handled than the tongue lesions. This success probably reflects accessibility for resection rather than triumphant surgery per se. Two patients (one buccal mucosa; one tongue) wore permanent tracheostomy tubes; and in two, permanent gastrostomy was necessary.

The hypopharynx patient underwent multiple operations in stages plus x-ray therapy, was never free of cancer, but lived nearly nine years!

The adamantinoma patients were all adequately resected with no recurrence at 2 years, 6½ years, and 9 years, respectively, and all can eat and talk satisfactorily.

Our results show 33% five-year survivals in tongue, 40% in the buccal mucosa group, and five-year survivals in the alveolar ridge group have not been followed long enough to establish rate. Survival rates do not include the five patients who died immediately after operation.

The postoperative deaths clearly indicate overenthusiasm for surgical therapy cases (four out of five) well beyond the scope of surgical cure or decent surgical palliation.

Conclusion

The study shows that good results can be expected in properly chosen patients with well-planned radical surgical maneuvering. It also indicates that there is a limitation to the use of surgery and, regardless of interest, one must employ radiation when extensive manipulation is necessary. Resection of the soft palate and hypopharynx in the extensive cases has produced disastrous results in four of our patients. The commando procedure has been attended with good cure rate averages and fair functioning results.

Ralph F. Bowers, MD, Chief, Surgical Service, Kennedy Veterans Administration Hospital, Memphis 15, Tenn.

REFERENCES

1. Baud, J.: End Results of Radiotherapy of Cancer of the Tongue, Amer J Roentgen 63:701-711 (May) 1950.

2. Cade, S.: Treatment of Cancer of the Tongue, Amer J Roentgen 63:716-718 (May) 1950.

3. Sellers, A. H.: A Statistical Review of Intra-Oral Cancer, Canad Med Ass J 83:157-159 (July 23) 1960.

4. Martin, H. E.; Munster, H.; and Sugarbaker, E. D.: Cancer of the Tongue, Arch Surg 41:888-963 (Oct) 1940.

5. Martin, H.; Del Valle, B.; Ehrlich, H.; and Cahan, W. G.: Neck Dissection, Cancer 4:441-499 (May) 1951.

6. Slaughter, D. P.: Surgical Management of Intra-Oral Cancer, Amer J Roentgen 73:605-610 (April) 1955.

7. Ward, G. E.; Edgerton, M. T.; Chambers, R. G.; and McKee, D. M.: Cancer of the Oral Cavity and Pharynx and Results of Treatment by Means of the Composite Operation (in Continuity With Radical Neck Dissection), Ann Surg 150:202-220 (Aug) 1959.

8. Southwick, H. W.; Slaughter, D. P.; and Trevino, E. T.: Elective Neck Dissection for Intraoral Cancer, AMA Arch Surg 80:905-909 (June) 1960.

9. Kremen, A. J., and Arhelger, S. W.: Early Cancer of the Oral Cavity With Special Reference to Cancer of the Tongue, Postgrad Med 27:422-427 (March) 1960.

10. Kremen, A. J.: Cancer of the Tongue: Surgical Technique for Primary Combined en Bloc Resection of Tongue, Floor of Mouth, and Cervical Lymphatics, Surgery 30:227-240 (July) 1951.

11. Slaughter, D. P., and Southwick, H. W.: En Bloc Resection of Cancer of the Mouth and Cervical Lymphatics With Preservation of the Mandible, Ann Surg 136:957-963 (Dec) 1952.

12. Bernier, J. L.: Manual for the Differential Diagnosis of Oral Lesions, St. Louis: The C. V. Mosby Company, 1942, p 178.

13. Ash, C. L., and Millar, O. B.: Radiotherapy of Cancer of the Tongue and Floor of the Mouth, Amer J Roentgen 73:611-619 (April) 1955.

14. Lampe, I.: Radiation Therapy of Cancer of the Buccal Mucosa and Lower Gingiva, Amer J Roentgen 73:628-638 (April) 1955.

15. Wookey, H.; Ash, C.; Welsh, W. K.; and Mustard, R. A.: Treatment of Oral Cancer by Combination of Radiotherapy and Surgery, Ann Surg 134:529-540 (Oct) 1951.

Successful Resection of Syphilitic Aneurysm of Aortic Arch

GILBERT B. BRADHAM, MD
AND
JULIAN T. BUXTON, JR., MD
CHARLESTON, SC

It is well inferred that symptoms caused by syphilitic aneurysms of the aortic arch are probably of only two years' duration, their limitation being imposed by death of the patient. Kampmeier [3] examined 188 such cases and found that only 18 of these lived longer than two years.

In the past 12 years, there has been a vigorous attempt by surgical means to alter this unfavorable prognosis. In 1958, DeBakey, Cooley, Crawford, and Morris [1] reported seven years experience involving 50 aneurysms of the aortic arch, 35 of which were syphilitic in origin. Their operative mortality was 56%. This mortality figure is thought still generally representative by Gaertner, Spencer, and Bahnson [2] who reviewed the subject in 1962.

It is because of this high mortality and because of the technical aspects of such surgery that we wish to present a single case of syphilitic aneurysm of the aortic arch and innominate artery that was successfully resected without need of cardiopulmonary bypass.

Report of a Case

A 67-year-old Negro female was admitted to the Medical College Hospital on May 25, 1962, having a one-year history of a progressively enlarging mass in her right neck which was accompanied by progressively intense pain. She recently had experienced hemoptysis.

The patient was normally developed, but showed evidence of recent weight loss. Vital signs were normal. There was a large pulsatile mass occupying the right anterior supraclavicular space and appearing to erode the sternoclavicular juncture. There was pain on abduction of the right arm. There was an apical grade 2 diastolic heart murmur.

Laboratory data included hemoglobin of 8.4 gm% with microcytic hypochromic indices, a positive serology, and a prothrombin time 50% of normal.

Submitted for publication Feb 5, 1963.

Fellow in Surgical Cardiology, University of California in Los Angeles (Dr. Bradham); Instructor in Surgery, Department of Surgery, Medical College of South Carolina (Dr. Buxton).

From the Department of Surgery, Medical College of South Carolina.

Supported in part by the John A. Hartford Foundation.

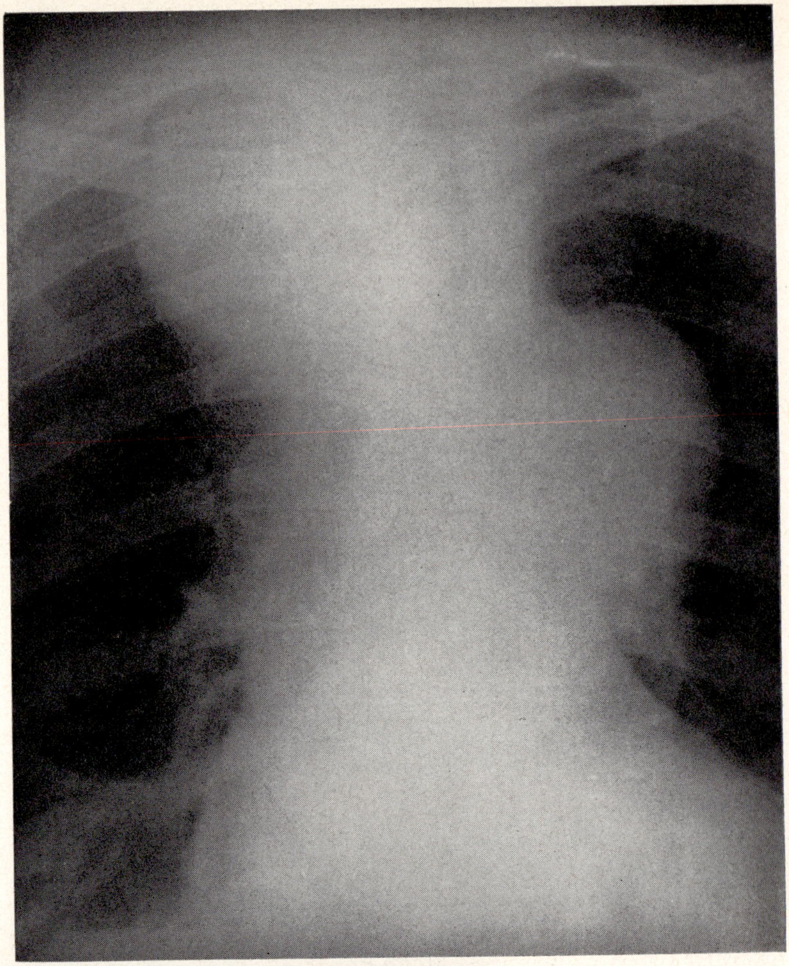

Fig 1.—Preoperative chest film showing large aneurysm in the superior mediastinum.

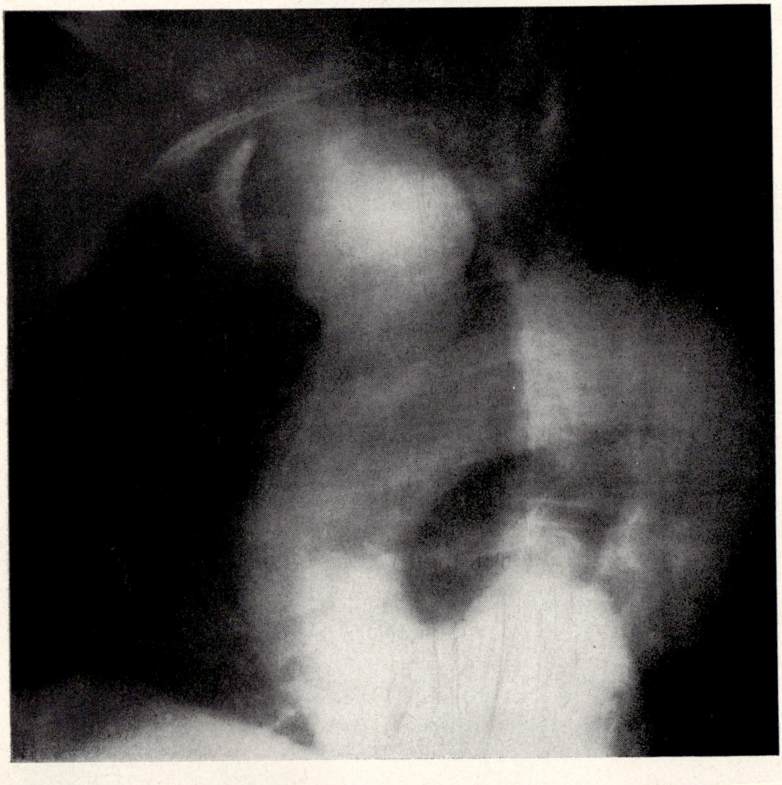

Fig 2.—Angiocardiogram demonstrating aneurysm arising from the arch of the aorta at the innominate artery area.

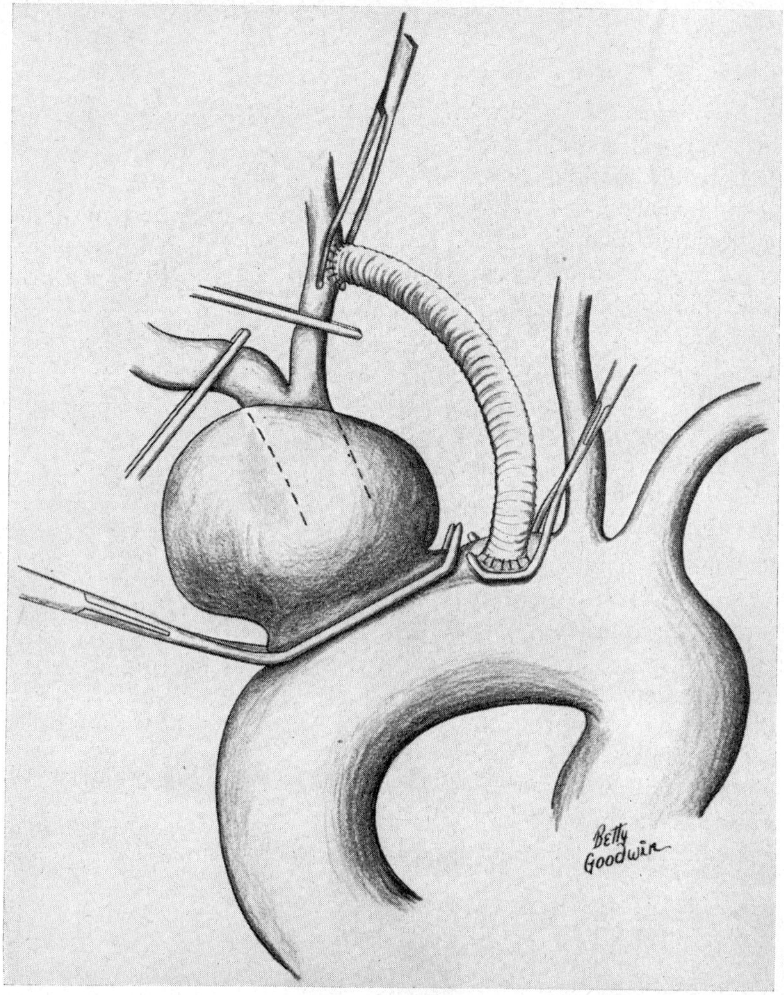

Fig 3.—Artist's conception of operating procedure shows normal innominate artery stretched over the aneurysm posteriorly.

Chest films, (Fig 1) chest fluoroscopy, barium swallow, and angiocardiograms (Fig 2) revealed an aneurysm of the ascending aortic arch and innominate artery. An EKG was interpreted as showing first degree A-V block with possible old anterior myocardial infarction.

The patient was prepared for surgery and on June 1, 1962, an incision in the right neck was made in continuity with a median sternotomy. An $8 \times 10 \times 12$ cm aneurysm was found arising from the aortic arch and involving the proximal two thirds of the innominate artery. With aid of partial occlusion clamps, a Teflon shunt was placed from the distal aortic arch to the right common carotid artery. A large Satinsky clamp was then used to partially occlude the proximal aortic arch and isolate the base of the aneurysm. The common carotid artery proximal to the shunt and the right subclavian artery were then occluded and the aneurysm was resected (Fig 3).

The clamped aortic wall was closed, and the remaining innominate artery was reimplanted at a more proximal site in the arch. The Teflon shunt was left in, and blood appeared to flow through the shunt, the entire common carotid artery, and the subclavian artery. A nodule was palpated in the right lobe of the thyroid, and a partial thyroidectomy was performed. A subsequent pathological report was benign adenoma of thyroid and perivascular round-cell infiltration in aortic wall compatible with syphilitic origin.

The patient did well except for tachycardia in the early postoperative course. She was discharged on the 19th postoperative day, asymptomatic and afebrile. She has been followed since and is apparently fully recovered.

Comment

The technique in the case presented was uncomplicated and carried few unusual operative risks. No cardiopulmonary bypass was necessitated, and, therefore, clotting problems, exposure to large amounts of foreign blood, and operative time and extent were minimized. Partial occlusion of the aortic arch is well tolerated so long as left ventricular strain or breaking off of a luminal plaque is not encountered. Shunting of blood to the common carotid by partial occlusion of distal arch and common carotid can be easily accomplished without marked diminution of flow through either vessel. Persistent tachycardia during the early postoperative course did occur in the patient presented, and this was thought to be due to dislodgement of a portion of plaque into a coronary despite gradual closure of clamps on the aortic wall. This is felt to be the greatest danger present at operation.

Gaertner, Spencer, and Bahnson pointed out the inadvisability of operating upon patients with extensive lesions of the arch unless that patient is in severe distress. They are more optimistic regarding patients with well localized lesions of the arch who are in otherwise good general health. We feel that the case presented certainly falls within this latter category, and that her successful operation was due to this fortunate circumstance.

The contribution of one such case is thought sufficient to strengthen categorization of such lesions and to lend optimism towards their surgical treatment.

Summary

A case of excision of an aneurysm of the ascending aortic arch and the successful reestablishment of arterial supply to the arm and head is presented.

The technical details are discussed, and the need of preoperative categorization of lesions of the arch to predetermine operative prognosis is stressed.

Julian T. Buxton, Jr., MD, Vascular Laboratory, Roper Hospital, 300-310 Calhoun St, Charleston 16, SC.

REFERENCES

1. DeBakey, M. E.; Cooley, D. A.; Crawford, E. S.; and Morris, G. C., Jr.: Aneurysms of the Thoracic Aorta: Analysis of 179 Patients Treated by Resection, J Thorac Surg 36:393, 1958.

2. Gaertner, R. A.; Spencer, F. C.; and Bahnson, H. T.: Current Status of Surgery of the Lesions of the Aortic Arch, Progr Cardiov Dis 4:373, 1962.

3. Kampmeier, R. H.: Saccular Aneurysm of the Thoracic Aorta: A Clinical Study of 633 Cases, Ann Intern Med 12:624, 1938.

Myxoma of the Left Atrium

Presenting as an Embolus to the Femoral Artery

RICHARD W. HIBNER, MD
HOWARD F. CORBUS, MD
AND
HARLAN F. FULMER, MD
FRESNO, CALIF

Introduction

Intracardiac myxoma is a rare tumor, initial manifestations of which may be life-threatening or fatal. Peripheral embolization is one such manifestation which, if recognized and acted upon promptly, may lead to the successful treatment of this unusual disorder.

Less than 250 cases of intracardiac myxoma have been reported in the medical literature. Prichard [1] reviewed 128 cases in 1951, and in 1959 Padhi [2] added 90 more. Antemortem diagnosis of this tumor has been reported only during the last decade. The first successful removal of such a tumor was reported in March, 1955, by Crafoord,[3] and since that time 50 or more additional cases have appeared in the literature. Silverman [8] and associates reviewed embolization as a manifestation of intracardiac myxoma and reported a patient who succumbed to this complication. Three cases [4-6] have been reported in which the diagnosis has been established by embolectomy followed by successful removal of the tumor (Table). A fourth such patient is described below.

This paper was presented at the Stanford Surgical Society meeting, Palo Alto, Calif, Nov 10, 1962.

From the department of vascular and general surgery (Dr. Hibner) and the department of internal medicine (Dr. Corbus), Fresno Medical Group; from the department of pathology, St. Agnes Hospital (Dr. Fulmer).

Report of Case

The patient was a 41-year-old housewife whose past history was devoid of major illnesses. On rare occasions she had experienced night cramps in the right calf and had been aware of numbness in the right lower extremity after prolonged periods of sitting, but she had never had intermittent claudication. She was not aware of ever having had a heart murmur, cardiac arrhythmia, or symptoms of congestive heart failure. She had undergone a complete physical examination just two weeks prior to this illness and no abnormalities had been encountered. While swimming in a mountain lake at Yosemite National Park on Aug 24, 1962, severe pain and numbness in both legs and feet began abruptly. The symptoms started at four o'clock in the afternoon. She was taken to the Lewis Memorial Hospital in Yosemite Valley where the diagnosis of acute arterial occlusion of the right lower extremity was made, and she was immediately transferred to the St. Agnes Hospital in Fresno by ambulance. Upon arrival, she complained of severe pain in the right leg and inability to move this extremity. During the trip the pain and numbness in the left leg had disappeared.

On physical examination the blood pressure was 132/80, pulse 60, respiration 16, and temperature 98.6 F (37.0 C). The heart appeared to be in normal sinus rhythm and was not enlarged to percussion. No murmurs were heard. Significant physical findings were limited to the lower extremities. The right calf was somewhat swollen. The right leg was cool to touch distal to the lower thigh. The patient

Myxoma Diagnosed by Embolectomy With Successful Tumor Removal

Author	Age, Sex	Site of Embolus
Beanlands	8, F	Femoral artery
Zuidema	38, F	Bilateral popliteal artery
Differding	12, M	Left popliteal & right common femoral arteries
Hibner	42, F	Common femoral artery

was unable to move the right foot. Both femoral pulses were easily felt. The popliteal, dorsalis pedis, and posterior tibial pulses were present on the left and absent on the right. No venous filling or capillary pulsation was noted in the right foot. The right lower leg was anesthetic to pin prick.

The hemoglobin was 10.8 gm with a hematocrit of 33 vol%. The white blood cell count was 8,800 with 16% bands, 75% neutrophils, 7% lymphocytes, and 2% monocytes. The specific gravity of the urine was 1.016 and it was negative for protein and reducing substances. Six to eight white cells and one to three red cells per high-power field were seen in the centrifuged microscopic sediment on a voided specimen. A portable chest x-ray taken on the morning after admission was normal, and the electrocardiogram was normal.

Two hours after admission and 7½ hours after the onset of symptoms, the patient was taken to the operating room.

Under spinal anesthesia, the right popliteal artery was exposed by an anterior-medial approach. Heparin was injected distally and the artery was isolated and opened. No thrombus was encountered and none could be suctioned proximally from the superficial femoral artery. There was no bleeding from the arterial incision. The right common femoral artery was then exposed and pulsations were seen proximal to the point of bifurcation of the superficial femoral and the profunda femoral arteries. As the area of apparent occlusion was incised, a pale gray-yellow gelatinous mass oozed from the incision and was removed. It measured approximately 2 × 1 × 0.8 cm. Strong pulsations were then noted in the remainder of the femoral artery and in the popliteal artery. Through the popliteal incision, three small similar appearing emboli were removed by suction from the distal popliteal artery and from the anterior and posterior tibial arteries. Good back flow was obtained from the distal popliteal artery, and circulation appeared to be re-established into the tibial arteries.

Antibiotics and heparin were administered postoperatively, and for 24 hours she appeared to be doing well. The right foot was pink and warm and displayed good venous filling despite absence of pedal pulses. She did well until 24 hours after operation at which time she experienced severe pain in her right foot, which became cold, mottled, and cyanotic. Examination disclosed that the previously palpable pedal pulses in the left foot had disappeared. Spinal anesthesia was administered without improvement. It was presumed that another shower of tumor emboli had been released from the left atrium.

Urgent open heart surgery seemed in order, and the patient was transferred by ambulance to the University of California Hospital in San Francisco, where a fortunate cancellation in the surgical schedule permitted an operation a few hours after admission. Using the open technique with extracorporeal circulation, and with induced ventricular fibrillation, a large myxoma weighing 17.5 gm was successfully removed from the left atrium (Fig 1). The right popliteal artery was re-explored through the old wound, and several bits of thrombus and tumor were removed from the tibial arteries by suction with a return of circulation to the right foot. Continuous epidural anesthesia was administered for 24 hours. Postoperatively, she did well, circulation to the right foot was re-established, and she was discharged to her home approximately two weeks after admission to the University of California Hospital.

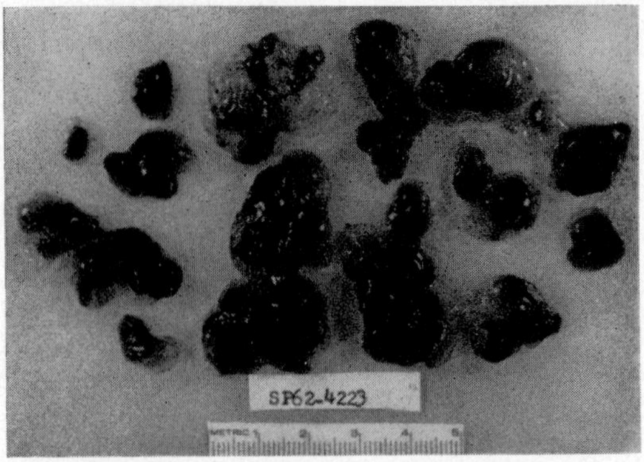

Fig 1.—Particles of the myxoma tumor removed from the left atrial septum. Total weight of tumor tissue is 17.5 gm.

Etiology

Although the neoplastic origin of intracardiac myxomas has been challenged in the past, the evidence at the present time supports this concept. Prichard[1] summarizes this as follows:

> Most of the tumors are much larger than thrombi, and far less cellular. [Myxomas] occur for the most part in hearts free of other disease. There is usually no evidence of damage to account for thrombosis. Almost all the myxomas are found in the atriums, especially the left, while thrombi occur with . . . equal frequency in the atriums and the ventricles. Most atrial thrombi are in the auricular appendage, and myxomas are not found in that location. There are no convincing intermediate stages between a frank thrombus and a myxoma, even in the pedunculated and ball valve thrombi found in the atriums. There is no evidence of stratification in myxomas, although almost all thrombi show it.

Fischer and Hellstrom[7] report more direct supporting evidence for the neoplastic concept of cardiac myxomas based on histochemical studies. Identical reactions were found in the umbilical cord, cutaneous

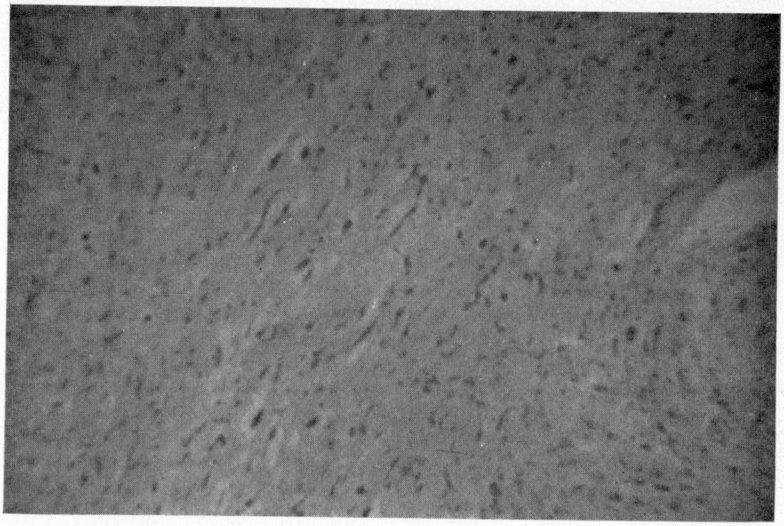

Fig 2.—Myxoma tumor cells. Reduced 31% from mag × 10.

myxoma, and cardiac myxoma with all giving positive reactions for acid mucopolysaccharide. This may be demonstrated in thrombi also, but only at sites of early organization of granulation tissue; it is absent in older organized fibrous thrombi. In contrast, acid mucopolysaccharide is demonstrated in all areas of myxoma.

Electronmicroscopy studies [5] have shown a cellular composition clearly distinct from that seen in organized thrombus.

Still unexplained is the precise histogenesis of this myxomatous tissue. Both Fischer and Hellstrom [7] and Prichard [1] have studied atrial septa and fossa ovalis in normal adult and infant hearts without finding myxomatous tissue. Both call attention to the increased amount of connective tissue in this area compared with the remainder of the heart. Possibly this accounts for the preponderance of myxomas at this site. This tumor of primitive mesenchyme may be derived from septal connective tissue gone awry.

Pathology

Primary cardiac tumors are so infrequent that they may be considered pathological curiosities. Limburner * records four cases (0.05%) in 8,500 autopsies at Mayo Clinic. Myxomas account for 35% to 50% of these primary tumors.[7] Strauss and Merliss [13] report eight cardiac myxomas in an analysis of

* In Friedberg, C. K.[12]

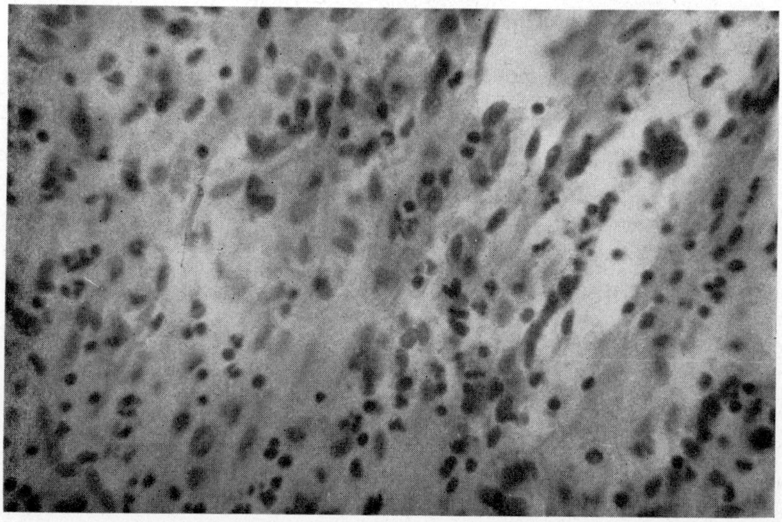

Fig 3. — High - power magnification of myxoma tumor cells.

480,331 autopsies for an incidence of 0.0017%.

Seventy-five per cent of myxomas are located in the left auricle, typically attached to the atrial wall of the fossa ovalis. Less frequent sites are right auricle and left ventricle.

Characteristically, a cardiac myxoma is a pedunculated mass varying from a minute size incidentally discovered at autopsy to one nearly filling the atrium. It is lobular with a smooth villous surface and has a glistening myxoid appearance. The color varies from white to yellow-white to tan, and the consistency varies from gelatinous to firm.

Microscopically, the tumor consists of myxomatous stroma containing variable numbers of stellate and spindle cells and many capillaries, which may have prominent endothelial cells (Fig 2 and 3). Some areas may be more dense with collagen, less cellular and less vascular. Areas of hemorrhages, hemosiderin, thrombus, and leukocytic infiltration may be seen.

Diagnosis

Intracardiac tumors may defy antemortem or preoperative diagnosis, either because they remain asymptomatic prior to some catastrophic event, such as the case herein reported, or because they may be indistinguishable clinically from rheumatic heart disease with mitral stenosis. The signs and symptoms which mimic rheumatic heart disease are a consequence of obstruction of the mitral valve and a partial obliteration of the left atrial cavity. The following features may be helpful in differential diagnosis: (*a*) the presence of mitral murmurs which change from day to day or with change in position; (*b*) episodes of syncope or extreme dyspnea which are related to changes in posture; and (*c*) sudden unexplained worsening of the clinical course.

Peripheral embolization from an intracardiac myxoma may produce a clinical picture resembling subacute bacterial endocarditis. The absence of splenomegaly, fever, and bacteremia may be helpful in this difficult differential diagnosis.

Finally, the occurrence of embolization from either the right or left atrium in the absence of auricular fibrillation may be an important diagnostic feature.

The present case emphasizes the importance of considering the diagnosis of intracardiac tumor in a patient with a sudden arterial occlusion without obvious cardiac abnormality or extensive vascular disease. In the presence of coronary or generalized atherosclerosis, embolization from a mural thrombus or sudden arterial occlusion due to atherosclerosis might well be indistinguishable on clinical grounds from embolization from a myxoma. Bizarre and perplexing neurological disorders have resulted from cerebral embolization.

The similarity of this condition and mitral stenosis is emphasized in a report by Padhi,[2] who noted that in 43 patients with a confirmed diagnosis of intracardiac myxoma, 27 had the diagnosis established at the time of atrial exploration for mitral stenosis. Angiocardiography is the procedure of choice where the diagnosis is suspected, although simple x-ray examinations may be extremely helpful if a double atrial shadow or calcification within the tumor is present. Increased pulmonary markings secondary to pulmonary hypertension may be present.[9]

It has been suggested by Wassermill [10] that phonocardiography may be a useful diagnostic procedure, and Isley and Reinhardt [11] have reported the demonstration of a right atrial myxoma on scintogram of the chest.

Treatment

When a case of intracardiac myxoma manifests itself as a peripheral embolus, emergency embolectomy is indicated. At surgery, the diagnosis of a myxoma embolus can easily be made by gross inspection of the semitransparent gelatinous-appearing tissue. If the diagonsis of intracardiac myxoma is made at surgery, the case becomes a surgical emergency in that open-heart surgery should be performed as soon as possible. In the case reported in this paper, the patient was transferred to a hospital where open-heart surgery was performed on the basis of a diagnosis made at the time of embolectomy and without benefit of a microscopic diagnosis.

Since the development of the pump oxygenator and extracorporeal circulation, at least 50 cases of successful removal of intracardiac myxoma have been reported in the medical literature. Differding and associates [6] stressed the importance of deliberately inducing ventricular fibrillation to prevent serious embolization from a friable left atrial tumor mass. This technique was successfully employed in this case.

Summary

An unusual case of intracardiac myxoma presenting with an embolus to the common femoral artery in a previously healthy patient is reported. This is the fourth recorded case in which the intracardiac tumor was diagnosed by embolectomy and the patient survived open-heart surgery. Similar successfully treated patients have been fortunate in that embolization has occurred in a location accessible to embolectomy. When intracardiac myxoma is suspected, angiocardiography is indicated. The current therapy of this disease is open-heart surgery using extracorporeal circulation with induced ventricular fibrillation.

Richard W. Hibner, MD, Fresno Medical Group, 1300 N Fresno St, Fresno, Calif.

REFERENCES

1. Prichard, R. W.: Tumors of the Heart: Review of the Subject and Report of 150 Cases, AMA Arch Path 51:98, 1951.

2. Padhi, R. K.; Kelly, H. G.; and Lynn, R. B.: Intra-Atrial Myxoma: Review of Literature and Report of a Right Atrial Myxoma Diagnosed Preoperatively and Successfully Treated, Canad J Surg 2:414, 1959.

3. Crafoord, C.: Discussion on Mitral Stenosis and Mitral Insufficiency, in Proceedings of the International Symposium on Cardiovascular Surgery, held at the Henry Ford Hospital, Detroit, Michigan, March, 1955, edited by C. R. Lam, Philadelphia: W. B. Saunders Company, 1955.

4. Beanlands, D. S.; Roy, D. L.; Doland, F. G.; and Share, S. J.: Myxoma of the Left Atrium, Canad Med Ass J 83:715, 1960.

5. Zuidema, G. D.; Burke, J. F.; Villegas, A. H.; and Scannell, J. G.: Surgery of Atrial Myxoma, New Eng J Med 264:1016 (May 18) 1961.

6. Differding, J. T.; Gardner, R. E.; and Roe, B. B.: Intra-Cardiac Myxomas With Report of Two Unusual Cases and Successful Removal, Circulation 23:929 (June) 1961.

7. Fischer, E. R., and Hellstrom, H. R.: Evidence in Support of the Neoplastic Nature of Cardiac Myxoma, Amer Heart J 60:630, 1960.

8. Silverman, J.; Olwin, J. S.; and Graettinger, J. S.: Cardiac Myxomas With Systemic Embolization, Circulation 26:99-103 (July) 1962.

9. Solomon, M.: Interstitial Pulmonary Fibrosis Secondary to Pulmonary Venous Hypertension: Report of Case Due to Myxoma of Left Atrium, JAMA 174:464-467 (Oct 1) 1960.

10. Wassermill, M.; Warkentin, O. L.; and Rovin, A.: Myxoma of the Left Atrium: Phono-Cardiographic Study of Three Cases, Circulation 25:50-56 (Jan) 1962.

11. Isley, J. K., and Reinhardt, J. F.: Intra-Cardiac Myxoma Demonstrated on a Vascular Scan, Amer J Roentgen 88:70-73 (July) 1962.

12. Friedberg, C. K.: Diseases of the Heart, ed 2, Philadelphia: W. B. Saunders Company, 1956.

13. Strauss, R., and Merliss, R.: Primary Tumors of the Heart, Arch Path 39:74, 1945.

Renal Hypertension, Heart Failure, and Azotemia

Report of a Case Treated Successfully by Nephrectomy

DAVID E. KLEIN, MD
AND
LESTER PERSKY, MD
CLEVELAND

Frequent reports have appeared in the urological literature dealing with the diagnosis and treatment of renal hypertension.[1-6] Emphasis has been placed on clinical history, intravenous pyelography, divided function studies, renal angiography, and more recently the radioisotope renogram.[7] Unexplained flank pain followed by the abrupt onset of severe hypertension naturally alerts the physician to the possibility of segmental or main renal artery thrombosis or embolism, but more often the history is less suggestive or unremarkable. Intravenous pyelograms and tests of total renal function are frequently normal, and divided function studies are subject to considerable error, in both performance and interpretation. Renal angiography, while important in the ultimate preoperative evaluation of the patient with suspected renal hypertension, has certain attendant hazards and should not be used as a routine diagnostic procedure.

In the preoperative evaluation of the patient with renal hypertension it has generally been emphasized that total renal function should be normal or near normal.[2,8] Those patients with azotemia, and hence evidence of bilateral renal functional impairment, have not been considered candidates for nephrectomy. Grob, however, has commented that total renal function may be significantly decreased without precluding surgical benefit by nephrectomy.[9] The following case clearly illustrates this unusual situation.

Report of Case

A 58-year-old retired engineer was admitted to Cleveland Veterans Administration Hospital on Dec 18, 1960, because of severe chest pain. Fourteen years previously he had a myocardial infarct, after which he required moderate salt restriction, digitalis, and occasional mercurial diuretics. Five years previously he passed a right ureteral calculus, and intravenous pyelograms demonstrated normal kidney size bilaterally. Blood pressure had been normal

Submitted for publication Feb 13, 1963.

Department of Urology, Western Reserve University School of Medicine, and the Cleveland Veterans Administration Hospital.

during repeated visits to his physician. Exertional angina had been relieved by nitroglycerin tablets taken once or twice weekly. Increasing restlessness several months before admission was treated with barbiturates. Two weeks previously he experienced increasing angina with overt signs of congestive heart failure. Two days before admission severe, intermittent, nonradiating substernal pain was unrelieved by nitroglycerin.

Physical examination revealed an anxious male in no acute distress. Blood pressure was 250/140 mm Hg; the remaining vital signs were unremarkable. Xanthelasma were present over both eyelids, a small hemorrhage was seen in the left optic fundus, and vascular changes were minimal. Moderate cardiomegaly with scattered inspiratory rales at the lung bases was detected. The abdominal aorta was pulsatile, and an arterial bruit was audible anteriorly left of the umbilicus and in the left flank. The peripheral vessels were tortuous and calcific.

The hematocrit was 55%; white cell count 17,600 with 43% neutrophils and 55% lymphocytes. Urine specific gravity was 1.013, albumin 1+, sugar negative, with 10-15 red blood cells, 2-4 white blood cells, and several hyaline casts per high-power field. Serum creatinine was 2.0 mg/100 cc, blood urea nitrogen 21 mg/100 cc, and phenolsulfonphthalein excretion 25% in 15 minutes. Serum transaminase values were within normal range. Electrocardiogram showed a remote inferior wall infarct, digitalis effect, and first-degree atrioventricular block. Chest film revealed pleural fluid at the left base.

Intravenous pyelogram revealed tortuosity and calcification of the abdominal aorta, a normal right upper urinary tract, and poor excretion from a small left kidney. Left retrograde pyelogram showed a normal collecting system. Translumbar aortography revealed marked arteriosclerotic changes of the abdominal aorta and stenosis of the proximal left renal artery with poststenotic dilatation (Fig 1).

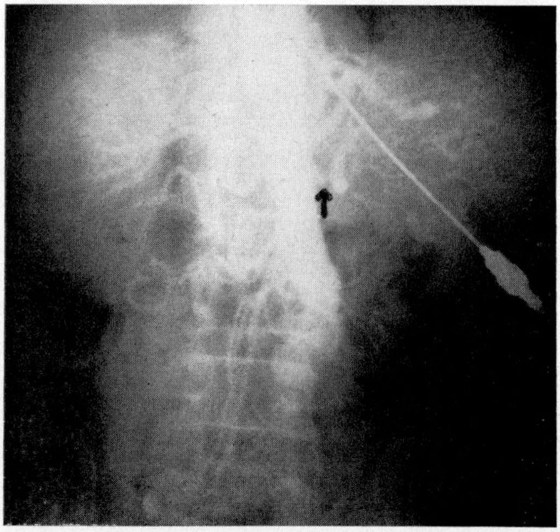

Fig 1

Sodium and Creatinine Concentrations

		Sodium, mEq/Liter	Creatinine, Mg/100 Cc
A.	Left	46	161
	Right	18	100
B.	Left	15	298
	Right	6.1	144

Prior to aortography divided function studies were performed. On two occasions inadequate flow rates and excessive leakage around the ureteral catheters precluded accurate clearance studies and volume measurements. Separated sodium and creatinine concentrations, however, were obtained as shown in the Table.

Radio-isotope renogram using I^{131}-labeled iodohippurate (Hippuran) showed a normal vascular spike on the right and a flattened curve on the left, suggesting diminished arterial flow on this side.

Despite bed rest, salt restriction, diuretics, and antihypertensive medications, occasional chest pain and mild congestive failure persisted. The patient was restless, frequently dyspneic and diaphoretic, and complained of marked weakness. Serial electrocardiograms suggested subendocardial ischemia and left ventricular strain. Slowly the urea nitrogen and serum creatinine increased until values reached 49 and 3.8 mg/100 cc, respectively (Fig 2). On the 27th hospital day a left nephrectomy was performed. No pulse was palpable in the left renal artery, which contained a large atheromatous plaque with adherent thrombus in its most proximal portion. The atrophic contracted kidney weighed 106 gm and on sectioning revealed widespread ischemic tubular atrophy, arterial nephrosclerosis and pyelonephritis.

Postoperatively the patient was normotensive, and one week later blood urea nitrogen and creatinine values were within normal range. Angina and heart failure improved dramatically, and at this writing, 16 months after surgery, he remains normotensive, having reassumed his prehospitalization status.

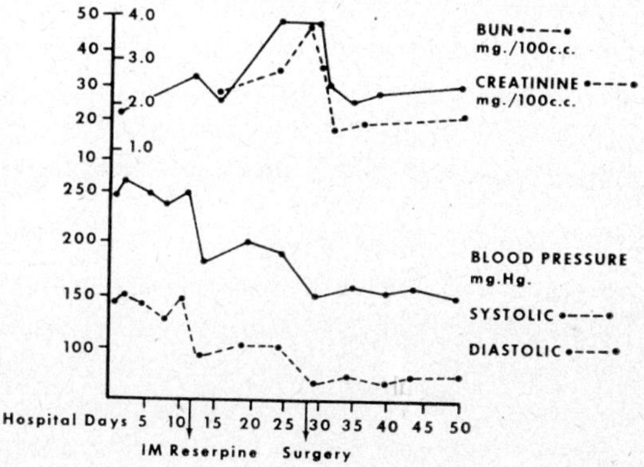

Fig 2

Comment

When of brief duration, relief of hypertension may slow advancement of nephrosclerosis and occasionally even allow for some return of function. Imber and Clymer described a 34-year-old male with abrupt onset of malignant hypertension, proteinuria, impaired concentrating ability, and a blood urea nitrogen level of 30 mg/100 cc.[10] Intravenous and retrograde pyelograms demonstrated a small poorly functioning right kidney with normal collecting system. No indigo-carmine excretion from the right was observed after 20 minutes. At surgical exploration a kinked renal artery secondary to fibrous bands was found, and nephrectomy resulted in immediate return to normotensive levels, with less rapid but definite improvement in renal function. There were no morphologic changes found in the removed kidney, probably attesting to the brevity of the process.

Margolin, Merrill, and Harrison reported a 37-year-old male with segmental infarction associated with aneurysm and thrombosis of the right renal artery.[11] Although polyuria, albuminuria, and impaired concentrating ability were present, diminution in total function preoperatively was limited to a maximum specific gravity of 1.018, the urea nitrogen level at this time being 9 mg/100 cc. Deming noted a 28-year-old female with malignant hypertension, polyuria, and albuminuria due to partial occlusion of the left renal artery.[12] Removal of an atrophic kidney improved both blood pressure and renal function.

Moyer, Heider, Pevey, and Ford have clearly documented this problem in five cases of malignant hypertension due to renal artery occlusion.[13] All demonstrated advanced retinopathy and acute onset of symptoms. Divided function studies showed absence of urine flow from the occluded kidney and reduced inulin clearances from the less affected "hypertensive" kidney. In two cases, with blood urea nitrogen values of 70 and 82 mg per 100 cc, nephrectomy relieved the hypertension and subsequent improvement in renal hemodynamics occurred. One patient, in whom an arterial homograft was used, had no demonstrable return of function from the affected side, but filtration rate and blood flow in the contralateral kidney improved dramatically, and the urea nitrogen dropped from 70 to 30 mg per 100 cc.

Our patient is older than those previously reported. Onset was abrupt, with persistent diastolic pressures in the range of 120 to 150 mm Hg. Leukocytosis, albuminuria, and impaired urine concentrating ability were seen on admission. The rise in urea nitrogen and serum creatinine, while the patient was receiving optimal medical care, indicated severe bilateral renal impairment, although complete separated function studies were not performed. It is possible that congestive failure, and treatment required thereof, contributed to the moderate azotemia. Sodium and creatinine concentrations in the urine failed to reveal a significant disparity between kidneys. Because of his precarious cardiovascular status, only at the urging of attending physicians was a left nephrectomy performed. An atrophic kidney with thrombotic occlusion of the left main renal artery was found. The postoperative course was characterized by a prompt return to previous normotensive state and reasonable renal function.

This case again suggests that depressed function of the unaffected kidney may be due to acute reversible vascular damage rather than chronic deterioration. Sudden hypertension in this patient aggravated a cardiovascular apparatus which was marginally compensated and produced bilateral renal functional impairment. Amelioration of the hypertension following nephrectomy apparently reversed this process. When total impairment is present, functional deterioration is potentially reversible, providing increased sympathetic vasoconstriction has not provoked progressive renal failure.

Summary

Renal hypertension associated with thrombotic occlusion of a main renal artery is reported in a 58-year-old male. Angina, mild congestive failure, azotemia, and severe diastolic hypertension were benefited after nephrectomy. It is again emphasized that bilateral renal functional impairment, especially when of recent onset and of moderate degree, does not always preclude surgical approaches in the treatment of diagnosed renal hypertension.

Drs. Alan Yoho, Sheldon Sidell and Paul Wisenbaugh, Western Reserve University, University Hospitals and Cleveland Veterans Administration Hospital, Dr. John E. Williams, and Dr. Norman Shumway assisted in this report.

David E. Klein, MD, 11811 Shaker Blvd. Cleveland 20, Ohio.

REFERENCES

1. Smith, H. W.: Unilateral Nephrectomy in Hypertensive Disease, J Urol 76:685, 1956.

2. Connor, T. B.; Berthrong, M.; Thomas, W. C.; and Howard, J. E.: Hypertension Due to Unilateral Renal Disease, With a Report on a Functional Test Helpful in Diagnosis, Bull Hopkins Hosp 100:241-276, 1957.

3. DeCamp, P. T., and Birchall, R.: Recognition and Treatment of Renal Arterial Stenosis Associated With Hypertension, Surgery 43:134, 1958.

4. McDonald, D. F.: Individual Renal Clearance in Diagnosis of Hypertension of Renal Origin, J Urol 86:289-294, 1961.

5. Straffon, R. A., and Garcia, A. M.: A Clinical Evaluation of the Radioactive Diodrast Renogram as a Screening Test in Hypertension, J Urol 83: 774-781, 1960.

6. Stokes, J. M.; Wohltmann, H.; and Carlson, E.: Coarctation of the Abdominal Aorta and Renal Artery Stenosis Corrected by Surgical Treatment: The Importance of Individual Renal Function Tests in Selection of Proper Management, Ann Surg 152:856-860, 1960.

7. Winter, C. C.; Maxwell, M. H.; Rockney, R. E.; and Kleeman, C. R.: Results of the Radioisotope Renogram and Comparison With Other Kidney Tests Among Hypertensive Individuals, J Urol 59:674, 1959.

8. Yendt, E. R.; Kerr, W. K.; Wilson, D. R.; and Jawarski, Z. F.: The Diagnosis and Treatment of Renal Hypertension, With Special Reference to a Case of Hypertension Due to Stenosis of Both Renal Arteries, Amer J Med 28:169, 1960.

9. Grob, D.: Diagnosis and Management of the Curable Forms of Hypertension, Advance Intern Med 10:219-258, 1960.

10. Imber, I., and Clymer, R.: Obstruction of Renal Artery Producing Malignant Hypertension, New Eng J Med 252:8, 1955.

11. Margolin, E. G.; Merrill, J. P.; and Harrison, J. H.: Diagnosis of Hypertension Due to Occlusions of the Renal Artery, New Eng J Med 256:581, 1957.

12. Deming, O. B.: Association of Polyuria and Albuminuria With Hypertension of Unilateral Renal Origin, Arch Intern Med 93:197-204, 1954.

13. Moyer, J. H.; Heider, C.; Pevey, K.; and Ford, R. V.: The Effect of Treatment on the Vascular Deterioration Associated With Hypertension, With Particular Emphasis on Renal Function, Amer J Med 24:177, 1958.

Special Article

A Proposed Glossary of Cancer

HAYES MARTIN, MD, NEW YORK

Pliny the Elder (23-79 AD) is reported to have found the following epitaph on a Roman tombstone: "He died by reason of the confusion of the doctors." While such an epitaph might never be inscribed and seldom justified today, it can hardly be denied that some semantic confusion by the doctors is nevertheless still with us in medical parlance and writing.

The human factors in the art of healing are so many and varied as to preclude medicine from ever becoming an exact science to the same degree as mathematics, chemistry, or physics. There is no good reason, however, why medical nomenclature and terminology should not be so exact that the reader or the listener might know literally what is meant, and what is intended to be included as well as what is to be excluded. Medical editors might well insist that authors say precisely what they mean in terms understood by all, rather than a somewhat irresponsible resort to a Humpty-Dumpty policy: "When I use a word, it means exactly what I choose it to mean, neither more nor less" (*Alice in Wonderland*).

During the past quarter century there has been a steady increase in interest and activities in the cancer problem by both the layman and the physician. This specific interest has come to surpass the general concern regarding tuberculosis and poliomyelitis, which at one time were major preoccupations of public health. The latter diseases are now amenable to almost complete control, while cancer, next to atomic war, remains the bête noire of human survival.

Scientific knowledge may be defined as the accumulation, coordination, and application of proven facts. As such knowledge concerning cancer grows, one may confidently expect increasingly rapid progress in the form of new and better methods of treatment and the eventual discovery of the cause and specific method of cure. If such progress is to be made with the greatest possible speed, a prime requisite is an orderly and exact recording and reporting of clinical and laboratory observations or, in other words—facts. Such reporting is not possible without a literal and uniform nomenclature and terminology. Unfortunately, medical reports and even dictionaries (including the medical variety) are often inconsistent, contradictory, and confusing. But, after all, the compilers of dictionaries have little recourse other than common usage, which would naturally be authoritative provided that it be logical, consistent, and uniform. It is with this purpose in mind that the following glossary of cancer is proposed.

Submitted for publication Feb 19, 1963.

Attending Surgeon (Emeritus), Memorial Hospital.

Glossary

Cancer.—A long-accepted inclusive term for all forms of malignant neoplasia, eg, "carcinoma," "epithelioma," "sarcoma," "lymphoma," "leukemia," "malignant melanoma," "endothelioma," "mesothelioma." All of these basic root terms (except melanoma) designate the tissue from which the cancer arises. In order to avoid tiresome alliteration, there are a number of acceptable synonyms for *cancer,* such as *malignant tumor* (growth, neoplasm), or where the antecedent is plain, simply *tumor, growth, lesion, disease,* etc. With the latter usage the inclusion of the adjective *malignant* to the terms *lesion* or *disease* is redundant.

The term *cancer* is perfectly respectable. The public accepts and uses it. It is in no sense a "dirty word." Some otherwise forthright medical writers and even speakers before medical audiences nevertheless appear to find the term too crude and inelegant for polite usage and, therefore, resort to ostensibly more refined and erudite euphemisms, such as *a malignancy* or *malignant disease.*

Carcinoma (never a synonym for cancer) *and Sarcoma.*—These as well as the other basic root terms had best seldom if ever be employed without a specific qualifying prefix (eg, squamous carcinoma, adenocarcinoma, basal cell carcinoma, papillary carcinoma, lymphosarcoma, reticulum cell sarcoma, neurosarcoma, periosteal osteogenic sarcoma, et al). There would rarely be any justification for such titles as "Carcinoma of the Breast" or "Carcinoma of the Tongue," where there is no intent or purpose to exclude from the report all other possible forms of malignant neoplasms of the respective organs. Properly the title should have read simply, "Cancer of the Breast" or "Cancer of the Tongue." Later in the text under a section on pathology, the author would find ample occasion to discuss the exclusive (if any) occurrence of the epithelial cancers and their specific subvarieties.

Carcinogen(ic)(esis) and Cancerigen(ic)-(esis).—Although the meaning of these respective terms should be plain to all, one often hears or reads of a cancer researcher referring to a "carcinogen" as producing some form of "sarcoma." It should be obvious that a *carcinogen* can cause only *carcinoma,* while the responsible agent in the causation of a sarcoma, if it need be specifically defined, requires some other term. The etymologically sound term "cancerigen," which has the additional authority of long though possibly not common usage, would not only be proper but an entirely adequate substitute for the tiresome, repetitious "carcinogen," where no such restriction is intended. If there were actually any great need for the term "carcinogen," then logically there should be an equal need for collateral terms such as "sarcomagen," "lymphomagen," "leukemogen," or even "melanomagen."

Malignant—Malignant Disease—Malignant Lesion.—From *Webster's New International Dictionary of the English Language,* second edition, 1943:

Malignant (adj.) . . . 1. Rebellious against God or against a government. 2. Having a fateful influence . . . 3. Poisonous; deleterious . . . 4. Disposed to do harm . . . 5. (Med.) tending or threatening to produce death. Curiously enough, there is no reference either in the 1927 or 1943 Editions to *malignant disease* as a synonym for cancer.)

If one relies on the foregoing, the term *malignant* has many applications in medicine as well as in human behavior, animals, plants, forces of nature, etc. In medicine, any disease "tending or threatening to produce death" therefore may be rightly termed *malignant.* Diseases of the heart (the number one cause of death), such as coronary occlusion, valvular insufficiency, et al, are consequently more malignant than cancer. Moreover, since there is a definite percentage of recovery and cure both in heart disease and cancer, the distinction of being the most malignant must go to such lethal diseases as tetanus and rabies, practically always fatal within a few days, or to such lingering, invariably fatal afflictions as multiple sclerosis, Parkinson's disease, and lupus erythematosus, for which there are no remedies to date. By contrast, basal cell carcinoma (a form of cancer and therefore logically included in the malignant disease category) is seldom a cause of death and certainly less malignant than hemophilia. Other diseases ordinarily considered to be benign, such as perforated gastric ulcer or perforated appendiceal abscess (actually highly malignant lesions), are certainly much more malignant than let us say papillary carcinoma of the thyroid.

In the case of Pope John XXIII, is it not a curious commentary that up until the day of his death, some newspapers should continue to report that the Vatican authorities had not as yet disclosed whether the Holy Father's disease was "malignant or benign"?

Malignant Tumor or Malignant Neoplasm.—From the practical standpoint these terms had probably best be accepted as proper synonyms for *cancer,* although strictly speaking, such "benign" neoplasms as bulky adenomas of the thyroid or hypertrophy of the prostate are certainly malignant if they progress to a fatal issue.

Malignant Biopsy or Malignant Biopsy Specimen.—These common solecisms are at least a minor offense to good literary taste. Surely a biopsy is always made for a humane purpose and in itself can hardly be termed a "malignant" act. The specimen which is even bacteriologically sterile after immersion in formalin or alcohol is certainly among the most innocuous objects on earth. It would be proper to speak of a biopsy of a suspected malignant tumor, but (of all horrors!) hardly of a "malignant biopsy."

Malignancy.—When used as a synonym for cancer, this malapropism is inexcusable, and here one must take issue with *Webster's New International Dictionary of the English Language* (second edition, 1943) which has come under the malign influence of some modern medical writers.

> Malignancy. 1. state or quality of being malignant . . . 2. (a) virulence . . . (b) the state of having a malignant tumor . . . (c) a malignant tumor; as a malignancy of the breast.*

Actually, except in the medical definition, the term is defined by Webster's as being an abstraction, expressing a quality or characteristic of an action, an object, a plant, a person, a disease, or a neoplasm. As an abstraction it cannot properly be used to define a concrete object. When used in reference to a neoplasm, *malignancy* is of course by far the most significant characteristic, along with its other less significant properties such as size, shape, color, microscopic appearance, etc. One may correctly speak only of the *malignancy of a tumor,* or of any other disease, or of an act of human behavior. How ridiculous it would be to speak of the "American Malignancy Society," the "American Society for Malignancy Research," or the "National Malignant Disease Society."

Operable and Inoperable.—These malapropisms are among the most objectionable because they so often serve as a convenient excuse for inaction in those cancer cases in which, despite their advanced state, there may be an excellent chance of cure by prompt and competent surgery, which may nevertheless be of a more radical nature than a timid, less experienced, or less competent surgeon cares to undertake. In such cases the chance of cure is often lost, and "palliative" treatment in the form of radiation is given. More often than not such treatment is more palliative to the bad conscience of the incompetent or timid surgeon than to the sufferings of the patient.

Actually, any disease case is operable if a surgeon is willing to make the attempt and the patient gives consent. The question of *operability* (if that term of doubtful propriety were to be used) should be determined only by the patient's best interests and by a competent surgeon. The only *truly inoperable* cases are those in which the patients refuse to give consent, where facilities for adequate surgery are lacking, or when no competent surgeon is available. The alternatives for these terms are discussed in the following section.

Resectable (in toto) or Nonresectable (in toto).—On the Head and Neck Service at Memorial Hospital, the terms "operable" and "inoperable" are not used in conferences. A growth is either *resectable* or *nonresectable,* with the tacit meaning of *in toto.* In many instances, although a growth is *not resectable in toto,* it may nevertheless be "operable" in the sense that a subtotal resection of a bulky, bleeding, infected, and painful tumor may give great relief for such complications as dyspnea, dysphagia, hemorrhage, pain, etc, and thereby prolong life. Other cases certainly become "operable" when ligation of arteries for hemostasis, tracheostomy, gastrotomy, esophagostomy, colostomy, cystostomy, or neurotomy are performed to relieve complications of cancer.

Biopsy.—(cf. necropsy). This term defines the process of examining a portion of tissue removed from a living subject. It includes the taking, or detachment, of the specimen, its immediate immersion in a fixative fluid (formalin in most cases), its submission with clinical data to a pathology laboratory for further processing, ending in the preparation of a stained slide, and finally its interpretation by the microscopist. There-

* Such a definition appears here for the first time in Webster's.

fore, the surgeon does not "take a biopsy." He rather takes a specimen for a biopsy. From the practical standpoint, one might say that he "makes a biopsy," although he actually only initiates the process by taking a specimen for the subsequent longer process.

Glands.—This term is one of the most likely to confuse and mislead in discussions on cancer. The tendency for most forms of cancer to disseminate widely more often through the lymphatics than through the blood stream makes the lymph nodes the subject of prime importance in the discussions of the clinical aspects of cancer. The term "glands" as applied to lymph nodes arose in English when the cervical lymph nodes (often affected by scrofula or tuberculosis) were not differentiated from the true cervical glands, seven in number, ie, the three paired salivary glands and the thyroid and, if one wishes to pursue the point to absurdity, the sweat and sebaceous glands of the skin of the neck. The French have no such difficulty; lymph nodes are called *les ganglions* in differentiation from *les glandes.* The German *Knoten* or *Lymphknoten* likewise differentiates the two forms of anatomic structures. In English and American medical literature, the misuse of the term has sometimes resulted in such ludicrous sequences with a few sentences or paragraphs as "a glandular cancer . . . of the thyroid gland . . . metastasized to the cervical glands." Sometimes the term "glands" is used as a synonym for "metastases," and an author may report that in such and such a percentage of cases "there were no glands" or "no glands were present"—*mirabile dictu* and surely a most unusual anomaly.

The modern concept of the lymph nodes as the source of production of certain antibodies can hardly hold to be a justification for persisting in the ancient and confusing "glands" or "lymph glands" rather than *nodes* or *lymph nodes.*

Summary

The following abridgement is intended for the convenience of and usage by those medical writers and medical editors who may find themselves in agreement with the logic of the foregoing discussion.

Cancer.—An inclusive term for all forms of malignant neoplasia. Synonyms—malignant growth, malignant tumor or, where the antecedent is plain, simply growth, tumor, lesion. ("Malignancy," "malignant disease," and "carcinoma" should not be used as synonyms for cancer.)

Carcinoma.—(cf. sarcoma, lymphoma, leukemia, melanoma, et al). A cancer arising from epithelial tissues. This term alone, like its collaterals (sarcoma et al), should seldom if ever be used without qualifying prefixes (eg, squamous carcinoma, neurosarcoma). In most instances where the term "carcinoma" is used alone and nonspecifically, the all-inclusive term *cancer* is to be preferred.

Malignancy.—An abstraction, a property of many diseases, of which cancer is one. It is ungrammatical and incorrect when used as a synonym for cancer.

Malignant Disease.—Incorrect when used as a synonym for cancer. Cancer is not the only malignant disease, nor is it even the most malignant.

Biopsy.—A long and somewhat involved process, beginning with the removal of tissue from a living subject and ending with the microscopist's interpretation. A surgeon, therefore, does not *take* a biopsy. He simply initiates the process by taking a specimen for biopsy.

Operable and Inoperable.—The true definitions of these terms actually depend mainly on the patient's consent or lack of consent to an operation or the absolute lack of facilities for surgery. It is too often used as a feeble excuse and face saver for inaction in advanced cases of cancer where there is a chance of cure by competent surgery.

Resectable and Nonresectable (in toto).—Wholly necessary descriptive terms which are not in all cases synonymous with the conventional meaning of the terms operable and inoperable.

Hayes Martin, MD, 737 Park Ave, New York, NY.

Correspondence

FOR WHOM THE BELL TOLLS

To the Editor: In the paper, "Closure of Boxing Lacerations Between Rounds" (Arch Surg 86:295 [Feb] 1963), the author correctly emphasizes the paradox of a fighter who is ahead on points losing by a technical knockout because of a facial laceration. Would it be invidious to point out a greater paradox, that of a plastic surgeon whose art is primarily directed not at preventing or correcting deformity but at permitting a contestant to continue longer in the meat grinder than might otherwise be possible?

It should also be noted that the author shares with John Boyle O'Reilly (O'Reilly, J. B.: Ethics of Boxing and Manly Sport, Boston: Ticknor & Co., 1888.), that ancient admirer of John L. Sullivan, the myth that padded gloves reduce the chances of injury to the participants. There is little doubt that gloves are a protection to the wearer's hands rather than to his opponent's head or body. As such, they permit more forcible blows to be delivered without incapacitating the essentially fragile fist.

Eugene G. Laforet, MD
1180 Beacon Street
Brookline, Mass

To the Editor: With pleasure I counter. It would seem the questions come more from book knowledge than ring experience but are still of theoretical interest. A response gives the opportunity to jab, hook, and cross to the heart of this problem with some pertinent and concrete suggestions which should be considered for enforcement by the AMA.

For me the serious paradox is not a boxer losing on a butt or even a plastic surgeon's suture prolonging a competition. It is that America, once individualistic, competitive, and rugged, is looking to a softer way, generally in a slide toward the welfare state and specifically in such cries as the one for the abolition of boxing. Why boxing? Why not car or motorcycle racing, football, mountain climbing, or any sport that poses a reasonable hazard?

Those who have boxed know that it is a great sport, a character builder, and a developer of not only physical fitness but courage. Every young man should be taught the art, and the sport should be encouraged on an amateur level toward Olympic championships. It is also important that control of professional boxing be undertaken by an impartial central committee to reduce corruption and increase medical supervision.

Head injuries, not lacerations, pose the serious danger, and to reduce this hazard without emasculating the sport there should be the following: (1) some form of compulsory head gear; (2) abolition of hand taping; (3) use of larger and better constructed gloves; (4) mandatory eight count; (5) out after two times down in one round; (6) enforced suspension of injured boxers; (7) more alert and closer coordination between referees and ring physicians during contests, facilitated by a signal (buzzer) to call temporary halts for closer examination of a boxer's condition.

As for the danger of padded gloves, of course it depends on the amount of padding and its distribution. Bare fist fighting is impractical because of the high incidence of fractured hands and lacerated faces. Slight padding, as in the present eight ounce gloves, is more dangerous especially when the gloves are wet. Heavier padding as in 12-16 ounce gloves (20 ounces for Sonny Liston) reduces the lethal punching power, the effect of a direct blow, and the danger of the rabbit punch over the kidney. At the same time the larger gloves increase the boxer's defense potential. Then if points also were awarded for making an opponent miss, so that the skill of feinting and blocking was encouraged, the sport again would revert back to the manly art of self-defense.

D. Ralph Millard, Jr., MD
2121 Biscayne Boulevard
Miami 37, Fla

Post-Traumatic Vasospasm: Role of Thermal Measurement

STEPHEN W. MEAGHER, MD
BOSTON

Physicians fail to recognize post-traumatic vasospasm of the upper extremity because of its low incidence, the minor nature of the original injury in many patients, and the absence of obvious physical findings in some patients. The nature of post-traumatic vasospasm is poorly understood beyond the realization that sympathetic activity in the involved area is abnormal after an injury. This abnormality is characterized by one or more of the symptoms of pain, coldness, and weakness, or the signs of rubor, edema, impaired motor power, and increased pseudomotor activity.

Patients with post-traumatic vasospasm are erroneously thought to be malingerers or in possession of a low pain threshold in response to a minor injury. As a result, treatment is not given or the treatment prescribed is either improper or woefully inadequate. Unfortunately, these circumstances lead to a period of drifting from one physician to another in search of relief; the patient remains incapable of performing productive work and sustains a significant economic injury to complicate his course.

Measurements of skin temperature with a very sensitive thermister have provided scientific evidence that blood flow is diminished, thereby leading to a correct diagnosis and appropriate treatment. In addition, the thermister provides data to assist in evaluating the effectiveness of treatment of post-traumatic vasospasm.

Prior to investigating the application of thermal measurement to a large variety of hand problems, readings were taken at random in 100 healthy, working controls. In no case did the variation between a fixed point on one hand and the same point on the other hand exceed one degree Fahrenheit.

The two cases which follow adequately demonstrate the value of thermal measure-

Submitted for publication Dec 18, 1962.

Associate visiting surgeon, First (Tufts) Surgical Service, Boston City Hospital.

From the Hand Service, Boston City Hospital, and the Department of Surgery, Tufts University School of Medicine.

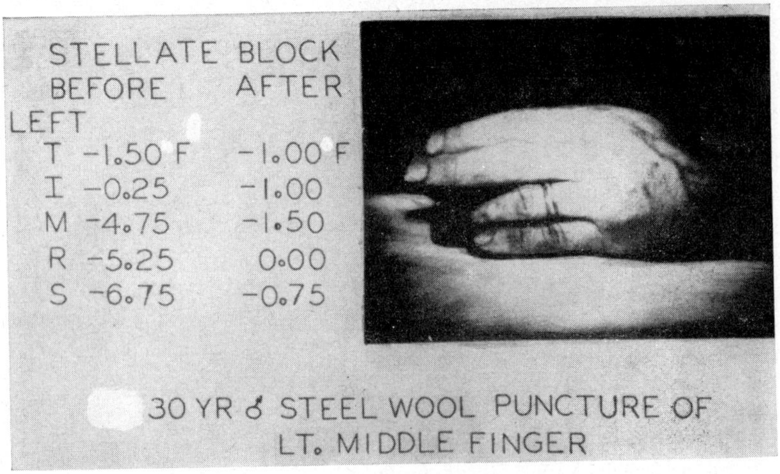

Fig 1.—Measurements of the skin temperature of the thumb (*T*), index (*I*), middle (*M*), ring (*R*), and small (*S*) fingers before and after a stellate ganglion block are listed. Measurements are expressed as net degrees Fahrenheit of coldness of the left hand as compared to the corresponding parts of the normal right hand.

ments in determining and documenting the diagnosis in patients who are afflicted with post-traumatic vasospasm.

Report of Cases

CASE 1.—A 30-year-old male grocery clerk sustained an injury to his left middle finger on steel wool while working on April 21, 1962. An infection ensued in the digit; incision and drainage were carried out twice by his physician. On another occasion, he was hospitalized for five days for treatment of cellulitis in the same digit.

Since the time of injury, he had experienced sensitivity to cold, redness of the hand on exposure to cold, weakness in grasping, and pain in the left middle finger extending to the elbow. Except for a two-week period following the injury, he had not missed work in spite of his disability.

He was told by the plant physician that his weakness and pain were to be expected and no special treatment was prescribed to relieve his symptoms. Fig 1 lists the net degrees Fahrenheit of coldness in the left thumb (*T*), index (*I*), middle (*M*), ring (*R*), and small (*S*) fingers compared to the normal right hand when he was first seen. A left stellate ganglion block was administered. Within five minutes coldness, pain, and weakness were relieved entirely. In Fig 1, thermister measurements taken after the block reveal that the temperatures of all digits of the left hand had risen to within the normal limit of variation except for one half of one degree Fahrenheit of abnormality in the left middle finger.

The relief of symptoms lasted for two months. At the end of this period a partial return of symptoms required a second stellate ganglion block; complete relief was obtained.

CASE 2.—A 24-year-old male factory worker was cleaning a machine when he was struck on the dorsum of the left wrist by a falling steel roller on Sept 5, 1962. An x-ray of the left hand and wrist did not reveal any abnormality. A 1 cm break in

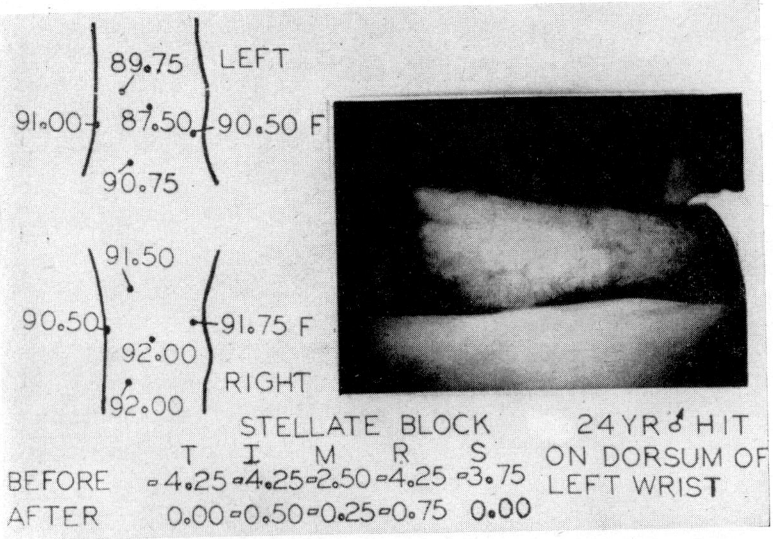

Fig 2.—Below, the net degrees Fahrenheit of coldness of the digits of the left hand compared to the normal right hand are given before and after a stellate ganglion block. The thermal readings on the line drawings of the dorsal left and right wrists demonstrate a persistent cold spot on the dorsum of the left wrist at the site of trauma as compared to the normal right wrist.

the skin did not require suturing. On Sept 10, 1962, the patient was told by a physician in an insurance company clinic that he had recovered and was ready to return to work, in spite of his complaint of severe pain over the dorsum of the left wrist.

When he was seen on Sept 13, 1962, the left hand was held in a protected position with the wrist extended and the digits in midflexion. Grasp was almost nonexistent due to pain in the wrist; the fingers could only be actively flexed to within 2½ in of the proximal palm; an attempt to passively flex the digits caused very severe pain in the wrist; the left hand was colder than the right hand, and perspiration was more abundant on the left hand.

Fig 2 reveals a significant net coldness in all digits of the left hand. Therefore, a left stellate ganglion block was administered; within several minutes the temperature of all of the digits of the left hand was within the limit of normal variation of one degree Fahrenheit. Normal temperatures have persisted in the digits up to the present time. Motor power of grasping showed marked improvement, the hand was warm; freedom of movement of the small joints was very much improved; the pain over the dorsum of the wrist was moderately relieved but persisted. Therefore, thermister measurements were taken over both wrists; these revealed a significant cold spot at the site of injury that had not completely yielded to the effect of the stellate block on blood flow. These measurements appear in the diagram of Fig 2.

In both of these patients, the thermister provided data of great value in determining the correct diagnosis and management. The thermister also provided a means of measuring the effectiveness of treatment, especially in the second patient on whom measurements demonstrated a small area of persistent vasospasm corresponding with the area of persistent pain.

Summary

The role of thermal measurement in determining the diagnosis of post-traumatic vasospasm is demonstrated in two patients. In both patients, the initial data indicated the necessity for a stellate ganglion block. In addition, thermal readings provided a scientific method of measuring the effectiveness of treatment.

Stephen W. Meagher, MD, 520 Commonwealth Ave, Boston 15, Mass.

Vein Grafts in the Venous System

An Experimental Evaluation of Autogenous Veins Used as Bypass Implants

HENRY HAIMOVICI, MD
NICOLA ZINICOLA, MD
MEHDI NOORANI, MD
AND
PAUL W. HOFFERT, MD
NEW YORK

End-to-end implantation of a graft is the most commonly used procedure for vein implants in the venous system. In contrast to the growing literature on this method of venous grafting,[1] no information is available on the end-to-side implants.

Since in some clinical conditions it might be necessary to carry out a bypass procedure around veins involved by thrombosis or neoplastic invasions, its experimental investigation appeared desirable.

The present study was therefore designed to evaluate the fate of such grafts and was carried out in two venous areas: the jugular and the inferior vena cava.

Methods and Material

Fifty-six adult mongrel dogs weighing 10 to 19 kg were used. The procedures were performed under intravenous anesthesia with pentobarbital (Nembutal) (12 mg/kg body weight).

Fresh autogenous grafts were used in all experiments and secured from the right external jugular vien. A four-stay suture technique[2] was always used for the end-to-side implantation of the graft. The length of the longitudinal phlebotomy in the host veins, at the site of the implantation, ranged from 0.7 cm to 1.0 cm. The type of anastomosis consisted of a continuous over-and-over stitch, employing 5-0 arterial silk. Great care was exercised to excise the adventitia from both graft and host at the site of implantation. Frequent irrigations with heparin solution of the veins were used routinely. Penicillin and streptomycin were administered for the first three postoperative days.

Phlebography, using 50% diatrizoate (Hypaque), was carried out periodically, one to two weeks postoperatively and then four months later, just prior to the sacrifice of the animal. Evaluation of the results was finally made by excision of the graft and pathologic study.

Results

The results will be considered separately for the two sites of implantation of the bypass graft.

Submitted for publication Jan 9, 1963.

Trainees in Vascular Surgery, supported by grant No. HTS-5260 from the National Heart Institute, United States Public Health Service(Dr. Zinicola, Dr. Noorani).

From the Henry L. and Lucy Moses Surgical Laboratories and the Vascular Service, Surgical Division, Montefiore Hospital.

TABLE 1.—*Results of Bypass Grafts Into the Jugular Vein*

State of Host Veins	No. Dogs	Thrombosed		Patent	
		No.	Duration, Days	No.	Duration, Days
Excision	6	1	8	5	117
Ligation	6	1	10	5	140
Intact	6	2	9	4	140

Jugular Vein

Through a vertical midline incision in the neck both external jugular veins were isolated. A segment measuring 8 to 10 cm of the right jugular was excised and immediately implanted into the left side.

Three series of experiments, each one including six dogs, were carried out in the jugular vein bypass, as indicated in Table 1. The host jugular vein was either: *a*) excised; *b*) ligated at both ends, or *c*) left intact. The results of these experiments are summarized in Table 1. In the first two series, five out of six, or 83.3%, of the grafts remained patent as determined 117 to 140 days later by phlebography and anatomical examination. In the third series, four, or 66.6%, of the grafts remained patent as determined 140 days later. Thrombosis of the graft usually occurred within eight to ten days after implantation.

The over-all incidence of thrombosis in the jugular bypass group was four out of 18, or 22.2%. The apparent cause for the thrombosis was: *a*) technical error of the proximal anastomosis in one; *b*) infection of the wound in one; and *c*) fibrous reaction surrounding the graft in two.

Phlebographic illustrations of the above three techniques are shown in Fig 1, 2, and 3. Several interesting observations were made, some of which were applicable either to all series or only specifically to a given one.

Thus, from the phlebograms taken one to two weeks postoperatively, it was apparent that initially all grafts were narrower than the host vein. Later phlebographic examination uniformly disclosed return of the diameter of the graft to its original size.

In the series with the excision of the host vein, the bypass graft appeared to be similar to an end-to-end implant (Fig 1). In the series with ligation at both ends, the shunting appeared quite clearly on the phlebogram (Fig 2). Finally, in the cases with the intact host vein, the blood flow through the shunt appeared to be diminished (Fig 3*A*). In these cases, temporary occlusion of the host vein

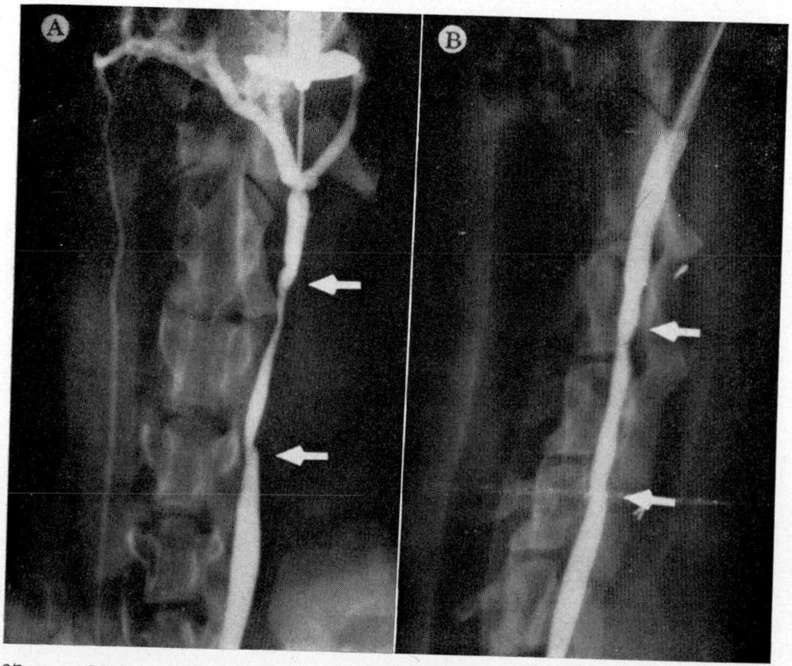

Fig 1.—*A*, phlebogram showing a patent autogenous vein bypass in the jugular vein eight days after its implantation. The bypassed host vein was excluded by excision. *B*, phlebogram of the same case taken 117 days after implanation of the graft.

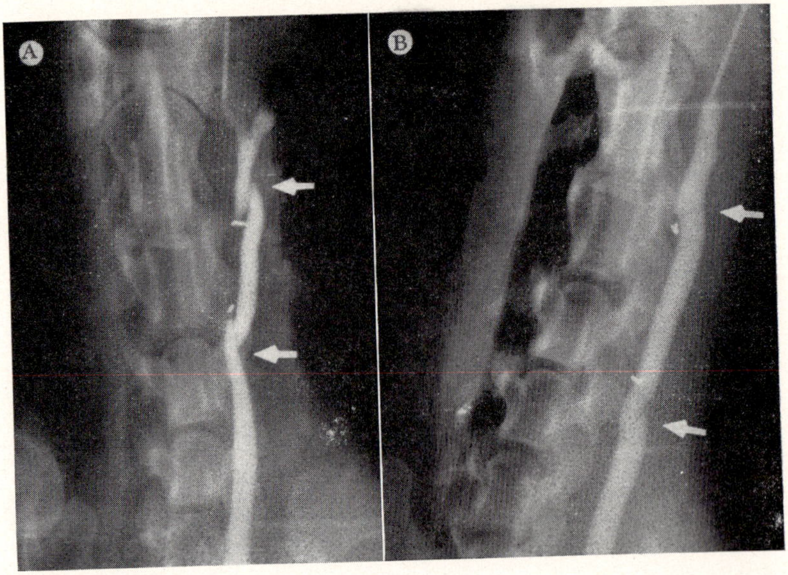

Fig 2.—*A*, phlebogram of a patent autogenous vein bypass in the jugular vein nine days after its implantation. The bypassed host vein was excluded by placing ligatures at both ends. *B*, phlebogram of the same case taken 140 days after implantation of the graft.

resulted in increased flow through the graft (Fig 3*B*).

Inferior Vena Cava

The infrarenal inferior vena cava and the right iliac vein were exposed through a transperitoneal midline abdominal incision. Implantation of the graft proceeded from the right iliac vein to the inferior vena cava. The right iliac vein, in all but five cases, was interrupted or excised between its junction with the left iliac and the distal anastomosis of the graft. Exclusion of this segment of the vein was deemed necessary to avoid a cul-de-sac which might lead to thrombus formation.

The experiments in this group were divided into two series: A) the animals which received no anticoagulants, and B) those with anticoagulants (Table 2).

A. *Without Anticoagulant Therapy.*—In this series, the right common iliac vein was either left intact (5 cases) or interrupted by excision or ligations (14 cases). In the latter

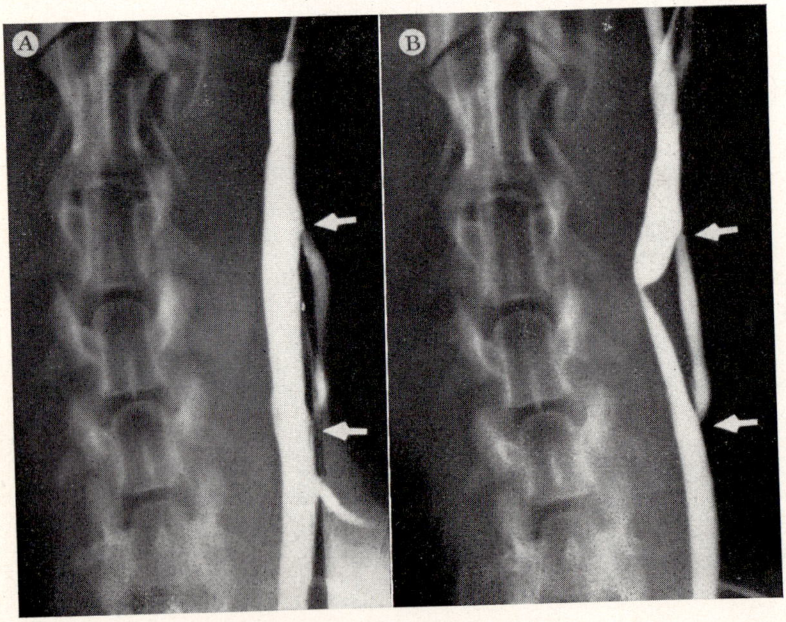

Fig 3.—*A*, phlebogram of a patent autogenous vein bypass in the jugular vein eight days after its implantation. The bypassed host vein was left intact. Note moderate opacification of the shunt in contrast to the host vein. *B*, phlebogram of the same case taken 140 days after implantation of the graft. Note that occlusion of the host vein resulted in increased opacification of the graft.

TABLE 2.—*Results of Bypass Grafts Between Right Iliac Vein and Inferior Vena Cava*

		Thrombosed		Patent	
Anticoagulants	No. Dogs	No.	Duration, Days	No.	Duration, Days
No	19	18	9	1	188
Yes	9	5	11	4	9
	11	7	120	4	120

series, one ligation was placed just above the distal anastomosis and the other below the junction of the two common iliac veins.

The results of this series are summarized in Table 2. Only one out of the 19 cases showed a patent graft 188 days postoperatively as disclosed by phlebography and anatomical examination. Thrombosis of the graft in the 18 cases occurred between 3 and 14 days after its implantation. The site of thrombosis was the distal anastomosis in 15 cases, and the entire graft in 3. In all 18 instances, marked fibrosis surrounded the distal anastomosis and extended occasionally around the lower half of the graft, but it never involved the caval anastomosis.

B. *With Anticoagulant Therapy.*—Anticoagulants were administered either only postoperatively or both pre- and postoperatively.

In the *first group,* which includes nine dogs, heparin and warfarin sodium (Coumadin)* were administered immediately postoperatively. After the second day, when the prothrombin time disclosed a therapeutic anticoagulant level, heparin was discontinued. In this group anticoagulation was maintained for one week. Duration of observations ranged from 9 to 11 days.

Of the nine dogs, four or 47.3% showed patency of the graft, while in the remaining five, a thrombus was found at the lower anastomosis. The clot extended from the iliac up to the anastomosis without invading the graft itself. In addition, as in the previous series, marked fibrosis surrounded the lower anastomosis and the initial segment of the graft. The cause for the failure was not clear

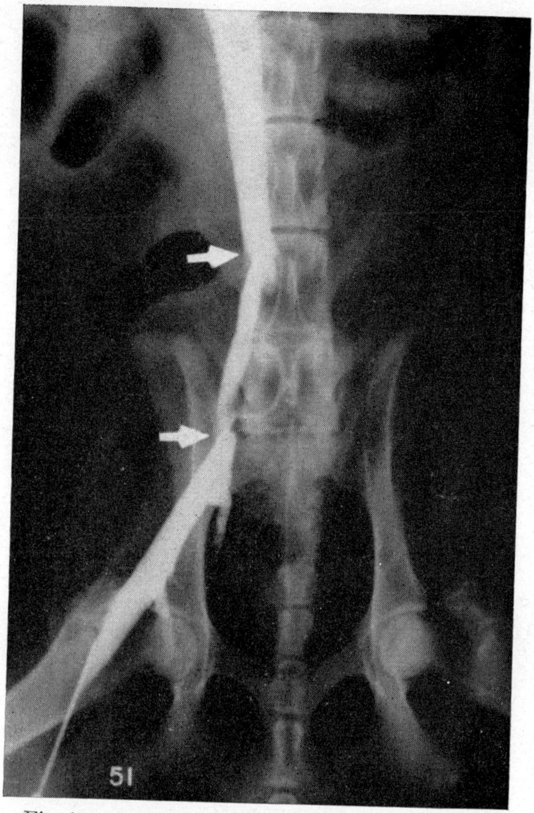

Fig 4.—Inferior vena cavagram showing a patent autogenous vein bypass graft 120 days after its implantation between the right iliac and the infrarenal segment of the inferior vena cava.

in four cases, except that the anticoagulation therapy may not have been quite effective in the first few hours. In the fifth case the presence of some adventitia in the suture line could possibly account for the thrombosis.

Fig 4 illustrates a patent bypass on the vena cavagram taken 120 days postoperatively. Fig 5 demonstrates the development of collateral circulation after failure of the graft as shown by the vena cavagram taken nine days after its implantation.

In a *second group* of 12 dogs, warfarin sodium was administered 24 to 36 hours prior to surgery (1.5 mg/kg body weight) and also for one week after surgery. The average control prothrombin time was seven seconds. At the time of surgery and 24 hours postoperatively its average levels were, respectively, 17 and 38 seconds. Postoperative intra-abdominal hemorrhage occurred in one

* Coumadin was supplied by Endo Laboratories, Inc.

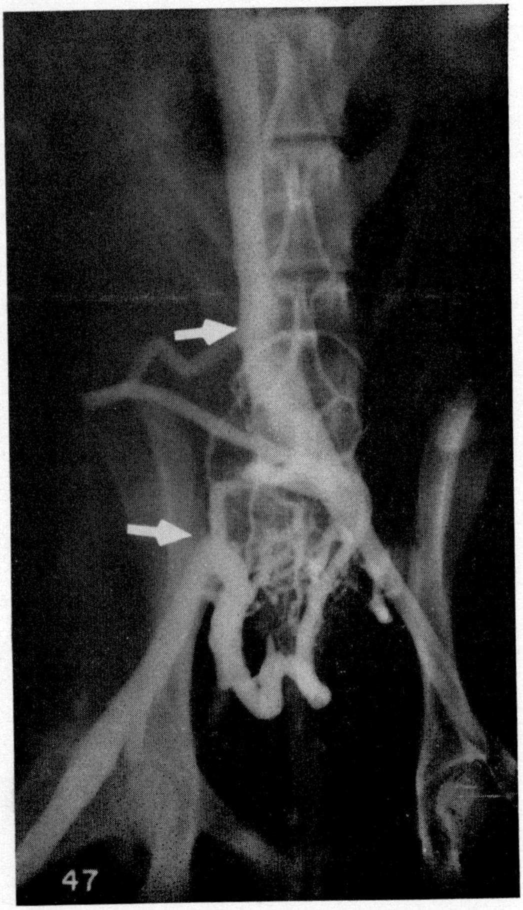

Fig 5.—Inferior vena cavagram taken nine days after implantation of a bypass graft between the iliac and inferior vena cava. It shows marked development of collateral circulation due to thrombosis at the distal end of the graft.

dog only and was fatal on the fourth day despite a fresh blood transfusion. His highest prothrombin time reached 75 seconds 48 hours after surgery.

In the remaining 11 dogs, the results as disclosed by phlebography four months postoperatively are indicated in Table 2. Of 11 grafts only four, ie 36.3%, were patent after that period of time, although one week postoperatively phlebographic evaluation showed six out of 11, ie 55.5%, of the grafts to be patent. These data indicate no significant difference in patency rate between the two series, the one receiving both pre- and postoperative anticoagulants and the other only postoperative.

Comment

From the foregoing data it is clear that the fate of an autogenous venous bypass graft in the venous system is distinctly different according to the site of its implantation. Comparison of these data on bypass grafting with those on end-to-end anastomosis found in the literature shows that while the methods of implantation do not seem to have any influence on the fate of the jugular grafts, they distinctly seem to have a significant bearing upon those used in the inferior vena cava.

Thus in the jugular, in our series, the over-all graft patency was 77.8% as compared to an average of 82% for the end-to-end anastomosis (the range of percentage varying from 58 to 90.9) found in the literature.[3-5]

In the inferior vena cava, the difference in the rate of patency between the bypass and the end-to-end procedures is quite striking. Using the bypass technique without anticoagulants, the percentage of patency was merely 5.5, while with anticoagulants the late results displayed a patency rate of 36.3%. In contrast to these results, most of those obtained with the end-to-end technique show an over-all high percentage of success,[3-5] ranging from 80% to 100%. However, even with the end-to-end technique, Collins et al [6] in a series of eight inferior vena cava reimplants reported five patent grafts after three weeks, two after six weeks, and none after four months. The divergent results obtained by the above investigators reemphasize the fact that failures of these grafts are more frequent the longer the observation period. In our series with initial anticoagulation, after a comparative four-month period the rate of patency was 36.3%.

While the results obtained by various investigators with venous implants in the inferior vena cava are variable, those in the jugular vein have yielded uniformly greater rate of success. The reason for the difference in the incidence of patency of the bypass venous grafts in the two sites, although not entirely clear, may be accounted for by the different circulatory factors involved in these two areas. In the jugular region, the isogravitational venous flow is very likely an important factor in preventing stasis. In contrast, the antigravitational flow prevailing in the inferior vena cava may explain the stasis and the high percentage of thrombosis in this type of graft implantation. Increased pressure in a venous bed has been shown to enhance patency of the grafts.[7] Thus, in experimental vein grafting in the portal system, an increased pressure led to almost uniform success not only with autogenous but also with homologous veins as well as with other substitutes.[8] Also in the inferior vena caval system and femoral vein, Schauble et al [5] were able to demonstrate the favorable influence of increased pressure upon the patency of the venous graft. Likewise, Bryant et al [3] utilizing the artificial production of an A-V fistula have shown the latter's role in enhancing the patency from 0% in the control group to 75% when the above pressure factor is brought into the picture.

In the inferior vena cava, the low flow rate, low pressure, and the fibrous reaction around the graft appear to play here even a greater role than in the direct grafts as factors leading to thrombosis. Use of anticoagulants appears to have overcome these factors in a relatively fair percentage of cases. Although the validity of the usefulness of anticoagulants may be questioned due to the short-term of their use, it should be pointed out that our previous experience and that of others [8] has shown that the critical period of a venous implant does not exceed one week. Beyond this period anticoagulation protection is usually no longer necessary.

Summary

Autogenous vein bypass grafts in the jugular and inferior vena cava were studied in the dog.

The high percentage of patency in the bypass graft of the jugular is similar to that of the end-to-end implants reported in the literature.

In contrast to this venous bed, in the inferior vena cava almost uniform thrombosis occurred without the use of anticoagulants. When the latter therapy was applied, patency was obtained in about half of the cases in the first week and in about a third after four months.

The low pressure, low flow rate, and reactive fibrosis are thought to account for thrombosis in the inferior vena cava bypass grafts.

Results with anticoagulants suggest their possible beneficial effect upon maintaining the patency of these grafts.

Ruthven Ferreira, Alphonso Henry, and Kendrick McCord gave technical assistance.

Henry Haimovici, MD, 862 Park Ave, New York 21, NY.

REFERENCES

1. Zinicola, N., and Haimovici, H.: Grafts in the Venous System: An Experimental and Clinical Evaluation; Review of the Literature, in preparation.

2. Haimovici, H.: A Four-Stay Suture Technique for End-to-Side Arterial Anastomosis, Surgery 47:266-267, 1960.

3. Bryant, M. F., Jr.; Lazenby, W. D.; and Howard, J. M.: Experimental Replacement of Short Segments of Veins, AMA Arch Surg 76:289-293, 1958.

4. Earle, A. S.; Horsley, J. S.; Villavicencio, J. L.; and Warren, R.: Replacement of Venous Defects by Venous Autografts, AMA Arch Surg 80:119-124, 1960.

5. Schauble, J. F.; Anlyan, W. G.; and Postlethwait, R. W.: A Study of Grafts in the Venous System, AMA Arch Surg 78:288-292, 1959.

6. Collins, H. A.; Burrus, G.; and DeBakey, M. E.: Experimental Evaluation of Grafts in the Canine Inferior Vena Cava, Amer J Surg 99:40-44, 1960.

7. Rousselot, L. M.: Autogenous Vein Grafts in Splenorenal Anastomosis, Surgery 31:403-410, 1952.

8. Symbas, P. N.; Foster, J. H.; and Scott, H. W., Jr.: Experimental Vein Grafting in the Portal Venous System, Surgery 50:97-106, 1961.

Intentional Hemodilution

Use of a Rotating Disc Oxygenator Primed With Acid Citrate Dextrose Blood and Low Molecular Weight Dextran: A Preliminary Report

SARIEL G. G. ABLAZA, MD; GEORGE T. RABER, BS; GUMERSINDO BLANCO, MD; DRYDEN P. MORSE, MD; ALBERTO ADAM, MD; AND HENRY T. NICHOLS, MD, PHILADELPHIA

In the performance of open-heart surgery, a low-prime oxygenator is desirable. This solves problems associated with blood procurement and reduces reactions resulting from multiple blood transfusions. Neptune [1] was the first to utilize acid citrate bank blood (ACD) and isotonic saline in priming his system. Zuhdi,[2] Long,[3] DeWall,[4] and Cooley [5] have performed intentional hemodilution perfusion using either low molecular weight dextran (LMWD) or 5% dextrose in water as priming material.

The oxygenators used by these groups were variations of the basic bubble oxygenator. The rotating disc oxygenator which, in our hands, has proved hematologic advantages, however, can also be used with a low priming volume. This is accomplished by incorporating a Gebauer internal heat exchanger in the oxygenator and using LMWD and ACD blood for priming the extracorporeal circuit.

The purpose of this communication is to describe our experiences in using this system in the performance of open-heart surgery.

Materials and Method

Thirty patients underwent open-heart surgery utilizing this technique (Table 1). There were 17 congenital and 13 acquired heart lesions. Sixteen patients were female and 14 were male, ranging in age from 4 to 58 years. Body weight in adults varied from 46 to 80 kg (102 to 177 lb) and in children varied from 13 to 56 kg (29 to 124 lb).

Submitted for publication Jan. 22, 1963.

From the Deborah Hospital, Browns Mills, NJ, and the Department of Thoracic Surgery, Hahnemann Medical College and Hospital, Philadelphia.

The extracorporeal circuit employed consisted of a rotating disc oxygenator and roller pumps. Prior to the availability of the 13-inch and 17-inch internal heat exchangers, a Harrison-Brown type of external heat exchanger was incorporated into the circuit. The venous drainage was siphoned into a reservoir which also collected cardiotomy low-pressure suction. The arterial blood was pumped into a femoral artery.

The choice of oxygenator size depended on the total blood flow calculated on the basis of 50 cc

TABLE 1.—*Patients Undergoing Open-Heart Surgery*

No.	Age, Sex	Diagnosis
1	5, M	Ostium primum with cleft mitral valve
2	11, F	Atrial septal defect—secundum
3	17, F	Atrial septal defect—secundum
4	13, M	Atrial septal defect—secundum
5	4, F	Atrial septal defect with total anomalous pul. drainage
6	13, M	Atrial septal defect with total anomalous pul. drainage
7	4, M	Pulmonic stenosis with patent ductus arteriosus
8	15, M	Pure valvular pulmonic stenosis
9	37, F	Pure valvular pulmonic stenosis
10	5, M	Pure valvular pulmonic stenosis
11	9, F	Pure valvular pulmonic stenosis
12	17, F	Pure valvular pulmonic stenosis
13	12, M	Congenital aortic stenosis
14	15, M	Supravalvular aortic stenosis
15	4, F	Acyanotic tetralogy of Fallot
16	39, F	Cyanotic tetralogy of Fallot
17	20, M	Cyanotic tetralogy of Fallot
18	14, M	Pure mitral insufficiency
19	38, M	Mitral insufficiency (reoper) valve replacement
20	37, F	Mitral stenosis, valve replacement
21	58, F	Mitral stenosis, valve replacement
22	44, M	Mitral stenosis
23	39, F	Mitral stenosis
24	29, F	Mitral stenosis
25	35, F	Mitral stenosis
26	42, M	Mitral stenosis
27	33, M	Mitral stenosis
28	40, F	Mitral stenosis
29	42, M	Mitral insufficiency (major), mitral stenosis (minor)
30	28, F	Mitral insufficiency (major), mitral stenosis (minor)

TABLE 2.—*Proportion of ACD Blood and LMWD Used for Priming the Different Sizes of Oxygenators*

Oxygenator Size (In)	Patient Wt (Kg)	Maximum Flow Capacity (Cc/Min)	Priming Volume: W/Internal Heat Exchanger ACD Blood (Cc)	Priming Volume: W/Internal Heat Exchanger LMWD (Cc)	Priming Volume: W/External Heat Exchanger ACD Blood (Cc)	Priming Volume: W/External Heat Exchanger LMWD (Cc)
13	Up to 30	3,000	2,000	500	2,500	500
17	Up to 60	4,000	1,500	1,000	2,000	1,000
21	80 kg and above	5,000	2,000	1,000	2,500	1,000

per kilogram per minute. Table 2 shows the amount of ACD blood and LMWD used with the various sizes of oxygenators utilizing either internal or external heat exchangers. The use of an internal heat exchanger reduced the priming volume by 500 cc.

Rheotran,* 15% dextran in 5% dextrose, was used as a diluent. The amount used was calculated on the basis of 20 cc per kilogram. This amount is slightly more than one third of the daily fluid requirement of patient. With the exception of two cases, we limited the total amount of Rheotran used to 1,000 cc in adults regardless of weight.

ACD blood collected in plastic bags one to four days prior to the operation was added to the calculated amount of Rheotran. Neither calcium nor heparin was added to this blood.

For total heparinization, 2.5 mg of heparin per kilogram was given to the patient intravenously. This was neutralized at the end of bypass with an equal amount of hexadimethrine bromide (Polybrene).

An indwelling Foley urethral catheter was used routinely. This was inserted after induction of anesthesia and removed 48 hours postoperatively.

Hemoglobin and hematocrit, bleeding time, clotting time, and platelet count were determined prior to bypass. Hemoglobin and hematocrit were determined again after cessation of bypass, after neutralization of heparin, and for three consecutive hours following the patient's return to the recovery room. These determinations were repeated on the first and third postoperative days. Platelet count, bleeding time, clotting time, and prothrombin time were determined again after the neutralization of heparin.

Sodium, potassium, calcium, chloride, and carbon dioxide combining power were determined preoperatively, after the patient's return to the recovery room, and on the first and third postoperative days. An additional calcuim determination was obtained five minutes after the start of bypass.

Urinary output was measured during bypass and every hour for the first eight hours postoperatively. The total 24-hour and 48-hour urinary outputs were also measured.

The total postoperative chest drainage was measured, and the chest tubes were routinely removed after 48 hours.

Results

The results of operative procedures on the various intracardiac lesions in this series are summarized in Table 3.

Bypass.—Actual blood flow always exceeded calculated blood flow (Table 4). The mean perfusion pressure was generally low in children and relatively high in adults. This was seen in spite of high flows in the former and moderately increased flows in the latter. Disc revolutions ranged from 50 to 120 per minute. Even with slow disc revolutions, oxygenation of blood appeared adequate. Temperature during bypass ranged from 26 to 38 C. Three patients had spontaneous hypothermic arrest, and eight patients had cardiac arrest after cross-clamping of the aorta. Those with spontaneous arrest converted to normal rhythm on rewarming. Only three out of the eight patients who arrested after cross-clamping of the aorta converted to preoperative rhythm after restoration of coronary flow. Five fibrillated after removal of the aortic clamp and had to be electrically defibrillated. Three patients fibrillated at the beginning of bypass and persisted throughout the operation. Only one of these three patients converted spontaneously. Two were defibrillated electrically. Except for two patients in whom the aorta was clamped, those with acquired heart disease did not fibrillate or have cardiac arrest.

* Low molecular weight dextran manufactured by Pharmachem Inc., Bethlehem, Pa; av molecular weight: 40,000; viscosity: 0.19.

TABLE 3.—*Results of Operative Procedures on Intracardiac Lesions*

	Operation	No.	Deaths
Congenital lesions			
Atrial septal defect			
A. Secundum	Primary suture	3	0
B. Primum	Suture of cleft mitral valve and Teflon patch repair of ASD	1	0
C. With total anomalous pulmonary venous drainage	Extracardiac anastomosis of PV confluens and LA, direct suture of ASD and ligation of left superior vena cava	2	0
Pulmonic stenosis			
A. Pure valvular	Pulmonary valvulotomy	5	0
B. Associated with patent ductus arteriosus	Valvulotomy and ligation of PDA	1	0
Aortic stenosis			
A. Valvular	Aortic commissurotomy	1	0
B. Supravalvular	Teflon patch graft	1	1 *
Tetralogy of Fallot			
A. Acyanotic	Total correction	1	0
B. Cyanotic	Total correction plus Teflon roof to right ventricular outflow tract	2	0
		17	1
Acquired lesions			
Pure mitral stenosis	Mitral commissurotomy,	7	0
	Starr valve replacement	2	0
Pure mitral insufficiency	Starr valve replacement,	1	0
	cross polar plication of posterior and anterior annulus	1	0
Major mitral insufficiency and minor mitral stenosis	Mitral commissurotomy and annulus plication	2	0
		13	0
Total		30	1

* The single death in this series occurred seven days after surgery as a result of acute massive hemorrhage due to a Staphylococcus infection with necrosis of the aortic suture line.

TABLE 4.—*Blood Flow: Actual and Calculated*

No.	Wt (Kg)	Calculated Flow (Cc/Min)	Actual Flow (Cc/Min)	Mean Perfusion Pressure (Mm Hg)	Duration of Bypass (Min)
1	20	1,400	2,800	35	60
2	27	1,900	2,600	50	35
3	50	2,500	3,300	50	40
4	31	1,600	1,700	45	35
5	13	650	1,800	20	80
6	25	1,250	2,800	30	80
7	17	850	1,600	30	55
8	56	3,000	3,200	40	17
9	51	2,550	3,000	70	15
10	23	1,100	2,200	30	20
11	24	1,200	3,000	20	25
12	55	2,650	3,500	70	15
13	33	1,650	2,600	30	25
14	55	2,750	3,300	20	65
15	14	700	1,400	30	90
16	50	2,500	3,500	30	170
17	46	2,275	2,800	40	90
18	38	1,900	3,200	40	72
19	79	4,000	4,400	50	135
20	64	3,200	4,000	50	115
21	60	3,000	4,400	40	90
22	77	3,850	4,500	30	35
23	50	2,500	4,000	65	45
24	61	3,050	3,400	60	35
25	59	2,950	3,500	70	40
26	66	3,300	4,000	50	60
27	80	4,000	4,200	40	55
28	63	3,150	3,600	60	33
29	71	3,500	4,000	70	65
30	62	3,100	3,500	80	50

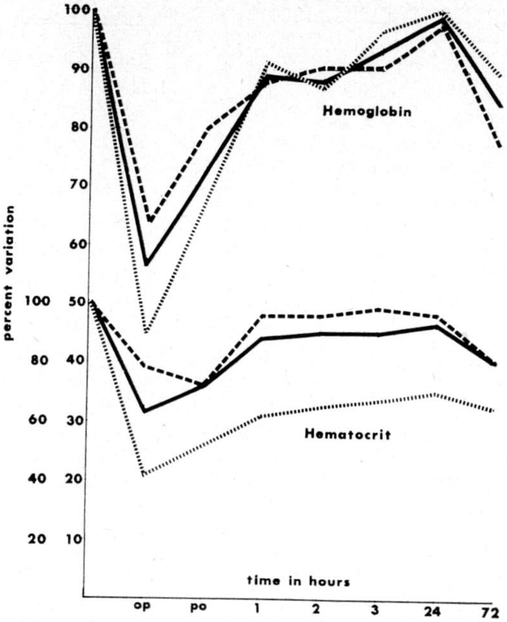

Fig. 1.—Per cent change in hemoglobin and hematocrit. Broken line represents lowest variation; solid line, mean variation of entire group; and striped line, highest variation.

Total bypass time ranged from 15 minutes to 170 minutes.

Hematologic Studies.—A definite and constant pattern was noted regarding the hemoglobin and hematocrit (Fig 1). There was a sharp drop of both values during bypass followed by a return to normal levels within two hours after the operation. This indicates effective but transient hemodilution. The bleeding time, clotting time, and prothrombin time remained within normal limits. Platelet count showed a transient drop and reversion to normal levels in 24 hours. There was no unusual bleeding problem associated with this temporary fall.

Electrolyte Studies.—There was a moderate drop in both the sodium and the chloride levels which persisted up to the third postoperative day. Potassium levels remained within normal limits. The carbon dioxide combining power was slightly reduced. Calcium values taken five minutes after the start of bypass dropped slightly in 15 patients and remained normal in 15 patients. Determinations repeated one to two hours after termination of bypass, however, showed all values to be normal. No incidence of tetany was seen. In those cases where intravenous calcium was given after bypass, the values were temporarily increased.

Urinary Output.—During perfusion, minimal or no urinary output was observed. Within 30 to 45 minutes after the cessation of bypass, rapid excretion of urine began (Fig 2). This continued for two hours. A period of relative oliguria then ensued which lasted for 24 hours. Then, 36 to 48 hours after operation, normal urinary output was observed. No renal shutdown or persistent oliguria was seen in this series.

Postoperative Blood Loss.—The total postoperative chest drainage ranged from 50 cc to 600 cc with an average loss of 283 cc.

Comment

The rotating disc oxygenator can be easily adapted to intentional hemodilution. Obvi-

Fig. 2.—Average uninary output of 30 patients. Note the rapid excretion of urine during the renal flush period.

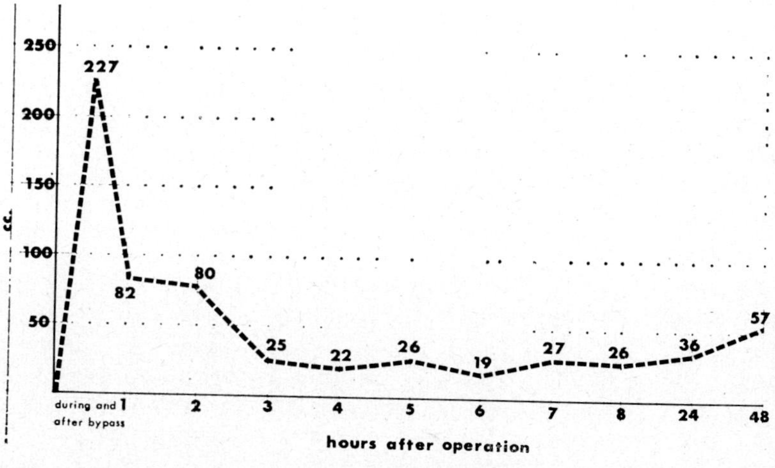

ously the priming volume has to be partly satisfied by blood. The use of small amounts of citrated blood, however, is not considered a disadvantage.

An average of four pints of blood was needed. In patients in whom the 17-inch oxygenator with an internal heat exchanger was used, only three pints of blood were needed (Table 2).

It is preferable to use ACD blood drawn the day before surgery, but the period of collection of blood can be extended to four days. This is particularly helpful when rare types of blood are needed. ACD blood was not reconstituted as recommended by Foote [6] because of the small amounts used. Clinical citrate intoxication was not seen. Calcium gluconate was given in four cases after the cessation of bypass only because myocardial contractions were not strong and there was a low blood pressure apparently not related to hypovolemia.

Low molecular weight dextran is an excellent diluent. It has been shown to increase systemic blood flow, decrease peripheral resistance, and decrease blood viscosity.[7] In this series actual blood flow constantly exceeded calculated blood flow. Frequently it was twice this calculated amount. Long and associates [3] used a flow of 25 to 30 cc per kilogram in association with moderate hypothermia. This was not feasible with the perfusion apparatus we have used. Venous return was greatly increased, and considerable amounts of blood accumulated in the oxygenator and venous reservoir. This necessitated increasing the inflow rate up to a certain point to accommodate the excessive venous return. In four instances, blood had to be withdrawn from the circuit because the oxygenator and venous reservoir could not contain the augmented venous return. To avoid this, a larger venous reservoir with a capacity of 3,000 cc was used.

Even with high flows and slow disc revolution, however, oxygenation of the blood appeared adequate. This was thought to be due to thinner filming of blood with consequent greater exposure and oxygen uptake of the red cells.

The initial low mean pressure seen to occur generally with children may be related to decreased blood viscosity and lowered peripheral resistance. In adults, the mean perfusion pressure was generally high even with only moderate increase in flow rates. It was also noted that in children, at the end of perfusion, only small amounts of blood accumulated in the oxygenator and venous reservoir at the termination of bypass. In adults, greater amounts of blood remained in the oxygenator and venous reservoir at the termination of bypass. This blood was returned to the patient in small amounts until a balance was achieved.

In the beginning of this study, moderate hypothermia was instituted by utilizing cold blood and dextran. Cooling was so rapid that cardiac arrest or ventricular fibrillation occurred shortly after the initiation of bypass. This was avoided by using warmed blood and gradual buildup to complete bypass. If cross-clamping of the aorta to obtain a quiet bloodless heart became necessary, gradual cooling to the desired temperature level was done. For short bypass or when cross-clamping of the aorta was not necessary, near normal temperature was maintained from the onset of bypass. When arrest occurred due to hypothermia, spontaneous conversion to normal sinus rhythm was seen with rewarming. The myocardium was flaccid during the entire duration of bypass. Even with prolonged hypothermic arrest the relative myocardial rigor seen with the regular perfusion was not noted. This greatly facilitated exposure of the intracardiac lesion. Furthermore, cardiac resuscitation was not difficult, and invariably vigorous cardiac contractions were seen soon after resumption of a regular beat. Studies are now being undertaken to determine if this is related to improved myocardial metabolism.

There were no bleeding problems. On the contrary, the total postoperative chest drainage was less than the usual. This is thought to be due to better neutralization of heparin inasmuch as with the use of ACD blood, in contrast to heparinized blood, the total amount of heparin given to the patient is less.

It may also be due to direct influence of LMWD on the coagulation mechanism.

The rapid excretion of urine seen 30 to 45 minutes after cessation of bypass, which we have designated as the renal flushing period, is due to osmotic diuresis exerted by the LMWD. Two hours postoperatively a state of equilibrium is probably reached, and the usual postoperative stage of relative oliguria ensues. No attempt was made to correct this. The patients received the usual postoperative intravenous fluid of 5% dextrose in water containing antibiotic. As was mentioned earlier, 36 to 48 hours later, urinary output returned to normal levels.

The patients were alert and well oriented after coming out of anesthesia. This may be a reflection of good cerebral perfusion.

Gelin [8] has shown that intravascular aggregation of red cells can be prevented by the use of LMWD. He attributes this to a reduction of blood viscosity due to hemodilution. Bernstein [9] suggested that this effect may be due to the increased negativity of the red cells. Both mechanisms are probably responsible for the reduction of intravascular clumping of red cells which may also protect the cerebral capillaries. This suggests that LMWD could prevent cerebral damage.

Summary and Conclusions

1. The rotating disc oxygenator with an internal or external heat exchanger is readily adaptable to a hemodilution technique using ACD blood and LMWD.

2. The amount of blood required to prime the oxygenator is reduced to three or four pints.

3. The use of unreconstituted ACD blood collected within a four-day period prior to surgery was shown to be feasible. No clinical evidence of citrate intoxication was observed.

4. There was no significant alteration of the hematologic or electrolyte patterns. Urinary output was good, and postoperative blood loss was less than usual.

5. No difficulties were encountered in the conduct of bypass. The augmented venous return appeared to be adequately oxygenated, and the rotating disc oxygenator returned the blood to the patient in high flow rates.

6. The relaxed state of the myocardium during bypass allowed good exposure of the underlying lesion and facilitated surgical repair.

Miss Theo M. Shemanski, RN, provided technical assistance.

Henry T. Nichols, MD, Department of Thoracic Surgery, Hahnemann Medical College and Hospital, 230 N Broad St, Philadelphia 2, Pa.

Addendum

Since submission of this manuscript about 150 more patients have been operated with this technique.

REFERENCES

1. Neptune, W. B.; Bougas, J. A.; and Panico, F. G.: Open Heart Surgery Without the Need for Donor-Blood Priming in the Pump-Oxygenator, New Eng J Med 263:111, 1960.

2. Zuhdi, N.; McCollough, B.; Carey, J.; and Greer, A.: Double-Helical Reservoir Heart-Lung Machine, Arch Surg 82:320, 1961.

3. Long, D. M., Jr., Sanchez, L.; Varco, R. L.; and Lillehei, C. W.: The Use of Low Molecular Weight Dextran and Serum Albumin as Plasma Expanders in Extracorporeal Circulation, Surgery 50:12, 1961.

4. DeWall, R. A., and Lillehei, C. W.: Simplified Total Body Perfusion, JAMA 179:430, 1962.

5. Cooley, D. A.; Beall, A. C., Jr.; and Grondin, P.: Open Heart Operations With Disposable Oxygenators, 5 Per Cent Dextrose Prime, and Normothermia, Surgery 52:713, 1962.

6. Foote, A. V.; Trede, M.; and Maloney; J. V., Jr.: Experimental and Clinical Study of the Use of A.C.D. Blood for Extracorporeal Circulation, J Thorac Cardiov Surg 42:93, 1961.

7. Drake, C. T.; Macalalad, F.; and Lewis, C. J.: Effect of Low Molecular Weight Dextran Upon Blood Flow During Extracorporeal Circulation, J Thorac Cardiov Surg 42:735, 1961.

8. Gelin, L. E., and Löfström, B.: A Preliminary Study on Peripheral Circulation During Deep Hypothermia, Acta Chir Scand 108:402, 1955.

9. Bernstein, E. F.; Castaneda, A.; Evans, R. L.; and Varco, R. L.: Alterations in Red Blood Cell Charge With Extracorporeal Circulation, Surg Forum 13:193, 1962.

Intentional Hemodilution

NAZIH ZUHDI, MD; JOHN CAREY, MD; JAMES CUTTER, MD; LLOYD RADER, MD;
AND ALLEN GREER, MD, OKLAHOMA CITY

After the publication of our early reports on hemodilution perfusion,[1-4] Cooley et al [5] suggested its usefulness for expediency in pulmonary embolectomy and recently used it routinely for total body bypass.[6] DeWall and Lillehei [7] and DeWall et al [8] constructively elaborated on this subject.

Our comparative studies of two series of patients who had open-heart surgery with the aid of extracorporeal circulation using blood primes or 5% dextrose in water primes did not reveal the superiority of either method.[9] The unfavorable theoretical and experimental attributes of blood primes did not materialize in our small series of patients. It is possible that the use of low priming volumes has obviated some of them, and it is conceivable that with larger series these disadvantages will become apparent. However, these studies demonstrated that 5% dextrose in water primes compare favorably with the conventional and traditional blood primes. This report is a brief analysis of 180 consecutive clinical perfusions using the principle of intentional hemodilution with 5% dextrose in water primes. A series of patients in whom blood replacement of the usual blood loss from the surgical field was either delayed until the termination of perfusion or not given at all if considered safe is not included in this presentation.

Method

The oxygenator is a scaled-down DeWall-Lillehei bubble oxygenator.[10] The double helical reservoir heart-lung machine [11] is primed with 5% dextrose in water using the formula: weight in kilograms × 16 ml.[12] This is pumped into the patient as his own blood is being drained by gravity into the oxygenating tube producing intentional hemodilution.[3] Moderate internal hypothermia from 25 to 30 C as measured in the midesophagus is accomplished by countercurrently pumping water at 4 C through the inner helix. Water at 45 C is used during the warming phase. The flow rates of 20 ml per kilogram of body weight per minute are not changed during the entire period of cardiopulmonary bypass and provide a priming volume to flow rate per minute ratio of 0.8. Partial perfusion is used during the cooling phase to 30 C and during the warming phase when feasible. Warming is stopped at about 33 C. At the termination of perfusion, the contents of the heart-lung machine are returned to the patient. An average of 3 mg of heparin per kilogram of body weight are given intravenously prior to cannulation and an equivalent amount of hexadimethrine bromide (Polybrene) or protamine sulfate at the termination of perfusion. Blood loss from the surgical field is replaced, as it occurs, with citrated blood.[1] The majority of patients in this series received nitrous oxide as the primary anesthetic agent supplemented with minimal quantities, 0.3 and 0.5 vol %, of halothane vapor for maintenance.

Results

1. *Mean Arterial Pressure.*—The mean arterial pressure during total body bypass is usually between 40 mm Hg and 50 mm Hg. It is more uniform and predictable than the mean arterial pressure in our series of blood primes. The average maximum oxygen arteriovenous difference in 14 consecutive patients was 9.8 vol %.

2. *Cerebral Complications.*—Awakening is usually immediate, and patients respond to verbal commands. One patient failed to regain consciousness, an incidence of 0.55%. Her total perfusion time and total body bypass time were at the upper limits of the range of the survivors. She had open mitral valvuloplasty for a recurrent mitral stenosis and insufficiency.

Interpretation of cerebral manifestations and actual brain damage following perfusions

---

Submitted for publication June 17, 1963.

Department of Anesthesiology, Mercy Hospital (Dr. Cutter); Resident in Surgery, St. Anthony Hospital (Dr. Rader).

TABLE 1.—*Cerebral Complications Following Hemodilution Perfusion*

No. of Patients	Cereb Death	Cereb Complic	Outcome
180	1 (0.55%)	13	Complete recovery

is difficult. There were eight instances of minor and five instances of major cerebral manifestations. Minor complications include difficulty in focusing, hallucinations, loss of minor modalities of coordination, and short periods of confusion. Major complications include pareses, convulsions, unresponsiveness, and prolonged periods of disorientation. One of the patients with major complications had a previous history of grand mal seizures, and another one had been treated for schizophrenia. The remaining patients recovered without overt clinical findings at the present time (Table 1).

3. *Urinary Studies.*—There was one case of renal shutdown, an incidence of 0.55%. Recovery occurred without dialysis. The amount of urine output in the first 24 hours was satisfactory and averaged 31.92 ml per kilogram of body weight per 24 hours. It was usually higher in the second 24 hours. Albuminuria (31.3%) and microscopic hematuria (67.3%) were reversible within one to three days (Table 2).

4. *Acid-Base Balance.*—Plasma bicarbonate concentrations in blood corrected to a pH of 7.4 by the use of Peters and Van Slyke formula were performed prior to and at the end of perfusion in 14 patients. The average base deficit was 3.42 mEq per liter, the range being from +0.27 to −8.79. No attempt was made to correct this deficit, and it did not correlate with the clinical course (Table 3).

5. *Hemolysis Data.*—The average rise in plasma hemoglobin following a standard

TABLE 2.—*Urinary Studies Following Hemodilution Perfusions*

Urine Output During Initial 48 Hr Ml/Kg/24 Hr	Albuminuria	Micro Hematuria
35.65	31.3%	76.3%

mechanical fragility test [12] performed before and after hemodilution cardiopulmonary bypass in four patients was 22.1 mg%. Following an average perfusion of 60 minutes, the average rise in plasma hemoglobin in 33 consecutive patients was 13.9 mg%, with a range from 2.8 to 83.4 mg% (Table 3).

6. *Changes in Blood Elements.*—There is a decrease in the number of platelets in the postoperative count ranging from 114,000 to 410,000 per cubic millimeter, with an average of 206,000, the preoperative value being 371,000 per cubic millimeter. There are no significant alterations in the coagulation time, prothrombin time, prothrombin consumption time, and fibrinogen levels (Table 3).[42]

7. *Postoperative Chest Drainage.*—Postoperative chest drainage in 77 patients, a good index of over-all hemostasis, ranged

TABLE 3.—*Positive and Negative Changes in Studies Performed Prior to and Following Hemodilution Perfusions*

Bicarbonate deficit (mEq/liter)	−3.42
Platelet (count/cu mm)	−135,000
Lee-White coagulation time (min)	−1 min 04 sec
Fibrinogen (mg %)	+14
Prothrombin time (sec)	+0.19/14
Prothrombin consumption time (sec)	−7.3
Postoperative blood loss (ml/kg body weight)	12

− indicates a postoperative value which is smaller than the preoperative value by the indicated figure;
+ indicates a postoperative value which is larger than the preoperative value by the indicated figure.

from 0 ml to 39 ml per kilogram of body weight over an average period of 37.8 hours [12] (Table 3).

8. *Clinical Tabulation.*—The results in this series of 180 consecutive patients are tabulated in Tables 4 and 5. Table 6 provides the range and mean values of age, weight, perfusion time, and complete body bypass time of the survivor group.

Comment

The neurological findings of Brown et al [13] on dogs being subjected to low-flow perfusions are significant, but transposition of animal data to humans may be misleading. Immediate awakening and excellent clinical response indicate that probably human and

TABLE 4.—*Congenital Cardiac Defects Corrected With Hemodilution Perfusion*

Type of Defect	No. of Patients	No. Living
Atrial septal defect	35	35
Ventricular septal defect	41	37
Pulmonary stenosis	17	14
Tetralogy of Fallot	6	3
Aortic stenosis	6	6
Supravalvular aortic stenosis	3	3
Atrioventricularis communis	3	1
Drainage of right pulmonary venous trunk into inferior vena cava	1	1
	112	100 (89.2%)

animal anatomic arrangements and tolerances of physiologic limits and tissue perfusion are dissimilar. Galletti and Brecher [14] point out that the irreducible "structural metabolism" required for keeping cerebral tissue alive is 20% of what is needed for functional activity. This is confirmed by the work of Andreason and Watson [15] and Cohen and Lillehei.[16] This figure is lower in young animals [17] and during hypothermia. Our cerebral complications could be due to a poor myocardial contraction in the early postperfusion period resulting in brain ischemia, to air emboli trapped in the left side of the heart, or to fat embolization from cardiotomy suction blood,[18] rather than due to the low flow rates. Signs of temporary or permanent neurologic damage are reported with other types of oxygenators and higher flow rates.[14] Calcium, antifoam, and fibrin are unlikely causes. The electroencephalogram did not prove to be a useful tool in forewarning of cerebral complications.

Moderate internal hypothermia permits safe reduction of metabolic and oxygen requirements, not associated with the limitation of external hypothermia, profound hypothermia, or perfusion alone. Gollan et al [23] and Sealy et al [24] are among the early investigators to point out the safety of combining moderate internal hypothermia and total body perfusion. DeWall and Lillehei found the average maximum arteriovenous oxygen difference to be 7.1 vol% at 30 ml per kilogram of body weight per minute.[7] There is no evidence for deficient utilization of oxygen or disruption of blood-brain barrier during moderate internal hypothermia.[25] In 31 patients, DeWall and Lillehei found that accumulation of excess lactic acid, a representation of the metabolic response to hypoxia,[26] averaged 2.99 mM per liter and readily reversed after the hemodilution hypothermic perfusion.[8]

TABLE 5.—*Acquired Cardiac Defects Corrected With Hemodilution Perfusion*

Type of Defect	No. of Patients	No. Living
Mitral stenosis and insufficiency	60	54
Mitral valve replacement	2	2
Aortic stenosis including aortic replacements	5	1
Myocardial disease	1	0
	68	57 (83.8%)

TABLE 6.—*Range and Mean Values of General Data on 148 Patients of Survivor Group of Patients Having Hemodilution Perfusion*

No. of Patients	Age, Yr	Wt, Kg	Perfusion Time, Min	Total Body Bypass Time, Min
148	13 Mo-58	7.9-77.30	22-189	11-118
	18	42.84	61.18	33.01

The average bicarbonate deficit in our patients of 3.42 mEq per liter is within the range of reported loss of buffer base [19-22] with other types of perfusions using higher flow rates. The acid-base balance is more decisively affected by the postperfusion cardiopulmonary status than by the type of perfusion system used. Moderate internal hypothermia is a useful and not an essential modality of intentional hemodilution. It slows the "tempo," and the consequent low flow rates mean a slower blood turnover per minute.

Tissue perfusion is related to peripheral vascular resistance and to blood viscosity. Peripheral vascular resistance has been found by various observers to be elevated during moderate hypothermia.[28,29] In dogs, the degree of elevation has been found to be directly related to the magnitude of depression of body temperature with either barbiturate or ether anesthesia.[30] Studies on humans cooled to a range of 31 C to 32.5 C revealed a mean increase in total peripheral resistance of 89% in seven of ten subjects.[31] The failure of the remaining three subjects to show an increase may be related to the inconsistence of anesthetic methods and agents employed in the study; for in humans, at least, various responses in circulatory dynamics are produced not only by different anesthetic agents but also by changes in the depth of anesthesia with a single agent.

Although no alterations in circulatory dynamics have been ascribed to nitrous oxide, halothane has been found both clinically and experimentally to produce peripheral vascular dilatation and a consequent fall in peripheral vascular resistance.[32-35] Controlled studies during halothane anesthesia in humans have shown conflicting results which probably reflect the differences between light and deep anesthesia. In one study of ten adults during light halothane anesthesia no consistent changes in peripheral resistance were found.[36] Another study of 13 subjects during moderately deep halothane anesthesia revealed a mean fall in total peripheral resistance of 18%.[37]

Considering the minimal concentration of halothane vapor employed in this series of patients, it is unlikely that a significant reduction in peripheral resistance results from this agent as compared with the magnitude of change in the opposite direction induced by hypothermia. In addition, the concentration of dissolved halothane in blood and tissues is rapidly reduced during circulatory bypass because only 100% oxygen, rather than an anesthetic mixture, is utilized for gas exchange in the pump oxygenator. It would be anticipated, then, that any halothane-induced vasodilatation would be dissipated by the time hypothermia had been induced.

DeWall et al [8] measured relative viscosities of blood and of blood diluted with 5% glucose in water, taken from a patient when her esophageal temperature was 30 C. This sample was then tested in vitro throughout the temperature range from 37 C to 10 C. The viscosity of diluted blood remains lower. Reemtsma and Creech [27] believe that hemodilution with dextran may lower blood viscosity by lowering the hematocrit, even though it is more viscous than blood.

The degree of intentional hemodilution should be limited. Perfusing a patient with one third to one half of his daily fluid requirements is well tolerated. This amount of priming volume is adequate for substantially higher flow rates than the ones we use. Experimentally, this fluid does remain for the most part in circulation for about 60 minutes.[3] Longer periods of perfusion were not studied. However, a more severe degree of hemodilution may lead to tissue anoxia and poor perfusion.[9]

The usual blood loss from the surgical field is replaced with banked citrated blood. Because of the decrease in the red blood cell count inherent in hemodilution perfusion, a delay in or omission of this blood replacement may prove injurious to the vital organs.[9] In ideal cases, open-heart surgery with hemodilution perfusion may be performed without the use of any blood before, during, or after surgery.[12] When postoperative chest drainage is in excess of the expected limits, a bleeding vessel or cardiotomy incision, rather than a defect in the coagulating mechanism, is more likely to be the cause. Early re-exploration is recommended.

The use of 5% dextrose in water as a definitive prime inducing hemodilution permits better tissue perfussion and oxygenation, particularly during hypothermia, which predisposes to increased blood viscosity, increased peripheral resistance, and capillary stagnation. Long et al [38] advocated the use of low molecular weight dextran in order to prevent sludging of blood that occurs during total body perfusion. It is axiomatic that other blood substitutes have been and will be advocated. Five per cent dextrose in water is of simple composition, has been extensively studied, and may have some protective action on the myocardium.

The use of blood when not needed should give us some concern. In his Nobel Prize lecture in 1930, Karl Landsteiner elaborated on his concept of the individual differences in human blood. This applies to the red blood cells as well as to the other elements, including proteins. Anaphylactoid responses, major and minor blood incompatibilities, renal complications, and hepatitis are still present, even though greatly reduced through acquired knowledge. An analysis of 33,090 blood transfusions given between 1953 and 1959 at St. Anthony Hospital in Oklahoma City revealed an average of one reaction for every 131 transfusions. There were five deaths related to transfusions, a fatality incidence of 1:6,615.[39] In addition, there is a decrease in pH of donor blood that occurs after its collection, due to an accumulation of lactic acid from anaerobic glycolysis.[40] This may be important in individuals with cyanotic congenital heart disease with uncompensated metabolic acidosis under ambulatory conditions.[41]

The safety, efficiency, and feasibility of blood substitute primes are demonstrated. Theoretical and experimental advantages of blood substitute primes are such that they are bound to become evident as our series enlarges.

Summary

Hemodilution perfusions induced by complete 5% dextrose in water primes of the heart-lung machine are safe, efficient, and physiologic. Blood substitute primes do away with many of the theoretical and experimental disadvantages of blood and of pooled blood. Minor and major incompatibilities, acidosis, renal complications, hepatitis, sludging, and sequestration of blood are among such complications. The simplicity of such a perfusion system is attractive.

Nazih Zuhdi, MD, 430 NW 12th St, Oklahoma City 3, Okla.

REFERENCES

1. Zuhdi, N.; McCollough, B.; Carey J.; and Greer, A.: The Use of Citrated Banked Blood for Open Heart Surgery, Anesthesiology 21:496-501, 1960.

2. Zuhdi, N.; McCollough, B.; Carey, J.; and Greer, A.: Double-Helical Reservoir Heart-Lung Machine: Designed for Hypothermic Perfusion; Primed With 5% Glucose in Water; Inducing Hemodilution, Arch Surg 82:320-325, 1961.

3. Zuhdi, N.; McCollough, B.; Carey, J.; Grieger, C.; and Greer, A.: Hypothermic Perfusion for Open Heart Surgical Procedures: Report on the Use of a Heart-Lung Machine Primed With 5% Dextrose in Water, Inducing Hemodilution, J Int Coll Surg 35:319-326, 1961.

4. Zuhdi, N., in discussion of Chardack, W. M., et al: Correction of Complete Heart Block by a Self-Contained and Subcutaneously Implanted Pacemaker, J Thorac and Cardiov Surg 42:827-828, 1961.

5. Cooley, D. A.; Beall, A. C., Jr.; and Alexander, J. K.: Acute Massive Pulmonary Embolism, JAMA 177:283-287, 1961.

6. Cooley, D. A.; Sealy, A. C.; and Grondin, P.: Open Heart Operations With Disposable Oxygenators, 5% Dextrose Prime, and Normothermia, Surgery 52:713-719, 1962.

7. DeWall, R., and Lillehei, C. W.: Simplified Total Body Perfusion: Reduced Flows, Moderate Hypothermia, and Hemodilution, JAMA 179:430-434, 1962.

8. DeWall, R. A.; Lillehei, R.; and Sellers, R.: Hemodilution Perfusions for Open Heart Surgery, New Eng J Med 266:1078-1084, 1962.

9. Zuhdi, N.; Carey, J.; Sheldon, W.; and Greer, A.: Comparative Merits and Results of Blood Primes and 5% Dextrose in Water Primes of Heart-Lung Machines: Analysis of 250 Patients, J Thorac Cardiov Surg, to be published.

10. DeWall, R. A.; Warden, H. E.; Varco, R.; and Lillehei, C. W.: The Helix Reservoir Pump Oxygenator, Surg Gynec Obstet 104: 699-710, 1957.

11. Zuhdi, N.; McCollough, B.; Carey, J.; and Greer, A.: Hypothermic Total Body Cardiopulmonary Bypass: Experimental and Clinical Studies, J Okla Med Ass 53:514-516, 1960.

12. Zuhdi, N.; Carey, J.; and Greer, A.: Hemodilution for Body Perfusion, J Okla Med Ass 56:88-107, 1963.

13. Brown, I., in Surgery of the Chest, edited by J. H. Gibbon, Philadelphia: W. B. Saunders Company, 1962, p. 738.

14. Galletti, P. M., and Brecher, G. A.: Heart-Lung Bypass, New York: Grune & Stratton, Inc., 1962, p. 232.

15. Andreason, A., and Watson, F.: Experimental Cardiovascular Surgery, Brit J Surg 39:548-551, 1962.

16. Cohen, M., and Lillehei, W.: A Quantitative Study of the "Azygos Factor" During Vena Caval Occlusion in the Dog, Surg Gynec Obstet 98:225-232, 1954.

17. Kabat, H., and Dennis, C.: The Resistance of Young Dogs to Acute Arrest of the Cephalic Circulation, Proc Soc Exp Biol Med 42:534-537, 1939.

18. Caguin, F., and Carter, M.: Fat Embolization With Cardiotomy Using Cardiopulmonary Bypass, J Thorac Cardiov Surg, to be published.

19. Lim, R.; Rehder, K.; Harp, R. A.; Dawson, B.; and Kirklin, J. W.: Circulatory Arrest During Profound Hypothermia Induced by Direct Blood-Stream Cooling: Experimental Study, Surgery 49:367-374, 1961.

20. Bjork, V. O.: Effective Blood Heat Exchanger for Deep Hypothermia in Association With Extracorporeal Circulation, but Excluding Oxygenator, J Thorac Cardiov Surg 40:237-252, 1960.

21. Young, W.; Sealy, W.; Brown, I.; Smith, W.; Callaway, H.; and Harris, J.: Metabolic and Physiologic Observations on Patients Undergoing Extracorporeal Circulation in Conjunction With Hypothermia, Surgery 46:175-184, 1959.

22. Starr, A.: Oxygen Consumption During Cardiopulmonary Bypass, J Thorac Cardiov Surg 38:46-56, 1959.

23. Gollan, F.; Blos, P.; and Schuman, H.: Exclusion of Heart and Lungs From Circulation in the Hypothermic Closed Chest Dog by Means of a Pump Oxygenator, J Appl Physiol 5:180-190, 1952.

24. Sealy, W.; Brown, I.; Young, W.; Stephen, R.; Harris, J.; and Merritt, D.: Hypothermia, Low Flow, Extracorporeal Circulation and Controlled Cardiac Arrest for Open Heart Surgery, Surg Gynec Obstet 104:441-450, 1957.

25. Pollard, H. S., Jr.; Fleischaker, R. J.; Timmes, J. J.; and Harlson, K. E.: Blood Brain Barrier Studies in Extracorporeal Cooling and Warming, J Thorac Cardiov Surg 42:772-781, 1961.

26. Huckabee, W. E.: Relationship of Pyruvate and Lactate During Anaerobic Metabolism: I. Effects of Infusion of Pyruvate or Glucose and of Hyperventilation, J Clin Invest 37:244-254, 1958.

27. Reemtsma, K., and Creech, O.: Viscosity Studies of Blood, Plasma and Plasma Substitutes, J Thorac Cardiov Surg 44:674-680, 1962.

28. Jude, J. R.; Haroutunian, L. M.; and Folse, R.: Hypothermic Myocardial Oxygenation, Amer J Physiol 190:57, 1957.

29. Hegnauer, A. H., and D'Amato, H. E.: Oxygen Consumption and Cardiac Output in Hypothermic Dog, Amer J Physiol 178:138-142, 1954.

30. Bigelow, W. G.; Lindsay, W. K.; and Greenwood, W. F.: Hypothermia, Its Possible Role in Cardiac Surgery: An Investigation of Factors Governing Survival in Dogs at Low Body Temperatures, Ann Surg 132:849-866, 1950.

31. Rose, J. C.; McDermott, T. F.; Lilienfield, L. S.; Porfido, F. A.; and Kelly, R. T.: Cardiovascular Function in Hypothermic Anesthetized Man, Circulation 15:512-517, 1957.

32. Black, G. W., and McArdle, L.: Effects of Halothane on Peripheral Circulation in Man, Brit J Anaesth 34:2-10, 1962.

33. Burnap, T. K.; Galla, S. J.; and Vandam, L. D.: Anesthetic, Circulatory and Respiratory Effects of Fluothane, Anesthesiology 19:307-320, 1958.

34. Hall, L. D., and Forbes, H. N.: Respiratory and Cardiovascular Effects of Fluothane in Dogs, Anesthesiology 19:339-352, 1958.

35. Mauzan, J. E.; Hanna, C.; and Abajian, J.: Effect of Halothane on the Heart, Anesthesiology 23:156-158, 1962.

36. Wenthe, F. M.; Patrick, R.; and Wood, E. H.: Effects of Anesthesia With Halothane on the Human Circulation, Anesth Analg (Cleveland) 41:381-390, 1962.

37. Deutsch, S.; Linde, H. W.; Dripps, R. D.; and Price, H. L.: Circulatory and Respiratory Actions of Halothane in Normal Man, Anesthesiology 23:631-638, 1962.

38. Long, D. B., et al: Use of Low Molecular Weight Dextran and Serum Albumin as Plasma Expanders in Extracorporeal Circulation, Surgery 50:12-28, 1961.

39. Bricker, E.: Blood Transfusions, Obstet Gynec 18:439-442, 1961.

40. Callaghan, J. C.; Fraser, R. S.; Brorkin, J.; and Stewart, A. G.: "The Acid Base Aspects of Extracorporeal Circulation," in Extracorporeal Circulation, edited by J. D. Allen, Springfield, Ill: Charles C Thomas, Publisher, 1958, p 179.

41. DeWall, R. A.; Warden, H. E.; Melby, J. C.; Minot, H.; Varco, R. L.; and Lillehei, C. W.: Physiological Responses During Total Body Perfusion With a Pump-Oxygenator: Studies in 120 Patients Undergoing Open Cardiac Surgery, JAMA 165:1788-1792, 1957.

42. Zuhdi, N.; Carey, J.; and Greer, A.: Hemodilution and Coagulation Factors in Extracorporeal Circulation, J Thorac Cardiov Surg 43:816-821, 1962.

New Iodine Compound for Degerming Skin Surface

CHARLES L. GERACI, MD
REDWOOD CITY, CALIF

For the past several years the most generally accepted method of degerming the skin surface in preparation for surgical procedures has involved the preliminary scrubbing of the skin with a soap or detergent containing the bacteriostatic agent hexachlorophene, followed by a wash using either tincture or solution of a quaternary ammonium compound, usually benzalkonium chloride. With the awareness during the past few years of an increasing number of postoperative wound infections of serious nature, often involving organisms which are resistant to conventional forms of therapy, the medical literature has reflected a renewal of the search for more effective skin preparation techniques and substances. This has no doubt been spurred on by the general feeling that the offending organisms involved in most postoperative wound infections are probably not brought in extraneously but are much more likely harbored on and in the surface of the patient's skin. Numerous investigators [10,11,14] have corroborated the fact that sterilization of the skin is highly improbable, and that after decontamination of the skin the remaining organisms may rise to the surface of the cut skin, multiply, and inoculate themselves into the body along the incision made by the surgeon. For this reason Price [11,14,15] has introduced the term "degermation" to indicate the process by which the bacterial counts of the skin are lowered.

During the past 15 years a large volume of clinical experience has been accumulated in the use of hexachlorophene as a surgical preparation material throughout this country. Hexachlorophene has continued to be effective and is generally well accepted. Nevertheless it is far from being a complete germicide, and therefore research to find a compound that will fullfill these requirements continues. Benzalkonium chloride is well known to be effective against Gram-positive and Gram-negative organisms, but there has been no agreement regarding its effect on spore-

Submitted for publication Feb 4, 1963.
From the Surgical Section of Sequoia Hospital.

forming organisms. Similarly, there is no good evidence available as to the effectiveness of hexachlorophene against acid-fast bacteria, bacterial spores, spirochetes, fungi, or viruses.[5,11] In addition, it has been demonstrated by Price and others that the presence of organic matter, especially blood serum, greatly hampers the activity of hexachlorophene soaps as well as benzalkonium chloride.[9,11,16]

Preparations containing iodine have long been known to be extremely effective as bactericidal agents, but iodine in both solution and tincture was long ago virtually given up as a method of skin preparation because of the high incidence of skin sensitivity to iodine. Iodine first began to receive some attention as a skin disinfectant in 1905, due to the work of Senn.[11] In fact the chief use of iodine has always been just for that purpose. Tincture of iodine was generally recommended because the alcohol facilitated penetration and spreading. The outstanding features of iodine as a germicide have been recognized since the beginning of its use. It is a rapidly acting disinfectant with maximal bactericidal and minimal bacteriostatic properties. Iodine exhibits the broadest spectrum against pathogens of any antiseptic known. It has accepted lethal action against bacilli, cocci, spores, spirillae, fungi, yeasts, viruses, rickettsia, protozoa, and helminths.[3,4] However, the use of iodine, though a very effective skin antiseptic, results in almost inevitable skin irritation if the iodine is allowed to remain on the skin for any sustained period. Medrek and Litsky,[11] in 1957, reported toxicity for skin occurring in four of 25 patients (about 15%.) This toxicity of iodine for skin has been fairly well determined to be due to the presence of free iodine in contact with the skin surface, and it depends, in direct relationship, on the concentration of the iodine. Tinctures or solutions of iodine weak enough to preclude skin sensitivity have been conversely found to be too weak to have effective germicidal properties.

Very recently there has been considerable interest regenerated in the study of so-called "iodophores," complexed mixtures of iodine with cationic, anionic, or nonionic detergents. These substances appear to have at least twofold advantages. The detergents act as very effective skin cleansing agents, and in addition the iodine present is bound to the detergents in such a way that it is released in active form only very slowly. Thus its activity is spread out over a long period of time, and its toxicity for the skin is greatly reduced. This type of compound has been produced for use as surgical skin preparations and as scrub solutions by several manufacturers. Numerous authors have investigated the in vitro properties of these iodine substances and the in vivo evidences of their activity,[1,3,4,6,10,12] but the literature concerning their practical effectiveness is still meager, probably due to the fact that they have been in use for such a short period of time.

This paper deals with studies of a new complexed iodine skin degerming agent, Surgidine,* which was developed to meet the specific need for a nonirritating, nonstaining bactericidal agent. This substance has a pH of 4, and consists of iodine, complex fatty amido compound (the fatty group being derived from coconut oil), polyoxyethylated fatty alcohol, and polyoxyethylated vegetable oil, in an aqueous system. It is both nonionic and cationic, the cations being derived from the complex amido ampholyte. This substance contains 2% iodine of which 1.2% is titratable with sodum thiosulfate. The titratable portion is regarded as the available iodine. The remaining 0.8% is in the form of iodides. This substance may be broadly defined as an iodophor, an iodine carrier, or a complexed iodine. As has been noted above, elemental iodine is both a primary irritant and a skin sensitizer. Strong solutions of elemental iodine and alcohol may cause burns on the skin because the alcohol evaporates, leaving concentrated iodine on the skin. Complexed iodine does not evaporate, iodine remains in a dilute form, with consequent virtual elimination of the iodine burn and

* Supplied by Continental Laboratories, Palo Alto, Calif.

skin staining. This appears to be true in both the aqueous complexed systems and those mixed with alcohol in reasonable ratios.

This particular study of the complexed iodine preparation, Surgidine, involved skin cultures taken from patients before skin preparation, after preparation, and after operation when prepared with the substance. At the hospital involved in this study the preparation of skin prior to surgery for the past 12 years has been scrubbing of the operative area for five minutes with a solution of hexachlorophene (pHisoHex) and water, followed by a wash of the same area with a 1 to 1,000 solution of benzalkonium chloride. It was decided that the experiment should be set up so that preparation of patients using the complexed iodine would be done in a roughly similar manner: eg, the skin of the operative area would be scrubbed for five minutes with a solution of the complexed iodine, Surgidine, followed by a wash of the same area with tincture of Surgidine supplied separately by the manufacturer.

The Experiment

Fifty patients were prepared in the usual manner with hexachlorophene and solution of benzalkonium chloride as described above, and 50 patients were prepared with Surgidine, both solution and tincture. The surgeons scrubbed from three to five minutes in the usual manner, using either hexachlorophene and water or Surgidine solution. It was hoped in this manner to compare the relative effectiveness of each method of skin preparation, using skin cultures as hereinafter described:

For the hexachlorophene preparations, swabs moistened in phosphate-buffered saline containing 1% polysorbate (Tween) 80, and stored in 5 ml of this substance prior to plating, were rubbed briskly over a 1 inch by 2 inch area of skin adjacent to the operative site, (*a*) before the skin preparation was begun, (*b*) after skin preparation but before beginning the operation, and (*c*) after completion of the operation. Tube dilution colony counts were made for total counts, and were plated on human blood (for Gram-positive cocci) and on MacConkey's medium (for Gram-negative bacilli). For the Surgidine preparations swabs moistened in phosphate-buffered saline containing 5% sodium thiosulfate, and stored in 5 ml of this solution prior to plating, were rubbed briskly over a 1 inch by 2 inch area of skin adjacent to the operative area in the same manner as for the hexachlorophene preparations.

TABLE 1.—*Surgidine*

Operation	Min	Cultures (Staphylococci Only) Preprep	Postprep	Postop
Vein stripping	170	30,000	NG	NG
Herniorrhaphy	60	5,000	NG	NG
Rad. mastectomy	110	NG	NG	NG
Herniorrhaphy	50	1,000	NG	NG
Exc. pilonidal sinus	45	500,000	1,500	1,600
Herniorrhaphy	90	5,400	50	400
Thyroidectomy	150	110	NG	NG
Herniorrhaphy	40	1,500	NG	NG
Herniorrhaphy	60	8,250	NG	300
Herniorrhaphy	75	50	50	NG
Exc. pilonidal sinus	37	188,000	NG	NG
Open red. ankle	60	50	NG	NG
Laminectomy	90	NG	NG	NG
Exc. toe nodule	20	1,800,000	50	NG
Exc. tibial chondroma	40	400	NG	NG
Hernia and orchidopexy	105	7,750	450	3,700
Finger amputation	40	350	NG	NG
Red. humeral fracture	30	200	NG	NG
Heel cord lengthening	105	50	NG	600
Exc. ganglion cyst	35	NG	NG	NG
Tibial biopsy	30	120,000	50	50
Meniscectomy	30	350	NG	50
Femoral stapling	20	400	NG	NG
Neurolysis	25	250	NG	NG
Exc. neuroma	50	50	NG	NG
Tendolysis	30	NG	NG	NG
Exc. breast tumor	15	600	NG	NG
Appendectomy	75	200	400	250
Cholecystectomy	90	500	NG	NG
Vein stripping	180	100	NG	50
Gastrectomy	160	NG	NG	NG
Herniorrhaphy	105	11,000	NG	550
Thyroidectomy	100	100	NG	1,750
Herniorrhaphy	105	22,500	NG	750
App. abscess	67	10,000	NG	200
Gastrectomy	180	NG	NG	NG
Patellectomy	60	NG	NG	NG
Thyroidectomy	65	350	NG	NG
Portocaval shunt	254	500	50	NG
Rad. vulvectomy	210	400	NG	NG
Exc. breast tumor	60	50	NG	NG
Enterotomy	90	1,600	50	NG
Cholecystectomy	120	150	NG	50
Epig. herniorrhaphy	50	NG	NG	NG
Colectomy	300	550	NG	NG
Appendectomy	30	100	NG	NG
Herniorrhaphy	114	1,300	550	100
Exc. ovarian cyst	70	50	NG	50
Exc. fingernails	20	NG	NG	NG
Thyroidectomy	78	NG	NG	NG

Patients involved were chosen at random though not strictly alternately, as the procedures were carried out by only three surgeons in a large active general hospital. In general an attempt was made to use cases which were anticipated to last more than 30 minutes and not involve drainage of large contaminated wounds or abscesses. Otherwise it was planned to secure a complete range of type of operation and age groups, and in this way it was hoped to obtain a relative, though admittedly rough, comparison of the general effectiveness of the new skin preparation as compared with the standard

TABLE 2.—*Hexachlorophene (pHisoHex)*

Operation	Min	Cultures (Staphylococci Only) Preprep	Postprep	Postop
Umb. herniorrhaphy	40	1,000	NG	NG
Herniorrhaphy	135	24,000	1,800	14,000
Hemorrhoidectomy	30	8,000	1,750	5,000
Splenectomy	150	3,000	50	NG
Herniorrhaphy	41	1,000	300	200
Vein stripping	150	100	NG	50
Bil. orchidopexy	85	5,600	350	7,000
Exc. breast tumor	45	NG	NG	NG
Herniorrhaphy	60	11,250	NG	300
Herniorrhaphy	105	66,000	61,500	130,000
Hemorrhoidectomy	30	4,200,000	6,450	1,750
Colostomy	115	64,000	300	150
Ileal bypass	270	4,000	1,250	NG
Cholecystectomy	140	100	NG	950
Vagotomy	107	750	50	NG
Herniorrhaphy	47	7,000	NG	400
Appendectomy	60	50	NG	NG
Vein stripping	75	450	NG	50
Gastrectomy	190	37,000	50	5,000
Ileocolectomy	190	NG	NG	200
Hydrocelectomy	83	100,000	2,800	100
Splenectomy	125	50	NG	50
Colotomy	95	1,000	NG	NG
Herniorrhaphy	70	200	NG	600
Bowel obstruction	115	1,250	1,100	2,450
Thoracotomy	115	4,500	NG	NG
App. & herniorrhaphy	80	72,500	300	50
Thyroidectomy	80	8,750	50	NG
Exc. granuloma	55	2,150	NG	50
Herniorrhaphy	47	1,000	NG	NG
Perf. appendectomy	60	1,500	NG	50
Herniorrhaphy	65	4,750	NG	NG
Thyroidectomy	104	550,000	3,350	2,700
Gastrectomy	215	NG	100	NG
Vein stripping	200	5,500	7,000	NG
Cholecystectomy	95	500	NG	50
Rad. mastectomy	50	50	NG	3,450
Appendectomy	30	2,700	100	NG
Appendectomy	50	60,000	NG	NG
Choledochostomy	180	350	NG	NG
Colectomy	240	NG	NG	NG
Herniorrhaphy	67	130,000	50	100
Herniorrhaphy	43	50	100	NG
Lap. and liver biopsy	35	600	200	NG
Herniorrhaphy	62	9,500	NG	50
Cholecystectomy	60	6,450	550	NG
Herniorrhaphy	98	NG	NG	NG
Herniorrhaphy	30	4,000	550	NG
Mastectomy-oophorectomy	120	3,600	50	NG
Herniorrhaphy	62	700	NG	NG

method under normal, everyday operating conditions in a community type hospital. It was fully realized that bacterial counts obtained of skin cultures do not reflect the true microbial population of the skin. The organisms that may be in the glandular ducts and hair follicles have not been counted in any of the studies presently employed. It must be remembered that what is being measured in a study such as this are the organisms removed from the skin, but what is of importance are the organisms which remain on or in the skin.

Results

Complete listing of the entire 100 cases is shown in Tables 1 and 2, the cases prepared with Surgidine and with hexachlorophene and solution of benzalkonium chloride. Fig 1 is an attempt to display graphically the range of the postoperative *Staphylococcus* colony counts in patients prepared with both Surgidine and hexachlorophene. It can be seen that the number of postoperative sterile cultures was considerably greater in Surgidine-prepared patients than in those prepared with hexachlorophene and benzalkonium chloride. Roughly 70% of Surgidine-prepared patients showed sterile postoperative *Staphylococcus* cultures with none culturing more than 10,000 colonies per unit area. Half of the hexachlorophene-treated patients showed sterile cultures; the other half cultured staphylococcal colonies to over 100,000 per unit area.

The number of sterile cultures in each group was thought to be of some significance, and this is demonstrated in Table 3. The number of negative *Staphylococcus* cultures before the preparation, after the preparation, and at the end of the operation are tabulated directly and also as a percentage of 50 cases with each agent. Of some significance is the demonstration that after preparation with Surgidine 40 patients had negative cultures for *Staphylococcus* and 25 patients had negative cultures with hexachlorophene.

Fig 2 graphically illustrates the reduction in the average *Staphylococcus* colony counts in patients being prepared with both substances, both as to number of positive cultures and as to a percentage of the pre-preparation colony count. It can be seen from the chart that before preparation the number of positive cultures is high in both groups of patients, but after the preparation 25% of Surgidine-prepared patients had positive cultures to any degree, whereas 56.8% of hexachlorophene-prepared patients had positive cultures to any degree. The average postpreparation staphylococcal colony count as a percentage of the prepreparation colony count was seen to be 0.5% with Surgidine-

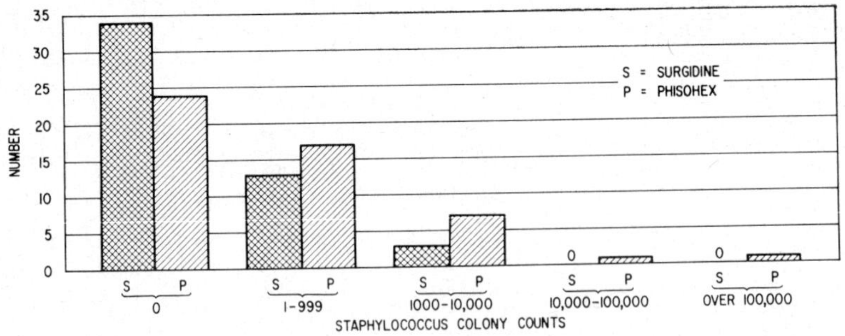

Fig 1.—Average postoperative *Staphylococcus* colony counts.

treated patients, and 2.9% with hexachlorophene-treated patients.

I felt that the average postoperative *Staphylococcus* colony count related to operative time would be of some significance, and this is demonstrated in Table 4. It can be seen from this Table that patients grouped into operating times from one hour to more than two hours were quite similar in both groups. However, the average *Staphylococcus* colony counts were considerably higher in all categories in the group of patients prepared with hexachlorophene and solution of benzalkonium chloride. It was found that one particularly high colony count significantly raised the average for the group in which the hexachlorophene was used. There is some evidence to indicate that a few individuals harbor a bacterial flora that is resistant to the action of hexachlorophene.[16] If the single high colony count after the preparation with hexachlorophene is deleted, the average staphylococcal colony count was 533 after the preparation and 894 at the end of the surgical procedure. In both instances it was still considerably higher than in those patients prepared with Surgidine.

It was of great interest to note that studies of Table 1 and 2 indicated that the ten negative skin cultures obtained before preparation on patients in the Surgidine group were negative throughout the entire study, whereas only three negative cultures obtained before preparation on hexachlorophene-prepared patients were negative throughout the study. However, 13 positive cultures after hexachlorophene preparation turned negative by the end of the operation, and only four cultures after Surgidine preparation

Table 3.—*Negative Staphylococcus Cultures, Before Prep, After Prep, and After Operation (as a Percentage of 50 Cases With Each Agent)*

	Surgidine		Hexachlorophene	
	No.	%	No.	%
Before prep	10	20	5	10
After prep	40	80	25	50
At completion of operation	34	68	25	50
Total cases	50	100	50	100

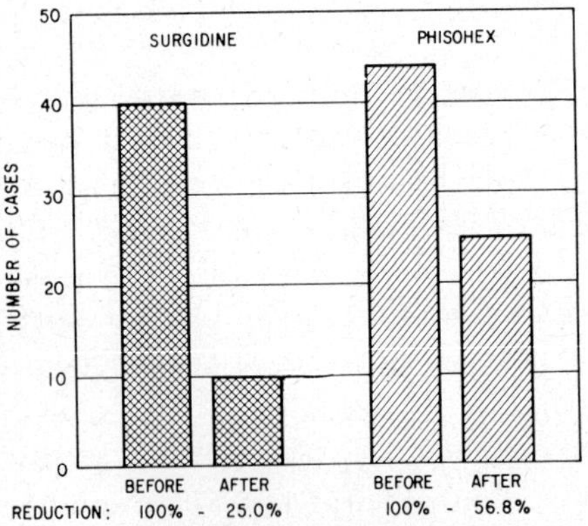

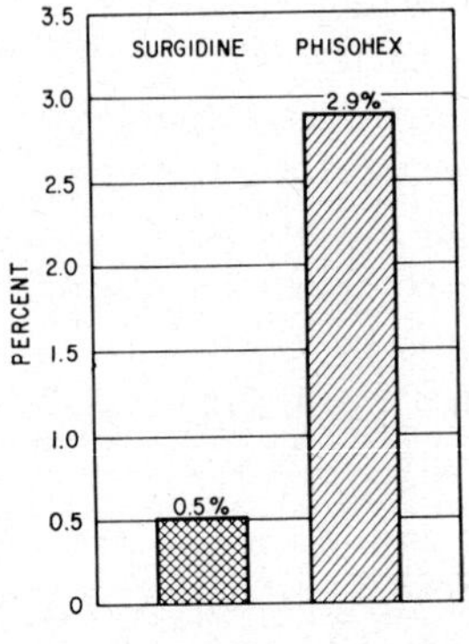

Fig 2.—*Left,* reduction of average *Staphylococcus* colony count, before preparation to after preparation, positive cultures. *Right,* average postpreparation *Staphylococcus* colony count as a percentage of prepreparation colony counts.

TABLE 4.—*Average Postoperative Staphylococcus Colony Count Related to Operation Time*

	Surgidine		Hexachlorophene	
Length of Operation	No. of Cases	Av Count	No. of Cases	Av Count
Under 1 hr (15-55 min)	19	90	14	775
1-2 hr (60-115 min)	22	390	23	6,250
2 hr & up (120-300 min)	9	11	13	1,562
All operations	50	210	50	3,495

turned negative after the operation. This finding appeared to lend credence to the previously noted evidence that hexachlorophene appears to exert a lasting antibacterial effect and requires a significant period of time in contact with the bacteria in order to enhance its effectiveness.[4,11,16]

Comment

Though substances containing hexachlorophene and washes with solutions of water and quaternary ammonium compounds have been standard skin preparation materials for patients undergoing surgery over the past 15 years, there has been some evidence that these substances are not complete germicides, and the search for a more effective skin degerming agent is a continuing process. Compounds containing iodine in solution or tincture, long known to be extremely effective as skin antiseptics, were given up many years ago for this use because of the high incidence of skin sensitivity to iodine. Recently the development of newer compounds containing iodine, known as iodophors, iodine carriers, or complexed iodines, has reopened the study of iodine as a skin disinfectant. Iodine is generally conceded to be a bactericide of the broadest spectrum, having lethal action against bacilli, cocci, spores, spirillae, fungi, yeasts, viruses, rickettsias, protozoa, and helminths. Certain of the complexed iodine materials have proved themselves extremely effective as skin degerming agents, and in addition have shown virtually no toxicity for skin.

The subject of this present study, Surgidine, was originally developed specifically as a skin preparation material to meet the need for a nonirritating, nonstaining bactericidal agent. Prior to the institution of the use of Surgidine at this hospital, the work of Dahlsrud[2] was reviewed, in which 1,054 presurgical preparations, 3,162 surgical scrubs, 3,080 patient baths, and 124,200 staff hand washings were carried out, with no known development of irritation, sensitivity, toxicity, or cutaneous burning observed in any of the 1,184 human subjects involved in this study, either with topical application or under dressings and casts. Similarly the work of Krupp, in which the hands of 18 subjects were inoculated with *Staphylococcus aureus* and *Escherichia coli* suspensions and then the hands washed in Surgidine, hexachlorophene and nonmedicated soap, after which skin cultures were taken, was reviewed. It was found, on the basis of Krupp's study, that four times as many *S aureus* colonies and 143 times as many *E coli* colonies remained after scrubbing with hexachlorophene solution as after scrubbing with Surgidine. It was decided, on the basis of these studies, to conduct the practical experiment described above with its results, and the evidence obtained indicated Surgidine to be a safe and effective skin preparation material.

Conclusion

On the basis of preliminary investigations done by Dahlsrud and by Krupp, a new complexed iodine substance, Surgidine, has been studied under normal, everyday operating conditions in an attempt to determine its comparative effectiveness as a skin preparation material. One hundred patients were used for the study, taken as nearly alternately as possible to cover a complete range of surgical operations. Fifty patients were prepared with a standard preparation at this hospital, hexachlorophene (pHisoHex) and water, followed by a wash of solution of benzalkonium chloride. Fifty patients were prepared using Surgidine, followed by a wash of tincture of Surgidine. Skin cultures were taken before preparation, after preparation, and at the end of the operation on each patient. The *Staphylococcus* cultures were reduced to 25% of their prepreparation level, after preparation with Surgidine, and to 56.8% of the prepreparation level with patients prepared with hexachlorophene. The average postoperative *Staphylococcus* colony counts were 210 for patients prepared with Surgidine, and 30,495 for patients prepared with hexachlorophene. After preparation 40 cultures were negative for *Staphylococcus* in patients prepared with Surgidine, whereas in the similar study on patients prepared with hexachlorophene 25 had negative cultures after preparation and 25 at the completion of the operation.

In this study no attempt was made to correlate the incidence of wound infection with the skin preparation used, as this small series of cases was deemed insufficient for such a study. However, it should be reported that one postoperative wound infection did occur in this hundred patients, after closure of a small bowel fistula, in a patient prepared with Surgidine.

On the basis of the above results this new substance appears to be a safe, effective, and esthetically acceptable surgical preparation material with skin degerming properties at least equal to and probably superior to those of the common materials now in use in this country.

Charles L. Geraci, MD, 1303 San Carlos Ave, San Carlos, Calif.

REFERENCES

1. Boswick, J. A.; Kissell, E.; and Metzger, W. I.: Laboratory and Clinical Studies of a New Presurgical Skin Antiseptic, 3:6 (Nov) 1961.

2. Dahlsrud, H. A.: Clinical Evaluation of a New Anionic: Non-Ionic Iodophor as a Surgical Scrub, to be published.

3. Frisch, A. W.; Davis, G. H.; and Krippaehne, W.: Skin Degerming Agents With Special Reference to a New Cationic Iodophore, Surg Gynec Obstet 107:442 (Oct) 1958.

4. Goldenberg, I. S.; Haley, L. D.; and Higashi, G. I.: An Evaluation of an Iodine Preoperative Scrub Detergent, Surg Gynec Obstet 114:329 (March) 1962.

5. Goodman, L. S., and Gilman, A. Z.: Pharmacological Basis of Therapeutics, ed 2, New York: The Macmillan Company, 1955, pp 1075-1112.

6. Joress, S. M.: A Study of Disinfection of the Skin: A Comparison of Povidone-Iodine With Other Agents Used for Surgical Scrubs, Ann Surg 155:296 (Feb) 1962.

7. Krupp, M. A.: Personal communication to the author, 1962.

8. Knudsin, R. B.: Investigations on Dynamics of Bactericidal Action of Two Quaternary Ammonium Salts, Arch Surg 81:789 (Nov) 1960.

9. Malizia, W. F.; Gangarosa, E. J.; and Goley, A. F.: Benzalkonium Chloride as a Source of Infection, New Eng J Med 263:800 (Oct 20) 1960.

10. Mannix, H., Jr., and Dineen, P.: "Germicides" for Skin Preparation Before Surgery, Arch Surg 83:752 (Nov) 1961.

11. Medrek, T. F., and Litsky, W.: Surgical Antiseptics: Collective Review, Surg Gynec Obstet 104:209 (March) 1957.

12. Miller, J. M.; Jackson, D. A.; Callies, C. S.; and Johnson, H. R.: The Microbicidal Property of a New Iodophor Antiseptic Solution, Milit Med 126:441 (June) 1961.

13. Price, P. B.: The Bacteriology of Normal Skin: A New Quantitative Test Applied to a Study of the Bacterial Flora and Disinfectant Action of a Mechanical Cleansing, J Infect Dis 63:301, 1938.

14. Price, P. B.: "Surgical Antiseptics," in Antiseptics, Disinfectants, Fungicides, and Chemical and Physical Sterilization, edited by G. F. Reddish, Philadelphia, Lea & Febiger, Publishers, 1954.

15. Price, P. B.: Ethyl Alcohol as a Germicide, Arch Surg 38:528 (March) 1939.

16. Price, P. B.: Fallacy of a Current Surgical Fad: The Three-Minute Preoperative Scrub With Hexachlorophene Soap, Ann Surg 134:476 (Sept) 1951.

17. Roberts, E. S., and Russell, M.: Two Methods of Preparing Patients' Skin for Surgery, Arch Surg 82:426 (March) 1961.

Carcinoma of the Bile Ducts

E. LEE STROHL, MD
WILLIAM H. REED, MD
WILLIS G. DIFFENBAUGH, MD
AND
RAYMOND E. ANDERSON, MD
CHICAGO

Carcinoma of the major extrahepatic and intrahepatic bile ducts, although infrequently encountered, merits consideration in every patient having obstructive jaundice. The correct preoperative diagnosis is seldom made. The operative diagnosis is difficult because of the limited anatomical boundaries and the difficulty of thorough exploration of the ductal system. Malignant tumors of the ducts produce complete obstruction early in the course of the disease, in most instances. The proximity of the vital structures permits the tumors to grow to an inoperable state in a short period of time following the onset of symptoms.

Submitted for publication Feb 4, 1963.

From the Department of Surgery, Cook County Hospital, University of Illinois College of Medicine, and Presbyterian-St. Luke's Hospital.

This study concerns malignant tumors of the extrahepatic and intrahepatic ducts, exclusive of the ampulla of Vater. Each tumor was histologically verified at operation or autopsy. In 1941, Kirschbaum and Kozoll [1] reported the findings regarding these tumors in 13,330 postmortem examinations from Cook County Hospital, Chicago. Our review concerns the bile duct tumors found at surgery or on postmortem examination at Cook County Hospital, Chicago, subsequent to that report.

Historical Data

Courvoisier,[2] in 1890, stated that carcinoma of the bile ducts was first described in 1508. Durand Fardel,[3] nevertheless, is credited with reporting the first case of carcinoma of the bile duct, in 1840. In 1878, Schueppel [4] described the first case of carcinoma of the hepatic duct. Musser,[5] in 1889, wrote the first comprehensive review on the subject and added 18 cases of his own. In 1890, Courvoisier [2] collected 13 cases of primary carcinoma of the hepatic and common bile ducts. Baudoin,[6] in 1896, was the first surgeon to carry out hepatocholangioenterostomy for carcinoma of the bile ducts. Ulizinski,[7] in 1902, performed the first segmental resection for carcinoma of the bile ducts; however, the patient died within a few days. W. J. Mayo [8] reported a block resection of a primary carcinoma of the common bile duct, in 1903. Subsequent reports of block resection have been published by Cattell,[9] Garlock,[10] Jackson and Caylor,[11] Dragstedt, Julian, Allen, and Owens,[12] Brunschwig and Bigelow,[13] and Pickrell and Blalock.[14] Stewart, Lieber, and Morgan,[15] in 1940, reviewed the world literature through 1936. Their report documented 98 cases, and they added six cases of their own. In 1957, Sako, Seitzinger, and Garside [16] collected 564 cases from the literature during the years 1933 through 1954. They added six cases from their own experience. Large series of cases have since been reported by Kuwayti, Baggenstoss, Stauffer, and Priestley [17] from the Mayo Clinic, Glenn and Hill,[18] Thorbjarnarson,[19] Todd,[20] Lippman, McDonald, and Longmire,[21] as well as many individual case reports.[22-50]

Incidence

Kirschbaum and Kozoll [1] found 52 cases of carcinoma of the extrahepatic bile ducts in 13,330 autopsies at the Cook County Hospital, Chicago, an incidence of 0.39%. Sako, Seitzinger, and Garside [16] quoted an incidence of 0.01% to 0.458% in autopsy material collected from the literature. Neibling, Dockerty, and Waugh [53] found a malignant lesion of the bile ducts in one of every 210 operations on the biliary tract. Glenn and Hill [18] noted that carcinoma of the bile ducts is less common than carcinoma of the gallbladder, the ratio being one to five. Thorbjarnarson,[19] at Cornell University Medical Center, found 31 carcinomas of the bile ducts to every 90 carcinomas of the gallbladder, and to every 20 carcinomas of the ampulla of Vater.

Etiology

Cholelithiasis is, probably, a contributing factor in the pathogenesis of carcinoma of the bile ducts, just as it is probably a contributing factor in the pathogenesis of carcinoma of the gallbladder. Stewart, Lieber, and Morgan [15] found associated gallstones in 20.2%; Sako, Seitzinger, and Garside [16] in 38.7%; and Neibling, Dockerty, and Waugh [53] in 57% of patients having carcinoma of the bile ducts. Eleven of our 26 patients had associated gallstones, and three of the patients had stones in the bile ducts in addition to stones in the gallbladder.

Willis [54] postulated that there is a conversion of bile acids to methylcholanthrene, which may have carcinogenic action in susceptible persons. Sternberg and Popper et al [55] produced a carcinoma of the bile ducts in animals after the long-term feeding of Aramite,* an alkylating agent. The production of carcinoma of the ducts was an incidental finding in studies on the toxic effects of the drug. Gupta [56] produced carcinoma of the ducts with thioacetamide. Grott [57] reported a high incidence of carcinoma of the bile ducts in association with *Giardia lamblia* infections. Reports have appeared of carcinoma of the bile ducts developing in experimental animals by injections of human bile and carcinogenic extracts.[58-60] Okinaka, Nakao, Ibayaski, Nakaidsumi, Kakehi, and Sugimura [61] reported a case of biliary tract carcinoma which developed 11 years after the injection of thorium dioxide suspension (Thorotrast) for cholangiography. Roberts and Carlson [62] reported a similar case of carcinoma which developed 17 years after the injection of thorium dioxide suspension. Dick [63] suggested that some carcinomas of the bile ducts originate in benign papillomas. Zenker [64] and Rolleston [65] have supported such a theory. Cases of benign papillomas of the ducts have been reported,[66-71] as well as

* Sulfurous acid 2-(*p-tert.*-butylphenoxy)-1-methylethyl 2-chlorethyl ester.

multiple papillomas of the ducts.[72,73] Schmug[74] reported eight cases of malignancy of the ducts associated with papillomas of the ducts. He states that there was no apparent relationship between the papillomas and the carcinomas in seven of the eight cases. Booher and Pack[36] state that carcinomatous changes are frequently found in the stalks of the papillomas present in the ducts. On the contrary, papillary carcinoma of the extrahepatic bile ducts is rare, accounting for less than 5% of carcinomas of the ducts.

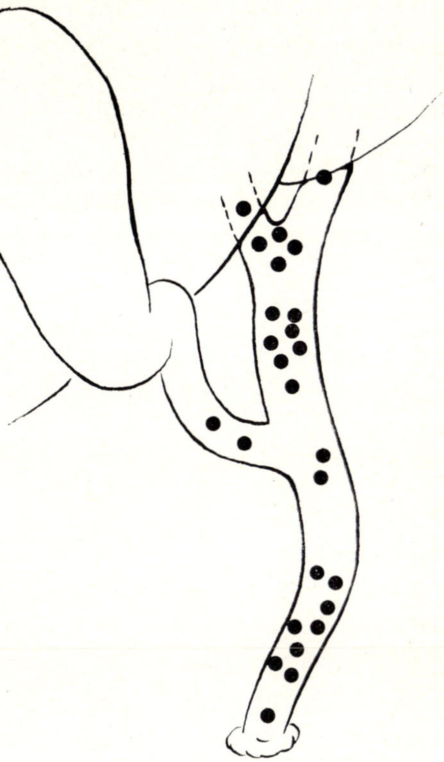

Fig 1.—Diagram of the location of the 26 bile duct tumors in the present series.

Pathology

Gross examination reveals the tumors to be nodular or scirrhous, diffusely infiltrating, or papillary. The most common type is a firm, circumscribed, grayish tan, nodular tumor. The tumor occludes the duct, partially or completely. The bile ducts proximal to the tumor are markedly dilated.

The diffusely infiltrating type of tumor produces a string-like stricture of the duct, which simulates inflammatory stricture. Such a tumor poses a difficult problem for the surgeon in differentiating between stricture and tumor.[75,76]

Papillary lesions are found less frequently. They invade and obstruct the lumen of the ducts. Such tumors may cause intermittent obstruction. There is no particular segment of the ducts which is specifically selective for a single type of tumor.

The distribution of the lesions in our series is illustrated in the diagram (Fig 1). Sako, Seitzinger, and Garside[16] listed the hepatic ducts as the site in 47, the common hepatic ducts in 79, the common bile duct-cystic duct junction in 137, the cystic duct alone in 34, and the lower common bile duct in 203 cases.

Carcinoma infiltration develops frequently in the submucosa of the bile ducts. Half of our patients revealed extension of the tumor, or widespread metastases at the time of autopsy examination. The pattern of the tumor spread reflected no tendency of the tumor to spread locally, before metastasizing to the regional lymph nodes. In three of our cases there were metastases in the regional lymph nodes and to the peritoneum, with no evidence of involvement of the structures immediately adjacent to the bile ducts. Gross tumor thrombi were noted in one case. In four patients, ascites was present, and, in each of these patients, thrombi were present in the portal vein. In each of the patients having metastatic disease, the symptoms had been present for at least three months prior to the hospital admission. In those patients without metastases, the symptoms had been present for less than one month. There was no difference in the survival time of the two groups.

Thorbjarnarson[19] found no metastases at operation or autopsy in 57% of his cases. Ransom,[77] in 30 autopsies with a clinical diagnosis of carcinoma of the pancreas, found one fourth of the group to have primary carcinoma of the bile ducts. Five of these eight lesions were localized and would have been amenable to radical resections. Metastases

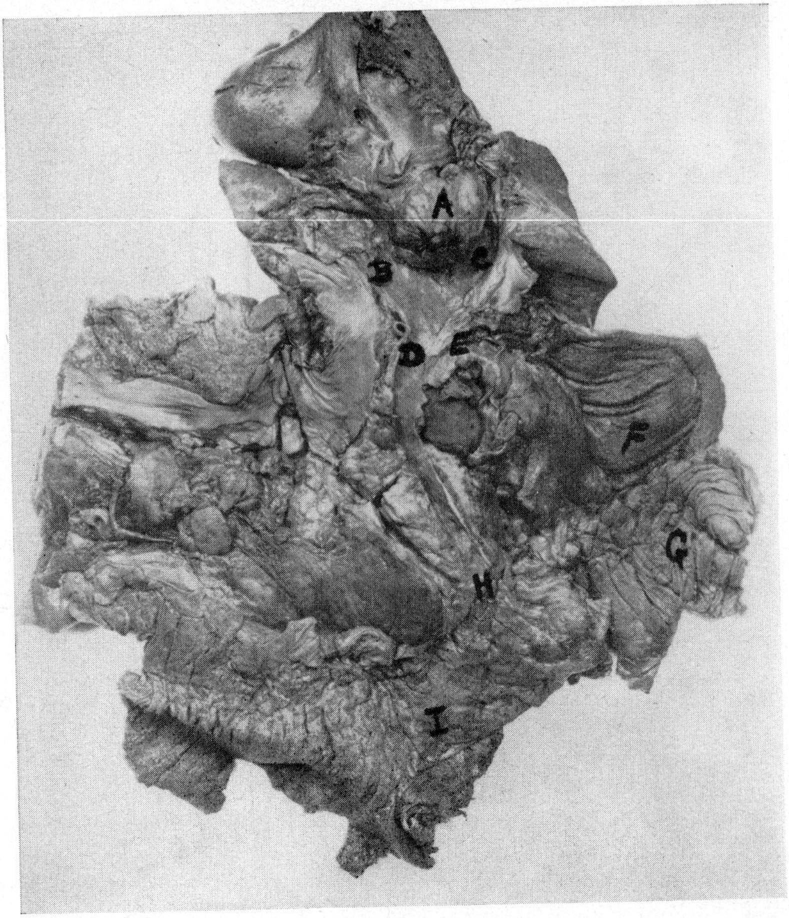

Fig 2.—Autopsy specimen of a papillary carcinoma at the bifurcation of the right and left hepatic ducts: *A*, papillary carcinoma; *B*, left hepatic duct; *C*, right hepatic duct; *D*, common bile duct; *E*, cystic duct; *F*, gallbladder; *H*, ampulla of Vater; *G*, and *I*, bowel and duodenum.

were present in 63% of the cases of Neibling, Dockerty, and Waugh,[53] in 45.8% of Stewart, Lieber, and Morgan,[15] and in 76.7% of the cases reported by Kirschbaum and Kozoll.[1]

Fig 3.—Photomicrograph showing the cellular structure of the papillary carcinoma illustrated in Fig 2; (Reduced 41% from mag × 198).

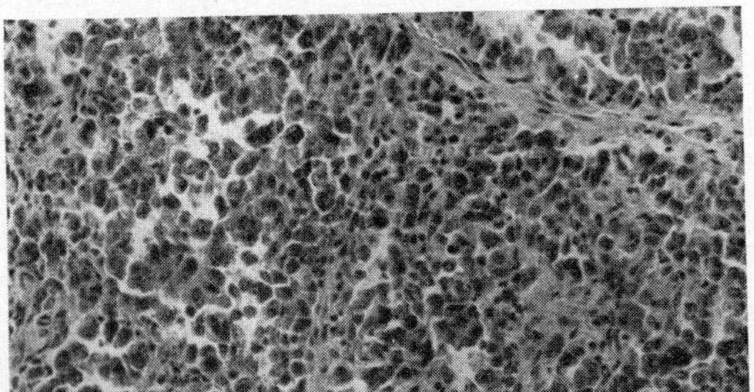

Squamous cell carcinoma and sarcoma botryoides of the bile ducts have been reported.[78,79]

Age and Sex

The majority of reports reveal a larger number of males than females having carcinoma of the ducts, in the ratio of three to two. This figure differs from carcinoma of the gallbladder, where females outnumber males four to one.

In our 26 cases, 18 were male and 8 were female, a two to one ratio. Sako, Seitzinger, and Garside [16] reported a ratio of three females to two males, and Neibling, Dockerty, and Waugh [53] reported a series of 90 cases with 48 males and 42 females.

Our youngest patient was a male 43 years of age and the oldest a male age 84 years. The average age of the 26 patients was 70.1

years. Sixteen of the 26 patients were over 65 years of age.

Symptoms and Clinical Findings

A characteristic feature of carcinoma of the bile ducts is the rapid onset of symptoms. In our series, the interval between the onset of symptoms and the hospital admission ranged between one and eight weeks. Jaundice was present in 20 of our patients, or 76%. It was noted early in the course of the disease and was progressive in character. In a patient having papillary carcinoma the jaundice can be intermittent. In our series, the icteric index was elevated between 80 and 300 units, with an average of 169 units. Pruritus is frequently a very distressing early symptom. If the pruritus precedes the jaundice, this is strongly suggestive of extrahepatic obstruction.[80-81] We had such an experience recently. A 70-year-old female consulted her physician because of a pruritus at night. The examination revealed a slight jaundice, which became more prominent rapidly. Three weeks after the onset of the pruritus, abdominal exploration revealed an extensive carcinoma at the junction of the right and left hepatic ducts with invasion of the liver and the regional lymph nodes. Deep jaundice with little or no pruritus suggests intrahepatic obstruction.

Pain was a prominent symptom in 13 of our patients, or 50%. It was of the intermittent, colic type, rather than the constant, deep-seated right upper quadrant pain, often encountered in carcinoma of the gallbladder. The pain has been ascribed to distention of the ducts, as well as to invasion of the nerves in and about the ducts.

Weight loss was a prominent symptom. Thorbjarnarson [19] found weight loss early in the course of the disease in his patients.

A palpable liver is usually present and is rarely tender.

Diagnosis

The diagnosis is rarely made early and seldom prior to the onset of jundice.

Operative cholangiograms may be of help. Kantor, Evans, and Glenn [82] found eight

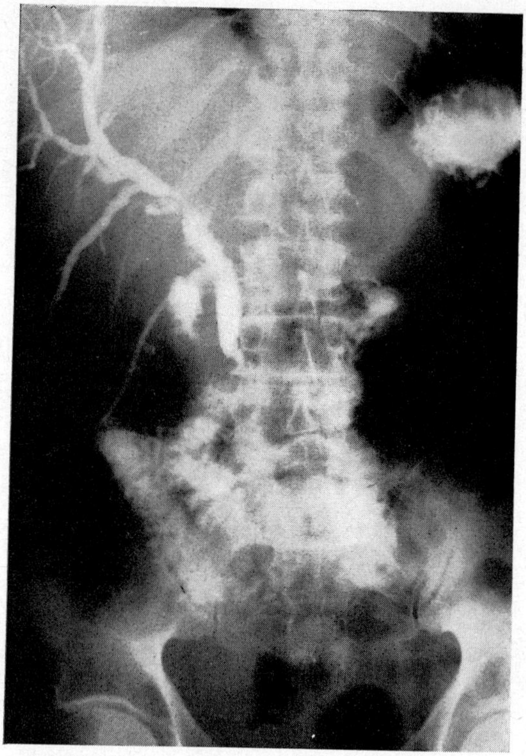

Fig 4.—Cholangiogram of a carcinoma obstructing the left hepatic duct.

cases of tumor in 116 operative cholangiograms. Evans and Mujahed [83] described cholangiographic changes in carcinoma of the bile ducts. Larsen [84] studied the cholangiographic findings in postmortem cholangiograms which were taken in patients having bile duct carcinoma.

Cytological examination of the duodenal contents may be of value in the preoperative diagnosis. Dreiling, Nieburg, and Janowitz [85] described three common duct carcinomas which showed positive duodenal cytology. Wenger and Raskin [86] described five cases of carcinoma of the bile ducts, three of which showed positive duodenal cytology.

Treatment

The surgical management of carcinoma of the bile ducts depends upon the location of the tumor. The tumor occurring high in the hepatic ducts, at the hilus of the liver, can rarely be removed. In addition, palliative decompression is difficult to carry out. In the

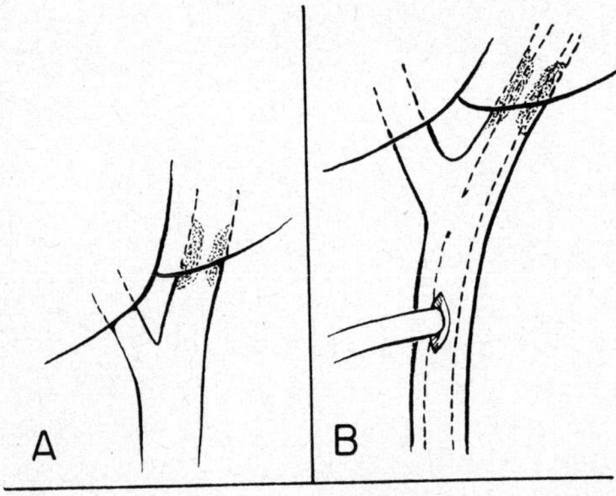

Fig 5.—Diagram of carcinoma of the left hepatic duct bridged by a rigid tube to allow bile drainage.

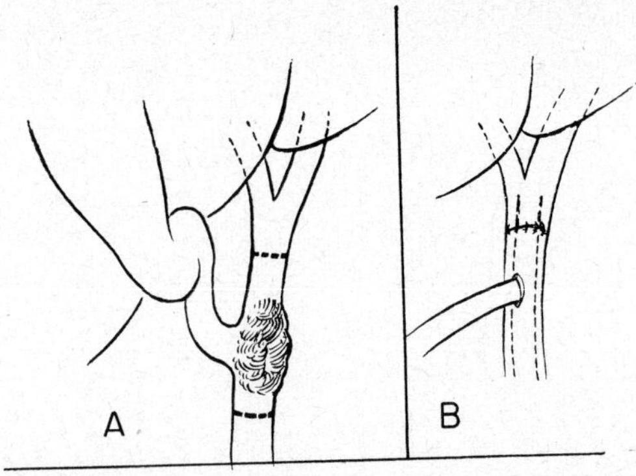

Fig 6.—Diagram of primary resection of a carcinoma of the common duct with end-to-end anastomosis.

occasional patient, decompression may be possible by the introduction of a cannula or a T-tube through the tumor and into the proximal ducts. The Longmire procedure is seldom feasible, or advantageous, although short-term relief has been reported after its use.[87]

Tumors of the central portion of the ducts are more amenable to surgical resection. Resection and end-to-end anastomosis has been successfully carried out by a number of surgeons. Garlock [10] and Leiter [88] had a five-year survival after such a procedure. When resection results in too great a loss of bile duct structure for primary anastomosis, a loop of jejunum may be interposed. Wallensten and Fries [46] reported success in two cases in which this method was utilized. A Roux en Y loop of jejunum may be used to bridge the gap. Cholecystojejunostomy or cholecystoduodenostomy may be the operation of choice when the tumor is bulky and the prognosis is poor. Barnes and Zarr [89] used the cystic duct and the ampulla of the gallbladder to bridge the gap in the common bile duct after resection of a tumor.

Tumors located in the lower portion of the common bile duct were difficult to distinguish from tumors of the pancreas. Pancreaticoduodenostomy may be the procedure of choice. However, instances of local resection with reimplantation of the pancreatic and

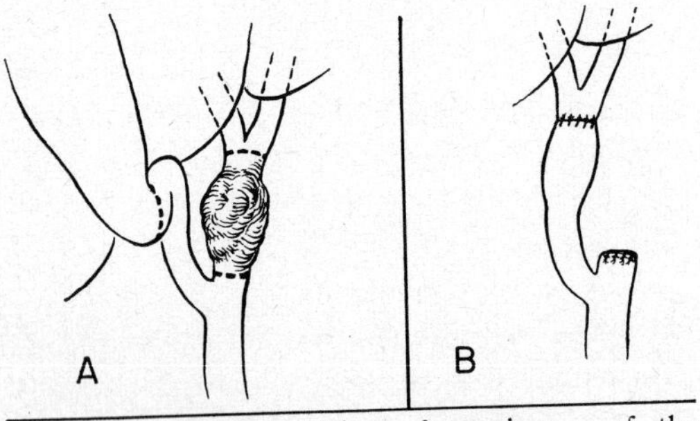

Fig 7.—Primary excision of carcinoma of the bile duct with bridging of the gap by anastomosis of the ampulla of the gallbladder to the proximal common bile duct (Barnes and Zarr).

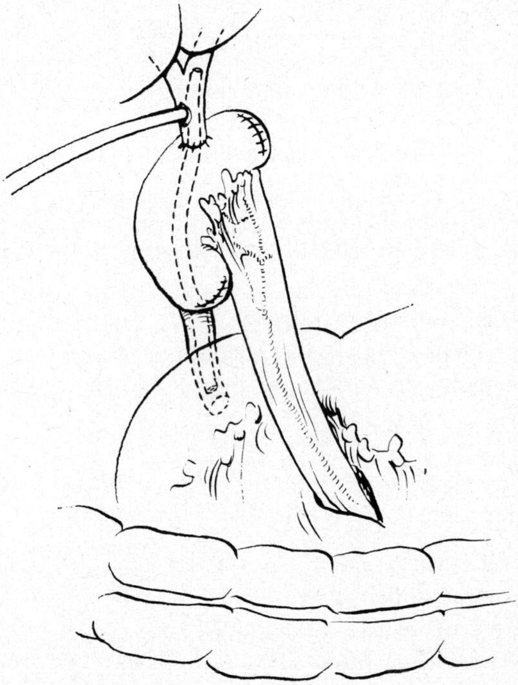

Fig 8.—Primary excision of carcinoma of the common duct and bridging of the gap with a segment of jejunum attached to its mesentery (Wallensten and Fries).

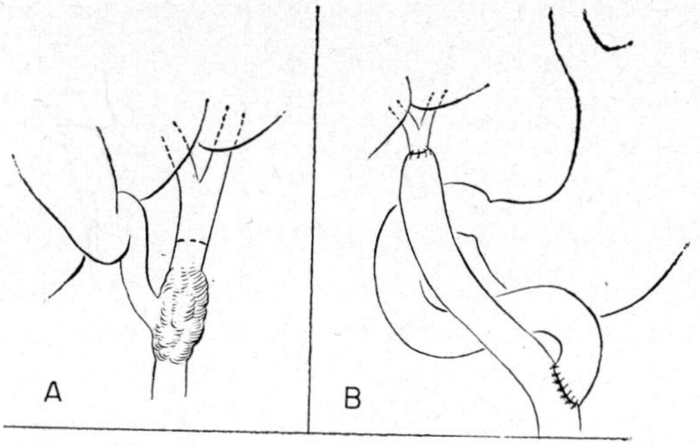

Fig 9.—Primary excision of common duct carcinoma and anastomosis of the proximal common duct stump to a Roux en Y loop of jejunum.

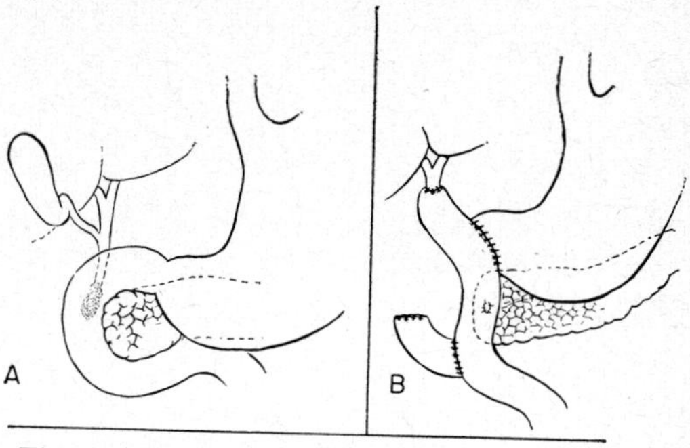

Fig 10.—Pancreaticoduodenectomy for carcinoma of the lower portion of the common bile duct.

bile ducts have been reported with long-term survival.

Surgery without relief of the jaundice hastens the death of the patient. If bile can be diverted into the intestinal tract by a palliative procedure, the patient may obtain distinct relief from the pain, pruritus, and jaundice for a short interval of time. An occasional patient may survive for several years after such a procedure.

Ariel and Pack [90] treated 14 patients having carcinoma of the biliary tract with intravenous I^{131} rose bengal with definite palliation in nine of the 14 patients.

External drainage procedures are unsatisfactory. The problems created by diversion of fluids and electrolytes become insurmountable in a short interval of time.

Results of Surgery

In 1944, Pickrell and Blalock,[14] after a review of the literature, summarized the attempts at operative removal and the results obtained in surgery for carcinoma of the bile ducts. Kehr,[91] in 1903, resected a tumor, and the patient survived for 27 months. Quénu, in 1909,[92] reported 18 radical resection patients, four of whom lived for 6 months to 4½ years. Pallin, in 1921,[93] resected a tumor, and the patient lived for 11 months, dying of causes other than carcinoma. No tumor was found at autopsy. Pickrell and Blalock [14] had one patient with a radical resection who lived for five years and another patient who survived for seven months.

Garlock [10] reported a patient who had a local resection with primary anastomosis in 1939. The patient lived for five years. Grayton Brown's [38] patient survived for ten months after resection and Roux en Y anastomosis. Altemeier, Gall, and Zinninger [76] listed two patients with sclerosing carcinoma of the intrahepatic ducts, who lived for 3½ and 5½ years after bypass operative procedures. Keeley and Schairer [87] had a patient who survived for nine months after a Longmire procedure. Lippman, McDonald, and Longmire [21] reported nine radical operations, with five patients surviving for six months to seven years. Thorbjarnarson [19] had a survival for 39 months after radical resection. Neibling, Dockerty, and Waugh [53] described one block resection patient who survived for 26 months. Dennis and Varco [94] noted two patients who survived 12 months and 15 months after resection. Siler and Zinninger [95] had a 16-month survival after pancreatoduodenectomy. Warren, Cattell, Blackburn, and Nora [96] mention a radical resection patient living for eight years, another for six years, and six patients living from one to five years. Booher and Pack [36] performed, with success, a radical resection 51 months after a local resection of a carcinoma of the bile ducts.

There are reports of long-term survival after palliative operations of a short-circuiting nature. Marshall [97] reported a 51-month survival after a cholecystogastrostomy. Goldenberg [98] reported a six-year survival after a palliative procedure. Walters and

Snell [99] mention a four-year survival after a palliative procedure. One of the Cook County Hospital patients is living after a drainage procedure and uracil mustard therapy.

Comment

The results of surgery in carcinoma of the bile ducts are discouraging. Despite the fact that the tumors, in general, are slow-growing and metastases may not have developed, death is usually due to obstruction of the bile flow. A considerable number of these tumors will, at postmortem examination, be found to be technically resectable. This observation should encourage the surgeon in his future attempts at curative resection. An aggressive surgical approach is the only hope of cure. When curative resection cannot be performed, diversion of bile into the gastrointestinal tract is of paramount importance for the relief of symptoms. This can be accomplished in the majority of patients. Surgery, without relief of bile duct obstruction, serves only to hasten the patient's death.

Summary

Carcinoma of the bile ducts merits consideration in every person having obstructive jaundice, particularly in the elderly patient.

The most common type of bile duct carcinoma is a firm, circumscribed, nodular tumor obstructing the duct. No metastatic involvement is present in about 50% of the patients having bile duct carcinoma.

Pruritus and jaundice, which progress rapidly, are the most prominent symptoms.

Pain, intermittent, or of the colic type, is present in one half of the patients.

Treatment should accomplish resection of the tumor, if at all possible. Failing resection, some method to relieve the obstruction and deliver bile into the gastrointestinal tract is a necessity. External drainage procedures are unsatisfactory.

Paul Szanto, MD, Chairman, Department of Pathology, Cook County Hospital, assisted in the preparation of this paper.

E. Lee Strohl, MD, 122 S Michigan Ave, Chicago 3, Ill.

REFERENCES

1. Kirschbaum, J. D., and Kozoll, D. C.: Carcinoma of the Gallbladder and Extrahepatic Bile Ducts: Clinical and Pathological Study of 117 Cases in 13,330 Necropsies, Surg Gynec Obstet 73:740-754 (Nov) 1941.

2. Courvoisier, L. G.: Casuistisch-statistische Beiträge zur Pathologie und Chirurgie der Gallenwege, Leipzig, Germany: F. C. W. Vogel, 1890.

3. Fardel, D.: Quoted by Renshaw, K.: Malignant Neoplasms of the Extrahepatic Biliary Ducts, Ann Surg 76:205-221 (Aug) 1922.

4. Schueppel, H.: Quoted by Renshaw, K.: Malignant Neoplasms of the Extrahepatic Biliary Ducts, Ann Surg 76:205-221 (Aug) 1922.

5. Musser, J. H.: Primary Cancer of the Gall-Bladder and Bile-Ducts, Boston Med Surg 121: 525-529, 1889.

6. Baudoin, C. E.: Quoted by Deaver, J. B., and Ashurst, A. P. C.: Surgery of the Upper Abdomen: II. Surgery of the Gallbladder, Liver, Pancreas, and Spleen, Philadelphia: P. Blakiston's Son & Co., 1913, vol 24, p 409.

7. Ulizinski, M.: Quoted by Pickrell, K. L., and Blalock, A.: The Surgical Treatment of Carcinoma of the Common Bile Duct, Surgery 15:923-937 (June) 1944.

8. Mayo, W. J.: "Malignant Disease of the Common Bile Duct," in Mayo, W. J., and Mayo, C. H.: A Collection of Papers Published Previous to 1909, Philadelphia: W. B. Saunders Co., 1912, p 401-406.

9. Cattell, R. B.: Successful Resection of Carcinoma of the Bile Duct, Surg Clin N Amer 23:747-752 (June) 1943.

10. Garlock, J. H.: Primary Carcinoma of the Common Bile Duct: Resection, End-to-End Anastomosis, Ann Surg 110:474-479 (Sept) 1939.

11. Jackson, C. E., and Caylor, H. D.: Adenocarcinoma of the Common Bile Duct With Resection and Anastomosis of the Hepatic Duct to the Cystic Duct and Cholecystogastrostomy, Amer J Surg 71:696-701 (May) 1946.

12. Dragstedt, L. R.; Julian, O.; Allen, J. G.; and Owens, F. M.: Implantation of the Hepatic Duct Into the Duodenum or Stomach, Surg Gynec Obstet 77:126-129 (Aug) 1943.

13. Brunschwig, A., and Bigelow, R. R.: Advanced Carcinoma of the Extrahepatic Bile Ducts: Cholangiocholecystocholedochectomy, Ann Surg 122:522-528 (Oct) 1945.

14. Pickrell, K. L., and Blalock, A.: The Surgical Treatment of Carcinoma of the Common Bile Duct, Surgery 15:923-937 (June) 1944.

15. Stewart, H. L.; Lieber, M. M.; and Morgan, D. R.: Carcinoma of the Extrahepatic Bile Ducts, Arch Surg 41:662-713 (Sept) 1940.

16. Sako, K.; Seitzinger, G. L.; and Garside, E.: Carcinoma of the Extrahepatic Bile Ducts: Review

of the Literature and Report of Six Cases, Surgery 41:416-437 (March) 1957.

17. Kuwayti, K.; Baggenstoss, A. H.; Stauffer, M. H.; and Priestley, J. T.: Carcinoma of the Intrahepatic and Extrahepatic Bile Ducts Exclusive of the Papilla of Vater, Surg Gynec Obstet 104: 357-366 (March) 1957.

18. Glenn, F., and Hill, M. R., Jr.: Extrahepatic Biliary Tract Cancer, Cancer 8:1218-1225 (Nov-Dec) 1955.

19. Thorbjarnarson, B.: Carcinoma of the Bile Ducts, Cancer 12:708-713 (July-Aug) 1959.

20. Todd, M. C.: Carcinoma of the Extrahepatic Bile Ducts, Western J Surg 64:536-539 (Oct) 1956.

21. Lippman, H. N.; McDonald, L. C.; and Longmire, W. P., Jr.; Carcinoma of the Extrahepatic Bile Ducts, Amer Surg 25:819-826 (Nov) 1959.

22. Irons, H. S., Jr.: Carcinoma of the Cystic Duct: Case Reports of Successful Resection, Surgery 38:396-401 (Aug) 1955.

23. Erler, C.: Unusual Abnormalities of the Intra and Extrahepatic Bile Ducts with Cholelithiasis and Carcinoma of the Bile Ducts, Zbl Allg Path 10:448, 1951.

24. Coleman, J. U.: Adenocarcinoma of the Common Bile Duct, Canad Med Ass J 75:576-579 (Oct 1) 1956.

25. Finkelberg, W. O.: Carcinoma of the Common Duct: Two Cases, Minnesota Med 38:28-29 (Jan) 1955.

26. Paulino, F.: Carcinoma of the Gallbladder and Extrahepatic Bile Ducts, Rev Brasil Cirurg 25: 1-2 (Jan 1) 1953.

27. Steeper, J. R.: Tumors of the Extrahepatic Biliary Tract, J Int Coll Surg 24:180-191 (Aug) 1955.

28. Pera Blanco-Morales, C., and Viñuela Herrero, A.: Carcinoma primitivo del colédocho (Primary Carcinoma of the Choledochus), Rev Clin Esp 56:39-42 (Jan 15) 1955.

29. Chrismer, R.; Lambermont, J.; and Droze, C.; Primary Carcinoma of the Common Duct: Semeiologic Study, Acta Gastroent Belg 19:495-520 (July) 1956.

30. Shanmugaratnam, K.: Primary Carcinoma of the Liver and Bill Tract, Brit J Cancer 10:232-246 (June) 1956.

31. Prohaska, J. V.; Nelsen, T. S.; and Evans, S. O.: Radical Surgery in Advanced Carcinoma of Intra-Abdominal Organs: Therapeutic Achievements, AMA Arch Surg 73:671-681 (Oct) 1956.

32. Laszlo, V.: Primary Carcinoma of the Bile Ducts, Zbl Chir 82:899-905 (June) 1957.

33. Mortier, G.: Scirrhous Carcinoma of the Main Bile Duct With Intrahepatic Metastases, Belg T Geneesk 15:1158-1162 (Nov 1) 1959.

34. Penrod, R.: Carcinoma of the Bile Ducts, Gaz Med France 67:555-559 (March 10) 1960.

35. Keiss, G.: Primary Carcinoma of the Extrahepatic Bile Ducts, Wien Klin Wschr 72:301-304 (April 29) 1960.

36. Booher, R. J., and Pack, G. T.: Recurrent Cancer of the Common Bile Duct and Periampullary Region, AMA Arch Surg 64:224-237 (Feb) 1952.

37. Reiffenscheid, M.: Carcinoma of the Extrahepatic Biliary Tract: New Viewpoints on Etiology, Therapy, and Prognosis, Munechen Med Wschr 101:272-275 (Feb) 1959.

38. Brown, G.: Surgical Removal of Tumors of the Hepatic Ducts, Postgrad Med J 16:79-85 (Aug) 1954.

39. Brown, G., and Myers, N.: Surgical Approach for Resection of Tumor of the Hepatic Ducts, Aust New Zeal J Surg 23:308-312 (July) 1954.

40. de Mello, J. B.: Primary Carcinoma of the Extrahepatic Bile Ducts, Rev Ass Med Brasil 5: 441-446 (Dec) 1959.

41. Gautier, R.; Bonnet-Eymard, J.; and Coupie, G.: Neoplasms of the Upper Bile Ducts: Intrahepatic Bilio-Intestinal Shunt, Mem Acad Chir (Paris) 86:680-683 (Oct 12) 1960.

42. Finzi, R.: Neoplasms of the Extrahepatic Biliary Tract, Minerva Gastroent 6:84-98 (April-June) 1960.

43. Massot, P.: Neoplastic Jaundices and Cancers of the Biliary Tract: Anatomical Localizations and Anatomopathology, Rev Prat 10:2451-2458 (Sept 11) 1960.

44. Goinard, P., and Pelissier, C.: Surgical Exploration of Tumors of the Vaterian Ampulla and Carcinoma of the Common Bile Duct, Rev Prat 10:2487-2491 (Sept 11) 1960.

45. Roix, G.; Baumel, H.; Vidal J.; and Badosa, J.: Carcinoma of the Hepatic Duct and Choledochus Offsite Between Nodular Forms and Extensive Forms, Ann Chir 14:923-928 (Aug) 1960.

46. Wallensten, S., and Fries, B.: Reconstruction of the Common Duct With an Isolated Jejunal Segment Following Choledochal Resection for Carcinoma, Acta Chir Scand 119:417-421 (Sept 26) 1960.

47. Brenen, R. B.: The Surgery of Malignant Disease of the Extrahepatic Bile Ducts and Head of the Pancreas, Irish J Med Sci 424:137-155 (April) 1961.

48. Bullen, R. A., and Amogalan, A.: Primary Tumors of the Bile Ducts, Rev Esp Enferm Apar Dig 20:127-165 (Feb) 1961.

49. Method, H. L., and Douglass, T. C.: Carcinoma of the Extrahepatic Bile Ducts: Two Cases, Quart Bull Northwest Univ Med Sch 28:304-307, 1954.

50. White, R. J.: Carcinoma of the Larger Bile Ducts, Exclusive of the Papilla of Vater, Ann Surg 149:762-772 (May) 1959.

51. Saypol, G. B.: Carcinoma of the Extrahepatic Bile Ducts Exclusive of the Papilla of Vater, New York J Med 51:1049-1053 (April 15) 1951.

52. Brown, D. B.; Strang, R.; Gordon, J.; and Hendry, E. B.: Primary Carcinoma of the Extrahepatic Bile-Ducts, Brit J Surg 49:22-28 (July) 1961.

53. Neibling, H. H.; Dockerty, M. B.; and Waugh, J. M.: Carcinoma of the Extrahepatic Bile Ducts, Surg Gynec Obstet 89:429-438 (Oct) 1949.

54. Willis, R. A.: Some Aspects of the Carcinomata of the Biliary Tract, Med J Aust 2:340-344 (Oct 10) 1942.

55. Sternberg, S. S.; Popper, H.; Oser, B. L.; and Oser, M.: Gallbladder and Bile Duct Adenocarcinoma in Dogs After Long-Term Feeding of Aramite, Cancer 13:780-789 (July-Aug) 1960.

56. Gupta, D. N.: Production of Carcinoma of the Bile Ducts With Thioacetamide, Nature (London) 175:257 (Feb 5) 1955.

57. Grott, J. W.: Lambliaza jako mozliwy cznnik chorobotworczy (Lambliasis in Etiology of Cancer of Biliary Tract), Medycyna 843-846 (Nov 21) 1938.

58. Fortner, J. G.: Experimental Bile-Duct Cancer Possibly Induced by Bile of Humans With Bile-Duct Cancer, Cancer 8:683-686 (July-Aug) 1955.

59. Steiner, P. E.: A Carcinogenic Extract From Human Bile and Gallbladders, Proc Soc Exp Biol Med 51:352-383 (Dec) 1942.

60. Lauber, W., and Danneberg, P.: Zur Morphologie der durch p-Dimethylamino-azobenzol erzeugten Leberveränderungen und Tumoren bei der Ratte (Morphology of p-Dimethylamino-azobenzal-Induced Liver Changes and Tumors in Rats), Z Krebsforsch 61:327-345, 1956.

61. Okinaka, S.; Nakao, K.; Ibayaski, H.; Nakaidsumi, M.; Kakehi, H.; and Sugimura, T.: A Case Report of the Development of Biliary Tract Carcinoma 11 Years After the Injection of Thorotrast, Amer J Roentgen 78:812-818 (Nov) 1957.

62. Roberts, J. C., Jr., and Carlson, K. F.: Hepatic Duct Carcinoma 17 Years After the Injection of Thorium Dioxide, AMA Arch Path 62:1-7 (July) 1956.

63. Dick, J. C.: Carcinoma of the Lower End of the Common Bile Duct, Brit J Surg 26:757-763 (April) 1939.

64. Zenker, H.: Der primäre Krebs der Gallenblase und seine Beziehung zu Gallensteinen und Gallenblasennarben, Deutsch Arch Klin Med 44:159-184, 1888-89.

65. Rolleston, Sir Humphrey, and McNee, J. W.: Diseases of the Liver, Gall-Bladder, and Bile-Ducts, Ed 3, London: Macmillan & Co., Ltd., 1929.

66. Bazin, A. T.: Benign Papilloma of the Common Duct, Ann Surg 92:658-662 (Oct) 1930.

67. Moore, S. W.; McElwee, R. S.; and Romiti, C.: Benign Tumors of the Biliary Tract, JAMA 150:999-1002 (Nov 8) 1952.

68. Zaslow, J., and Lorry, R. W.: Obstructive Jaundice Due to Benign Tumors of the Extrahepatic Bile Ducts: Case, J Int Coll Surg 15:212-218 (Feb) 1951.

69. Rogers, R. E.: A Papillary Cystadenoma of the Common Hepatic Duct, Canad Med Ass J 55:597-599 (Dec) 1946.

70. Gerber, A.: Retention Cyst of the Liver Due to Bile Duct Polyp, Ann Surg 140:906-910 (Dec) 1934.

71. Hultén, O.: On Precancerous Bile Duct Tumors, Acta Chir Scand 119:122-125 (June 30) 1960.

72. Eiss, S.; DiMaio, D.; and Caedo, J. P.: Multiple Papillomas of the Entire Biliary Tract, Ann Surg 152:320-324 (Aug) 1960.

73. Boerner, P.: Papillomatosis of the Intrahepatic and Extrahepatic Biliary Tracts, Z Krebsforsch 63:474-480, 1960.

74. Schmug, G. E.: So-Called Papillomas of the Gallbladder, Amer J Surg 96:296-301 (Aug) 1958.

75. Hess, R., and Werthermann, A.: Primary Stenosing Cholangitis: Its Relation to Carcinoma, Gastroenterologia (Basel) 88:305-311, 1957.

76. Altemeier, W. A.; Gall, E. A.; Zinninger, M. M.; and Hoxworth, P. I.: Sclerosing Carcinoma of the Major Intrahepatic Bile Ducts, AMA Arch Surg 75:450-461 (Sept) 1957.

77. Ransom, H. K.: Carcinoma of the Pancreas and Extrahepatic Bile Ducts, Amer J Surg 40:264-281 (April) 1938.

78. Farianacci, C. J.; Fairchild, J. F.; Sulak, M. H.; and Gillpatrick, W.: Sarcoma Botryoides Form of Embryonal Rhabdomyosarcoma of the Common Bile Duct: Two Cases, Cancer 9:408-417 (March-April) 1956.

79. Horn, R. C., Jr.; Yakon, C. W. C.; and Koop, E. E.: Rhabdomyosarcoma (Sarcoma Botryoides) of the Common Bile Duct: Report of a Case, Cancer 8:469-477 (March-April) 1955.

80. Flandreau, R. H.; Weber, J. M.; and Baird, W. F.: Obstructive Jaundice: The Problems of Differential Diagnosis in a Patient With Carcinoma of the Major Intrahepatic Ducts, Gastroenterology 33:978-984 (Dec) 1957.

81. Lombardi, A. A.: Jaundice as a Symptom of Biliary Cases, Bull NY Med Coll 17:17-20, 1954.

82. Kantor, H. G.; Evans, J. A.; and Glenn, F.: Cholangiography: Critical Analysis, AMA Arch Surg 70:237-252 (Feb) 1955.

83. Evans, J. A., and Mujahed, Z.: Roentgenographic Aids in Diagnosis of Neoplasms of Liver and Extrahepatic Ducts, JAMA 171:7-11 (Sept 5) 1959.

84. Larsen, K. A.: Malignant Lesions Affecting the Bile Ducts in the Post-Mortem Cholangiogram, Acta Path Microbiol Scand 51:24-46, 1961.

85. Dreiling, D. A.; Nieburg, H. E.; and Janowitz, H. D.: The Combined Secretin and Cytology Test in the Diagnosis of Pancreatic and Biliary Tract Carcinoma, Med Clin N Amer 44: 811-815 (May) 1960.

86. Wenger, J., and Raskin, H. F.: The Diagnosis of Carcinoma of the Pancreas, Biliary Tract, and Duodenum by Combined Cytologic and Secretory Methods, Gastroenterology 34:1009-1017 (June) 1958.

87. Keeley, J. L., and Schairer, A. E.: Intrahepatic Cholangiojejunostomy (Longmire Procedure) in Carcinoma of Intrahepatic Bile Ducts, AMA Arch Surg 75:21-27 (July) 1957.

88. Leiter, H. E.: Carcinoma Involving the Common Bile Duct: Report of Four Cases of Successful Resection, Surgery 22:627-647 (Oct) 1947.

89. Barnes, J. P., and Zarr, L. L.: Resection of the Common Hepatic Duct for Papillary Adenocarcinoma, Surg Gynec Obstet 84:427-434 (April) 1947.

90. Ariel, I. M., and Pack, G. T.: The Treatment of Inoperable Cancer of the Biliary System With Radioactive (I^{131}) Rose Bengal, Amer J Roentgen 83:474-490 (March) 1960.

91. Kehr, H.: Ein Fall von ausgedehnter Resektion des Ductus choledochus und hepaticus wegen Carcinoma choledochi mit nachfolgender Ektomie der Gallenblase und Hepatiko-Duodenostomie, Muenchen Med Wschr 50:101, 1903.

92. Quénu, E.: De l'opération radicale dans le cancer des voies biliaries, Rev Chir Orthop 29:245-266, 1909.

93. Pallin, G.: Das Carcinom des Ductus Hepatico-choledochus und seine chirurgische Behandlung (Cancer of bile ducts), Bruns Beitr Klin Chir 121:84-137, 1920.

94. Dennis, C., and Varco, R. L.: Neoplastic Biliary Obstruction, Surg Gynec Obstet 20:72-81 (July) 1946.

95. Siler, V. E., and Zinninger, M. M.: Surgical Treatment of Carcinoma of the Ampulla of Vater and Extrahepatic Bile Ducts, Arch Surg 56:199-223 (Feb) 1948.

96. Warren, K. W.; Cattell, R. B.; Blackburn, J. P.; and Nora, P. F.: A Long-Term Appraisal of Pancreaticoduodenal Resection for Peri-Ampullary Carcinoma, Ann Surg 155:653-662 (May) 1962.

97. Marshall, J. M.: Tumors of the Bile Ducts, Surg Gynec Obstet 54:6-12 (Jan) 1932.

98. Goldenberg, I. S.: Carcinoma of the Bile Ducts, Amer J Surg 86:292-300 (Sept) 1955.

99. Walters, W., and Snell, A. M.: Diseases of the Gallbladder and Bile Ducts, Philadelphia: W. B. Saunders Company, 1940, p 478.

Whole-Body Hypothermia in Ammonia Intoxication

Effect on Monkeys With Portacaval Shunts

GEORGE D. ZUIDEMA, MD
WALTER D. GAISFORD, MD
RICHARD S. KOWALCZYK, PhD
AND
EARL F. WOLFMAN, JR., MD
ANN ARBOR, MICH

Hepatic coma is a serious complication of advanced liver disease. It may occur secondary to hemorrhage from gastroesophageal varices, after operation for portal decompression, or in the final stages of hepatic decompensation. The prognosis varies with the severity of the underlying liver disease and the recuperative powers of the liver.

Although the metabolic derangements associated with hepatic coma are not completely known, elevated levels of blood ammonia are found with reasonable consistency.[1,2] This has been recognized since 1896 when Nencki and Pawlow[3] related blood ammonia elevations with meat intoxication. McDermott and Adams,[4] Mann et al,[5] and Levine and Rigler[6] showed that blood ammonia levels often rose after portacaval anastomosis.

Protein digestion in the gastrointestinal tract is a major source of ammonia. The products of digestion, including ammonia, are absorbed and carried by the portal vein. The normal liver can readily detoxify ammonia by converting it to urea. The liver damaged by disease or bypassed by portal-systemic collateral veins cannot, however, manage efficient detoxification. As a result increased amounts of ammonia reach the systemic circulation. Portacaval anastomosis permits ammonia-rich portal blood to enter the systemic circuit directly. Patients with massive hemorrhage from gastroesophageal varices have a large volume of protein entering the gastrointestinal tract where intestinal microorganisms aid in its digestion, with liberation of ammonia.

Keirle et al[7] studied the effect of hypothermia on blood ammonia levels in normal dogs and in two patients with cirrhosis and elevated blood ammonias. The present study was undertaken in Eck fistula monkeys in which experimental ammonia intoxication was induced by administering whole blood by nasogastric tube.

Materials and Methods

Seven *Macaca mulata* monkeys weighing 3-5 kg were used. End-to-side portacaval shunts were created by a previously described method. The animals were allowed seven days to recover prior to study. They were then anesthetized with thiamylal (Surital) (23 mg/kg), and an endotracheal tube was inserted and connected to a respirator. Outdated human bank blood was administered by nasogastric tube (40 ml/kg), and blood ammonia levels were determined hourly for eight hours. Rectal temperatures were monitored continuously and ranged between 96 and 99 F. Blood urea nitrogen determinations were made before each experiment and hourly during each run. Thirty and 45 minute sulfobromophthalein (Bromsulfalein) retention tests were made before each experiment and at four and eight hours during the experiment. The animals were permitted to recover for five to seven days. The experiments were then repeated under whole-body hypothermia, with rectal temperatures

Submitted for publication Feb 4, 1963.

John and Mary R. Markle Scholar in Academic Medicine, United States Public Health Service Career Development Awardee, AM K3 13,702 (Dr. Zuidema).

From the Department of Surgery, University of Michigan Medical School.

Supported by USPHS grant No. H4260 C-3, USPHS grant No. 05269, and US Army Contract DA 49-007-MD 1016.

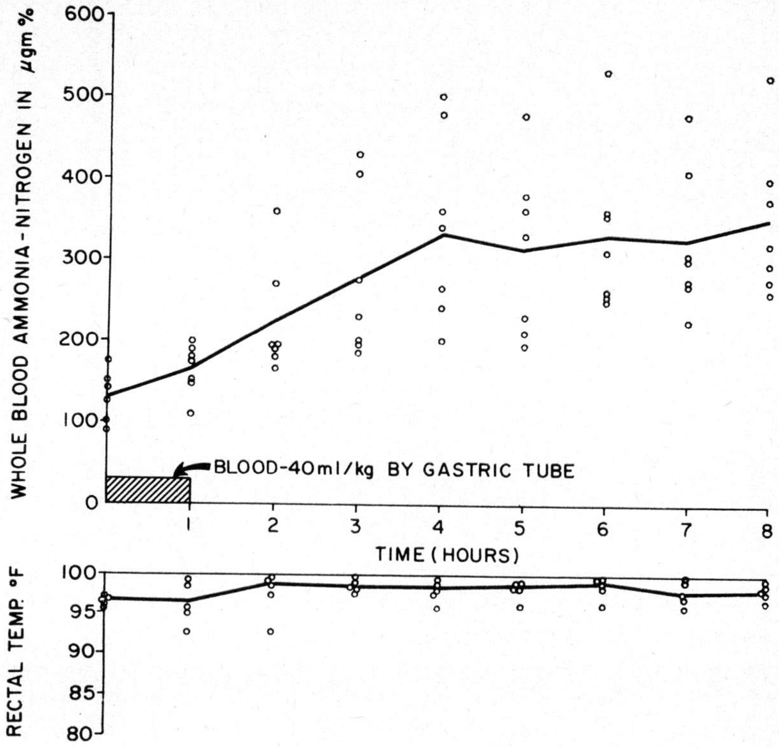

Fig 1.—Whole blood ammonia nitrogen values in seven normothermic monkeys with end-to-side portacaval shunts after administration of whole blood (40 ml/kg) by gastric tube. All animals were anesthetized and maintained with endotracheal tubes and assisted respiration. Rectal temperatures shown.

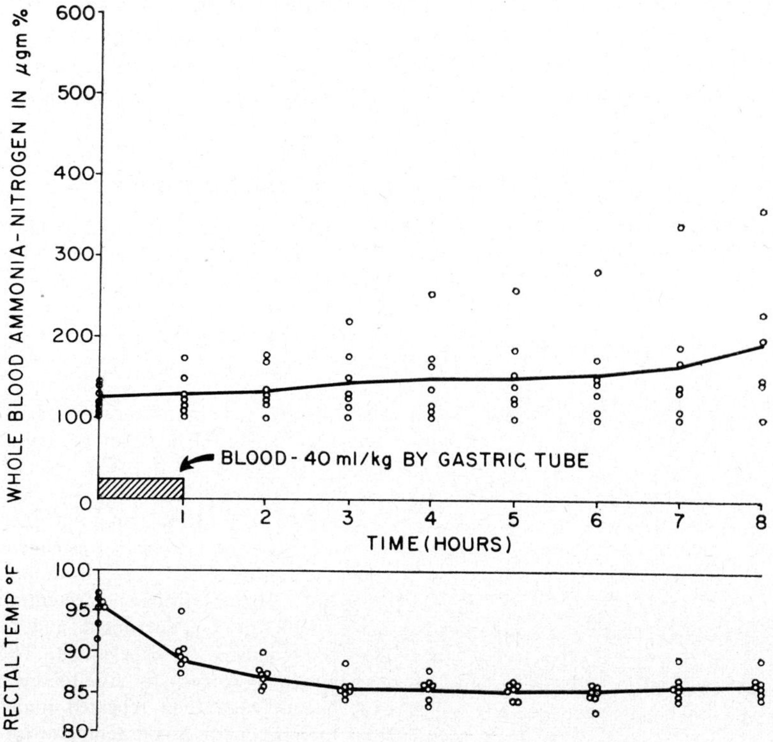

Fig 2.—Whole blood ammonia nitrogen values in seven hypothermic monkeys with end-to-side portacaval shunts after administration of whole blood (40 ml/kg) by gastric tube. All animals were anesthetized, maintained with endotracheal tubes and assisted respiration, and under whole body hypothermia. Mean rectal temperature was maintained at approximately 86 F.

Table 1.—*Statistical Treatment of Blood Ammonia Data*

	0	1	2	3	4	5	6	7	8
Normothermic animals, mean blood NH_3 values	130	166	226	275	342	313	333	326	351
Hypothermic animals, mean blood NH_3 values	125	130	137	146	153	154	156	170	198
Mean difference	5	36	89	129	189	159	177	156	153
Standard deviation		27.5	55	78	89	83	84	88	88.5
Value of t_{12}		2.47	2.98	2.98	3.99	3.61	3.99	3.36	3.29
Value of P		<0.05	<0.02	<0.02	<0.01	<0.01	<0.01	<0.01	<0.01

maintained at 86±2 F. All blood samples were taken from the inferior vena cava by polyethylene catheters inserted via the femoral vein.

Blood urea nitrogen and sulfobromophthalein retention tests were performed by standard laboratory methods. Blood ammonia determinations were made by the modified microdiffusion method of Conway.*

Results

Fig 1 displays the blood ammonia levels in seven normothermic, anesthetized monkeys with end-to-side portacaval shunts after administration of whole blood by gastric tube. There is a gradual rise during the first three hours, after which the curve plateaus at approximately 300μg %-350μg %. This mean curve averages about 75μg % lower than a similar curve obtained from unanesthetized monkeys with end-to-end shunts as previously reported from this laboratory.[10]

Fig 2 shows the blood ammonia levels observed in seven anesthetized monkeys with end-to-side portacaval shunts under whole-body hypothermia. The mean level remains approximately at baseline, gradually rising about 70μg % late in the course of the eight-hour experiment. Statistical treatment of these data is shown in Table 1.

Blood urea nitrogen determinations showed no consistent or significant changes in either control or experimental animals (Table 2).

The 30- and 45-minute sulfobromophthalein retention tests were consistently higher in the hypothermic, anesthetized animals. Table 3 lists control data obtained the day prior to each experiment and results obtained four hours after the beginning of the experiment. Control values ranged from 0%-10% retention. The 45-minute retentions were elevated above 10% in only two animals under hypothermia. Thirty-minute retentions were elevated above 10% in seven animals under hypothermia.

* Described in Reif[8] and Natelson.[9]

Table 2.—*Monkeys With End-To-Side Portacaval Shunts: Blood Urea Nitrogen Values, Mg%*

Hour	0	1	2	3	4	5	6	7	8
Monkey 1-6a									
Normothermic	26	22	23	22	21	24	24	25	30
Hypothermic	33	26	29	25	26	22	25	28	26
Monkey 1-8									
Normothermic	16	12	15	16	21	23	25	31	34
Hypothermic	18	17	16	18	17	18	20	18	21
Monkey 1-11									
Hypothermic	25	22	20	19	21	17	16	14	14
Monkey 1-12									
Normothermic	35	41	51	31	32	33	32	34	34
Hypothermic	18		14	15	15	13	12	13	12
Monkey 1-13									
Hypothermic	29	27	25	25	25	24	22	23	26
Monkey 1-15									
Normothermic	13	14			14				
Hypothermic	20		16				18	28	20
Monkey 1-16									
Normothermic	26	25.8			30.0				45.1
Hypothermic	20		16		20.5				24.5

TABLE 3.—*Sulfobromophthalein Retention, %, Controls and at Four Hours*

	30 Minutes			45 Minutes		
Monkey	Normal (Day Prior to Experiment)	Normothermic, Anesthetized	Hypothermic, Anesthetized	Normal (Day Prior to Experiment)	Normothermic, Anesthetized,	Hypothermic, Anesthetized
1-6a	8	3	12	6	2	8
1-8	2	9	29	0	2	15
1-12	7	16	21	—	2	7
1-15	3.6	4	19	2.2	2	7
1-16	2	—	11.3	1	—	4
1-7	7	4	—	6	—	—
1-11	6	—	12	3	—	5
1-13	10	—	18	8	—	15

Comment

Eiseman, Owens, and Swan [11] and Clauss et al [12] have reported that whole-body hypothermia can be used with good results during operations on patients with cirrhosis. Hypothermia is known to reduce enzymatic activity and bacterial metabolism [13,14] and might therefore be beneficial in the treatment of ammonia intoxication.

Keirle et al [7] studied the effects of hypothermia on blood ammonia levels in normal anesthetized dogs given whole blood (50 ml/kg) by gastric tube. They found that there was a reduction and delay in the production and absorption of ammonia in the gastrointestinal tract and that the normal, hypothermic liver at 88 F was capable of detoxifying ammonia. They applied the technique clinically in two patients, both of whom responded to this treatment.

It is difficult to produce ammonia intoxication in normal dogs, for the normal liver has great capacity for converting ammonia to urea, even under conditions of hypothermia. This experiment was undertaken, therefore, to obtain objective data on Eck fistula monkeys, simulating the clinical condition as closely as possible.

The slight increase in sulfobromophthalein retention occurring under hypothermia confirms the previous observation of Brauer.[15] The significance of this increase is unclear, but it is likely that it reflects biliary stasis rather than depressed hepatocellular function.

Our data show significantly decreased levels of blood ammonia in all animals protected by whole-body hypothermia. A number of factors might contribute to this result. Hypothermia probably produces decreased bacterial digestion of protein and impaired enzymatic activity within the bowel.[16] As a result ammonia production and absorption might be impaired. The metabolism of ammonia by peripheral tissues may also be altered by whole-body hypothermia, although the liver apparently retains its ability to detoxify ammonia.

There is no evidence that hypothermia decreases intestinal motility to any marked degree. The stool of several animals in both control and experimental groups contained blood at the end of the experiment. No significant amount of blood was retained in the stomachs of animals in either group.

Direct translation of these experimental data to the clinical situation must be done with care. Many patients with ammonia intoxication of the "exogenous type" are conscious in the early stages when hypothermia would be expected to be of greatest help. Shivering occurs in these patients, and it is not feasible to avoid this by using anesthesia and tracheal intubation. Chlorpromazine has been widely employed to prevent shivering in patients undergoing hypothermia for other reasons. Because of its possible hepatic effects, however, we have hesitated to recommend its use in patients with liver disease. With these reservations it would appear that whole-body hypothermia might find application in the patient with hepatic coma, as part of a broader therapeutic program designed to control variceal hemorrhage, sterilize the bowel, and prevent the continued absorption of ammonia from the intestine.

Summary

Whole-body hypothermia has been shown to reduce significantly the levels of blood ammonia following administration of whole blood by gastric tube to Eck fistula monkeys.

Blood urea nitrogen values were not elevated in either control or experimental animals during the experiment.

Sulfobromophthalein (Bromsulfalein) retention was only slightly increased under whole-body hypothermia.

Mrs. Mary Clapp gave technical assistance, and Margaret M. Fletcher, MD, did the statistical treatment of the experimental data.

George D. Zuidema, MD, Department of Surgery, University of Michigan Medical School, Ann Arbor, Mich.

REFERENCES

1. Bessman, S. P., and Bessman, H. N.: The Cerebral and Peripheral Uptake of Ammonia in Liver Disease With an Hypothesis for the Mechanism of Hepatic Coma, J Clin Invest 34:622, 1955.

2. Pearlman, D. M.: The Effect of Glutamate Administration on Blood Ammonia Level and Its Correlation With Clinical Status in Patients With Hepatic Coma, Surg Forum 6:364, 1955.

3. Nencki, M., and Pawlow, J. P.: Arch Exp Path Pharmakol 32:161, 1896, and 37:26, 1896, cited by Folin, O., and Denis, W.: Protein Metabolism From the Standpoint of Blood and Time Analysis: II. The Origin and Significance of the Ammonia in Portal Blood, J Biol Chem 11:161, 1912.

4. McDermott, W. V., Jr., and Adams, R. D.: Episodic Stupor Associated With an Eck Fistula in the Human, With Particular Reference to the Metabolism of Ammonia, J Clin Invest 33:1, 1954.

5. Mann, J. D.; Bollman, J. L.; Huizenga, K. A.; Farror, T.; and Grindlay, J. H.: Blood Ammonia, Experimental and Clinical Study in Abnormalities of the Liver and Portal Circulation, Gastroenterology 27:399, 1954.

6. Levine, R. S., and Rigler, S. P.: Studies on the Ammonia Tolerance Curve in Dogs With Portacaval Shunts, Surg Forum 8:235, 1957.

7. Keirle, A. M.; McGloin, J. J.; Buben, R. W.; and Altemeier, W. A.: Blood Ammonia: Experimental and Clinical Reduction by Hypothermia, Arch Surg 83:348-355, 1961.

8. Reif, A. E.: The Ammonia Content of Blood and Plasma, Anal Biochem 1:351-370, 1960.

9. Natelson, S.: Microtechniques of Clinical Chemistry for the Routine Laboratory, Springfield, Ill: Charles C Thomas, Publisher, 1959, p 484.

10. Zuidema, G. D.; Gaisford, W. D.; Rakolta, G.; Fletcher, M. M.; Burton, W. D.; and Child, C. G., III: Comparative Blood Ammonia Studies in Dogs and Monkeys, Arch Surg 85:776-782, 1962.

11. Eiseman, B.; Owens, J. C.; and Swan, H.: Hypothermia in General Surgery, New Eng J Med 255:750, 1956.

12. Clauss, R. H.; Junker, R. D.; Browning, L. D.; and MacFee, W. F.: Hypothermia for Portacaval Shunts, Ann Surg 150:99, 1959.

13. Wotkyns, R. S.; Kirose, H.; and Eiseman, B.: Prolonged Hypothermia in Experimental Pneumococcal Peritonitis, Surg Gynec Obstet 107: 363, 1958.

14. Fedor, E. J.; Fisher, B.; and Fisher, E. R.: Observations Concerning Bacterial Defense Mechanisms During Hypothermia, Surgery 43:807, 1958.

15. Brauer, R. W.: "The Effect of Hypothermia on the Isolated Perfused Rat Liver," in The Physiology of Induced Hypothermia: Proceedings of a Symposium, October 1955, Division Medical Sciences, National Academy of Sciences, National Research Council, pp 235-242.

16. Welch, H. F.; Affifi, R.; and Rosano, C. L.: Effect of Hypothermia on Blood Ammonia Formation, Surgery 50:390-394, 1961.

Effect of Simulated Gallstones on Guinea Pig Gallbladders

M. H. SIMMERS, MD
AND
EILEEN PODOLAK, MS
LOS ANGELES

Introduction

Cancer of the gallbladder and gallstones have been considered for many years to be in some way related. There is still, however, no exact knowledge of the relationships which prevail. Because the sequence of formation is unknown, both have been considered precursors of the other, while some have suggested a simultaneous development.

With the belief in the etiological relationship between biliary calculi and carcinoma, many authors [1,4,12,16,19,37,38] have advocated cholecystectomy in cases of cholelithiasis as a prophylactic measure. This reasoning seems to be borne out by the high percentage of gallbladders with carcinoma that are found to contain gallstones, the reported percentage varying from 54% to 91%.* When studies were made of gallbladders removed because of cholelithiasis, however, only 10% were found to show carcinoma.† It is on the basis of this low percentage that Kramer[22] states that if calculi were a causative factor in carcinoma of the gallbladder, the incidence of carcinoma would be much higher. Derman et al [8] state that gallbladder carcinoma is not related to the presence of gallstones, and there is, therefore, no justification for the prophylactic removal of a gallbladder containg stones for the purpose of preventing malignancy.

This history of the study of the connection between gallstones and cancer of the gallbladder dates back to 1918 when Lazarus-Barlow [23] stated that gallstones found in cases of primary carcinoma showed considerable amounts of radium. He implanted stones removed from humans into the gallbladders of nine rabbits: three as controls and six with radium placed in them. He found simple foreign-body reactions in the gallbladders of the controls, with irregular proliferative columnar epithelial changes in the others. One may have had columnar-cell carcinoma with liver metastasis, others had questionable carcinoma. Kazama,[20] in 1922, placed pebbles in the gallbladders of guinea pigs and other animals and produced various reactions, including 26 carcinomas in 98 animals; none of the animals lived over four months. In 1924, Leitch [24] placed gallstones, pebbles, pitch, and melted wool fat (lanolin) into the gallbladders of guinea pigs. Wool fat produced no reaction, whereas the solid foreign bodies all produced epithelial activity. He concluded that the stimulus was not chemical and that the eight cancers found in 40 guinea pigs were mechanically induced. In 1932, Burrows [6] placed biliary calculi from noncancerous humans into gallbladders of 47 guinea pigs. Of the 33 followed, 31 showed epithelial proliferation with penetration and the other two were still alive at the

Submitted for publication Feb 6, 1963.

California College of Medicine, Oncology Laboratory.

This research was supported by an American Cancer Society grant E-112.

* References 13, 16, 17, 22, 30, 34-37, 39-41.

† References 4, 5, 8, 11, 17, 19, 21, 30, 39, 41.

time of writing. He found suggestions of early malignant change, but cancer was not produced; the changes were largely inflammatory. In 1939, Mohardt[25] reviewed the literature and expressed the belief that gallstones were causative agents of gallbladder carcinoma, due to the frequency with which calculi were found in cases of primary cancer of the gallbladder and the experimental production of cancer by the insertion of foreign bodies into the gallbladders of animals. In their study in 1947, Petrov and Krotkina[27] placed a variety of sterile hard foreign bodies into the gallbladders of guinea pigs which reacted with hyperplastic growth. Of 100 animals, 52 had epithelial hyperplasia, 5 showed malignant tumors, and 4 of these showed metastases. In 1950, Desforges et al[10] placed glass beads, cholesterol pellets, and 3-methylcholanthrene-cholesterol pellets into 32 guinea pigs. Within 1 to 41 weeks none showed carcinoma. They concluded that the gallbladder of the guinea pig is extremely resistant to the development of cancer and that the role of foreign bodies in the pathogenesis of carcinoma of the gallbladder in the guinea pig is not as direct as was thought.

In 1955, Fortner[14] placed methylcholanthrene pellets in the gallbladders of dogs and cats. He found cancer in none of the cats dying in three to ten months postoperatively. Five of the six cats, with survival times of 23 months or longer, had primary carcinoma of the gallbladder, whereas one cat had none after 32 months.

In 1957, Zeppa and Womack[43] used an injection technique to introduce methylcholanthrene, dimethylbenzanthracene, cholesterol, croton oil, and particles of human gallstones into the gallbladders of mice, with no resultant carcinoma.

In 1948 Fortner[15] questioned whether cancer of the gallbladder had ever been produced by irritation with a foreign body and denied that there was proof of a causal relation between gallstones and cancer. On theoretical grounds he postulated the existence of a carcinogen produced by, or excreted by, the liver. The chemical similarity between some carcinogenic hydrocarbons and natural steroids was noted, the in vitro conversion of cholesterol and bile acids to methylcholanthrene was pointed out, and attention was called to the carcinogenicity of cholesterol and bile acids for the subcutaneous tissues of mice, and of estrogens for the liver of hamsters. Fortner suggested that gallstones may only localize or potentiate biliary carcinogens or may even form after the cancer.

In 1959, Baim et al[2] implanted methylcholanthrene pellets in the gallbladders of 50 hamsters. Of these, 25 subsequently received a course of treatment with estradiol, injected subcutaneously. Of the 39 hamsters which survived longer than one month, 12 of the 19 which received the methylcholanthrene pellet showed biliary cancer and 12 of the 20 which received both the pellet and the course of estradiol treatment showed biliary carcinoma. More recent work by Fortner[16] with methylcholanthrene pellets in the gallbladders of five dogs resulted in a papillary adenocarcinoma in one and marked papillary hyperplasia in a second after 58 months. The other three showed neoplastic growth after 79 months.

Cancers of the gallbladder and bile ducts have been produced experimentally in dogs without direct manipulation of the gallbladder as reported by Sternberg et al in 1960.[33] A miticide, Aramite, containing as the active agents a mixture of 2(*p*-tert-butylphenoxy)isopropyl 2-chlorethyl sulfite and bis 2-(*p*-tert-butylphenoxy)isopropyl sulfite, was fed to dogs in amounts calculated to range from 828-1,429 ppm in the diet over a period of 3½ years. Fifteen of 19 animals autopsied after 462 to 1,220 days of the diet had one or more carcinomas of the biliary tract, of which nine were in the gallbladder and unaccompanied by gallstones. Earlier, Nelson and Woodard[26] noted adenocarcinomas of the entire biliary tract in dogs fed *o*-aminoazotoluene for 30 to 62 months.

We present this report on further experiments done in an attempt to clarify the significance of the association between gallstones and cancer of the gallbladder. Guinea pigs were used in these experiments because they are highly resistant to carcinogens and are rarely known to form gallbladder carcinomas spontaneously.[7,10,24,27,31,32]

Materials and Methods

Young male and female guinea pigs were obtained from a local breeder. Pellets made from beeswax containing 5% suspension of various substances or beeswax alone were implanted in their gallbladders. When two materials were put into a pellet, 5%, by weight, of each substance was used. The pellets were formed in a pellet-molding machine, and each weighed approximately 0.1 gm. The suspensions used were calcium carbonate, ground glass, and methylcholanthrene. In other experiments pellets of these substances plus cholesterol were implanted, as well as pellets of 5% cholesterol alone. Some animals were implanted with plain beeswax pellets, and others were operated upon and no pellets implanted.

Because of the reported association between cholelithiasis and hypothyroidism,[42] and between thyroid activity and some cancers,[9,18,28,29] guinea pigs were surgically thyroidectomized, and immediately after this their gallbladders were implanted with a methylcholanthrene pellet. We have no positive proof that thyroidectomy was complete although slides were made in all cases to prove the removal of thyroid tissue.

The animals were anesthetized with pentobarbital sodium given intraperitoneally and supplemented by ether inhalation if necessary. Aseptic surgical technique was used. A right upper midrectus incision approximately 1.5-2 cm long permitted delivery of the gallbladder. The gall bladder was incised, the pellet inserted, and the gallbladder closed with a running suture of 5-0 chromic catgut on an atraumatic needle. The abdomen was closed by 3-4 interrupted sutures of No. 40 black cotton thread through all layers but the skin. The skin was closed by several interrupted sutures of the same thread. No dressing was used on the wound. With few exceptions, healing was uncomplicated. The animals were maintained in cages with Purina guinea pig chow and water given ad libitum. After death they were autopsied, and slides were made of the gallbladder and other areas of interest. It was originally intended to allow the animals to live out their normal life-span, but an epidemic of pneumonia occurred and killed the entire colony. This epidemic began 958 days after the first operation and 802 days after the last implantation. The time from the beginning of the epidemic until the death of the last animals was 35 days. The longest postoperative survival of any animals was 924 days.

Results

The Table summarizes the results of our experiments. First, there were no carcinomas found. All animals showed some degree of inflammation with scarring and fibrosis. Minimal reaction followed sham operations. The pure beeswax (Fig 1) pellet caused some inflammation, scarring, and mucosal proliferation; three of the eight gallbladders in this

Summary of Results

Group	No. Animals in Group	Range of Survival & Av Survival (Wk)	Mucous Membrane Proliferation	Pseudo-adenoma	Osseous Metaplasia	Minimal Reaction	Cancer
Beeswax only	8	27-127 Av 85	5			3	0
Calcium carbonate	10	25-106 Av 85	8	2	1	2	0
Calcium carbonate & cholesterol	8	13- 80 Av 68	2			6	0
Glass	11	5-125 Av 66	7			4	0
Glass & cholesterol	9	13- 82 Av 62	6			3	0
Methylcholanthrene	11	23-130 Av 72	9	2	4	2	0
Methylcholanthrene & cholesterol	10	19- 78 Av 54	9	1		1	0
Methylcholanthrene & thyroidectomy	17	2- 65 Av 39	10	2	2	7	0
Cholesterol only	9	11-132 Av 64	8			1	0
Sham	14	41-113 Av 72	4			10	0

All of the specimens showed some foreign-body reaction with inflammatory changes, scarring, and fibrosis (minimal reaction). Columns 4-6 list the additional significant changes.

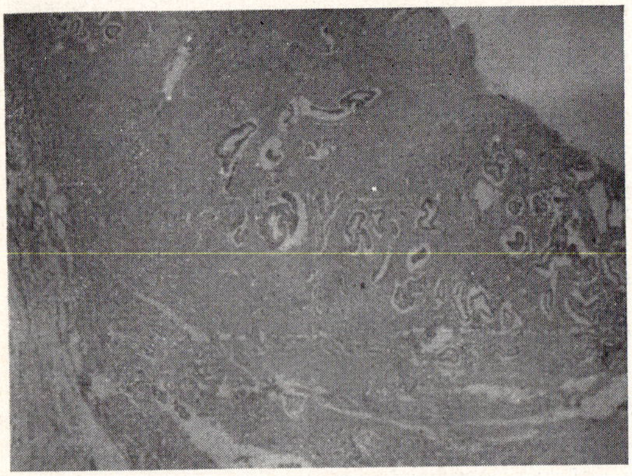

Fig 1.—Pure beeswax pellet showing thickening of gallbladder wall, fibrosis, and some mucosal proliferation. Reduced 23% from mag approx × 20.

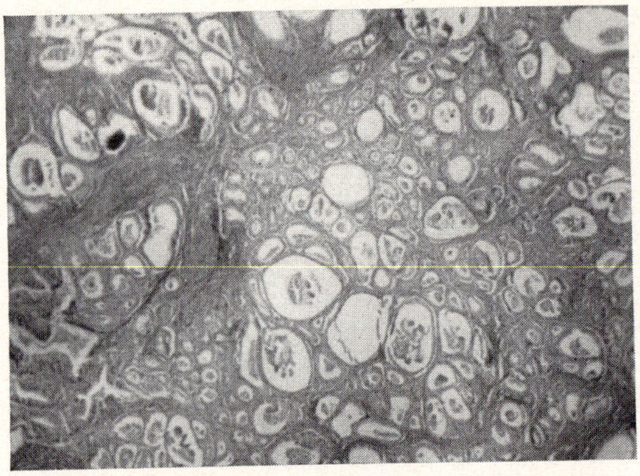

Fig 2.—5% calcium carbonate pellet. Shows marked mucosal hyperplasia and proliferation (pseudoadenoma). Reduced 23% from mag approx × 20.

group were classified as essentially normal (minimal reaction in Table).

Calcium carbonate pellets resulted in considerable scarification and some glandular proliferation. In two there were adenomatous changes which were not considered to be true neoplasia (Fig 2). One specimen showed osseous metaplasia.

Reaction to the pellets containing 5% cholesterol and 5% calcium carbonate showed less scarification and hyperplasia than was seen with beeswax alone. This difference may be related to the average postoperative time of 67.5 weeks for the latter and 85 weeks for the control pellet. This difference of almost 20 weeks may have been important in the development of hyperplasia. The time element appears to be important since most proliferative responses occurred after 74 weeks. One of the most proliferative lesions encountered was associated with the group in which the pellet consisted of 5% ground glass. This occurred after 28 weeks—a relatively short postoperative period. None of the others in this group showed as exuberant a growth so that this example cannot be considered representative. The remainder showed fibrosis and low-grade inflammatory lesions, not unlike those seen in other categories.

The pellets of 5% cholesterol and 5% ground glass excited an exudative and hyperplastic reaction in the early postoperative stages (Fig 3). Generally, these manifestations subsided and were replaced by dense scar tissue.

A 5% cholesterol pellet (Fig 4) elicited almost as much proliferative response as any stimulus and can be regarded as essentially

Fig 3.—5% cholesterol and 5% ground glass exhibiting marked mucosal proliferation and scarring. Reduced 23% from mag approx × 20.

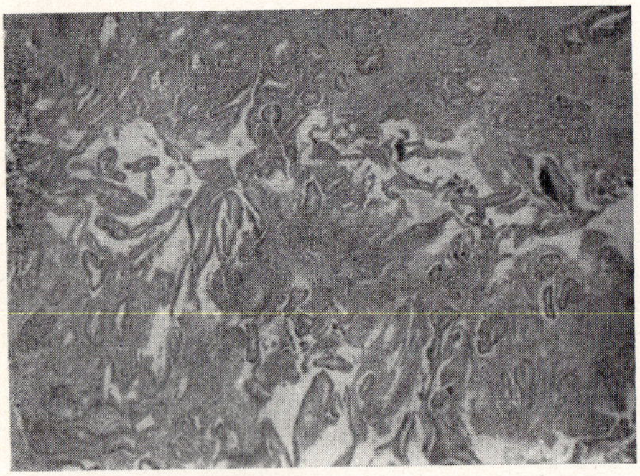

Fig 4.—5% cholesterol pellet demonstrates mucosal proliferation, thickening of gallbladder wall, scarring, and fibrosis. Reduced 23% from mag approx × 20.

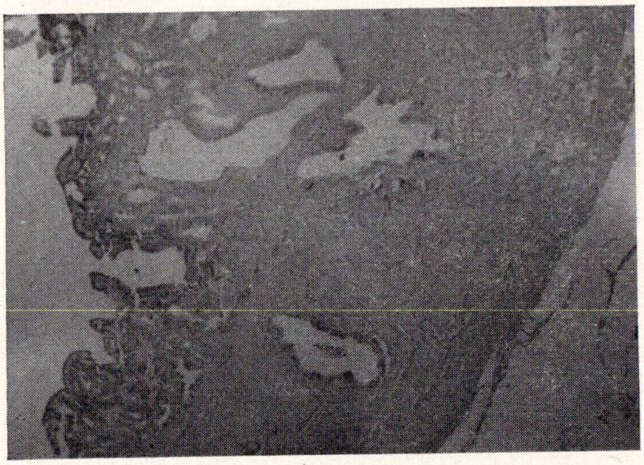

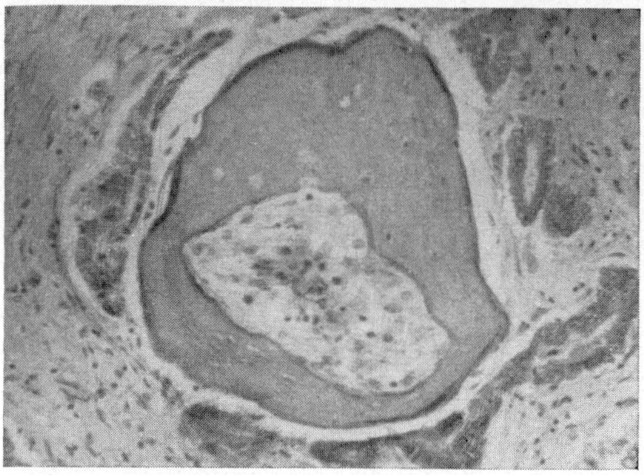

Fig 5.—Osseous metaplasia following implantation of a methylcholanthrene pellet. This occurred in six specimens containing 3-methylcholanthrene. Reduced 23% from mag approx × 60.

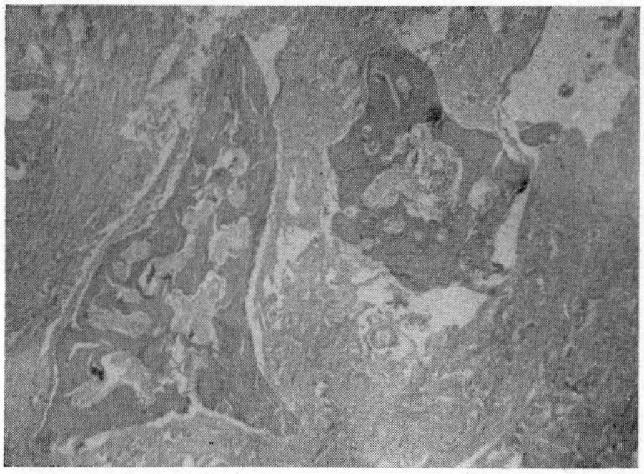

Fig. 6.—Extensive osseous metaplasia accompanying a methylcholanthrene pellet. Reduced 23% from mag approx × 60.

as potent as the other agents used. No frank malignancies were produced, but one case showed considerable nuclear aberration in addition to proliferation. This specimen was obtained after 11 weeks. As in the other groups, the longer the period of time elapsing between implantation and study, the more likely that simple scarification remained as the dominant sign of injury.

There were several in the group of combined 5% methylcholanthrene and thyroidectomy, or 5% methylcholanthrene alone, which revealed focal osseous metaplasia in areas of fibrosis (Fig 5 and 6). The addition of thyroidectomy was no more successful in producing cancers than was 5% methylcholanthrene alone or the stimuli provided by the other substances. This group also showed adenomatous hyperplasia or pseudoadenomatous proliferation in four of 28 animals (14%).

In the group in which 5% methylcholanthrene and 5% cholesterol pellets were used the response was usually moderate or severe. Fibrosis dominated, but adenomatous reactions were also encountered. The average postoperative survival was 53.8 weeks, a relatively short period. Apparently these agents were quite effective in initiating tissue responses.

Comment

Generalizing from the pathologic changes recounted, there is a tendency for an evolution of response. Initially there is an exudative and proliferative reaction which varies in intensity and which is gradually replaced by scar tissue. This inflammatory reaction occurs with all types of pellets and even with the sham operation. It is the reaction to the foreign body, be it ground glass or suture material, and occurs in every animal operated upon. Following the initial acute reaction there is a hyperplasia and proliferation of the mucosa. This may occur to a degree we have termed pseudoadenomatous. Despite the not uncommon wild appearance of this mucosal proliferation, the cell nuclei remain within a normal range of size. Mitoses are rare, and no frank criteria of malignancy have been seen. Accompanying the mucosal hyperplasia is a thickening of the muscular layer with fibrosis and scarring. In general there seems only a loose relationship between the degree of tissue response and the content of the pellet. All substances implanted, including the plain beeswax pellet, showed an occasional intense response. Our impression is that the most intense proliferative reactions occurred when methylcholanthrene was one constituent of the pellet. An interesting observation is the degree of osseous metaplasia seen. In the entire series bone formation occurred in the gallbladders of seven animals (Fig 5 and 6), six of which had pellets containing methylcholanthrene, and the seventh was seen with a pellet containing calcium carbonate. These findings substantiate the opinion of Bridges [3] that nonspecific initiation and trauma is responsible for heterotopic ossification. The hypothesis that calcium is a specific inductor of bone formation is not supported by our finding of but one instance of bone formation among 18 animals implanted with pellets containing calcium carbonate alone (ten animals) or in combination with cholesterol (eight animals). Of the materials used by us the methylcholanthrene is the most carcinogenic and was associated with all but one case of bone formation.

Thyroidectomy seemed to have no influence on the reaction of the gallbladder to the pellets (methylcholanthrene), possibly because the average life-span of 39 weeks in this group was the shortest of any; the next shortest average age for any group was 54 weeks for the methylcholanthrene-and-cholesterol group.

Because of the failure to induce cancer in any of our animals even after as much as 132 weeks of exposure to as potent a cancer producer as methylcholanthrene and because of the similarity of tissue reaction to all of the foreign materials, we are inclined to the view, expressed by Fortner,[14] that more than local exposure of the gallbladder mucosa to cancer-producing situations is involved in the carcinomatous transformation. New experiments, which we hope to do, are suggested by this view.

Conclusions

Others have failed to produce cancer in the gallbladder of guinea pigs by local implantation of foreign bodies other than those known to be extremely potent cancer producers, eg, radioactive materials and pure methylcholanthrene.

Despite the variety of materials used by us and exposures to 132 weeks, no cancers were found.

The frequent presence of stones in the gallbladders of humans with cancer of this organ does not prove a causal connection.

Cancers of the gallbladder have been experimentally produced by the feeding of certain chemicals in the absences of any foreign bodies of the gallbladder.

The above four observations recommend the conclusion that the most plausible explanation for the cause of gallbladder cancer may reside in the perverted metabolism of some substances excreted in bile. The gallstones so often found associated with gallbladder cancer may be only coincidental, but may, by mechanical irritation, act synergistically to enhance the chemical carcinogenesis.

Dr. Raymond L. Teplitz assisted in reading the slides.

M. H. Simmers, MD, Director, Oncology Laboratory, California College of Medicine, 1721 Griffin Ave, Los Angeles 31, Calif.

REFERENCES

1. Arner, O., and Von Schreeb, T.: Carcinoma of the Gallbladder, Acta Chir Scand 116:477-483, 1959.

2. Baim, G. O.; Allen, P. B. R.; Silbermann, O.; and Kowalewski, K.: Induction in Hamsters of Biliary Carcinoma by Intracholecystic Methylcholanthrene Pellets, Cancer Res 19:93-96, 1959.

3. Bridges, J. B.: Experimental Heterotopic Ossification, Int Rev Cytol 8:253-278, 1959.

4. Brown, P. F., Jr. and Dixon, P. K., Jr.: Complications of Gallstones, J Med Ass Georgia 48:455, 1959.

5. Burdette, W. J.: Carcinoma of the Gallbladder, Ann Surg 145:832-847, 1957.

6. Burrows, H.: An Experimental Inquiry Into the Association Between Gallstones and Primary Cancer of the Gallbladder, Brit J Surg 20:607-629, 1932-1933.

7. Cohrs, P.; Jaffe, R.; and Meessen, H., editors: Pathologie der Laboratoriumstiere, Berlin: Springer-Verlag, 1958, vol 2, p 493.

8. Derman, H.; Gerbarg, D. S.; Kelly, J .H.; Pauker, S.; and Singer, J.: Are Gallstones and Gallbladder Carcinoma Related? JAMA 176:450-451, 1961.

9. Desaive, P.: Observations cliniques en faveur de l'existence de relations entre la fonction thyroïdienne et le comportement de cancers hétérologues, Acta Chir Belg 55:25-49, 1956.

10. Desforges, G.; Desforges, J.; and Robbins, S. L.: Carcinoma of the Gallbladder: An Attempt at Experimental Production, Cancer, 3:1088-1096, 1950.

11. Donhauser, J. L.: Primary Carcinoma of the Gallbladder, AMA Arch Surg 77:918-924, 1958.

12. Etala, E.: [Primary Cancer of the Gallbladder], Arch Ital Mal Appar Dig 26:5-34, 1959.

13. Feller, N., and Mordechai, I.: Primary Carcinoma of the Gallbladder, Israel Dapim Refuim, 18:122-128, 1959.

14. Fortner, J. G.: The Experimental Induction of Primary Carcinoma of the Gallbladder, Cancer 8:689-700, 1955.

15. Fortner, J. G.: An Appraisal of the Pathogenesis of Primary Carcinoma of the Extrahepatic Biliary Tract, Surgery 43:563-571, 1958.

16. Fortner, J. G., and Leffall, L. D.: Carcinoma of the Gallbladder in Dogs, Cancer 14:1127-1130, 1961.

17. Gerst, P. H.: Primary Carcinoma of the Gallbladder, Ann Surg 153:369-372, 1961.

18. Grad, B.; Berenson, J.; and Coplan, L.: The Influence of Hyper- and Hypothyroidism on the Incidence of Lymphogenous Leukemia in A. K. R. Mice, Proc Amer Ass Cancer Res 2:20, 1955.

19. Horwitz, A., and Rosensweig, J.: Carcinoma of the Gallbladder—A Real Hazard: Summary of 20 Cases, JAMA 173:234-236, 1960.

20. Kazama, Y.: Studies on the Artificial Production of Tumors in Viscera, Jap Med World 2:309-312, 1922.

21. Kozoll, D. D.; Dwyer, G.; and Meyer, K. A.: Pathologic Correlation of Gallstones, AMA Arch Surg 79:514-536, 1959.

22. Kramer, A.: Das Gallenblasenkarzinom, Munchen Med Wschr 102:2082-2087, 1960.

23. Lazarus-Barlow, W. S.: An Attempt at the Experimental Production of a Carcinoma by Means of Radium, Proc Roy Soc Med 11:1-17, 1918.

24. Leitch, A.: Gallstones and Cancer of the Gallbladder: An Experimental Study, Brit Med J 2: 451-454, 1924.

25. Mohardt, J. H.: Carcinoma of the Gallbladder: Collective Review, Surg Gynec Obstet 69: 440-451, 1939.

26. Nelson, A. A., and Woodard, G.: Tumors of the Urinary Bladder, Gallbladder and Liver in Dogs Fed O-Aminoazotoluene or p-Dimethyl-Aminovasobenzene, J Nat Cancer Inst 13:1497-1510, 1953.

27. Petrov, N. N., and Krotkina, N. A.: Experimental Carcinoma of the Gallbladder, Ann Surg 125:241-248, 1947.

28. Relation of Thyroid Function to Cancer, CA 7:115, 1957.

29. Newsletter, CA 8(2):V, 1958.

30. Schneiderbaur, A., and Lhotka, E.: [Gallbladder Carcinoma], Wien Med Wschr 111:331-336, 1961.

31. Shimkin, M. B., and Mider, G. B.: Carcinogenesis in Guinea Pig, Cancer Res 1:751-752, 1941.

32. Shimkin, M. B., and Mider, G. B.: Induction of Tumors in Guinea Pigs With Subcutaneously Injected Methylcholanthrene, J Nat Cancer Inst 1:707-725, 1941.

33. Sternberg, S. S.; Popper, H.; Oser, B. L.; and Oser, M.: Gallbladder and Bile Duct Adenocarcinomas in Dogs After Long Term Feeding of Aramite, Cancer 13:780-789, 1960.

34. Strauch, G. O.: Primary Carcinoma of the Gallbladder: Presentation of 70 Cases From The Rhode Island Hospital and a Cumulative Review of the Last 10 Years of the American Literature, Surgery 47:368-383, 1960.

35. Strohl, E. L., and Diffenbaugh, W. G.: Carcinoma of the Gall Bladder, AMA Arch Surg 70:772-781, 1955.

36. Tabet, B. J.: Primary Carcinoma of the Gallbladder: Report of 47 Cases, Amer J Surg 100:365-371, 1960.

37. Thorbjarnarson, B., and Glenn, F.: Carcinoma of the Gallbladder, Cancer 12:1009-1015, 1959.

38. Thorbjarnarson, B.: Carcinoma of the Gallbladder, Letters to the Journal, JAMA 177:530-531, 1961.

39. Torvik, A., and Hoivik, B.: Gallstones in an Autopsy Series, Acta Chir Scand 120:168-174, 1960.

40. Van Zandt, I. L.: Carcinoma of the Gallbladder, Texas J Med 36:616-617, 1941.

41. Warren, R., and Balch, F. G., Jr.: Carcinoma of the Gallbladder: The Etiological Role of Gallstones, Surgery 7:657-666, 1940.

42. Worter, J., and Weill, J. P.: Lithiase biliare et hypothyroidie, Schweiz Med Wschr 87:101-105, 1957.

53. Zeppa, R., and Womack, N. A.: Carcinoma of the Gallbladder: Attempt at Experimental Induction, Southern Med J 50:1267-1271, 1957.

Surgical Aspects of Histoplasmosis

WILLIAM A. GRYBOSKI, MD
RICHARD R. CRUTCHER, MD
JAMES B. HOLLOWAY, MD
PORTER MAYO, MD
RICHARD H. SEGNITZ, MD
AND
BEN EISEMAN, MD
LEXINGTON, KY

Although the pathogenesis,[1,2] epidemiology,[3-5] and clinical manifestations[6-10] of histoplasmosis have been extensively reviewed, relatively few studies have been made of the surgical implications of this disease. Noteworthy exceptions are the reviews of Forsee,[11] Takaro,[12] Curry,[13] Polk,[14] and others.[15-35] There are but 370 surgical cases in these studies in which there has been either histologic or cultural identification of the organism.

The purpose of this paper is to review the clinical experience in three private hospitals in Lexington, Ky, over a five-year period with 51 cases of proven pulmonary and mediastinal histoplasmosis. The indications for surgery are reviewed, the proven safety of conservative resection without chemotherapy demonstrated, and the benefits of the Gomori methenamine silver stain (GMS) illustrated for identification of the infecting organism.

Materials and Methods

The records of the three private hospitals* in Lexington, Ky, were reviewed for the five-year period from 1957 to 1962. Eleven cases had a coded pathologic diagnosis of histoplasmosis. A further review was made of 55 cases diagnosed as nonspecific granuloma. The original blocks of these granules were recut and restained with Gomori methenamine silver stain[36-38] and studied for evidence of histoplasmosis. Forty of these 55 restained specimens (73%) revealed easily identified *Histoplasma capsulatum* organisms. Fig 1 is illustrative of a lesion termed a nonspecific granuloma after examination with a hematoxylin and eosin stain and the same lesion prominently showing the organism when stained with the GMS method.

Pertinent clinical, radiologic, and laboratory data concerning the 51 proven cases of surgically resected histoplasmosis were recorded.

Results

There were 34 males and 17 females in this study, whose ages ranged from 2½

Submitted for publication Feb 13, 1963.
From the Department of Surgery, the University of Kentucky Medical School.
This work was supported by United States Public Health grant HE 06738-02.

* St. Joseph, Good Samaritan, and Central Baptist.

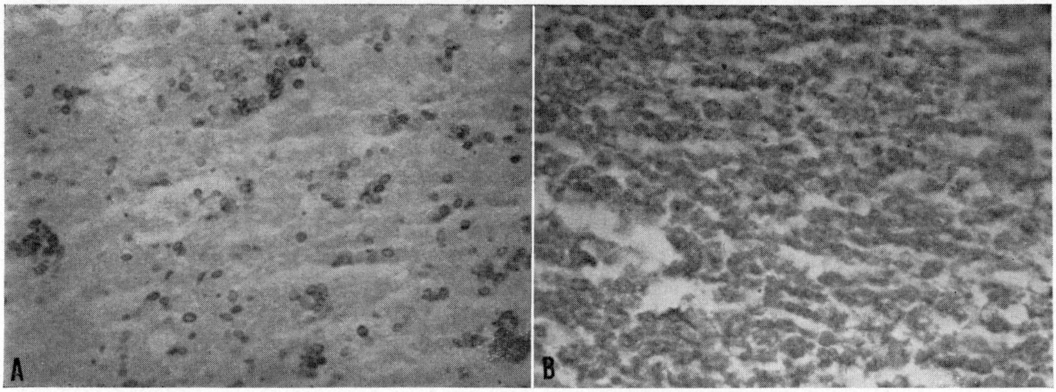

Fig 1.—*A*, hematoxylin and eosin stain; *B*, Gomori methenamine silver stain.

years to 72 years (mean 42 years). Forty-nine were Caucasian whites, and two were Negroes. Table 1 shows the age of these patients by decades. Forty-one (80%) of the cases were in the third through the sixth decades.

The presenting symptoms are listed in Table 2. Twenty-two (43%) were asymptomatic at the time of operation and gave no history of previous respiratory infections. Seven patients had two major complaints and are included in the table. Cough was a major complaint in 16 (31%). Seventeen of 33 (51%) cases of localized pulmonary lesions were asymptomatic compared to only two of 18 (11%) of the remaining lesions. The initial complaint of chest pain present in three patients was described as vague, diffuse, with occasional radiation to the shoulder but could not be related to the location or pathology of the lesion. Four patients presented with increasing dyspnea. One of these patients, with a solitary nodule, had long-standing asthma which most likely accounted for the dyspnea. The three remaining patients were those with a cavity, a localized pulmonary lesion, and bullous emphysema with associated histoplasmosis granuloma. Of the four patients who presented with hemoptysis, three had endobronchial histoplasmosis and one had a cavity. Four patients had coexisting significant pathology in the pulmonary parenchyma. Three had associated tuberculosis and the fourth squamous cell carcinoma.

Five patients presented with a superior mediastinal mass. One was a 2½-year-old white male who had classical signs of superior vena cava obstruction. Another was a 13-year-old white boy with a cough of six years' duration. The other symptomatic patient with a mediastinal mass had fever, general fatigue, and was suspected of having lymphoma. The other two patients with superior mediastinal masses were asymptomatic.

TABLE 1.—*Age by Decades*

Decade	No. Cases
1-10	1
11-20	2
21-30	9
31-40	9
41-50	13
51-60	9
61-70	6
70	2

TABLE 2.—*Presenting Symptoms*

Symptoms	No.
Asymptomatic	22 (43%)
Cough	16 (31%)
Hemoptysis	5
Dyspnea	4
Chest pain	3
Weight loss	2
Fever	2
Hoarseness	1
Wheeze	1
Tracheal tickle	1
Recurrent pneumonia	1
Superior caval obstruction	1
General fatigue	1

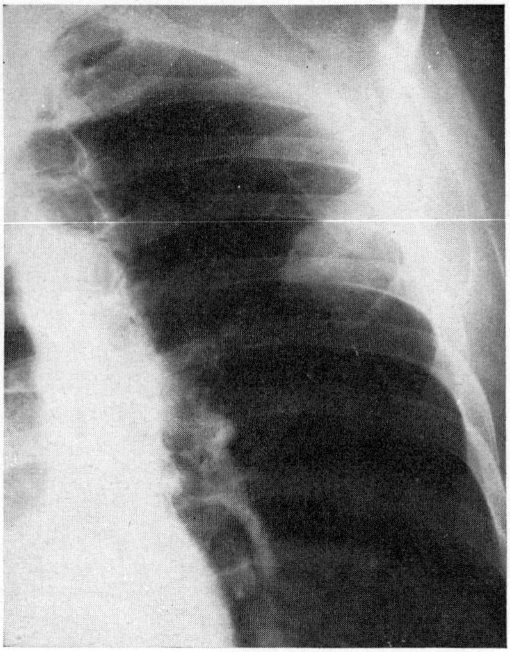

Fig 2

Histoplasmin skin tests and intermediate PPD were performed on 36 of the 51 cases (70%). The histoplasmin skin test was positive in 30 (83%); being negative in four patients with localized pulmonary lesions,

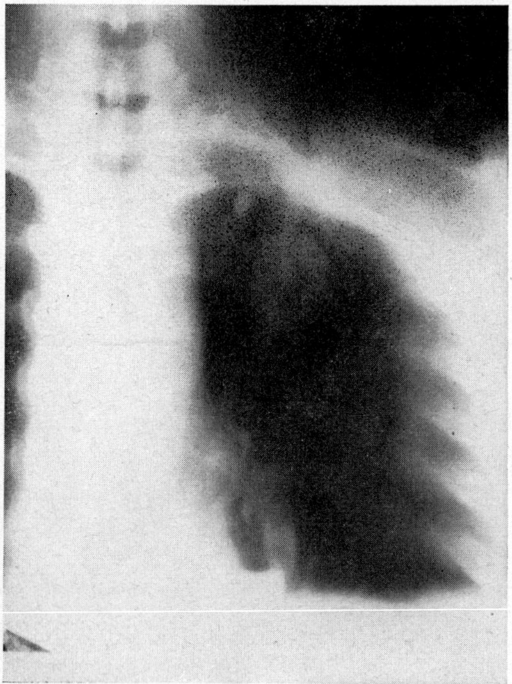

Fig 4

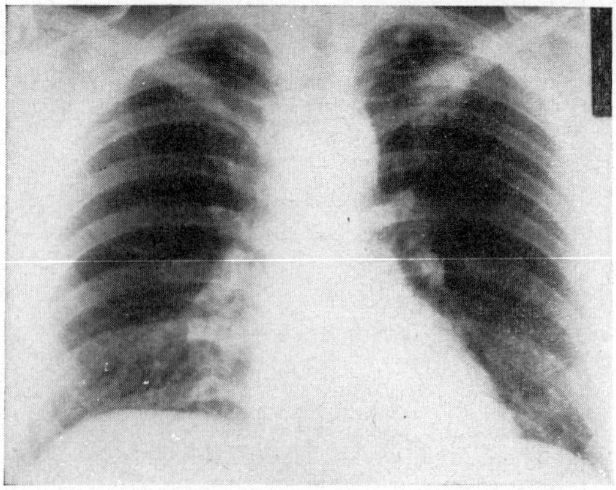

Fig 3

one patient with an infiltrative lesion, and one with a cavity. The intermediate PPD was positive in 16 (44%).

A definite preoperative diagnosis was seldom made from the x-ray. Thirty-three (65%) of the cases appeared as solitary spherical lesions (Fig 2, 3), which were clinically sufficiently suspect to warrant thoracotomy. Cavitary lesions (Fig 4), nonresolving infiltrating lesions (Fig 5), "middle lobe syndrome" (Fig 6), and mediastinal lymphadenopathy (Fig 7 and 8) exemplify the protean radiologic patterns of this disease. Fig 9 is an intravenous angiogram of one patient (Fig 8) who presented with superior caval obstruction and shows filling of the azygos system and complete obstruction of the superior vena cava.

Radiologic evidence of calcification occurred in seven cases. Six of these were

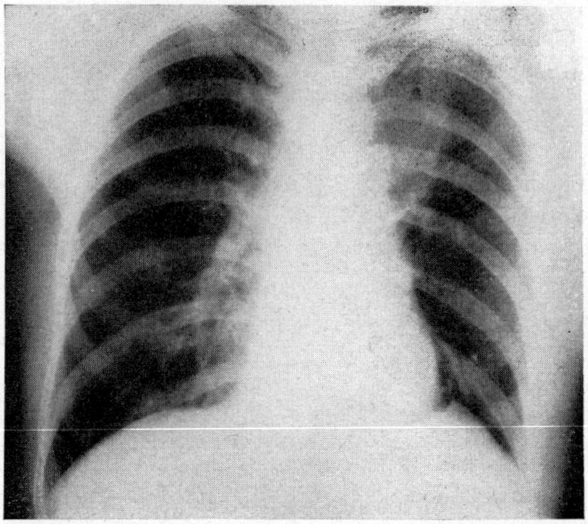

Fig 5

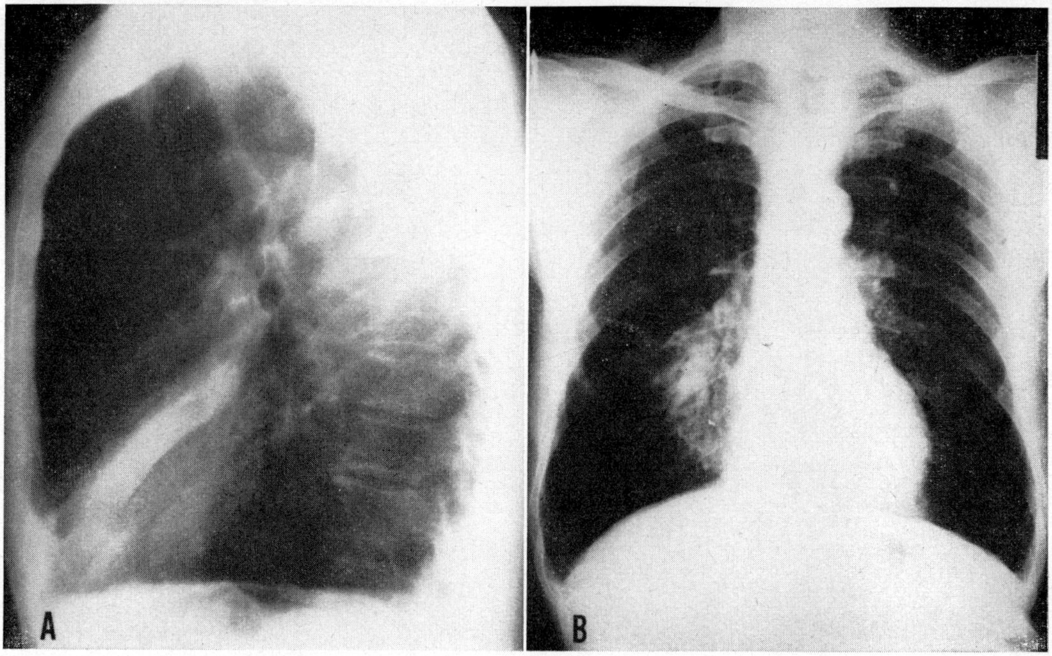

Fig 6.—*A*, posteroanterior view; *B*, lateral view.

calcified solitary nodules. One enlarged calcified lymph node presented as a superior mediastinal mass.

Three cases (6%) are presumed to have associated tuberculosis and histoplasmosis. In two, the acid-fast organisms were identified on preoperative sputum smears, but in neither case was acid-fast organism identified on histologic section or cultured from the resected specimen. The third case had a positive postoperative culture for tuberculosis.

Table 4 shows the lobar distribution of the intrapulmonary lesions. It will be noted that 33 solitary pulmonary lesions are distributed throughout all lobes. The cavitary disease was limited to the upper lobes, three on the right and two on the left. Eighteen of 42 cases (43%) of lesions had their location in the middle and lower lobes. Four infiltrative lesions all occurred on the left side, three being in the left upper lobe. These lesions were clinically and radiologically indistinguishable from tuberculosis.

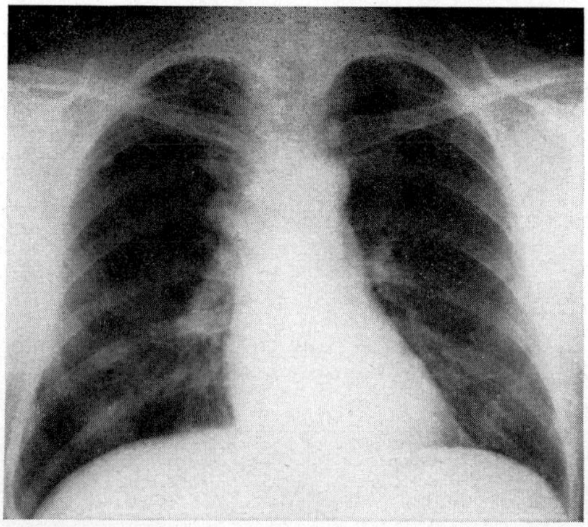

Fig 7

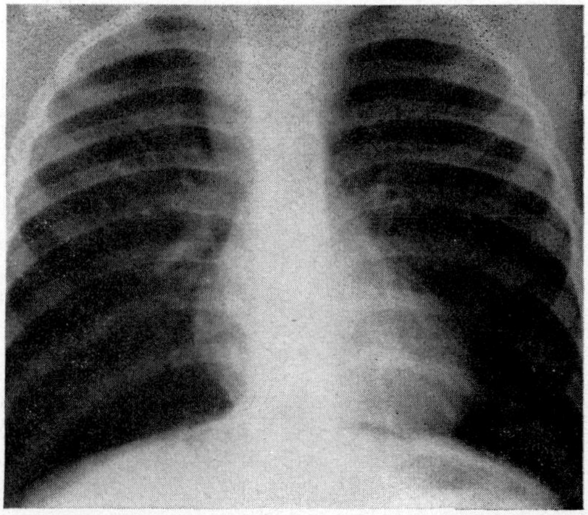

Fig 8

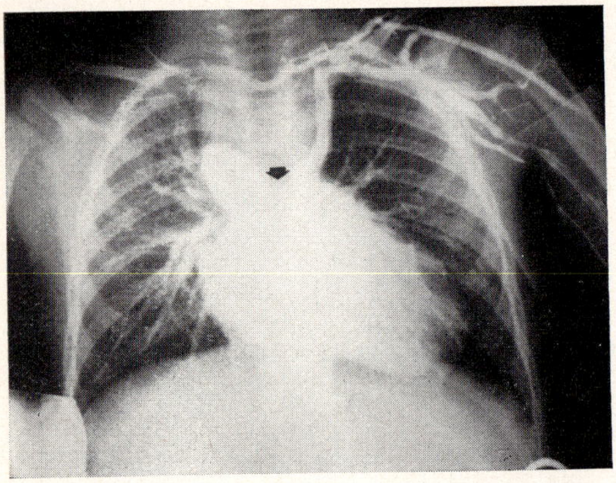

Fig 9

Table 5 correlates the operative procedure with the type of lesion encountered in these 51 cases. In no case was a resection more extensive than lobectomy required. It was noted by the operating surgeon that pleural adhesions and enlarged mediastinal nodes were very seldom found. In a high percentage of cases there were miliary nodules, both satellite to the main lesion and scattered throughout other lobes. Varying types of operative procedures were carried out in the five cases of cavitary disease without sequelae. Wedge resection was carried out in 29 of the 33 cases of localized pulmonary nodules, and in 6 of these multiple wedges were performed. One lobectomy and three incisional biopsies were carried out for infiltrative lesions which were impossible grossly to differentiate from carcinoma. Lobectomy in one and decortication in the other were performed for middle lobe syndrome. The two patients with bullous emphysema, pneumothorax, and associated histoplasma granuloma were treated by lobectomy in one case and by resection of blebs in the other.

The histopathology of the lesions was one of granuloma with varying degrees of caseation necrosis, fibrosis, epithelial cells, and calcification. The microscopic picture was usually indistinguishable from tuberculosis or other granulomas. In no case was the organism cultured preoperatively. Postoperative culture data of the lesion for fungus organisms was carried out in 34 patients. In only one case, a 2½-year-old white male with superior vena cava obstruction secondary to enlarged superior mediastinal nodes, was the organism isolated. The localized pulmonary lesion varied in size from 0.6 cm to 5.4 cm (mean 2.6 cm). The

TABLE 3.—*Radiologic Appearance*

	No	% Cases
Nodule	33	65
Cavity	5	10
Infiltrate	4	8
Bullous emphysema with granuloma	2	3.5
Mediastinal mass	5	10
Middle lobe syndrome	2	3.5

TABLE 4.—*Lobar Distribution of Lesions*

Location *	Nodule	Cavity	Infiltrate	Total
RUL	10	3		13
RML	1			1
RLL	9 (B6-5)			9
LUL	6	2	3	11
LLL	7		1	8
Total cases	33	5	4	42

* RUL: right upper lobe; RML: right middle lobe; RLL: right lower lobe; LUL: left upper lobe; LLL left lower lobe.

TABLE 5.—*Operation Procedure*

	Lobectomy	Wedge	Excision	Segmental Resection	Decortication
Cavity	2	2		1	
Nodule	3	29		1	
Infiltrate	1	3			
Mediastinal mass			5		
Middle lobe syndrome	1				1
Bullous emphysema	1	1			
Totals	8	35	5	2	1

cavities ranged from 1.3 cm to 3.0 cm (mean 2.0 cm). Two of the cavities had relatively thick walls.

There was one postoperative death (2%), which occurred in a 51-year-old white male with bullous emphysema associated with histoplasma granuloma, who died due to respiratory insufficiency after excision of blebs. There were no other postoperative complications.

No preoperative or postoperative antifungal chemotherapy was used in this series. The clinical results of all cases except the postoperative death were excellent. A recurrence of reactivation of generalized histoplasmosis was not noted. Follow-up of the five cases with mediastinal nodes, from three months to three years, revealed no evidence of recurrence or fibrosing mediastinitis.

Comment

In the United States approximately thirty million persons have been infected with histoplasmosis.[9] Lexington, Ky, a city of 75,000 population, is in the middle of a highly endemic area, thus accounting for the unique experience of 51 histologically proven cases available within a five-year period. A common drawback to previous studies of pulmonary granulomas has been the difficulty in positive identification of the etiologic agent.[23-27] Characteristically, investigators have been able to identify the organism in between 55% to 77% of the cases [23-27] with the use of special stains. A definite preoperative diagnosis is seldom made in this disease because of the varied clinical manifestations as well as the difficulty in culturing the organism. We were able to culture the organism in only one of 51 cases. This is similar to the reported experience of others [13,28,32] who were able to isolate the organisms in less than 5% of cases in which localized pulmonary nodules were found. Because of this fact it is suggested that the organisms may be nonviable within these granulomas. The benign postoperative course in these cases may partially be explained by dormancy, or nonviability of the organisms. A higher percentage of positive cultures are obtained in cases with chronic, progressive histoplasmosis, pre- and postoperatively.[17,31,34,35] This correlates well with a higher incidence of postoperative complications in this group.

The histoplasmin skin test was positive in 83% of this series which is in keeping with the results of Rubin et al [31] and Loewen et al.[35] The test is of relatively little value in this, as in other endemic areas, where from 50% to 80% of the population have a positive skin test. Further to complicate the picture is the fact that from 10% to 20% of patients with a current or previous histoplasmosis infection will have an anergic response to the antigen.[31,35] In a series of 369 skin tests performed on thoracic surgical patients in Lexington, the histoplasmin skin test was positive in 238 (64.5%), and the intermediate or second strength PPD was positive in 168 (45.5%).[39]

Pulmonary calcification has been shown to be more closely related to a positive histoplasmin skin test than to a positive PPD.[40] Although only 14% of x-rays in this series revealed evidence of calcification, Peterson and Christie [41] reported pulmonary calcifications in 87.4% of patients with a positive histoplasmin skin test as opposed to only 18.8% with a positive PPD. Over 40% of routine chest x-rays in endemic areas will show evidence of the characteristic laminated or stippled calcification.[42]

As has been stated, three cases in the present series had associated tuberculosis. Of significance is the fact that intrapulmonary histoplasmosis, unlike tuberculosis, does not have a predilection for the upper lobes. Rubin et al [31] and Polk et al [14] isolated both organisms, either culturally or histologically, in 15% to 20% of cases. When in the preoperative period there is any doubt, persistent search for both organisms should be carried out, so that specific preoperative chemotherapy can be administered.

Although chronic progressive and disseminated histoplasmosis has a poor prognosis,[31,35,43,44] the majority of cases have a benign clinical course, and the question obviously arises as to the indications for surgery in this disease.

Table 6 is a composite summary of 370 previously reported surgical cases of proven histoplasmosis and the 51 cases reported within this study. Because of the repeated and overlapping reports from the Army hospitals only the last composite summary of 100 proven cases is included in the table. Certain manifestations of this disease clearly require surgical intervention.

I. *Cavitary and Infiltrative Disease.*—Seventy-five cases of cavitary and infiltrative disease have been reported with ten postoperative deaths, a mortality rate of 13%. The postoperative complications included four bronchial pleural fistulas and one postoperative empyema. Three patients revealed reactivation or persistent disease postoperatively. In the present series of nine cases, there were no postoperative deaths or complications. The indications for surgery in

TABLE 6.—*Surgical Histoplasmosis*

Author *	Yr	No. Cases	Pathology	Postop Complications
Bunnell & Furcolow (19)	1948	1	Mass	BPF † Postop death
Wilson & Duryea (20)	1952	1	Infiltrate	Reactivation postop
Sutliff et al (18)	1953	6	5 cavity 1 mass	1 relapse
Matthiesen (21)	1954	3	3 nodules	None
MacInnis (22)	1955	1	Broncholithiasis	None
Davis et al (23)	1956	39	Nodules	—
Howson et al (24)	1956	1	Cavity	None
Hughes (17)	1956	7	6 cavity 1 nodule	6 of 7 asymptomatic 1 postop empyema
Polk et al (14)	1957	21	13 cavities 2 bronchiectasis 2 mass 1 nodule 2 destroyed lung 1 middle lobe	3 postop deaths
Sweany et al (25)		34	—	—
Zimmerman (26)	1957	19	Nodules	—
Baum & Schwarz (15)	1958	11	5 "coin" 5 nodes 1 cavity	None
Greendyke & Emerson (27)	1958	20	20 nodules	None
Baum et al (29)	1958	1	Bronchiectasis Broncholithiasis	
Walker & James (30)	1959	1	Cavity	Persistent disease
Rubin et al (31)	1959	19	Infiltrate & cavity	4 postop deaths
Takaro et al (12)	1959	11	6 nodule 4 cavity 1 cavity with BPF	1 postop death
Segal et al (28)	1959	67	Nodules	—
Curry & Weir (13)	1958	100	69 nodules	6 hemothorax
Forsee & Pfotenhauer (11)	1960		13 multiple of diffuse	1 space
Puckett (32)	1955		10 mediastinal	1 reactivation
Hopeman (33)	1962		8 pulmonary & mediastinal	1 pneumonitis Empyema with BPF-1
Chessman et al (34) (Mayo Clinic)	1960	9	5 cavity 4 nodule	None
Loewen et al (35)	1960	5	5 cavity	1 postop death
Conrad et al (7)	1960	2	2 cavity	None
Beatty et al (16)	1962	12	10 cavity 1 nodule 1 node	4 BPF
Gryboski et al	1962	51	5 cavity 33 nodules 4 infiltrate 5 mediastinal mass 2 middle lobe 2 blebs with granuloma	1 postop death

* Parentheses indicate reference numbers.
† BPF: bronchopleural fistula.

cavitary histoplasmosis in general should parallel those used for pulmonary tuberculosis. There is ample clinical and pathologic evidence to indicate that cavitary histoplasmosis would indicate poor tissue response to the disease and a threat of subsequent progression. Because this group of patients has the poorest prognosis and highest incidence of complications, it is our feeling that pre- and postoperative amphotericin B chemotherapy is indicated if known cavitary histoplasmosis is to be surgically resected.

II. *Solitary Pulmonary Nodule.*—The operative intervention in localized pulmonary lesions has been well reviewed.[23,45-47] There is now overwhelming evidence that no clinical diagnostic means is available to differentiate a benign from a malignant peripheral pulmonary lesion, and indeed one of our patients did have an associated histoplasma granuloma and squamous cell carcinoma. The advisability of excising isolated, discrete, noncalcified or minimally calcified pulmonary lesions need not be re-emphasized. There have been 235 localized pulmonary histoplasma lesions previously described as reviewed in Table 6 to which we have added 33 cases. This total of 268 cases represents two thirds of all surgically excised cases of histoplasmosis. There were no postoperative complications in this series, and only one minor complication was reported in previous studies [11] when solitary histoplasma lesions of this type were excised. This clinical experience obviously re-emphasizes the benignity of surgical resection of localized histoplasmosis granuloma. The high recorded incidence of wedge resection in this and previous studies indicates that conservation of pulmonary tissue is perfectly justified. Despite the known fact that these lesions are often surrounded by satellite nodules, cutting across involved pulmonary tissue does not apparently disseminate the disease. Such lack of spread serves to emphasize the advisability of conservatism in the surgical excisional management of this disease.

III. *Mediastinal Mass.*—Enlarged mediastinal lymph nodes need be removed only when they occur as a mass which is clinically and radiologically indistinguishable from mediastinal tumors or when complications of these nodes arise. Peabody et al [48] in a series of over 200 mediastinal tumors found 25 granulomas, seven of which were due to *Histoplasma capsulatum* and 11 were nonspecific granuloma. In light of our experience, one wonders what percentage of these 11 nonspecific granulomas would be positive for *Histoplasma capsulatum* if stained with the Gomori methenamine silver technique. Enlarged mediastinal lymph nodes may present the complications of superior caval obstruction,[15,49] esophageal obstruction,[50,51] or encroachment on the tracheal-bronchial tree. Occasionally symptomatic and radiologically proven mediastinal masses secondary to histoplasmosis may decrease in size during an observation period, with regression in symptoms and size, radiologically. Contrary to the reports of others,[52-54] fibrosing mediastinitis was not an indication for surgical intervention in this series. The present study would indicate that such mediastinal involvement must be rare if not more frequently noted in an endemic area where from 50% to 80% of the population has a positive histoplasmin skin test. The present case of superior vena cava obstruction, like that of Baum et al,[29] responded to surgical excision of the node with decompression of the superior vena caval.

IV. *Middle Lobe Syndrome.*—There have been four previous reported cases of the middle lobe syndrome due to enlarged lymph nodes involved with histoplasmosis as shown in Table 6. The case presented here constitutes the fifth. Lobectomy, without postoperative complications or mortality, was carried out for the atelectatic and destroyed lobe in all cases. That more cases of middle lobe syndrome secondary to enlarged histoplasma lymph nodes have been reported is surprising.

V. *Bronchiectasis.*—Although there are no cases of bronchiectasis in this series, Polk et al [14] and Baum et al [29] have documented the association of histoplasmosis with bronchiectasis. It must be exceedingly rare.

VI. *Bullous Emphysema.*—It is difficult to evaluate the association of histoplasma granuloma and bullous emphysema as noted in two cases by Puckett [32] and two cases in our series. Both diseases are common and their coexistence is probably fortuitous.

Summary and Conclusions

A five-year surgical experience with 51 proven cases of pulmonary and mediastinal histoplasmosis has been reviewed. There was one postoperative death and no other postoperative complications in this series.

Of these, 40 (78%) were diagnosed as granuloma, type unknown, until the sections were stained according to the Gomori methenamine silver technique and the *Histoplasma capsulatum* organisms definitely identified. It is therefore recommended that this stain routinely be employed for examination of pulmonary and mediastinal granulomas where the etiologic organism cannot otherwise be identified.

The indications for surgical intervention in pulmonary and mediastinal histoplasmosis consist of cavitary disease, middle lobe syndrome, and obstruction of the vena cava and other structures within the mediastinum. The vast majority of such lesions, however, were removed for diagnostic differentiation from carcinoma either as a solitary peripheral or mediastinal mass.

Surgical conservatism without specific chemotherapy has been entirely satisfactory in resecting localized pulmonary histoplasmosis. No evidence of dissemination was noted after wedge resection in this series. Chronic progressive histoplasmosis, as indicated by cavity and infiltrative disease, justifies the preoperative and postoperative use of systemic amphotericin B.

On the basis of this and the previously recorded experience of others a surgical approach to pulmonary histoplasmosis is described.

Dr. James Packer, Department of Pathology, University of Kentucky Medical Center, reviewed the histological sections; Dr. David H. Chipps (Central Baptist Hospital), Dr. James T. McClellan (St. Joseph Hospital), and Dr. Harold E. Resinger (Good Samaritan Hospital) made the permanent blocks of tissue available.

William A. Gryboski, MD, Department of Surgery, University of Kentucky, Lexington, Ky.

REFERENCES

1. Vivian, D. N.; Weed, L. A.; McDonald, J. R.; Clagett, O.; and Hodgson, C. H.: Histoplasmosis: Clinical and Pathological Study, Surg Gynec Obstet 99:53, 1954.

2. Straub, M., and Schwarz, J.: Healed Primary Complex in Histoplasmosis, Amer J Clin Path 25:727, 1955.

3. Kokko, U. P.; DeHaven, H.; and Guiglia, T.: Histoplasmin Reactivity in Three Kentucky Areas, J Kentucky Med Ass 55:797, 1957.

4. Furcolow, M. L.; Schubert, J.; Tosh, F. E.; Doto, I. L.; and Lynch, H. J., Jr.: Serologic Evidence of Histoplasmosis in Sanatoriums in the USA, JAMA 180:109, 1962.

5. Manos, N. E.; Ferebee, S. H.; and Kerschbaum, W. F.: Geographic Variation in the Prevalence of Histoplasmin Sensitivity, Dis Chest 29:649, 1956.

6. Furcolow, M. L.: The Clinical Diagnosis of Histoplasmosis, Postgrad Med 20:349, 1956.

7. Conrad, F. G.; Saslaw, S.; and Atwell, R. J.: The Protean Manifestations of Histoplasmosis as Illustrated in 23 Cases, AMA Arch Intern Med 104:692, 1959.

8. Peeples, W. J., and Spence, M. J.: Pulmonary Cavitation Due to Histoplasma Capsulatum, Amer Rev Tuberc 69:111, 1954.

9. Loosli, C. G.: Histoplasmosis, J Chronic Dis 5:447, 1957.

10. Prior, J. A.; Saslaw, S.; and Cole, C. R.: Experiences With Histoplasmosis, Ann Intern Med 40:221, 1954.

11. Forsee, J. H., and Pfotenhauer, M.: Surgical Management of Focalized Pulmonary Histoplasmosis, JAMA 173:878, 1960.

12. Takaro, T.; Walkup, H. E.; and Mathews, J. H.: The Place of Excisional Surgery in the Treatment of Pulmonary Mycotic Infections, Dis Chest 36:19, 1959.

13. Curry, F. S., and Weir, J. A.: Histoplasmosis: A Review of 100 Consecutively Hospitalized Patients, Amer Rev Tuberc 77:749, 1958.

14. Polk, J. W.; Cubiles, J. A.; and Buckingham, W. W.: The Surgical Treatment of Chronic Progressive Pulmonary Histoplasmosis, J Thorac Cardiov Surg 34:323, 1957.

15. Baum, G. L., and Schwarz, J.: Pulmonary Histoplasmosis, New Eng J Med 258:677, 1958.

16. Beatty, O. A.; Levene, N.; Saliba, A.; and Coelho, J.: Surgical Therapy of Chronic Pulmonary Histoplasmosis With and Without Amphotericin B, J Thorac Cardiov Surg 44:228, 1962.

17. Hughes, F. A.: "Surgical Treatment of Chronic Pulmonary Histoplasmosis," in Transactions of 15th Conference on the Chemotherapy of Tuberculosis, US Veterans Administration, Department of Medicine and Surgery, 1956, p 313.

18. Sutliff, W. D.; Hughes, F.; Ulrich, E.; and Burkett, L. L.: Active Chronic Pulmonary Histoplasmosis, AMA Arch Intern Med 92:571, 1953.

19. Bunnell, I. L., and Furcolow, M. L.: A Report of Ten Proven Cases of Histoplasmosis, Public Health Rep 63:299, 1948.

20. Wilson, H. M., and Duryea, A. W.: Pulmonary Histoplasmosis: Report of a Case Long Considered Tuberculous Improved by Acti-Dione, Dis Chest 21:346, 1952.

21. Matthiesen, D. E.: The Surgical Significance of Solitary Circumscribed Lung Nodules in Histoplasmosis, Amer Rev Tuberc 69:829, 1954.

22. MacInnis, F. E.: Broncholithiasis and Histoplasmin Sensitivity, Missouri Med 52:868, 1955.

23. Davis, E. W.; Peabody, J. W.; and Katz, S.: The Solitary Pulmonary Nodule: A Ten-Year Study Based on 215 Cases, J Thorac Cardiov Surg 32:728, 1956.

24. Howson, C. R.; Brewer, L. A.; Oatway, W. H.; and Rouff, E. A.: Progressive Pulmonary Histoplasmosis With Bilateral Resection and Chemotherapy, Ann Intern Med 44:985, 1956.

25. Sweany, H. C.; Gorelick, D.; Coller, F. C.; and Jones, J. L.: Pathologic Findings in Benign Pulmonary Histoplasmosis, Dis Chest 34:119, 1958.

26. Zimmerman, L. E.: Some Contributions of the Histopathologic Method to the Study of Fungus Diseases, Trans NY Acad Sci 19:358, 1957.

27. Greendyke, R. M., and Emerson, G. L.: Occurrence of Histoplasma Pulmonary Nodules in Non-Endemic Area, Amer J Clin Path 29:36, 1958.

28. Segal, E. L.; Starr, G. F.; and Weed, L. A.: Study of Surgically Excised Pulmonary Granulomas, JAMA 170:515, 1959.

29. Baum, G. L.; Bernstein, I. L.; and Schwarz, J.: Broncholithiasis: Produced by Histoplasmosis, Amer Rev Tuberc 77:162, 1958.

30. Walker, W. J., and James, E. C.: Pulmonary Histoplasmosis, Canad Med Ass J 81:486, 1959.

31. Rubin, H.; Furcolow, M. L.; Yates, J. L.; and Brasher, C. A.: The Course and Prognosis of Histoplasmosis, Amer J Med 27:278, 1959.

32. Puckett, F. T.: Pulmonary Histoplasmosis, Amer J Surg 90:92, 1955.

33. Hopeman, H.: in Fifteenth Annual Symposium on Thoracic Diseases, Fitzsimmons General Hospital, US Army, 1962, p 121.

34. Chessman, R. J.; Hodgson, C. H.; Bernatz, P. E.; and Weed, L. A.: Surgical Resection in Treatment of Histoplasmosis, Dis Chest 37:356, 1960.

35. Loewen, D. F.; Procknow, J. J.; and Loosli, C. G.: Chronic Active Pulmonary Histoplasmosis With Cavitation, Amer J Med 28:252, 1960.

36. Gridley, M. F.: Stain for Fungi in Tissue Sections, Amer J Clin Path 23:303, 1953.

37. Grocott, R. G.: Stain for Fungi in Tissue Sections and Smears Using Gomori's Methenamine-Silver Nitrate Technique, Amer J Clin Path 25:975, 1955.

38. Peabody, J. W., Jr.; Murphy, J. D.; and Seabury, J. H.: Demonstration of Fungi by Periodic Acid-Schiff Stain in Pulmonary Granulomas, JAMA 157:885, 1955.

39. Crutcher, R.: Personal communication to the authors, Lexington, Ky.

40. Santag, L. W., and Allen, J. E.: Lung Calcifications and Histoplasmin-Tuberculin Skin Sensitivity, J Pediat 30:657, 1947.

41. Peterson, J. C., and Christie, A.: Histoplasmosis and Pulmonary Calcifications, Amer Rev Tuberc 57:361, 1948.

42. Serviansky, B., and Schwarz, J.: Calcified Intrathoracic Lesions Caused by Histoplasmosis and Tuberculosis, Amer J Roentgen 77:1034, 1957.

43. Furcolow, M. L.: Course and Prognosis of Untreated Histoplasmosis, JAMA 177:292, 1961.

44. Parsons, R. J., and Zarafonetis, C. J. D.: Histoplasmosis in Man: Report of Seven Cases and a Review of 71 Cases, Arch Intern Med 75:1, 1945.

45. Meckstroth, C. V.; Andrews, N. C.; and Klassen, K. P.: Surgery for Solitary Lesions of the Lung, AMA Arch Surg 69:220, 1954.

46. Storey, C. F.; Grant, R. A.; and Rothmann, B. F.: Coin Lesions of the Lung, Surg Gynec Obstet 97:95, 1953.

47. Hood, R. T., Jr.; Good, C. A.; Clagett, O. T.; and McDonald, J. K.: Solitary Circumscribed Lesions of the Lung, JAMA 152:1185, 1953.

48. Peabody, J. W., Jr.; Brown, R. B.; Davis, E. W.; Katz, S.; and Cannon, A.: Surgical Implications of Mediastinal Granulomas, Amer Surg 25:357, 1959.

49. Garamella, J. J.; Stutzman, F. L.; Varco, R. L.; and Jensen, N. K.: Subcarinal Mediastinal Granulomas Causing Esophageal Obstruction, J Thorac Cardiov Surg 30:187, 1955.

50. Moore, T. C.: Esophageal Obstruction Due to Mediastinal Granuloma, J Thorac Cardiov Surg 37:127, 1959.

51. Gillespie, J. G.: Superior Vena Cava Obstruction in Childhood: Report of a Case Secondary to Histoplasmosis, J Pediat 49:320, 1956.

52. Salyer, J. M.; Harrison, H. N.; Winn, D. F.; and Taylor, R. R.: Chronic Fibrous Mediastinitis and Superior Vena Cava Obstruction Due to Histoplasmosis, Dis Chest 35:364, 1959.

53. Knox, L. C.: Chronic Mediastinitis, Amer J Med Sci 169:807, 1925.

54. Tubbs, O. S.: Superior Vena Cava Obstruction Due to Chronic Mediastinitis, Thorax 1:247, 1946.

Primary Nonspecific Ulceration of the Small Bowel

MILTON R. WATSON, MD, SAN JOSE CALIF

Introduction

Primary or simple ulcer of the small intestine occurring beyond the duodenum is rare. The lesion includes single ulcers within the jejunum and ileum of unknown etiology. This lesion is to be differentiated from the type of ulceration occurring in regional enteritis as shown in Table 1. About 170 cases of simple ulcer of the small intestine have been reported in the world's literature. The purpose of this paper is to report two additional cases from the Department of Surgery at Santa Clara County Hospital and briefly to review the literature.

Historical Background

Baille was the first to report an ulcer of the small intestine in 1805. Morrin reported 85 cases occurring before 1931.[10] Evert et al reviewed an additional 31 cases between 1931 and 1944,[4] and Morlock et al reported 32 cases from the Mayo Clinic up to 1956.[9] Sporadic cases have since been reported in the literature.

Submitted for publication Feb 18, 1963.

Resident in General Surgery (Dr. Watson).

Department of Surgery, Santa Clara County Hospital.

Incidence

Simple ulcer of the small intestine is known to occur at all ages, the range being from 1 to 77 and the average age being 43. Seventy-five per cent of cases are found in males.

Etiology

Numerous theories have been advanced to explain the etiology of simple ulcer of the small bowel. A few investigators feel that the ulcer is of inflammatory origin while others believe that the ulcer develops in heterotopic gastric mucosa in the intestine. Other authors postulate that the ulcer may be caused by a foreign body, eventually evacuated through the intestinal canal. The fact that ulceration is usually situated in the vicinity of the duodenojejunal flexure or of the ileocecal aperture suggests that mechanical factors might be important in the etiology of this disease.[6] Finkbiner et al recently presented three case reports of ulceration and perforation of the small intestine due to

TABLE 1.—*Comparison of Simple Ulcer With Regional Enteritis*

	Simple Ulcer	Regional Enteritis (12) *
Number of ulcers	Usually single	Multiple
Thickening of bowel wall	Adjacent to and beneath ulcer	Diffuse thickening of entire involved segment
More than one segment of bowel involved?	No	Yes, not uncommonly there may be skip areas
Formation of fibrous tissue	Mild, in chronic &/or healing ulcers	Marked
Narrowing of bowel lumen	Usually eccentric	Concentric narrowing
Regional node involvement	Rarely	Almost always
Involvement of surrounding mesentery	None	Extensive
Granuloma formation	Rare; occasional foreign-body type giant cells	Almost always
Proliferation of endothelial cells within the lymphatics of the bowel wall	Absent	Characteristically present

* Parenthesis indicates reference numbers.

necrotizing arteriolitis. In all three cases a collagen disease contributed to the pathologic process of focal necrosis of the bowel, ulceration, perforation, peritonitis, and death. Histologically, acute fibrinoid necrosis was found to involve the walls of submucosal arterioles in the segment of bowel affected.[5]

Teicher et al postulate that these ulcerations may be secondary to vascular changes that originate within the mesentery. In one of the four cases reported, microscopic examination of adjacent bowel mesentery demonstrated thrombotic occlusion of several of the larger veins and arteries with partial organization of the thrombi.[14]

Signs, Symptoms, and Diagnosis

Barnett summarized 148 cases from the literature through 1958.[1] In 49 of these cases there was information regarding symptomatology and physical findings. Crampy abdominal pain was present in 46 instances, vomiting in 15, diarrhea in 10, and rectal bleeding in 5. Physical signs are variable depending on whether or not perforation or obstruction has occurred.

The diagnosis is usually made at the time of surgical exploration or at postmortem examination. X-ray studies for the most part have failed to reveal these ulcerations in the small bowel. The ulcer can occasionally be delineated by instilling barium through a long tube that is well into the small bowel.[11]

Pathology

Primary ulcers have been reported to occur throughout the small intestine. There is no relationship to mesenteric attachment. The ulcers range in size from 0.3 to 4.0 cm in diameter. They are oval or annular with well-defined edges; the bases are covered with reddish granulation tissue. The surrounding mucosa may be locally edematous. In cases with multiple ulcers, various degrees of healing have been noted.[9] Microscopically the ulcer appears much like the typical peptic ulcer.[7] The base is covered with a thin layer of fibrin and leukocytes. The muscularis mucosa is replaced by granulation tissue and infiltrated with plasma cells and leukocytes. There is varying involvement of the muscular layers. The amount of fibrous connective tissue present around the edges and beneath the granulation tissue indicates the degree of chronicity.

Complications

The complications of simple ulcer of the small intestine are usually the first clinical sign of the disease process. These consist of perforation, obstruction, and gastrointestinal bleeding. In Table 2 a review of 151 cases from the literature demonstrates the complications encountered.[3,4,9,10]

Contrary to numerous earlier reports, acute perforation is now not the chief complication of this disease. It is felt that earlier surgical intervention encounters the disease process before occurrence of perforation. However, localized perforation associated with obstruction is present in about one third of cases.

TABLE 2.—*Review of Cases from Literature*

	Obstruction	Bleeding	Perforation
Literature to 1944	8	10	102
Evert et al (4) *			
Morrin (10)			
Mayo Clinic	21	10	4
Brown & Pemberton (3)			
Evert et al (4)			
Morlock et al (9)			
Santa Clara County Hospital	2	—	—
Total	31	20	106

* Parentheses indicate reference numbers.

Treatment and Mortality

Treatment of choice for this condition has been surgical resection of the involved segment of bowel.[9] The extent of local bowel fixation is never serious enough to require surgical bypass. At the time of exploration the existence of malignancy cannot be ruled out in many instances.

Review of the literature reveals rather wide variance in mortality statistics. In Morrin's series of 85 cases prior to 1931, the mortality rate was 66%.[10] Evert's summary of 45 cases included a mortality rate of 47%. Present-day death rate is about 11%, possibly, in part, because of earlier surgical intervention before perforation and peritonitis occur.[9,13]

Report of Cases

Case 1.—A 74-year-old white female was admitted to the hospital on March 1, 1962, with a long history of vague abdominal pain and constipation. On the day of admission there was onset of crampy abdominal pain and vomiting. Physical examination revealed a diffusely tender, distended abdomen without guarding, rebound, or abnormal bowel sounds. Temperature was 98 F (36.7 C).

Admission white blood cell count was 6,500 with 71% polymorphonuclears and 29% lymphocytes. Initial x-ray films of the abdomen revealed partial small bowel obstruction.

The patient was treated with parenteral fluids and Miller-Abbott tube for the next two days without noticeable improvement. Repeat x-ray films with barium instillation into the Miller-Abbott tube demonstrated a considerable amount of fluid and gaseous distention of the small bowel with absence of gas and contrast material in the colon. This was felt to be compatible with small bowel obstruction, with the point of obstruction in the ileum.

On March 4, 1962, the abdomen was opened and the small bowel found to be massively distended. A constricting lesion 1 cm in length was found in the ileum 4 ft from the ileocecal valve with proximal dilatation and distal collapse of the small bowel. Bowel gas could be passed through the lumen only with much pressure. No regional nodes were noted. A 6 cm segment of ileum containing the lesion was resected.

The segment of resected small bowel contained a circular ulcer 1 cm in its longitudinal width. The base was granular and brown, and the surrounding mucosa appeared to be only slightly edematous. The borders of the ulcer were well delineated. Sections of the lesion revealed an ulcer eroding into a thickened, sclerotic, very vascular, chronically inflamed submucosa (Figure). This was felt by one pathologist to represent a spreading hemangioma, producing secondary mucosal ulceration. The patient has done well postoperatively.

Case 2.—A 65-year-old white male was hospitalized on March 12, 1962, complaining of crampy abdominal pain, nausea, and vomiting. Four days prior to admission the patient had numerous loose stools. Past history included known syphilitic aortitis with aneurysm of the descending aorta, cardiomegaly, and congestive heart failure.

Physical examination revealed a distended tympanitic and diffusely tender abdomen, with high pitched bowel sounds. A left inguinal hernia was easily reducible. The temperature was 99 F (37.2 C).

White blood cell count was 9,900 with 81% polymorphonuclears, 17% lymphocytes, and 2% band forms. X-rays of the abdomen revealed multiple

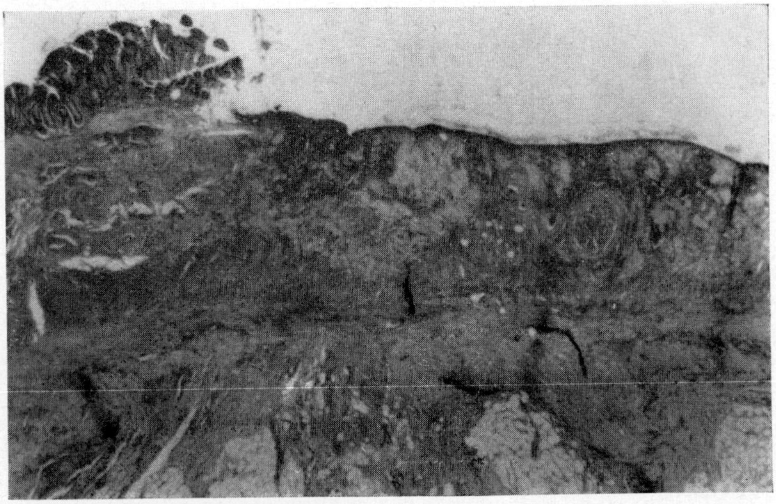

A microscopic section through the ulcer and adjacent, normal appearing mucosa (case 1).

dilated loops of small bowel with fluid levels, consistent with an organic small bowel obstruction. A barium meal added no further information.

After adequate replacement of fluid and electrolyte losses, an exploratory laparotomy was done on March 13, 1962. The entire small bowel was markedly dilated from the ligament of Treitz to a point 6 in from the ileocecal valve. At this level in the ileum, there was an inflammatory circumferential lesion 0.5 cm in width, associated with slight thickening of the bowel wall. A patent lumen appeared to be present through the inflammatory lesion, but the small bowel distal to this was entirely collapsed. No other lesions were noted. A decompression enterostomy was performed in the proximal ileum, and the lesion was biopsied, taking a wedge of bowel wall in its longitudinal direction.

The section of tissue biopsied was oval and measured $1.0 \times 0.4 \times 0.4$ cm in its various diameters. The specimen was bright red-gray in color and moderately soft in consistency. Multiple sections revealed severe inflammation involving all layers. The mucosal layer was ulcerated with an abundant number of acute and chronic inflammatory cells and red blood cells in the submucosal layer. Pathological diagnosis was that of chronic nonspecific inflammation with ulceration of the terminal ileum.

The patient did well in the immediate postoperative period. He was readmitted to the hospital on May 13, 1962, and died during this admission from acute pulmonary edema. Postmortem examination was done. The small bowel was opened and appeared entirely normal without evidence of residual inflammation or ulceration.

Summary

Primary nonspecific ulceration of the small bowel is a rare disease with only about 170 cases reported in the literature. The cause of this entity is as yet not determined. The symptoms are often a manifestation or result of the complications, including perforation, obstruction, and bleeding. The most frequently encountered symptoms are crampy abdominal pain, vomiting, diarrhea, and rectal bleeding. Pathologically the lesion is much like a peptic ulcer, is found to involve both ileum and jejunum, and is usually single. The treatment of this disease consists of resection of the involved segment of bowel. There is a low recurrence rate, and the present mortality rate is about 11%.

Milton R. Watson, MD, c/o Stanley P. Rigler, MD, Chief, General Surgery Service, Santa Clara County Hospital, South Bascom Avenue, San Jose 28, Calif.

REFERENCES

1. Barnett, W. O.: Primary Non-Specific Ulceration of the Small Intestine, Amer J Surg 96:679-683 (Nov) 1958.

2. Bartholomew, L. G.: Review of Lesions of the Small Intestine, Gastroenterology 36:232-233 (Feb) 1959.

3. Brown, P. W., and Pemberton, J. deJ.: Solitary Ulcer of the Ileum and Ulcer of Meckel's Diverticulum, Ann Intern Med 9:1684 (June) 1936.

4. Evert, J. A.; Black, B. M.; and Dockerty, M. B.: Primary Nonspecific Ulcers of the Small Intestine, Surgery 23:185-200 (Feb) 1948.

5. Finkbiner, R. B., and Decker, J. P.: Ulceration and Perforation of the Intestine Due to Necrotizing Arteriolitis, New Eng J Med 268:14-18 (Jan) 1963.

6. Hangos, G.: Nonspecific Ulcer of the Small Intestine, Gastroenterology 37:318-320 (Sept) 1959.

7. Horwitz, F.; Paradny, R.; and Baronofsky, I. D.: Primary Non-Specific Ulceration of the Small Intestine, J Mount Sinai Hosp NY 27:308-312 (May-June) 1960.

8. Koenig, R. P.: Acute Primary Ulcer of the Small Intestine, Ohio Med J 56:495-496 (April) 1960.

9. Morlock, C. G.; Goehrs, H. R.; and Dockerty, M. B.: Primary Nonspecific Ulcers of the Small Intestine: Clinicopathologic Study of 18 Cases With Follow-Up of 14 Previously Reported Cases, Gastroenterology 31:667-682 (Dec) 1956.

10. Morrin, F. J.: Spontaneous Perforation of Primary Jejunal Ulcers, Irish J Med Sci 6:198 (May) 1931.

11. Palmer, H. D., and Koneman, E. W.: Non-Specific Ulcers of Small Intestine, Rocky Mountain Med J 57:86-91 (Nov) 1960.

12. Rappaport, H.; Burgoyne, F. H.; and Smetana, H. F.: The Pathology of Regional Enteritis (Differentiation from Simple Non-Specific Ulcer of Ileum and Jejunum), Milit Surg 109:479 (Oct) 1951.

13. Scudamore, H. H.: Recent Advances in Diseases of the Small Intestine, J Iowa Med Soc 49:563-564 (Sept) 1959.

14. Teicher, I.; Arlen, M.; Muehlbauer, M.; and Allen, A. C.: The Clinical Pathological Spectrum of Primary Ulcers of the Small Intestine, Surg Gynec Obstet 116:196-202 (Feb) 1963.

Visceral Lesions in Acute Pancreatitis

An Experimental Study

LUCIANO DOS REIS, MD, COIMBRA, PORTUGAL

Several functional disorders have been found in patients with acute pancreatitis. Bockus[1] reported pathologic sulfobromophthalein (Bromsulphalein) retention associated with that disease in many patients. Howard[2] also found abnormal liver function tests in several people afflicted by the same disease. Colp and Dreiling[3] made similar observations.

Anatomical lesions have also been described by several writers. Fisher and McCloy[4] reported hepatic lesions in 11 out of 14 cases of acute pancreatitis, consisting of biliary thrombi, sometimes associated with hepatic necrosis and hemorrhage. Howard[2] and Edlund[5] mention similar cases. Besides the liver, other viscera have been found to be affected during acute pancreatitis. Necrosis of the renal tubules, mainly at the lower nephron, was observed by Ferris, Lynn, Cain, and Baggenstoss.[6] Vogel[7] reported cerebral, cardiac, adrenal, and ovarian lesions found at autopsy of a case of acute pancreatitis.

We attempted to reproduce similar lesions experimentally in several groups of animals, which are reported below.

Material and Methods

In these experiments we used 31 dogs divided into four groups. All animals were anesthetized by means of intravenous thiopental (Pentothal or Trapanal).

The first group consisted of 12 mongrel dogs weighing between 7 and 13 kg. A midline abdominal incision was made on each animal, the accessory pancreatic duct was dissected out, ligated distally, and catheterized with a polyethylene tube. Six cubic centimenters of bile collected from the animal's gall bladder at the time of surgery were then injected into the accessory pancreatic duct, with immediate production of acute hemorrhagic pancreatitis in every case, as was proved at gross examination and by pancreatic biopsy. The polyethylene tube was then removed and the accessory duct ligated proximally to the opening previously made. In this group, two animals died on the fourth day, two on the third, two on the second, and six either died or were sacrificed on the first day after production of acute pancreatitis. All animals were autopsied and fragments of every viscus removed for histological examination.

The second group included eight animals, weighing between 6 and 9 kg. Four of these had a laparotomy done, and an infusion of trypsin solution (30 mg into 300 cc of 5% dextrose in water) was injected into one of the splenic veins, running for a period of approximately three hours. All the animals died or were sacrificed 24 hours after the operation. The other four animals in this group had a similar injection given into the common carotid artery (30 mg of trypsin in 200 cc of 5% dextrose in water), after surgical exposure of that artery. Three of these animals were sacrificed 24 hours and one dog 48 hours postoperatively.

The third group consisted of six dogs, weighing between 5.5 and 10 kg. All of them had a laparotomy done, with exposure and catheterization of the accessory pancreatic duct and injection of six cc of sterile normal saline into that duct. Of these animals only one developed acute pancreatitis, as proven by biopsy and autopsy. Three animals were sacrificed 24 hours and three animals 48 hours after the pancreatic injection of saline.

The fourth group consisted of five dogs, weighing between 7.5 and 10 kg. After laparotomy and dissection of the accessory pancreatic duct, a polyethylene tube, 10 cm long and 1 mm wide was inserted into the duct and tied. This tube drained pancreatic fluid into the peritoneal cavity through several lateral holes. Total omentectomy was also done in all these dogs to avoid the omentum wrapping itself around the tube and obliterating its holes. One animal died 28 hours postoperatively; the others were sacrificed between four and seven days postoperatively.

Submitted for publication Feb 20, 1963.

Fellow, Calouste Gulbenkian Foundation, Lisbon, Portugal.

This work was done at the Instituto de Patologia Geral, University of Coimbra (Director, Prof Mário Trincão).

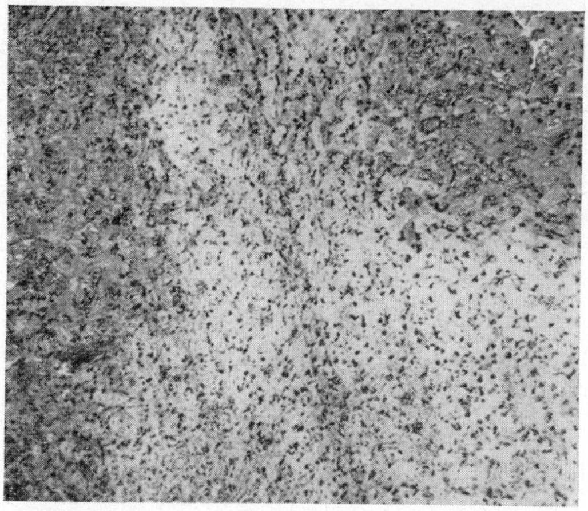

Fig 1.—Dog 36; Liver, 24 hours after production of bile pancreatitis: large necrotic areas. Hematoxylin and eosin; × 100.

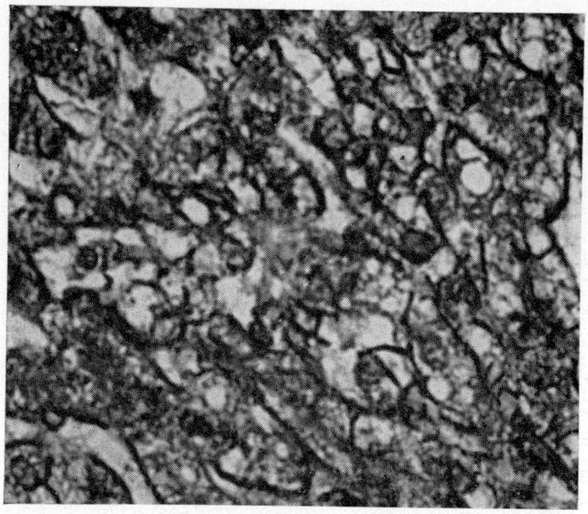

Fig 2.—Dog 67; Liver four days after production of bile pancreatitis: vacuolation of cells of cords of Remak. Hematoxylin and eosin; × 450.

Results

The first group of animals showed constantly typical histological lesions of acute hemorrhagic pancreatitis as a consequence of the intraductal injection of bile.

Hepatic lesions were found in every animal (Fig 1 and 2). They were mild in eight dogs and consisted of congestion of the centrolobular veins and of the vessels of the spaces of Kiernan, together with congestion of the intralobular capillaries; edema of the spaces of Disse, frequently with considerable disorganization of the cords of Remak; small interstitial hemorrhagic foci (four animals); cellular changes consisting of intracellular pigment, polikarinosis, pyknosis, vacuolation of the cytoplasm; hyperplasia and swelling of the Kupffer cells. Four animals had more advanced lesions, reaching hepatic necrosis.

The heart of four dogs in this group showed degenerative myocardial foci (Fig 3 and 4): the cytoplasm in these foci was discolored, yellowish-gray when stained with hematoxylin and eosin, and frequently granular; no striation was apparent in these fibers; many nuclei were pyknotic. Some of the fibers looked like having been emptied of their cytoplasm and were formed by their sarcolema only.

All animals in this group showed mild

Fig 3.—Dog 66; Heart, four days after production of bile pancreatitis: many groups of myocardial fibers are turgid, grayish in color, frequently without striation and with pyknotic nuclei. Hematoxylin and eosin; reduced 16% from mag × 450.

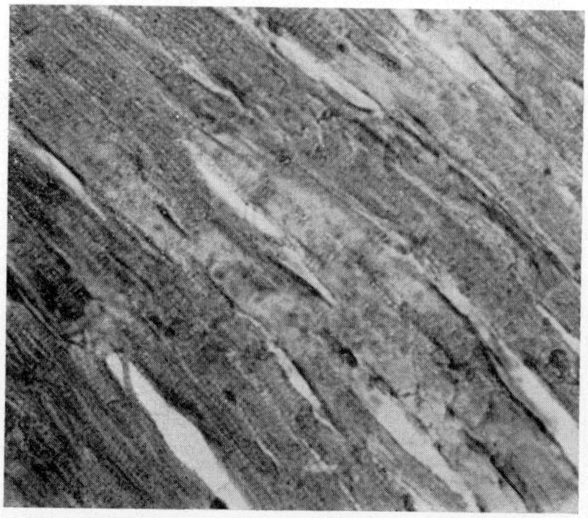

Fig 4.—Dog 22; Heart, 22 hours after production of bile pancreatitis: degenerative myocardial changes. Hematoxylin and eosin; reduced 16% from mag × 100.

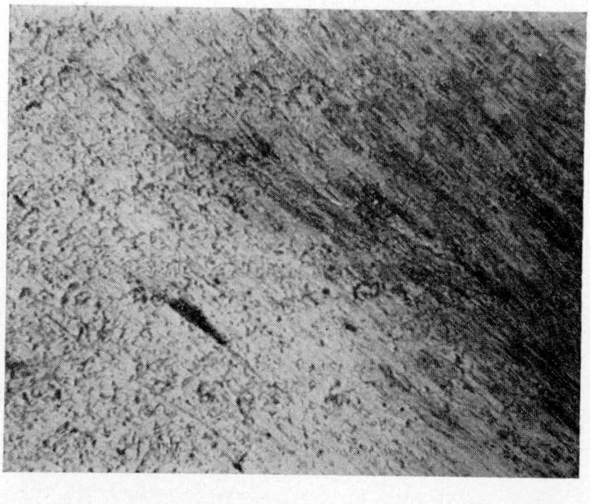

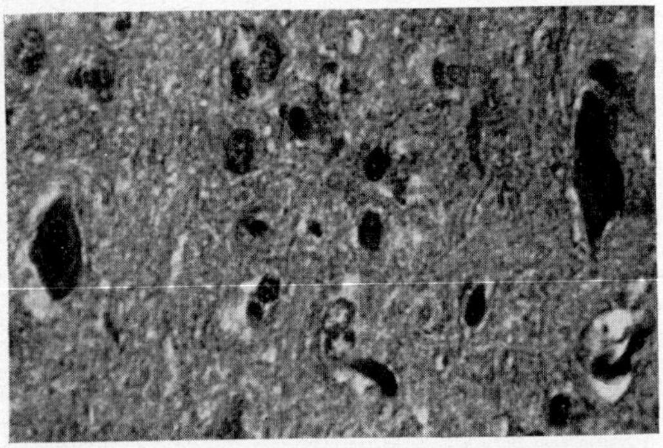

Fig 5.—Dog 60; Brain, about 40 hours after production of bile pancreatitis: two nervous cells with nuclear pycnosis. Hematoxylin and eosin; reduced 11% from mag × 450.

brain congestion and edema. Six animals had also degenerative changes of central nervous cells (Fig 5), consisting of nuclear pyknosis and cytoplasmic basophilia, the cytoplasm being either homogenized or granular; some cells contained granules of abnormal pigment. Myelin changes were not found.

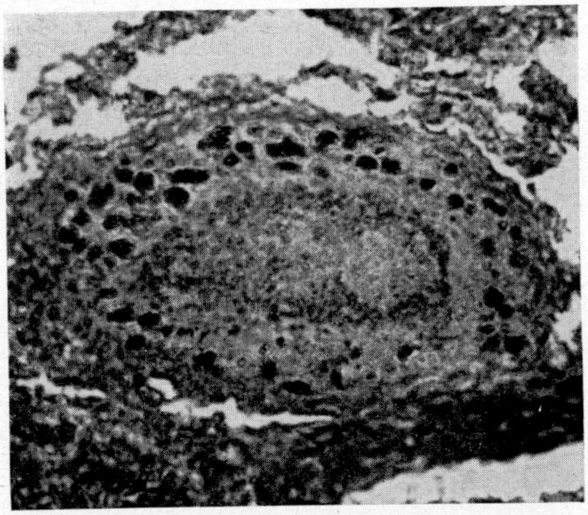

Fig 6.—Dog 18; Liver, about 40 hours after injection of trypsin solution into the splenic vein: a necrotic vessel. Hematoxylin and eosin; reduced 6% from mag × 450.

Significant lesions were not observed in the other viscera.

The four dogs in the second group, which were injected with trypsin into the splenic veins, also developed visceral lesions. The liver (Fig 6) was severely affected in two animals, showing wide areas of necrosis and hemorrhage. The other two animals showed

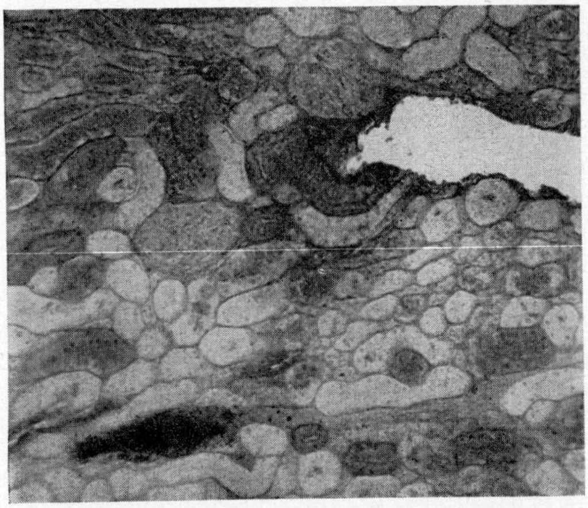

Fig 7.—Dog 18; Kidney: necrosis of renal tubules. Hematoxylin and eosin; × 100.

milder hepatic lesions as in the previous group. The pancreas of one animal had hemorrhagic and necrotic foci, together with inflammatory infiltrates; another dog had small necrotic pancreatic foci.

Renal lesions were found in three of the four animals, and consisted of tubular necrosis and hemorrhagic foci (Fig 7).

Myocardial lesions (Fig 8 and 9) were also found in one animal and were entirely similar to those described in the previous group. The same kind of lesions was also found in the psoas muscle of one animal.

Cerebral changes were observed in two animals and were similar to the lesions found in the first group.

The other four animals in the second group, injected into the carotid artery,

Fig 8.—Dog 18; Heart: degenerative changes of myocardial fibers. Hematoxylin and eosin; reduced 16% from mag × 450.

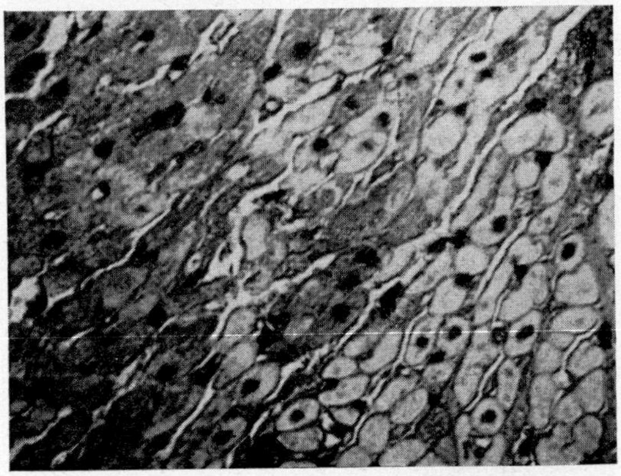

showed visceral changes as follows. The liver had congestion and edema of the spaces of Disse in two animals; polykarynosis and intracellular pigment were present in three dogs; one other animal had hyperplasia and swelling of the Kupffer cells. The heart showed myocardial changes in one animal which were similar to those previously described. One other animal had central nervous cell changes also similar to those reported in the previous animal groups.

Some of the six animals in the third group also presented visceral lesions. One animal had acute pancreatitis with necrosis and hemorrhage, and this same dog had also hepatic necrosis, myocardial degenerative foci and central nervous cell damage. The other five dogs in this group did not develop acute pancreatitis, but only mild pancreatic edema and congestion. The liver of these dogs never showed far advanced lesions, however there was polykarynosis, edema of the spaces of Disse, and intracellular pigmentation in three of them. Degenerative changes of the central nervous cells similar to those found in the previous groups were present in two of these animals, and one had myocardial lesions still entirely similar to those found in previous animals.

The fourth group, consisting of five animals with pancreatic drainage into the peritoneal cavity, had also some visceral lesions. Every animal showed hepatic changes:

Fig 9.—Dog 18; Heart: degenerative changes of myocardial fibers. Hematoxylin and eosin; reduced 16% from mag × 450.

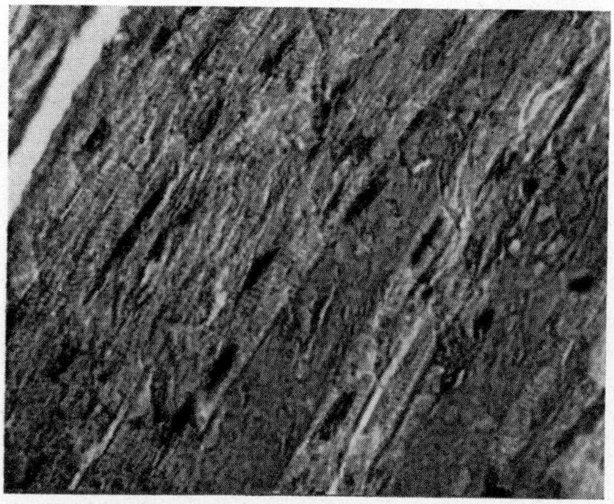

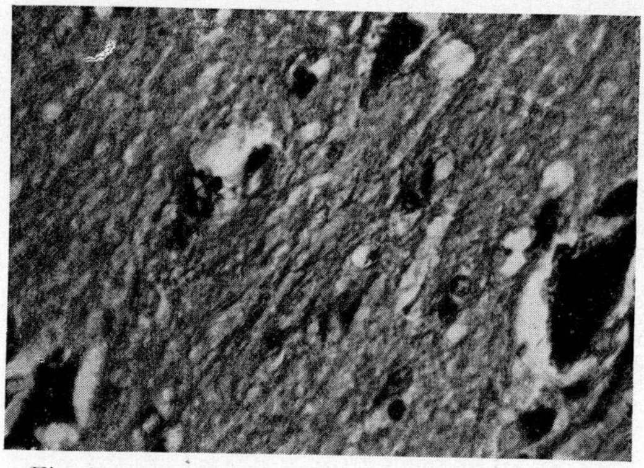

Fig 10.—Dog 103; Brain: three nervous cells showing homogenized, basophilic cytoplasm and pyknotic nuclei. Hematoxylin and eosin; reduced 24% from mag × 450.

vacuolation of the hepatic cells, congestion, edema of the spaces of Disse, polykarynosis, intracellular pigment; picnosis and interstitial hemorrhage were present in two animals. One dog had myocardial degenerative changes, similar to those described above. Three animals had degenerative changes in some central nervous cells (Fig 10).

In all animals of the first, third, and fourth groups, serum amylase determinations were carried out and found constantly elevated.

Comment

In every case of experimental bile pancreatitis, as was shown by the study of these animals, there were hepatic lesions, as well as lesions of the myocardium in one third and brain cell changes in half of them. The myocardial lesions are particularly interesting in that they correspond closely to those described in human material by Vogel.[7]

The visceral lesions found in acute pancreatitis might be produced by a toxic substance originating in the necrotic pancreas,[2,4] or by enzymatic action also originating in the pancreas.[2,5,8,9] Shock could possibly play a role in the formation of some lesions, mainly renal.[6]

That pancreatic enzymes can cause lesions in living tissue has been found by several writers.[10-13] Our second group of animals also showed lesions that were the result of direct action of trypsin, and these lesions were entirely similar to those found in bile pancreatitis.

In order to induce the liberation of pancreatic enzymes in the absence of shock or pancreatic necrosis, the third and fourth groups of experiments were carried out. One of the dogs in the third group still developed acute hemorrhagic pancreatitis; some of the other five animals in this group, and some of the dogs in the fourth group, however, developed visceral lesions which were similar to those found either in association with bile pancreatitis or with the injection of trypsin, all in the absence of acute pancreatitis.

The only factor that seems to be a common denominator in all these experiments as far as the production of visceral lesions is concerned is probably the presence of circulating enzymes, and especially trypsin.

Summary

Looking for the presence of visceral lesions associated with acute pancreatitis, the author produced a bile pancreatitis in 12 dogs, and found hepatic, myocardial, and brain cell changes in many of the animals. Similar lesions and kidney necrosis were found in animals injected with trypsin.

Hepatic, myocardial, and cerebral changes of the same kind were also found in animals which were made to have pancreatic enzymes in circulation; this was accomplished in two groups of animals, one with intraductal injection of saline, the other with drainage of pancreatic fluid into the peritoneal cavity.

Circulating pancreatic enzymes, especially trypsin, are possibly responsible for the lesions found.

Prof Renato Trincão reviewed the pathology slides; Dr. Ermelinda Gaspar gave technical assistance.

Luciano dos Reis, MD, R. Antero de Quental, 55 Coimbra, Portugal.

REFERENCES

1. Bockus, H. L.: Acute Inflammation of the Pancreas, Gastroenterology 34:467, 1958.

2. Howard, J. M.: Symposium on Recent Advances in Surgical Physiology of Pancreatitis: Surgical Physiology of Pancreatitis, Surg Clin N Amer 29:1789, 1949.

3. Colp, R., and Dreiling, D. A.: "The Pancreas," in Zimmerman, L. M., and Levine, R.: Physiologic Principles of Surgery, Philadelphia: W. B. Saunders Company, 1957, p 665.

4. Fisher, E. R., and McCloy, D.: Hepatic Lesions of Acute Hemorrhagic Pancreatitis: Their Nature and Pathogenesis, Surgery 37:213, 1955.

5. Edlund, Y.: Acute Necrosis of the Pancreas: An Analysis of Clinical Material, Acta Chir Scand 99:497, 1950.

6. Ferris, D. O.; Lynn, T. E.; Cain, J. C.; and Baggenstoss, A. H.: "Fatal Postoperative Pancreatitis," in Collected Papers of the Mayo Clinic and Mayo Foundation, Philadelphia: W. B. Saunders Company, 1957, 49:94.

7. Vogel, F. S.: Cerebral Demyelination and Focal Visceral Lesions in a Case of Acute Hemorrhagic Pancreatitis With a Consideration of the Possible Role of Circulating Enzymes in the Causation of the Lesions, AMA Arch Path 52:355, 1951.

8. Bernard, A.: Essai de Synthèse sur la Pathogénie de la Pancréatite Aiguë, (Synthetic Essay on the Pathogenesis of Acute Pancreatitis) Biol Med (Paris) 48:522, 1959.

9. Bernard, A.: Pancréatite Aiguë: la Part de l'Histamine dans la Génèse de Certains de ses Symptômes, (Acute Pancreatitis: The Role of Histamine in the Origin of Certain of its Symptoms) Arch Mal Appar Dig 48:714, 1959.

10. Reis, L. dos: Etiopatogenia e Fisiopatologia da Pancreatite Aguda, Coimbra: Coimbra Editora, 1960.

11. Powers, S. R.; Brown, H. H.; and Stein, A.: The Pathogenesis of Acute and Chronic Pancreatitis, Ann Surg 142:690, 1955.

12. Stein, A. A.; Powers, S. R.; and Brown, H. H.: Experimental Hemorrhagic Pancreatitis: New Concepts of Pathogenesis, Ann Surg 143:508, 1956.

13. McCune, W. S., and Stanbro, W. W.: Visualization of the Pancreas by Aortography, Ann Surg 150:561, 1959.

Radical Pancreatoduodenectomy and Portal Vein Resection

Report of Two Successful Cases With Transplantation of Portal Vein

SAKAE ASADA, MD
HIROYUKI ITAYA, MD
KAZUO NAKAMURA, MD
TAMOTSU ISOHASHI, MD
AND
SUSUMU MASUOKA, MD
OSAKA, JAPAN

The resectability rate of the carcinoma located in the head of the pancreas has been discouragingly low as illustrated by the rate of 14.1% in Porter's series [9] and 10% in Moore's report.[8] The main reason for this low rate is apparently its anatomical situation in the vicinity of the portal vein. Early involvement of the portal vein has made such a lesion inoperable in most cases. It is natural to deduce, therefore, that a block resection of the tumor and the portal vein together, supplemented by appropriate reconstruction of the portal system, would greatly improve the rate of resectability of carcinomas in this particular area.

Our efforts in the experimental laboratory aimed at the solution of this problem have resulted in a reasonably safe and clinically applicable method of resection and reconstruction of the portal vein using a portal vein homograft preserved in a 70% alcohol solution and a technique of temporary simultaneous occlusion of the superior mesenteric artery.[5] The success of this experimental work encouraged us to perform more radical operations for carcinomas occurring in the area mentioned.

This report is concerned with two cases of carcinoma of the stomach which occurred around the head of the pancreas and were successfully removed by the portal vein resection and reconstruction technique.

Submitted for publication Feb 21, 1963.

Professor of Surgery, (Dr. Asada), Associate Professor of Surgery, (Dr. Itaya), Instructor in Surgery, (Dr. Nakamura), Osaka Medical College.

From the Department of Surgery, Osaka Medical College.

Report of Cases

CASE 1.—A 48-year-old female had a subtotal gastrectomy (Billroth I) for carcinoma of the stomach on Jan 16, 1959, with uneventful recovery from operation. Since January, 1961, the patient complained of vomiting and frequent belching, accompanied by weight loss, and was admitted to the Osaka Medical School Hospital on Feb 9, 1961.

On admission, the patient showed an emaciated and anemic appearance. Blood pressure was 120/70 mm Hg. A fist-sized, clearly delineated hard mass fixed to the retroperitoneum was felt at the center of the abdomen. Laboratory examination revealed RBC 368×10^4, Hgb content 68%, WBC 5,600, albumin and casts in urine, positive occult blood in stool, serum protein 8.0 gm/dl, A/G 0.68, cephalin-cholesterol flocculation (CCF) (+), Thymol turbidity test (TTT) 3, Takata-Ara 9, CoR R4,* Meulengracht 3. The gastrointestinal barium examination revealed a stenotic area extending from the site of the previous gastroduodenal anastomosis to the descending part of the duodenum. These findings strongly suggested recurrence of the carcinoma of the stomach, and exploration was performed on Feb 10, 1961.

Under endotracheal ether anesthesia combined with a moderate hypothermia of 29 C (rectal temperature), the abdominal cavity was entered through a median laparotomy. The tumor was located in the proximal portion of the duodenum, extending to the head of the pancreas and partly adhering to the transverse colon. Aiming at total removal, the tumor was dissected out, together with adjacent organs which included the lower half of the remaining stomach, the common bile duct, the duodenum, and the head and body of the pancreas. However, a firm adhesion between the tumor and the superior mesenteric vein necessitated leaving a part of the tumor attached to the vein. After removal of the main mass, the remaining tumor tissue was removed by resecting the involved part of the superior mesenteric vein under simultaneous occlusion of the superior mesenteric artery and the portal vein. The continuity of the portal system was re-established by an end-to-end anastomosis of a 2 cm long portal vein homograft which had been preserved in 70% alcohol solution for six months. The gastrointestinal tract was reconstructed according to Child's technique. In addition, a hemicolectomy on the right side was performed to remove the adhering part of the transverse colon (Fig 1).

The time duration of the total occlusion of the portal vein was 31 minutes, during which time the blood pressure, pulse rate, and respiration remained fairly stable. Pre- and postocclusion biopsies revealed a slight dilation of the Glisson's capsule in the liver and an extensive venous congestion in the jejunum. Studies on the resected specimen revealed a carcinoma simplex, originating from the site of the previous gastroduodenal anastomosis and infiltrating the tissue of the pancreas head.

The immediate postoperative course was complicated by abnormal ECG changes, namely, frequent premature ventricular beats associated with a depressed ST-T segment and inverted T wave, which were controlled by oxygen inhalation and nitroglycerin. A bloody diarrhea appeared on the third postoperative day and lasted for a week, probably due to the venous stasis of the intestine during the portal vein occlusion. Except for a decrease in the serum protein level the liver function remained within normal limits. The patient looked all right until the 18th postoperative day when she suddenly died. Though a complete autopsy examination was not permitted, the cause of death was judged to be a cardiac arrest due to coronary insufficiency. A local postmortem examination was permitted, and the transplanted homograft of the portal vein was found to be entirely patent with a smooth internal surface. No thrombus or shrinkage was seen (Fig 2). An intimate union between the

* Cobalt reaction.

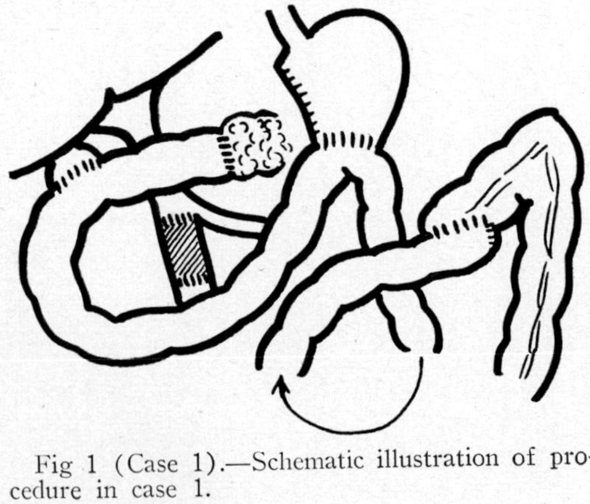

Fig 1 (Case 1).—Schematic illustration of procedure in case 1.

Fig 2 (Case 1).—A photograph showing the smooth internal surface of the completely patent homograft of the portal vein, obtained at autopsy 18 days after transplantation. No thrombus is seen.

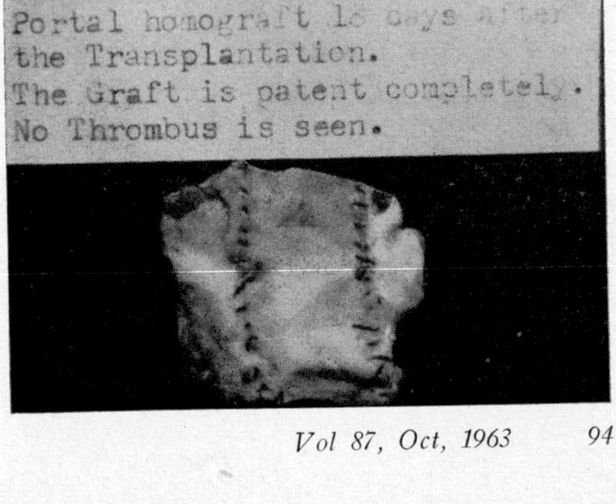

graft and the host vein covered with a newly developed intima was confirmed by histology.

CASE 2.—A 44-year-old male was admitted to the Osaka Medical School Hospital on March 19, 1962, with a diagnosis of carcinoma of the stomach. His main symptoms consisted of epigastric fullness, melena, and emaciation.

On admission, the patient was pale and had a malnourished appearance. His blood pressure was 128/68 mm Hg. A fist-sized, hard, irregular nodular mass was palpable in the upper right quadrant of the abdomen. The mass was not clearly delineated, and it was fixed to the surrounding tissue. Laboratory examination revealed RBC 382×10^4, Hgb content 60%, Hct 39.6%, WBC 6,400, SGOT 13, SGPT 21, Blood ammonia 1.2μg/ml, negative finding in urine sulfobromophthalein (SBP) 5% (30 min), CCF negative, TTT 1, Takata-Ara negative, CoR R4, Meulengracht 2, serum protein 6.4 gm/dl, AG 1.5, positive occult blood in stool. The gastrointestinal barium examination demonstrated a filling defect and a loss of motility in the pyloric area.

Exploration was performed on April 6, 1962, under general anesthesia combined with hypothermia. The tumor was located in the anterior wall of the antrum, extending to the duodenum and the head of the pancreas. Because of the absence of lymphatic metastasis or intraperitoneal dissemination, a combined gastroduodenopancreatectomy was decided upon. However, an attempt to dissect the tumor mass from the portal vein had to be abandoned on encountering inaccessible adhesion. A concomitant resection of the portal system was imperative if a total resection of the tumor was intended. This was accomplished in the same fashion as in case 1. Under occlusion of the superior mesenteric artery and the portal vein, the portal vein including the main stem of the superior mesenteric vein was resected to an extent of 2.5 cm. Vascular continuity was re-established by an end-to-end anastomosis, using nylon sutures, of a

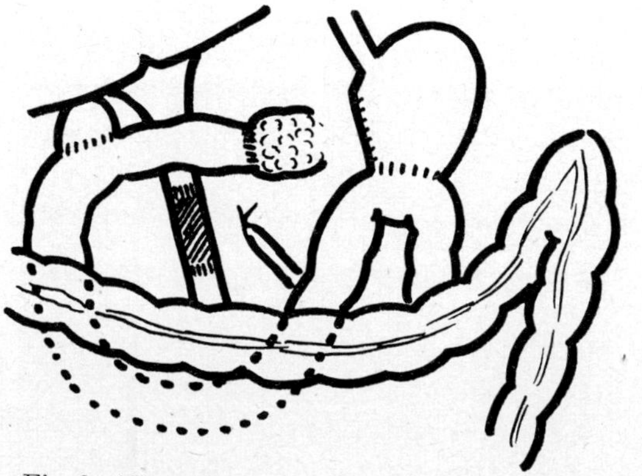

Fig 3. (Case 2).—Schematic illustration of procedure in case 2.

Postoperative Laboratory Findings, Case 2

	7 Days After Op.	1 Month After Op.	3 Mo After Op.
RBC	450×10^4	535×10^4	417×10^4
Hgb content	65%	73%	67%
WBC		3,000	3,000
Serum protein	6.4 gm/dl	7.0 gm/dl	4.4 gm/dl
A/G	0.5	0.5	0.6
Icterus index	14	7	14
CCF	—	++	+++
TTT	1	2	7
CoR	R2	R3	R8
Takata-Ara reation	0	0	8
Blood ammonia	1.2μg/ml	1.0μg/ml	
SGOT	13	12	
SGPT	21	14	

3.0 cm long homograft preserved in a 70% alcohol solution for a year. The gastrointestinal tract was reconstructed according to Child's technique (Fig 3). The time duration of the complete occlusion of the portal vein was 59 minutes. No significant change in blood pressure, pulse rate, or respiration was observed during or after the occlusion. Gross and microscopic examination of the specimen revealed a large mass of carcinoma simplex in the pyloric region involving the head of the pancreas. The portal vein was firmly adherent to the tumor mass but not remarkably constricted or invaded by the tumor cells.

The immediate postoperative course was uneventful except for a bloody diarrhea which began on the fourth postoperative day and lasted four

Fig 4 (Case 2).—A portography showing the patency of the transplanted graft 21 days after operation.

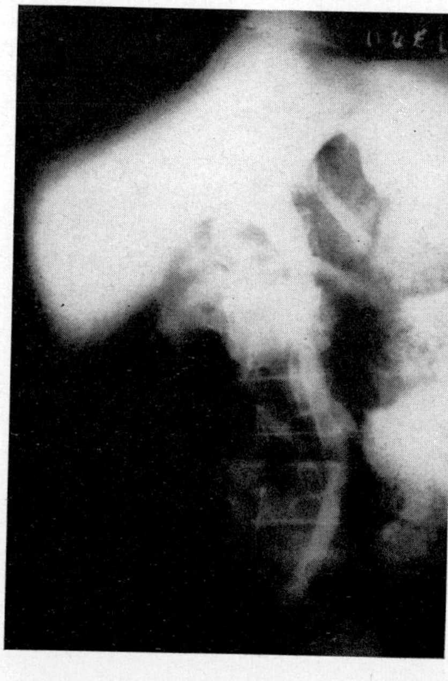

days. Postoperative laboratory findings are summarized in the Table. On the 21st postoperative day, the patient had to be re-explored for adhesive obstruction of the intestine. This was treated successfully with ileocolostomy and cecostomy. At this time, the portal vein pressure measurement and portography could be performed. The pressure was 170 mm H_2O and the portography revealed perfect patency of the anastomosis (Fig 4). Eighty days after the initial operation, the patient developed a jaundice, and then the liver function gradually deteriorated. An abdominal mass began to be palpable. On the 124th day after the initial operation the patient died.

Postmortem examination revealed metastatic lesions in the lungs, liver, and intestine. The peritoneum showed a picture of carcinomatous peritonitis. The transplanted portal vein graft was found to have been compressed and narrowed by carcinomatous infiltration into the surrounding tissues. However, the internal surface was clear and patent without thrombus formation.

Comment

For the procedure of pancreatoduodenectomy necessitating resection of a portion of the portal vein, Child [1] advocates a two-stage operation: first, ligation of the portal vein, and then, after restoration of a sufficient collateral circulation, resection of the head of the pancreas together with the portal vein. For the treatment of carcinomas, however, a procedure with two-stages is a definite disadvantage. Furthermore, there may be ill effects from the hemodynamic alteration in the portal circulation after ligation of the portal vein. McDermott [7] recommends a one-stage resection with establishment of an Eck fistula, a procedure approved by Hubbard,[4] Moore [8] and Zimmermann.[11] Yet this procedure, also, is not recommended because of the possibility of its causing postoperative complications such as impaired liver function or Eck syndrome.

The ideal solution to this problem would seem to be resection and reconstruction of the portal vein by graft transplantation so that blood from the portal system can reach the liver. When approximation of the divided ends can be made without difficulty, a simple anastomosis of the divided ends may be undertaken (Moore and Ure,[8] Dennis and Varco,[3] Waugh and Giberson,[10] Kikuchi [6]).

We have found in the experimental laboratory that a practical method of occluding the portal vein is simultaneous occlusion of the superior mesenteric artery and moderate general hypothermia (29-30 C [84.2-86.0 F]): portal vein occlusion up to 60 minutes can thus be achieved quite safely, allowing a deliberate operative technique. In the two cases reported in this paper, the time duration of the portal vein occlusion was 31 minutes and 59 minutes, respectively, without any significant change in blood pressure, pulse rate, or respiration. The only attributable symptom was the bloody diarrhea lasting several days after operation which need not be considered serious from the point of postoperative care.

A comparative study of various types of grafts—synthetic, arterial homografts, systemic venous homografts, and portal venous homografts—was carried out in our laboratory using dogs. Each of the homografts was preserved in a 70% alcohol solution. Among these grafts, the portal venous homograft was the most satisfactory, showing a long-term patency in six out of eight dogs, including two dogs in which the patency of the graft was observed as long as seven and eight months.[5] These favorable results are probably due to the fact that the portal venous homograft can retain its shape, is of suitable size, and induces a less severe tissue reaction which might be a cause of late stenosis or obstruction (usually one month or later). An interesting fact is that in spite of a considerable amount of purulent discharge from the wounds, suggesting a leakage of bile or pancreatic juice and contamination of the graft, the graft was able to sustain its patency. The portal vein homograft preserved in a 70% alcohol solution appeared to be more resistent to infection than any other synthetic graft, including one made of Teflon. Daniel [2] recognized a high patency rate with fresh autogenous vein grafts placed in dogs, but, as a matter of practice, it is too difficult to get this type of graft large enough to use in portal vein reconstruction in humans.

Summary

In this paper, two successful cases of portal vein resection and transplantation for carcinoma occurring in the area of the head of the pancreas were reported. As far as we know, this is the first report of this type of procedure applied to humans, and the results of the application of this technique should broaden the indications for the surgical treatment of carcinoma of the head of the pancreas.

Kazuo Nakamura, MD, Department of Surgery, Osaka Medical School, Takatsuki-shi, Osaka, Japan.

REFERENCES

1. Child, C. G., III; Holswade, G. R.; McClure, R. D., Jr.; Gore, A. L.; and O'Neill, E. A.: Pancreaticoduodenectomy With Resection of the Portal Vein in the Macaca Mulatta Monkey and in Man, Surg Gynec Obstet 94:31, 1952.

2. Daniel, W. W.: Bridging Defects in the Canine Portal and Superior Mesenteric Veins With Plastic Tubes and Vascular Grafts, Cancer 5:1041, 1952.

3. Dennis, C., and Varco, R. L.: Survival for More Than Five Years After Pancreatoduodenectomy for Cancers of the Ampulla and Pancreatic Head, Surgery 39:92, 1956.

4. Hubbard, T. B.: Carcinoma of the Head of the Pancreas: Resection of the Portal Vein and Portacaval Shunt, Ann Surg 147:935, 1958.

5. Itaya, H.; Asada, S.; Date, M.; Nishimoto, K.: Morino, M.; and Kasagawa, O.: Experimental Studies on the Re-Establishment of Portal Flow After En Bloc Portal Resection With Pancreaticoduodenectomy, Bull Osaka Med Sch 6:76, 1960.

6. Kikuchi, S.: A Clinical and Experimental Study on the Management of Portal Vein During Pancreaticoduodenectomy, Tohoku J Exp Med 64:121, 1956.

7. McDermott, W. V., Jr.: A One-Stage Pancreatoduodenectomy With Resection of the Portal Vein for Carcinoma of the Pancreas, Ann Surg 136:1012, 1952.

8. Moore, G. E., and Ure, B.: One-Stage Pancreatoduodenectomy With Resection of the Superior Mesenteric Vein, Surgery 35:734, 1954.

9. Porter, M. R.: Carcinoma of the Pancreatico-Duodenal Area: Operability and Choice of Procedure, Ann Surg 148:711, 1958.

10. Waugh, J. M., and Giberson, R. G.: Radical Resection of the Head of the Pancreas and of the Duodenum for Malignant Lesions, Surg Clin N Amer. 37:965, 1957.

11. Zimmermann, B.: in discussion on Rhoads, J. E.; Zintel, H. A.; and Helwig, J. Jr.: Results of Operations of the Whipple Type in Pancreaticoduodenal Carcinoma, Ann Surg 146:667, 1957.

Pancreatic Ducts and Postoperative Pancreatitis

THOMAS R. KELLY, MD
AND
MARLIN L. TROYER, MD
AKRON, OHIO

Sixty years ago, Opie[1] presented his "Common Channel" theory of the etiology of acute hemorrhagic pancreatitis. The anatomy of the pancreatic ductal septem has been the subject of numerous studies ever since this first report.

We have been interested in the anatomy of the ducts of the pancreas relative to the pathogenesis of postoperative pancreatitis. Postoperative morbidity and mortality after injury to pancreatic ducts and arteries have been well documented in the literature.[2-9] The purpose of this report was to study the anatomy of the pancreatic ducts and to demonstrate their variants. The distal portion of the common bile duct and the pancreatic ducts are located anatomically in an inaccessible location to the surgeon, and it is therefore important that the anatomical variants be thoroughly understood if injury to these structures is to be avoided.

Submitted for publication Feb 25, 1963.

From the Surgical Research Department of The Akron City Hospital.

Materials and Methods

The material in this study consisted of 50 fixed specimens consisting of pancreas, antrum of stomach, duodenum, and terminal common bile duct removed en bloc from autopsies of the department of pathology. Twenty of the specimens were studied by the vinyl acetate cast technique. The glands were injected utilizing one of the following three ports: (1) the entrance of the duct of Wirsung into the ampulla, (2) the main duct in the pancreatic tail after partial transection of the gland, and (3) the common bile duct after suturing the duodenal mucosa at the papilla. This last location was found to be the most satisfactory since it facilitated identification of the ducts of Wirsung and Santorini. A 40% solution of vinyl acetate plastic in acetone was injected by means of a 10 cc syringe through an 18-gauge cannula. The injection was continued until a regurgitation of the material was noted, usually 5-7 cc of the plastic was needed to obtain a satisfactory specimen. The injected specimen was allowed to stand suspended in water for about 24 hours and then placed in 10% potassium hydroxide solution for digestion. After 36 hours the cast was lifted from the digested soft tissues of the gland and allowed to dry. The casts were friable and necessitated careful handling during the experiment. To assure the integrity of the casts for accurate

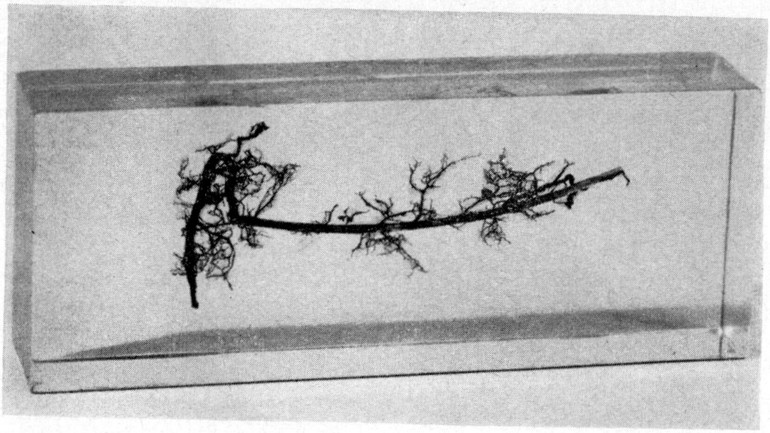

Fig 1.—Vinyl acetate cast of the pancreas embedded within bioplastic.

study they were embedded in a clear bioplastic (Fig 1).

Thirty of the specimens were studied by gross dissection. The main pancreatic duct of Wirsung was located in the neck of the gland where the pancreatic tissue overlies the superior mesenteric vessels. At this level the duct approaches the dorsal surface of the gland and is readily found usually about midway between the cephalic and caudal borders at a depth of 2-3 mm in the gland substance.[2] Once located the duct was easily traced both toward the tail of the gland and toward the duodenum. In both of these regions it was found to be nearer the dorsal than the ventral surface of the gland. The accessory duct of Santorini was most quickly reached by working along the ventral surface of the main duct beginning at the neck and proceeding towards the duodenum.

In order to clearly understand the anatomy of the ducts and their variants described in this study, one must review the embryologic development of the pancreas.[3] Since the pancreas develops by separate outgrowths, of which one is directly from the duodenum and the other from the lower end of the diverticulum for the liver (Fig. 2*A*), it should of course have two ducts. The dorsal pancreatic anlage, growing directly from the dorsal wall of the duodenum is normally carried toward the ventral mesentery by differential growth of the duodenum and expands in this ventral mesentery to form the major portion of the pancrease (Fig 2*B*). The ventral anlage, from the hepatic diverticulum, grows directly into the ventral mesentery and forms a large portion of the head of the pancreas.

These two parts normally fuse together to form the definitive pancreas, and the ventral duct typically anastomoses with the dorsal duct and takes over from this duct the drainage of the body and tail of the pancreas (Fig 2*C*). Thus, under usual circumstance, the ventral pancreatic duct becomes the

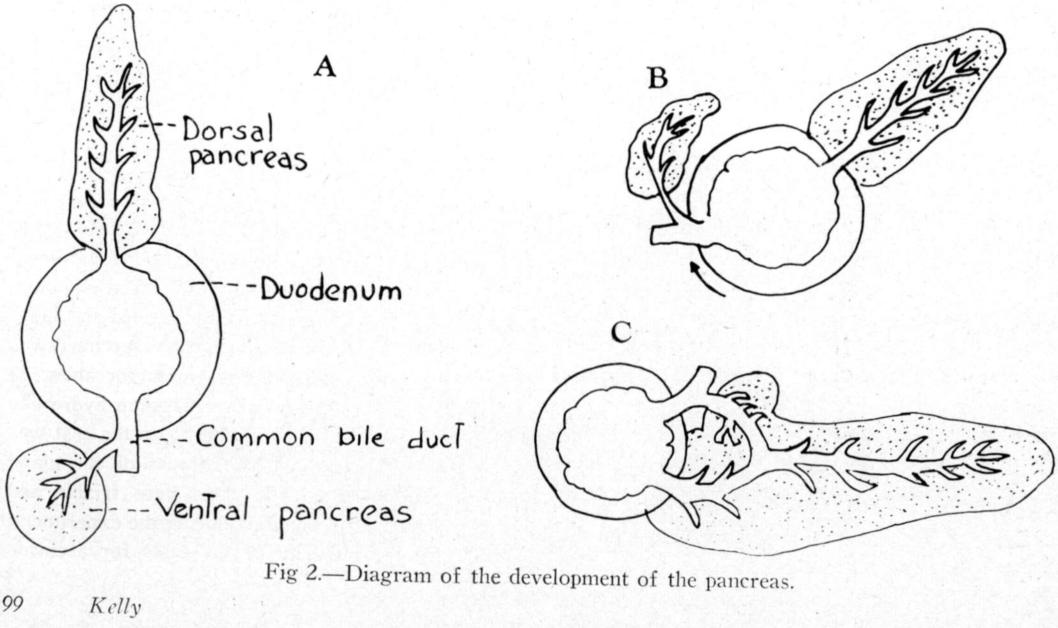

Fig 2.—Diagram of the development of the pancreas.

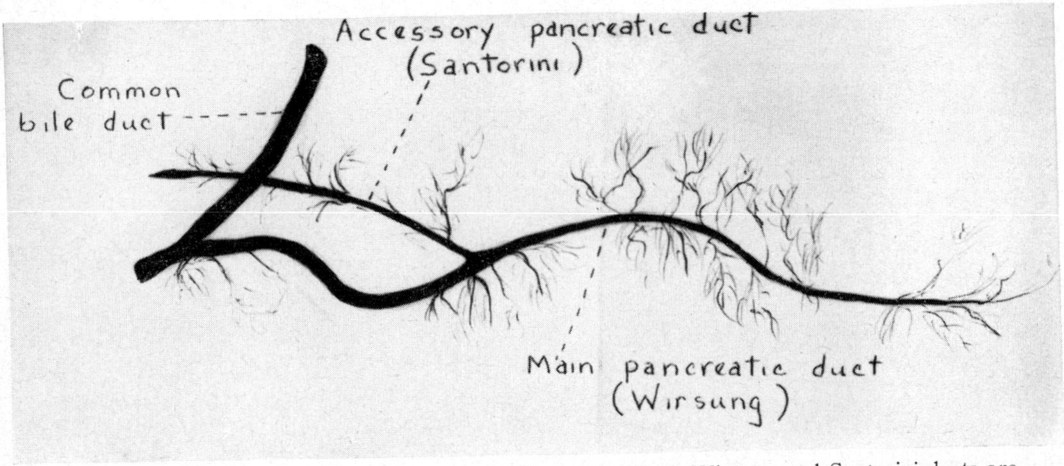

Fig 3.—Drawing of a cast from a 45-year-old woman. Both Wirsung and Santorini ducts are present.

chief pancreatic duct, or duct of Wirsung, which is normally far larger than the dorsal pancreatic duct and drains the major portion of the pancreas. The lesser pancreatic duct, or duct of Santorini, normally drains primarily simply the upper and more anterior portion of the head of the pancreas, the portion of the head to which it originally gave rise, and/or it may become atresic toward its duodenum end. Variations in the development of the anastomosis between the two ducts is the common cause of departures from the usual relations.

Results

In the 50 glands subjected to gross dissection and injection technique, the main pancreatic duct of Wirsung was found to be the largest duct and emptied through the ampulla of Vater in 47 (94%) cases as shown in Fig 3 and 4. The incidence of intraglandular communication between the major and minor ductal system was 90%. In only five instances could no demonstration of communication between the two ducts be found. In three (6%) specimens the accessory pancreatic duct was the sole duct and emptied through the accessory papilla (Fig 5). The accessory pancreatic duct was patent and opened through an accessory papilla in 35 (74%) of the 47 cases in which the ampulla of Vater was the main excretory outlet of the gland. Thus, it was found that a patent accessory papilla existed in 76% of cases and that it was capable of transmitting pancreatic juice in varying amounts.

Clinical Significance

Acute postoperative pancreatitis is a tragic and somewhat inexplicable accompaniment

Fig 4.—Drawing of a cast from a 60-year-old man. The duct of Wirsung is present. No Santorini duct was present.

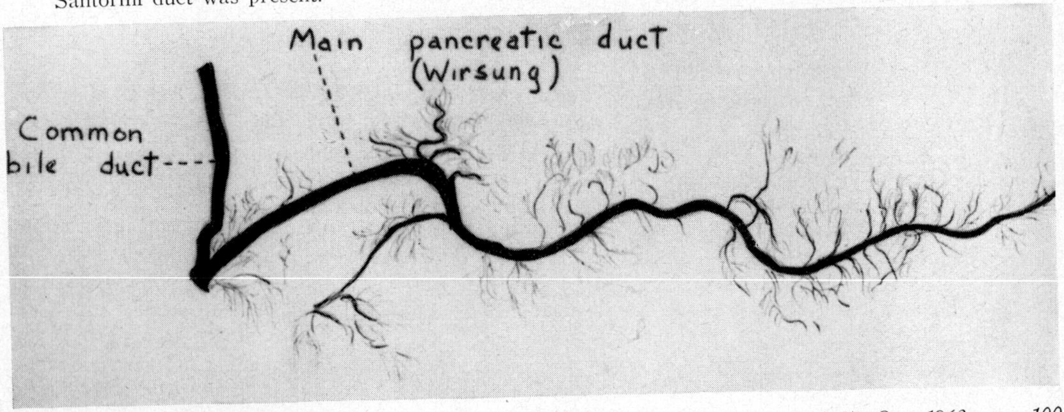

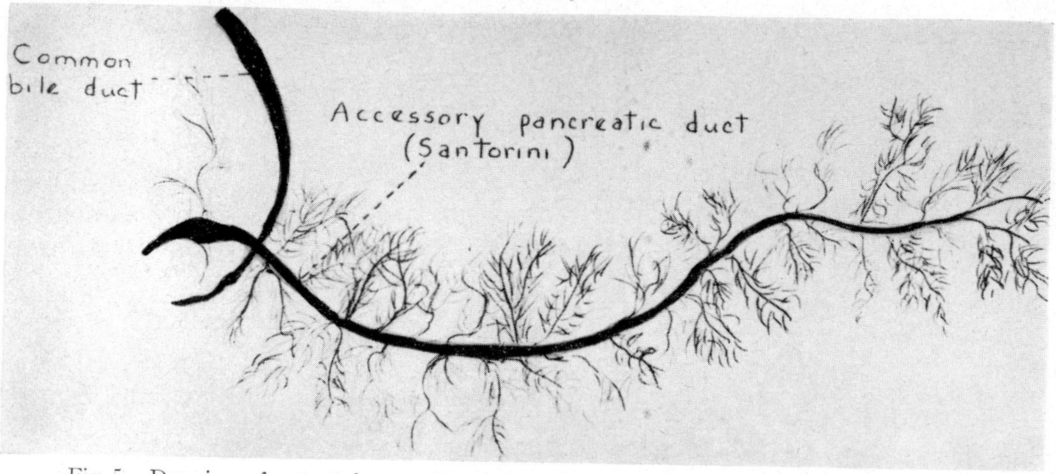

Fig 5.—Drawing of a cast from a 48-year-old man. Note the large duct of Santorini with outlet cephalad to the common bile duct. No duct of Wirsung was demonstrated.

of surgical operations. The disease is fortunately seen infrequently in postoperative patients, but when it occurs the patient has approximately a 50% chance of survival.[4] Pancreatic ductal and arterial injuries have been emphasized by many researchers as significant etiologic factors in the pathogenesis of the postoperative pancreatitis. Dunphy [5] stated that the posterior pancreaticoduodenal artery and the duct of Santorini are particularly vulnerable to injury when the duodenum is mobilized during gastrectomy. Schmieden and Sebening [6] related that 11 of 91 acute pancreatic affections following gastric operations were caused by ligation of the duct of Santorini. Millbourn [7] concluded that in 50% of cases there is some risk of injury to the duct of Santorini in separating the ulcerated duodenum from the head of the pancreas, and that in 10% of individuals such an injury may have serious consequences. Stuart and Jordan [8] stated that scarring caused by a posterior penetrating ulcer predisposes to injury of the pancreatic duct during dissection of the first portion of the duodenum. Boles [9] reported 30 cases of postoperative pancreatitis and emphasized the consequence of damage to the duct of Santorini during duodenal mobilization.

As a result of this study it is apparent that the accessory pancreatic duct is a functional part of the pancreatic duct system emptying at the accessory papilla in 76% of cases. In fact, in 6% of the cases, the accessory duct was the main duct of excretion for the pancreas. Kleitsch [10] found that a patent accessory papilla existed in 70% of his injected specimens. In 10% of his cases the accessory duct was the main duct of excretion for the pancreas and emptied through the accessory papilla.

The consequence of injury to the duct of Santorini will vary widely and depends upon the size of the duct and its relative functional importance.[11] Ligation of the duct of Santorini when it is small and when it arborizes with the main pancreatic duct is unquestionably of minor significance. In those instances in which the duct of Santorini is the main excretory duct of the pancreas, 6% in this study, ligation would undoubtedly result in pancreatitis.

Finally, since the accessory pancreatic duct is small and virtually impossible to demonstrate at the operating table, it is more practical to identify landmarks to assist in avoiding injury to this structure. As Kleitsch [10] pointed out, it is not safe to dissect the duodenum distal to the area of the duodenal bulb. This area can be identified at the operating table as that point in the duodenum where the gastroduodenal artery passes below and the common bile duct passes behind (Fig 6).

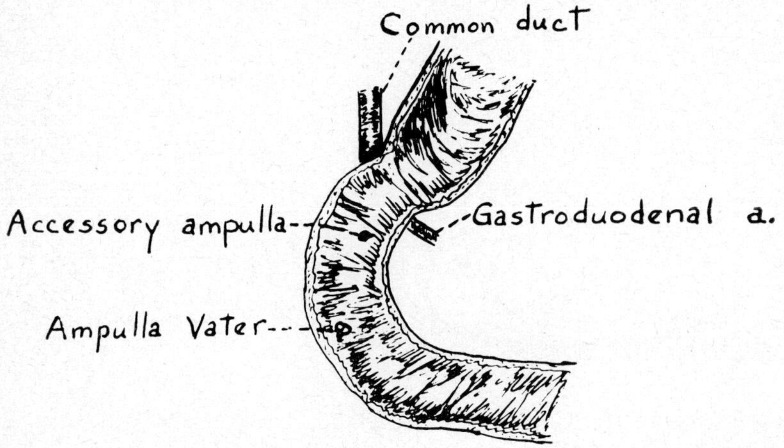

Fig 6.—A diagram showing important landmarks in gastrectomy. It is not safe to dissect the duodenum from the pancreas below the area of the common bile duct above and the gastroduodenal artery below.

Summary and Conclusions

The anatomy of the pancreatic ducts and their variants have been studied by vinyl acetate casts and gross dissections.

The embryologic development of the pancreas from dorsal and ventral anlagen is discussed.

The accessory duct of Santorini was found to be patent in 76% of cases and the sole duct of excretion in 6% of cases.

The possible dangers of a severe postoperative pancreatitis developing as a consequence of damage to the duct of Santorini should be fully appreciated by all general surgeons.

Thomas R. Kelly, MD, 503 Ohio Building, Akron 8, Ohio.

REFERENCES

1. Opie, E. L.: Etiology of Acute Hemorrhagic Pancreatitis, Bull Hopkins Hosp 12:182, 1901.

2. Rienhoff, W. F., and Pickrell, K. L.: Pancreatitis, Arch Surg 51:205, 1945.

3. Hollinshead, W. H.: Anatomy for Surgeons: Vol 2. The Thorax, Abdomen, and Pelvis, New York: Paul B. Hoeber, Inc., Medical Book Department of Harper & Row, Publishers, 1961, p 433.

4. Ponka, J. L.; Landrum, S. E.; and Chaikof, L.: Acute Pancreatitis in the Postoperative Patient, Arch Surg 83:475, 1961.

5. Dunphy, J. E.; Brooks, J. R.; and Achroyd, F.: Acute Postoperative Pancreatitis, New Eng J Med 248:445, 1953.

6. Schmieden, V., and Sebening, W.: Surgery of the Pancreas, Surg Gynec Obstet 46:735, 1928.

7. Millbourn, E.: On Acute Pancreatic Affections Following Gastric Resection for Ulcer or Cancer and the Possibilities of Avoiding Them, Acta Chir Scand 98:1, 1949.

8. Stuart, J. R., and Jordan, P. H., Jr.: Unusual Complications of Subtotal Gastric Resection, AMA Arch Surg 74:459, 1957.

9. Boles, E. T., Jr.: Postoperative Pancreatitis, AMA Arch Surg 73:710, 1956.

10. Kleitsch, W. P.: Anatomy of the Pancreas, AMA Arch Surg 71:795, 1955.

11. Warren, K. W.: Acute Pancreatitis and Pancreatic Injuries Following Subtotal Gastrectomy, Surgery 29:643, 1951.

Gastric Ulcers—Management

SIGMOND H. NADLER, MD
BUFFALO

The treatment of patients with gastric ulcers has been debated by internists and surgeons for many years. It is agreed by all, however, that a gastric ulcer is a potentially malignant lesion, but there is no foolproof method of deciding which ulcers will become malignant, which are already malignant, or which will remain benign.

The purpose of this paper is to evaluate the radiological and laboratory findings along with the treatment and pathological diagnoses in a group of patients with gastric ulcers in an attempt to decide the manner in which this lesion should be managed.

The study period includes all patients in whom a diagnosis of gastric ulcer was made at Roswell Park Memorial Institute, Buffalo, from Jan 1, 1950, through Dec 31, 1962.

Criteria

1. All patients were required to have a diagnosis of primary gastric ulcer made by radiographic techniques.
2. All patients treated surgically were required to have follow-up at Roswell Park Memorial Institute.
3. All surgical diagnoses had to be confirmed pathologically.

Material

Two hundred patients with gastric ulcers were seen at Roswell Park Memorial Institute during the years from 1950 through 1962.

Sex: Males comprised 139, or 69.5%, and females 61, or 30.5%, of the series.

Age: The most common age group involved was from ages 50-59 with 58 cases, or 29% of the patients. The next most common was the 60-69-year-old group with 54, or 27%, of the cases.

Radiological and Laboratory Findings

Radiological examination, consisting of an upper gastrointestinal series using barium, interpreted 106 of the ulcers as benign, 49 cases as malignant, and in 45 cases no comment was made. The most common location of the ulcer was on the lesser curvature of the stomach in the antral area.

Cytological examination of gastric contents was performed by use of gastric wash-

Submitted for publication March 4, 1963.

Department of Surgery, Roswell Park Memorial Institute, New York State Department of Health.

ing specimens in 45 cases. In only two of these cases were the washings interpreted as being positive for the presence of malignant cells, and in both of these cases the ulcers proved to be malignant on subsequent pathological examination of surgical specimens. Even more important, however, is the fact that both of these cases were called benign radiologically.

A gastric analysis was performed in 77 of the 200 cases. In only 16 instances was there absence of free acid in the specimen. Absence of free acid was present in 12 cases which were found subsequently to be benign ulcers and in four cases of proven malignancy by pathological examination of a surgical specimen.

Treatment

The treatment received by a patient was divided into the categories of medical only, medical plus surgical, surgical only, and none at all. Medical therapy consisted of diet, antispasmodics, etc for varying intervals of time, depending on the discretion of the attending physician. Surgical therapy usually consisted of a subtotal gastric resection, with occasionally just a local excision of the ulcer being performed. If after local excision was performed the ulcer was determined to be malignant pathologically a subtotal gastric resection was done. Medical plus surgical therapy was that treatment comprising three weeks to three months of strictly medical therapy followed by surgery because of a lack of response of the lesion to medical treatment only. No therapy was given to patients who refused it or wished to be treated by their own physician.

Seventy-seven patients received medical treatment only. Fifty-five of these cases were diagnosed as benign ulcers radiologically, five were diagnosed as malignant ulcers, and in seventeen cases no opinion was given. In no instance did any of these patients subsequently have treatment for a malignancy of the stomach.

Seventeen patients were treated with combined medical and surgical techniques. By x-ray ten were called benign lesions, five malignant, and in two cases no opinion was offered. Four of the ten "benign" cases and two of the five "malignant" cases by radiographic technique demonstrated carcinoma in the ulcer after pathological examination of the surgical specimen.

Surgical therapy alone was given to 79 cases. These were composed of 30 radiographically benign ulcers, 29 malignant, and 20 cases in which no comment was made. Six of the 30 "benign" and 2 of the 29 "malignant" cases actually showed carcinomatous changes in the ulcer pathologically.

The remaining 27 cases of this series were given no treatment either because they were referred back to their own physician and were not seen at Roswell Park Memorial Institute again, or because of a refusal of or lack of returning for therapy. Eleven of these cases were called benign ulcers, ten were read as malignant, and in six no comment was made. None of these patients later returned to Roswell Park Memorial Institute with carcinoma of the stomach.

Pathology

Pathological examination was done, of course, only in those patients upon whom a surgical procedure was performed. Of the 96 surgical specimens received, carcinoma of the stomach was demonstrated in 14, or 14.6%. This is 7% of the total number of cases seen, however.

Of the 40 cases classified as benign preoperatively and then treated by a surgical procedure, ten demonstrated carcinoma on pathological examination of the surgical specimen. Four malignancies were found in the 34 cases called malignant ulcers preoperatively and then treated eventually with surgery. No evidence of malignancy was found in any of the 22 cases in which no radiographic comment had been made as to benignity of malignancy prior to surgery.

This was a 25% radiological margin of error on the "benign" lesions treated surgically and only 11.8% accuracy in those lesions called "malignant" and treated surgically. The over-all radiologic error was 10/106 "benign" radiographic cases, 45/49 "malignant" radiographic cases, and 0/45 "no comment" cases, or 9.4%, 91.8%, and 0% respectively. There was a complete radiographic technique error rate, therefore, in 55/200 cases or 27.5%.

None of the patients whose surgical specimen was diagnosed as a benign gastric ulcer pathologically returned at a later date with carcinoma of the stomach. In addition, no patient in whom a malignancy had been diagnosed and then was treated either medically or surgically, and the specimen found to be benign, returned with a gastric carcinoma at a later date.

The pathological classification of the 14 malignant ulcers was done by using the modifications of Dukes classification as suggested by Kirklin, Dockerty, and Waugh, in 1949, and with the additional modification as suggested by Astler and Coller in 1953. These criteria were as follows: Type A, lesions limited to the mucosa; Type B_1, lesions extending into the muscularis propia, but not penetrating it, with negative nodes; Type B_2, lesions penetrating the muscularis propria, but with negative nodes; Type C_1, same as B_1, but with positive nodes; Type C_2, same as B_2, but with positive nodes. In addition, a Class D was added to constitute lesions in which distal organ or tissue involvement was present, treated, and the lesion considered curable.

Three of the gastric ulcers with carcinoma were classified as B_1 lesions. There was one B_2, two C_1, and one D lesion. The most common classification was the C_2 group with seven cases.

All but two of the malignant ulcers were located on the lesser curvature of the stomach. The most common location for these lesions was the antrum with six cases. Three malignancies were present in both the cardia and the body of the stomach.

Peritoneal washings, using normal saline were obtained in 5 of the 14 malignant ulcer cases in the attempt to find free tumor cells in the peritoneal cavity. In no instance were these cells demonstrated.

As can be seen from the basic classification, 10 of the 14 cases had lymph node involvement by carcinoma.

Results

As stated earlier none of the 186 patients proven by follow-up, either medical or surgical, to have had benign disease returned with gastric carcinoma at a later date. In the group of 14 patients with malignancy present in the ulcer, only two are presently alive, with only one of these two patients having lived over five years postoperatively. The other patient is still within the first postoperative year. The single five year survivor was a patient in whom the ulcer was diagnosed as a malignant one radiographically and in whom the pathological classification was given as Dukes C_1. In the other living patient the Dukes classification was B_1, and this patient was interpreted as having a benign ulcer preoperatively.

One of the operative cases which proved to be a carcinoma had a palliative resection only because it was known that residual tumor remained at the time of completion of the surgical procedure.

Ten of the 12 recurrences of tumor occurred in the first three years after pathological diagnosis, three the first postoperative year, one in the second, and six in the third.

Discussion

The treatment of gastric ulcers has been debated for many years and most likely will not be completely resolved for some time yet. It is well known, however, that malignancy definitely plays a role in this lesion as compared to the rarity of carcinoma being present in a duodenal ulcer.

As can be seen from this study, the use of radiologic techniques is not completely infallible. Even in the best hands, a margin of considerable error is possible. The high incidence of error in the "malignant" group in this series of cases could possibly be attributed to the orientation of the radiologists at Roswell Park Memorial Institute to malignant disease. The combination of radiological interpretation with corresponding laboratory findings can also have its pitfalls. The use of cytological findings, however, may tend to prevent some of the errors in diagnoses in the future.

It has been repeatedly documented that the over-all five year survival rate for patients with gastric carcinoma is somewhere around 10%. Medical personnel and organizations, well known for their fine medical backgrounds, have urged earlier diagnosis and treatment not only in gastric malignancies, but also in the treatment of all forms of cancer.

In this series of 200 gastric ulcer cases, it was seen that 7% proved to be actual gastric carcinoma. In this group the survival rate was very poor, as is evidenced by the fact that only two of the 14 patients are now alive without recurrence of disease, with only one patient living five years postoperatively. Whether or not the survival rate could be increased by earlier treatment of the malignancy would be an entirely separate study, but from all previous studies of malignant disease, it would probably prove to be extremely worthwhile.

Many of the lesions pathologically proved to be rather far advanced, with lymph node spread, as was mentioned earlier. Some of these patients had had both medical and surgical therapy combined. It is possible that the delay prior to surgery was too long and that some of these patients might have been saved if better methods of diagnosis were available or if a more positive approach to the treatment of gastric ulcers was taken.

Although the incidence of 7% malignancy in gastric ulcers is not overwhelming it is very noteworthy, for the prognosis for carcinoma of the stomach that has metastasized is essentially nil. In the face of such a poor prognosis for patients with gastric carcinoma an aggressive approach to a possible malignant lesion should be taken even though the mortality rate for gastric resection is approximately 3%. It is true that, as in all surgical procedures, there is some associated morbidity, but with the realization that there is a good possibility of carcinoma being present in the ulcer this has to be discounted immediately. The realization that surgery is the only known method, at this time, for establishment of an absolute diagnosis of the true nature of a gastric ulcer must be accepted. The incidence of malignancy in this lesion does not allow for temporization.

Therefore, recommendations for the treatment of gastric ulcers consist of:

1. Diagnosis of the gastric ulcer by radiographic techniques.
2. Cytological study of gastric contents.
3. Gastric resection, either subtotally or locally, as the situation warrants.

Sigmond H. Nadler, MD, Department of Surgery, Roswell Park Memorial Institute, New York State Department of Health, Buffalo, NY.

REFERENCES

1. Astler, V. B., and Coller, F. A.: The Prognostic Significance of Direct Extension of Carcinoma of the Colon and Rectum, Ann Surg 139:846, 1954.

2. Brown, P. M.; Cain, J. C.; and Dockerty, M. B.: Clinically "Benign" Gastric Ulcerations Found to be Malignant at Operation, Surg Gynec Obstet 112:82, 1961.

3. Kirklin, J. W.; Dockerty, M. D.; and Waugh, J. W.: The Role of the Peritoneal Reflection in the Prognosis of Carcinoma of the Rectum and Sigmoid Colon, Surg Gynec Obstet 88:326, 1949.

4. Palumbo, L. T., and Sharpe, W. S.: Gastric Ulcer: Is It Benign or Malignant? Arch Surg 85:705, 1962.

Repair of Traumatic Fistulas of the Parotid Duct

A. STEPHEN MOREL, DMD, MD
AND
ALAN FIRESTEIN, DDS
NEW YORK

Many ingenious methods for primary repair of the severed parotid duct have been suggested.[1-14] All of these have in common the passing of a dowel or hollow tube through the cut ends of the duct and approximation with fine sutures. Baron[15] in 1961 described a method of ligation of the parotid duct for the correction of salivary fistula. However, not since 1917 has the problem of secondary surgical repair of parotid duct fistula and sialocele been reviewed in the literature. Morestin,[1] at that time, after an extensive experience with war injuries, described various methods of dealing with this distressing problem.

This paper deals with a method of converting a chronic external salivary fistula or sialocele into an intraoral fistula with the preservation of parotid gland function.

Anatomy

The parotid gland is the largest of the salivary glands and is located mainly in the retromandibular fossa. It extends medially to the styloid process and posteriorly to the mastoid process and sternocleidomastoid muscle. Anteriorly, the gland contacts the posterior border of the ramus of the mandible and the medial pterygoid muscle. A superficial portion of the gland extends anteriorly on the lateral surface of the jaw and masseter muscle.

The parotid duct, or Stensen's duct (Figure, *A*), is located at the intersection of a horizontal line extending from the tragus of the ear to a point midway between the upper lip of the ala of the nose. Very often, an accessory parotid duct joins the main duct as it crosses the masseter muscle. At the anterior border of the masseter muscle, the duct passes through the fat pad of the cheek and penetrates the buccinator muscle, opening into the oral cavity opposite the second upper molar teeth (Figure, *B* and *C*). As the duct crosses the outer portion of the masseter muscle, it lies close to the zygomatic and buccal branches of the facial nerve. It is at this point that the duct is most superficial and susceptible to injury.

Submitted for publication March 5, 1963.

Departments of General and Maxillofacial Surgery of Beekman-Downtown Hospital.

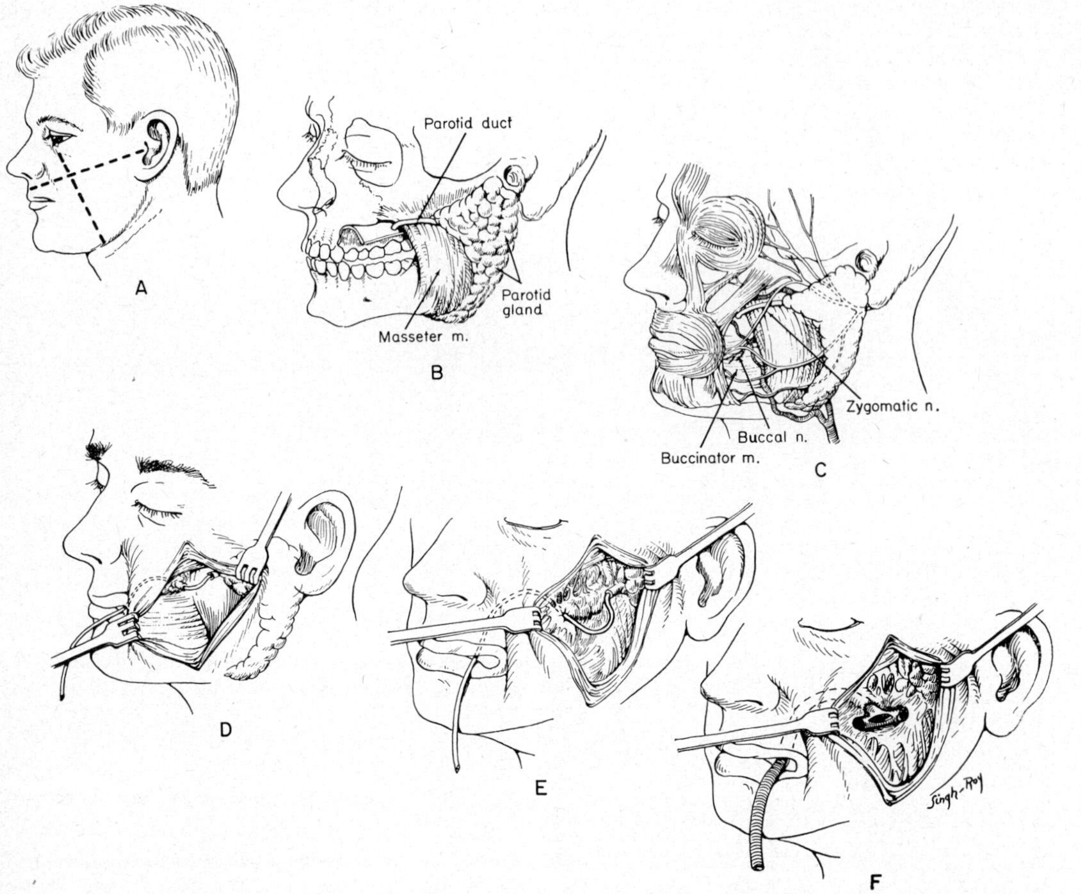

A, topographical demonstration of the location of the parotid duct; *B*, anatomic relationship of the parotid duct to the masseter muscle and oral mucosa; *C*, demonstrates the common relation of the zygomatic branch of the facial nerve to the parotid duct; *D*, method of primary duct repair with a polyethylene catheter threaded through the cut ends; *E*, method of formation of intraoral fistula when distal end of duct is not available; *F*, method of formation of intraoral fistula where cut ends of duct are obscured within the walls of a sialocele.

Report of Cases

Case 1.—A female, aged 19, was admitted to the Beekman-Downtown Hospital on March 27, 1959, after an automobile collision in which she was thrown against a shattered windshield. Deep lacerations of the left face were sutured in the emergency room. Two days later a clear discharge was noted on the left check. A salivary amylase of 533 confirmed the presence of a salivary fistula.

On April 7, 1959, exploration of the left cheek wound was carried out. Upon careful inspection, fragments of shattered glass were found. The proximal end of the severed parotid duct was easily located. The distal end was markedly irregular, scarred, and imperforate. There was a 3 cm loss of duct length. For this reason an end-to-end anastomosis was impossible. Consequently, a fine polyethylene catheter was threaded into the proximal duct and brought into the mouth around the lateral border of the masseter muscle through a mucosal stab wound (Figure, *E*). It was then fixed to the buccal mucosa by a silk suture. The free end of the catheter was taped to the external skin of the face. Careful layer closure of the incision was performed. Suture and catheter were left in place for seven days before removal. The patient has subsequently remained asymptomatic, with demonstrable salivary flow throughout the intraoral salivary fistula.

Case 2.—A male, aged 44, was admitted to the Beekman-Downtown Hospital on Aug 11, 1961. His history revealed a knife wound on Aug 3, 1961, at which time he suffered a laceration of the left cheek. This was sutured in the hospital emergency room. The patient later noticed swelling of the left cheek and profuse discharge of clear fluid through the suture line. At the time of surgical exploration of the wound (Sept 20, 1961), a 3 cm cavity, with marked fibrosed walls over the left masseter muscle, was found. It was filled with approximately 15 cc of thick mucoid saliva. Because of marked scarring, the ends of the severed parotid duct could not be located. An internal fistulization of the sialocele was performed by placing a small T-tube *in situ* and carrying the long limb through a stab wound in the buccal mucosa and out through the mouth (Figure, *F*). The T-tube was left *in situ* for 14 days and subsequently removed. At follow-up 15 months later, there was continued salivary flow through the internal fistula, with no episode of difficulty or pain of the left parotid gland reported.

Comment

Case 1 presents a situation where the distal remnants of the duct were already obliterated by scar at the time of surgery. Consequently, a fine polyethylene catheter was threaded into the proximal end of the duct and brought around the lateral border of the masseter muscle into the mouth through a stab wound in the buccal mucosa.

In Case 2 neither proximal nor distal ends of the severed duct could be identified because of very extensive scarring and sialocele formation. It was apparent, because of the saliva formation, that the parotid gland was actively secreting. Therefore, a T-tube was used to drain the scarred space with the formation of an intraoral salivary fistula.

Trauma to the parotid gland from a direct blow usually causes no damage and generally requires little more than closure of the parotid capsule with replacement of the skin over it. Trauma and injury to the parotid duct, however, should be considered whenever there are lacerations of penetrating facial wounds. It is usually possible, and certainly desirable, to treat injuries by recognition and primary repair (Figure, *D*).

In a fresh wound it is often possible to see the cut ends of the duct. In cases where severance of the duct is uncertain, a fine polyethylene catheter may be passed through the osteum into the duct until it appears in the wound. Mucosal folds often obscure the ostium; however, it will appear if the surrounding area is dried and then catheterized. A dye, such as methylene blue, may be used to outline the os. To facilitate tubal passage by straightening the duct, the cheek should be pulled outward.[14]

The masseteric portion of the duct is the area most frequently injured and is the easiest portion to repair, since it is relatively straight and immobile and has tough, elastic walls. As the duct approaches the parotid gland, repair becomes more difficult. The walls are thinner here and begin to branch; they are also hidden by the overhanging portion of the gland. It is at this point that related injuries to both gland and duct may damage the branches of the facial nerve (Figure, *C*).

Perhaps one of the reasons for neglect of secondary parotid duct repairs is based upon the existence of six "major" salivary glands, so that when one gland is not functioning, only a proportionate degree of emphasis is placed upon its importance.[8] However, loss of the parotid gland due to extirpation, obstruction, or atrophy will cause facial asymmetry, particularly when there is associated facial nerve paralysis.

The two basic approaches for correcting an extraoral fistula resulting from a lacerated duct are 1) primary repair over a dowel and 2) transference of fistulas from external to internal.

These methods are preferable to use of radiation, surgical extirpation of the parotid gland, or ligation of the duct. For even under the most careful circumstances, radiation is always a hazard and is not recommended unless all other methods are of no avail. Extirpation is a major surgical procedure with unwarrented risk to the facial nerves. Although surgical ligation is an effective means of dealing with persistent or recurring external salivary fistulas,[16] its major drawback is atrophy of the gland with resultant cosmetic defect and loss of physiologic function.

Summary

The importance of early recognition of trauma and injury to the parotid duct so that primary repair may be instituted has been stressed.

In cases of delayed repair of an external parotid duct fistula, we believe that the best methods for repair are those which permit continued physiologic functioning of the parotid gland. To these ends, it is believed that meticulous anatomic repair over some form of dowel, such as a polyethylene catheter, is to be preferred. When this is impossible because there are no patent duct ends, a method of changing an extraoral fistula into an intraoral fistula is of great value. Two successful cases of secondary repair are reported here.

A. Stephen Morel, 245 Henry St, Brooklyn 1, NY.

REFERENCES

1. Morestin, H.: Contribution à l'étude du traitment des fistules salivaires consecutives aux blessures de guerre, Bull Soc Chir Paris 43:845-855, 1917.

2. Dickenson, A. M.: Injuries to Stenson's Duct, New York State J Med 27:548, 1927.

3. Tees, F. J.: Primary Repair of Injuries to the Parotid Duct, Canad Med Ass J 16:145-146, 1926.

4. Glascock, H., and Glascock, H., Jr.: Repair of Traumatic Fistulas of Stenson's Duct, Surg Gynec Obstet 65:355-356, 1937.

5. Wallace, F. T.: Primary Repair of the Parotid Duct, Amer J Surg 70:412-413, 1945.

6. Newman, S. C., and Seabrook, D. B.: Management of Injuries to Stenson's Duct, Ann Surg 124:544-556, 1946.

7. Goodall, R. E., and Flanders, S. E.: Successful Primary Repair of Lacerated Stensen's Duct, Surgery 21:865, 1947.

8. Seeley, R. C.: Maxillofacial Injuries, Amer J Surg 73:551-563, 1947.

9. Sparkman, R. S.: Primary Repair of Severed Parotid Duct, Ann Surg 129:652, 1949.

10. Sparkman, R. S.: Laceration of Parotid Duct, Ann Surg 131:743-753, 1950.

11. White, J. E.: Primary Repair of Parotid Duct Injuries, J Nat Med Ass 42:232-234, 1950.

12. Bornstein, L. A., and Simon, B. E.: Successful Primary Repair of Severed Parotid Duct, Plast Reconstr Surg 6:217-227, 1950.

13. Perkins, R. B., and Ward, D. E.: Parotid Duct Wounds and Injuries, Replacement of Portion by Plastic (Polyethylene) Tube, N Carolina Med J 14:122-123, 1953.

14. Kazangian, V. H., and Converse, J. M.: The Surgical Treatment of Facial Injuries, Baltimore: The Williams & Wilkins Company, 1959, p 99-102.

15. Baron, H. C.: Surgical Correction of Salivary Fistula, Ann Surg 153:545-554, 1961.

16. Baron, H. C., and Ober, W. B.: Parotid Gland Atrophy, Arch Surg 85:1042, 1962.

Lethal Properties of a Rapidly Polymerizing Adhesive

Product Used in Nonsuture Surgery

DONALD T. LEWERS, BS
JORGE O. JUST-VIERA, MD
AND
GEORGE H. YEAGER, MD
BALTIMORE

Introduction

Distinct progress towards sutureless surgery followed the discovery of the adhesive properties of cyanoacrylates by a group of investigators in 1959.[1] A year later Nathan and co-workers [2] described the effectiveness of methyl 2-cyanoacrylate in the nonsuture closure of incisions in the aorta of dogs. Currently, the surgical potential of these adhesives is being defined. Encouraging reports include the nonsuture repair of blood vessels and bronchi, sutureless intestinal anastomosis, the treatment of mandibular fractures in dogs, the closure of skin incisions, and renal and hepatic hemostasis.[3-9]

It is important to investigate fully both the advantages and disadvantages of any experimental product intended for humans. The purpose of this report is to present the results of injecting methyl 2-cyanoacrylate, supplied by the Borden Company as AD/here, into Swiss albino mice. The results indicate that methyl 2-cyanoacrylate is toxic to small laboratory animals.

Methods

Detailed accounts of the physical properties of methyl 2-cyanoacrylate are available in the references cited and need not be repeated. AD/here contains the pure liquid monomer without plasticizers. This cement polymerizes at room temperature without requiring solvents or an added catalyst. Due to rapid polymerization, accurate small amounts of adhesive are best administered only with a dis-

Submitted for publication March 9, 1963.

Pangborn Fellow in Peripheral Vascular Diseases (Dr. Just-Viera).

From the Department of Surgery, University of Maryland School of Medicine.

Supported by grants from the American Cancer Society and the Pangborn Foundation.

posable plastic tuberculin syringe. The doses of adhesive injected in the different groups of mice were 0.1 cc, 0.2 cc, and 0.3 cc. Dosages less than 0.1 cc could not be measured accurately and were not employed. Absence of a nontoxic diluent handicapped the injection of lesser amounts of the liquid monomer; however, small quantities of the solid polymer can be suspended in saline.

Two- to six-month-old Swiss albino mice and white laboratory rats served as experimental animals. The following groups of animals received the monomer by injection:

Group 1.—In 24 mice, 0.2 cc of the adhesive was injected intrahepatically. During injection some cement unavoidably spilled into the peritoneal cavity. It proved impossible to confine the material to the liver. Injection was performed after laparotomy following pentobarbital (Nembutal) anesthesia. This was unnecessary in most other groups.

Group 2.—Three groups of 30 mice each were injected intraperitoneally with 0.1, 0.2, and 0.3 cc of adhesive, respectively. The exact destination of the adhesive was confirmed by autopsy. In all mice the adhesive was found free in the peritoneal cavity. No adhesive gained access to the bowel lumen.

Group 3.—In 37 mice, 0.2 cc of cement was injected subcutaneously. Prior to injection, aspiration of the subcutaneous site assured that no adhesive entered blood vessels.

Group 4.—After pentobarbital anesthesia this group of 20 mice underwent laparotomy. Addition of saline to 0.2 cc of monomer resulted in a solid mass of polymer 30 minutes later. This was placed intraperitoneally and the incision was closed with 5-0 silk.

Group 5.—In order to determine whether increasing age rendered animals less susceptible to the toxic properties of the adhesive, five weanlings and five six-month-old mice simultaneously received injections of adhesive totalling 0.2 cc.

Group 6.—This group consisted of 20 rats. The lethal dose administered to the mice expressed in terms of body weight guided the determination of the dosage injected into rats. Two equal groups of ten rats each received intraperitoneally 0.005 cc and 0.01 cc per gram of body weight, respectively.

Group 7.—Control groups of mice corresponded to each experimental group. Saline substituted the adhesive. Twenty mice received 0.2 cc of isotonic saline subcutaneously, 30 mice received 0.2 cc of isotonic saline intraperitoneally, and 10 mice received 0.2 cc of isotonic saline intraperitoneally after pentobarbital anesthesia and after laparotomy.

All groups underwent daily examination. They were housed in mice cages, in small groups, and received routine animal farm feed. Whenever death occurred, autopsy was performed as soon as possible afterwards.

The results were grouped into four categories:

1. Death occurring within 24 hours of the injection.
2. Death occurring between 24 and 48 hours after injection.
3. Death supervening after 48 hours but before one week after injection.
4. Survivors. In this study it was considered that mice surviving more than one week did not die of acute toxic effects secondary to implantation of the adhesive.

Results

Group 1.—A mortality of 100% resulted in those mice receiving 0.2 cc of the adhesive intrahepatically. Of these, 66.6% were dead within 24 hours (Table 1, A).

Group 2.—Those mice receiving the plastic intraperitoneally had ruffled coats 10 to 12 hours after the injection. The animals

TABLE 1.—*Mortality Resulting From Injection of 0.2 CC of Methyl 2-Cyanoacrylate*

Site of Injection	Dose, Cc	No. of Mice	Dead Within 24 Hr No.	Dead Within 24 Hr %	Dead 24-48 Hr No.	Dead 24-48 Hr %	Dead 48 Hr-1 Wk No.	Dead 48 Hr-1 Wk %	% Dead 1 Week
A. Intrahepatically in Swiss Albino Mice After Laparotomy and Nembutal Anesthesia									
Liver		24	16	66.6	0	0	8	33.3	100
B. Intraperitoneally in Unanesthetized Swiss Albino Mice									
Intraperitoneal	0.1	30	11	36.6	11	36.6	5	16.6	90
	0.2	30	21	70.0	0	0	7	23.3	93.3
	0.3	30	29	96.6	1	3.3	0	0	100
		90	61	67.7	12	13.3	12	13.3	94.4
C. Subcutaneously in Unanesthetized Swiss Albino Mice									
Subcutaneous	0.2	37	0	0	0	0	2	5.4	5.4

TABLE 2.—*Mortality Resulting From Intraperitoneal Injection of 0.2 CC of Prepolymerized Methyl 2-Cyanoacrylate in Swiss Albino Mice*

No. of Mice	Dead 24 Hr		Dead 24-48 Hr		Dead 48 Hr-1 Wk		% Dead
	No.	%	No.	%	No.	%	
20	17	85	2	10	1	5	100

were quiet and huddled in the corners of their cages but were easily irritated. This appearance continued until death. The survivors regained their normal appearance in four or five days.

In a total of 90 mice injected intraperitoneally with varying doses of cement, the over-all mortality was 94% (Table 1, B).

The plastic was uniformly lethal within 48 hours in 30 mice given 0.3 cc of methyl 2-cyanoacrylate intraperitoneally. Those mice receiving 0.2 cc intraperitoneally showed a 94% mortality after one week, and of those injected with 0.1 cc intraperitoneally, 90% died within one week.

Although the minimum lethal dose remains unknown, greater survival with the lower dose suggests that it is being approached.

Group 3.—A marked decrease in mortality resulted in the group of mice injected subcutaneously as compared with the animals receiving plastic by other routes. The total mortality was 5.4% in 37 mice, and all the succumbing animals died between 48 hours and one week after injection (Table 1, C).

Group 4.—In 20 mice, 0.2 cc of the fully polymerized plastic was injected intraperitoneally. One week later, all the animals were dead. The polymerization reaction itself is no longer suspect as responsible for death (Table 2).

Group 5.—Age did not affect the results of adhesive injection. Both groups of different ages, five weanlings and five six-month-old mice, that received 0.2 cc of plastic died within 48 hours.

Group 6.—Methyl 2-cyanoacrylate is lethal to other laboratory animals in addition to mice. Two groups of ten white rats each received 0.005 cc/gm and 0.01 cc/gm of body weight intraperitoneally. They showed a mortality of 80% and 90%, respectively (Table 3).

Group 7.—Sixty mice served as controls for the intraperitoneal and subcutaneous injections, for pentobarbital anesthesia and laparotomy. They received saline instead of plastic, and all survived (Table 4).

Comment

These results demonstrate the lethality of injecting methyl 2-cyanoacrylate into the peritoneal cavity of mice and rats. The reaction of the animals following injection of the adhesive suggests that the mechanism of death, undefined at present, is a systemic one. Several possibilities appear worthy of discussion.

Certainly, death could result from electrolyte imbalance. The fluid and electrolyte levels of body fluids after the rapid polymerization of the monomer in the peritoneal cavity remain undetermined. Autopsied mice, however, presented normal amounts of peritoneal fluid. Confirmation of this hypothesis awaits more complete studies of the changes associated with polymerization of plastics in tissues.

TABLE 3.—*Mortality Resulting From Intraperitoneal Injection of Methyl-Alpha-Cyanoacrylate in White Laboratory Rats*

Amount Injected	No. of Rats	% Dead 24 Hr	% Dead 24-48 Hr	% Dead 48 Hr-1 Wk	% Dead 1 Wk
0.005 cc/gm	10	0	10	80	90
0.01 cc/gm	10	40	30	10	80

TABLE 4.—*Control Animals: Results of Injection of 0.2 CC of Isotonic Saline in Swiss Albino Mice*

Site	No. of Mice	% Dead in 1 Wk
Subcutaneous	20	0
Intraperitoneal	30	0
Intraperitoneal, after pentobarbital anesthesia and after laparotomy	10	0

Autopsy of the mice also ruled out fatal bowel obstruction by demonstrating patent bowel lumens and absence of bowel distention. Although cultures were not obtained, lethal peritonitis appears improbable in these mice. Autopsy yielded no evidence of peritonitis, and the adhesives are self-sterilizing.

The difference in mortality between the groups of mice injected subcutaneously and those injected intraperitoneally suggests that possibly the absorption rate and detoxification capacity of each site determine survival.

The addition of plasticizers accounts for much of the toxicity observed after the implantation of plastics. However, the adhesive used here supposedly contains only the pure monomer. Nathan and co-workers [2] found that the tissue reaction observed in their experiments with AD/here did not result from the plasticizer which the original form of AD/here contained. These studies point to the monomer as responsible for toxicity.

Two previous studies described the tissue reaction noted after implantation of methyl 2-cyanoacrylate in the liver and the kidney.[8,9] This constitutes a most important disadvantage. Histological examination was carried out at varied intervals of time from three hours to 11 months after implantation. The observed reaction consists of an initial large focal area of acute necrosis and hemorrhage following application of the plastic over the cut surface. The parenchyma immediately underlying this area shows acute congestion. A marked inflammatory response occurs during the first 24 hours. By two weeks, organization of the necrotic area begins. Young fibroconnective tissue and foreign-body cells appear. Connective tissue begins to encapsulate the adhesive about this time. After one month the adhesive becomes completely circumscribed by connective tissue and foreign-body granulomas. A chronic inflammatory response predominates. Between 2 and 11 months after application of the adhesive, fibrosis around the plastic increases. The chronic inflammatory reaction gradually decreases with a diminution of foreign-body granulomas. In the kidney, calcification appears, and squamous epithelium presumably from the incised calyceal system may line the inner wall of the fibrotic capsule to the adhesive.

If the lethal dose per unit of body weight given to these laboratory animals is extrapolated to dogs or man, the amount of adhesive necessary for surgical use remains far below the amount producing death in this study. The adhesive will probably be needed in minute amounts for clinical use but the disquieting presence of toxicity and of a significant tissue reaction urges extreme caution when implantation of this adhesive is entertained in humans.

The absence of studies related to the tumor-producing potential of this particular

TABLE 5.—*Summary of Results Obtained in Control Animals and Those Receiving Methyl 2-Cyanoacrylate by Various Routes*

Site, Dose	No. of Animals	% Dead 24 Hr	% Dead 24-48 Hr	% Dead 48 Hr-1 Wk	% Dead 1 Wk
Controls, 0.2 cc saline, all routes	60	0	0	0	0
Liver, 0.2 cc	24	66.6	0	33.4	100
Intraperitoneal, all doses	90	67.7	13.3	13.3	94.3
Subcutaneous, 0.2 cc	37	0	0	5.4	5.4
Prepolymerized, 0.2 cc intraperitoneally	20	85	10	5	100
Rats:					
0.005 cc/gm	10	0	10	80	90
0.01 cc/gm	10	40	30	10	80

plastic constitutes an additional source of concern. Such experiments are under way in our laboratory with the full realization that it is difficult to transpose results obtained in animals to humans. The fact that histologically the plastic diminishes with the passage of time and disappears points out the glaring lack of knowledge related to the field of plastic metabolism and the need for further research in the metabolism of implanted plastics.

At present, methyl 2-cyanoacrylate appears to be a valuable experimental starting point for the ultimate development of a reliable, nontoxic plastic of sufficient tissue adherence to permit nonsuture surgery.

Summary

Recent studies have defined the experimental value of methyl 2-cyanoacrylate as a new rapidly polymerizing, promising adhesive. It now appears that the use of this plastic presents the disadvantage of a significant tissue reaction as well as a possible lethal effect at least in small laboratory animals.

A large portion of this work was performed under the immediate direction of Dr. Harlan I. Firminger. Mrs. Anne Johnson and Mr. George E. Moore gave technical assistance.

George H. Yeager, MD, Professor of Clinical Surgery, University Hospital, University of Maryland, Baltimore 1, Md.

REFERENCES

1. Coover, H. W., Jr.; Joyner, F. B.; Shearer, N. H.; and Wicker, T. H., Jr.: Chemistry and Performance of Cyanoacrylate Adhesives, Soc Plast Eng J 15:413, 1959.

2. Nathan, H. S.; Nachlas, M. M.; Solomon, R. D.; Halpern, B. D.; and Seligman, A. M.: Nonsuture Closure of Arterial Incisions Using a Rapidly-Polymerizing Adhesive, Ann Surg 152:648, 1960.

3. Healey, J. E., Jr.; Clark, R. L.; Gallager, H. S.; O'Neill, P.; and Sheena, K. S.: Nonsuture Repair of Blood Vessels, Ann Surg 155:817, 1962.

4. Healey, J. E., Jr.; Sheena, K. S.; Gallager, H. S.; Clark, R. L.; and O'Neill, P.: The Use of a Plastic Adhesive in the Technique of Bronchial Closure, Surg Forum 13:153, 1962.

5. O'Neill, P.; Healey, J. E., Jr.; Clark, R. L.; and Gallager, H. S.: Nonsuture Intestinal Anastomosis, Amer J Surg 104:761, 1962.

6. Lighterman, I., and Farrell, J. J.: Treatment of Experimentally Induced Mandibular Fractures with Plastic Polymers, Surg Forum 13:466, 1962.

7. Fischl, R. A.: An Adhesive for Primary Closure of Skin Incisions, Plast Reconstr Surg 30:607, 1962.

8. Just-Viera, J. O.; Puron-del Aguila, R.; and Yeager, G. H.: Control of Hemorrhage From the Liver Without the Use of Sutures or Clamps: Preliminary Report, Amer Surg 28:754, 1962.

9. Just-Viera, J. O.; Puron-dell Aguila, R.; and Yeager, G. H.: Experimental Control of Renal Hemorrhage by the Use of a Rapidly Polymerizing Adhesive, presented at the Southern Surgical Association Meeting, Boca Raton, Fla, 1962.

Left Superior Vena Cava With Anomalous Inferior Vena Cava

Report of a Case With Associated Atrial Septal Defect and Pulmonic Stenosis, Successfully Corrected

T. SUNADA
K. INADA
M. NAKANISHI
AND
Y. KOMOTO
OKAYAMA, JAPAN

Persistent left superior vena cava has been merely a medical curiosity until recent years because it is uncommon and has little influence on hemodynamics. However, recent advances in cardiac surgery have brought the condition to prominence. It is important to recognize its existence before open heart surgery, for special arrangements have to be made for venous cannulation to get a completely dry field during total bypass.

Eight cases of congenital heart disease associated with persistent left superior vena cava were found in about 400 cases of congenital heart disease encountered in the Second Surgical Division of Okayama University Medical School. The superior vena cava was present on both sides in seven; in the case reported here, only a left superior vena cava was present with an absent normal inferior vena cava. Associated anomalies, atrial septal defect and pulmonic stenosis, were corrected under direct vision with the aid of extracorporeal circulation.

Report of Case

An eight-year-old boy was admitted to the hospital with complaints of shortness of breath and cyanosis on exertion. He was known to have heart disease since birth. He has had frequent episodes of respiratory infection, and development was retarded. He became gradually inactive during the last year, and six months prior to admission the parents noticed cyanosis and squatting on exertion.

Physical examination revealed an alert boy, rather small for his age. There was neither

Submitted for publication March 11, 1963.

Professor of Surgery (Dr. Sunada); Assistant Professor of Surgery (Dr. Inada); Assistant in Surgery (Dr. Nakanishi, Dr. Komoto).

From the Second Surgical Division, Okayama University Medical School.

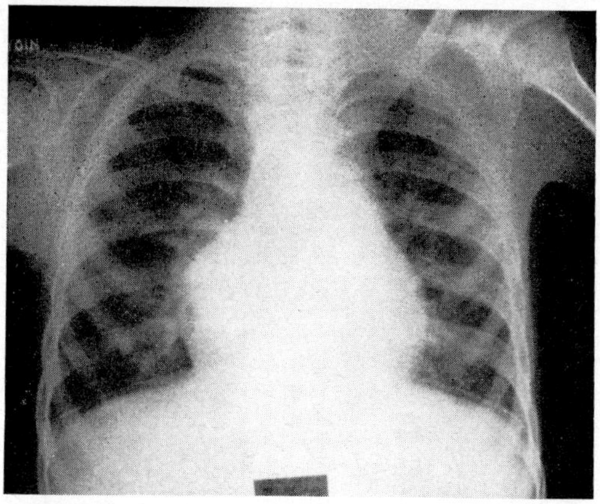

Fig 1.—Chest roentgenogram showing marked prominence of right heart margin suggestive of hypertrophy of the right atrium.

cyanosis of the lips nor clubbing of the fingers. The thoracic cage showed severe pigeon breast deformity. Cardiac impulse was not prominent and a definite thrill was palpable in the second intercostal space along the left sternal border. A harsh, grade 3-4 systolic murmur was audible all over the precordium, maximal at the pulmonic area. The second pulmonic sound was diminished.

Chest roentgenogram revealed a slightly enlarged heart displaced to the right (mesocardia). Enlargement of the right atrium was noticeable, and bronchovascular markings appeared to be increased (Fig 1).

Electrocardiogram was interpreted as right axis deviation and right ventricular hypertrophy.

The cardiac catheter via the right cubital vein entered the right atrium via the coronary sinus through a persistent left superior vena cava and was advanced into the left atrium through an atrial septal defect. The catheter via the right saphenous vein entered the left superior vena cava through the left inferior vena cava and was then advanced into the coronary sinus, right atrium, and left atrium in that order. Pressure in the right ventricle was markedly elevated, suggesting the existence of a pulmonic stenosis, although it was not possible to advance the catheter into the pulmonary artery. The hepatic vein was found to enter the right atrium at the place where normally the inferior vena cava joins.

Fig 2.—Angiocardiogram clearly showing the left superior vena cava. Cardiac catheter is present in anomalous inferior vena cava.

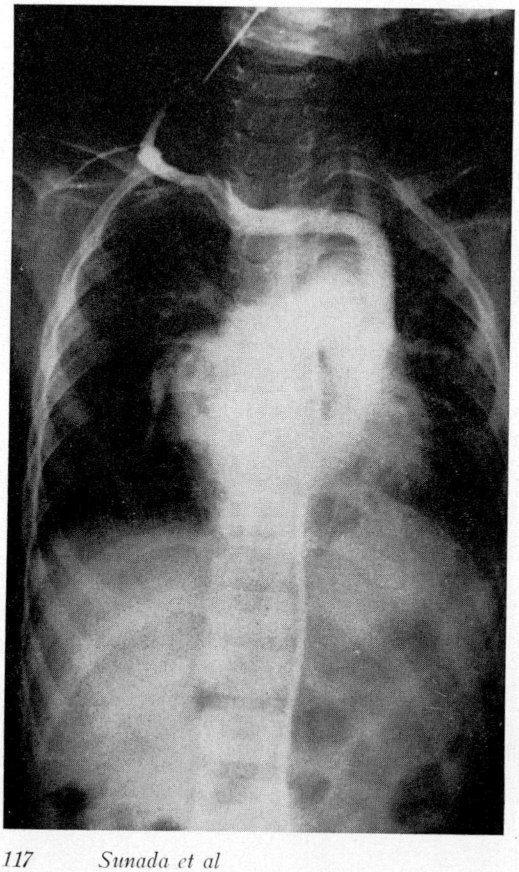

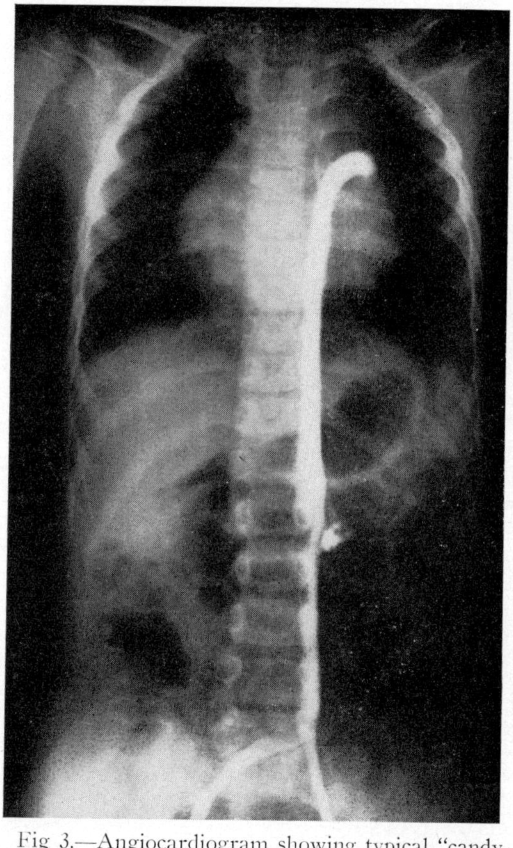

Fig 3.—Angiocardiogram showing typical "candy cane" appearance of anomalous inferior vena cava.

Angiocardiography via the right external jugular vein demonstrated a persistent left superior vena cava and absence of the right (Fig 2). Angiocardiography via both external iliac veins disclosed the absence of a normal inferior vena cava. To compensate for the absent inferior vena cava there was an enlarged hemiazygos which emptied into the left superior vena cava (Fig 3).

Operation for atrial septal defect and pulmonic stenosis was undertaken using extracorporeal circulation. A median sternotomy revealed a moderately enlarged and hypertrophied right ventricle and a prominent pulmonary artery measuring 2.8 cm in diameter compared to a relatively small aorta. No remnant of a right superior vena cava was found. The left superior vena cava and the markedly enlarged hemiazygos vein, which joined and communicated with a moderately distended coronary sinus, were found at the posterior aspect of the left atrium.

After the superior and inferior vena cava were dissected for cannulation, a catheter was introduced into the hepatic vein through the right atrial wall. A second catheter was introduced into the coronary sinus through the right atrial wall and advanced into the left superior vena cava. A third catheter was introduced into the inferior vena cava via the right external iliac vein. After venous and arterial cannulations were completed, bypass was begun. Right atriotomy revealed a large atrial septal defect of the secundum type, which was closed by a continuous suture.

After the atriotomy was closed, the pulmonary artery was incised and the fused pulmonic valve was widely opened. During complete total bypass, it was necessary to occlude the inferior vena cava intermittently near its junction with the left superior vena cava to get a completely dry operative field.

The postoperative course was complicated by intrathoracic bleeding which was controlled by thoracotomy eight hours after the first operation. On the second postoperative day the patient developed tonic, then clonic, convulsions simulating the Jackson type of epilepsy which was controlled by muscle relaxants and barbiturates. He tolerated these complications very well and made a rapid recovery after these episodes. He was discharged from the hospital on the 39th postoperative day in good condition. Follow-up examination two months later revealed no cardiac murmur.

Comment

Persistence of the left superior vena cava results from failure of obliteration of the left anterior cardinal vein at the early developmental stage of the heart. Development of the inferior vena cava is more complex compared to the superior vena cava. The variations in this developmental anomaly and the many terms for the same condition have made the subject confusing.

Persistent left superior vena cava in association with congenital heart disease is being recognized as not so rare, especially since cardiac catheterization and angiocardiographic studies have been widely used in the investigation of cardiac diseases. The incidence of left superior vena cava in congenital heart disease is said to be around 3%-4%.[1-3] However, most of them are bilateral superior vena cava, as were 39 of 46 cases in Campbell's series.[2] On the other hand, unilateral left superior vena cava is rare. Only 33 cases, including autopsy cases, had been reported up to 1954 according to Holmes.[4]

Anomalous inferior vena cava with azygos continuation or with hemiazygos continuation (Anderson [5]) is less common than persistent left superior vena cava. Kjellberg [6] gave its incidence as 0.45% (3/668), Loogen [7] as 0.2% (2/1,000) and Anderson [5] as 0.6% in congenital heart disease. Anderson collected 41 cases of this anomaly from the literature including 16 cases of his own series. The azygos vein was developed as a substitute for inferior vena cava in 18 of the cases and the hemiazygos vein in 8 cases. Of the 41 cases, there were only two where unilateral left superior vena cava and anomaly of inferior vena cava were associated. The azygos vein, as a substitute for the inferior vena cava, communicated with the right atrium in both of them. The reported case is considered to be an unusual one in this respect.

Anomalous vena cava is now an important subject from the practical point of view, for open heart surgery is becoming a routine operation in large hospitals. Kirklin [8] found 22 cases of persistent left superior vena cava at the correction of ventricular septal defects among a total 320 cases. Sirak [9] encountered five cases of this condition among 63 cases of atrial septal defect and discussed methods for cannulation of the anomalous vena cava.

It is considered easy to introduce a cannula into the left superior vena cava via the coronary sinus through the right atrial wall in our experience. However, special consideration was required for venous cannulation in the present case.

It is difficult to predict the existence of this anomaly in plain roentgenograms, although Gensini [10] emphasized the widening of the upper mediastinal shadow and Fraser [3] points out the presence of a crescentic shadow passing from the upper left border of the aortic arch toward the middle third of the left clavicle in the posteroanterior film. One should always bear this possibility in mind at the time of right heart catheterization.

Summary

A case of an anomaly of both the superior and inferior vena cava, associated with atrial septal defect and pulmonic stenosis, is reported. The superior vena cava was present only on the left side; it continued as the coronary sinus and terminated in the right atrium. The hemiazygos vein enlarged and developed as the substitute for the inferior vena cava which joined the left superior vena cava. The hepatic vein entered separately the right atrium. Associated anomalies were corrected under direct vision with extracorporeal circulation. Attention is called to anomalies of the vena cava associated with congenital heart disease, and a technique for venous cannulation in cardiopulmonary bypass is briefly discussed.

Kiyoshi Inada, MD, Assistant Professor of Surgery, Okayama University Medical School, Okayama, Japan.

REFERENCES

1. Abbott, M. E.: "Congenital Cardiac Disease," vol IV of Osler's Modern Medicine, Philadelphia: 1927.

2. Campbell, M., and Deucher, D. C.: The Left-Sided Superior Vena Cava, Brit Heart J 16:423, 1954.

3. Fraser, R. S.; Dvorkin, J.; Rossall, R. E.; and Eidem, R.: Left Superior Vena Cava, Amer J Med 31:711, 1961.

4. Holmes, T. W., Jr.: Unilateral Left Superior Vena Cava: Incidence and Technique for Cardiopulmonary Bypass, J Thorac Cardiov Surg 44:253, 1962.

5. Anderson, R. C.; Adams, P., Jr.; and Burke, B.: Anomalous Inferior Vena Cava With Azygos Continuation (Infrahepatic Interruption of the Inferior Vena Cava), J Pediat 59:370, 1961.

6. Kjellberg, S. R.; Mannheimer, E.; Rudhe, U.; and Johnson, B.: Diagnosis of Congenital Heart Disease, ed 2, Chicago: The Year Book Medical Publishers, Inc., 1959, p 12.

7. Loogen, F., and Rippert, R.: Anomalien der grossen Körper- und Lungenvenen, Z Kreislaufforsch 47:677, 1958.

8. Kirklin, J. W.; McGoon, D. C.; and DuShane, J. W.: Surgical Treatment of Ventricular Septal Defect, J Thorac Cardiov Surg 40:763, 1960.

9. Sirak, H. D.: The Repair of Interatrial Defects Through a Right Anterolateral Thoracotomy: A Method for Controlling a Persistent Left Superior Vena Cava, Amer J Surg 100:455, 1960.

10. Gensini, G.; Caldini, P.; Casaccio, F.; and Blount, S. G.: Persistent Left Superior Vena Cava, Amer J Cardiol 4:677, 1959.

Popliteal Aneurysm With Osteochondroma of the Femur

LT GASPAR W. ANASTASI, MC, USN
CAPT HASKELL M. WERTHEIMER
MC, USN
AND
LT JAMES R. BROWN, MC, USN
ST ALBANS, NY

This paper might have been more accurately entitled "An Unusual Complication of the Twist," for it was shortly after doing "the twist" that the patient began to complain of pain in the popliteal fossa.

Arterial aneurysms of the lower extremity occur infrequently. Mills, at the Mayo Clinic, reported an incidence of only 3.5% in 396 cases of aneurysms.[1] Even so, the popliteal artery is the vessel most commonly the site of peripheral aneurysm formation.[2] The commonest etiologic factor in such aneurysms is arteriosclerosis.[3] In 100 cases reviewed by Gifford, Hines, and Janes,[4] 32 cases were associated with arteriosclerosis, 3 with syphilis, 1 with mycotic infection, and 1 with trauma. No case of popliteal aneurysm associated with osteochondroma or exostosis of the femur was reported by this group of investigators. Brailsford,[5] in his radiology textbook, makes references to a case; however, a detailed case report does not appear in the literature until 1953 when Milroy Paul[6] described a case. Only four other cases have been reported since that time (see Table).

The mechanism of production of such a false aneurysm needs explanation. It has been postulated[7] that a deflection in the femoral vessel due to the presence of an osteochondroma on the femur leads to eventual eroding of the vascular wall. This slow eroding process plus some form of vigorous exercise, such as "the twist" or, as Hudson reported in his case,[8] vigorous bicycling may lead to the formation of either a popliteal aneurysm or an arteriovenous (AV) fistula.

These patients usually present with the complaint of pain and swelling in the popliteal area. There may also be inter-

Submitted for publication March 14, 1963.

Resident in Surgery (Lt Anastasi); Chief of Surgery (Capt Wertheimer); Department of Radiology (Lt Brown).

From the Departments of Surgery and Radiology, United States Naval Hospital.

The opinions expressed herein are those of the authors and do not necessarily reflect the views of the Navy Department.

Previous Cases of Popliteal Aneurysm Associated With Osteochondroma of the Femur

Author *	Age, Yr & Sex	History & Physical Findings	Dorsalis Pedis Pulse	Predisposing Factors	Treatment
Brailsford (5)	19, F	Not given			
Paul (6)	21, M	Painful swelling behind knee for 17 days, multiple osteochondromas	None	No trauma or exercise	Endo-aneurysmorrhaphy & excision of osteochondroma
Chirls (7)	12, M	Pain for 2 wk., single osteochondroma	Diminished	No trauma or exercise	Resection of aneurysm & excision of exostosis
Hudson (8)	14, M	Pain for 2 wk., multiple osteochondromas	Good	Vigorous bicycling	Suture rent in vessel & resection of exostosis
Lesser (10)	14, M	Pain for 6 yr., single osteochondroma	None	Fractured osteochondroma	End-to-end anastamosis & resection of exostosis
Denman (11)	9, M	Pain for 3 mo., multiple congenital osteochondromas	Good	Vigorous exercise'	End-to-end anastamosis & resection

* Parentheses indicate reference numbers.

mittent claudication and the absence of any history of trauma. The physical findings might reveal a pulsating mass in the popliteal fossa and the absence of an ankle pulse. If left untreated, pressure on the popliteal vessel due to the aneurysm might well lead to gangrene. A more common occurrence is the formation of a thrombus. Embolic phenomenon has also been reported. Lord [9] states that the possibility of rupture and eventual death of the patient also exists. A popliteal aneurysm, according to Janes and associates,[4] is a sinister harbinger of a medical catastrophe in which neither the patient nor his physician should rest easily until this threat to life and limb is surgically extirpated or obliterated. In view of the formidable complications, proper surgical treatment becomes exigent.

Over the years, many surgical procedures have been attempted for the correction of this condition. Two procedures which have weathered the test of time are the Matas procedure and simple ligation of the vessel. Matas performed the first endo-aneurysmorrhaphy in 1881. According to Lord, the Matas procedure in his cases was reserved for those patients with no demonstrable dorsalis pedis pulse. The remainder of his cases were treated with resection of the aneurysm and the use of a venous graft. The treatment in the case presented here was simple excision of the aneurysm, removal of the exostosis, and closure of the defect in the vessel wall with suitable suture material.

Arteriography is an important adjunct in diagnosis of these lesions. Diagnosis made on the basis of the patient's complaints and his physical findings was, in the five reported cases of popliteal aneurysms due to osteochondroma, always confirmed with femoral arteriography. In our case, films from the femoral arteriogram on anterior-posterior projection demonstrated displacement of the popliteal artery laterally just as it passes through the adductor canal with a fine jet of contrast material originating from its medial margin (Fig 1). Films of the popliteal region were taken at a rate of two per second for a period of six seconds. On the film presented in Fig 2, we see that there is a direct relation between the aneurysm and the exostosis. The method of percutaneous arteriography employed has been in almost constant use at the St. Albans Naval Hospital since its introduction in 1958. In 206 such procedures done at this hospital, transient spasm was noted in approximately ten cases, but only in one case was it of significant severity so that a temporary sympathetic block had to be performed. There were no permanent sequelae in any of these cases.

Report of a Case

The patient, a 41-year-old white male, was admitted to the St. Albans Naval Hospital with a four day history of swelling and pain in the left popliteal area exacerbated by walking and straightening of the left leg. The only pertinent finding in the past

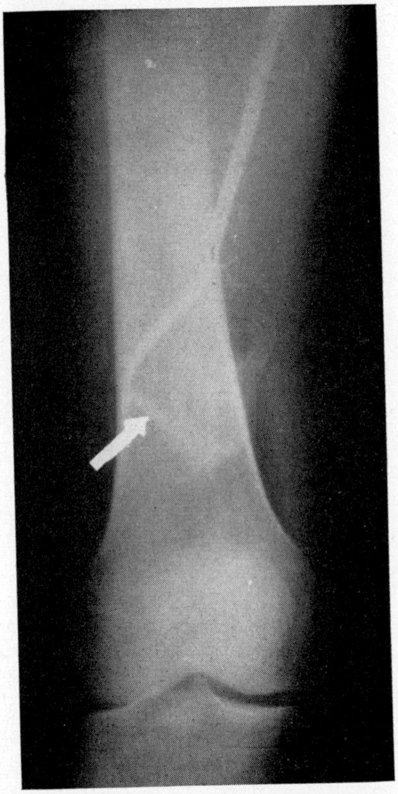

Fig 1.—The artery is well visualized with contrast material and is displaced laterally in the region of the exostosis. A fine jet of contract material is seen to escape from the medial wall of the artery (arrow).

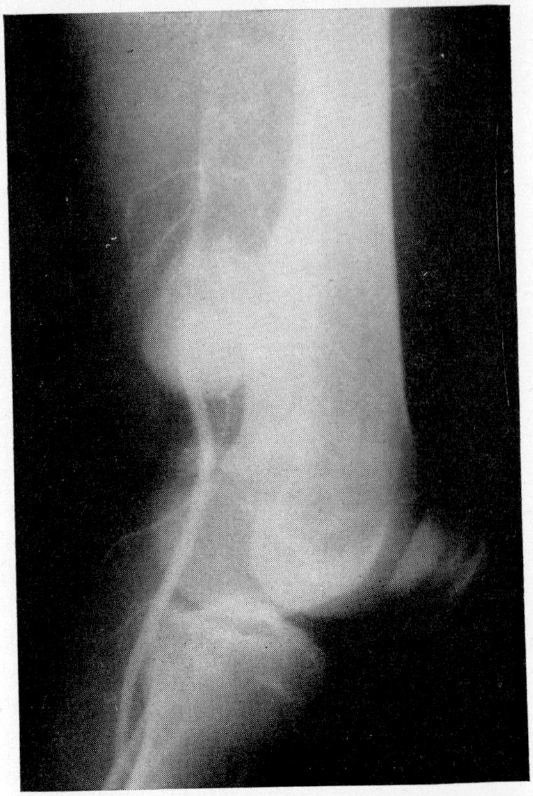

Fig 2.—Lateral film with contrast filled artery and aneurysmal sac.

history was that ten days prior to admission he was at a party where he was doing "the twist." Two days after doing this dance, he states he felt pain in the left knee. No other history of trauma could be elicited.

The physical examination revealed a Caucasian male in good health. There was a pulsating mass in the left popliteal area which exhibited a bruit on auscultation. The left leg was swollen but no calf tenderness was elicited. There were good ankle pulses. A plain film revealed a bony exostosis on the posteromedial margin of the distal femur (Fig 3). An arteriogram of the femoral artery was done subsequently and revealed a popliteal aneurysm and osteochondroma of the femur.

Operation was performed on the tenth hospital day when it became apparent that the popliteal mass was enlarging. Under spinal anesthesia, an inverted S-shaped incision was made along the posteromedial aspect of the left leg. Dissection was done in the area of Hunter's Canal. Once the false aneurysm and the vessels were identified, tapes were placed on the vessels above and below the aneurysm. The aneurysm sac was then dissected free and excised. A small perforation in the vessel opposite the osteochondroma was repaired with 5-0 black arterial silk. The bony lesion was removed with an osteotome. Erosion of that area of the exostosis which was in contact with the artery was noted (Fig 4). The leg was immobilized with a posterior splint. Postoperatively the ankle pulse remained good. The patient was ambulating by the 12th postoperative day. The remainder of his recovery was essentially uneventful.

Summary

Popliteal aneurysm associated with osteochondroma of the femur is discussed. A relationship between vigorous exercise such as doing "the twist" and the formation of such an aneurysm is reported.

A review of the literature discloses six other cases of popliteal aneurysm associated with osteochondroma.

The diagnosis and surgical treatment are discussed.

Lt G. W. Anastasi, MC, USN, US Naval Hospital, St. Albans, LI, 25, NY.

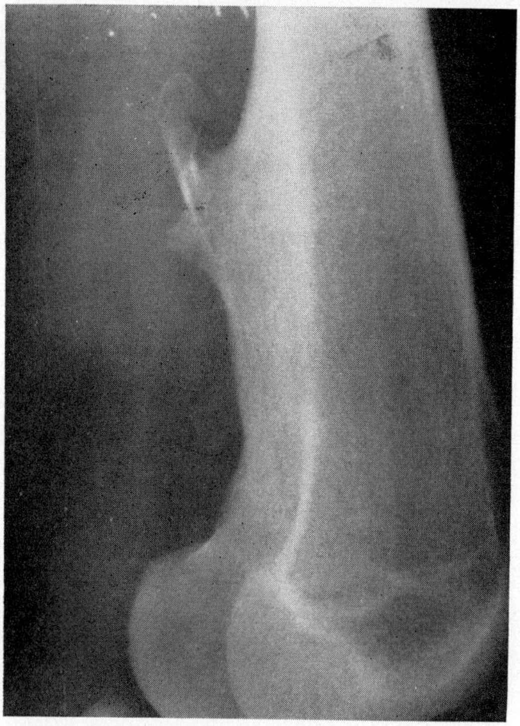

Fig 3.—Large exostosis on posteromedial surface of lower end of femur. The lower component shows localized erosion and sharpening. It is associated with a large soft tissue density.

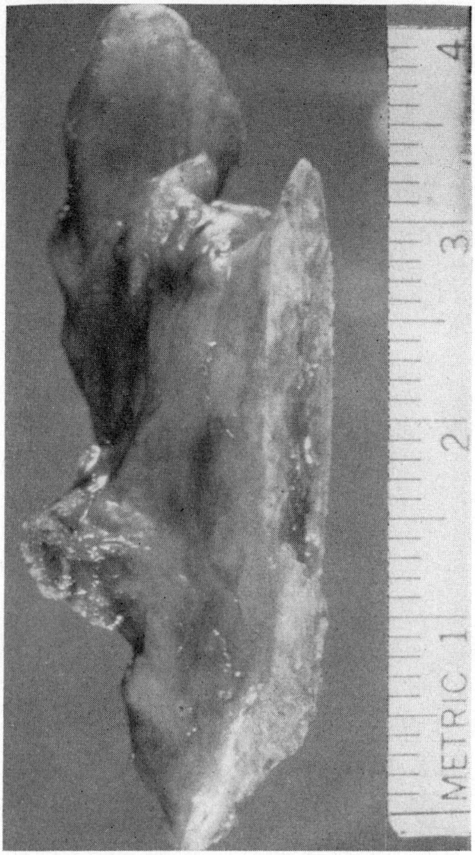

Fig 4.—Gross specimen removed at time of surgery reveals the exostosis with its cartilagenous cap. There is an obvious erosion and sharpening of the tip with loss of most of the cartilagenous cap.

REFERENCES

1. Mills, J. H., and Horton, B. T.: Clinical Aspects of Aneurysms, Arch Intern Med 62:949, 1938.

2. Lloyd, J. T.: Traumatic Peripheral Aneurysms, Amer J Surg 93:755-764, 1957.

3. Crawford, E. S.; DeBakey, M. E.; and Cooley, D. A.: Surgical Considerations of Peripheral Arterial Aneurysms, AMA Arch Surg 78:236-238, 1959.

4. Gifford, R. W., Jr.; Hines, E. A., Jr.; and Janes, J. M.: An Analysis and Follow-Up Study of 100 Popliteal Aneurysms, Surgery 33:284-293, 1953.

5. Brailsford, J. F.: Radiology of Bones and Joints, ed 5, Baltimore: The Williams & Wilkins Company, 1953, p 241.

6. Paul, M.: Aneurysm of the Popliteal Artery From Perforation by a Cancellous Exostosis of the Femur: Report of a Case, J Bone Joint Surg (Amer) 35B:270-271, 1953.

7. Chirls, M.; Litchman, H.; and Grant, A. D.: Osteochondroma of the Femur Involving the Popliteal Artery: Case Report, Bull Hosp Joint Dis 22:150-152, 1961.

8. Hudson, O. C.: Traumatic Aneurysm of the Popliteal Artery Due to Osteochondroma, Amer J Surg 90:528-530, 1955.

9. Lord, J. W., Jr.: Clinical Behavior and Operative Management of Popliteal Aneurysms, JAMA 163:1102-1106, 1957.

10. Lesser, A. J., and Greeley, C. E.: Femoropopliteal Arteriovenous Aneurysm Caused by Fractured Osteochondroma of the Femur, JAMA 167:1830-1832, 1958.

11. Denman, F. R.; Shindler, T. O.; Hampton, J.; and Hanson, L.: Aneurysm of the Popliteal Artery Caused by Osteochondroma of the Femur, J Bone Joint Surg (Amer) 41A:1526-1528, 1959.

Low-Flow Fail-Safe Intra-Arterial Infusion

THOMAS S. NELSEN, MD; EDWIN H. EIGENBRODT; AND MALCOLM A. BAGSHAW, MD, PALO ALTO, CALIF

Since the original description by Duff, Sullivan, et al [1] of intra-arterial infusion treatment of inoperable tumors of the head and neck, many methods and schedules of this type of therapy have been developed. These techniques have been applied largely to patients with inoperable head and neck tumors or with inoperable cancer in the pelvis. Recent work has produced several antitumor agents which are effective, at least temporarily, in controlling growth of tumors in man as well as in animals. Most of these agents have serious systemic toxicity, and great caution is required in their use to prevent undesired complications. The introduction of an antitumor agent into the arterial circulation of the tumor offers several distinct advantages, the greatest of which is the several-fold increase in concentration of the agent in the blood supplying the tumor as compared with the concentration in the general circulation. This relative concentration increase is approximately inversely proportional to the size of the vascular bed being infused. Furthermore, if a systemic antagonist to the agent exists, it is possible to enhance the antitumor effect by administering the chemical antagonist to the agent in question and increasing the local dose commensurately. When a suitable antagonist is available this technique tends to reduce the incidence of serious systemic complications due to agent toxicity while preserving the local effect on the neoplasm.

Anatomically, two regions of the body lend themselves admirably to local intra-arterial tumor infusion therapy. The portions of the neck and face supplied by the external carotid artery contain many neoplasms that are beyond treatment with the usual surgical or radiotherapeutic techniques; many inoperable pelvic tumors are encompassed by the distribution of the hypogastric arteries. In all of our cases, the chemotherapeutic agent, methotrexate (amethopterin) has been used as the antitumor agent in doses of 50 mg or more daily with concomitant administration of 24 mg daily of calcium leucovorin (Citrovorum Factor) (divided into four equal intramuscular doses) as a systemic antagonist. Five to ten milligrams (average daily dose) of heparin in the infusate avoids clotting within the catheters. Because of the demonstrated failure of chemotherapeutic techniques, in either isolated perfusion or infusion, to provide long-term palliation it was considered that most inoperable tumors might be best treated with concurrent radiotherapy and intra-arterial chemotherapy with the hope that the resultant antitumor effect would be additive or superadditive. This required the development of a technique of infusion which would allow daily transport of the patient anywhere in the hospital (eg, to radiotherapy) without causing difficulty with the pumping system or clotting within the catheters.

In the ten years since Sullivan's description, several methods of infusion of antitumor agents have been developed and described. Gravity infusion has been successfully employed by elevation of the fluid reservoir high enough to overcome the arterial pressure in the catheter.[2] This technique is the simplest and cheapest method and avoids the possibility of air embolism inherent in most pumping systems. It requires that the drug be diluted into relatively large volumes of solution and, in most hos-

Submitted for publication March 14, 1963.

From the departments of Surgery and Radiology, Stanford University.

This work was supported by USPHS grant No. 61-94-C5838.

pitals, that special provision be made for the great elevation of the reservoir necessary to overcome the arterial pressure. This has been accomplished by modification of the room ceiling, placement of the reservoirs in a stairwell, etc. It has been customary to assign special nurses to observe such reservoirs, often not visible from the patient's bed. Transport of patients being infused by gravity is difficult at best and usually requires temporary disconnection of the system with the possibility of complications.

The alternative techniques largely involve the use of devices, such as the Bowman or Barron pumps,[3] that propel the fluid through tubing indirectly with mechanical fingers or rotors. The major difficulties found with these pumping systems are high cost, serious danger of air embolism if the reservoir becomes empty, more frequent blowout of connections with resultant hemorrhage, somewhat critical tubing requirements to prevent back flow, pump failure, noise, and in the case of the larger pumps, restriction of the patient to his bed or to a portion of his room during the course of the infusion which often lasts for several weeks. On the other hand, pumping systems provide relatively constant flow rates, an important feature. Recently, Skinner et al[4] described an infusion method using a pneumatic pump compressing a closed, fluid-filled system which has many advantages, particularly simplicity and economy. A constant flow rate is difficult to obtain from such a system without large volumes of solution and a relatively large air reservoir or frequent pneumatic adjustment.

The following requirements are considered desirable for an ideal intra-arterial infusion system at the present time.

1. The equipment should be designed to provide fail-safe operation. Complications due to mechanical failure, electrical failure, or human error should be prevented by proper design. Under no circumstances should the mechanism be capable of producing air embolism. Hemorrhage due to mechanical failure should be impossible.

2. The infusion system should be small, lightweight, easy to operate, and transportable to provide patient mobility, be easily observed by physician, nurse, and patient, and be usable in any hospital room without disturbance of other patients.

3. The flow rate of the infusate should be constant regardless of arterial pressure, line voltage, reservoir level, change of cross sectional area of the tubing, or other variables.

4. The flow rate should be as low as is consistent with uniform delivery of drug to allow dilution of the drug with the patient's blood rather than electrolyte solution and to allow even distribution of drug throughout the vascular bed.

The following method was developed with the above criteria in mind.

Method

The surgical techniques for insertion of the infusion catheters have been well reviewed by Sullivan. Our preference is for introduction of the catheter into the external carotid artery under direct vision through the stump of the divided superior thyroid artery. The catheter material of choice has been polyvinyl tubing of 0.044 in. inside diameter in 8 ft. lengths to provide patient mobility. The tubing is introduced into the external carotid artery approximately 1 cm so that its tip is well below the orifices of

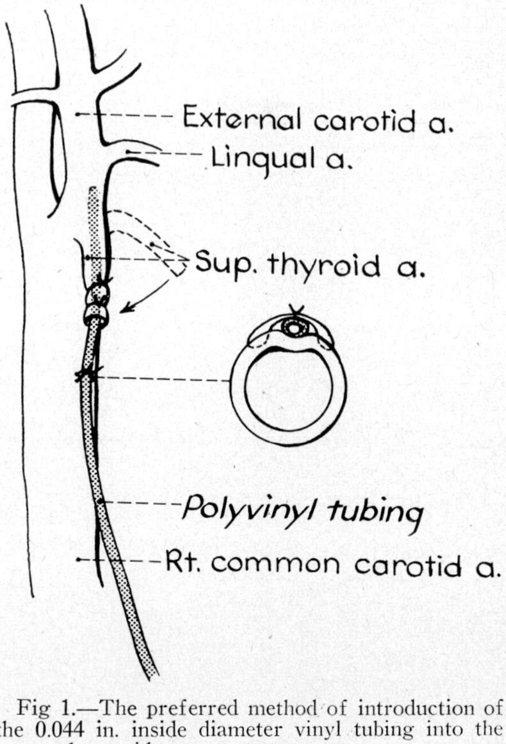

Fig 1.—The preferred method of introduction of the 0.044 in. inside diameter vinyl tubing into the external carotid artery.

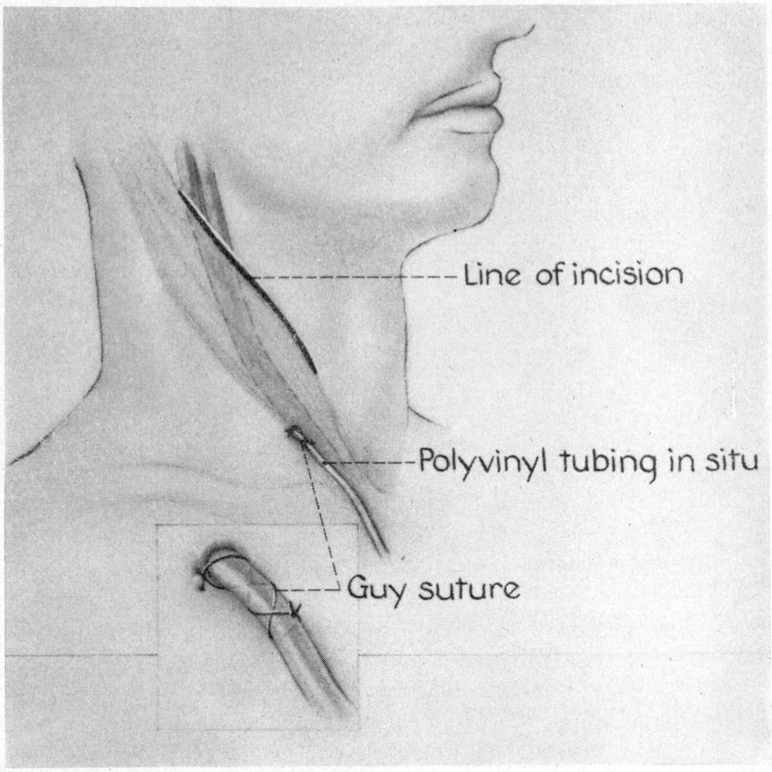

Fig 2.—Details of surgical wound and separate exit wound for infusion catheter.

the other branches of the external carotid artery. Anchor sutures are always placed to avoid subsequent change of position (Fig 1). If the superior thyroid artery cannot be cannulated, a small arteriotomy is made in the external carotid at the level of the superior thyroid artery origin. The tubing is led separately through the tissues and skin of

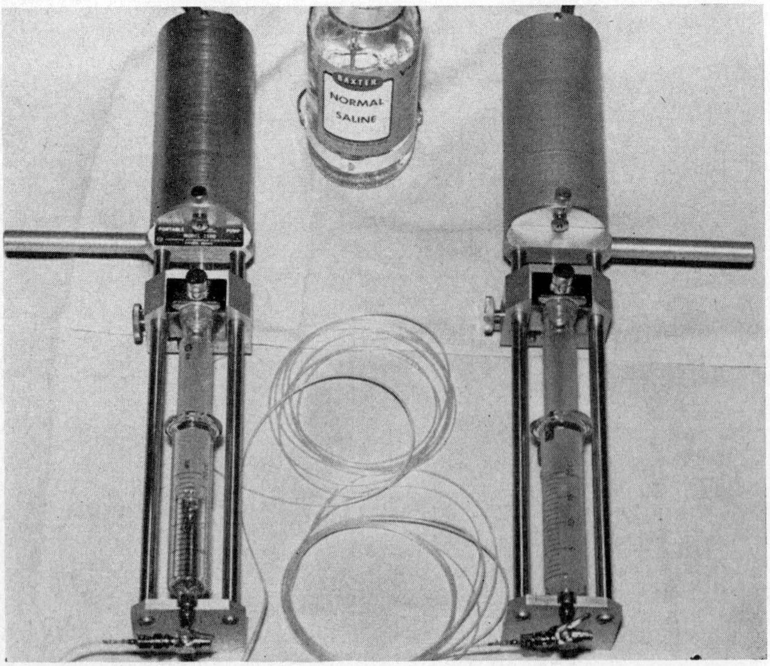

Fig 3.—Pumps, syringes, connections, reservoir, and tubing for bilateral intra-arterial infusion.

the neck with a trochar (a No. 13 needle) away from the surgical wound, and a guy suture is placed in the skin (Fig 2). This has permitted better healing of the surgical wounds.

If circumstances mitigate against direct surgical exposure of the carotid arteries, retrograde introduction of the catheters through the superficial temporal arteries has proved efficacious. This method provides much less security of placement due to variation in length of vessels and/or tubing, even if the initial placement is considered correct by angiography or fluorescein distribution studies.

For pelvic neoplasms, the catheters are introduced into the hypogastric arteries by direct arteriotomy and secured in position with sutures of vascular silk.

Each catheter is attached to a No. 18 blunt needle and connected to a 20 ml syringe through a three-way stopcock, all fittings be-

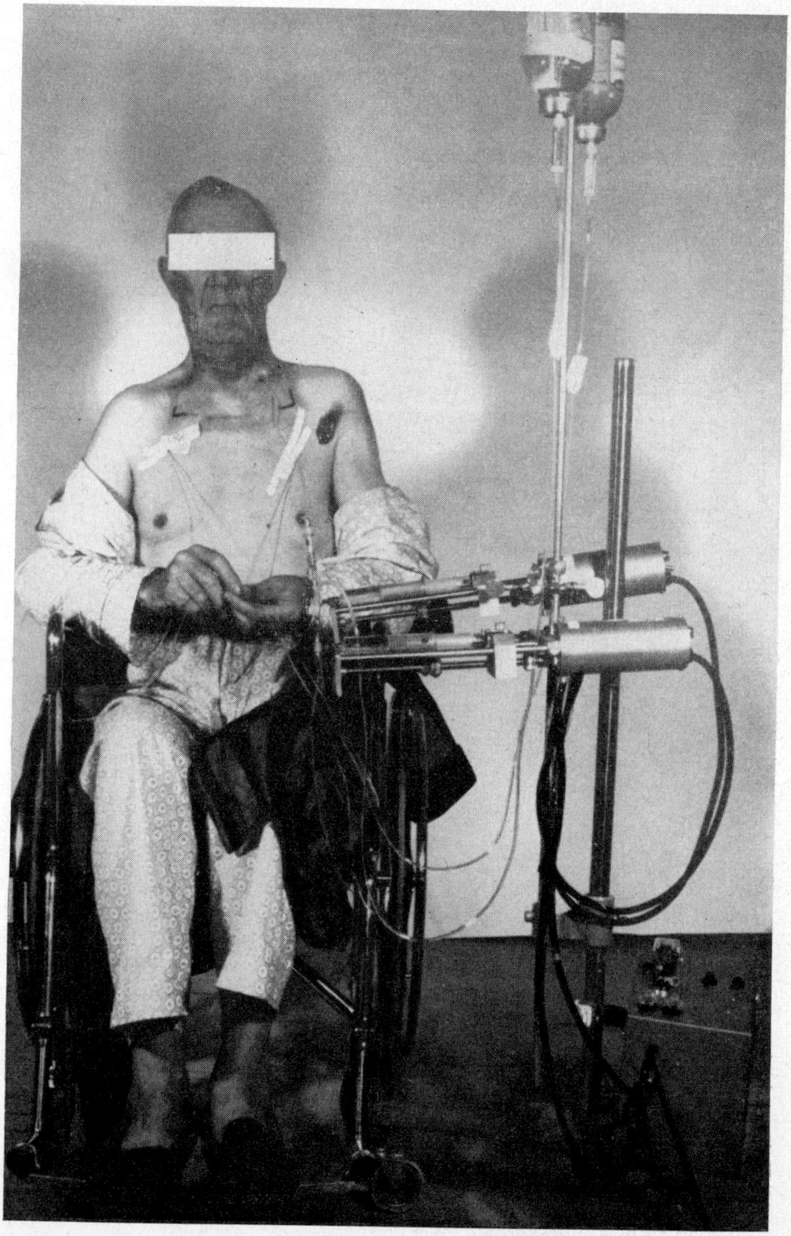

Fig 4.—Patient undergoing intra-arterial infusion treatment. The pumps, reservoirs, and emergency power supply are mounted on an ordinary intravenous standard.

ing of the Luer-Lok type. A bottle of sterile saline containing 40 mg/liter of heparin is attached to the third connection of the three-way stopcock. This saline reservoir is used for flushing as well as for filling the syringes during periods when antitumor drug is not being infused.

The syringe becomes the cylinder and piston of the infusion pump by placement in a mechanical drive system * powered by a synchronous motor (Fig 3). This mechanism delivers approximately 2.5 ml/hr from a 20 ml syringe through reduction gears. The pumps are quiet, require only a few watts of power, and run at a constant rate. Adjustable limit stops prevent syringe breakage or leakage if personnel fail to refill the syringe each eight hours. The light weight and small size of the system allow attachment of pumps and reservoirs to intravenous standards in regular use. An emergency automatic switching power supply is mounted on the base of the stand to allow uninterrupted operation of the pumps during transport or accidental disconnection of electric power (Fig 4).

One to three days after insertion we confirm the placement of the catheters by injecting 1-2 cc of fluorescein sodium in each catheter and observing the distribution with an ultraviolet light source. Arteriography at the time of surgery is used only in exceptional circumstances. For patients undergoing bilateral infusion the daily dose of methotrexate (50 mg/day) is divided into equal parts and placed in two syringes which are inserted into the pumps each morning. The usual treatment schedule we use is to give the methotrexate over an eight-hour period during the day. During the rest of the 24-hour period heparinized saline from the reservoirs is used to fill the syringes. The catheters are withdrawn on the ward upon completion of therapy.

* Model No. 1100 Harvard Apparatus Co.

Comment

During the past 18 months, this technique has been employed in the treatment of 23 patients without major complication. We have been pleased to find that patients and equipment can be well cared for by the regular floor nurses. The simplified design and auxiliary power source provide patient freedom of motion comparable to that of patients on long-term intravenous therapy. The patients treated have received from 500 mg to 2,000 mg (10 to 40 treatment days) of methotrexate as a course of chemotherapy, usually combined with radiotherapy. Other chemotherapeutic agents have not been used. Although one breakdown in the pumping apparatus occurred, because of the fail-safe design of the drive mechanism no complication ensued. Evaluation of the efficacy of this treatment program will be published after a suitable observation period has elapsed.

Summary

A simple, reliable, low-flow technique for constant rate intra-arterial infusion utilizing mechanical pumps is described. This technique has now been used in 23 patients without serious complication.

Thomas S. Nelsen, MD, Department of Surgery, Stanford Medical Center, Palo Alto, Calif.

REFERENCES

1. Duff, J. K.; Sullivan, R. D.; Miller, E.; Ulm, A. H.; Clarkson, B. D.; and Clifford, P.: Antimetabolite-Metabolite Cancer Chemotherapy Using Continuous Intra-Arterial Methotrexate With Intermittent Intramuscular Citrovorum Factor, Cancer 14:744 (July-Aug) 1961.

2. Nahum, A. M., and Rochlin, D. B.: Regional Arterial Chemotherapy of Cancer of the Head and Neck, Surg Gynec Obstet 115:478-483 (Oct) 1962.

3. Sullivan, R. D.; Miller, E.; and Sikes, M. P.: Antimetabolite-Metabolite Combination Cancer Chemotherapy, Cancer 12:1248 (Nov-Dec) 1959.

4. Skinner, D. B.; Herbst, L.; Austen, W. G.; and Raker, J. W.: A Simplified Technique of Intra-Arterial Infusion for Regional Chemotherapy, Surg Gynec Obstet 115:242-244 (Aug) 1962.

Acute Carpal Tunnel Syndrome

Median Artery Thrombosis as Cause

PRESTON J. BURNHAM, MD
SALT LAKE CITY

Anatomy

The carpal canal or tunnel conducts the long flexor tendons and the median nerve from the anterior compartment of the forearm into the central compartment of the palm. It is bounded by the volar transverse carpal ligament (flexor retinaculum) anteriorly and an arch formed by the carpal bone on the other three sides. On the radial side the ligament is attached to the tubercle of the navicular and the ridge on the greater multangular and, on the ulnar side, to the pisiform and the hook of the hamate. The ligament is continuous along its proximal margin with the deep fascia of the forearm, and it merges distally with the palmar fascia.

This tunnel is, therefore, bounded by inelastic ligamentous tissue and bone. The close mechanical tolerance in this tunnel gives rise to increased pressure upon its contents when enlargement of any of the enclosed tissue by edema of trauma or disturbance of homeostasis occurs, when there is encroachment of the tunnel space by overgrowth or dislocation of bone into it, extensive thickening of the ligament, or by neoplasms that may invade the tunnel confines.

The causes of this syndrome are legion and may be grouped under some general headings:

Intrinsic

Edema of the nerve due to:

1. External trauma
2. "Internal" trauma (repetitive motions of wrist)
3. Peripheral neuritis
4. Edema of pregnancy or of menstrual cycle

Pathologic condition of the nerve:

1. Tumor

Extrinsic

Pressure on the nerve by:

1. Ganglion
2. Other tumor or tissues in the area
3. Rheumatoid arthritis
   (*a*) Proliferative synovitis

Idiopathic

The structure most sensitive to pressure in the tunnel is the median nerve. According to the amount of pressure upon it and the length of time that it has been extant there will be abnormal nerve signs distal to the ligament from paresthesias over the thumb, index, long, and ring fingers, and the palm and weakness in the thenar muscles to complete anesthesia and wasting of the thenar muscles.

Treatment has consisted in splinting of the wrist to prevent further trauma and to allow subsidence of edema, the injection of hydrocortisone, and the severance of the entire volar transverse carpal ligament. The latter is obviously the only treatment for mechanical encroachments and usually becomes the ultimate treatment when trials with hydrocortisone fail.

Report of Case

This is a report of acute thrombosis occurring in a persisting median artery in the carpal tunnel that illustrates an unusual cause of the syndrome and presents supporting evidence for the need of early diagnosis and immediate operation.[1]

Submitted for publication March 18, 1963.

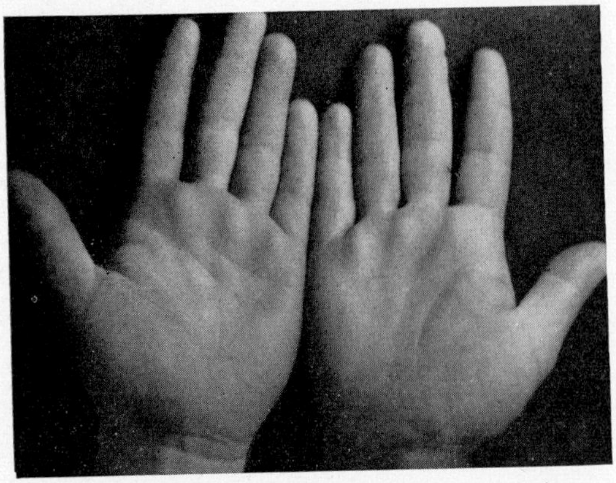

Fig 1.—Hand of patient two weeks after thrombosis of persisting median artery.

On April 28, 1961, a male short-order cook, age 31, was referred for diagnosis and treatment five days after the sudden onset of paresthesias of the median nerve distribution in the right hand which occurred while handling heavy pans. For the first two or three days there was swelling over the midline of the flexor surface of the wrist which had subsided by the time he was seen.

There was an impression of fullness in the palm and moderate tenderness (Fig 1). Sensation was reduced over the volar surface of the thumb, index, and long fingers, and most of the volar surface of the ring finger. Function of the thenar intrinsic muscles was reduced by approximately 50%. X-ray examination was interpreted as normal.

Because of the acute onset and objective findings he was advised to have immediate surgical relief, but he could not return until May 8, 1961, when the transverse volar carpal ligament was sectioned.

Entering the carpal tunnel a persistent median artery was found. Beneath the ligament, the entire artery was enlarged, edematous, and thrombosed (Fig 2). Sections are shown in Fig 3.

Fig 2.—Entire specimen of artery.

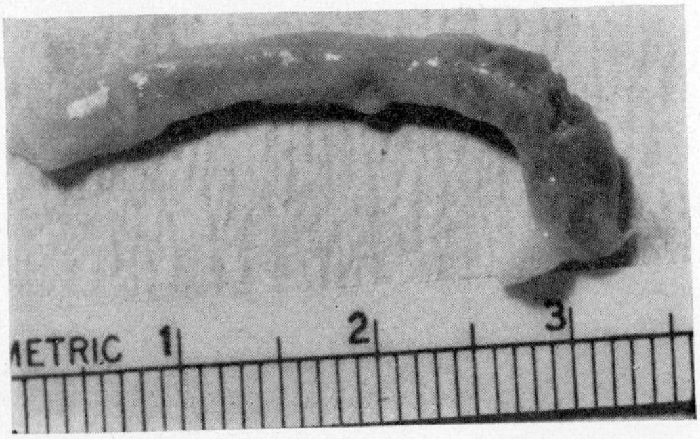

Relief of discomfort was present postoperatively. Complete return of normal sensation and muscle strength occurred in two to three weeks.

Further examination revealed a pulsating median artery in the left wrist too. McCormack[2] reported the presence of persistent median artery in 4.43% of 750 cadavers.

Comment

The pathology in the case herein described was not diagnosed preoperatively, though it should have been and might have been had I had the possibility of the presence of such an artery in mind. The persisting median artery in the other forearm was easily palpated. Had not the severity of the discomfort brought about early operation it is conceivable that delay would have resulted in irreversible damage to the nerve.

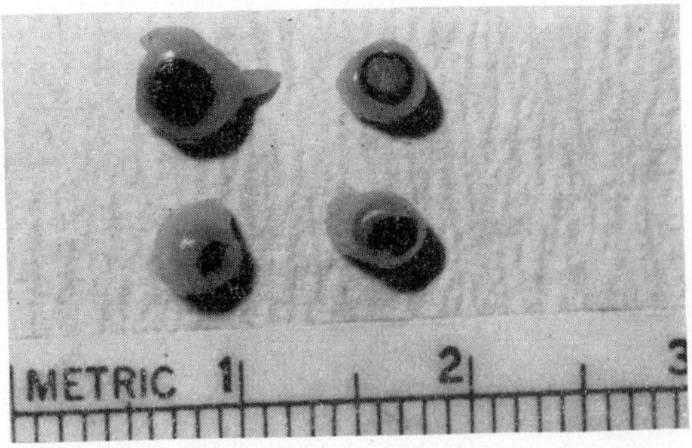

Fig 3.—Cross section of thrombosed artery.

It is suggested, therefore, that this cause of the carpal tunnel syndrome should be easily diagnosed at the patient's first visit and that surgical relief be not delayed.

Preston J. Burnham, MD, 508 E South Temple, Salt Lake City, Utah.

REFERENCES

1. DeAbreau, L. B., and Moreira, R. G.: Median-Nerve Compression at the Wrist, J Bone Joint Surg (Amer) 40:1426-1427 (Dec) 1958.

2. McCormack, L. J.; Cauldwell, E. W.; and Anson, B. J.: Brachial and Antebrachial Arterial Patterns, Surg Gynec Obstet 95:43-54 (Jan) 1953.

Cartilage Speeds Healing in Diabetic Wounds

MICHAEL R. GOLDING, MD
LAWRENCE K. OBERLANDER, BS
AND
IRVING F. ENQUIST, MD
BROOKLYN

Prudden and his collaborators have consistently shown an acceleration of wound healing in normal rats by the topical application of digested bovine cartilage powder, or by the subcutaneous implantation of cartilage pellets at a distance from the wound.[9] Prior work in our laboratory has shown that the healing of sutured incised wounds is impaired in animals with alloxan diabetes, and that this impairment may be partially or completely corrected by adequate control of the diabetic state.[11,12]

It seemed appropriate, therefore, to determine whether or not locally applied bovine cartilage powder would correct the healing defect in poorly controlled diabetic animals.

Methods

Male albino Wistar rats weighing from 150 to 200 gm were used. The normal blood sugar values in this strain range from 65 to 120 mg%. Diabetes was induced in animals which had been fasting for 48 hours by intraperitoneal injection of alloxan (150 mg/kg), one hour following a subcutaneous injection of 0.2 units of regular insulin. The blood sugar levels in the animals following this preparation ranged from 70 to 658 mg%. Only animals with levels above 200 mg% were considered to be diabetic and were used in the studies.

The test wound was made in the following manner. The animals were anesthetized with intraperitoneal pentobarbital, and under sterile conditions the skin and subcutaneous tissue of the upper abdomen was incised in the midline. A 4 cm vertical incision was made through the musculofascial wall and peritoneum in the left upper quadrant. This incision was then repaired with seven interrupted sutures of 0000 silk, placed exactly 0.5 cm apart and 0.5 cm from the edges. The subcutaneous tissue and skin was then closed separately as one layer with a continuous suture of 00000 silk. In those animals receiving cartilage, 25 mg of acid pepsin-digested bovine cartilage powder was applied to the sutured musculofascial wound with a standard powder atomizer before the skin was closed.

Wound healing was evaluated in the following manner. All animals were sacrificed on the seventh postoperative day with intraperitoneal pentobarbital. The skin and subcutaneous tissue of the abdomen

Submitted for publication March 20, 1962.

Department of Surgery, State University of New York Downstate Medical Center.

Supported by a grant (A-3609) from the National Institute of Arthritis and Metabolic Diseases, United States Public Health Service.

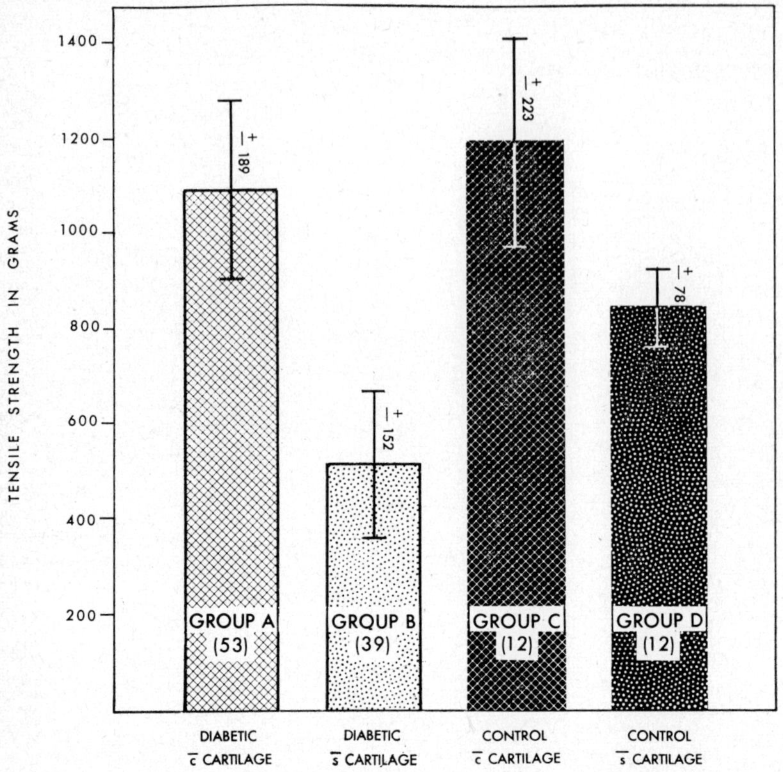

Mean tensile strengths of wounds in all animals. One standard deviation from the mean is plotted with each figure.

was reflected from the midline, and the entire musculofascial abdominal wall was excised. Three transverse strips, each 1 cm wide, were cut from the wound in such a fashion that each strip contained two of the previously placed sutures, as well as intact abdominal wall opposite the incision. The tensile strength of each strip was determined by suspending it in a motor driven tensiometer capable of recording the breaking force with considerable accuracy (±5 gm). The mean of the three readings from each animal was used in calculating the results.

Results

Four groups of animals were studied: group A (53 animals)—rats with alloxan diabetes, wounds treated with cartilage powder; group B (39 animals)—rats with alloxan diabetes, wounds *not* treated with cartilage powder; group C (12 animals)—normal rats, wounds treated with cartilage powder; group D (12 animals)—normal rats, wounds *not* treated with cartilage powder.

The mean tensile strengths of the wounds can be seen in the Figure. There is a significant increase in the wounds treated with cartilage powder, both in the diabetic and normal animals ($P = < 0.001$ in both groups).

Comment

Most surgeons are aware of the problems in healing to be encountered when operating upon diabetic patients. However, most of these problems are associated with operations performed in areas with insufficient arterial blood supply, or in well-vascularized areas in patients with improperly controlled diabetes. Modern surgeons expect no increased wound problems when operating upon the arms, trunk, or abdomen of diabetic patients under good control.[2] Certainly, the healing defect in animals with alloxan diabetes is readily corrected with proper diabetic control.[11]

Lattes [5] was first to recognize that cartilage powder applied to healing wounds would reverse the inhibition of fibroplasia induced by cortisone. It was soon noted that this striking local effect of cartilage not only was effective against the actions of cortisone, but also enhanced wound healing in animals in a normal metabolic and endocrine state.[7] This acceleration of wound healing, produced by heterologous cartilage, was shown to increase the tensile strength 20% at postoperative day seven.[7] Histologically, an increase in reticulin fibers and a less conspicuous increase in collagen fibers were noted.[6]

Inoue [4] tested a number of materials, many of them similar to cartilage in chemical structure, for the repair-stimulating effect shown by cartilage powder. None was found to exert a demonstrable benefit, and some actually exerted a deleterious effect upon wound healing. It has been concluded, therefore, that cartilage powder contains a highly specific material which accelerates wound healing.

Prudden [9] has recently shown the acceleration of healing by subcutaneous implantation of cartilage pellets at a distance from the wound, and more recently Prudden [10] and Houck [3] have shown the same effect from the injection of isotonic saline extracts of cartilage powder. The exact chemical nature of the factor responsible has not yet been found, but it is logical to believe that accurate chemical dissection of the cartilage powder will result in its identification. When this is accomplished, clinical use in patients with suspected healing difficulties seems mandatory.

Summary and Conclusions

The experiment reported confirms the stimulating effect of local cartilage powder on the gain in tensile strength of sutured, incised wounds, in normal rats.

Local cartilage application has also effected an acceleration of wound healing in animals with poorly controlled alloxan diabetes, a condition associated with deficient healing.

Irving F. Enquist, MD, State University of New York, Downstate Medical Center, 450 Clarkson Ave, Brooklyn 3, NY.

REFERENCES

1. Forscher, B. K., and Cecil, H. C.: Biochemical Studies of Acute Inflammation, Arch Biochem 70:367, 1957.

2. Greene, J. A.; Swanson, L. W.; and Jacobs, C. A.: Control of Diabetes Mellitus: Relation to the Healing of Clean and Infected Wounds and to Incidences of Infection in Clean Wounds, JAMA 115:1518, 1940.

3. Houck, J. C., and Vickers, K.: The Inhibition of Inflammation and the Acceleration of Tissue Repair by Cartilage Powder, Surgery 51:632, 1962.

4. Inoue, T.: The "Cartilage Effect" on Healing Wounds: A Study of the Specificity of the Phenomenon, Arch Surg 82:432, 1961.

5. Lattes, R.; Martin, J. R.; Meyer, K.; and Ragan, C.: Effect of Cartilage and Other Suspensions on Reparative Process of Cortisone Treated Animals, Amer J Path 32:979, 1956.

6. Paulette, R. E., and Prudden, J. E.: Studies on the Acceleration of Wound Healing With Cartilage: II. Histologic Observations, Surg Gynec Obstet 108:406, 1958.

7. Prudden, J. F.; Nishihara, G.; and Baker, L.: The Acceleration of Wound Healing With Cartilage, Surg Gynec Obset 105:283, 1957.

8. Prudden, J. F.: The Stimulation of Wound Healing With Heterologous Cartilage, Transplant Bull 5:14, 1958.

9. Prudden, J. F.; Inoue, T.; and Ocampo, L.: Subcutaneous Cartilage Pellets, Arch Surg 85:245, 1962.

10. Prudden, J. F.; Gabriel, O.; and Allen, B.: The Acceleration of Wound Healing, Arch Surg 86:157, 1963.

11. Rosen, R. G., and Enquist, I. F.: The Healing Wound in Experimental Diabetes, Surgery 50:525, 1961.

12. Rosenthal, S.; Lerner, B.; DiBiase, F.; and Enquist, I. F.: Relation of Strength to Composition in Diabetic Wounds, Surg Gynec Obstet 115:437, 1962.

Severity of Renal Injury Incident to Abdominal Aortography

Effect of Concentration of Contrast Solution

DUNCAN A. KILLEN, MD
AND
JOHN H. FOSTER, MD
NASHVILLE, TENN

Previous studies reported from this laboratory have revealed that a standardized injection of sodium acetrizoate 70% (Urokon) into the canine abdominal aorta results in renal damage.[3,4] It seems necessary that a critical amount of contrast medium gain access to the renal parenchyma during aortography to produce renal injury severe enough to result in azotemia.[3] This report concerns further definition of the nephrotoxic potential of abdominal aortography, especially as regards the concentration of the injected solution.

Method

Adult mongrel dogs served as test animals. A standardized abdominal aortic injection technique was used.[4] The injections were made 1 cm below the origin of the left renal artery in the supine animal at laparotomy. Veterinary pentobarbital sodium (Nembutal) was used for anesthetization. The actual injection was accomplished by manual evacuation of the bolus of contrast medium from a syringe through a No. 18 gauge venipuncture needle. Four groups of animals were prepared for injection of the following concentrations and volumes of contrast medium: (1) 15 cc of 35% sodium acetrizoate; (2) 7.5 cc of 70% sodium acetrizoate; (3) 30 cc of 35% sodium acetrizoate; and (4) 15 cc of 70% sodium acetrizoate. An attempt was made to deliver the entire bolus within the same time span regardless of volume and concentration of the solution injected. The injection in each instance was completed within five seconds.

Quantitation of nephrotoxicity was based upon the course of the serum nonprotein nitrogen during the first week after injection. Serum nonprotein nitrogen determinations were performed prior to intra-aortic injection of sodium acetrizoate and on alternate days, beginning on the second postinjection day. A rise of the nonprotein nitrogen to levels beyond 45 mg% was arbitrarily categorized as azotemia.

Results

A total of 29 animals (body weights varied from 8.0 kg to 18.5 kg) were used in this study. Only 23 animals survived to permit postinjection evaluation of renal function. The incidence of azotemia following aortic injection of the various solutions of sodium acetrizoate is recorded in the Table. The relationship of amount (per unit body weight) of sodium acetrizoate injected to the incidence of azotemia is shown in the Figure. The incidence of azotemia following injection of a total amount of 5.25 gm of sodium acetrizoate (Urokon) and 10.5 gm of sodium acetrizoate was 36% and 58%, respectively. The incidence of azotemia following injection of the 35% solution of sodium acetrizoate and the 70% solution of sodium acetrizoate was 17% and 82%, respectively. Thus, it is noted that the extent of renal injury can be correlated more closely with the concentration of sodium acetrizoate than with the total amount of the organic iodide infused into the aorta. It is also noted that the concentration of the solution is more critical than the total amount of agent in-

Submitted for publication March 20, 1963.

Instructor in Surgery (Dr. Killen); Associate Professor of Surgery (Dr. Foster).

From the S. R. Light Laboratory for Surgical Research and the Department of Surgery, Vanderbilt University School of Medicine.

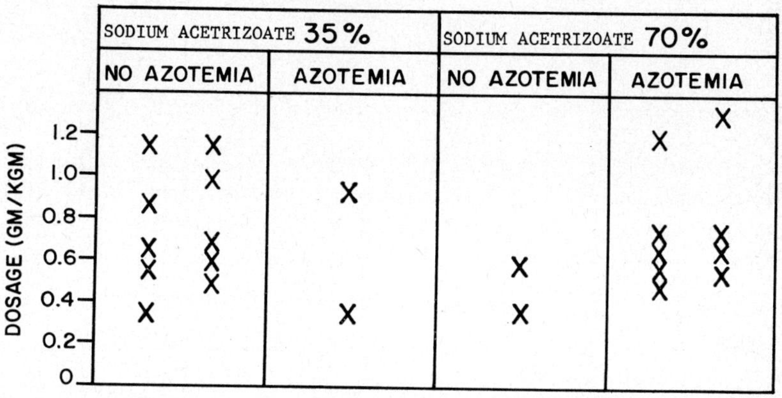

The incidence of azotemia (NPN greater than 45 mg%) following injection of 35% and 70% solutions of sodium acetrizoate. The ordinate represents the amount (per kilogram body weight) of sodium acetrizoate injected. It is noted that the incidence of azotemia can be correlated more closely with the use of the more concentrated solution than with the greater dosage of sodium acetrizoate injected during aortography.

jected in determining the early postinjection mortality (Table).

Comment

The technique of aortic injection as performed in this study was designed to deliver a massive amount, relative to body weight, rapidly into the aorta in the region of the renal artery orifices. Thus, a bolus effect is created so that the contrast medium is swept undiluted by the blood into the renal artery. Under such circumstances the renal parenchyma is subjected to perfusion by a greater amount of the contrast agent when the more concentrated solution (70% solution) is used. Had the injection of either 5.25 gm or 10.5 gm of sodium acetrizoate been performed slowly over a long but uniform period of time, perhaps the difference in concentration would not be so critical as regards nephrotoxicity; for under these circumstances, the same amount of sodium acetrizoate would be delivered per unit time into the renal arteries regardless of the concentration of the solution injected into the aorta.

Under the conditions of the experiments performed the more concentrated solution of sodium acetrizoate carries a much higher nephrotoxic potential. The higher osmolarity of the more concentrated solution does not seem to be critical in the mechanism of renal injury since other angiographic contrast media with osmolarities comparable to that of sodium acetrizoate 70% do not cause such severe renal damage when injected into the canine aorta in the standard manner used in this study.[2,4,7] There is evidence that the toxic effects of sodium acetrizoate upon the renal parenchyma is a cytotoxic rather than primarily a vasomotor reaction.[4,5] The enhancement of the renal damage by an increase in concentration of sodium acetrizoate suggests a mass action effect in this cytotoxic reaction.

Clinical studies have also emphasized the importance of the high concentration of contrast solutions injected into the aorta in the production of renal injury during aortography. The survey of complications of abdominal aortography reported by McAfee in 1957 revealed renal injury to be the most

Incidence of Azotemia and Mortality Following Aortic Injection of Sodium Acetrizoate (Urokon)

Dosage of Na Acetrizoate Injected: Conc (%)	Vol (Cc)	Gm	No. Animals	Survived for Evaluation	Mean NPN Increase	Animals Azotemic *	Mortality
35	15	5.25	6	6	8.7	1	1
70	7.5	5.25	6	5	47.	3	3
35	30	10.5	6	6	4.8	1	1
70	15	10.5	11	6	49.	6	8

* Postinjection NPN greater than 45 mg %.

frequently encountered severe complication.[6] The over-all tabulation revealed that 39 instances of renal injury were incurred during the performance of 13,207 procedures, an incidence of 0.3%. In at least 96% of these procedures contrast solutions of 70%-75% concentration (weight by volume) were used, and in 55% of the procedures sodium acetrizoate 70% was the contrast medium employed. The incidence of renal injury when a volume of contrast medium greater than 40 cc was injected was 1.0%. The incidence of renal damage following inadvertent direct renal artery injection was 12.5%. The higher incidence of renal injury following direct renal artery injection as compared to the incidence of injury following injection of a large volume of contrast medium into the aorta suggests that the momentarily high concentration of contrast medium in the renal artery is more critical in the production of renal damage than is the total amount of contrast medium instilled in the aorta. A review of the clinical instances of renal damage following aortography reported by Crawford et al revealed that as small a volume as 35 cc of sodium acetrizoate 70% injected into the abdominal aorta has been followed by renal damage.[1] McAfee cited one instance of temporary impairment of renal function following injection of only 10 cc of sodium acetrizoate 70% directly into a renal artery.[6] The relative amounts of sodium acetrizoate 70%, on the basis of volume per unit body weight, used in the clinical instances of renal injury incident to sodium acetrizoate aortography have been within the general range of that used in this study.[1,3]

Unfortunately, the quality of radiologic definition of renal vessels during renal angiography is also dependent primarily upon the concentration of the contrast medium within the renal vessels at the time of x-ray exposure. Thus, the greater the radiocontrast obtained in renal vessels during renal angiography, the greater is the potential for renal injury. Fortunately certain other angiographic contrast media in concentrations greater than 70% are not as toxic to the kidney as is sodium acertizoate 70% (ie, diatrizoate salts and sodium iothalamate).[2,4,7] Direct perfusion of sodium acetrizoate 70% into the renal arteries is hazardous. In the performance of translumbar or retrograde catheter aortography, it is difficult to be absolutely certain of avoiding direct perfusion of a renal artery.

John H. Foster, MD, Department of Surgery, Vanderbilt University School of Medicine, Vanderbilt University Hospital, Nashville 5, Tenn.

REFERENCES

1. Crawford, W. E.; Beall, A. C., Jr.; Moyer, J. H.; and DeBakey, M. E.: Complications of Aortography, Surg Gynec Obstet 104:129, 1957.

2. Foster, J. H., and Killen, D. A.: Experimental Appraisal of a New Angiographic Contrast Medium, Surg Gynec Obstet 113:234, 1961.

3. Killen, D. A.; Foster, J. H.; and Scott, H. W., Jr.: Toxic Reactions Incident to Urokon Aortography as Related to the Volume of Contrast Medium Injected, Ann Surg 155:472, 1962.

4. Killen, D. A., and Lance, E. M.: Experimental Appraisal of the Agents Employed as Angiocardiographic and Aortographic Contrast Media: II. Nephrotoxicity, Surgery 47:260, 1960.

5. Killen, D. A., and Lance, E. M.: Experimental Appraisal of the Agents Employed as Angiocardiographic and Aortographic Contrast Media: IV. Physical and Chemical Properties, Amer J Surg 102:512, 1961.

6. McAfee, J. G.: A Survey of Complications of Abdominal Aortography, Radiology 68:825, 1957.

7. Sessions, R. T.; Winfrey, E. W.; Killen, D. A.; and Foster, J. H.: Experimental Evaluation of a New Angiographic Contrast Medium, Surg Gynec Obstet 115:187, 1962.

Ceramic-Plastic Material as a Bone Substitute

LYMAN SMITH, MD
ELGIN, ILL

Introduction

The era in which we live has been described by engineers as The Materials Age. It is marked by a bewildering variety of materials developed since the turn of the century at an exponential rate. As surgeons, we are familiar with the metallurgical advances which have given us corrosion resistant alloys, as well as the many developments in the chemistry of plastics, which in some instances have been found to be useful in surgery. Another field of materials—ceramics—has also had tremendous growth in the last 20 years. Ceramic materials are now produced which have considerable strength and impact resistance, as well as great chemical resistivity. The latter characteristic is of prime interest to the surgeon, as the most important property of any surgical material is in its inertness in the environment of human tissue. Although strong, these new ceramic materials have the disadvantage of being extremely rigid. Attempts to produce a ductile ceramic material could follow either of two approaches—one being to alter the microstructures; the other being the formation of a combination or alloy of a ceramic with a more ductile substance. The latter approach has been accomplished by producing a ceramic which has a true interconnecting porosity. This ceramic body has then been impregnated with a close-bonding epoxy resin, thus producing a material which retains the hardness and corrosion resistance of ceramics, but also demonstrates resilience and adequate strength.*

Method of Production

A mixture was made consisting of alumina (Al_2O_3), silica (SiO_2), calcium carbonate ($CaCO_3$), and magnesium carbonate ($MgCO_3$). A so-called green body was then formed by a method commonly used in ceramic production, known as slip casting.

Submitted for publication March 25, 1963.

Assistant Professor of Orthopedic Surgery, Northwestern University Medical School.

* The ceramic-plastic material was developed by Joseph F. Estes and Helmut Bruchmann of The Haeger Potteries, Inc., Dundee, Ill; R. J. Cowles of Arthur D. Little, Inc., Cambridge, Mass; and myself.

This green body was placed in a furnace, and the temperature slowly raised to about 2,000 F for some hours. During this period, the magnesium carbonate decomposed to magnesium oxide and carbon dioxide gas and the calcium carbonate decomposed into calcium oxide and carbon dioxide gas. Since the individual particles of calcium carbonate and magnesium carbonate were small and thoroughly dispersed throughout the green body, the carbon dioxide gas produced by the decomposition thereof upon heating was also thoroughly dispersed and formed small individual cells that were uniformly distributed and of substantially uniform size. As the carbon dioxide gas formed was further heated, it passed from cell to cell and eventually to the surface of the body. Since about one third of the starting materials, on a dry basis, were carbonates, the green body had a high porosity of about 65% thereof by volume. This so-called prefired body was then finally fired at a temperature of about 2,700 F. The final porosity was controlled by controlling the firing temperature—the lower the firing temperature the higher the porosity and the higher the firing temperature the lower the porosity. In other words, with the higher temperatures, the ceramic body shrank more and thus produced the lower porosity. Porosities ranging from 6% to about 65% by volume of the fired ceramic member were achieved.

Four-inch ceramic bars of varying porosity were impregnated with a liquid aromatic epoxy resin of the diepoxide 0 type mixed with a hydroxy-aliphatic amine hardener. A bar was placed in a casting chamber from which air was evacuated by a water inspirator. The liquid resin and hardener were mixed at 50 C and run into the evacuated chamber. After the mixture had flooded the ceramic piece, positive pressure was applied and the part cooled. To insure complete curing of the resin, the bar was finally baked at 120 C for three hours. The method was successful in completely impregnating the ceramic bar as could be calculated by weight changes and by direct observation following destructive tests.

Cured epoxy resins are particularly inert to most chemicals and solvents as compared with other organic plastic materials. Methylene chloride, a halogenated hydrocarbon, is one solvent that slowly attacks the surface of epoxy formulated parts. Before the final temperature cure at 120 C for three hours is applied to the impregnated ceramic, there is a period just after impregnation when the resin is most susceptible to this solvent. It can be applied in various degrees of time and agitation to effect a complete surface removal of the impregnant. Once the resin has been completely cured, contact with the solvent would be necessary for some days. Fig 1 is a specimen which was dipped for three to five minutes in methylene chloride solvent after impregnation and before curing. It demonstrates a leaching away of the surface resin to a depth of 50 to 70 mils.

Examinations of the Material

Flexural Strength and Modulus of Elasticity.—Bars of the impregnated ceramic were prepared measuring 4×½×¼ inch. The bars varied in porosity from 6% to 65% by volume. The bar to be tested was supported at each end and a load applied from

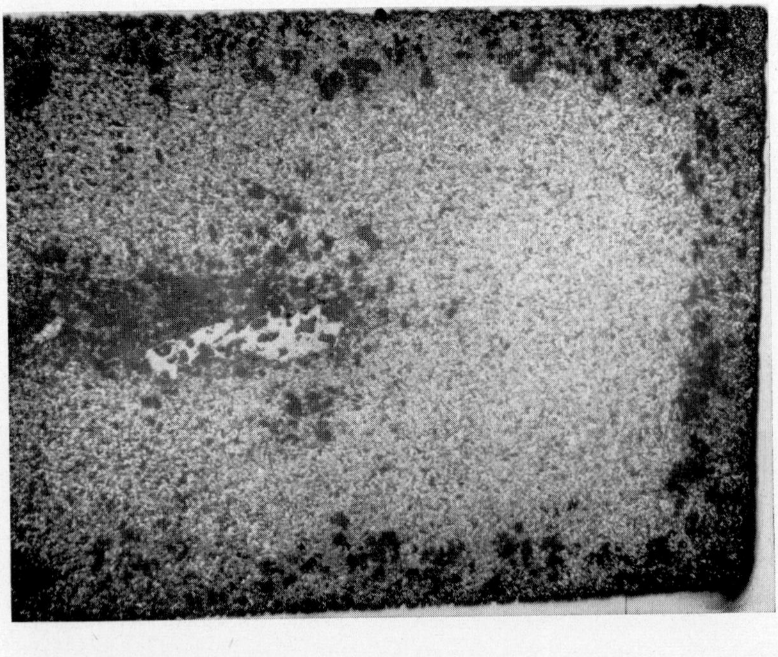

Fig 1.—An impregnated ceramic bar after surface leaching. Reduced 58% from mag × 11.

above at the center on a table model "Instron" machine. The crosshead was lowered at the rate of 0.2 inch per minute, and an automatic recording of the deflection produced in the test bar was made. From the readings obtained, flexural strength in pounds per square inch (psi) was calculated as well as the modulus of elasticity (resistance to bending) for each sample. Both figures varied with the degree of porosity of the sample. A bar of 46% porosity was chosen as ideal because its modulus of elasticity was approximately the same as bone (3.0×10^6 psi) and its flexural strength was 12,000 psi, as compared to an average wet bone sample of 11,000 psi.

Resistance to Aging.—Test bars measuring 4½×½×¼ inch were placed in isotonic saline solution in glass tubes, and the tubes were sealed with the volume of air therein equal to the volume of the saline solution. The bars were then aged at elevated temperatures for varying periods of time. Three series of tests were run at 124 C, 149 C, and 190 C. The tubes were opened and a maximum bending stress for each bar expressed in psi was determined, by utilizing the test method described above. The value of flexural strength obtained on each test bar was graphed, and then, by extrapolation, the length of time it would take to reduce the flexural strength of the material to 8,000 psi at body temperature of 37 C (98.6 F) could be calculated. This age life was determined to be about 2×10^8 hours, or 23,000 years.

Abraison Resistance.—A machine was used that provided a fresh abradent surface with each cycle of movement of a pressure head. A water-proof Carborundum silicone carbide paper was moved at a rate of five inches per minute under a one-fourth-inch diameter abradent head at a pressure of 100 pounds per square inch. The change in thickness due to abrasion was recorded as the movement of an electric displacement sensing device attached to the head of the abrader. The impregnated ceramic was abraded for 10,000 cycles as was a polished piece of Vitallium. The results are graphed in Fig 2 and show that the impregnated ceramic wore

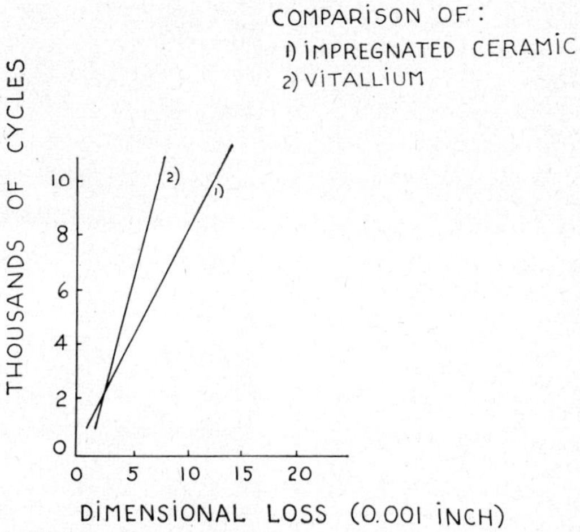

Fig 2.—Comparison in abrasion of impregnated ceramic and Vitallium.

less than the Vitallium for the first 3,000 cycles and was almost equal in continued cycles. As a further test, the abradent paper was removed and a piece of human bone with a hyaline cartilage face cut to one-fourth-inch diameter was mounted for movement against a piece of the impregnated ceramic. The cartilage was wetted every 1,000 cycles with two drops of synovial fluid. After 24,000 cycles, the impregnated ceramic had no change in its surface, while the cartilage sample lost 0.012 inch, most of which was removed during the first 10,000 cycles.

Hardness.—The hardness of an impregnated porous ceramic structure is difficult to define. Considered as a continuous surface structure rather than as each of two components, it was thought best to test the hardness by methods ordinarily used on metal. A Wilson-Rockwell instrument was used to test the material using a one-eighth-inch and a one-sixteenth-inch ball penetrator. The superficial hardness was found to vary inversely in accordance with the degree of porosity. The ceramic alone retained a hardness of 94 to 97 up to 28% porosity, as compared to a finding of 99 on Vitallium sample. The impregnated ceramic in the 50% porosity range showed a value of 83.

Pore Size.—Microscopic studies have shown the pores in a 46% porosity body to average 18μ in diameter with some up to 25μ (Fig 3).

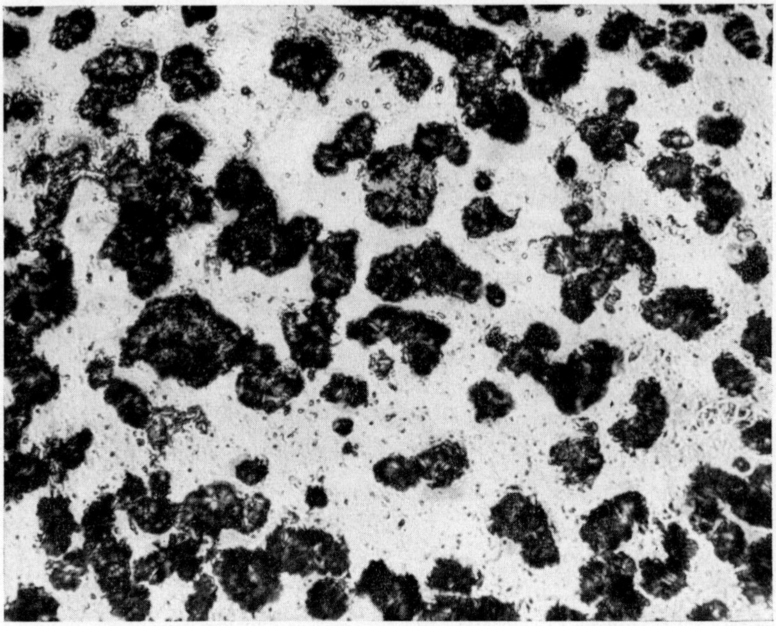

Fig 3.—Pore size and distribution in a ceramic body of 46% porosity. Reduced 58% from mag × 210.

Fatigue.—Fatigue studies are being made on the material. The early results are good within the range of failure of the material. It is known that Vitallium will fatigue at about 40% of its failure strength; stainless steels fatigue at 45% to 50% of their failure strength. On the basis of preliminary data, it appears that the impregnated ceramic fatigues at 50% to 55% of its failure strength, although it should be realized that the failure strength of this material is well below that of metal.

Compression.—An Eicher type stainless steel hip prosthesis was duplicated out of this material. The stainless steel prosthesis weighed 1 lb 2 oz; the ceramic-plastic prosthesis weighed 11 oz. Each prosthesis was placed under compression in a universal tensile-testing machine. The stainless steel prosthesis failed by plastic deformation at approximately 550 lb; the impregnated ceramic failed by fracture at 608 lb. The results are graphed in Fig 4.

Resistance to Chemicals.—The impregnated ceramic has been tested by immersing a piece in aqua regia for 24 hours at room temperature. No weight loss was recorded, and the same lack of reaction was found when the material was placed in 50% sodium hydroxide at body temperature for 48 hours.

Animal Studies

Methods.—Forty-two White Satin rabbits weighing an average of nine pounds have been used.† At irregular intervals, implants of the epoxy resin, the porous ceramic, and the impregnated ceramic have been placed in subcutaneous tissues, skeletal muscle, and knee joints. Operations were done under pentobarbital sodium (Nembutal) anesthesia plus 1% procaine locally.

† This work was aided by a grant from the Committee for the Advancement of Research, Sherman Hospital, Elgin, Ill.

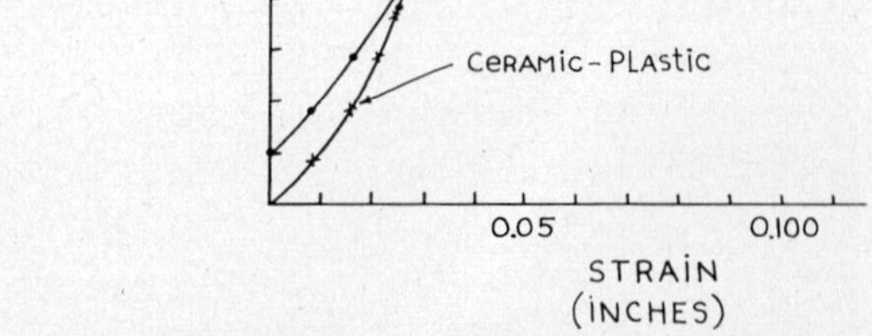

Fig 4.—Compression test on stainless steel and ceramic-plastic hip prostheses (Eicher type).

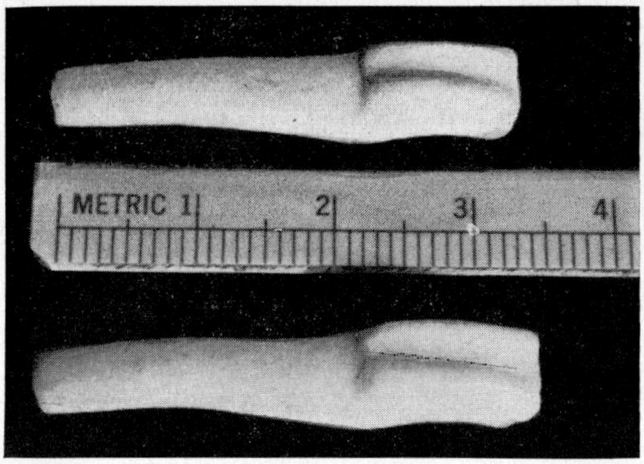

Fig 5.—Prosthesis used to replace the superior articular surface of the femoral condyles.

Fig 5 is a photograph of a ceramic-plastic prosthesis shaped for insertion into the knee joint replacing the anterior portion of the femoral condyles in articulation with the patella. At operation, the knee joint was approached from the lateral aspect, and the patella and its tendinous attachments were dislocated medially. The anterior portion of the femoral condyles was removed by an oscillating saw to a point just short of the weight-bearing area and the prothesis loosely laid into the cavity, the stem being pushed proximally up the medullary canal. The patella was then reduced into apposition with the prosthesis (Fig 6), and the wound was closed in layers after irrigation with saline solution. Some of the prostheses were surface leached of the plastic before insertion; others were not. The rabbits were kept out of doors in narrow cages 20 feet long with food and water at alternate ends to encourage activity. They were sacrificed at irregular intervals.

Results.—Three anesthetic deaths were encountered. Three postoperative deaths occurred at various times due to pneumonia, and three knee joints were grossly infected. Six fractured femurs into and proximal to the prosthesis were seen.

Fig 7 is a photograph of a transverse section taken through a prosthesis and femur three weeks after operation. The prosthesis was found tight in its bed, held so by cancellous bone and fibrous tissue grown in firm apposition to it. It was removed from the femur by chiseling. This firm apposition of bone to prosthesis has been a constant feature of all knees examined. Fig 8 shows the adherence of bone and fibrous tissue to a 40-day implant. The bone was allowed to dry and shrink away from the prosthesis, but close adherence is demonstrated even though in this prosthesis the epoxy had not been leached from its surface.

To date, six months have been the longest a leached prosthesis has been in place before autopsy. The knee of that rabbit showed no limitation of motion. On opening the joint, there was no increase in synovial fluid, the capsule was not bound down, and there were no intra-articular adhesions. The articular

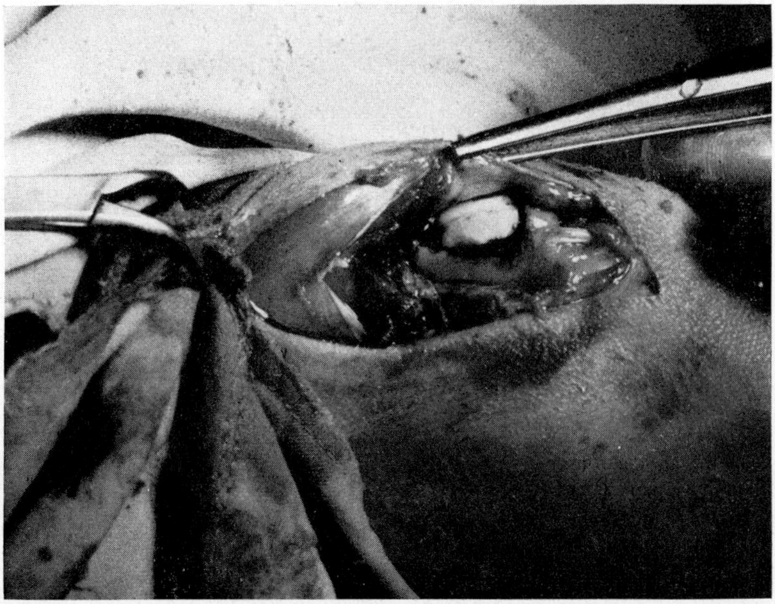

Fig 6.—The prosthesis has been laid loosely in place and the patella reduced in apposition to it.

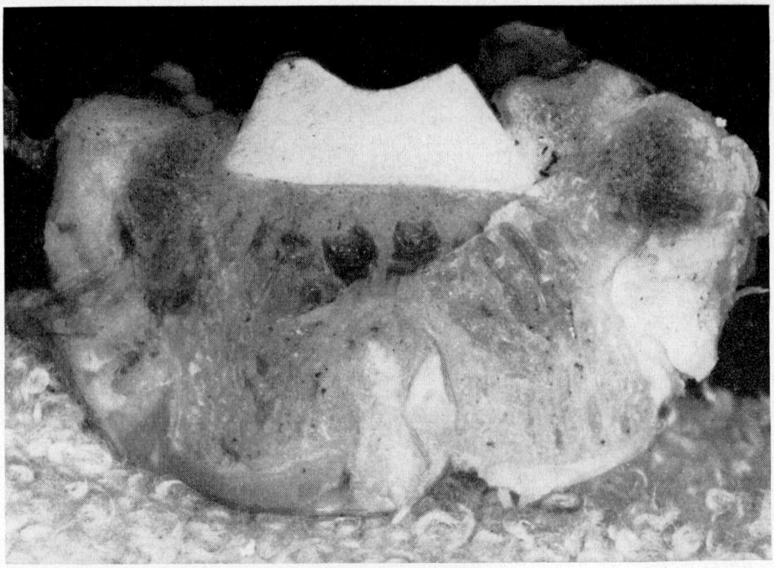

Fig 7.—Transverse section through femur and prosthesis three weeks after operation.

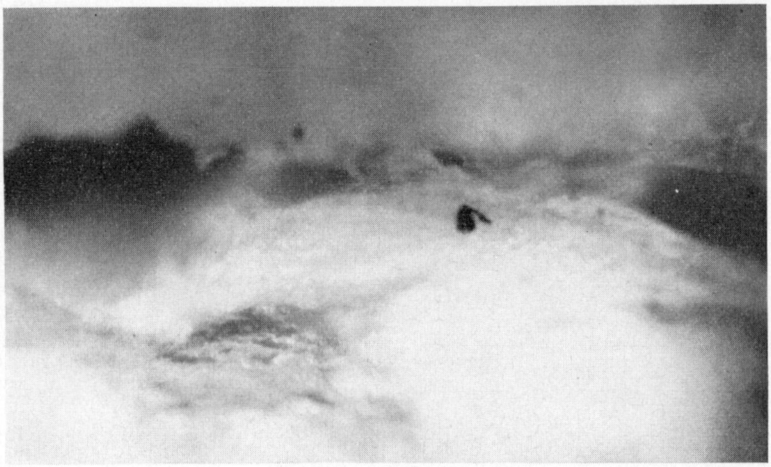

Fig 8.—Adherence of tissue to a 40-day implant. Reduced 11% from mag × 36.

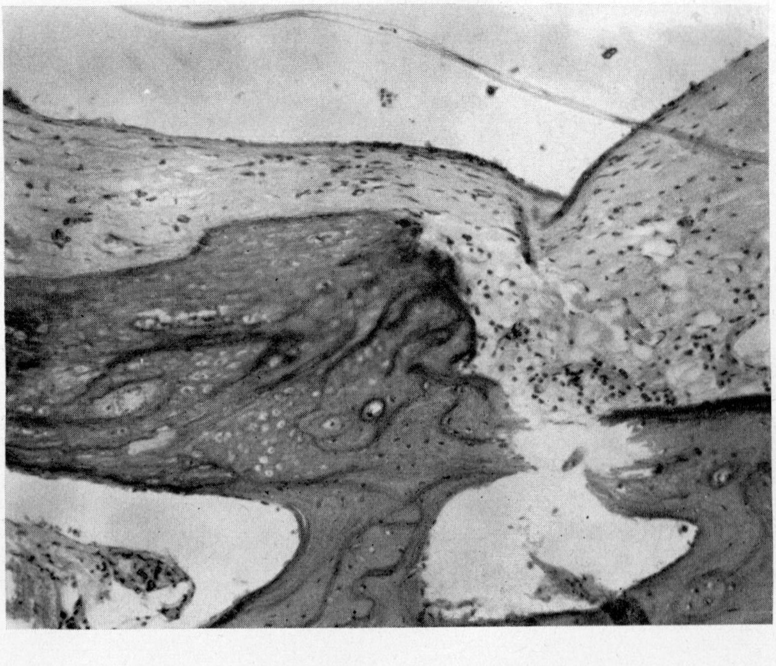

Fig 9.—Section from bed beneath an implant in place six months. Reduced 11% from mag × 100.

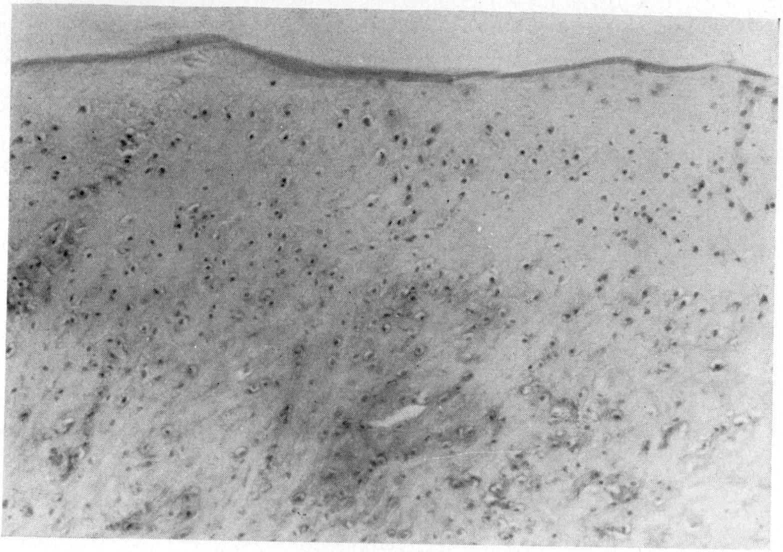

Fig 10.—Articular cartilage of patella after six months apposition to the prosthesis. Reduced 11% from mag × 100.

cartilage was everywhere shiny and glistening. The prosthesis was firmly held in its bed by new bone and could not be removed until the femur was decalcified. Fig 9 is a section taken through a corner of the bed showing dense, relatively acellular fibrous tissue merging with osteoid and orderly trabeculae of lamellar bone. Fig 10 is a section through the articular cartilage of the patella showing no surface reaction to wear against the prosthesis. Fig 11 is the x-ray appearance of the knee at the time of insertion of the prosthesis, and Fig 12 is the same knee six months later. There is considerable endosteal calcification in the medullary canal about the peg of the prosthesis, and the bone trabeculae of the host appear to be interwoven with the substance of the prosthesis.

Fig 11.—Lateral view of knee joint a few hours after insertion of a prosthesis.

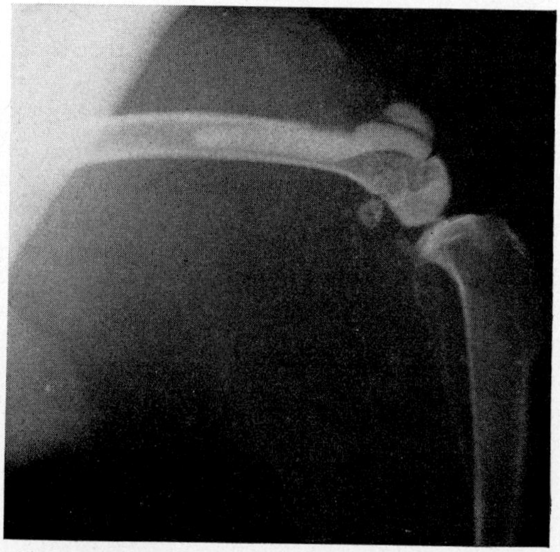

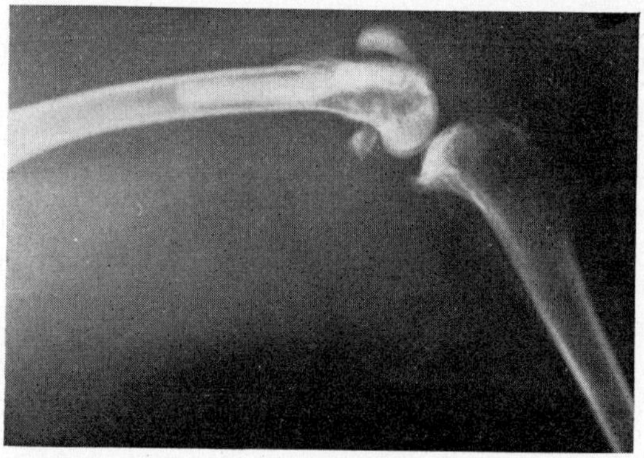

Fig 12.—The same knee joint as in Fig 11 six months later.

Fig 13 is a section from tissue immediately adjacent to a seven-week subcutaneous implant of epoxy resin. The implant was approximately the size of a shirt button and was freely movable. The section shows a thin layer of mesothelial cells overlying a loose areolar tissue. There are no giant cells or collection of polymorphonuclear leukocytes indicating an inflammatory reaction.

The pieces of the porous ceramic and the impregnated ceramic after leaching, which had been embedded in skeletal muscle, were examined after three to nine weeks. They were found to be tightly bound in place by

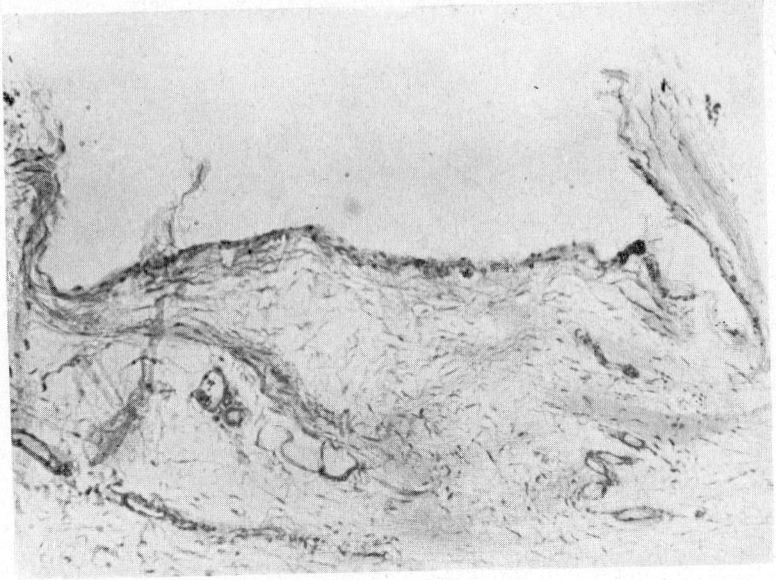

Fig 13.—Tissue surrounding a subcutaneous implant of epoxy resin after seven weeks. Reduced 14% from mag × 100.

fibrous tissue and normally colored muscle fibers in contrast to the synovial-like sheath found around similarly embedded inert metal alloys. In these instances, and in the case of the closely bound knee prosthesis, it has been assumed that fibrous tissue and perhaps bone had invaded the open pore structure. Such ingrowth has been demonstrated with polyvinyl sponge implants.[4] The ceramic is too hard to cut with the microtome, so thin sections have been prepared by grinding on sandpaper. Examination of these sections has been disappointing in that no fibrous tissue or bone has been seen. However, it is possible that soft tissues have been pulled out of the pores in the grinding process. Other methods of preparation are being attempted.

Comment

This material has been developed in the belief that it may act as a better substitute for bone than the metal alloys in common use. These alloys are almost ten times as strong and approximately ten times as stiff as the bone they are called upon to replace or to immobilize. On bending, there is a relative movement between the flexible bone and the rigid alloy which sets up high localized stresses on certain areas, and at these points bone is absorbed. The impregnated ceramic of 46% porosity has the same modulus of elasticity as bone and will bend symmetrically with it, thus avoiding such stresses.

The prime reason the 18-8 stainless steel and the cobalt-chromium molybdenum alloys have been used in surgery is their relative resistance to corrosion. Macrocorrosion is common with stainless steels,[1] and microcorrosion is seen with all types of metal alloys, including Vitallium.[2] This latter type consists in the deposition of metallic elements in the tissues around implants, but its significance is not known. Galvanic corrosion of alloys in the body, an electrochemical phenomena, is not seen in ceramic and plastic materials, which is the reason for their common use in industry for insulation. Some alloys and metals protect themselves from chemical corrosion by the formation of a thin layer of oxides on their surfaces; ceramic materials are commonly oxides, and could be loosely stated to have "already corroded." The epoxy resin used to impregnate the porous ceramic is also chemically inert. The structure of this class of polymers suggests that ether linkages are the only bonds other than the carbon to carbon. Ether linkages are among the most stable known to organic chemists so it follows that these resins are highly resistant to attack by various solvents, acids, and alkalis.

Epoxy shares its chemical inertness with other types of plastics, but was chosen over them because of its unique ability to bond tightly to the ceramic. Most plastics would only act as fillers in the void cavities of the ceramic, contributing little to the flexural strength of the material. The resistance-to-aging test showed that this tight bond between the epoxy and the ceramic would not materially deteriorate with time and temperature.

Some chemically inert plastics have been found to be toxic in tissues, due to remnants of catalysts or to unreacted molecules of the components of the plastics themselves. The completely cured epoxies have been found nondeleterious to health by medical investigators of the major resin manufacturers. Regardless of the type of curing agent used, the cross-linked epoxy apparently does no harm when powdered and fed to rats in massive doses over long periods.[3] However, dermatitis has been reported in workers handling the liquid amine hardeners used in preparation of the plastic.

The impregnated ceramic is far weaker than the metal alloys but equal with the strength of bone. Its strength should be adequate as a substitute for bone if used in sufficient mass and properly engineered. It is hoped that this material will be re-enforced by the growth of soft tissue and bone into the surfaces which have been leached of epoxy.

Summary

A material developed for use as a bone substitute is described. It is a porous ceramic composed of the high-temperature reaction products of alumina, silica, and the oxides of magnesium and calcium. The honeycomb structure of the ceramic is impregnated with a close-bonding epoxy resin. The resultant material is as strong as bone and has the same modulus of elasticity, is light in weight, inert in rabbit tissues, resilient, hard, difficult to abrade, and is highly resistant to acids and alkalis.

Lyman Smith, MD, 1185 Dundee Ave, Elgin, Ill.

REFERENCES

1. Cohen, J., and Hammond, G.: Corrosion in a Device for Fracture Fixation, J Bone Joint Surg 41A:524-534, 1959.

2. Ferguson, A. B.; Laing, P. G.; and Hodge, E. S.: The Ionization of Metal Implants in Living Tissues, J Bone Joint Surg 42A:77-90, 1960.

3. Skeist, I: Epoxy Resins, New York: Reinhold Publishing Corporation, 1960.

4. Struthers, A. M.: An Experimental Study of Polyvinyl Sponge as a Substitute for Bone, Plast Reconstr Surg 15:274-289, 1955.

The Cast Syndrome

A Case Report

WILLIAM R. THOMPSON, MD
PROVIDENCE, RI

Profound gastric atony associated with epigastric pain, bloating, intermittent vomiting, and moderate to severe degrees of alkalosis following the application of a body cast is a syndrome that has been reported infrequently in the medical literature. The seriousness of the condition is clearly apparent from a review of the 11 published cases, in four of which the patient died. Dorph's [1] case report and review of the literature in 1950 served to establish the term "cast syndrome," and its various features were stressed later that year in an editorial by Leucutia.[2] The first case to fulfill the criteria for the cast syndrome as outlined by Dorph was reported by Willett [3] in 1878. Single case reports appeared subsequently by Buzzard (1880),[4] Kelling (1901),[5] and by Conley and Miller (1935).[6] Four of the five patients died, presumably from the effects of severe metabolic alkalosis. All of the patients were adolescents. Of these cases, in contrast to those later reported, none was operated upon.

Etiological factors that have been proposed as being of fundamental importance are primary paralysis of the stomach, reflex inhibition of the gastric motor mechanism, and mechanical obstruction of the third portion of the duodenum by compression of the superior mesenteric vessels against the aorta and vertebral column (Fig 1 and 2). That the latter mechanism has been accepted by many as the primary etiological factor is apparent from the more recent case reports. This syndrome in a 12-year-old boy treated successfully by duodenojejunostomy was reported by Kauffman and Gerbode [7] in 1951. They postulated that the increased lordosis caused by the cast led to a more acute angle between the aorta and superior mesenteric vessels, thus causing an obstruction of the third portion of the duodenum (Fig 2). Waddell et al [8] in 1955 reported a 12-year-old girl who developed extreme alkalosis and was operated upon when in critical condition. A dilatation of the stomach and

Submitted for publication March 28, 1963.

From the Department of Surgery, Rhode Island Hospital.

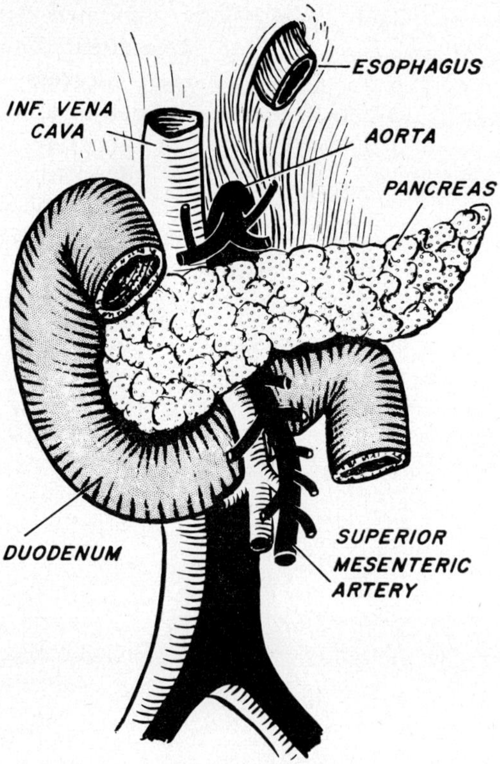

Fig 1.—Duodenum in relation to superior mesenteric artery.

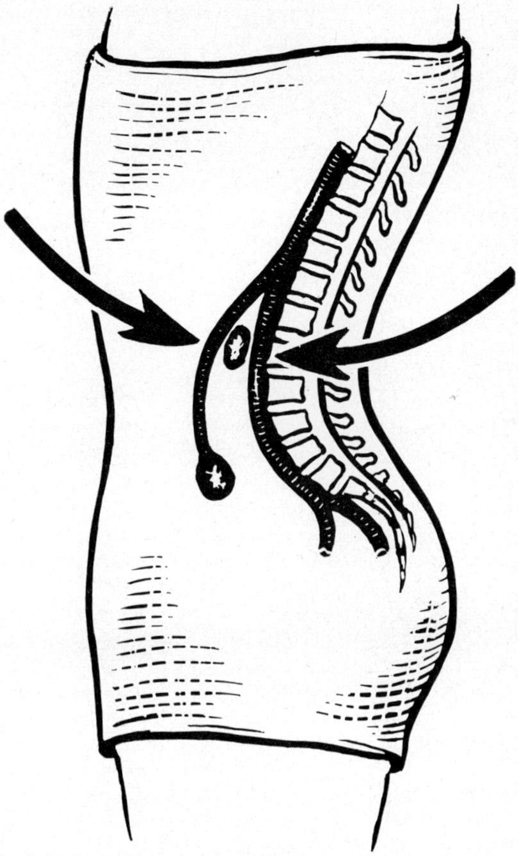

Fig 2.—Acute angle between aorta and superior mesenteric vessels, causing an obstruction of third portion of duodenum.

duodenum was detected down to the point where the superior mesenteric vessels crossed anteriorly. A transection of the ligament of Treitz was performed, gas passed through the previously obstructed area, and the patient improved thereafter. This would appear to be one of the first reports of the treatment of arteriomesenteric duodenal occlusion by transection of the ligament of Treitz as later popularized by Strong.[9] Their case, plus characteristic autopsy findings in two earlier reported cases, suggested to the authors that arteriomesenteric duodenal occlusion may be of prime importance as a causative factor of the cast syndrome.

In 1956, Rosenburg and Sampson [10] reported a case in a 16-year-old boy treated with a body spica because of a slipped femoral epiphysis. The obstruction was also felt to be on the basis of arteriomesenteric compression, and the patient did well after duodenojejunostomy. Kaiser et al [11] in 1960 reported three more cases with proximal obstruction following applications of body casts. The authors diagnosed arteriomesenteric duodenal obstruction in each of the cases, the diagnoses presumably being established by x-ray studies and confirmed at operation. Duodenojejunostomies were performed on all of these patients, and all survived, including a 67-year-old male, the only patient over 30 years of age ever reported. In this regard, if the acute angle between the superior mesenteric vessels and the aorta is accepted as a reason for obstruction, it follows that the younger age groups with more pliable spinal columns are more commonly affected. It is interesting to note that the patients in all of the last six published cases lived and underwent surgery for correction of their "obstruction." The patient reported in this paper was not operated upon but did survive.

Report of Case

An 18-year-old male was admitted to the Rhode Island Hospital on March 14, 1962, after an automobile accident. Roentgenograms revealed a moderately displaced transverse fracture of the midshaft of the left femur. There were no other serious injuries. The patient was treated in Russell's traction for 11 weeks. At the end of this time, a body spica, incorporating the entire left leg, was applied under general anesthesia. Forty-eight hours later, on June 7, he was discharged apparently well, although he complained of some fullness and tightness in the upper abdomen. Two days later he became anorexic, and then nausea plus intermittent vomiting developed. He became progressively lethargic and was readmitted acutely ill one week later. On examination the pulse rate was 150, and there was evidence of moderate dehydration. Through a window cut in the anterior portion of the cast, abdominal examination revealed only epigastric tenderness. The blood urea nitrogen had risen from a previous level of 7.0 mg% to 31.0 mg%, and the carbon dioxide combining power had risen to 31 mEq per liter. A nasogastric tube was inserted, and a large quantity of gas and coffee-ground material was aspirated. Copious amounts of dark brown fluid continued to flow from the Levin tube, requiring vigorous corrective intravenous therapy. The cast was removed and Russell's traction was reapplied. A gastrointestinal series demonstrated a large atonic stomach without evidence of ulceration. Barium passed into the slightly dilated duodenum only by gravity, and a four-hour film showed just a small amount of contrast material beyond the ligament of Treitz. A definite point of obstruction at the ligament was not demonstrated. After four days, transient improvement in the patient's general condition occurred. However, the ensuing five weeks were marred by exacerbations and remissions of gastric atony and vomiting requiring almost continual nasogastric suction. Periodic trials on oral fluids were unsuccessful. During this time, progressive weight loss occurred so that the young man—a tall, lean, asthenic type—lost a total of 45 lb (20.4 kg) from the time of the initial injury. An added problem was the slow healing of the fracture, necessitating maintenance in Russell's traction. Near the end of the five-week period another trial on oral fluids was given with success. Four days later traction was released and the patient was ambulated in a long leg brace and crutches. Further vomiting did not occur, and the diet was gradually progressed. A repeat gastrointestinal series was entirely within normal limits. The young man was finally discharged in mid-August, and when seen again in October, he had regained 35 lb (15.9 kg) and had not experienced any further adverse gastrointestinal symptoms.

Comment

Whether or not operation in this case was indicated is a moot point. Did the clinical situation as developed represent a form of gastric atony ascribed by Dragstedt [12] and other authorities to inhibition of the gastric motor mechanism, or was true organic obstruction present? It appeared reasonable that the initial loss of gastric tone was reflex in nature and could have been attributed to a combination of prolonged bed rest and gradual weight loss further aggravated by general anesthesia when the spica cast was applied. Anatomical factors then most likely came into play and contributed to duodenal occlusion. The increased lordosis resulting from the cast probably accentuated the acuity of the aortosuperior mesenteric angle, and weight loss may have converted the broad band containing the superior mesenteric vessels into a thin cord-like structure.

Dragstedt [12] has observed that a fine line across the third portion of the duodenum suggesting some degree of compression is not an unusual autopsy finding in the common forms of gastric dilatation. One might therefore reason that since most cases of gastric atony respond to conservative therapy with nasogastric tube suction and intravenous fluids, such areas of obstruction are usually overcome with the return of normal gastric and duodenal motor activity. Whether or not the majority of cases of the "cast syndrome" respond to such therapy is difficult to determine since it does appear that only the most severe cases have been published. The subject of the present report finally regained satisfactory gastric and doudenal motor activity after a prolonged period, but with early surgery his hospital course possibly could have been shortened.

An additional method of treatment has been suggested by Kaiser et al.[11] They have emphasized that positioning in the left lateral or prone position may aid in relieving the obstruction caused by the arteriomesenteric bundle. This maneuver could not be utilized in the case reported on because of the nature of the fracture and the form of the traction. When possible, however, repositioning plus the basic steps of cast removal, gastric decompression, and intravenous fluids should be given an adequate trial, reserving operation only for the most resistant cases.

Summary

A case of the "cast syndrome" has been reported and the pertinent literature briefly reviewed. Possible mechanisms responsible for its development plus treatment have been discussed.

William R. Thompson, MD, Senior Resident in Surgery, Rhode Island Hospital, Providence 2, RI.

REFERENCES

1. Dorph, M. H.: The Cast Syndrome, New Eng J Med 243:440, 1950.

2. Leucutia, T.: The Cast Syndrome, Editorial, Amer J Roentgen 64:1113, 1950.

3. Willett, A.: Fatal Vomiting Following Application of Plaster-of-Paris Bandage in Case of Spinal Curvature, St. Bartholomew's Hosp Rep 14:333, 1878.

4. Buzzard, T.: Case of Paraplegia from Pott's Disease: Treatment by Sayre's Jackett; Intestinal Obstruction, Death from Kink in Duodenum, Trans Clin Soc London 13:157, 1880.

5. Kelling, G.: Über den Mechanismus der acuten Magendilatation, Arch Klin Chir 64:393, 1901.

6. Conley, A., and Miller, D. S.: Acute Dilatation of Stomach With Perforation Following Body Cast Application, Industr Med 4:185, 1935.

7. Kauffman, R. R., and Gerbode, F.: Arteriomesenteric Duodenal Ileus, Stanford Med Bull 9:262, 1951.

8. Waddell, W. W., Jr.; McKay, B. M.; and Donegan, C. C., Jr.: Possible Cast Syndrome, J Bone Joint Surg (Amer) 37:597, 1955.

9. Strong, E. K.: Mechanics of Arteriomesenteric Duodenal Obstruction and Direct Surgical Attack Upon Etiology, Ann Surg 148:725, 1958.

10. Rosenburg, S. A., and Sampson, A.: The Syndrome of Mesenteric Vascular Compression of the Duodenum: Report of 11 Cases With Operative Correction, AMA Arch Surg 73:296, 1956.

11. Kaiser, G. C.; McKain, J. M.; and Shumacker, H. B., Jr.: The Superior Mesenteric Artery Syndrome, Surg Gynec Obstet 110:133, 1960.

12. Dragstedt, L. R.: "Acute Dilatation of Stomach," In Lewis' Practice of Surgery, Hagerstown, Md: W. F. Prior Company, vol VI, chap 10, pp 1-18.

Intraperitoneal Hemorrhage Due to Uterine Fibroid

Report of a Case in Late Pregnancy

FRANCIS A. AVOLA, MD
AND
JOHN P. GONNELLA, MD
MEDFORD, MASS

Exsanguinating intraperitoneal hemorrhage due to rupture of a subserosal vein of a fibroid tumor of the uterus is a very rare entity. The condition has been seen even less frequently in association with pregnancy, only four cases having been reported,[1] one of which occurred 36 hours after normal delivery. Despite the rarity of this clinical entity its recognition is extremely important since a fatality may ensue unless prompt surgical intervention is instituted. The following case recently encountered by us in a community hospital is, therefore, being reported.

Submitted for publication March 30, 1963.

Assistant Clinical Professor of Surgery, Tufts University Medical School; Visiting Surgeon, Lawrence Memorial Hospital and Malden Hospital; Associate visiting Surgeon, Boston City Hospital (Dr. Avola); Visiting Physician, Lawrence Memorial Hospital (Dr. Gonnella).

Report of a Case

A 31-year-old, white, primiparous female in the eighth month of a normal pregnancy was admitted to the Lawrence Memorial Hospital on Feb 5, 1960, with the chief complaint of sharp lower abdominal pain of several hours' duration associated with vomiting and general malaise. About 5½ hours prior to admission to the hospital the patient attempted to have a bowel movement which did not result in the emission of stools. While straining, she felt a very sharp, diffuse pain in the lower abdomen which did not localize anywhere. She immediately went to bed feeling weak and faint. She became nauseated and had several bouts of vomiting of stomach contents without evidence of blood. She had previously been completely asymptomatic, and there was no history of trauma or upper respiratory infection. About 14 years previously she had been hospitalized at a sanitarium because of pulmonary tuberculosis and had a right upper lobectomy. Since that time she had been followed at six-month intervals and had remained well. She was seen for the first time by her obstetrician only two weeks before the present admission, at which time physical examination was negative except for enlargement of the abdomen consistent with a normal pregnancy of eight months. Her expected date of confinement was March 10, 1960. The past history and systems reviewed were otherwise completely negative.

Physical examination revealed a pale, acutely-ill, 31-year-old, white woman. Blood pressure was 118/74; pulse, 110; respiration, 24; temperature, 99 F. The skin was cold and clammy. There was a well-healed right thoracotomy scar from the previous surgery. The positive findings were confined to the abdomen.

The abdomen was distended with an enlarged uterus, consistent with an eight-month pregnancy. There was diffuse tenderness throughout the abdomen. Peristalsis was moderately subdued. She complained of fullness in the abdomen above what had been present prior to the onset of the present illness. Palpation of the abdomen was hampered somewhat by the distended uterus, but definite increase in muscle resistance in the right lower quadrant was present. The fetal heart beat varied from 135 to 145 per minute. There was no vaginal discharge on examination. Rectal examination revealed the cervix to be closed. Stool specimen on the gloved finger was black, but the Guaiac test was negative. The patient had been taking iron. White blood cell count on admission was 21,600 cells per cu ml with a normal differential count. Hemoglobin was 9.9 gm, and hematocrit was 30%. Prothrombin time was 13.7 seconds, control 11.3 seconds. Urinalysis was negative.

The patient was transfused with 1,000 ml of whole blood and brought to the operating room with a preoperative diagnosis of massive intraperitoneal hemorrhage secondary to possible rupture of a right ovarian tumor or rupture of varicosity of broad ligament. Using spinal anesthesia supplemented by inhalation anesthesia, laparotomy was performed through a low midline incision. Immediately upon entering the peritoneal cavity a large quantity of dark liquid blood was encountered with massive clots in both lateral peritoneal gutters. About two liters of liquid blood was evacuated with suction, and the large clots were removed manually. Rapid exploration of the peritoneal cavity was then carried out. Occupying the entire right peritoneal gutter was a large kidney-shaped mass, measuring 15 by 10 by 8 cm. This mass was attached by a broad pedicle about 4 cm in diameter near the right cornu of the uterus. On the anterior surface of the mass near its upper pole there was a dilated subserosal vein which was oozing dark venous blood. Because the tumor fit rather snugly with its long axis in the right pericolic area and because of the rather broad-based pedicle, torsion of the pedicle of the tumor was not possible. No other source of bleeding was encountered. Removal of the tumor was accomplished by cutting across the base of the pedicle between crushing Kocher clamps. The defect on the side of the uterus was then closed over with a running chromic suture. Because of the vascularity of the pregnant uterus, each suture bled rather vigorously but subsided after applying several interrupted sutures and Gelfoam to the surface. After removal of the tumor it could be ascertained that both tubes and ovaries were quite normal. The abdomen was then closed in layers. Her condition remained quite stable during the operation.

Two postoperative transfusions of whole blood, 500 ml each, were given to restore the hematocrit to a near normal level for her expected delivery in four weeks. Except for a minor allergic reaction to one of the postoperative transfusions, convalescence was essentially uneventful. Pathologic report was benign leiomyoma of the previously stated dimensions. She was discharged home, improved, on Feb 15, 1960. On March 8, 1960, she was readmitted to the hospital, where on the following day she was delivered of a normal 6 lb, 11 oz (3.034 gm) girl. Her delivery was essentially normal, and she was again discharged home on March 15, 1960. The patient has had one other normal delivery since that time and has remained perfectly well with normal pelvic examinations.

Comment

Saidi et al,[1] in a review of the world literature in 1961, noted 46 cases in every instance of which the bleeding had occurred from torn and enlarged veins coursing over the surface of subserous fibroids. After excluding a number of cases which included ruptured vessel at the stalk of a pedunculated and twisted fibroid, evidence of infarction in the fibroid, and malignant or aseptic degeneration of the tumor with secondary hemorrhage, these authors reduced the total number of reported cases to 26.

In this patient the sudden straining effort at stool with the consequent rise in venous pressure apparently was enough to rupture the vessel. One can postulate a pre-existing weakness at the site of rupture with enlargement and stretching of the surface veins caused by the pressure of rapid growth of the fibroid under the persistent hormonal stimulus of pregnancy. Indeed, Sampson,[2] using injection studies found that the venous drainage of large uterine fibroids occurs by way of veins coursing over their surface and entering the supporting myometrium at the periphery of the tumor. Under these circumstances, anything which increases venous pressure suddenly (coughing, straining, stooping) may precipitate the final bleeding event, and direct trauma from an external source need not enter the picture at all. The difficulty of examining the abdomen in a patient with catastrophic bleeding with its attendent abdominal spasm and impending shock generally makes the diagnosis difficult to make preoperatively. In a pregnant woman, especially near term, the diagnosis is almost impossible to make by physical examination. Knowledge of a pre-existing uterine fibroid obtained during previous examinations certainly would be helpful. Treatment in the reported cases has usually consisted of supracervical hysterectomy. At times the configuration and position of the fibroid tumor lends itself to rather simple myomectomy. In cases where the condition of the patient is extremely poor and speed is of the essence, there should be no contraindication to simple ligation of the bleeding vein. In this particular patient the ease of removal of the fibroid because of its relatively narrow stalk prompted this mode of therapy. Had this tumor been incorporated within the wall of the fundus, cesarean section, followed by myomectomy could have been resorted to.

Francis A. Avola, MD, 10 High St, Medford 55, Mass.

REFERENCES

1. Saidi, F; Constable, J. D.; and Ulfelder, H: Massive Intraperitoneal Hemorrhage Due to Uterine Fibroids, Amer Obstet Gynec 82:367-374, 1961.

2. Sampson, J. A.: The Influence of Myomata on the Blood Supply of the Uterus, With Special Reference to Abnormal Uterine Bleeding, Based on the Study of 150 Injected Uteri Containing These Tumors, Surg Gynec Obstet 16:144, 1913.

Oxidized Regenerated Cellulose for Hepatic Hemostasis

GEORGE F. WRIGHT, MD
AND
R. ROBERT TYSON, MD
PHILADELPHIA

Introduction

Oxidized regenerated cellulose is a relatively recent addition to the surgeon's armamentarium for hemostasis. Its hemostatic and absorbable qualities have been attested to by several authors in recent articles.[1-5] There have also been several articles describing its chemical nature, the mechanism of solubility in human tissues, and, finally, the methods by which it stops bleeding.[1,5] Briefly, it is a polyanhydroglucuronic acid manufactured from a substantially pure α-cellulose.[5] Its specific hemostatic property apparently depends upon the formation of a coagulum consisting of cellulose acid and hemoglobin, and it has been demonstrated to be readily soluble in alkaline solution.[5]

It is our purpose to evaluate this hemostatic gauze experimentally with regard to the frequently trying problem of hepatic hemostasis and to comment on a few of our clinical experiences with this material to date.

Submitted for publication March 30, 1963.

Fellow of the American Cancer Society (Dr. Wright).

This study was supported by a grant from Johnson & Johnson, New Brunswick, NJ.

Methods and Procedures

Adult, medium-sized mongrel dogs were used. All operations were done under sterile conditions. Anesthesia consisted of 1 mg of intravenous sodium pentobarbital per pound body weight. Respirations were supported with endotracheal intubation and a respirator. All dogs received 600,000 units of procaine penicillin and 1.0 gm of streptomycin as the abdomen was being closed.

A. *Group A—Control.*—One half of the left posterior lobe of the liver was excised in three dogs and the abdomen then closed. In three hours the abdomen was reopened, and the blood in the peritoneal cavity was measured. The results are listed in Table 1.

B. *Group B—Hemostasis.*—This same procedure with the following modifications was then carried out in six additional dogs. First, the lobe was grasped between the index and middle fingers of the right hand as close to its hilum as possible, controlling hemorrhage by compression of the parenchyma until the gauze could be applied. Then after excision, a 4 $\times$ 8 inch piece of the gauze

TABLE 1.—*Group A—Control*

Dog No.	Wt (Lb)	Blood Loss	Death: Time	Death: Mode	Findings
1	22	Massive	2 hr	Died	475 cc blood in abd.
2	26	Massive	3 hr	Sac.	400 cc blood in abd.
3	21	Massive	3 hr	Sac.	400 cc blood in abd.

was doubly or triply folded and wrapped over the cut surface of the lobe, and compression was maintained over this for four-five minutes, in addition to the proximal compression. Usually one or two additional 2 × 3 inch pieces of the gauze were required to stop all oozing. No sutures were used to hold the gauze in place, and no other measures were used to control the hemorrhage. The results are listed in Table 2.

C. *Group C—Absorbability.*—The above procedure was then carried out in ten additional dogs, but these were not reopened in three hours. They were sacrificed at various times during the ensuing three months. Each animal had a complete autopsy at the time of death, all gross findings were noted, and specimens of the operative area were taken for microscopy. The results are briefly summarized in Table 3.

Comment

A. *Hemostatic Ability.*—Preliminary work in our laboratories had shown that the dog will survive without any therapy whatsoever after extensive liver trauma and secondary massive hemorrhage. Thus, we decided to use as the endpoint for our evaluation the amount of blood present in the peritoneal cavity at a specified time after completion of a standard amount of hepatic trauma. In the control group A this averaged approximately 400 cc. With the addition of the hemostatic gauze in group B blood loss averaged 40-50 cc at the time of appli-

TABLE 2.—*Group B—Hemostasis*

Dog No.	Wt (Lb)	Blood Loss	Death: Time	Death: Mode	Findings	Result
1	26	50 cc	3 hr	Sac.	15 cc serosanguineous fluid in abd. and gauze in place	Excellent
2	15	60 cc	3 hr	Sac.	15 cc serosanguineous fluid in abd. and gauze in place	Excellent
3	26	300 cc	3 hr	Sac.	75 cc blood and extensive clot around liver	Poor
4	26	75 cc	3 hr	Sac.	15 cc blood in abd. and gauze in place	Excellent
5	13	250 cc	3 hr	Died	75 cc blood in abd. and clot around liver	Poor
6	36	40	3 hr	Sac.	15 cc blood in abd. and gauze in place	Excellent

TABLE 3.—*Group C—Absorbability*

Dog No.	Wt (Lb)	Death: Time	Death: Mode	Findings	Result
1	20	3 da	Sac.	No blood or evidence of infection; gauze in place and brown in color	Excellent
2	20	4 da	Died	400 cc blood in abd.; gauze mixed with clot in LUQ	Poor
3	24	6 da	Died	No blood or evidence of infection; gauze in place, brown and friable; gross pneumonia with lung abscess	Excellent with regard to the gauze
4	18	10 da	Sac.	No blood or infection; gauze almost absorbed	Excellent
5	22	13 da	Sac.	Gross peritonitis with leaking abscess at operative area that contained pieces of gauze	Poor
6	36	21 da	Sac.	Gross peritonitis with leaking abscess at operative area that contained pieces of gauze	Poor
7	24	29 da	Sac.	No blood or infection in abd.; gauze absorbed; many adhesions in upper abdomen	Excellent
8	20	33 da	Died	No blood or infection in abd.; gauze partly absorbed; diffuse pneumonia	Excellent with regard to the gauze
9	15	70 da	Sac.	No blood or infection in abd.; gauze absorbed; adhesions in upper abdomen	Excellent
10	25	86 da	Sac.	No blood or infection in abd.; gauze absorbed; adhesions in upper abdomen	Excellent

cation, and at re-exploration only 15-20 cc of serosanguineous fluid was found in the peritoneal cavity in four of the six dogs. This indicated in these dogs that the gauze was an extremely effective hemostatic agent. In the remaining two dogs difficulties arose in controlling the hemorrhage prior to and during application, and a good result was not achieved. Under these conditions the gauze had a tendency to stick to wet instruments or gloves, and it could not be snugly contoured to the surface. In view of this, we would suggest, when possible, temporary proximal control of the bleeding and then some means of fixation such as sutures. This gauze, in contrast to other hemostatic materials currently available, does not fragment easily, but maintains its tensile strength for some time, and would lend itself well to this technique.

B. *Absorbability.*—Previous workers have described the rapid disappearance of this gauze in animals and humans, especially when it was placed in the peritoneal cavity.[1-5] Jantet and Rob,[3] however, demonstrated in rats that absorption from the liver was slower than from other sites and that encapsulation sometimes occurred. Absorption was complete in 10-14 days in all their animals except for one who developed an abscess and local peritonitis. In this animal the gauze was still visible at 15 days. Miller and Thomas[4] demonstrated in dogs that the gauze after being implanted in the liver was still demonstrable at ten days. No infection developed in their six dogs.

In our group of ten dogs, examined from three days to three months postoperatively, seven showed no further evidence of bleeding or infection in the peritoneal cavity although two of these died of pneumonia at 6 and 33 days. The gauze was recognizable grossly at ten days but not at 29 days. The sequence of events microscopically was initial minimal infiltration of the operative area by neutrophils and macrophages followed by fibroblastic organization. Granuloma production was evident at ten days, and the gauze appeared as a mass of pink-staining amorphous material reminiscent of fibrin. Fibrosis and foreign-body granulomatous reaction with giant cells was seen at 29 days and finally only fibrosis at 70 days.

One dog in this group died on the fourth postoperative day of massive hemorrhage at the operative site. This was most likely due to faulty application of the gauze and probably would have been prevented if some means of fixation had been used such as was suggested above.

Two dogs developed gross peritonitis secondary to ruptured abscesses at the operative site. The abscess cavities contained between 75 and 100 cc of pus and, in addition, several small pieces of gray-brown, soft material that undoubtedly represented the gauze. Cultures of these abscesses revealed *Pseudomonas.* Factors in the etiology of these infections include the use of relatively large amounts of the gauze several layers thick making absorption much more prolonged and the well-known fact that the dog's liver contains organisms itself that may be released into the peritoneal cavity.

C. *Clinical Experience.*—In view of these results, it seems pertinent to mention our limited clinical experience with this material to date. The gauze was used in five cases of hepatic trauma with intraperitoneal hemorrhage. Four of the cases can be considered excellent results. Hemorrhage was stopped quickly, and the postoperative course was uneventful. A fifth patient had blunt trauma to the abdomen causing multiple liver lacerations and massive intraperitoneal hemorrhage. Adequate control of the hemorrhage was achieved at the time of surgery with large amounts of the hemostatic gauze. Postoperatively, however, a wound infection developed that continued to drain for 40 days, finally extruding much of the gauze prior to healing. The patient subsequently recovered without any further difficulties. Thus, infection and nonabsorption can occur when this gauze is used for hepatic hemostasis.

Nevertheless, because of its excellent hemostatic ability and its relative ease of handling we feel that this hemostatic gauze definitely has a role in the difficult case of extensive hepatic trauma with massive hemorrhage, a frequently trying situation for the surgeon. Several recommendations seem in order, though, when using it, and these are: (1) use only as much material as absolutely needed, (2) attempt to obtain proximal control of the bleeding area to facilitate application, (3) use some means of fixation such as sutures, and (4) as in all traumatic surgery, maintain strict asepsis and remove all blood and devitalized tissue.

Summary

Experimental evaluation of oxidized regenerated cellulose in hepatic hemostasis has demonstrated that the material is effective in controlling hemorrhage from the liver. Further investigation has shown that infection and nonabsorption can occur. In spite of this we feel that the material has a definite role in the difficult case of hepatic trauma with hemorrhage, provided one uses only as much as is necessary and adheres to good surgical principles.

George F. Wright, MD, Department of Surgery, Temple University, School of Medicine and Hospital, Broad and Ontario Streets, Philadelphia, Pa.

REFERENCES

1. Lebendiger, A.; Gitlitz, G. F.; Hurwitt, E. S.; Lord, G. H.; and Henderson, J.: Laboratory and Clinical Evaluation of a New Absorbable Hemostatic Material Prepared From Oxidized Regenerated Cellulose, Surg Forum, 10:440-443, 1960.

2. Hurwitt, E. S.; Henderson, J.; Lord, G. H.; Gitliz, G. F.; and Lebendiger, A.: A New Surgical Absorbable Hemostatic Agent, Amer J Surg 100: 439-446, 1960.

3. Jantet, G. H., and Rob, C.: An Experimental and Clinical Investigation of a New Hemostatic Absorbable Gauze, Brit J Surg 48:270-271, 1960.

4. Miller, J. M., and Thomas, V. T.: The Use of Oxidized Regenerated Cellulose as a Hemostatic Agent in Dogs, Exp Med Surg 19:192-195, 1961.

5. Miller, J. M.; Jackson, D. A.; and Collier, C. S.: An Investigation of the Chemical Reactions of Oxidized Regenerated Cellulose, Exp Med Surg 19:196-202, 1961.

Nasogastric Tube and Pulmonary Ventilation

W. D. MACKAY, MB ABERD, AND N. A. MATHESON, MB ABERD, FRCS, FRCSE,
ABERDEEN, SCOTLAND

The belief is widely held that a nasogastric tube adversely affects pulmonary ventilation, interferes with coughing, and predisposes to postoperative atelectasis. This impression is undoubtedly in part responsible for the present tendency to avoid nasogastric suction after major abdominal operations.

Bevan (1961) measured the forced expiratory volume in one second before and after withdrawal of a nasogastric tube in eight patients after operation and found an improvement of 4% to 24% in seven. On these grounds, he claimed that removal of the tube benefited both breathing and coughing and helped to prevent postoperative pulmonary complications. Although these views may be justified, they are based on insufficient evidence; therefore, it seemed desirable to extend Bevan's (1961) investigation and to interpret the eventual results more rigorously. Accordingly, the effect of a nasogastric tube on pulmonary ventilation was assessed in a larger number of patients, both before and after operation.

Sequential analysis enables a comparison of pairs of observations to be concluded as soon as a definite positive or negative result emerges, and usually provides an economical method of conducting such a study. Therefore, the interpretation of the findings in the postoperative group was based on a sequential *t*-test (Armitage, 1960).

Methods

1. An unselected group of 24 patients who had undergone nasogastric suction for at least 24 hours after gastrointestinal operations was studied: Peak expiratory flow rate (PEFR) in liters per minute was measured with a Wright flowmeter (Wright and McKerrow, 1959) in each patient, before and 15 to 30 minutes after removing the tube. The small number of patients who were unable to cooperate in performing the test were not included in the study.

2. PEFR was measured immediately before, and 15 to 30 minutes after, passing a nasogastric tube in 27 unselected patients about to have a histamine test meal. In addition, vital capacity (VC) and forced expiratory volume in one second (FEV_1) were measured in 12 of these patients, using a nine-liter, water-sealed spirometer, with a two-speed kymograph.

In both groups the figure taken for the PEFR was the mean of six consecutive attempts and that for the VC and FEV_1 the mean of three readings. The spirometric volumes were corrected to body temperature, prevailing barometric pressure, and water vapor saturation (BTPS).

Results

The results in the postoperative group of patients were analyzed, as they became available, with a sequential *t*-test. Peak flow rates from each patient with and without the tube provided one pair of observations in each instance. When the numerical difference d between each pair was found, z was calculated from the formula:

$$z = \frac{(\Sigma d)^2}{\Sigma d^2}$$

where Σd is the cumulative sum of the difference for all the pairs so far recorded, and Σd^2 is the cumulative sum of the squares of these differences. If in the long run there is no difference, the mean μ of the values of d tends towards zero and therefore z remains low. If d increases with either a positive or negative sign z also increases, but is always positive because it is a function of $(\Sigma d)^2$.

It is convenient to specify sequential designs to detect predetermined mean differences μ with reasonable certainty by a quan-

Submitted for publication March 30, 1963.

Registrar in Surgery (Dr. Mackay); Lecturer in Surgery (Dr. Matheson).

Department of Surgery, University of Aberdeen.

tity δ_1 and if σ denotes the standard deviation of the distribution of *d*, then the selection of a suitable design is based on the equation:

$$\mu = \delta_1 \sigma$$

It follows that an estimate of σ permits the choice of an appropriate value of δ_1, and accordingly a suitable design. At the beginning of this study information about σ was not available; therefore, the first ten pairs of observations were completed and analyzed to give an approximate value of σ (12.46) and of the mean level of performance (132.3). Changes of less than 5% in PEFR were arbitrarily regarded as being clinically insignificant and an open design was chosen with $\mu/\sigma = \delta_1 = 0.7$. The value of μ from this formula, expressed as a percentage of the mean performance, is 6.6%. In other words, the design can detect with reasonable certainty a 6.6% change in PEFR if such a change exists.

In the Figure the vertical axis indicates the value of *z* and the horizontal the number of pairs of observations. The sample path is formed by successive values of *z* plotted on the chart: If this path crosses the upper boundary, a significant difference in either direction exists; but should it cross the lower boundary, a significant difference is not present. With this particular design the probability of erroneously reaching the outer boundary when $\mu = 0$ is 0.05, and the probability of detecting the predetermined difference when it exists is 0.95.

The lower boundary was crossed when 23 pairs of observations had been made: Therefore there is satisfactory evidence that the presence of a nasogastric tube after operation does not impair peak expiratory flow rate by as much as 6.6%. It *may* cause a smaller decrement, and this seems not unlikely from the initial tendency for the sample path to wander between the boundaries. We believe that such an impairment, if it exists, is clinically unimportant.

PEFR fell by 30% after nasogastric intubation in one of the 27 patients who were investigated before operation, but the mean flow rate of the group was 420 liters per minute under both conditions: The tube did not cause significant impairment in performance.

One of the 12 patients in whom VC and FEV_1 were measured showed a notable reduction in ventilatory capacity (Table). This patient's (patient 11) VC fell by 20% and his FEV_1 by 10%, but the performance of the remainder was unaffected by the tube and there was no significant difference in the results obtained from the group as a whole.

Comment

Apart from reduced efficiency of coughing, the main factors in the causation of postoperative atelectasis are said to be impaired ventilatory capacity, airway obstruction from bronchospasm, and increased bronchial secretions (Palmer and Sellick, 1953; Palmer,

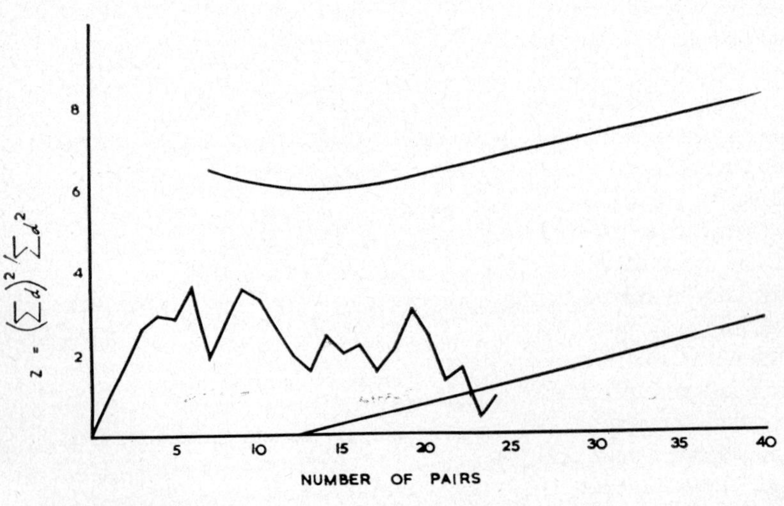

Sequential *t*-test open design. Critical value of $\mu/\sigma = \delta_1 = 0.7$.

*Comparison Between Basal Readings and Those With a Nasogastric Tube in Situ**

Patient No.	VC in Liters		FEV$_1$ in Liters	
	Basal	With NGT	Basal	With NGT
1	5.00	5.40	3.96	3.91
2	4.72	4.43	4.18	4.14
3	6.08	6.47	4.86	4.90
4	3.96	3.96	2.56	2.63
5	4.90	4.50	2.81	2.88
6	3.66	3.52	2.60	2.44
7	3.89	3.92	2.88	2.84
8	3.42	3.49	3.13	3.13
9	3.84	3.74	3.11	3.30
10	2.48	2.56	0.97	0.94
11	3.71	2.95	3.02	2.74
12	3.46	3.56	3.17	3.13
Mean	4.09	4.04	3.11	3.08

* Each volume is the mean of three estimations and has been corrected to BTPS. A significant difference does not exist.

1962). Notwithstanding recent attempts to estimate the force of coughing by measurements of intra-abdominal pressure (Egbert et al, 1961 and 1962), a method is not available to measure this force directly. However, coughing does depend to a large extent on rapid expulsion of air from the chest, and therefore peak expiratory flow rate should reflect coughing ability. If peak flow rate is adversely affected by any particular factor, the effectiveness of coughing must be reduced; but if peak flow rate is unaffected, coughing is probably unimpaired. We deduce that the presence of a nasogastric tube is unlikely to influence coughing ability postoperatively. Furthermore, the observation that a nasogastric tube does not affect the performance of conventional pulmonary ventilation tests preoperatively, or cause significant impairment after operation, indicates that neither is ventilatory capacity influenced nor bronchospasm induced. Finally, we know of no evidence that a nasogastric tube stimulates the production of bronchial secretions. Therefore, it would be surprising if the presence of a nasogastric tube affected the incidence of atelectasis, particularly in view of the marked reductions in ventilatory efficiency which follow abdominal operations for other reasons (Palmer, 1961). Nevertheless, objective evidence has recently been presented which suggests that some association exists between the nasogastric tube and respiratory complications: Grant et al (1962) in a retrospective study have found that patients over 60, who underwent prolonged nasogastric suction, had a higher incidence of complications than those decompressed with gastrostomy. Because we can neither confirm Bevan's (1961) findings nor support Farris and Smith's (1956) contention that the tube provoked "dislocation of the mechanisms involved in respiratory exchange," we suggest that the increased incidence depends on other factors; nasopharyngeal mucorrhea, and infection, and subjective unwillingness to cough may be some of the more important.

Summary

Peak expiratory flow rates were measured postoperatively before and after removal of a nasogastric tube. The results were analyzed by using a sequential *t*-test, a technique which proved useful in establishing the absence of a significant difference between the groups. The findings were similar in a group of preoperative patients, in whom vital capacity and forced expiratory volume in one second were measured, before and after passing a nasogastric tube. The relationship between the nasogastric tube and postoperative respiratory complications is discussed.

N. A. Matheson, MB, FRCS, Department of Surgery, University of Aberdeen, Foresterhill, Aberdeen, Scotland.

REFERENCES

1. Armitage, P., in Sequential Medical Trials, Oxford, England: Blackwell Scientific Publications, 1960.
2. Bevan, P. G.: Brit J Surg 49:126, 1961.
3. Egbert, L. D.; Tamersoy, K.; and Deas, T. C.: Anaesthesiology 22:882, 1961.
4. Egbert, L. D.; Laver M. B.; and Bendixen, H. H.: Surg Gynec Obstet 115:295, 1962.
5. Farris, J. M., and Smith, G. K.: Ann Surg 144:475, 1956.
6. Grant, G. N.; Elliot, D. W.; and Frederick, P. L.: Arch Surg 85:844, 1962.
7. Palmer, K. N. V.: Lancet 1:191, 1961.
8. Palmer, K. N. V.: J Roy Coll Surg Edin 7:110, 1962.
9. Palmer, K. N. V., and Sellick, B. A.: Lancet 1:164, 1953.
10. Wright, B. M., and McKerrow, C. B.: Brit Med J 2:1041, 1959.

Aneurysm of Splenic Artery With Calcification

JEHOOM YANG, MD
STEVEN J. SPINUZZA, MD
AND
R. KENNEDY GILCHRIST, MD
CHICAGO

Aneurysm of the splenic artery is an infrequent lesion. The diagnosis is rarely made from clinical symptoms alone. Rupture is attended by a very high mortality. However, if the lesion is diagnosed before rupture occurs, surgical treatment is usually uneventful and successful. We present a case which was diagnosed before rupture and was successfully treated surgically.

Report of a Case

A 53-year-old housewife, postmenopausal, healthy, was admitted to Ravenswood Hospital on March 24, 1962, for surgical treatment of a possible calcified aneurysm of the splenic artery. During her last admission the patient's chief complaint was a "fire ball in the stomach."

Present Illness.—In the past six to eight years, she had suffered from headache with nausea, occasional vomiting, bloating, and full sensation under the left costal margin which was associated with occasional pain in the back and shoulders.

About four years ago, while bending over, she felt a "twisting and knotting" sensation in the epigastrium, and she was momentarily breathless. She had had several attacks which were unaffected by diet. She complained of weakness, fatigue, insomnia, night sweats, and continued bloating in the left upper quadrant of the abdomen. She lost eight pounds of weight.

On March 5, 1962, she had a "flip-flop" sensation in the epigastrium and suddenly "a hot ball of fire" with radiating pain to the midepigastrium, the back, and across the shoulders, and she felt a "terrible" fullness in the epigastrium. The attack seemed to be relieved while she was lying flat on her back. The pain was not related to food intake. On March 6, 1962, gallbladder x-rays were normal. On March 12, 1962, she had another attack and was admitted to the hospital.

Past History.—She had had common childhood diseases and an appendectomy at the age of 14 years. She married at the age of 31 years, gravida II, para II.

Systemic survey was negative with the exception of frequent episodes of upper respiratory infection.

Physical Examination.—On her admission, the blood pressure was 112/78 mm Hg. The pulse was 80 and regular. The lungs revealed some coarse rales at the left base. The heart was negative.

Submitted for publication March 30, 1963.

From Department of Surgery, Ravenswood Hospital.

Resident in Pathology at Ravenswood Hospital; graduated, Chonnam University Medical College, Korea, 1958 (Dr. Yang).

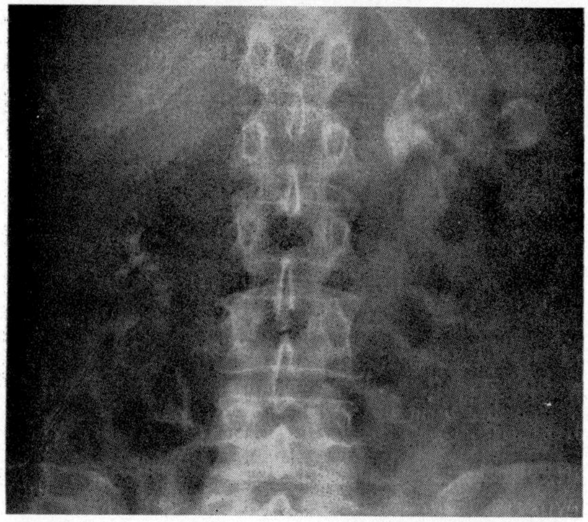

Intravenous pyelogram showing the round, somewhat eggshell-like shadow in the left upper quadrant.

There was slight tenderness in the left hypochondrium radiating to the left flank on palpation. No abnormal masses or bruit were detected. Pelvic examination was normal.

Laboratory Findings.—Blood and urine examinations were normal, and the Kahn test was negative as was the electrocardiogram.

Chest x-ray on March 14, 1962, revealed no significant findings. The gastrointestinal series on March 14, 1962, were negative. A 2.0 cm round calcification was present in the left upper quadrant, having the appearance of a vascular calcification, possible due to a calcified aneurysm of the splenic artery. On March 24, 1962, she still complained of a fullness and bloating in the epigastrium without physical change. The intravenous pyelogram on March 26, 1962, was normal, and the same calcified round mass was identified (Figure).

At operation on March 28, 1962, a thumb-sized, sharply localized, calcified aneurysm of the splenic artery at the hilum of the spleen was found. Overlying this, there was a thickened area of straw-gray-yellow substance which measured about 1.0 to 1.5 mm. There was no sign of any other pathology. The splenic artery was ligated proximal to the aneurysm, and the aneurysm and the spleen were removed.

Pathology Report.—Macroscopically the spleen was not remarkable, measuring 11.0 by 7.0 by 3.0 cm and weighing 135 gm. At the hilus of the spleen, a hard, calcified, round mass was encountered measuring up to 1.6 cm in diameter and was covered with a tough, gray-to-yellow membrane 0.5 mm thick. On both sides of the lesion, small veins and arteries entered the hilum of the spleen without lesions. Microscopically, the spleen was normal, and sections from the firm nodule showed a dilated, extensively hyalinized, and partly ossified arterial wall.

The postoperative course was uneventful. Subsequent to surgery, the patient was relieved of the abdominal pain and distress and discharged on April 12, 1962.

Comment

Incidence.—The splenic artery is a site for aneurysm within the abdomen along with the abdominal aorta and iliac arteries.[24,25] The incidence of aneurysm of the splenic artery at autopsy is 0.04% to 0.05% (Table 1).

Aneurysm of the splenic artery occurs two to three times as frequently in the female as in the male (Table 2). Other aneurysms occur more frequently in the male by a ratio of four or five to one.[4,14,25]

The ages range from 14 years to 88 years,[14,19] most common in the fifth decade.[25] There may be a relatively high incidence in the child-bearing period, which probably plays a role as to the initiating factor in the formation of the aneurysmal defect.[14,19]

TABLE 1.—*Incidence of Aneurysm of the Splenic Artery at Autopsy*

Author	Yr	No. of Autopsies	No. of Aneurysms	%	No. of Splenic Aneurysms	%
Emmerich *	1888	8,669	58	0.67	1	0.010
Bosdorf *	1898	3,108	93	3.00	7	0.230
Schroetter *	1898	19,300	200	1.04	4	0.020
Muller *	1902	10,360	184	1.78	9	0.090
Schroeder	1918	32,768	—	—	20	0.060
Garland	1921	4,100	—	—	3	0.070
Ophuls	1926	3,000	—	—	1	0.030
Guy	1936	1,500	—	—	1	0.070
Sperling	1940	33,810	393	1.17	7	0.020
Seids & Hauser	1941	13,874	—	—	4	0.029
Total		129,509	928	1.23	57	0.044

* Lindboe analyzed these four extensive surveys and found a 0.05% incidence of aneurysm of the splenic artery.

TABLE 2.—*Sex Incidence of Aneurysm of the Splenic Artery*

Authors		No. of Cases	No. in the Female (%)	No. in the Male (%)	Ratio
Baumgartner	(1924)	35 *	19 (54)	16 (46)	1.2:1
Sherlock	(1942)	117	75 (64)	42 (36)	1.8:1
Owens & Coffey	(1953)	190	127 (67)	63 (33)	2.0:1
Spittel	(1961)	61	46 (75)	15 (25)	3.0:1
Total		403	267 (66)	139 (34)	2.0:1

* Five of 40 cases were not included because of unknown sex.

Etiology and Pathogenesis.—Arteriosclerosis is the most common factor.[2,4,8,15,20,25] This degenerative change of the arterial wall provides weakened areas which may bulge with ease, even in the absence of increased blood pressure.[19] An older group of patients seem to be frequently involved by the factor (Table 3).

Developmental defect of the splenic artery is probably an important factor along with the arteriosclerosis. This is based on the demonstration or discovery of developmental failure, defect, or absence of a part of the blood vessel, the intima, or media.[3,4,7,11,12] Familial hemorrhagic telangiectasis and aneurysms of the circle of Willis might be associated with the splenic artery aneurysm.[6,19]

Embolus may be an important factor and may produce mycotic aneurysm of the splenic artery from vegetation of endocarditis,[2] involving a younger group of patients (Table 3).

Syphilis is a doubtful factor.[1,4,8,10,24] However, conclusive evidence of syphilitic panarteritis has been demonstrated.[14] Pregnancy not only may be an initiating factor, but may be the cause of rupture and/or increasing size of the pre-existing aneurysm of the splenic artery, providing an increase of intra-abdominal pressure,[15,26] which may cause a bulging of the degenerated, weakened, or congenitally defective wall of the splenic artery. Thus, pregnancy may be one of the most important factors which precipitate rupture of aneurysm of the splenic artery.[6,7,10,11,19] The lesion was more frequently found in multipara.[26]

Trauma, congestive splenomegaly, hypertension, and an arteriovenous communication should be considered as causative factors.[14,19,25]

Pathological Features.—The size of the aneurysm of the splenic artery, though variable, has averaged 3.0 cm in diameter, the largest one being 15.0 cm.[15]

The location of the aneurysm of the splenic artery is most commonly the main trunk of the artery [1,8,14]; only one third of the cases involved a branch. Involvement of both the trunk and a branch is much less frequent. Degenerative aneurysm seems to involve mostly the main trunk and occurs singly; only a quarter of the cases were multiple. Sherlock reported ten aneurysms of the splenic artery.[19]

Clinical Manifestations.—There are no specific symptoms for the splenic artery aneurysm, and many of the lesions are asymptomatic until rupture occurs. The onset is not obvious, and it is difficult to esti-

TABLE 3.—*Comparison of Etiologic Factors With Average Age Involved*

	Sherlock (1942), 117 Cases		Owens (1953), 190 Cases		Spittel (1961), 61 Cases	
Factors	%	Av Age	%	Av Age	%	Av Age
Arteriosclerosis	46	56	60	65	57.9	67
Congenital	8.2	41	10	30	28.9	58
Mycotic and embolitic	23	29	23	30	5.3	29
Trauma	5.4	—	3	35	2.6	34

mate the duration of the lesion; but there are several clinical manifestations which may suggest the presence of an aneurysm of the splenic artery and may be present from one day to many years.[1,8]

The symptoms produced by an aneurysm of the splenic artery are of two types: those occuring before rupture and those after rupture.

The most common symptom before rupture is abdominal pain, usually located in the epigastrium on the left upper quadrant with varying intensity from mild distress to colicky attack. These pains may be aggravated by change of posture, exercise, or bending. *Epigastric pain aggravated by bending or stooping is suggestive of a splenic artery aneurysm.*[13] The pain may radiate to the back, shoulders, the neck, and to the left arm, simulating a coronary attack, and radiate to the lower abdomen. Later it may localize in the right upper quadrant, simulating gallbladder disease and duodenal ulcer. The mechanism of the pain may be the adherence of the involved artery to the lesser curvature of the stomach which, by irritating the muscular wall of the stomach, produces pain similar to that of a gastric ulcer.[16] In association with the pain there are vague symptoms, most of which are referable to the gastrointestinal tract: nausea and vomiting, indigestion and dyspepsia, those of gastric or duodenal ulcer, or gallbladder disease. At times, there may be weakness and weight loss. A fullness with a bloating sensation in the epigastrium or in the left hypochondrium is one of the manifestations.

The incidence of rupture may be more than 40% of the cases,[1,2,14] and, when associated with pregnancy, it may exceed 80%.[14,20,26] The interval between the onset of the symptoms and rupture is from a few minutes or hours to months.

Occasionally, rupture may be the first manifestation of a silent aneurysm of the splenic artery. The rupture may occur as a single or one-stage rupture which is usually fatal, or a double or two-stage rupture.[3,7,10,18]

In the two-stage rupture, a retroperitoneal hematoma develops behind the lesser sac with the initial rupture producing a false aneurysm. At this time exacerbation of any symptoms and signs which have been previously present will occur. Then clotting occurs followed by a quiescent period which may last for a few hours or for several months. Sooner or later a secondary rupture of the false aneurysm will follow which will be fatal unless proper and prompt surgical treatment is instituted.[4] The rupture into the peritoneal cavity through the lesser sac and the foramen of Winslow is the most common [6,19]; next in occurrence is rupture into the stomach and the retroperitoneum. Zeluff reported a rupture into the left chest.[27]

The symptoms after rupture are usually those of an acute abdomen. The condition will simulate almost any acute disaster occurring within the abdomen, with sudden onset of the epigastric pain and a varying number of the signs of shock due to loss of blood. Among diagnoses to be considered are perforated peptic ulcer; acute pancreatitis; acute intestinal obstruction; volvulus; mesenteric infarction; tortion of the omentum; renal colic; cholecystitis; coronary thrombosis; during pregnancy, rupture of the uterus, ruptured ectopic pregnancy, and premature separation of the placenta.[19,23]

Physical Findings.—In our case, no significant findings were encountered except for some tenderness in the left hypochondrium and in the left flank. The abdominal tenderness, an important finding, may be occasionally severe, localized to the upper abdomen or to the left quadrant, and may be prominent if the lesion is large. There may be signs of shock, especially when the lesion ruptures. An abdominal mass may be palpated beside the spleen in the left upper quadrant. The mass may be pulsatile, but these findings are absent when the aneurysm is smaller. Splenomegaly may be present and may be a common finding.[14,18,19] Careful physical examination may disclose a bruit over the abdomen.[20] Occasionally, this bruit will be accompanied by a pulsatile tumor which may lead the examiner to suspect the presence of a splenic artery aneurysm.

Roentgenographic study is the most important diagnostic procedure and provides very valuable information.[25] If the lesion is calcified, x-ray findings may give the correct diagnosis.[15,24] Calcific deposits in an aneurysm of the splenic artery on a film present a round, oval, or eggshell-like shadow of increased density in the left upper abdomen.[4,15,17,19,21] The exact location of the calcific deposit may be determined by gastrointestinal series with contrast material or by urograms.

Fluoroscopy will show a pulsatile filling defect in the posterior wall of the stomach which is almost pathognomonic. Also, aortography is very valuable to confirm the diagnosis.[2,4,6,21,22] Lower reported one case accompanied by a pancreatic deficiency.[9]

Roentgenographically to be differentiated are calcified aneurysm of the renal artery, calcified *Echinococcus* cyst located in the left lobe of the liver or in the spleen, and calcified tuberculous lymph node in the mesentery, etc.[17]

The prognosis of aneurysm of the splenic artery varies with rupture of the lesion. The surgical mortality prior to rupture is 5% to 15%, and the mortality after rupture is over 75%.[2,5,10,14,19] When it ruptures into the gastrointestinal tract, it is usually fatal.[6] The only possibility of survival in cases of rupture of an aneurysm of the splenic artery lies in immediate proper surgical intervention. Recurrence seldom takes place, and if it does it may be fatal.[16]

Treatment of aneurysm of the splenic artery is surgical.[1,5,14] Once a diagnosis is made or is strongly suspected, prompt surgical intervention is essential. After ligation of the main trunk of the artery proximal to the aneurysm, as near the celiac axis as possible, splenectomy with removal of the aneurysm is performed.[10,14,15,17]

Summary

A case of aneurysm of the splenic artery is presented. It was calcified, diagnosed by x-ray, and confirmed by operation and pathologic examination.

Incidence of the lesion is 0.04% to 0.05% at autopsy and is two to three times more frequently seen in the female.

As to its pathogenesis, its association with arteriosclerosis, congenital defects, embolism, and intra-abdominal pressure (pregnancy) are emphasized.

There are no specific diagnostic symptoms and signs, though pain aggravated by bending or stooping is suggestive of its presence. X-ray examination is the most important aid in its diagnosis.

The diagnosis and surgical exploration for aneurysm of the splenic artery must be performed before rupture occurs because the mortality after rupture may exceed 75%. During pregnancy, special attention should be considered very carefully because of the very vague symptoms resembling many other diseases.

The treatment is excision of the aneurysm with splenectomy.

R. Kennedy Gilchrist, MD, 122 S Michigan Ave, Chicago 3, Ill.

REFERENCES

1. Baumgartner, E. A., and Thomas, W. S.: Aneurysm of the Splenic Artery, Surg Gynec Obstet 39:462, 1924.

2. Berger, J. S.; Forsee, J. H., and Furst, J. N.: Splenic Arterial Aneurysm, Ann Surg 137:108, 1953.

3. Chalmers, J. A.: Rupture of a Splenic Arterial Aneurysm as a Fatal Complication of Pregnancy, Brit J Surg 37:86, 1949.

4. Culver, G. J., and Prison, H. S.: Splenic Artery Aneurysm: Report on 17 Cases Showing Calcification on Plain Roentgenograms, Radiology 68:217, 1957.

5. Davis, B. F.: Aneurysm of the Splenic Artery: Operative Removal, JAMA 84:200, 1925.

6. Downs, C. R.; Hopeman, A. R.; Todd, W. A., Jr.; and Mathewson, C.: Aneurysm of Splenic Artery, Ann Surg 141:268, 1955.

7. Gillam, J. F. E.: Spontaneous Rupture of the Splenic Artery, Brit J Surg 36:203, 1948.

8. Hunt, E. L.: Aneurysm of the Splenic Artery: With Report of a Case With Rupture, Amer J Med Sci 176:195, 1928.

9. Lower, W. E., and Farrell, J. I.: Aneurysm of the Splenic Artery, Arch Surg 23:182, 1931.

10. Machemer, W. L., and Fuge, W. W.: Aneurysm of the Splenic Artery: Report of a Case and Review of the Literature, Arch Surg 39:190, 1939.

11. MacLeod, D., and Maurice, T.: Rupture of Branch of Splenic Artery Associated With Pregnancy, Lancet 1:924, 1940.

12. Nevin, S., and Williams, D. J.: The Pathogenesis of Multiple Aneurysms, Lancet 2:955, 1937.

13. Osborne, S. E.: Aneurysm of the Splenic Artery Simulating Cholecystitis, Lancet 1:1007, 1936.

14. Owens, J. C., and Coffey, R. J.: Aneurysm of the Splenic Artery, Including a Report of Six Additional Cases, Int Abstr Surg 97:313, 1953.

15. Palmer, T. H.: Aneurysm of the Splenic Artery, New Eng J Med 243:989, 1950.

16. Parsons, C. G.: A Case of Ruptured Aneurysm of the Splenic Artery With Recurrence, Brit J Surg 24:708, 1937.

17. Seids, J. V., and Hauser, H.: Aneurysm of the Splenic Artery, Radiology 36:171, 1941.

18. Shallow, T. A.; Herbert, P. A.; and Wagner, F. B.: Abdominal Apoplexy Secondary to Ruptured "Congenital" Aneurysm, Surgery 19:177, 1946.

19. Sherlock, S. P. V., and Learmonth, J. I.: Aneurysm of Splenic Artery With Account of Example Complicating Gaucher's Disease, Brit J Surg 30:151, 1942.

20. Sherwin, B., and Gardimer, H.: Aneurysm of the Splenic Artery, Ann Surg 131:599, 1950.

21. Steinberg, I., and Lord, J. W., Jr.: Splenic Artery Aneurysm: Diagnosis by Intravenous Abdominal Aortography, JAMA 174:74, 1960.

22. Steinberg, I.: Diagnosis of Aneurysm of the Hepatic and Splenic Arteries by Intravenous Abdominal Aortography, New Eng J Med 263:341, 1960.

23. Smith, W. R.: A Case of Ruptured Aneurysm of the Splenic Artery, JAMA 80:1692, 1923.

24. Sperling, L.: Aneurysm of the Splenic Artery, Surgery 8:633, 1940.

25. Spittel, J. A., Jr.; Fairbairn, J. F., II; Kincaid, O. W.; and ReMine, W. H.: Aneurysm of the Splenic Artery, JAMA 175:452, 1961.

26. Tomsykoski, A. J.; Stevens, R. C.; Izzo, P. A.; and Rodriquez, C. E.: Aneurysm of the Splenic Artery in Pregnancy, Amer J Obstet Gynec 66:1264, 1953.

27. Zeluff, G. W., and Parsonnet, V.: Ruptured Aneurysm of the Splenic Artery: Case Report With Discussion, Ann Intern Med 35:437, 1951.

Below-Knee Amputation in Patients With Diabetes Mellitus

M. A. BLOCK, MD, AND F. W. WHITEHOUSE, MD, DETROIT

Necrosis of large areas of the foot due to gangrene or infection, or both, related etiologically to occlusive vascular disease and neuropathy in patients with diabetes mellitus is a common problem. When amputation of the foot is indicated, it has often been considered necessary to amputate at the thigh level. Experience in recent years has proved to us that the below-knee amputation is usually feasible in these patients. The advantages of a below-knee level of amputation are several: walking with a prosthesis is easier, rehabilitation is facilitated, less strain is placed on a remaining foot, and even wheelchair and bed mobility is better.

This report deals with 40 patients for whom 43 below-knee amputations have been managed personally. The first operation, performed in 1955, resulted in the selection of the below-knee level in an increasing number of patients subsequently. Three of the patients have required bilateral below-knee amputations.

Conservative Attitude in Management of Foot Problems in Diabetes

We employ what we consider to be a conservative approach in the management of foot lesions in patients with diabetes mellitus. By this is meant the use of measures designed to permit healing of foot lesions even though considerable time may be required. Amputation has not been employed until large portions of the foot itself (at least a quarter of the foot usually) are destroyed by a nonlocalizing process of gangrene or infection, or both. Uncommonly, severe pain without extensive gangrene or uncontrollable sepsis forces an amputation.

Submitted for publication April 3, 1963.

From divisions of general surgery and metabolism, Henry Ford Hospital.

There are a number of common foot lesions in diabetics which may initiate necrosis. Callosities on the soles of the feet gradually enlarge, and walking results in pressure necrosis beneath them, culminating in infection, ulceration, gangrene, and large areas of tissue necrosis. The patient may precipitate infection by inept trimming of the callus with unsterile instruments. Web spaces between toes and ingrowing toenails, especially of the great toe, are common sites for initial infection. Areas of ulceration or gangrene may first appear on the heel, especially in patients with dry atrophic skin. Diabetic neuropathy is commonly present and results in loss of pain and temperature perception and alterations in position sense. Trauma to the foot may occur before the patient becomes aware of any injury. Extensive necrosis and infection often develop before a physician is consulted.

The first lesion may be frank gangrene evidently produced by the abrupt loss of arterial blood supply to the area. Of course, the feet of these patients characteristically show features of ischemia prior to the development of these areas of gangrene with or without associated infection. Furthermore, many of the elderly patients are incapable of or disinterested in conscientiously and intelligently following those measures needed to prevent these foot difficulties; ie, management of diabetes, cleanliness of feet, care of toenails and calluses, proper use of socks and shoes, weight control, proper foot rest, etc.

Patients seen with these lesions of infection with or without gangrene are usually placed on bed rest; cultures of the lesions are taken; and appropriate antibiotics are given. Moist saline compresses or soaks at room temperature are applied for short periods several times daily to facilitate cleanliness and drainage of lesions. Whirlpool baths are especially useful for these purposes after spreading infection is controlled. This is followed by exposure of the wound area to air or a bedside light. The damaged tissue is usually protected at other times by soft sterile dressings. Adhesive tape is not used to hold dressings in place. Abscesses are drained and irrigated when necessary. Necrotic and gangrenous tissue is debrided when the process appears sufficiently localized. Local debridement or surgery done too early will frequently precipitate wide extension of gangrene. Bone involved by infection is removed when the process appears localized. We have not found ointments or other preparations for local use to be of any value therapeutically, and on occasion such preparations may be harmful.

Occasionally toes are amputated or debrided off when the digits are destroyed and the destructive process is well localized to the toe. We have been reluctant to employ transmetatarsal amputation for patients with lesions localized to toes inasmuch as we have been satisfied with the efficacy of local measures for toe lesions and fear the relatively high failure rate of transmetatarsal amputations.

A considerable amount of time may be spent in employing conservative measures with the hope of obtaining healing of a foot lesion in these patients. The patients require care at home and often require hospitalization for one or several periods. However, most of the patients are not gainfully employed anyway and desire to avoid amputation if possible. Medical care costs have been minimized by utilizing home and outpatient care for the greatest portion of the illness. Outpatient care has been feasible and medically satisfactory for most patients.

Clinical Features of Patients Requiring Below-Knee Amputations

As is to be expected, most of these patients were elderly. The average age of the 40 patients at the time of amputation was 64 years, the range being from 36 to 82 years. There were 28 males and 12 females. The duration of recognized diabetes mellitus varied from 6 months to 30 years, the average being 12.5 years.

The severity of the diabetes varied considerably. Seven patients were managed by diet alone, and seven took an oral hypoglycemic agent; but 26 required insulin.

Previous operative procedures related to their feet and vascular problems of their extremities had been done in 19 patients. These included bilateral lumbar sympathectomy, aortograms, femoral arteriograms, and incision and drainage of abscesses of the foot as well as amputation of toes and one transmetatarsal amputation. Operative procedures carried out previously on the opposite foot and leg included incision and drainage of abscesses, toe amputations, two transmetatarsal amputations, and seven above-knee amputations. We are unimpressed by the therapeutic value of lumbar sympathectomy. We are unable to predict the conditions in which this procedure can be expected to improve the distal blood supply significantly. The operation certainly has not appeared to be of value when gangrene has occurred. Too often sympathectomy is done merely "to try something."

Aortography should be done in patients who appear to be possible candidates for reconstructive vascular surgery. In a few of the patients, especially the younger age group and those without evidence of widespread small blood vessel disease (retinopathy, nephropathy, neuropathy), these vascular procedures may facilitate healing of the foot lesions so that amputation can be avoided. However, many of these patients are not candidates for vascular surgery because of their poor general condition or because their vascular occlusive disease is too extensive. The small blood vessels distally are often the primary site of occlusive arterial disease in the patient with diabetes.[1]

In selecting patients for below-knee amputation, we depend more on gross features of the leg and foot than on the presence or absence of pulsations in the popliteal or more distal arteries. Of the 43 limbs for which a below-knee amputation was done, only 14 had palpable popliteal artery pulsations (Table 1). The remaining 29 patients had no arterial pulsations distal to the femoral artery in the groin, and in many of these patients the femoral artery pulsations were diminished. The presence of good pulsations in the popliteal artery obviously provides a better chance for healing of a below-knee amputation, but its absence should not eliminate a patient from consideration of a below-knee procedure. The texture of the skin and the presence of hair growth below the knee aid in evaluating the likelihood for healing of an amputation site below the knee. Extensive ulceration or infection of the leg itself may be seen in a few patients and may limit the chance of healing at the below-knee level. Short, extremely obese patients are marginal candidates for successful below-knee amputations and eventual rehabilitation with a prosthesis. Although it is difficult to ascertain with certainty how many patients in our group had significant diabetic neuropathy in the lower extremities, this seemed to be present in a high percentage.

In some instances the general condition of the patients, their weight, status of ambulation, and mental status were factors in making the decision regarding level of amputation, especially in situations that seemed to have a marginal chance for successful healing at the below-knee level. In some patients a later revision or reconstruction might not be tolerated. We have not started a below-knee amputation and then changed to a higher level at the same operation because of what appeared to be poor bleeding from cut surfaces. In our opinion oscillometric studies, differential skin temperatures, and similar determinations have added little in making the decision regarding level of amputation. Unless there are striking contraindications, we are inclined to proceed with a below-the-knee procedure.

TABLE 1.—*Preoperative Level of Arterial Pulsations Prior to Below-Knee Amputations*

Popliteal pulsations palpable	14
No pulsations below femoral artery palpable	29
Total	43

The 43 below-knee amputations were carried out usually (40 amputations) because gangrene, frequently complicated by infection, involved a large portion of the foot. In three, the amputation was done because of extensive necrosis of the foot from infection alone which had been present chronically and failed to respond to the usual conservative measures. Both of these patients had severe diabetic neuropathy. The original foot lesion started in a toe or toes in 34 instances, in the foot proper in four patients, in the heel in three cases, and in a bunion and a callus on the sole in one leg each. A number of patients had multiple areas of gangrene at the time of amputation.

The lesions eventuating in amputation had been present in these patients for periods varying from 1 month to 18 months. In the majority, the lesion had been present for three to six months. There were 14 patients hospitalized once previously for treatment of the foot lesion, and six were hospitalized twice previously for treatment of the lesion prior to the amputation. In a number of patients, the severity of the pain from the foot lesion made the patient request amputation. Amputation was delayed in others, however, because the patients refused surgery or even hospitalization, until pain or a foul necrotic mass made surgery mandatory.

It is of interest that conservative measures had been succesful in the treatment of previous ulceration, gangrene, or infection of the same foot in six of the patients. Also, similar lesions on the opposite foot had cleared with conservative measures in seven patients. However, contralateral above-knee amputations were necessary previously in seven patients, and two others had required contralateral transmetatarsal amputations. As previously noted, three of our 40 patients required bilateral below-knee amputations.

Techniques Employed in Below-Knee Amputation

Certain techniques in the below-knee amputation appear to us to be important in facilitating healing of the wound. Avoidance of bruising of the skin by instruments has been emphasized, as well as precise approximation of the skin edges. The skin flaps should not be too tight nor too loose. Dead space in the wound should be avoided. A tourniquet is not used.

The level of amputation is selected at three to four inches below the tibial tuberosity at the knee. It is possible to fit a prosthesis on a stump of two inches. The elected level of amputation is marked on each side of the leg, and long anterior and short posterior flaps are fashioned, after estimating proper dimensions for later accurate closure. The flaps consist of skin, subcutaneous tissue, and the fascia overlying the muscle below so that any interference with blood supply to the flaps is avoided as much as possible. The flaps are held with sponges in the hand rather than with instruments. They are reflected to the level selected for amputation. Muscle layers are then transected at a level a short distance distal to the selected level of amputation. Muscle then retracts a short distance proximally. Bleeding vessels are individually occluded with plain catgut ligatures. Large vessels are occluded with chromicized catgut or silk ligatures. The posterior tibial and peroneal nerves are isolated and sharply transected as high as feasible. The tibia is transected at the level selected for amputation. The fibula is divided at least an inch or so higher. The anterior portion of the tibia is beveled to avoid a sharp edge pressing on overlying skin.

After transection, hemostasis is ensured, and fragments of devitalized tissue that may be present are removed. We have not approximated muscle ends over the end of the stump in most of the patients inasmuch as survival of longer muscle ends often appears unlikely. It has been our practice to place a small rubber through-and-through drain in the wound, bringing the ends of the drain out both ends of the incision. It has seemed that the avoidance of collections of fluid and blood and the elimination of dead space which could prevent healing of the stump negate any disadvantages of the drain.

Probably the most important step in the operation involves the closure of the wound. It is our policy to carry out a primary closure. We have feared to permit raw surfaces to remain open and susceptible to infection, the occurrence of which would eliminate the possibility of healing at this level in these poorly vascularized tissues. We prefer to use fine monofilament stainless steel wire sutures. As many sutures are used as are necessary to obtain precise approximation of the skin edges at all points along the wound without tension. If the skin edges are not approximated at all points along the wound, the resulting raw surface may not be epithelialized or may become infected, thus nullifying the operation. It is enough to expect closely approximated skin edges to heal in these patients without asking the skin edges to serve as a base for epithelialization of grossly visible raw surfaces resulting from inaccurate approximation of the skin edges.

The amputation stump is wrapped loosely in soft bandages to avoid undue pressure on the wound. All possible measures are taken to avoid a flabby stump which will heal with difficulty or, when healed, will serve as a poor stump for a prosthesis. Antibiotics are usually administered postoperatively; most of these patients have been receiving antibiotics preoperatively. In some patients afflicted preoperatively with a septicemia or severe pain from foot lesions, a remarkable improvement in their general condition occurs soon after the operation is completed.

The patients are up out of bed as soon as feasible postoperatively. They are helped to sit up in bed the day following surgery and are up in a wheelchair for increasing periods each subsequent day. It is especially important to avoid a flexion contracture of the knee. Some patients keep the knee partially flexed even before the amputation because of pain. Placing the patient prone in bed intermittently assists in avoiding flexion contracture of the knee. It is important to initiate physical therapy exercises and crutch walking early. This can usually be done within several days after surgery. The drain in the wound is usually removed three to four days postoperatively. The skin sutures are left in place until there is evidence of strong union of skin edges. It has been our preference to err by leaving sutures in too long rather than too short a period. If permanent healing has not occurred when sutures are removed, skin edges may separate or a defect already present at the skin edges may enlarge as skin edges spread apart. This may result in a nonhealing wound and ultimate failure of the operation.

TABLE 2.—*Condition of Patients After Operation*

	No. Amputations
Ambulatory with prosthesis *	23
Wheelchair and crutch walking	7
Wheelchair †	10
Bedridden ‡	1
Too early postop to determine	2
Total	43

* Three bilateral amputees.
† Five bilateral amputees.
‡ Succumbed two months postop to diabetic nephropathy.

Postoperative Course of Patients With Below-Knee Amputations

Two of the 43 below-knee amputations failed to heal satisfactorily. The wound appeared to heal initially in one patient, but it was necessary to drain a hematoma in the wound two weeks postoperatively. This was one of the few patients in whom a drain was not placed in the wound at the time of surgery. Necrosis then developed in the anterior skin flap. A revision of the amputation stump was tried, but the wound later became infected and necrosis developed six weeks postoperatively. An above-knee amputation was finally carried out. The second patient died two months postoperatively of diabetic nephropathy without adequate healing of his wound.

There were two other below-knee amputations that were revised. One of these was revised not for poor healing but for pain in the stump thought to be a neuroma. The pain eventually disappeared. The other stump was revised because ulcerations developed over a bony prominence anteriorly whenever the patient ambulated normally with his prosthesis.

There were no operative deaths in the group. However, as mentioned above, one patient died two months postoperatively from renal failure due to diabetic nephropathy, never having been dismissed from the hospital.

Twenty-three patients became ambulatory with a prosthesis (Table 2). Three of these patients became ambulatory with a prosthesis on both lower extremities, two having had above-knee amputations previously on the contralateral extremity. These three patients were 56, 62, and 63 years of age, respectively. One of the 23 patients uses crutches to assist in ambulation with the prosthesis. One of the patients later had a contralateral below-knee and finally an above-knee amputation, and although he ambulated on a prosthesis after the first operation, he has not ambulated since the second amputation.

Sixteen patients were restricted for the most part to a wheelchair existence postoperatively, one of these patients requiring bilateral below-knee amputations and four contralateral above-knee amputations. However, seven of these 16 patients did walk with crutches part of the time.

There are 27 patients (who had a total of 30 below-knee amputations) still living of the total of 40 patients (Table 3). Follow-up periods ranged from 2 months to 5½ years. Twelve of the 14 deaths have been considered to be secondary to vascular insufficiency in vital organs; ie, myocardial infarcts, cerebrovascular accidents, or diabetic nephropathy (Table 4). The deaths occurred from two months to five years postoperatively. It is of interest that, in this series, the chance of the patient's succumbing later to vascular occlusive disease in a vital organ is greater than the chance that the patient will later require an amputation of the contralateral extremity.

The duration of hospitalization after the below-knee amputation averaged three to

TABLE 3.—*Postoperative Follow-Up Periods After Below-Knee Amputation*

	Living	Dead
Less than 6 mo	4	1
6-12 mo	5	2
12-18 mo	3	4
18-24 mo	0	1
2-3 yr	7	2
3-4 yr	7	1
4-5 yr	2	1
5-6 yr	2	1
Totals	30 *	13

* Includes three bilateral below-knee amputations.

four weeks. By the time of dismissal from the hospital, sutures were usually removed and the patients were ambulating whenever possible on crutches, including walking up and down steps. Various complications occurred postoperatively in 16 patients, including decubitus ulcers in two, urinary retention requiring transurethral resection of the prostate in two, urinary tract infection, gastric ulcer, thrombophlebitis, fecal impaction, and problems in control of the diabetes mellitus. Renal failure culminating fatally in one patient and failure of healing requiring reamputation have been previously mentioned.

Wound infection occurred in only two patients despite a high incidence of infection in the foot preoperatively. Crust formation along the wound edges occurred in three patients and delayed final healing. Local wound care and dressings are a very important aspect in the care of these patients. Dressings must not be placed so tight that tissues are constricted, or so loose that dressings come off. Avoidance of contamination of dressings and the wound from bowel movements is especially important.

TABLE 4.—*Cause of Deaths After Below-Knee Amputations*

	No.
From cerebrovascular accident	5
From myocardial infarct	4
From diabetic nephropathy	2
From other unrelated cause	1
Sudden death, cause not determined	2
Total	14

There are 18 patients who had no difficulty with the other extremity after the below-knee amputation; an additional seven patients could have no such difficulty because of a previous contralateral amputation (Table 5). Three of the 18 patients have never walked, however, for various reasons. Eight of the 18 patients have died.

There are 15 patients who have subsequently developed infection with or without gangrene in the contralateral foot. Six of these patients required hospitalization for treatment of the difficulty. Three of these patients required bilateral below-knee amputation, one finally requiring an above-knee amputation. The need for continuous alertness for foot lesions of the contralateral foot is obvious. Proper care of the remaining foot is mandatory.

TABLE 5.—*Status of Other Extremity Following Below-Knee Amputation*

	No. Patients
Other leg satisfactory	18
Infection, gangrene other foot *	11
Later below-knee amputation, other extremity	3
Later above-knee amputation, other extremity	1
Previous above-knee amputation, other extremity	7
Total	40

* In five, hospitalization required.

Two patients complained of some phantom limb sensations. However, this was never a significant problem in any of our patients.

Rehabilitation of Patients With Below-Knee Amputations

A majority of these patients present many difficult problems in care after recovery from the amputation. Their serious medical and socioeconomic problems remain and may be more serious than before. A conscientious active yet practical program should be arranged for each patient. This requires efforts by the patient and his family, the internist, surgeon, physiatrist, and social worker.

The eventual status of these patients depends on individual circumstances. Many

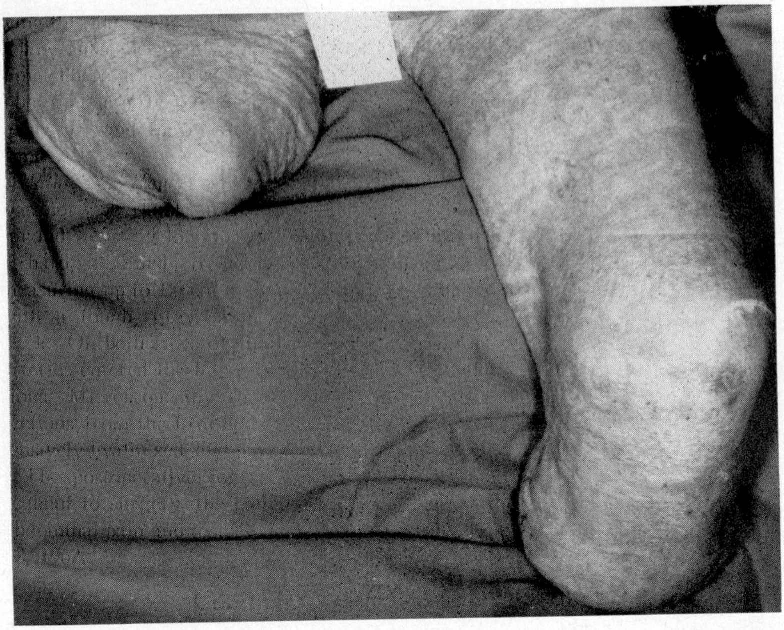

Patient with both an above-knee and below-knee amputation illustrates difference in length between the two levels.

of the patients had been in a wheelchair or even a bedridden status preoperatively because of physical handicaps as a result of previous strokes, senility, poor vision, weakness with lack of coordination and stability, obesity, etc. Others reach this status after an amputation because these factors become existent or because the condition of the contralateral foot prevents ambulation.

Nevertheless, the patient with a below-knee amputation does have a better chance for independence than the patient with an above-knee amputation (Figure). There is a greater likelihood of ambulation with a prosthesis. Even if a prosthesis is not feasible, the patient can move about in a wheelchair or bed with greater facility, especially if there has been or will be a contralateral amputation.

Early activity of the operated extremity, proper wrapping of the stump, avoidance of knee contractures, and instruction and help in crutch walking are considered important measures to be carried out during the first few days after the amputation.

Time and money is required for rehabilitation with a prosthesis. However, if it can be accomplished, money and time can be saved in the over-all future care of the patient. For most patients, measurement for the prosthesis is carried out about two months following the operation. They are then able to ambulate satisfactorily with the prosthesis by four to six months after the amputation. Readjustments and re-evaluation are required periodically.

Our institution is fortunate in that an Amputation Clinic has functioned with a very active schedule for many years; the physiatrist, orthopedist, physical therapist, social worker, and technician who manages the prosthetic appliances evaluate the patients frequently and plan their future program.

Remarks

Our experience to date with diabetic patients having extensive gangrene with or without associated infection of a foot requiring amputation has justified the below-knee level of amputation rather than the midthigh level in most instances. The patients have a better chance for self-mobilization. Although healing may be slow, it has been complete in nearly all patients. Success requires meticulous care in the surgical technique, in postoperative management, and in rehabilitation of the patients. It is of interest that during the period that the 43 below-knee amputations were performed we did 20 above-knee procedures. The above-knee procedures have been performed with decreasing frequency as the below-knee operation proved itself. Of 36 major amputations done during the last four years for patients with diabetes mellitus, only 6 were above-knee procedures and the remaining 30 were below-knee operations.

Other reports have also indicated satisfaction with the below-knee amputation in this group of patients.[2-4] Tolstedt and Bell[5] reported failure in ten of 35 patients and recommended arteriography in predicting which patients could have successful below-knee level amputations. The group of patients under consideration is far different, of course, from younger age patients requiring below-knee amputations for trauma. It does appear that below-knee amputations are more likely to heal when performed for gangrene of the foot developing in the patient with diabetes mellitus than in the patient with occlusive arterial disease without diabetes mellitus.

Summary and Conclusions

1. Experience with 43 below-knee amputations in 40 patients with diabetes mellitus is recorded.

2. Only one patient later required an above-knee amputation because of failure of healing at the below-knee level. This patient had a below-knee amputation on the contralateral leg that also required revision, not because of healing difficulty, but because of pain thought to be due to a neuroma. One other patient also required revision because of late ulceration due to pressure over a bony prominence when he was wearing the prosthesis.

3. Success requires meticulous technique in the operation, postoperative care, and rehabilitation.

4. In selection of patients for the operation, the gross appearance of the skin and leg and the presence or absence of hair growth at the leg level have been the most helpful criteria.

5. The advantages of the below-knee level over the midthigh level to the patient have warranted its continued use.

6. The majority of patients ambulated with a prosthesis postoperatively after the below-knee amputation despite many mitigating factors in the group of patients involved, including age, poor cardiovascular status, senility, poor vision, residual paralysis from strokes, and obesity.

M. A. Block, MD, Division of General Surgery, Henry Ford Hospital, Detroit 2, Mich.

REFERENCES

1. Goldenberg, S.; Alex, M.; Joshi, R. A.; and Blumenthal, H. T.: Nonatheromatous Peripheral Vascular Disease of the Lower Extremity in Diabetes Mellitus, Diabetes 8:261-273, 1959.

2. Silbert, S., and Haimovici, H.: Results of Midleg Amputations for Gangrene in Diabetics, JAMA 144:454-458, 1950.

3. Hoar, C. S., Jr., and Torres, J.: Evaluation of Below the Knee Amputation in the Treatment of Diabetic Gangrene, New Eng J Med 266:440-443, 1962.

4. Harris, P. D.; Schwartz, S. I.; and DeWeese, J. A.: Midcalf Amputation for Peripheral Vascular Disease, Arch Surg 82:381-383, 1961.

5. Tolstedt, G. E., and Bell, J. W.: Failure of Below-Knee Amputation in Peripheral Arterial Disease, Arch Surg 83:834-936, 1961.

Secretory Studies in Frozen Heidenhain Pouches

LAWRENCE E. SAVAGE, MD
L. STANTON STAVNEY, MD
JOHN K. STEVENSON, MD
HENRY N. HARKINS, MD
AND
LLOYD M. NYHUS, MD
SEATTLE

Since the advent of gastric freezing as a definitive treatment of duodenal ulcer at the University of Minnesota, considerable interest has evolved concerning this procedure. Wangensteen et al (1962)[6] have stated that local gastric hypothermia may produce a physiological gastrectomy since there is a marked reduction in acid secretion after freezing. Their laboratory investigations have demonstrated a total achlorhydria in three Heidenhain preparations with marked reduction in secretory responses in two other animals after the Heidenhain pouches were frozen. Similar data were obtained from other of their pouch preparations, and it eventually seemed feasible to apply the technique clinically.[2,3] In this regard it is estimated that 1,000 patients in the United States have currently undergone gastric freezing as definitive treatment of chronic duodenal ulcer.

Prior to any clinical evaluation of gastric freezing we have felt the necessity to fulfill two fundamental propositions in our experimental laboratory. In the first instance, gastric freezing must significantly reduce parietal cell activity and hence acid secretion in a high proportion of experimental animals. In the second circumstance, it must be unattended by serious complications and thus possess a wide margin of safety.

Submitted for publication April 22, 1963.

Instructor in Surgery (Dr. Savage); Assistant in Surgery (Dr. Stavney); Assistant Professor (Dr. Stevenson); Professor and Chairman (Dr. Harkins); Associate Professor (Dr. Nyhus).

From the Department of Surgery, University of Washington School of Medicine.

This study was supported by a grant-in-aid (A-2187) from the National Institutes of Health, Public Health Service; and the Vadheim Surgery Research Fund.

Methods

Twenty dogs weighing between 12 and 20 kg were utilized in the study. All of the animals were operated upon, and vagally denervated Heidenhain pouches were constructed. After a recovery period of three weeks, the animals were then studied by placing them in Pavlov stands for pouch collections. Throughout the experiment we have utilized two methods of secretory challenge, feeding and histamine. In most instances each animal had three or more feeding and histamine stands prior to freezing the pouch. Subsequent to each freezing the feeding and histamine stands were repeated. The feeding stimulus consisted of 200 gm of Gerber's liver fed to the animal after a 12- to 14-hour interval fast. The amount of histamine required to evoke a suitable secretory response varied from animal to animal. The usual range was 0.1 to 0.2 mg of histamine in water injected as a single dose subcutaneously. Maximum secretion invariably occurred within 45 minutes after the histamine was administered, with the pouch returning to a basal secretory state within two hours.

Collection Technique

We have utilized the collection technique of Burstall and Schofield[1] and find it highly advantageous in evaluating subtle changes in secretory patterns. It has been amplified in such a fashion as to enable the simultaneous study of a large group of animals. The essential feature of the collection system is the establishment of an open gravitational flow between the pouch and the reservoir pipette. This system

Fig 1.—*A,* exteriorization of a Heidenhain pouch prior to freezing. *B,* 150 ml of cooling solution has been introduced into the freezing balloon producing marked distention of the pouch. *C,* utilizing an inflow temperature of —20 C and an outflow temperature of —12 C the occurrence of frost is frequently evident after 15 minutes of freezing. *D,* extension of frost with increased firmness of the pouch is noted after 30 minutes of freezing. A needle thermistor has been placed into the pouch wall. *E,* generalized frost and pouch solidification after 45 minutes of freezing. *F,* freezing was discontinued after one hour, and, after a five-minute interval, the balloon was aspirated. Partial collapse of the pouch wall is noted.

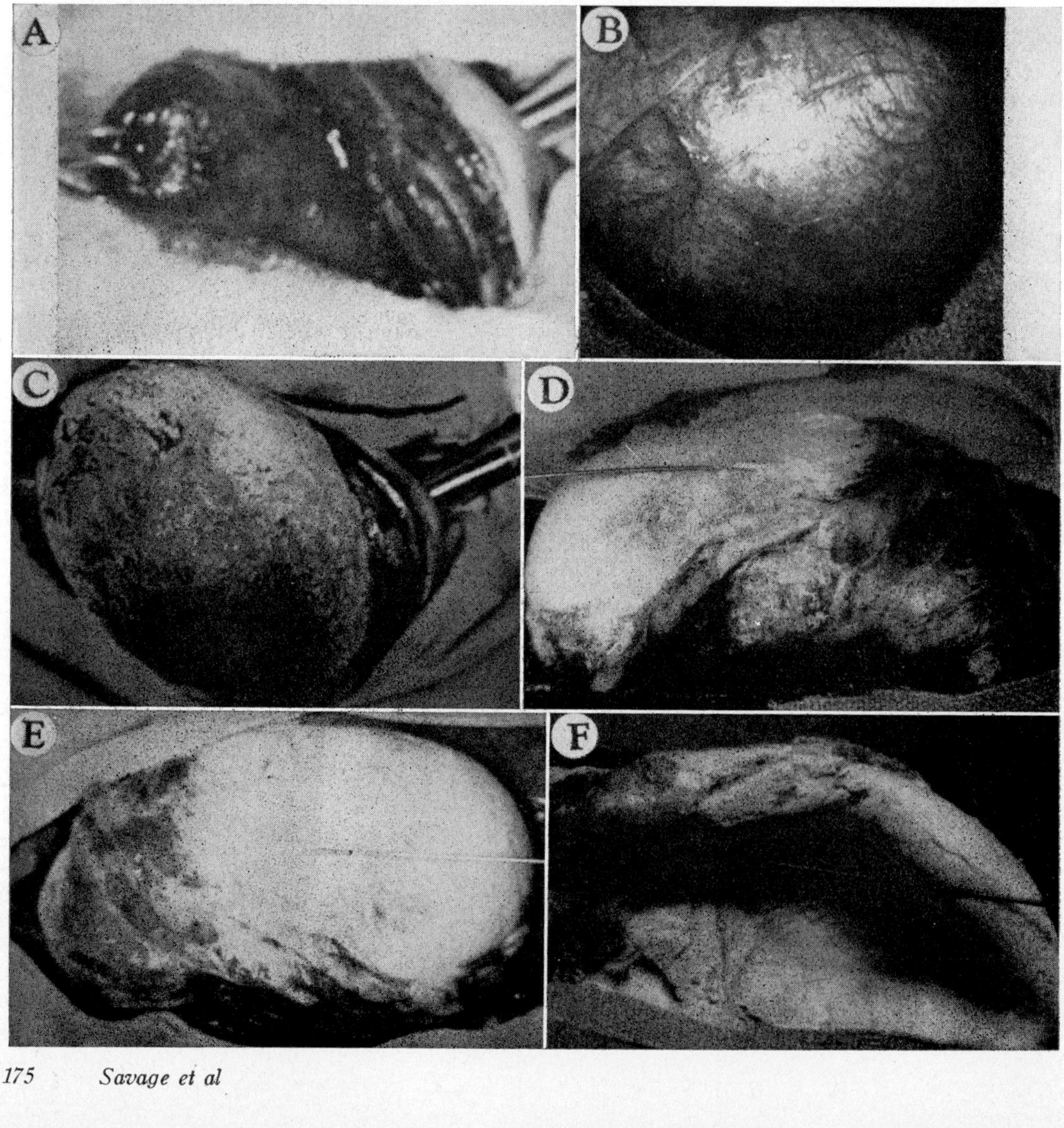

TABLE 1.—*Heidenhain Pouch Study*

Animals in study	20
Animals with frozen pouches	17
Animals completing secretion studies	14
Pouch freezings	25
Deaths from freezing	3
Deaths unrelated to freezing	3
Enteric-pouch fistulae subsequent to freezing	3

allows for gentle irrigation of the pouch and minimizes the possibility of overlapping samples. Every 15 minutes throughout the course of an experiment the secretory product of the pouch is titrated, enabling the accurate evaluation of acid secretory responses. The details of this collection technique have been recently described elsewhere.[5]

Mean histamine and feeding acid responses for each animal have been calculated and expressed in total milliequivalents before and after freezing. All data have been statistically analyzed by the "student" T-test, and P values noted.

Freezing Technique

After the completion of background studies each Heidenhain pouch was frozen, utilizing a Swenko Hypothermia machine with a latex finger cot attached to the two-way catheter, an inflow temperature ranging from —16 to —22 C. To secure maximum freezing of the entire pouch and to enable the monitoring of pouch wall temperatures, the pouches were exteriorized in eight animals through a celiotomy incision (Fig 1*A*). With the balloon in the pouch, it was filled with 150 to 250 ml of

TABLE 2.—*Histamine and Feeding Responses in 14 Heidenhain*

Animal	Before Freezing	After 1st Freeze	Change ‡	After 2nd Freeze	Change	After 3rd Freeze
L-2	H * 0.50	0.04	↓ 92% P >0.005			
	F † 0.81	0.02	↓ 98% P >0.005			
L-3	H 0.96	0.96	No significant change t=0	1.50	↑ 54%	
L-3x	H 0.64	0.84	↑ 31% t <0			
L-8	H 0.48	0.04	↓ 92% P >0.005			
	F 1.15	0.05	↓ 96% P >0.005			
L-10	H 0.40	0.48 2.54	No significant change	0.40 4.21	No significant change ↑ 66%	
L-12	H 0.14	0.14	No significant change			
L-13	H 0.75	0.72	↓ 4% No significant change	0.56	↓ 25% P >0.01	0.15
L-14	H 0.38	0.38	No significant change	0.38	No significant change	0.39
L-17	H 1.33	0.03	↓ 98% P >0.005			
	F 3.99	0.07	↓ 99% P >0.005			
L-20	H 0.46	0.22	↓ 52% P >0.05			
L-21	H 0.35	0.04	↓ 89% P >0.005			
	F 1.85	0.04	↓ 88% P >0.005			
L-22	H 0.61	0.44	No significant change			
L-26	H 1.30	0.81	↓ 38% P >0.005			
L-27	H 0.57	0.22	↓ 60% P >0.005			
	F 1.48	1.40	No significant change			

No. ofanimals: 14; No. of pouch freezes: 22.

Pouch freezing time: 50-60 min; inflow temp.: —15 to —22 C; outflow temp.: —10 to —14 C.

* H designates histamine.
† F designates feeding.
‡ Responses expressed in mean total mEq of two or more stands. All data analyzed statistically by "student" t-test and P values noted.

95% alcohol cooling solution (Fig 1*B*). In other animals the pouches were blindly distended by an equivalent amount of cooling solution. All animals were lightly anesthetized with intravenous pentobarbital (Nembutal). Fig 1, C, D, E, and F show the development of frost and the progression of freezing at 15-minute intervals. In those animals in which blind freezing was employed the pouches were easily palpable through the anterior abdominal wall as cold, solid spheres. Subsequent to celiotomy and freezing, the animals were returned to Pavlov stands after a three- to four-day recovery period. Animals whose pouches were frozen blindly were placed in stands for study 24 hours after freezing. All animals were evaluated two or three times weekly relative to the gastric secretory responses.

Pouches After Freezing

Change	After 4th Freeze	Change
↓ 80% $P >0$ 005	0.05	↓ 93% $P >0.005$
No significant change	0.31	No significant change

Postfreezing Acid Response	Reduced	8
	Unchanged	4
	Increased	2

Results

Seventeen Heidenhain preparations had their pouches frozen on 25 occasions (Table 1). The 14 animals which completed the study were summarized with regard to their secretory responses in Table 2. Dogs L-2, L-8, and L-17 presented strikingly reduced acid responses to a near achlorhydric state after one pouch freezing. Dog L-13 is of particular interest since a progressive decrease in acid response over a five-month period is demonstrated during which time the pouch was frozen on four occasions. The reverse of this pattern is noted in the responses of Dog L-14. This pouch was also frozen four times and demonstrates a persistently high acid response throughout a five-month period. In almost all animals in which feeding and histamine responses can be compared there is a close parallelism between the two. L-27 is an exception in which the histamine response is significantly reduced but the feeding response is curiously unaltered. Of the 14 animals, eight demonstrated significant lowering of their acid responses while the remaining six showed no effect of one or more pouch freezings. Achlorhydric patterns are typified by the responses noted in Fig 2 and 3, while Fig 4 demonstrates a continuing high level acid secretion after freezing. It is noteworthy that the three animals (L-2, L-8, and L-17) which were in a nearly achlorhydric state subsequent to freezing had their pouches frozen under direct vision through a celiotomy incision.

After a two-month period of achlorhydria the pouch from L-2 was removed and examined histologically. Representative sections suggested a decrease in the number of parietal cells. In addition, atrophic changes were noted in all tissue sections. Dog L-8 has remained essentially achlorhydric during the five months since its pouch was frozen.

The possibility that our freezing technique differs in some unrecognized manner from that of the originators of the method is to be considered. We did send one of our group (L.E.S.) to Minneapolis to observe the method for three days.

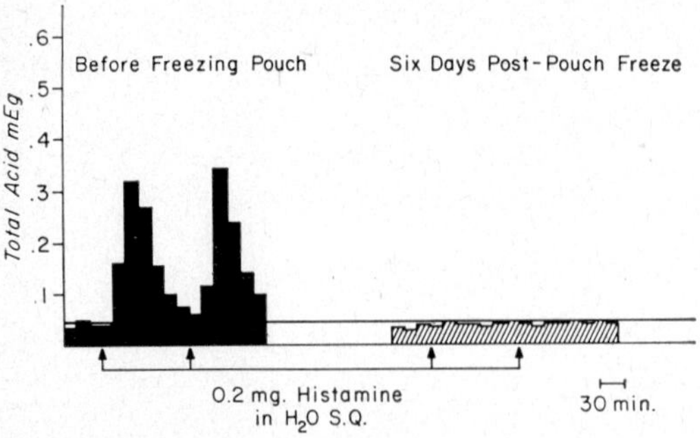

Fig 2.—Heidenhain pouch L-2: achlorhydric histamine response subsequent to pouch freezing.

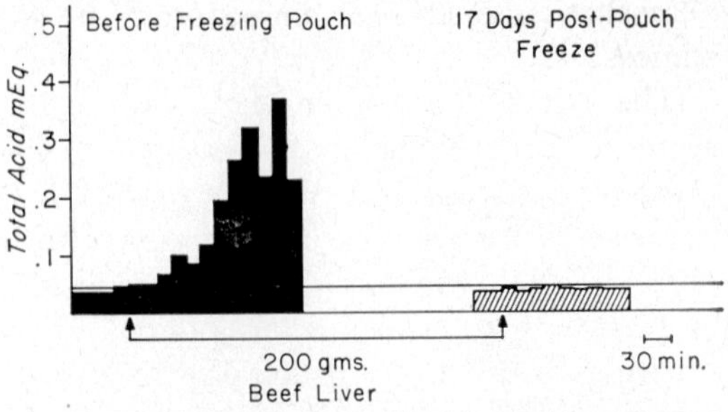

Fig 3.—Heidenhain pouch L-2: achlorhydric feeding response subsequent to pouch freezing.

Comment

Eight of 14 animals demonstrated significant reduction in acid secretion after freezing.

The mechanism responsible for reduced secretion patterns after freezing in these animals is doubtless dependent upon mucosal necrosis, fibrosis, atrophy, and decreased blood flow to the pouch. Effective freezing may precipitate all of these factors simultaneously (L-2, L-8, and L-17), or they may gradually become manifest over a considerable time interval subsequent to multiple freezing (L-13). If freezing acts in the intact stomach by producing either a "thermal vagotomy" or "thermal antrectomy," neither of these factors would be applicable to the Heidenhain pouch since in the one instance it is already vagotomized and in the other it contains no antrum.

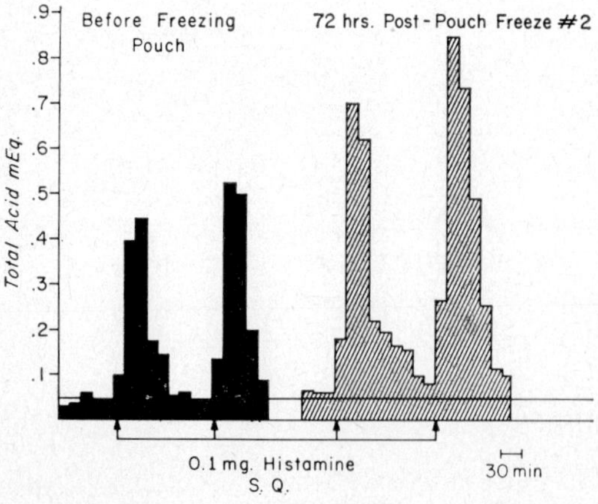

Fig 4.—Heidenhain pouch L-3: histamine response—acid secretion is increased 72 hours after the pouch was frozen a second time.

Of importance is the conformation of the freezing balloon to the pouch. Unless the pouch was distended to the point of bursting, we were invariably unsuccessful in adequately freezing pouches if monitored by needle thermistors in the pouch wall.

Of the several complications subsequent to freezing, hemorrhage was the most frequent and occurred in every instance. Gross bleeding was noted for three to seven days postfreezing.

That necrosis can occur is noted in Fig 5 which demonstrates a 3 cm necrotic area necessitating removal of the pouch from L-3 one month after it had been frozen a second time. Massive necrosis and hemorrhage occurring 12 to 18 hours subsequent to freezing were responsible for the death of three animals.

Another interesting complication evolved from this technique. We have encountered enteric-pouch fistulae in three animals,

Fig 5.—A 2 $\times$ 3 cm area of necrosis noted in a pouch three weeks after it was frozen.

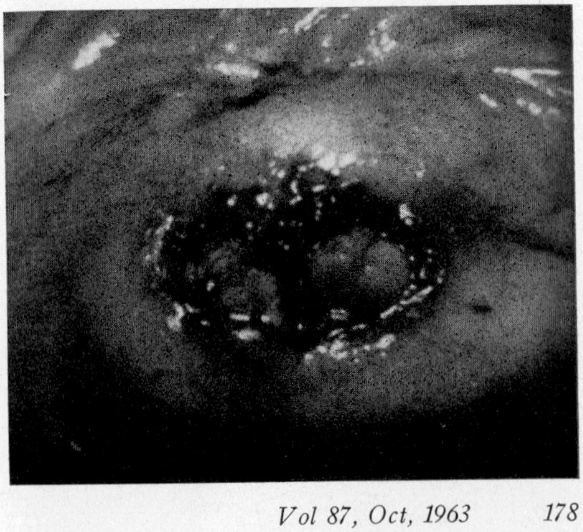

necessitating operative correction in all instances.

The partial success in diminishing acid secretion by freezing in this study is jeopardized to some extent by postfreezing sequelae. Pouch exteriorization with careful observation during the freezing period failed to prevent these sequelae. Blind cooling or freezing, as utilized in the clinical setting, increases the risk of rupturing the viscus (Richman and Anthony)[4] and decreases the effectiveness of the freezing process since adequate pouch distention is difficult to ascertain. There is an uneasy transition zone in which freezing may significantly reduce acid secretion or it may initiate massive necrosis, perforation, and hemorrhage. This zone is ill defined even if the variables of pouch distention and depth of freezing are minimized by pouch exteriorization. Unfortunately we have been unable to control the factors of pouch distention, depth of freeze, and length of freezing time in such a fashion as to produce a uniform result. Significant postfreezing complications have in themselves detracted from the secretory data relevant to reduced acid responses. For the present we are committed to the study of gastric freezing exclusively in the animal laboratory until we are ultimately convinced that the procedure is highly effective and possesses a wide margin of safety.

Summary

Seventeen animals underwent 25 freezings of their Heidenhain pouches with 14 survivors completing the secretion study.

Eight animals demonstrated greatly reduced acid secretion patterns after freezing, three of which were achlorhydric.

No change in acid response could be elicited in four animals, and in two there was a postfreeze increase.

Three animals died 12 to 18 hours postfreezing from massive necrosis and hemorrhage of the pouches.

Three animals developed enteric fistulae to their pouches subsequent to freezing.

Lloyd M. Nyhus, MD, Associate Professor, Department of Surgery, University of Washington School of Medicine, Seattle 5, Wash.

REFERENCES

1. Burstall, P. A., and Schofield, B.: Secretory Effects of Psychic Stimulation and Insulin Hypoglycaemia on Heidenhain Gastric Pouches in Dogs, J Physiol (London) 120:383-408, 1953.

2. Peter, E. T.; Bernstein, E. F.; Sosin, H.; Madsen, A. J.; Walder, A. I.; and Wangensteen, O. H.: Technique of Gastric Freezing in the Treatment of Duodenal Ulcer, JAMA 181:760-764, 1962.

3. Peter, E. T.; Bernstein, E. F.; Sosin, H.; Madsen, A. J.; Walder, A. I.; and Wangensteen, O. H.: The Role of Temperature in Controlling Gastric Digestion, JAMA 182:894-898, 1962.

4. Richman, A., and Anthony, D.: Experiences With Localized Gastric Hypothermia in Massive Upper Gastrointestinal Bleeding, Amer J Dig Dis 8:113-121, 1963.

5. Savage, L. E.; Stavney, L. S.; Nyhus, L. M.; and Harkins, H. N.: A Sensitive Technique for Gastric Pouch Collection, Surgery 53:474-476, 1963.

6. Wangensteen, O. H.; Peter, E. T.; Bernstein, E. F.; Walder, A. I.; Sosin, H.; and Madsen, A. J.: Can Physiological Gastrectomy be Achieved by Gastric Freezing? Ann Surg 156:579-591, 1962.

New Stent for Support of Veins in Arterial Grafts

VICTOR PARSONNET, MD; A. ATTAI LARI, MD; AND I. H. SHAH, MD, NEWARK, NJ

Although synthetic plastic vascular prostheses have been successful in the replacement of damaged and diseased arteries, particularly those of large caliber, there remains a gap in their performance and that of the theoretically ideal prosthesis. The defects that illustrate this gap include the failure of acceptance of the prosthesis as a normal host tissue, ultimate disruption of suture lines, lack of "normal" intima, absence of elasticity and vascular rebound of the vessel wall, and most significant, eventual thrombosis of the graft, particularly in vessels of small caliber.

The search for a more satisfactory prosthesis is in order because of the progressive change in clinical indications for blood vessel replacement. Resection of the aorta and its major branches with prosthesis replacement is largely successful; replacement of smaller arteries has a high incidence of failure even in the most competent hands. However, since clinical indications for replacement of small arteries have increased in step with refinements in diagnostic techniques, there is a real need for an ideal prosthesis in surgery of small, extracranial, coronary, renal, and peripheral arteries.

The fact that these defects in arterial replacement exist is demonstrated by the reported recent tendency to use autogenous veins as the material of choice in the replacement or bypass of small and medium size arteries. It is postulated that transplanted vascular tissue would be suitable for small arteries because of complete host acceptance and incorporation, maintenance of elasticity and tone of the graft, a smooth, normal intimal lining (except at the anastomosis), and long-term acceptability by the host tissues. Experience has shown, however, that vein grafts, too, become thrombosed in a significant number of cases, even in those cases ideally suited to surgery.[1]

Of the several factors that could account for the failure of vein grafts, the one that concerns this study is the frequent disproportion in size between artery and vein. At the time of transplantation the vein is often considerably wider than the host artery and will immediately dilate to its full width under arterial blood pressure. Such dilatation is likely to progress.[2] Even vein grafts that are at first isodiametric may gradually dilate. The result of such dilatation is the production of turbulent flow that leads to thrombosis of the graft.

A technique was, therefore, conceived that might prevent the initial disproportion of artery-vein diameter and subsequent graft dilatation. This consists of surrounding an autogenous vein graft with a loosely-knit plastic tube stent. Small adjustments in diameter of stent and vein to host artery could be made by changing the longitudinal tension of the stent much like a child's finger-trap toy (Fig 1).

Description of Stent

Scaffold tubes have been constructed of knitted monofilament fibers of polyethylene, polypropylene, and Teflon of varying widths, denier, and diameter.* The fabric is of

Submitted for publication April 5, 1963.

Hemodynamics Department, Newark Beth Israel Hospital.

Supported in part by grants from the Essex County Heart Association.

* These stents were developed by Prof. Thomas Edman of the Philadelphia College of Textiles and Science.

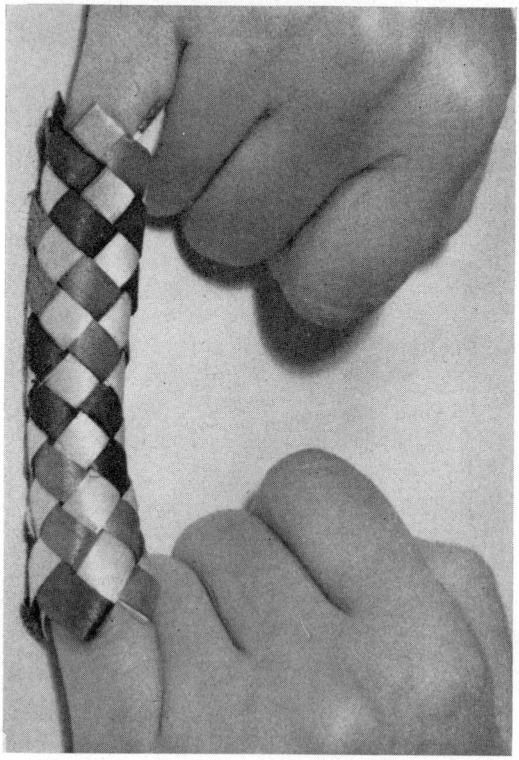

Fig 1.—Principle of adjustment of transverse diameter is similar to child's finger-trap toy. Increasing longitudinal tension decreased the transverse diameter.

plain tubular knit construction of 6-12 courses per inch and 12-18 wales per inch. It was knitted on a ten-cut flat-rib machine with laid-in selvage to start and bound off edge at the end to prevent raveling (Fig 2).

Method

Technique of Insertion.—Under sterile precautions a segment of the common carotid artery in dogs was excised and the cut ends stripped of adventitia for a few mm. A portion of external jugular vein was excised, reversed, and one end sutured end-to-end to the artery with 7-0 arterial silk suture. A scaffold of appropriate size was slid over the vein while the other remaining anastomosis was performed and blood flow established. The scaffold was then stretched lengthwise and attached to the host tissue or surrounding fascia with sufficient tension to provide a proper transverse diameter (Fig 3).

Tensile strength was measured by excising the involved segment at varying intervals of time after insertion and attaching it by appropriate size adapters to a pressure source. The intraluminal pressure was gradually raised with compressed air, and the bursting point measured with a specially constructed strain gauge transducer † attached to an Electronics for Medicine Recorder (Fig 4).

In a few cases angiography was performed in routine fashion to demonstrate functional dilatation of the venous segment. In one case the pressure gradient was measured across the graft while the diameter of the vein graft was altered by changing the longitudinal tension of the stent.

Microscopic sections were made of some of the removed specimens.

Results and Comment

Thrombosis of Grafts.—Thirty-five vein grafts were done, 25 with the stent and 10 without as controls. An initial study of 15 grafts, five with each of the test materials,

† Manufactured by Statham Electronics, Springfield, NJ.

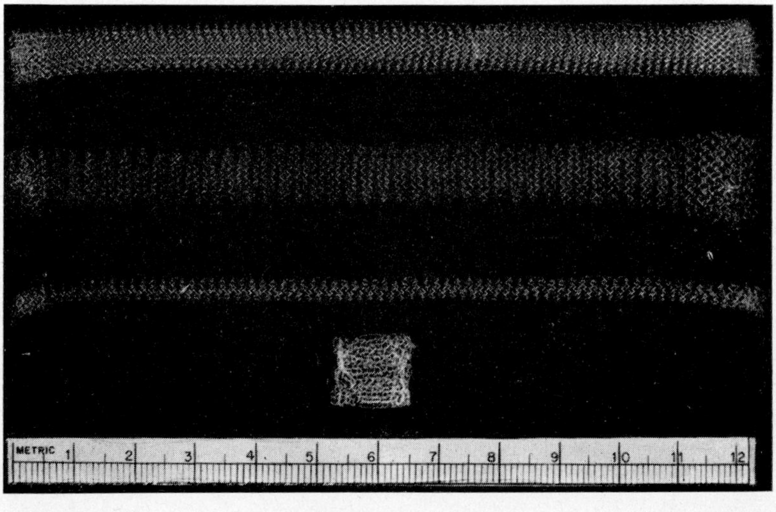

Fig 2.—Photograph of several types of polypropylene stent used in this study.

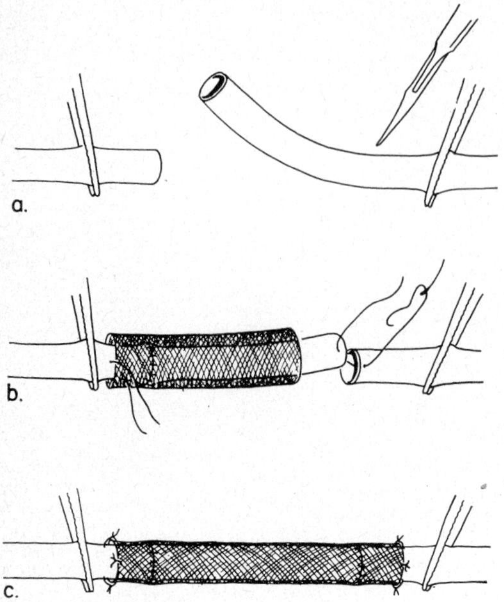

Fig 3.—Illustration of technique for insertion of vein graft and application of stent.

was performed. In this group there occurred the only thrombosis in the entire series, one of the veins with the Teflon stent. Therefore, only polypropylene stents were used, primarily because of simplicity of sterilization by autoclaving and of easy handling qualities (Table). Despite the fact that the host vessels were small, 2 to 4 mm in diameter, there was 100% patency in the control as well as test group. This can probably be explained by the continued improvement in technical facility of the surgeons since thrombosis was found more frequently in a series of vein grafts performed by the same surgeons several years ago.[3] Moreover, the grafts were not allowed to remain in situ as long as those in the earlier series. However, this low incidence of thrombosis does demonstrate that thrombosis is not produced by the stent.

Tissue Reaction.—After one week all the stents became densely incorporated in host fibrous tissue. This can be seen in the illustration where the stent can be discerned in the adventitia of the artery and vein completely surrounded by fibrous tissue (Fig 5). There was little tissue reaction to the polypropylene except for a mild foreign body giant cell reaction appearing very much the same as those illustrated by Usher and his co-workers in a recent study of polypropylene filaments (Fig 6).[4] Copious space between the fibers permits broad direct incorporation of the vein in the recipient tissues.

Prevention of Vein Dilatation.—It was demonstrated repeatedly at the time of vein graft insertion that the venous segment could be made isodiametric by altering longitudinal tension on the stent (Fig 7). Moreover, angiography performed at a later date revealed continued maintenance of a normal vein diameter on the supported side, and wide

Fig 4.—Photograph of apparatus used for measuring bursting point of graft.

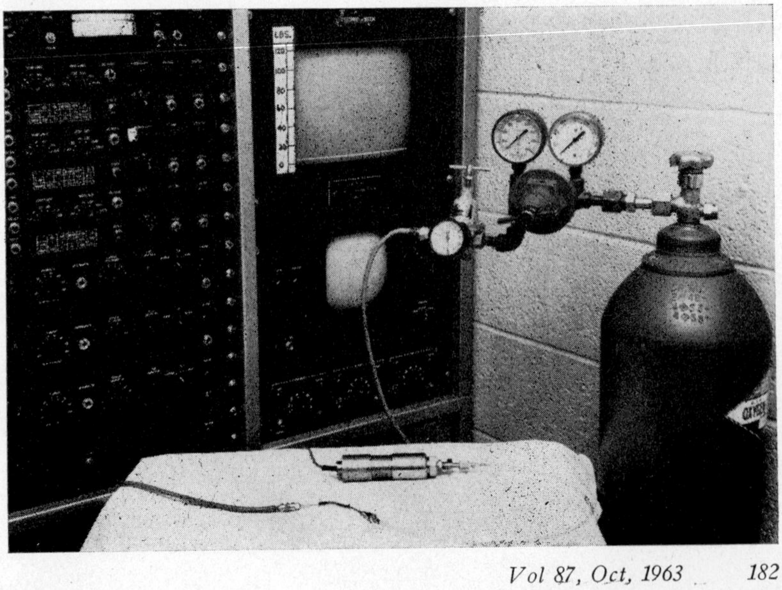

Comparison of Results

Procedure	Polypropylene With Stent	Polypropylene No Stent	Polyethylene	Teflon
Carotid vein graft	10	5	5	5
Patent	10	5	5	4
Carotid anastomosis	4	4		
Patent	4	4		
Abdominal aorta anastomosis	1	1		
Patent	1	1		
Total	15	10	5	5
Patent	15	10	5	4

dilatation on the nonsupported side (Fig 8). Dilatation did not occur in the supported side up to 63 days, the longest any stent was left in situ in this series. Whether or not maintenance of a normal vein diameter will affect the long-term patency of the graft remains to be seen. It is also not clear whether the unsupported side will continue to dilate although there is some evidence in the literature that further dilatation may occur.[2]

Pressure Gradient Across Graft.—In one graft only the effect of altering the vein diameter was tested by simultaneously measuring the blood pressure above and below the graft. It was found that a normal gradient was transmitted only when the graft was isodiametric but that the gradient fell when the vein was narrower or wider than host artery. This observation confirms those previously reported by the authors and many other investigators on the proper ratio of the diameter of host and transplanted vessel.

Tensile Strength of Vein and Anastomosis.—It has been reported by others that the

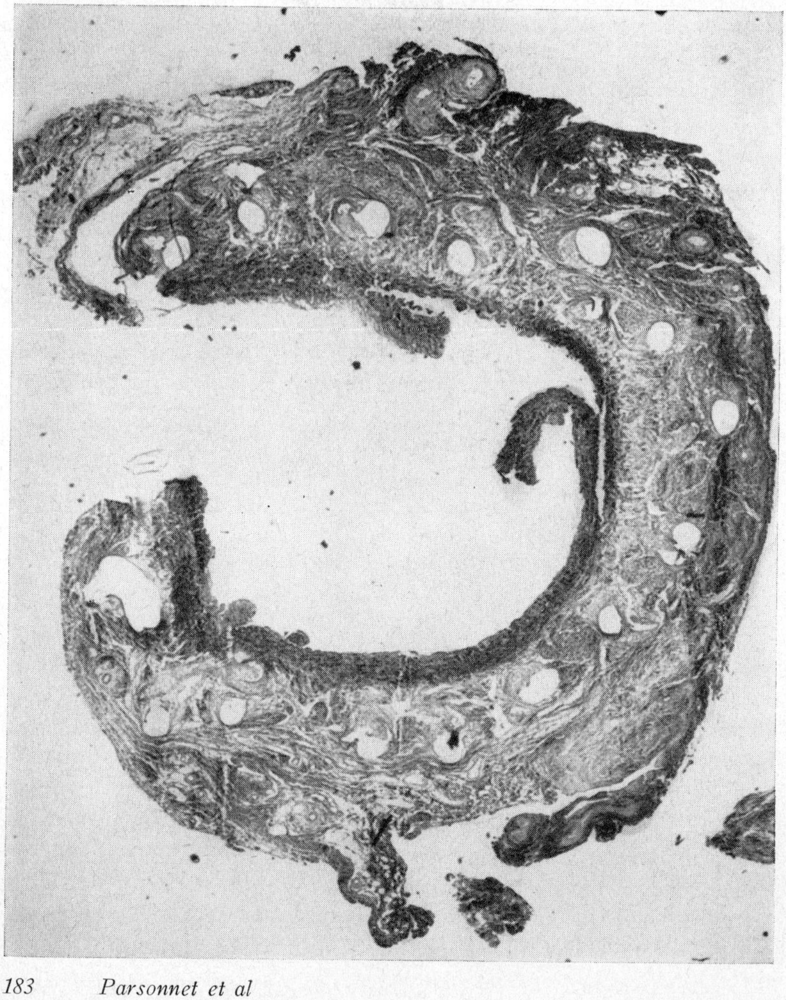

Fig 5. — Photomicrograph of vein graft surrounded by polypropylene stent in place 21 days. The fibers appear as large holes in the adventitia.

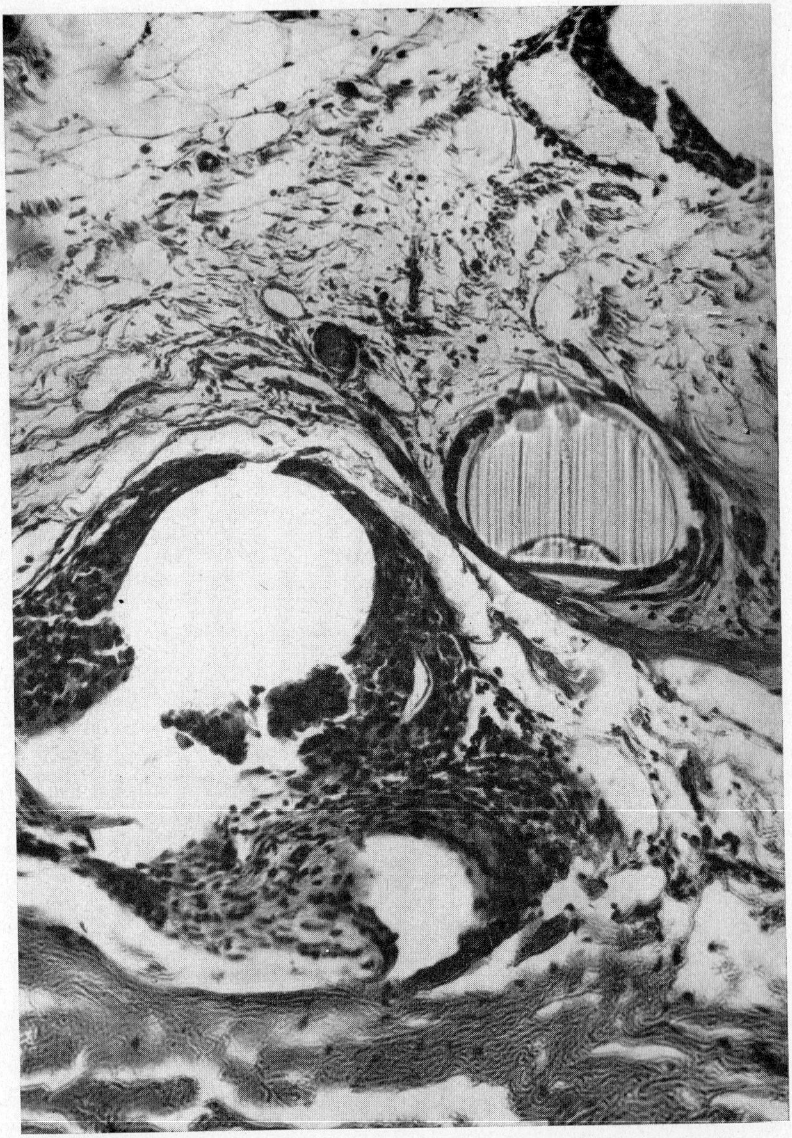

Fig 6.—Higher power photomicrograph of stent fiber with surrounding foreign-body giant-cell reaction.

healing of vascular anastomoses insofar as tensile strength is concerned is similar to healing wounds of skin and other tissues.[5,6] Standard tensiometer techniques have inherent defects especially in the reading of the end point, finding suitable methods of attaching the vessel to the weights and adjusting the results according to size and thickness of the excised segment of vessel. We developed the technique described above in the hope of mimicking intravascular phenomena more closely and finding a sharp end point easily (Fig 9). It is not clear exactly what this method measures, but, presumably, it is primarily a test of the strength of the surrounding collagen, particularly the collagen of the adventitia.

This assumption was suggested by the finding that both normal vein and artery burst at about 70-80 lb per square inch (PSI). Moreover, in no instance of the ten cases where measurement was performed did either a vein or anastomosis burst. The rupture always occurred in a point in the artery farthest from the grafted area where collagen of new scar tissue was most thin. After

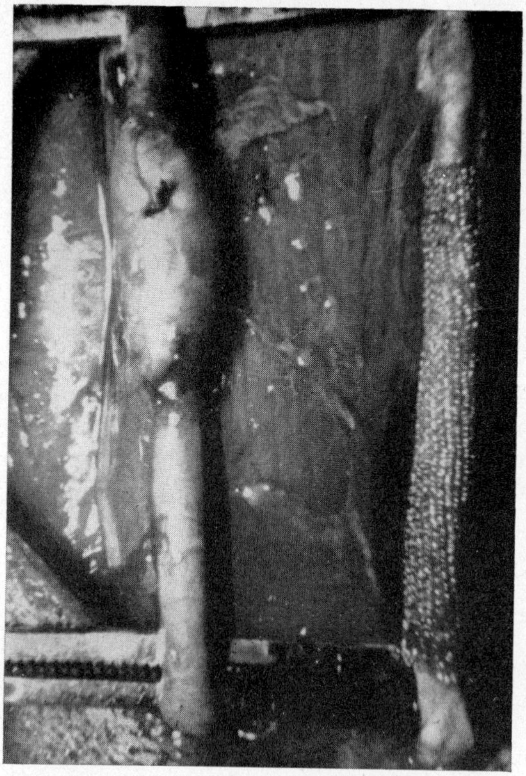

Fig 7.—Photograph of vein graft in situ, control on left, stent on right, showing prevention of initial vein dilatation.

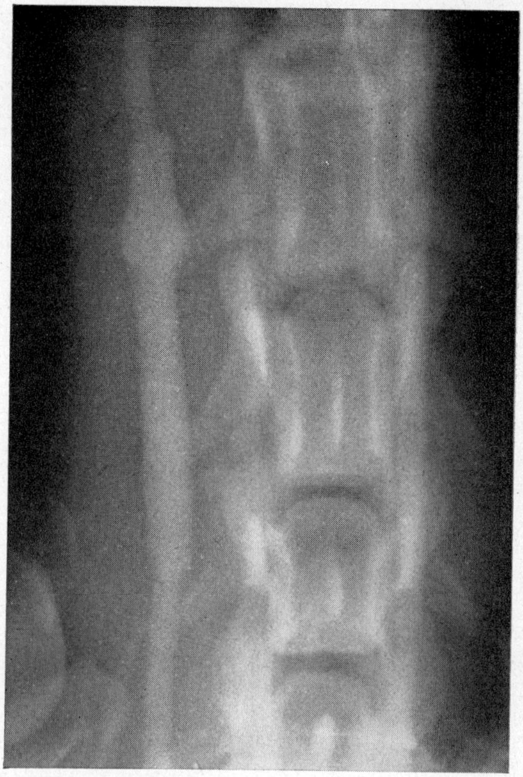

Fig 8.—Photograph of x-ray film of vein grafts three weeks after insertion. Note absence of dilatation and smooth patency of stent-supported vein (*right*).

seven days the bursting point was usually 135 PSI. Here again, this work is only in its preliminary phase, and more work is required to elucidate its meaning (Fig 10).

Implications of Study.—This study demonstrates that scaffold stents effectively prevent dilatation of arterialized veins. Presumably, if the stent itself can maintain its tensile strength and configuration *in situ* for prolonged periods, the beneficial results will persist. Hopefully, maintenance of a normal caliber will prevent thrombosis of autogenous vein grafts.

The dense incorporation of the stent fibers in fibrous tissues suggests that the principle of a surrounding scaffold might be useful in other clinical situations, particularly the support of deeply endarterectomized arteries,

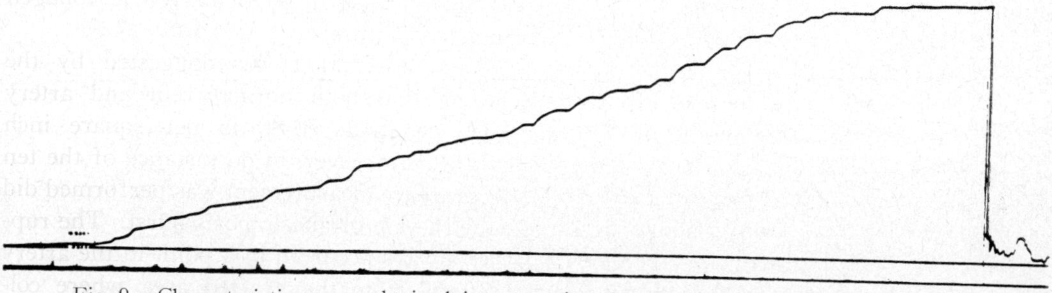

Fig 9.—Characteristic curve obtained in measuring bursting point. End point is at sudden drop to right of tracing.

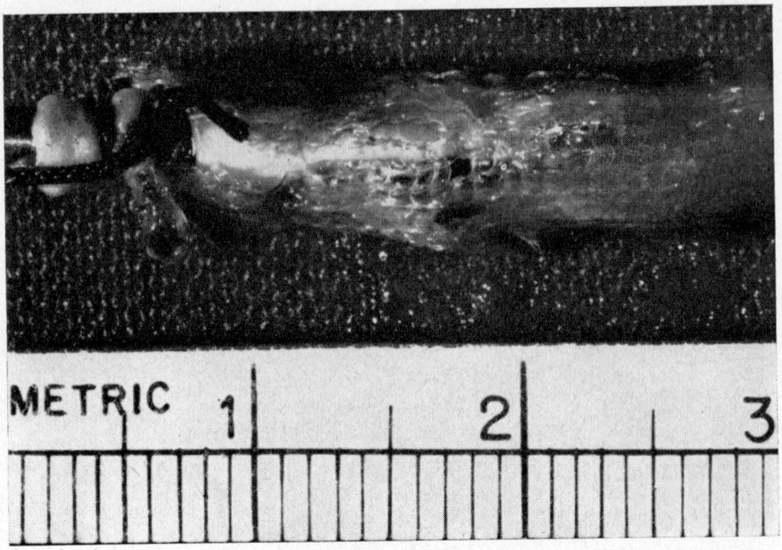

Fig 10.—Photograph of graft with rent outside of graft in normal artery.

precarious anastomoses of badly diseased vessels, and, perhaps, in the wrapping of unresectable aneurysms. The stent can also be used to support composite autogenous tissue grafts inserted in large arteries. We have recently inserted a composite vein graft supported by an external stent into the thoracic aorta of a dog with success.

Summary

A new external monofilament polypropylene tube stent has been devised to support arterial vein grafts. When used in autogenous vein grafts in the carotid artery of dogs it effectively prevents dilatation of the vein at the time of insertion of the graft for periods up to 63 days.

The stent material is accepted well by the host tissue; the wide space between the fibers allows broad incorporation of the transplanted vein in the recipient tissues.

No difference in tensile strength was noted between the supported and nonsupported vessels. In all cases, with or without the stent, the bursting point of the host artery was lower than the test area.

Of 25 grafts that were stent supported, all but one were patent for periods up to 63 days.

Victor Parsonnet, MD, Attending in Surgery, Newark Beth Israel Hospital, 201 Lyons Avenue, Newark 12, NJ.

REFERENCES

1. Dole, A. W., and Mahoney, E. B.: Autogenous Vein Grafts, and Related Aspects of Peripheral Arterial Disease, Springfield, Ill: Charles C Thomas, Publishers, 1959.

2. Sako, Y.: Prevention of Dilatation in Autogenous Venous and Pericardial Grafts in the Thoracic Aorta: An Experimental Study, Surgery 30:148, 1951.

3. Eslami, H.; Shah, I. U. H.; and Parsonnet, V.: Small Arterial Grafts: Factors Involved in the Prevention of Thrombosis, J Newark Beth Israel Hosp 14:14, 1963.

4. Usher, F. C.; Allen, J. E., Jr.; Crosthwait, R. W.; and Cogan, J. E.: Polypropylene Monofilament: A New, Biologically Inert Suture for Closing Contaminated Wounds, JAMA 179:780, 1962.

5. Hohf, R. P.: Tensile Strength of the Arterial-Prosthesis Anastomosis During Healing, Ann Surg 156:805, 1962.

6. Villegas, A. H.; Toll, G.; and Shaw, R. S.: Comparison of the Rate of Healing in Transverse and Longitudinal Aortotomies, J Thorac Cardiov. Surg 45:233, 1963.

Granular Cell Myoblastoma of the Breast

LEONARD STEIN, MD
BUFFALO

Granular cell myoblastoma is an uncommon tumor. More than 400 cases have been reported in the literature since its initial description by Abrikossoff in 1926. Granular cell myoblastoma of the female breast, however, must still be considered a rare tumor. Byrne and Deane [5] in 1960 were able to collect 27 reported cases occurring in the skin, subcutaneous tissue, and glandular tissue of the breast. My review of the literature to date has yielded a total of 31 acceptable cases (Table 1), eliminating two cases reported by Klemperer [19] which were not his own cases but reports of the cases of Abrikossoff and Meyer and one case reported by Cheatle and Cutler [6] which was reported to be a xanthoma by microscopic study. The granular cell myoblastoma morphologically has been confused with the xanthoma, but, in view of the microscopic report of xanthoma in this case, it would seem better to exclude it. Added are a case reported by Kirschner [18] in March, 1962, and four cases reported by Colberg and Hubay [8] in February, 1963.

Grossly these tumors appear as firm, sometimes hard, nodules of varying size, generally under 2 cm in diameter. At times the tumor

Submitted for publication April 8, 1963.

Senior Resident in Surgery, Buffalo General Hospital (Dr. Stein).

TABLE 1.—*Reported Cases of Granular Cell Myoblastoma of the Breast*

Author	Year	Cases
Abrikossoff	1931	1
Meyer	1932	1
Geschickter	1934	3
Gray & Gruenfeld	1937	1
Tuta & Schmidt	1942	1
Horn & Stout	1943	2
Haagensen & Stout	1946	5
Powell	1946	1
Simon	1947	1
Bangle	1952	3
Crawford & DeBakey	1953	1
Lowbeer	1953	1
Jernstrom & Fry	1956	1
Aulisio	1956	1
Schmidt, Ambler, & Wroth	1959	1
Byrne & Deane	1960	2
Kirschner	1962	1
Colberg & Hubay	1963	4
Stein	1963	4
Total		35

may appear to be well encapsulated and may be "shelled out" of the surrounding tissues. On cut section the surface is grey to greyish-yellow in color and may bulge slightly. Microscopically there are groups of acidophilic cells which may seem to be encapsulated (Fig 2) or may invade the surrounding tissue (Fig 1). The tumor cells may be well defined or appear as a syncytium. In accordance with Abrikossoff's classification, the cells may appear with or without striations.

Haagensen [14] stated that all the tumors of this type that he personally had seen were located in the medial quadrants of the breast, and he suggested a possible relationship between this localization and the pathogenesis of these tumors from muscle tissue. Experience with a tumor located in the midline of the breast in a personal case and reports of this tumor occurring in the outer quadrants of the breast have prompted this report. A search of the records of the Buffalo General Hospital has uncovered three additional cases.

Report of Cases

Case 1.—A 70-year-old white woman was admitted to the Buffalo General Hospital in 1954 with a painless mass in the right breast for two months.

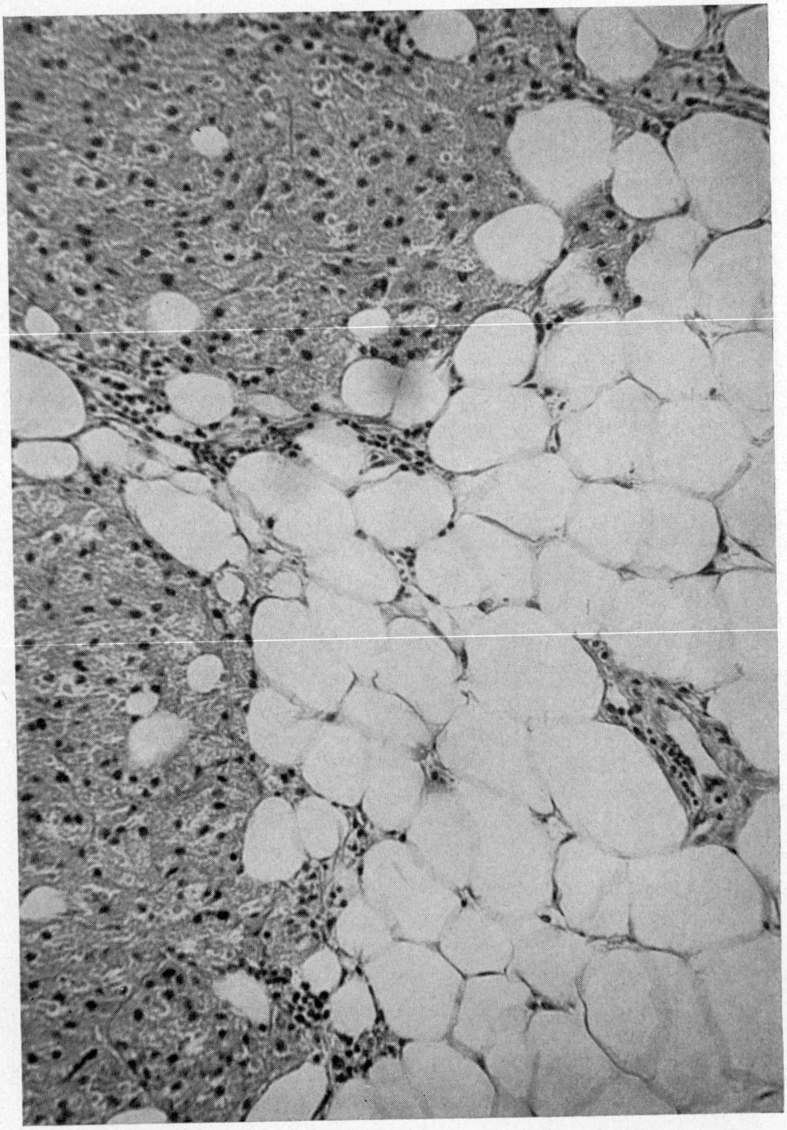

Fig 1 (Case 2).—Granular cell myoblastoma of the breast showing invasion of surrounding fatty tissue. Hematoxylin and eosin; reduced 7% from mag × 96.

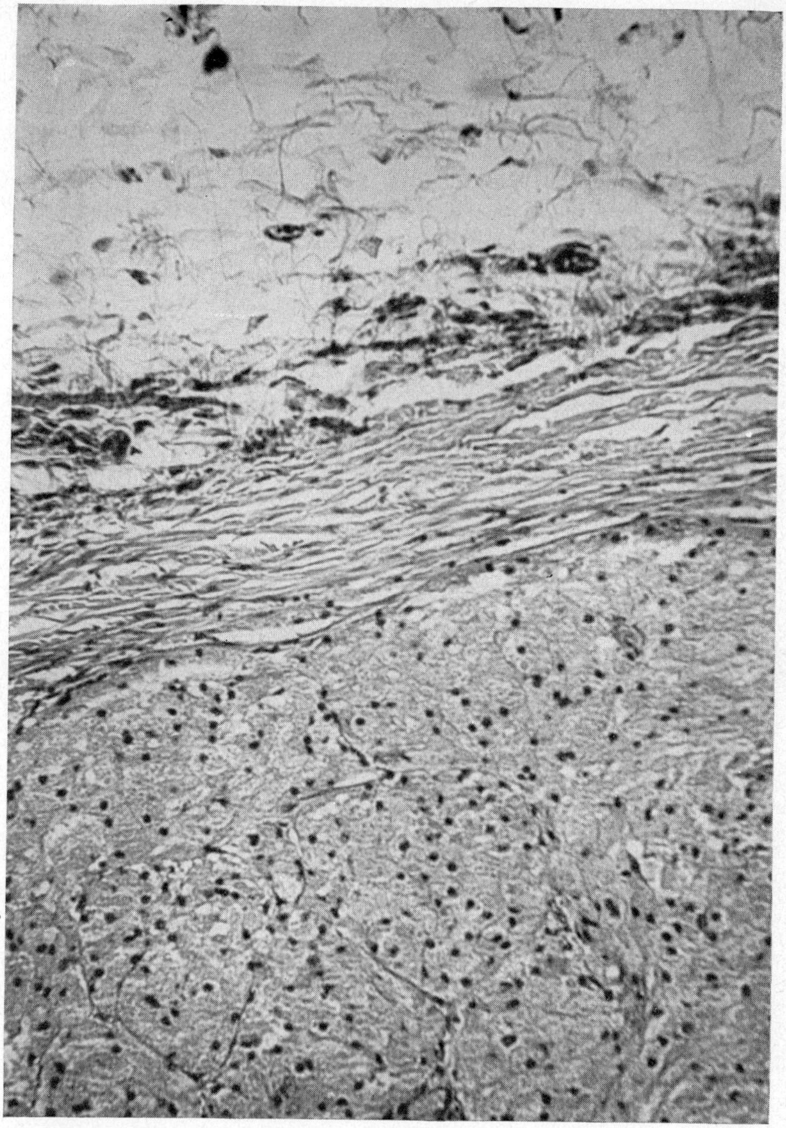

Fig 2 (Case 3).—Granular cell myoblastoma of the breast showing encapsulation. Hematoxylin and eosin; reduced 7% from mag × 96.

Physical examination revealed a pea-size mass in the subcutaneous tissue at the level of the second intercostal space at the midclavicular line. Excisional biopsy was performed, and the pathology report described a granular cell myoblastoma.

CASE 2.—A 21-year-old white woman was admitted to the Buffalo General Hospital in 1955 with a mass in the right breast for nine months which had increased slightly in size but was otherwise asymptomatic. Physical examination revealed a 1.5 × 1.5 cm mass in the subcutaneous tissue of the upper outer quadrant of the right breast 6 cm from the nipple. Excisional biopsy was performed, and the pathology report described a granular cell myoblastoma (Fig 1).

CASE 3.—A 51-year-old white woman was admitted to the Buffalo General Hospital in 1958 with an asymptomatic lump in the right breast for three weeks. Physical examination revealed a 2 cm subcutaneous nodule in the upper inner quadrant of the right breast 9 cm from the areola. Excisional biopsy was performed, and the pathology report read "granular cell myoblastoma" (Fig 2).

CASE 4.—A 21-year-old Negro woman was seen in the surgical clinic of the Buffalo General Hospital on April 30, 1962, stating that she had noticed a small lump in the right breast two weeks after her last menstrual period. The lump was asymptomatic. Physical examination revealed a 2 × 2 cm mass in the right breast located 2 cm above the areola and in line with the nipple. The mass was freely movable. There were no palpable lymph nodes. She was admitted to the hospital, where excisional biopsy was performed. The pathology

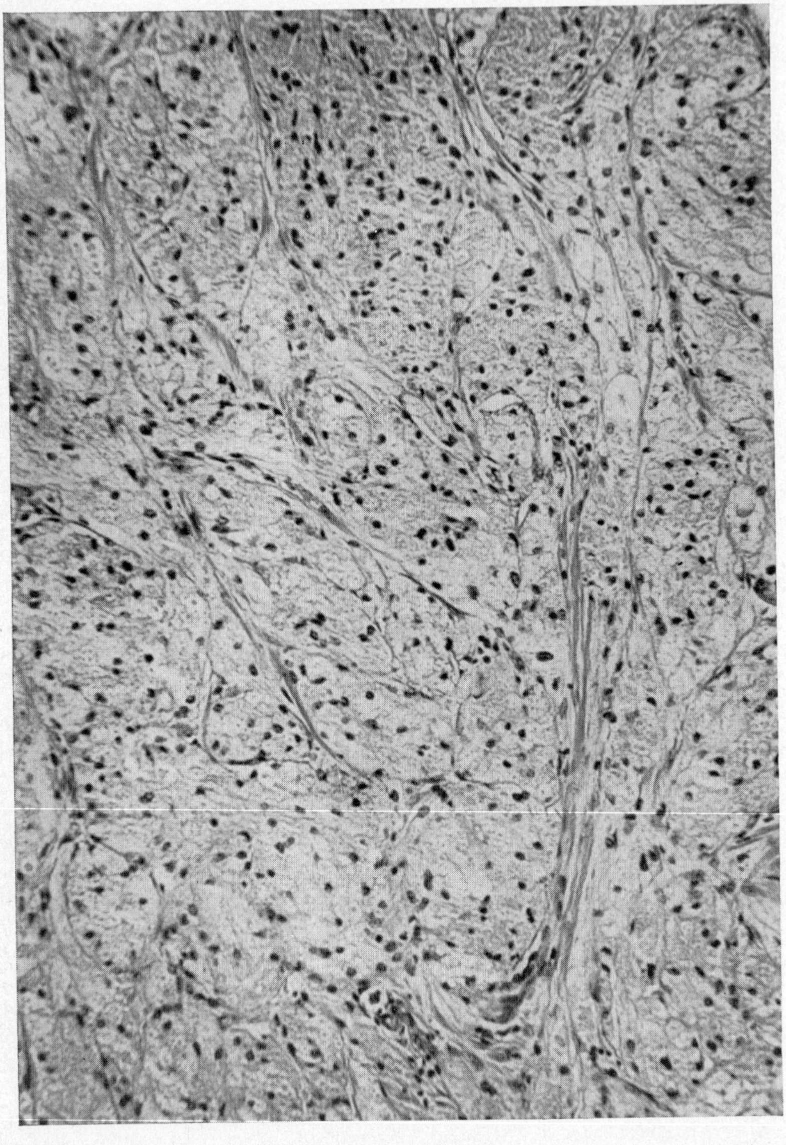

Fig 3 (Case 4).—Granular cell myoblastoma of the breast showing pseudolobulation. Hematoxylin and eosin; reduced 7% from mag ×96.

report read "granular cell myoblastoma" (Fig 3). She is being followed in the surgical clinic.

Comment

The pathogenesis of the granular cell myoblastoma is as yet unsettled. The first theories put forth related this tumor to origin in either muscle tissue or embryonic muscle tissue. However, this did not explain the occurrence of these tumors in areas devoid of muscular tissue, such as the breast. Other tissue cell origins have also been suggested including epithelium, myoepithelium, histiocytes, fibroblasts, vascular endothelium, and Schwann cells. Bangle[4] and Ashburn and Rodger[2] have championed the neural origin of these tumors and give convincing evidence.

Haagensen[14] has stated that, in his personal experience, granular cell myoblastomas of the breast have been located in the inner quadrants of the breast. He suggested that the origin of these tumors could be related to aberrant muscular tissue either from the platysma or from the sternal muscle. The occurrence of these tumors in other quadrants of the breast may argue for or against this possibility. As can be seen from Table 2, in

TABLE 2.—*Localization of Tumors Within the Breast*

Quadrant of Breast	No. Cases	%
Upper inner	8	48
Lower inner	3	18
Upper outer	4	22
Lower outer	0	0
Midline	2	12
	—	—
Total localized cases	17	100
Not stated	18	
	—	
Total cases	35	

approximately one half of the cases the precise localization of the tumors in the breast was not reported. In the other 17 cases, the localization was divided among all the quadrants except the lower outer quadrant, of which eight were located in the upper inner quadrant, three in the lower inner quadrant, four in the upper outer quadrant, and two in the midline of the breast above the nipple level. The majority of these tumors then indeed occur in the inner quadrants of the breast; however, they do occur elsewhere in approximately 34% of the cases. The only location in which the tumors have not been reported to occur is the lower outer quadrant. Haagensen has postulated that the tumors of the medial side of the breast could arise from either the sternal muscle or the platysma. It would seem that the platysma, taking its origin from the fascia of the deltoid and pectoralis major, could also give rise to the tumors arising in the upper outer quadrants of the breast and in the midline of the breast above the nipple line. Finding these tumors in the lower outer quadrant of the breast would tend to deny this muscular origin for these lesions; however, as yet there have been no reports of tumors in this location. Although the origin of the granular cell myoblastomas is still not settled, their various locations in the breast so far do not deny the possibility of muscular origin.

The granular cell myoblastomas are generally considered to be benign tumors, although malignant forms have been reported in such locations as the skin,[22] gluteal region,[1] and urinary bladder.[23] In these cases, the metastases have been both blood borne and lymphatic in nature. In Ravich's case with the primary site in the urinary bladder, the metastases were widespread, appearing in the prostate gland, liver, spleen, lymph nodes, right lung, pericardium, skull, vertebra, peritoneum, and pelvic tissues. Two cases of malignant myoblastomas of the breast have also been reported, one by Crawford and DeBakey [10] and one by Kirschner.[18] Metastases were present in one but not in the other. Crawford and DeBakey's patient succumbed to the disease with metastases present in the lung, liver, mesentery, and axilla. The primary lesion was located in the upper outer quadrant of the breast. In Kirschner's patient, the lesion was also located in the upper outer quadrant of the breast but there were no metastases. In the absence of metastases, cellular differences may aid in differentiating benign from malignant forms. In benign forms cell variation is minimal, and the nucleoli are said to be less prominent than in malignant forms. Ackerman and Phelps [1] have indicated that in benign forms the individual cells may be larger and the nucleoli smaller than in malignant forms. Other indications of possible malignancy are atypical cells and the presence of numerous mitotic figures. The accepted form of treatment for benign lesions is local excision. If the tumor is malignant, radical resection is indicated.

Summary

The literature concerning granular cell myoblastoma of the breast is reviewed, and four additional cases are added. The localization of these tumors within the breast and the possible relation to the origin of these tumors is discussed.

Dr. J. C. Brennan reviewed the slides of the cases here reported.

Leonard Stein, MD, c/o John R. Paine, MD, Chief of Surgery, The Buffalo General Hospital, 100 High St, Buffalo 3, NY.

REFERENCES

1. Ackerman, L. V., and Phelps, C. R.: Malignant Granular Cell Myoblastoma of the Gluteal Region, Surgery 20:511, 1946.

2. Ashburn, L. L., and Rodger, R. C.: Myoblastomas, Neural Origin, Amer J Clin Path 22:440, 1952.

3. Aulisio, A.: Un Case di Mioblastomioma Granulo-Cellulare della Mammella, Rass Int Clin Ter 36:479, 1956.

4. Bangle, R., Jr.: A Morphological and Histochemical Study of the Granular-Cell Myoblastoma, Cancer 5:950, 1952.

5. Byrne, J. J., and Deane, M. A.: Granular Cell Myoblastoma of the Breast, Amer J Surg 100:98, 1960.

6. Cheatle, G. L., and Cutler, M.: Tumours of the Breast: Their Pathology, Symptoms, Diagnosis, and Treatment, London: Edward Arnold (Publishers) Ltd, 1931, p 307.

7. Colberg, J. E.: Granular Cell Myoblastoma, Int Abstr Surg 115:205, 1962.

8. Colberg, J. E., and Hubay, C. A.: Granular Cell Myoblastoma: A Problem in Diagnosis, Surgery 53:226, 1963.

9. Crane, A. R., and Tremblay, R. G.: Myoblastoma, Amer J Path 21:357, 1945.

10. Crawford, E. S., and DeBakey, M. E.: Granular Cell Myoblastoma: Two Unusual Cases, Cancer 6:786, 1953.

11. Geschickter, C.: Tumors of Muscle, Amer J Cancer 22:378, 1934.

12. Gray, S. H., and Gruenfeld, G. E.: Myoblastoma, Amer J Cancer 30:699, 1937.

13. Haagensen, C. D., and Stout, A. P.: Granular Cell Myoblastoma of the Mammary Gland, Ann Surg 124:218, 1946.

14. Haagensen, C. D.: Diseases of the Breast, Philadelphia: W. B. Saunders Company, 1956, pp 277-282.

15. Horn, R. C., Jr., and Stout, A. P.: Granular Cell Myoblastoma, Surg Gynec Obstet 76:315, 1943.

16. Howe, C. W., and Warren, S.: Myoblastoma, Surgery 16:319, 1944.

17. Jernstrom, P., and Fry, K.: Granular Cell Myoblastoma of the Mammary Gland, Amer J Clin Path 26:1055, 1956.

18. Kirschner, H.: Über einen Fall von Maligne entartetem Myoblastenmyom der Mamma (On a Case of Malignant Degeneration of Myoblasticmyoma of the Breast), Bruns Beit. Klin Chir 204: 87, 1962.

19. Klemperer, P.: Myoblastoma of the Striated Muscle, Amer J Cancer 20:324, 1934.

20. Lowbeer, L.: "Granular Cell Myoblastomas" of Unusual Locations (Bronchus, Breast, Chest Wall), Amer J Path 29:611, 1953.

21. Murphy, G. M.; Dockerty, M. B.; and Broders, A. C.: Myoblastoma, Amer J Path 25: 1157, 1949.

22. Powell, E. B.: Granular Cell Myoblastoma, Arch Path 42:517, 1946.

23. Ravich, A.; Stout, A. P.; and Ravich, R. A.: Malignant Granular Cell Myoblastoma Involving the Urinary Bladder, Ann Surg 121:361, 1945.

24. Ross, R. C.; Miller, T. R.; and Foote, F. W., Jr.: Malignant Granular Cell Myoblastoma, Cancer 5:112, 1952.

25. Schmidt, E. C. H.; Ambler, J. T.; and Wroth, R. L.: Multiple Granular Cell Myoblastomas: Report of a Case, Maryland Med J 8:287, 1959.

26. Simon, M. A.: Granular Cell Myoblastoma, Amer J Clin Path 17:302, 1947.

27. Stout, A. P.: Granular Cell Myoblastoma of the Breast, J Missouri Med Ass 44:342, 1947.

28. Tuta, J. A., and Schmidt, F. R.: So-Called Myoblastoma, Arch Derm Syph 46:225, 1942.

Pulmonary Embolism

Historical Aspects

MICHAEL HUME, MD
NEW HAVEN, CONN

Even as Harvey's inspired concept of a "circulation" of the blood was based on a new interpretation of existing information (the anatomic presence of valves in the veins [10]), so the concept of "embolism" had to await a new interpretation of the implications of the circulation by Rudolf Virchow. The data upon which each concept was based were available to other brilliant scientists at the same (or earlier) times, and yet the implications had not been appreciated. In each instance the new concept arose from a combination of thorough familiarity with previous work, acute observation, a convincing experimental system, and a dedicated willingness to attack publicly the accepted precepts of the day. Any account of the development of recognition of pulmonary embolism and attempts to treat it is illuminated by wide contrasts, ranging from the spectacle of pulmonary embolectomy to the subtle influence of the vasomotor system on the dual circulation in the lung. In presenting some aspects of historical interest it is desirable, although not always easy, to consider the various "firsts" against the background of contemporary attitudes, both scientific and therapeutic, the impact of progress in other fields, and the capricious nature of the underlying disease process—still today a vexing problem in the diagnosis and, particularly, in the evaluation of treatment. These related aspects, considered with the historical events themselves, form a background against which the course of further development can be discerned a little more clearly.

Submitted for publication April 4, 1963.

Markle Scholar in Medical Science.

From the Department of Surgery, Yale University School of Medicine.

The Recognition of Pulmonary Embolism

It was Hunter whose observations anticipated an appreciation of thrombosis, although he believed the phenomenon which he saw to be a coagulation of lymph.[15] The development of the theory of inflammation of the veins after Hunter reached great proportions, and, as described by Cruveilhier,[9] inflammation of the veins was present under a variety of circumstances and was responsible for many, indeed most, pathological conditions. The concepts of his time paid particular attention to the inflammatory process in the vessel wall and appreciated thrombosis as a local phenomenon secondary to this inflammation. This was to be all changed by the observations of Rudolf Virchow who, as described by W. H. Welch, ". . . Between the years 1846 and 1856 constructed the whole doctrine of embolism upon the basis of anatomical, experimental and clinical investigations, which for completeness, accuracy and just discernment of the truth must always remain a model of scientific research in medicine." [33] He was able to show that not all thrombotic material in the pulmonary artery rose at the point where it was found at autopsy, and, by dissection of the pelvic veins and the veins of the lower limbs, he was able to demonstrate where fragments of clot arising in distal areas had migrated to the lung. By section of thrombi in the pulmonary artery he was able, as shown in the Figure, to differentiate between an embolus riding on the bifurcation of a pulmonary vessel and the encapsulating or secondary thrombus which propagated upon it but which was not associated with any capillary phlebitis. The clinical symptoms varied from none at all to dyspnea and sudden death, and the consequences of embolism were atrophy of the lung, pneumonia, gangrene, and infarction. He was the first to produce experimental pulmonary emboli, which he introduced into the veins of dogs, using fibrin, clot, muscle, and rubber, as well as producing air emboli, fat emboli, starch and metallic mercury emboli. He noted that embolic material passed through the right side of the heart without causing local symptoms. Infarction beyond emboli was hyperemic rather than anemic, which Virchow attributed to the dual circulation of the lung. Infection and necrosis occurred after experimental emboli, in contrast to emboli noted at autopsy, most of which were bland. This work, and the man himself, were summarized by Ackerknecht [1]:

> These early papers of Virchow reveal an unusual gift of observation, a phenomenal memory for retaining details of old observations and autopsies, and ability to remember them at the right moment, a very sharp logic, an extraordinary familiarity with the older and contemporary international medical literature, and an unlimited willingness to attack and criticize statements no matter by whom they were made.

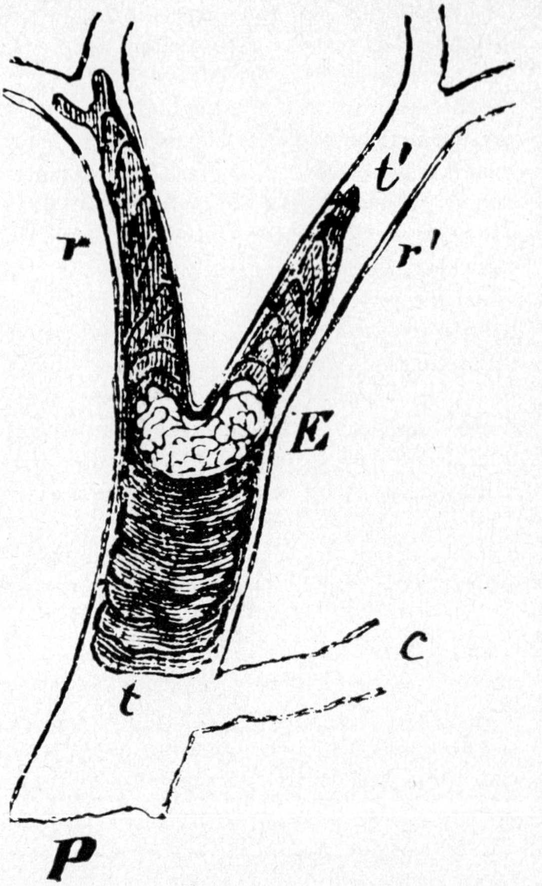

Embolus of pulmonary artery. *P* indicates middle-sized branch of pulmonary artery; *E*, embolus riding on the bifurcation of the artery; *t* to *t'*, the secondary (encapsulating) thrombus; *t*, the piece in front of the embolus extending to the next higher collateral vessel; *t'*, the piece behind the embolus, branching; *r* and *r'*, branches filled with clot which ends in a conical shape. From Virchow, R.: *Die Cellularpathologie,* Berlin: Verlag von August Hischwald, 1859, pp 444.

Mechanism of Death

Virchow and many after him appreciated that death from massive pulmonary embolism was due to asphyxia from obstruction of the main pulmonary artery. Dilation of the right side of the heart was noted in all experimental preparations, and when means were at hand to measure the pressure in several chambers at the same time, data were gathered which indicated that Virchow was correct in his assumption that reduced coronary flow was the cause of sudden death.

Megibow, Katz, and Steinitz [23] summarized the effects of pulmonary embolism with pea seeds, starch, and emboli made of Penrose tubing filled with fluid. They measured the rise in pulmonary artery pressure—perhaps for the first time in the closed chest preparation—the rise in venous pressure and the fall in femoral artery pressure which followed massive pulmonary embolization. They postulated that the mechanism of sudden death was related to coronary insufficiency caused by (1) diminished perfusion of the coronaries as the aortic pressure falls, (2) extravascular compression of the branches of the coronaries as they pass through the distended ventricular myocardium, and (3) resistance to flow in the coronary sinus and the thebesian veins due to the high right heart pressure. These factors causing coronary insufficiency would favor ectopic rhythms and ventricular fibrillation. The experiments of State and Salisbury [28] emphasized the critical effect of aortic pressure upon survival when the pulmonary artery is blocked by a balloon catheter. Animals made hypotensive by bleeding did not tolerate blockade, but if blood was rapidly returned into the aorta these animals could be resuscitated and tolerated the blockade as well as other animals initially normotensive or hypertensive. Although the cause of death in massive embolism is well explained by such experimental data, death after small emboli is noted occasionally and appears to demand a different explanation. A reflex mediated in the nervous system offers a plausible explanation, and considerable recent experimentation has been designed to demonstrate the role of vasomotor activity in the presence of small emboli.[25,36]

Diagnosis

Diagnosis of pulmonary embolism on the basis of physical examination and the great variation in these signs were known to Virchow. While Professor of Pathology at Berlin, he had a clinical service of his own and apparently ran it himself. The clinical diagnosis of less-than-massive pulmonary embolism was probably limited to cases having, besides chest findings, an obvious inflammatory phlebitis, varicose veins, or fracture in the lower extremity. New assistance in diagnosis was foreshadowed by the discovery of x-ray by William Roentgen in 1895 and the first use of the string galvanometer to record electric potential in the heart by William Einthoven in 1901. The earliest recorded report of the changes in the chest x-ray associated with acute pulmonary embolism is that of Wharton and Pierson [35] from the departments of Radiology and Gynecology at The Johns Hopkins Hospital. They noted small areas of pleural effusion blunting the costophrenic angles when small infarcts were present and larger opaque areas in the lungs when larger pulmonary vessels had been occluded. Subsequently, Nils Westermark [34] in 1938 described the radiolucency which corresponded to the area of diminished pulmonary artery perfusion following a major embolus and contrasted this clarified zone with the abrupt termination of the hilar vascular radicals medial to it. Undoubtedly, the most complete summary of radiographic and pathological material was reported by Aubrey O. Hampton and Benjamin Castleman [11] of the Massachusetts General Hospital, who obtained upright postmortem chest x-rays before commencing the autopsy. Besides defining the characteristics of infarcts of various size and the linear densities of a healed infarct, they described what they called "incomplete infarction" which was an area with rapidly disappearing consolidation in the lung following a clinical episode suggesting pulmonary embolism and proceeding to complete clearing as proved pathologically. They indicated that better appreciation of the x-ray findings would aid considerably in making a clinical diagnosis in uncertain cases.

Krumbhaar [18] was probably the first to record changes in the electrocardiogram in experimental occlusion of the pulmonary artery. This study was carried out on cats in the research laboratory of the Harvard Medical School during 1916, using a string galvanometer. The first clinical correlation of electrocardiographic findings in cases proved to have massive pulmonary embolism was reported by McGinn and White [21] in 1935.

Treatment

The treatment of embolism, particularly as foreshadowed in the management of suppurative thrombophlebitis, may be considered to go back to Hunter,[15] although the doctrine of embolism had not yet been born. He conceived that it would be desirable to compress externally a vein at a point central to the site of suppurative thrombophlebitis which he judged to be the source of septicemia in the soldier under his care. In 1902 Friedrich

Trendelenburg [31] reported the first successful control of puerperal infection by vein ligation and reviewed the previous vein ligation therapy for suppurative thrombophlebitis which dated, according to him, from the operation of Lee in 1865.[19] Trendelenburg was the first to ligate successfully the inferior vena cava,[17] gave his name to the positioning of an operative patient head down for pelvic surgery and to a test for incompetence of the venous valves, and revived the ligation of incompetent saphenous varices (first described by Paul of Aeginetus in the seventh century AD [27]). His most extraordinary contribution to surgery was undoubtedly the method for pulmonary embolectomy. This operation, which also bears his name, was presented to the German Surgical Congress on April 21, 1908, under the title "Operative Interference in Embolism of the Pulmonary Artery." [32] Diagnosis was possible, he pointed out, by relying on the clinical complex including collapse, pallor, cyanosis, pulselessness, and dyspnea, particularly when associated with previous operations involving the veins or the presence of evident thrombophlebitis, fracture, or varices. He further indicated that among nine cases studied, not all deaths occurred at once. In fact, only two were instantaneous, the other seven cases surviving from ten minutes to an hour, and in half of these cases more than 15 minutes were available to the surgeon. At the surgical congress he demonstrated the operative technique on a corpse and discussed the fact that complete occlusion of the pulmonary artery could be tolerated from 45 seconds to 2 minutes or partial occlusion for a longer period, enough to make the intra-arterial maneuver feasible for a surgeon as deft as he must have been. He proposed a T-shaped incision running transversely along the second rib and vertically along the left side of the sternum. The pleura was opened in the course of approaching the great vessels, which were surrounded by a rubber tube passed on a metal sound. This tube was used to elevate the pulmonary artery into the wound and to occlude it to reduce the flow during the embolectomy. A forceps was used to extract the embolic material, and the incision was closed with clamps as quickly as possible and the compressing tourniquet released. At the meeting he demonstrated healing of the pulmonary artery of a calf which had been sacrificed four months after successful removal of an experimental embolus 15 cm long, and he reported his own clinical experience which was limited to one unsuccessful case. In addition, he reported two operations performed in Leipzig in which the patients became pulseless during the operation but recovered after removal of pieces of embolus up to 34 cm in length. The first case survived 15 hours only to die in heart failure. The second died of hemorrhage from the internal mammary artery 37 hours postoperatively. It was not until 1924, however, that Kirschner [16] successfully performed pulmonary embolectomy. A. W. Meyer,[24] who had had a successful case, described an extrapleural approach and stressed the advantage of this modification. However, by the 1930's only seven successes had been reported in an experience of more than 300 operations, the tendency was to withhold the procedure until the patient's last breath, and discussions of its usefulness reflected more than a little pessimism.[5] Therapy soon became directed to vein ligation and anticoagulants, and interest arose in the detection of patients having an unusual susceptibility to thrombosis [4] and the prevention of postoperative embolism.

In 1934, John Homans reported the ligation of the femoral vein for pulmonary embolism secondary to bland phlebothrombosis.[12] He was probably one of the first to do so, and based the procedure on his observations of the type of quiet thrombosis in veins of the calf and popliteal area which he believed to be even more commonly the cause of embolism than acute, symptomatic ileofemoral thrombophlebitis—or phlegmasia alba dolens. This extension of the application of femoral vein ligation raised for the first time the possibility of surgical prophylaxis of pulmonary embolism and enjoyed a temporary popularity during the middle years of the 1940's. With the establishment of anticoagulant therapy, vein ligation became reserved for failures of anticoagulation and practically disappeared as prophylaxis. Ligation of the inferior vena cava and ovarian veins remained the treatment of choice for suppurative pelvic thrombophlebitis as described by Conrad Collins [6] of New Orleans.

It is noteworthy that William H. Welch's interest in thrombosis probably was communicated to William H. Howell, the physiologist with whom the young John McLean [22] discovered the anticoagulant property of heparin in 1916. Howell predicted the usefulness of such an agent in 1928.[13] This first anticoagulant was applied experimentally in Canada in 1936 and finally in patients by Murray and Best.[26] Reduction of mortality after pulmonary embolism by intravenous heparin was reported by them and from Scandinavia,[8] establishing its efficacy in treatment. Purification of bishydroxycoumarin (Dicumarol) from the anticoagulant agent in spoiled sweet-clover hay [20] and its use by the Mayo Clinic group [3] provided a more convenient agent for prophylaxis, and in 1949 Arthur W. Allen [2] was able to show from the Massachusetts General Hospital (the home of prophylactic vein ligation) that results with bishydroxycoumarin were better than with vein ligation.

No form of prophylaxis established complete control of the disease, however, and with the better methods of cardiac resuscitation attendant on the remarkable advances in cardiac surgery during the 1950's, success in pulmonary embolectomy was achieved for the first time in the Western hemisphere in the Massachusetts General Hospital in 1958.[29] This success foreshadowed a renewed application, and by 1961 the progress of the techniques of extracorporeal circulation had reached a point at which Denton A. Cooley and associates were able to take advantage of cardiopulmonary bypass and to report a successful pulmonary embolectomy with this aid.[7] With further refinements in pump apparatus, disposable presterilized tubing, and prepackaged small volume oxygenators, it is likely that partial cardiopulmonary bypass will be available at the bedside in the near future. Such a system would support arterial circulation and relieve the distention of the right side of the heart. If sufficiently compact, it could be transported with the patient for angiography of the pulmonary artery or to the operating suite where embolectomy could be carried out with the aid of the same partial bypass or with total bypass. The number of patients for whom this treatment can be effective is likely to be limited only by the length of time which they can survive before the arrival of the "crash wagon" and illustrates the desirability of further attention paid to emergency supportive measures during this interval. When the efficacy of thrombolytic enzymes is better established,[14] they can rationally be applied in any instance in which significant obstruction of the pulmonary bed exists, and, by using cardiopulmonary bypass, they may be applied in cases of massive embolism. Under such circumstances, pulmonary embolectomy could be reserved for the situation in which thrombolytic therapy was ineffective.

The development of these enzymes and the application of them and other forms of treatment, operative and otherwise, to pulmonary embolism will follow from research that combines clinical observation, animal experiment, and necropsy. This triad was enunciated in 1845 by Rudolf Virchow, in an attack upon the empiricism and romanticism that had befallen German medicine in those times, and was to serve him as a personal philosophy for research in the forthcoming discovery of the principles of pulmonary embolism.

Michael Hume, MD, Assistant Professor of Surgery, Yale University School of Medicine, 333 Cedar St, New Haven, Conn.

REFERENCES

1. Ackerknecht, E. H.: Rudolf Virchow—Doctor, Statesman, Anthropologist, Madison, Wis: University of Wisconsin Press, 1953, p 67.

2. Allen, A. W.: Management of Thromboembolic Disease in Surgical Patients, Surg Gynec Obstet 96:107-114, 1953.

3. Allen, E. V.; Hines, E. A.; Kvale, W. F.; and Barker, N. W.: The Use of Dicumarol as an Anticoagulant: Experience in 2307 Cases, Ann Intern Med 27:371-381, 1947.

4. Bancroft, F. W., and Stanley-Brown, M.: Postoperative Thrombosis, Thrombophlebitis and Embolism, Surg Gynec Obstet 54:898-906, 1932.

5. Churchill, E. D.: Mechanism of Death in Massive Pulmonary Embolism, Surg Gynec Obstet 59:513-517, 1934.

6. Collins, C. G.; Jones, J. R.; and Nelson, E. W.: Surgical Treatment of Thrombophlebitis: Ligation of the Inferior Vena Cava and Ovarian Veins; A Preliminary Report, New Orleans Med Surg J 95:324-329, 1943.

7. Cooley, D. A.; Beall, A. C., Jr.; and Alexander, J. K.: Acute Massive Pulmonary Embolism: Successful Surgical Treatment Using Temporary Cardiopulmonary Bypass, JAMA 177: 283-286, 1961.

8. Crafoord, C., and Jorpes, E.: Heparin as a Prophylactic Agent Against Thrombosis, JAMA 116:2831-2834, 1941.

9. Cruveilhier, J.: Anatomie pathologique du corps humain, Paris: Ballière, 1829-1842, vol 2, book 27.

10. Franklin, K. J.: William Harvey—Englishman, 1578-1657, London: MacGibbon and Kee, 1961.

11. Hampton, A. O., and Castleman, B.: Correlation of Postmortem Chest Teleroentgenograms With Autopsy Findings, With Special Reference to Pulmonary Embolism and Infarction, Amer J Roentgen 43:305-326, 1940.

12. Homans, J.: Thrombosis of the Deep Veins of the Leg, Causing Pulmonary Embolism, New Eng J Med 211:993-997, 1934.

13. Howell, W. H.: The Purification of Heparin and Its Clinical and Physiologic Reaction, Bull Hopkins Hosp 42:199, 1928.

14. Hume, M.: Thrombolysis of the Experimental Radioactive Pulmonary Embolus, New Eng J Med 264:471-475, 1961.

15. Hunter, J.: Observations on the Inflammation of the Internal Coat of Veins, Trans Soc Improvement Med Chir Knowledge (London) 1:18, 1793.

16. Kirschner, M.: Ein Durch die Trendelenburgische Operation geheilter Fall von Embolie der Artialen pulmonalis, Arch Klin Chir 133:312-359, 1924; described in J Thoracic Surg 5:1-17, 1935.

17. Krotoski, J.: Zur Venenunterbinding beziehungsweise Exstirpation bei der puerperalen Allgemeininfektion vom chirurgischen Standpunkt, Chirug 9:425-439, 1937.

18. Krumbhaar, E. B.: Electrocardiographic Changes Accompanying Acutely Increased Pressure Following Pulmonary Artery Ligature, Amer J Med Sci 187:792-794, 1934.

19. Lee: Med Times, 1865, p 777.

20. Link, K. P.: The Anticoagulant From Spoiled Sweet Clover Hay, The Harvey Lecture Series XXXIX, Lancaster, Pa: The Science Press Printing Co., 1944, pp 162-216.

21. McGinn, S., and White, P. D.: Acute Cor Pulmonale Resulting From Pulmonary Embolism, JAMA 104:1473-1480, 1935.

22. McLean, J.: The Thromboplastic Action of Cephalin, Amer J Physiol 41:250-257, 1916.

23. Megibow, R. S.; Katz, L. N.; and Steinitz, F. S.: Dynamic Changes in Experimental Pulmonary Embolism, Surgery 11:19-32, 1943.

24. Meyer, A. W.: The Operative Treatment of Embolism of the Lungs, Surg Gynec Obstet 50:891-898, 1930.

25. Moore, D. B.; Graff, R. J.; Lang, S.; and Pareira, M. D.: Studies on the Mechanism of Death in Pulmonary Microembolism, Surg Gynec Obstet 107:615-622, 1958.

26. Murray, G., and Best, C. H.: The Use of Heparin in Thrombosis, Ann Surg 108:163-177, 1938.

27. Oschner, A., and Mahorner, H.: Varicose Veins, St. Louis: The C. V. Mosby Company, 1939.

28. State, D., and Salisbury, P. F.: The Experimental Production of the Pulmonary Embolism Syndrome and the Effects of Variations of Systemic Arterial Pressure on Its Course, Surg Gynec Obstet 103:202-208, 1956.

29. Steenburg, R. W.: Warren, R.; Wilson, R. E.; and Rudolf, L. E.: A New Look at Pulmonary Embolectomy, Surg Gynec Obstet 107:214-220, 1958.

30. Sternberg, H., and Tamari, M.: Über den Einfluss der funktionellen Narkose und mechanischen Hirnausschaltung auf die Lungenkapillaren, Arch Exp Path Pharmakol 136:34-42, 1928.

31. Trendelenburg, F.: Über die chirurgische Behandlung der Puerperalen Pyämie, Muenchen Med Wschr 49:513-516, 1902.

32. Trendelenburg, F.: Operative Interference in Embolism of the Pulmonary Artery, Ann Surg 48:772-774, 1908.

33. Welch, W. H.: "Thrombosis and Embolism," in Allbutt, R. C.: A System of Medicine, New York: The Macmillan Company, 1901.

34. Westermark, N.: Roentgen Diagnosis of Lung Embolism, Acta Radiol 19:357-372, 1938.

35. Wharton, L. R., and Pierson, J. W.: Minor Forms of Pulmonary Embolism After Abdominal Operations, JAMA 79:1904-1910, 1922.

36. Widener, M. G., Jr., and Light, R. A.: Role of the Automatic Nervous System in the Control of the Pulmonary Vascular Bed: III. Further Studies in Experimental Pulmonary Embolism, Ann Surg 147:895-902, 1958.

Editorials

Kamongo and Anabolone

In the remarkable and complex system of checks and balances with which biological nature controls metabolism, many specific components have been biochemically identified, and some have been synthesized. We describe confidently specific enzymes, and enzyme "ases." We speak of diuretic and antidiuretic hormones. We think in terms of anabolism and catabolism. In the last instance, however, we have identified to date only one of the antagonists. The hormone of the thyroid gland, thyroxin, clearly speeds catabolism, presumably because of a generic widespread effect on the rate of metabolism of any and all cells. It catalyzes, somehow, the energy expenditure of the metabolic furnace, and it is not phylogenetically choosey. It works in any species. The target organ of the hormone is the complex of oxidative processes normally found in the biological activity of the cell's biochemical mechanics. But what of "anti-thyroid"? Who has identified it, this mysterious anabolic hormone? ("Anabolone.") Surely it must exist in nature to control metabolic rate, to hold thyroxin in control, and to elevate cellular metabolism above the level of a test tube of chemicals whose reaction rates are at the mercy only of temperature. Of course our homeostatic thermostatic mechanisms are vital to our brand of evolutional biochemistry which is geared to function only within a very small temperature span. When our internal milieu leaves this arena by significant deviations, our fires burn too fiercly to last, or smolder too slowly to support vital functions. We die.

But in the mammalian hibernators there is strong suggestion that some active biological agent is at work which permits very slow metabolic activity, at levels far below those tolerable by the nonhibernators. The "brown fat" of the hibernators has long been suspected but never positively convicted of elaborating such a specific agent. The principle is illusive, since no small effort has been expended on a world-wide basis in the study of the tissues of a ground hog and golden hamster. But these animals are very small.

I think the aestivators are even more to be admired in this respect. The word means "sleep in summer," and in practice this means that profound torpor is associated with very low cellular activity occurring in a relatively warm ambient environment, during which period the tissues survive and from which the animal can awaken to resume normal activity. Clearly his metabolic rate is suppressed by something other than temperature. Nor is he severely dehydrated. Often buried in mud or surrounded by cocoons, he neither eats nor drinks, only breathes; his water of oxidation more than matches that evaporated into the expired air. He simply must be metabolically under the control of "anabolone"! So why not look there for it?

The lungfish of Africa is a throwback to a cousin of some distant sea-dwelling ancestor of mammalian life. For 70 million years his adaptation to environment has never been changed. He surely has terrific survival value! He developed his air sac into a lung until he became an obligate breather when his regressing gills were no longer big enough to support his oxygen needs. Held indefinitely under water he will drown. If he had been able to develop his front fins into flippers, perhaps we would have had to accord him ancestral homage, but he didn't. He remained unchanged as the Ice Ages came and went. Only the coelecanth, known to still exist, is an older form of life.

The lungfish are a multitudinous clan spread widely over the world, but the best aestivators are those found in central Africa, *Protopterus annectens,* and *Protopterus aethiopicus.* Look in any direction from Lake Victoria and you will find a marsh or swamp they claim as home. And they grow to large size here, forty to sixty pounds worth, in fact. But the climate is a caution! In the rainy season it is very very wet on the high central plateau; but in the summer it doesn't rain for months, and the tropical sun dries the marshes to caked mud flats, as the streams wither and disappear under ground.

Then Kamongo * pulls his trick. Digging with his mouth and expelling the drying mud backward through his gills, he digs a den a couple of feet down with a round chimney leading to the open air. Then one day he curls up his tail over his shoulder, pokes his nose up his chimney, secretes a gelatinous material which hardens to an egg-shell cocoon, and slowly falls into a profound trance-like slumber. He moves no muscle save to breathe slowly. His metabolic rate falls to 15% of normal (ie, active). He stays this way for months. He has been known to live like this for almost two years!

With a clap of thunder the tropical torrents return to the cemented marsh. The cracks fill, and soon the water is pouring down his chimney. Kamongo must either wake up and swim to the surface or drown. Mother Nature wakes him up.

The ichthyologists have always been entranced with such goings-on. They have studied his every habit and have dissected him carefully. They describe large masses of brownish fat lying behind the coelomic cavity in the perirenal tissues. They say it slowly disappears as he sleeps, and they think it represents a major source of available energy for him during his long fast. Maybe it does.

But I think maybe it elaborates the hormone which suppresses his cellular metabolism. I think we should look closely at Kamongo and his "brown fat" which occurs, in a big fish, in handful amounts. And so also does a large agency of the government which concerns itself with the problems of space travel and which pricks up its ears at any mention of "suspended animation." It is interested in supporting biological investigation of the "brown fat" because perhaps Kamongo manufactures the universal antithyroid "anabolone." If so and we can identify it should we not call it "kamongone"?

Henry Swan, MD

* The native name for the lungfish.

Cardiac Denervation Effect in Hypoxia and Hypercapnia

Effect of Total Denervation on Cardiovascular Responses

LAZAR J GREENFIELD, MD
AND
PAUL A. EBERT, MD
BALTIMORE

The effects of hypoxia on the circulatory system involving changes in heart rate, cardiac output, and arterial blood pressure have received considerable attention. Most studies have been made in intact anesthetized dogs by varying the gas mixture used to ventilate the animal, and changes in cardiac function have been attributed to both the direct effect of oxygen deficit on the heart and to reflex neurogenic stimuli. Studies using separate perfusion systems for the systemic and cardiac circulations have shown little initial effect on the perfused heart with moderately hypoxic blood, whereas isolated perfusion of the carotid receptors with desaturated blood results in bradycardia during the period of hypoxia to the chemoreceptors.[3] Similarly, Austen and associates [1] have shown that systemic hypoxia could cause severe cardiac arrhythmia even when the heart was receiving fully oxygenated blood. It was originally shown by Harrison and coworkers [9] that thoracic sympathectomy did not alter the response of the dog to anoxia. Nahas [13] and associates later observed less change in heart rate and cardiac output in sympathectomized dogs. Other investigators also have reported different observations on the response of the heart to hypoxia or anoxia in animals that had thoracic and/or cervical sympathectomy. These conflicting results emphasize that regional sympathectomy does not completely interrupt the sympathetic pathways to the heart. Also, most of the sympathectomies were performed immediately before the experiment, and the heart still would contain a normal levarterenol content. Cooper [5] showed that catecholamine depletion of the heart did not occur until 72 hours after total denervation. Obviously the response of a totally denervated heart, which lacks levarterenol, to abnormal physiologic conditions will not be the same as the sympathectomized animal described above.

Studies of autotransplantation of the heart [10] have suggested that this totally denervated organ may not respond to altered physiologic states in the same manner as the normal intact heart. In fact, dogs with totally denervated hearts have been shown to have altered cardiovascular responses to hemorrhage and hypothermia.[8] Thus, it can be anticipated that the circulatory adjustments to abnormal states will be markedly different when homotransplantation of the heart is accomplished. Experimental animals with total extrinsic cardiac denervation are useful in predicting the response of the transplanted heart to circulatory and respiratory changes. In the present studies the effects of hypoxia and hypercapnia on the cardiovascular system were compared in normal dogs and ones with proved total extrinsic cardiac denervation as described by Cooper.[5]

Methods

Adult mongrel dogs were anesthetized with intravenous thiopental (25mg). A cuffed endotracheal tube was inserted and ventilation main-

Submitted for publication April 1, 1963.

From the Department of Surgery, The Johns Hopkins University and Hospital.

Table 1.—*Arterial Pressure, Heart Rate, and Myocardial Contractile Force Determined During*

Dogs	Mean Arterial Pressure Control	Mean Arterial Pressure 5 Min	Mean Arterial Pressure % Change	Myocardial Contractile Force, 5 Min % Change	Heart Rate Control	Heart Rate 5 Min	Heart Rate % Change	Mean Arterial Pressure 10 Min	Mean Arterial Pressure % Change	Myocardial Contractile Force, 10 Min % Change
Normal										
1	135	145	+7	+44	145	200	+38	142	+5	+16
2	120	140	+17	+62	110	175	+59	128	+7	+34
3	126	138	+9	+40	120	160	+33	120	—5	+12
4	110	125	+14	+35	135	180	+33	114	+3	+20
5	132	145	+10	+25	135	170	+26	145	+10	+10
6	116	137	+19	+25	125	175	+40	128	+10	+12
Average values			+13	+38			+38		+5	+17
Total Extrinsic Cardiac Denervation										
7	105	109	+4	+7	150	160	+7	109	+4	+10
8	100	104	+4	+9	110	115	+4	105	+5	+8
9	108	112	+3	+5	150	170	+13	108	0	0
10	110	115	+4	+14	140	135	—4	117	+6	+10
11	112	120	+7	+10	130	140	+8	115	+2	+10
12	95	100	+6	+15	110	105	—4	104	+10	+15
Average values			+5	+10			+4		+5	+9

tained by an intermittent positive pressure respirator. The left side of the chest was opened through the fourth intercostal space and a Walton-Brodie strain gauge arch sutured to the left ventricle to assess myocardial contractile force. A plastic catheter was inserted through a femoral artery and connected to a Statham transducer to measure aortic pressure. Myocardial contractile force, central aortic pressure, and lead II of the electrocardiogram were inscribed on a multichannel oscillograph.

The experiment was begun after the heart rate and aortic pressure had remained stable for ten minutes. During this control period the animal was ventilated with room air. Hypoxia was produced by ventilating the dog with a mixture of 10% oxygen and 90% nitrogen. Hypercapnia was induced, after an animal had been stable for 15

Table 2.—*Arterial Pressure, Heart Rate, and Myocardial Contractile Force Determined During*

Dogs	Mean Arterial Pressure Control	Mean Arterial Pressure 3 Min	Mean Arterial Pressure % Change	Myocardial Contractile Force, 3 Min % Change	Heart Rate Control	Heart Rate 3 Min	Heart Rate % Change	Mean Arterial Pressure 7 Min	Mean Arterial Pressure % Change	Myocardial Contractile Force, 7 Min % Change
Normal										
1	122	125	+2	—20	140	140	0	100	—5	—25
2	152	140	—8	—11	152	140	—8	120	—21	—24
3	160	150	—6	—21	130	125	—3	135	—16	—26
4	115	115	0	—13	135	127	—6	105	—7	—17
5	150	130	—13	—14	145	145	0	120	—20	—19
6	115	100	—7	—8	125	120	—4	96	—16	—20
Average values			—6	—15			—3		—14	—22
Total Extrinsic Cardiac Denervation										
7	150	150	0	—26	150	138	—8	140	—7	—34
8	140	135	—4	—22	160	145	—9	120	—14	—30
9	138	135	—2	—21	135	125	—8	125	—9	—26
10	155	135	—13	—14	125	117	—7	130	—16	—25
11	155	145	—7	—9	105	99	—5	138	—12	—16
Average values			—5	—18			—7		—9	—26

Ventilation with 10% Oxygen

Heart Rate		Arterial O_2, % Saturation	
10 Min	% Change	Control	5 Min
160	+10	99	83
140	+27	100	85
110	−9	100	81
145	+8	100	87
105	−15	98	85
130	+4	100	82
	+4		
150	0	100	84
100	−9	98	81
145	−3	99	88
135	−4	99	82
130	0	100	85
105	−9	99	84
	−3		

minutes, by ventilating the dog with a gas mixture of 20% oxygen, 6% carbon dioxide, and 74% nitrogen. Oxygen content of arterial blood was measured by the Van Slyke manometric technique during control periods and after five minutes of either hypoxia or hypercapnia. Hypoxia was maintained for a ten minute period, while the duration of hypercapnia was seven minutes. Observations were recorded during hypoxia and hypercapnia

Ventilation With 6% Carbon Dioxide

Heart Rate		Arterial O_2, % Saturation	
7 Min	% Change	Control	5 Min
128	−9	100	98
132	−13	97	98
117	−10	99	97
117	−13	98	98
129	−18	98	99
105	−17	97	98
	−13		
125	−17	99	98
127	−20	97	99
118	−20	100	97
115	−8	98	99
94	−11	98	97
	−14		

in both normal animals and in dogs previously subjected to total extrinsic cardiac denervation. Cardiac denervation was verified by neurogenic stimulation of sympathetic and parasympathetic pathways and by evaluating the response of the heart to intravenous 4-hydroxyphenethylamine (Tyramine) as previously described.[5]

Results

The observations recorded during hypoxia are shown in Table 1. The response of the normal dog to 10% oxygen ventilation was consistent. Arterial pressure rose an average of 13% in five minutes, myocardial contractile force increased an average of 38%, and the heart rate average elevation was 38%. After ten minutes the changes were not as marked; arterial pressure averaged 5% higher than control value, myocardial contractile force was an average of 17% above control, and the average heart rate was only 4% above the baseline value.

The effect of hypoxia on dogs with total extrinsic cardiac denervation was minimal. Mean arterial pressure rose an average of 5% at five minutes and was unchanged at ten minutes. Myocardial contractile force increased an average of 10% at five minutes and 9% after ten minutes. The heart rate increased an average of only 4% at five minutes and was 3% less than control levels after ten minutes of hypoxia.

Normal dogs and those with total cardiac denervation showed similar changes during ventilation with 6% carbon dioxide (Table 2). Both groups had a decrease in mean arterial pressure at three minutes, and a further drop was recorded at seven minutes. Heart rate and myocardial contractile force were decreased in both the denervated dogs (minus 14% and 26%, respectively) and the normal control animals (minus 13% and 22%). Oxygen saturation of the arterial blood showed no significant change during the ventilation with 6% carbon dioxide.

Comment

The initial cardiac acceleration response to hypoxia has been attributed mainly to increased activity of the sympathetic nervous system.[7,11,13] Some investigators[4] have thought that a delicate balance existed between the parasympathetic and sympathetic activity and that both systems were activated during hypoxia. Thus the response of the heart would be influenced by the most active system at any particular time. It has been difficult to know how much the direct effect of oxygen deficit on the heart participated in the early circulatory response to hypoxia, but myocardial depression only has been recognized after long periods of hypoxia.[7] The elevation of mean aortic pressure (+ 5%) observed after five minutes of hypoxia in the dogs with total extrinsic cardiac denervation probably was a result of sympathetic vasoconstriction of the peripheral circulatory system since only a 4% increase in heart rate occurred. Thus, increased cardiac output and peripheral vascular constriction, resulting from sympathetic activity, probably are responsible for the greater increase in aortic pressure recorded in the normal dogs. Both groups showed a reduction in heart rate after ten minutes of hypoxia as compared to the five-minute observation. This may represent some direct effect of reduced oxygen saturation on the heart, although it is doubtful that an arterial oxygen saturation of 80%-85% would depress the myocardium in such a brief period of time. In intact animals, parasympathetic activity has been suggested as the cause of this bradycardia rather than myocardial depression.[12]

Other investigators [2,13] have thought that the adrenal glands were in part responsible for the initial increased arterial pressure and tachycardia observed during hypoxia. From the present experiments it can be indirectly postulated that the adrenal gland has a very minor role in the initial cardiovascular response to moderate hypoxia. This is concluded because the dogs with cardiac denervation had a very minimal increase in heart rate (+ 4%) and myocardial contractile force (10%). If significant catecholamines were released during hypoxia a greater increase in heart rate and myocardial contractile force would have been anticipated since totally denervated hearts are highly sensitive to these compounds.[5] A release of catecholamines from sites within the myocardium can be excluded since denervated hearts are depleted of levarterenol. This, of course, is the reason for the sensitivity to levarterenol and why this drug must be administered with caution if it is used as a myocardial stimulant after the heart has been denervated.

Ventilation with 6% carbon dioxide resulted in similar circulatory changes in both the normal animals and those with totally denervated hearts. The effect of hypercapnia appears primarily to be direct myocardial depression with possibly some minimal peripheral vasodilatation. The decrease in myocardial contractile force accompanied by a proportionally smaller diminution of mean arterial pressure would suggest that peripheral vasodilatation was not the major circulatory adjustment. Also reflex parasympathetic activity, which causes peripheral vasodilatation, usually results in bradycardia, and this was not evident in the normal animals. The heart rate decreased 7% in the denervated dogs as compared to 3% in the normal animals. This would substantiate the direct depressive effect of hypercapnia on the heart.

These studies show that the initial circulatory adjustments during moderate hypoxia result from activation of peripheral receptors and the subsequent neurogenic reflexes imposed on the heart. Obviously the changes would be more profound if anoxia was produced, and these have been described by Woods.[14] Decreasing the oxygen saturation of the arterial blood from 99% to 83% does cause measurable changes in normal intact dogs that would be detectable clinically. When the heart is completely denervated, the circulatory changes, as measured by mean arterial pressure and heart rate, are less conspicuous and certainly are not specific enough to be diagnostic. If homotransplantation of the heart becomes a reality, the transplanted organ will by necessity be completely denervated. Thus, it can be anticipated that the effects of hypoxia will not be as obvious and that detection of the abnormal state will be more difficult, whereas, hypercapnia will result in depression of myocardial function that should be similar to the response of an animal with a normal intact neurocardiovascular system.

Summary

The physiologic responses to hypoxia and hypercapnia were compared in normal dogs and those with total extrinsic cardiac denervation. Both groups showed similar changes with hypercapnia, such as diminished mean aortic pressure, reduced heart rate, and a decrease in myocardial contractile force. During hypoxia the normal dogs showed the usual changes such as elevated arterial pressure, heart rate, and myocardial contractile force, whereas, only a minimal increase was noted in animals with total cardiac denervation. The possible mechanisms responsible for the altered responses after cardiac denervation are discussed.

Paul A. Ebert, MD, Department of Surgery, The Johns Hopkins Hospital, Baltimore 5, Md.

REFERENCES

1. Austen, W. G.; Ebert, P. A.; and Greenfield, L. J.: Mechanism of Cardiac Arrest in Acute Hypoxia, Surgery 53:784, 1963.

2. Baugh, C. W.; Cornett, R. W.; and Hatcher, J. D.: The Adrenal Gland and the Cardiovascular Changes in Acute Anoxic Anoxia in Dogs, Cir Res 7:513, 1959.

3. Bernthal, T.; Greene, W., Jr.; and Revzin, A. M.: Role of Carotid Chemoreceptors in Hypoxic Cardiac Acceleration, Proc Soc Exp Biol Med 76:121, 1951.

4. Bernthal, T., and Woodcook, C. C., Jr.: Responses of the Vasomotor Center to Hypoxia After Denervation of Carotid and Aortic Bodies, Amer J Physiol 166:45, 1951.

5. Cooper, T.; Gilbert, J. W., Jr.; Bloodwell, R. D.; and Crout, J. R.: Chronic Extrinsic Cardiac Denervation by Regional Neural Ablation, Circ Res 9:275, 1961.

6. Ebert, P. A.; Greenfield, L. J.; and Austen, W. G.: The Mechanism of Cardiac Arrest During Hypoxia, Surg Forum 13:187, 1962.

7. Gorlin, R., and Lewis, B. M.: Circulatory Adjustments to Hypoxia in Dogs, J Appl Physiol 7:180, 1954.

8. Greenfield, L. J.; Ebert, P. A.; Austen, W. G.; and Morrow, A. G.: The Effect of Total Cardiac Denervation on the Cardiovascular Responses to Hypothermia and Acute Hemorrhage, Surgery 51:356, 1962.

9. Harrison, T. R.; Blalock, A.; Pilcher, C.; and Wilson, C. P.: The Regulation of Circulation: VIII. The Relative Importance of Nervous, Endocrine, and Vascular Regulation in the Response of the Cardiac Output to Anoxemia, Amer J Physiol 83:284, 1927.

10. Hurley, E. J.; Dong, E., Jr.; Lower, R. R.; Hancock, E. W.; Stofer, R. C.; and Shumway, N. E.: An Approach to Extracorporeal Surgery of the Heart, J Thorac Cardiov Surg 44:776, 1962.

11. Korner, P. I.: Circulatory Adaptations in Hypoxia, Physiol Rev 39:687, 1959.

12. Korner, P. I., and Edwards, A. W. T.: The Immediate Effects of Acute Hypoxia on the Heart Rate, Arterial Pressure, Cardiac Output, and Ventilation of the Unanesthetized Rabbit, Quart J Exp Physiol 45, 113, 1960.

13. Nahas, G. G.; Mather, G. W.; Wargo, J. D. M.; and Adams, W. L.: Influence of Acute Hypoxia on Sympathectomized and Adrenalectomized Dogs, Amer J Physiol. 177:13, 1954.

14. Woods, E. F., and Richardson, J. A.: Effects of Acute Anoxia on Cardiac Contractility, Amer J Physiol 196:203, 1959.

Closure of an Established Potts Anastomosis

An Experimental Method

A. YUKSEL BOZER, MD; SAMUEL R. SCHUSTER, MD; AND EARL R. KIERNAN, MD, BOSTON

The surgical treatment of tetralogy of Fallot has passed through various phases. Initially, Blalock and Taussig[1] devised the subclavian pulmonary artery shunt which was followed by the Potts modification.[2] Thousands of these operations have been performed to the benefit of many patients.

Despite the rapid development of instruments and techniques for open heart surgery, the best initial surgical treatment of an infant severely troubled by a tetralogy of Fallot is still the establishment of a systemic pulmonary arterial shunt. With few exceptions most surgeons now favor the Blalock procedure (subclavian pulmonic anastomosis) because of the ease with which it can be taken down later when complete correction of the cardiac anomaly is undertaken. The problem confronting cardiac surgeons today is the management of patients with established Potts anastomoses who are now ready for total correction of their tetralogy.

The complete correction of tetralogy of Fallot with closure of the previously constructed Potts anastomosis has been reported.[3] The technical problems associated with the surgical closure of a Potts anastomosis by direct approach to the shunt via the left chest may lead to exsanguinating hemorrhage because of the technical problems associated with severe tissue reaction often found in the area of the shunt. There seems to be little question that the most reasonable approach is via the lumen of the pulmonary artery as described by Kirklin.[3] Our initial attempts to close Potts shunts in this manner, using hypothermia and total circulatory arrest, presented several problems.

Because of diversion through the aortic-pulmonary shunt, a large part of the hypothermic arterial output from the pump was returned almost immediately to the collecting system. As a result, cooling was very inefficient, and the pump time necessary to attain deep systemic hypothermia was prolonged.

Another problem apparent upon opening the pulmonary artery was the difficulty in differentiating the shunt orifice from the various orifices of the branches of the pulmonary artery. Furthermore, despite complete circulatory standstill, there was a persistent and annoying flow of blood from the aorta through the shunt making its visualization and closure more difficult.

Finally, air embolization to the brain via the open shunt is always a possibility.

For these reasons, we have developed experimentally a new method of closing a previously established Potts anastomosis through the open pulmonary artery either during cardiopulmonary bypass or prior to the onset of extracorporeal circulation.

Methods and Materials

A number 20, 22, or 24 rubber endotracheal catheter was modified by increasing the length of the inflatable cuff to 4 cm and having the cuff made of black rubber* (Fig 1). The small tube used for cuff inflation is within the larger lumen

Submitted for publication April 3, 1963.

From the Surgical Service, The Children's Hospital Medical Center, and the Department of Surgery, Harvard Medical School.

This work was supported by grants from the National Heart Institute, The American Heart Association, and the Massachusetts Heart Association.

* Manfactured by the Davol Rubber Co., Providence, RI.

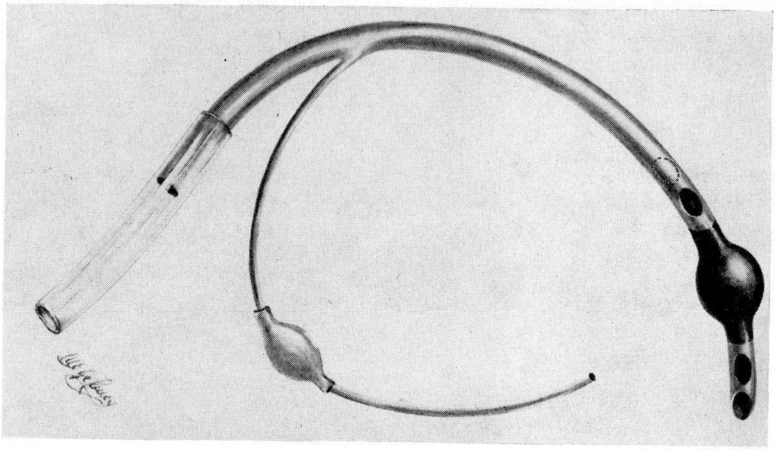

Fig 1.—Modified cuffed endotracheal tube used for occlusion of previously established Potts shunt during its closure via pulmonary arteriotomy.

of the catheter to insure that the cuffed tube will have a smooth round outer surface; in addition, two 3 × 6 mm openings in the tube were established proximal and distal to the inflatable cuff. Finally, the proximal end of the tube has been modified to adapt to the arterial line of the extracorporeal circuit.

Mongrel dogs weighing 15-25 kg, having had a Potts anastomosis established 1 to 30 days prior to this experiment, were anesthetized by intravenous pentobarbital (Nembutal) (30 mg per kilogram of body weight) and intubated for intermittent positive pressure respiration. The animals were placed in a supine position, and the left femoral artery and vein were cannulated for pressure recordings. The chest was entered thru a trans-sternal incision in the fourth interspace, and a crimped Teflon prosthesis (15 cm length by 8 mm diameter) was anastomosed to the ascending aorta. The venous sites for cannulation were prepared, umbilical tape

Fig 2.—Operative procedure for transpulmonary closure of Potts shunt during continued systemic perfusion with a pump oxygenator. Drawing *1,* shows modified cuffed endotracheal tube (see Fig 1) passing into the aorta thru a Teflon prosthesis which has been sewed to the aortic arch. Inflated black cuff occludes Potts shunt, while tube carries arterial input of pump. Drawing *2,* shows pulmonary orifice of Potts shunt thru pulmonary arteriotomy. This orifice is readily identified by means of black cuff pouting into it. Note that the main pulmonary artery has been occluded by a tourniquet, Drawing *3,* sutures being placed to close shunt. Drawing *4,* pulmonary arteriotomy closure.

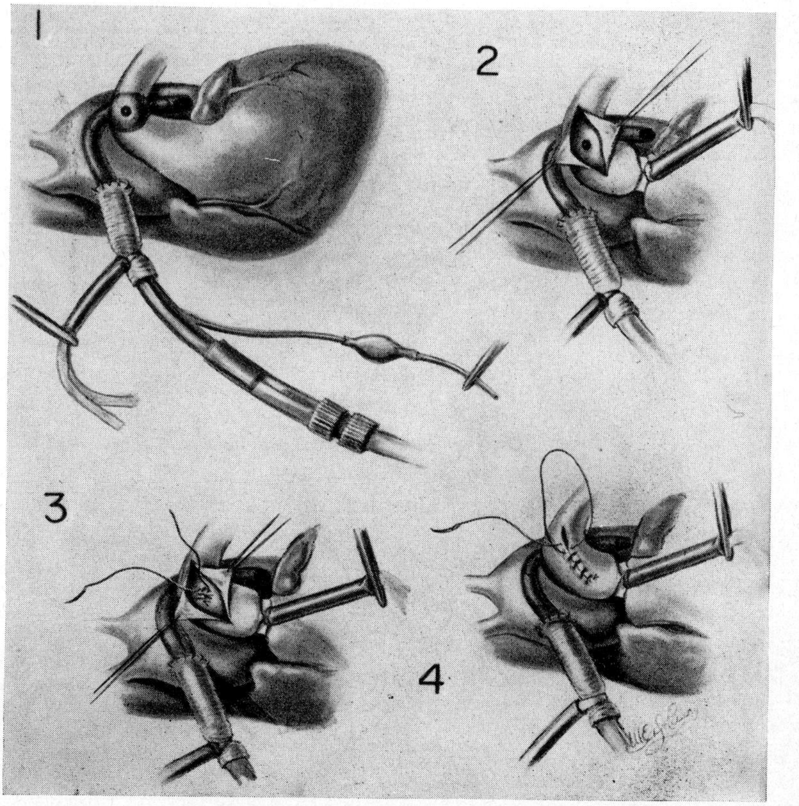

was passed around the base of the main pulmonary artery, and the left pulmonary artery was dissected distally as far as possible. Heparin was then administered in a dose of 1 mg per kilogram body weight and cannulization carried out.

Instead of directly connecting the arterial line of the pump to the crimped tube on the aortic arch, the modified cuffed endotracheal tube, described above, was introduced through this Teflon prosthesis into the aortic arch. Blood loss between the cuffed tube and inner wall of the Teflon prosthesis was prevented by means of an umbilical tape snugged down around the Teflon prosthesis. The cuffed tube was then advanced down the descending aorta so that the cuff lay below the estimated level of the previously established Potts anastomosis.

The closure of the Potts anastomosis may be carried out prior to the establishment of bypass, or during cardiopulmonary bypass.

When the closure of the Potts shunt is done during cardiopulmonary bypass, the intra-aortic cuffed tube serves as the arterial input catheter and is attached to the arterial side of the pump. Sump suckers are placed in both ventricles via their respective atria, the superior and inferior vena cava cannulated, and bypass established. The cuff on the catheter within the aorta is then inflated with 5-8 cc of saline, and the tube is slowly withdrawn until the Potts shunt has been sealed by the inflated cuff in the aortic lumen (Fig 2, drawing *1*). The obliteration of the shunt can be detected by the disappearance of the thrill and the decrease in volume of the blood being sucked out by the left ventricular sucker. At this point an umbilical tape about the base of the pulmonary artery is tightened (Fig 2, drawing 2), four stay sutures of atraumatic silk are placed as far distally on the presenting surface of the left pulmonary artery as possible, and an incision is made between them in the longitudinal axis of the artery.

If the cuffed tube has been properly positioned, there is no leak of blood into the operative field, although varying amounts of retrograde flow from the distal pulmonary artery will occur. The shunt orifice within the pulmonary artery is now closed under direct vision while the animal is continously being perfused; hypothermia, if desired, may be instituted at any time. The closure of the shunt opening is carried out with an appropriate number of 5-0 atraumatic interrupted silk sutures (Fig 2, drawings *3* and *4*). The inflated black rubber cuff within the aorta pouts into the shunt orifice and helps immeasurably in differentiating this opening from other branches of the pulmonary artery. Care must be taken, however, not to perforate the inflated cuff of the intra-aortic catheter as the sutures are placed. The margins of the shunt orifice hold sutures well because they are rigid and prominent as a result of healing reaction at this suture line. After the closure of the shunt, the cuff of the catheter is released, and if closure has been complete there will be no blood flooding the area. If leakage does occur, inflation of the cuff is repeated and additional sutures are placed. This procedure can be repeated an indefinite number of times until complete closure has been achieved.

Comment

In half of our animals the closure of the shunt was carried out during cardiopulmonary bypass as described above, systemic perfusion being maintained by way of the extracorporeal circuit diagramatically portrayed in (Fig 3 *A*). The advantage of this method is that hypothermia, if desired, may be instituted during this period of shunt closure. The disadvantage, of course, is the prolongation of total time on bypass.

In the other half of our animals, systemic circulation was maintained during shunt closure by the normally beating heart and the blood oxygenated autogenously by the right lung. This is possible because the intra-aortic

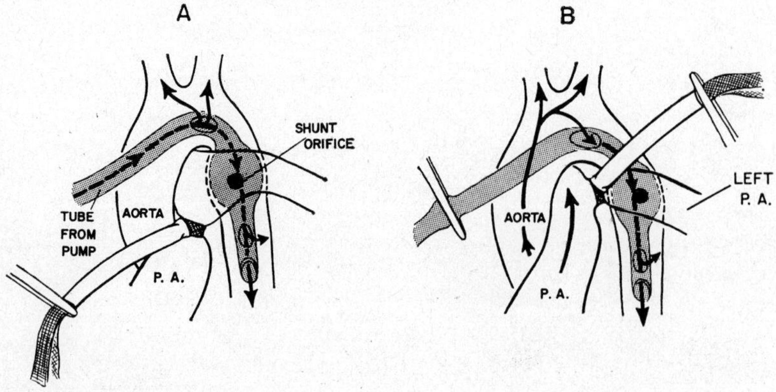

Fig 3.—*A*, portrayal of blood circulation thru modified tube while systemic circulation is maintained with a pump oxygenator during closure of Potts shunt. Note occlusion of main pulmonary artery. *B*, Circulation of blood thru aorta and tube; autogenous systemic perfusion and oxygenation is maintained during closure of Potts shunt. Note occlusion of left pulmonary artery only.

cuffed tube does not obstruct the aortic pathway, and the heart maintains normal systemic perfusion; the arterial blood from the left ventricle readily goes through the openings in the intra-aortic catheter proximal to the cuff and passes easily out the distal openings of the catheter to perfuse the remainder of the body. Oxygenation is maintained via the right lung, and hemorrhage from the open left pulmonary artery is avoided by having removed the umbilical tape from the base of the main pulmonary artery and instead occluding only the left pulmonary artery at its origin. This allows blood to flow in a normal manner to the right lung for oxygenation. This techniqce is demonstrated in Fig 3 *B*. This method is of particular advantage when the operator does not plan to use hypothermia during correction of the intracardiac defects, and, therefore, cardiopulmonary bypass is begun only after the shunt has been closed and the operator is prepared to go ahead with correction of the tetralogy. Bypass is established exactly as portrayed in Fig 3 *A*. By this method total "pump time" is reduced since the pump oxygenator is utilized only during correction of the intracardiac defects.

Results

A total of 12 dogs were operated upon during the course of these experiments. The initial six dogs were acute experiments in which extracorporeal circulation was utilized during the closure of the shunt. There appeared to be little difficulty with this technique, and in each case an adequate shunt closure was obtained.

The last six animals had closure of the shunt without the use of cardiopulmonary bypass. These were not planned as acute experiments, and five of these six animals have survived one month to 1½ years since surgery, with no evidence of a recurrent shunt. The sixth animal was inadvertantly not heparinized and died, presumably as a result of multiple emboli originating from a thrombus which had formed in the intra-aortic catheter.

The interpretation of shunt patency was based in each case on a clearly audible preoperative shunt murmur.

Summary

An experimental method for closing a previously established Potts anastomosis via a pulmonary arteriotomy while maintaining systemic perfusion has been described. The advantages of the technique are:

1. Time on the pump may be decreased by closing the shunt prior to establishment of cardiac bypass.

2. If bypass is started during closure of the shunt, this pump time may serve for the establishment of hypothermia to be used during later correction of the intracardiac defects.

3. Using this technique, the shunt orifice is occluded during its closure, and therefore the possibility of air emboli via the shunt is avoided.

4. The presence of the readily identifiable black rubber cuff within the lumen of the shunt orifice during its closure helps in the differentiation of this opening from the orifices of the various branches of the left pulmonary artery.

We wish to extend our thanks to Mrs. Denise Pav for her invaluable assistance in the completion of these experinents.

Samuel R. Schuster, MD, The Children's Hospital Medical Center, 300 Longwood Ave, Boston 15, Mass.

REFERENCES

1. Blalock, A., and Taussig, H. B.: The Surgical Treatment of Malformations of the Heart in Which There Is Pulmonary Stenosis or Pulmonary Atresia, JAMA 128:189-202, 1945.

2. Potts, W. J.; Smith, S.; and Gibson, S.: Anastomosis of the Aorta to a Pulmonary Artery: Certain Types in Congenital Heart Disease, JAMA 132:627-631, 1946.

3. Kirklin, J. W., and Devloo, R. A.: Hypothermic Perfusion and Circulatory Arrest for Surgical Correction of Tetralogy of Fallot With Previously Constructed Potts' Anastomosis, Dis Chest 39:87-91, 1961.

Stenosis of Trachea Resection and End-to-End Anastomosis

Report of Two Cases

LAURENCE MISCALL, MD
JOHN B. McKITTRICK, MD
ROCCO P. GIORDANO, MD
AND
RICHARD B. NOLAN, MD
JAMAICA, NY

Stenosis of the trachea, a frequent aftermath of both injury and disease, presents a formidable challenge to the surgeon. A variety of corrective methods have not yielded uniformly satisfactory results.* This report of successful resection and end-to-end anastomosis in two cases is submitted as an addition to the total experience that begins to justify a change in previous attitude.

Many facts attest to the rationale of this approach. Reports of success with immediate repair of complete division of the trachea or major bronchi without subsequent stricture formation are not uncommon.† Those few who have survived such trauma without this treatment have developed, almost invariably, some degree of stricture. When this has been incomplete and distal to the carina, recurrent infection usually has required major pulmonary resection. Healing with complete postcarinal obstruction has caused variable degrees of pulmonary insufficiency proportional to the volume of lung excluded and the time and duration thereof. It is no accident that the ability to recognize early and repair immediately such major injuries has been followed by improved results. Furthermore, the possibility of substituting lobectomy for pneumonectomy in some poor risk lung cancer patients by using segmental bronchial resection and end-to-end anastomosis is well known to all. While this may not qualify as the best cancer surgery, it still indicates that the method is an acceptable surgical procedure. In the trachea stenosis has generated more serious problems quite resistant to solution. A permanent tracheostomy not only holds no happy future for the patient but also has real immediate and long-term risks. Complete obstruction below a point of possible by-pass by tracheostomy is not consistent with life. Incomplete stenosis at such a point not only obstructs respiration but with recurrent infection causes severe

Submitted for publication April 3, 1963.

From the Thoracic and Cardiovascular Service (Triboro Hospital) of The Queens Hospital Center, Jamaica, NY.

* References 4, 6, 8, 12-15, 25, 27, 29, 33.

† References 2, 3, 13, 16, 20, 24, 31, 32.

pulmonary damage not amenable to surgical or other treatment until the basic defect can be corrected. A variety of procedures has been employed to accomplish this. The benefits of dilatation have been uniformly temporary with inevitable subsequent deterioration. Repair by partial or complete circumferential excision of the defect and plastic reconstruction using foreign material has failed. Retained secretions, erosion into adjacent structures, infection, and collapse have contributed to this course.[6,8,11,12,17,23,27] The dismal outlook for these two young patients with complete stenosis of the lower cervical trachea prompted us to use resection and end-to-end anastomosis in perference to these older methods. The results have been very satisfactory.

Report of Cases

CASE 1.—This six-year-old girl was first admitted to the Queens Hospital Center on Sept 4, 1960. A total lack of positive findings permitted early release to her home. One week later she was readmitted in coma after an onset with visual difficulty, convulsions, severe dyspnea, and cyanosis. Severe respiratory obstruction demanded immediate tracheostomy. The first attempt with incision of the third ring did not permit insertion of a No. 3 tube due to obstruction in the distal airway. Through a second incision at a lower level, it was readily inserted and provided an excellent airway. The definition of the local pathology was postponed to permit placement in a respirator. After two hours in it, normal spontaneous respiration was resumed with the disappearance of all signs and symptoms. In twelve hours she was ambulatory. One week later any attempt to modify or remove the tracheostomy tube precipitated acute respiratory distress. On Nov 4, 1960, bronchoscopy under general anesthesia administered through the tracheostomy showed that the trachea terminated above it in a blind end covered by apparently normal mucosa. The point of obstruction was confirmed by tracheogram (Fig 1 and 2).

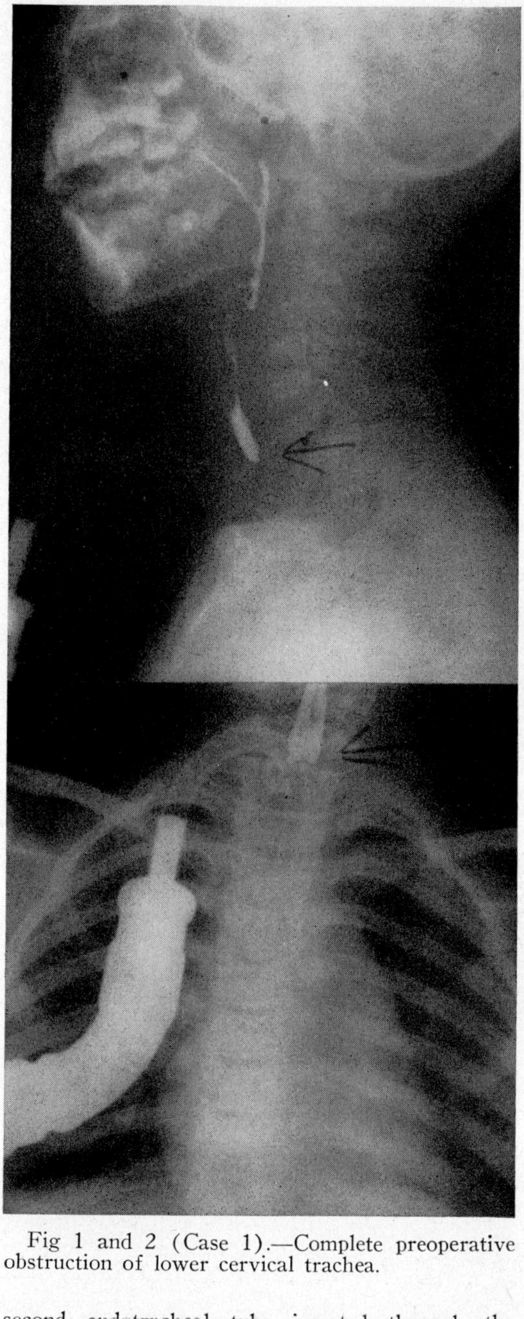

Fig 1 and 2 (Case 1).—Complete preoperative obstruction of lower cervical trachea.

On Nov 21, 1960, under anesthesia administered through the tracheostomy, exposure was obtained through a combined collar and sternal splitting incision. Scar tissue in the area of the obstruction required sharp dissection adjacent to the tracheal wall to obtain mobilization and avoid injury to surrounding structures. The rest of the trachea from the cricoid to carina was easily freed by blunt dissection without opening either pleural space. The area to be resected (3.5 cm) including the site of obstruction and of tracheostomy was outlined. A second endotracheal tube inserted through the larynx to the point of obstruction accurately located its upper limit. Silk sutures were then placed both above and below the intended sites of tracheal division to prevent later retraction. The trachea was first circumferentially divided above the point of obstruction through practically normal tissue. After hyperventilation through the tracheostomy tube, it was removed, and the segment of trachea from above the obstruction to below the tracheostomy was excised by a second circumferential in-

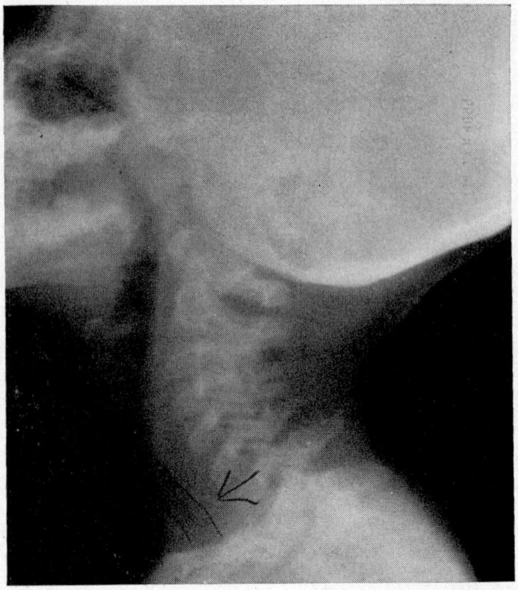

Fig 3 (Case 1).—Normal airway (accentuated) six months after operation.

cision. This was accomplished in a short time and anesthesia resumed by advancing the second endotracheal tube across the surgical defect into the lower trachea. The tension sutures permitted easy approximation of the ends which were then anastomosed around the tube using fine interrupted silk sutures through rings and full wall thickness reinforced by additional adventitial sutures. The distal tracheal traction sutures were brought out through the wound to facilitate tracheostomy should it be necessary at a later date. A tracheostomy was not done since, after withdrawal of the anesthesia tube, the repair site remained competent. It was hoped also that its lack might reduce the risk of infection and foreign-body reaction conducive to recurrent stricture. The wound was closed in layers with interrupted silk after insertion of a soft rubber drain. Recovery in a high humidity atmosphere was rapid. Primary union permitted removal of the sutures in five days. Bronchoscopy three weeks later revealed a normal tracheal lumen. Follow-up one year later shows no evidence of abnormality (Fig 3). The details of the operative procedure are illustrated by Fig 7.

The pathological report is of interest. The tracheal lumen is occluded above the tracheostomy by a diaphragm approximately 0.3 cm in thickness, composed of firm, white tissue. The mucosa and submucosa is edematous and infiltrated with large numbers of lymphocytes and plasma cells. Multinucleated giant cells are present and many contain a refractile foreign body best visualized with polarized light. The cartilagenous rings appear essentially normal. One small fragment of cartilage is proliferating in the submucosa. Although an exact etiology was not established by the sections, it was felt that some type of crystalline foreign body accounted for a chronic inflammatory process and fibrosis. The small fragments of cartilage proliferating in the submucosa may have resulted from traumatic displacement.

Case 2.—This 22-year-old white female was injured in a motor accident in November of 1961. A right-sided pneumothorax with mediastinal emphysema was treated with tube drainage. Severe respiratory obstruction appeared ten days later due to granulation tissue at the site of an unrecognized posterior laceration of the trachea at the thoracic inlet. This was treated by a tracheostomy and then

Fig 4 and 5 (Case 2).—Preoperative tracheal obstruction similar to case 1.

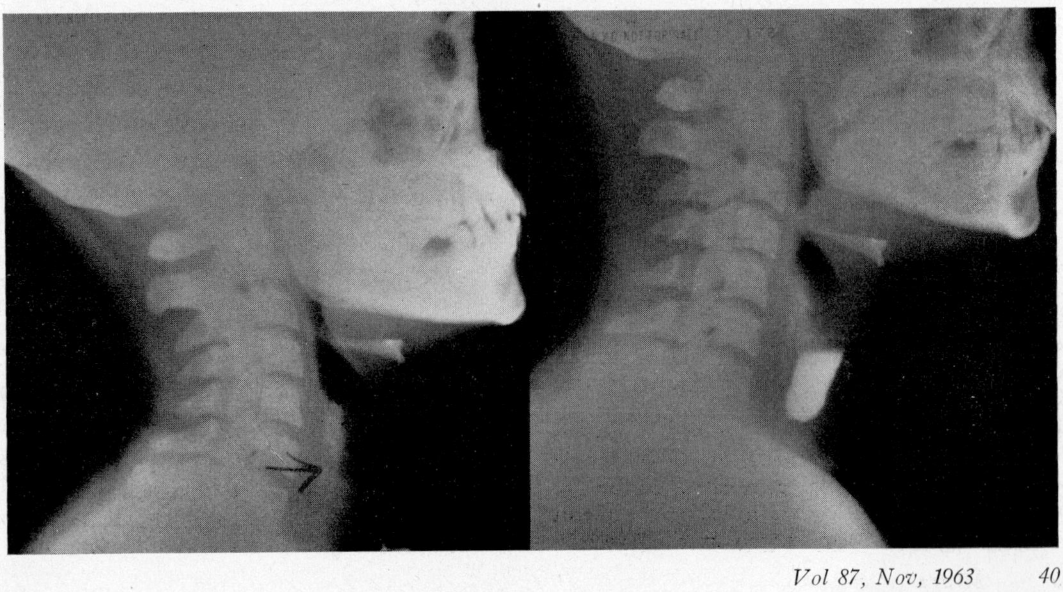

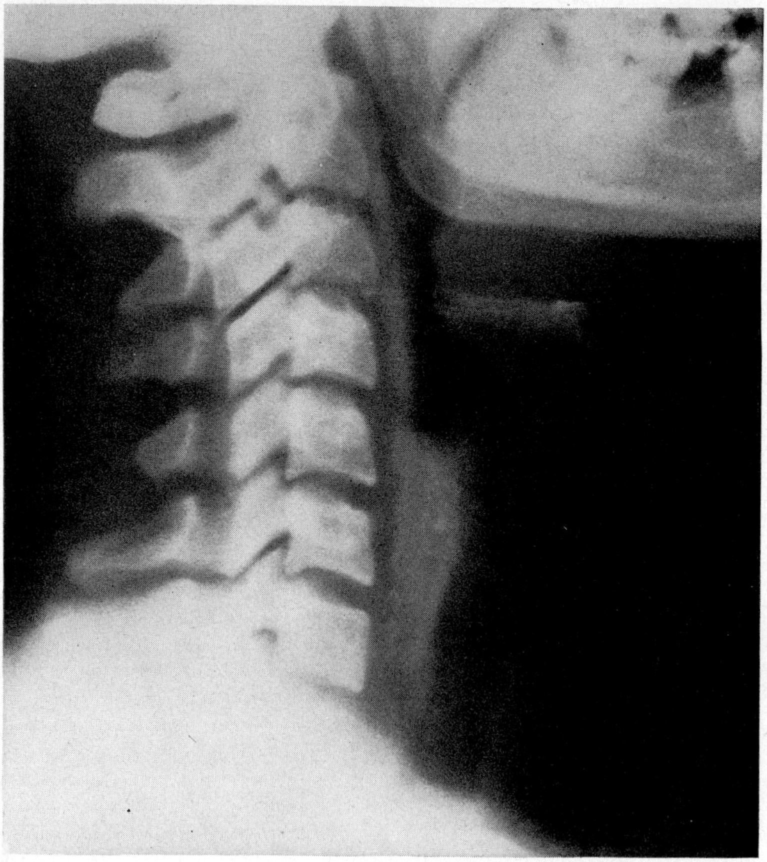

Fig 6 (Case 2).—Normal airway six months after operation.

repair of the laceration through a cervical approach. One month later endoscopy demonstrated complete obstruction of the trachea due to excessive granulation tissue. At this time she was discharged from the original hospital to permit the inflammatory reaction to subside before definitive care. After transfer to Triboro Hospital on March 12, 1962, endoscopy under general anesthesia again demonstrated complete tracheal obstruction about 3 cm below the cords. Fairly normal mucous membrane was present. A tracheogram (Fig 4 and 5) illustrates a situation similar to case 1. After another six weeks to permit further resolution she was readmitted on April 19, 1962, with all wounds well healed and only minimal reaction around the tracheostomy. On April 27, 1962, five months after original injury, 4 cm of trachea were resected from above the point of obstruction to below the tracheostomy site. The adhesions between adjacent structures were much firmer than in case 1 due in part likely to the delayed attempt to suture the laceration. The difficulty in mobilization of the structures required much sharp dissection and resulted in two small rents in the membranous portion of the trachea below the line of resection. These, however, were successfully repaired with fine interrupted silk sutures. Operation was completed in the same manner detailed in case 1. A tracheostomy was not done. A high humidity atmosphere with aerosolized shrinking agents maintained an effective airway. Penicillin and streptomycin held infection to a minimum. She made an uneventful recovery and was discharged from the hospital on May 18, 1962, 21 days after operation. She now shows no evidence of obstruction six months later (Fig 6).

Pathological examination showed a complete fibrous stricture covered by edematous mucous membrane without the refractile bodies noted in case 1.

Comment

Increasing experience indicates that the treatment of stenosis of the trachea may wisely be revised. Each successful case adds more evidence which justifies the definitive approach of resection and anastomosis, especially since other older methods have been so ineffective. In both patients wide exposure permitted easy mobilization of the entire

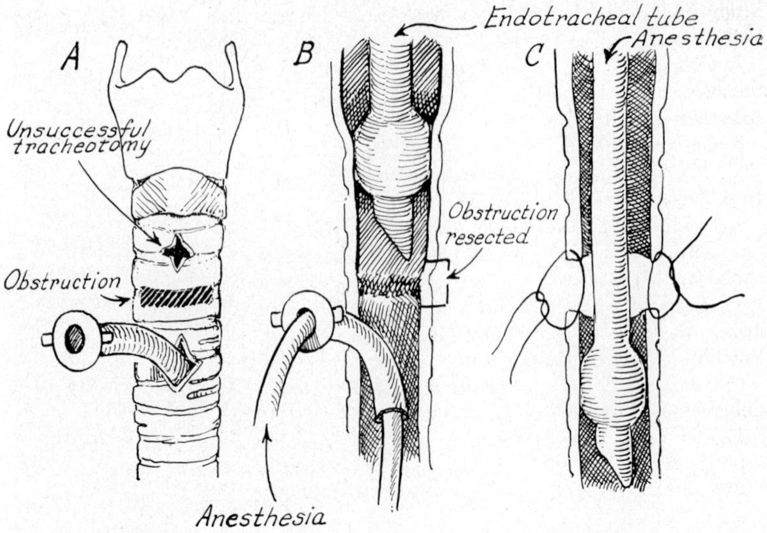

Fig 7 (Case 1).—Details of operation. The area from above the obstruction to below the tracheostomy was resected in both patients.

trachea which was sufficient for wide resection and accurate reanastomosis without tension. Even more extensive resection could have been completed without severely increasing the tension at the site of suture, which is probably the most important factor in the success of this operation.[5] The use of through and through interrupted fine silk sutures has not been followed by any adverse reaction. Repeated examination including bronchoscopy has not demonstrated any actual or relative loss of airway diameter at the anastomotic site. In addition, subsequent angiocardiography has shown that the mobilization and stretching of the trachea to overcome the surgically created defect has not disturbed the normal architectural relations of the pulmonary circulation and bronchi. The benign postoperative course attests to the safety of the method, provided adequate precautions have been planned to meet all emergencies before, during, and after operation. These have been described in detail in the case reports.

Of particular interest in case 1 is the pathological report which yields no clue to the origin of the obstructive lesion. A congenital origin aggravated by trauma and infection is suspected.

Summary

The pertinent facts which may influence the use of resection and reanastomosis for tracheal stenosis in preference to other methods have been reviewed.

Two cases with successful use of the method are reported to encourage others to use it in the attempt to improve results.

Although we have been prepared to use pneumoperitoneum to decrease tension at the suture line we did not find it necessary in these two patients.

A more aggressive effort to detect bronchial and tracheal injuries followed by primary repair would lower significantly the incidence of these stenotic lesions.

Laurence Miscall, MD, 11 E 68th St, New York, NY.

REFERENCES

1. Barclay, R. S., et al: Tracheal Reconstruction Without the Use of Grafts, Thorax 12:177, 1957.

2. Binet, J. P., and Aboulker, P.: A Case of Tracheal Stenosis After Tracheostomy: Resection and Suturing of the Trachea With Recovery, Mem Acad Chir 87:39-42 (Jan) 1961.

3. Beskin, C. A., and Rouge, B.: Rupture-Separation of the Trachea Following a Closed Chest Injury, J Thoracic Surgery 34:392, 1957.

4. Borrie, J.: Tracheal Stenosis in Infancy, Thorax 15:64, 1960.

5. Cantrell, J. R., and Folse, J. R.: The Repair of Circumferential Defects of the Trachea by Direct Anastomosis: Experimental Evaluation, J Thorac Cardiov Surg 42:589, 1961.

6. Clagett, O. T.; Grindlay, J. W.; and Moersch, H. J.: Resection of the Trachea: An Experimental

Study and Report of a Case, Arch Surg 57:253, 1948.
7. Colgan, F. J., and Keats, A. S.: Subglotic Stenosis: A Cause of Difficult Intubation, Anesthesiology 18:265, 1957.
8. Cummins, C. F. A., and Waterman, D. H.: The Management of Tracheal Stenosis With a Case Report, Dis Chest 31:375, 1957.
9. Erich, J. B.: Treatment of Extensive Cicatricial Stenosis of the Larynx or Trachea, Arch Otolaryng 41:344, 1945.
10. Ferguson, D. J.; Wild, J. J.; and Wangensteen, O. H.: Experimental Resection of the Trachea, Surgery 28:597, 1950.
11. Gebauer, P. W.: Plastic Reconstruction of Tuberculous Bronchostenosis With Dermal Grafts, J Thorac Surg 19:604, 1950.
12. Gebauer, P. W.: Reconstructive Tracheobronchial Surgery, Surg Clin N Amer 36:893 (Aug) 1956.
13. Gray, R. A.; Howard, J. M.; Harrison, W. H.; and Couves, C. M.: Injuries of the Trachea, AMA Arch Surg 76:138, 1958.
14. Greenberg, S. D.: Tracheal Reconstruction: An Experimental Study, Arch Otolaryng 72:565, 1960.
15. Grindlay, J. H.; Clagett, O. T.; and Moersch, H. J.: Resection and Anastomosis of the Trachea: An Experimental Study, Ann Otol 58:1225, 1949.
16. Hood, R. M., and Sloan, H. E.: Injuries of the Trachea and Major Bronchi, J Thorac Cardiov Surg 38:458, 1959.
17. Keshishian, J. M.; Blades, B.; and Beattie, E. J., Jr.: Tracheal Reconstruction, J Thorac Surg 32:707, 1956.
18. Kiriluk, L. B., and Merendino, K. A.: An Experimental Evaluation in the Dog of Bronchial Transplantation, Bronchial, Tracheal and Tracheobronchial Resection With Reconstruction, Ann Surg 137: 490, 1953.
19. Lazo, V. V.: Resection of the Cervical Part of the Trachea in Cancer of the Thyroid Gland, Vop Onkol (Eng) 3 (5):634, 1957.
20. LeJeune, F. J., and Owens, N.: Chronic Laryngeal Stenosis, Ann Otol 44:354, 1935.
21. Longmire, W. P., Jr.: Repair of Large Defects of the Trachea, Ann Otol 57:875, 1948.
22. Maisel, B., and Dingwal, J. A.: Primary Suture of the Divided Cervical Trachea, Surgery 275:726, 1950.
23. Michelson, E.; Soloman, R.; Maun, L.; and Ramirez, J.: Experiments in Tracheal Reconstruction, J Thorac Cardiov Surg 41:748, 1961.
24. Nach, R. L., and Rothman, M.: Injuries to the Larynx and Trachea, Surg Gynec Obstet 76: 614, 1943.
25. Pacheco, C. R.; Rivero, O.; and Porter, J. K.: Experimental Reconstructive Surgery of the Trachea, J Thorac Surg 27:554, 1954.
26. Rob, C. G., and Bateman, G. H.: Reconstruction of the Trachea and Cervical Esophagus, Brit J Surg 37:202, 1949.
27. Ross, R. R.: Repair of Tracheal and Esophageal Defect by Use of a Pedical Graft, Surgery 39:654, 1956.
28. Rush, B. F., and Cliffton, E. E.: Experimental Reconstruction of the Trachea With Bladder Mucosa, Surgery 40:1105, 1956.
29. Serrano, A.; Ortiz-Monasterio, F.; and Andrade-Pradillo, J.: Reconstruction of the Cervical Trachea: A Technique to Obtain a Permanently Patent Airway, Plast Reconstr Surg 24:333, 1959.
30. Schmidt, H. W.; Erich, J. B.; and Edwards, J. E.: Trauma to the Trachea, Dis Chest 37:262, 1960.
31. Scott, G. D.: Extensive Cut-Throat With Complete Laceration of the Trachea and Esophagus, JAMA 90:689, 1928.
32. Shaw, R. R.; Paulson, D. L.; and Kee, J. L., Jr.: Traumatic Tracheal Rupture, J Thorac Cardiov Surg 42:281-297, 1961.
33. Sonn, M. L., and Klein, S. H.: Primary Anastomosis of the Trachea After Resection of a Wide Segment: An Experimental Study, J Mount Sinai Hosp NY 25:211, 1958.
34. Sparger, C. F.; Polley, V. B.; and Lane, J. D.: Resection of the Intrathoracic Trachea in a Case of Tracheal Tumor, Amer J Surg 97:354, 1959.
35. Strandness, D. E.; Gustafson, I. J.; and Payne, J. T.: Surgical Resection of the Thoracic Trachea: An Experimental Study in Dogs, J Thorac Surg 34:269, 1957.
36. Work, W. P., and McCoy, E. G.: Surgical Repair of the Cervical Trachea Following Trauma: A Case Report, Ann Otol 65:573, 1956.

Prognosis in Deep Venous Thrombosis

R. S. PHILLIPS, MB, ChB, FRCSE
CLEVELAND

The management of gravitational ulcers and the "bottle leg" present many problems. Much time is given over to the treatment of the conditions both in hospital wards and out-patient departments. Recurrence of ulceration is only too common.

The pathogenesis of the condition now seems clear. A previous thrombosis in the deep veins of calf or thigh can be incriminated with certainty in the vast majority. Bauer,[1] who has done much work in this field, found that 80% of his patients, attending because of gravitational ulceration, gave a history of such a thrombosis. Dodd and Cockett[6] believe that 75% of patients who have had a thrombotic incident suffer subsequently from edema, induration, ulceration, or bursting leg pain.

The time that elapses before the patient has symptoms may be such that the original incident has been forgotten, and, indeed, a deep venous thrombosis may be silent, particularly in the bilateral case.

What happens then in these patients and their venous systems during this interim period? The object of this investigation is to study the clinical and phlebographic picture of a group of patients some two or three years after the thrombotic incident, comparing them with the findings in a group with the fully developed gravitational ulcer syndrome.

Submitted for publication April 3, 1963.

Orthopedic Research Fellow, Cleveland Metropolitan General Hospital, formerly Department of Surgery, Western General Hospital, Edinburgh, Scotland.

Material

There were six patients, all female, in the late group with the fully developed gravitational ulcer syndrome, of average age 42 years. Twenty-two patients, 16 male and 6 female, constitute the recent group under study, their average age being 55 years. In this latter group, 20 developed a venous thrombosis within a few days of a surgical operation and 2 during conservative treatment for fracture of the femoral shaft. In the late group five were post-partum in origin and one consequent upon trauma to the limb. The period of time which had elapsed since thrombosis was 10.3 and 2.3 years, respectively.

In the recent group Table 1 shows the evidence of acute thrombosis and the treatment prescribed.

In this group, the right limb was involved in 12 patients and the left in 10, whereas in the late group, the right and left limbs were involved in three occasions each.

Method of Study

In both groups an adequate history was taken both from the patient and from a review of his or her previous case records. A careful clinical

TABLE 1.—*Recent Group*

Evidence of Original Incident				
Calf Pain and Tenderness	Pyrexia	Edema	Limb Discoloration	Pulmonary Embolus
21	6	7	1	4

Treatment	
Anticoagulants	Supportive Therapy Only
20	2

examination of the limbs and of the cardiovascular system was made. All patients underwent ascending phlebography. Where possible both legs were done and not just the one considered to have been the site of thrombosis.

The following is the method adopted for phlebography and is a modification of that described by Bauer.[1]

1. The patient lies supine on the x-ray table with the limb exposed from toes to groin.

2. A soft rubber tourniquet is wrapped round the limb at the level of the malleoli to occlude the superficial veins.

3. A sphygmomanometer cuff is wound round the thigh at as high a level as possible.

4. 20 ml of 45% sodium diatrizoate (Hypaque Sodium) is drawn into a syringe containing 1,000 units of heparin.

5. After skin cleansing, a vein on the dorsum of the foot is punctured and 4-5 ml of diatrizoate are injected to ensure initial filling of the deep venous system.

6. The pneumatic tourniquet is then inflated to midway between systolic and diastolic pressures, and the remainder of the diatrizoate is injected over the next 10-15 seconds.

7. On completion of injection, two anteroposterior and two lateral stereoscopic films are taken as rapidly as possible, after which the tourniquets are released.

8. The limb is elevated and massaged to avoid stagnation of the radiopaque material.

Of a total of 54 phlebograms done, apart from minor bruising at the injection site, the only complication was superficial thrombophlebitis in one patient which responded readily to conservative measures.

Results

Table 2 presents the clinical findings in both groups of patients. In the late group all had symptoms and signs of a fairly severe nature, though in only four had progression to ulceration occurred. However, these patients had received intensive therapy to heal, control, or prevent ulceration.

In the recent group ten only were symptomless. Of the other 12, symptoms and signs were as yet minimal enough not to have caused the patient to seek hospital treatment, although one or two were wearing elastic stockings prescribed by their own

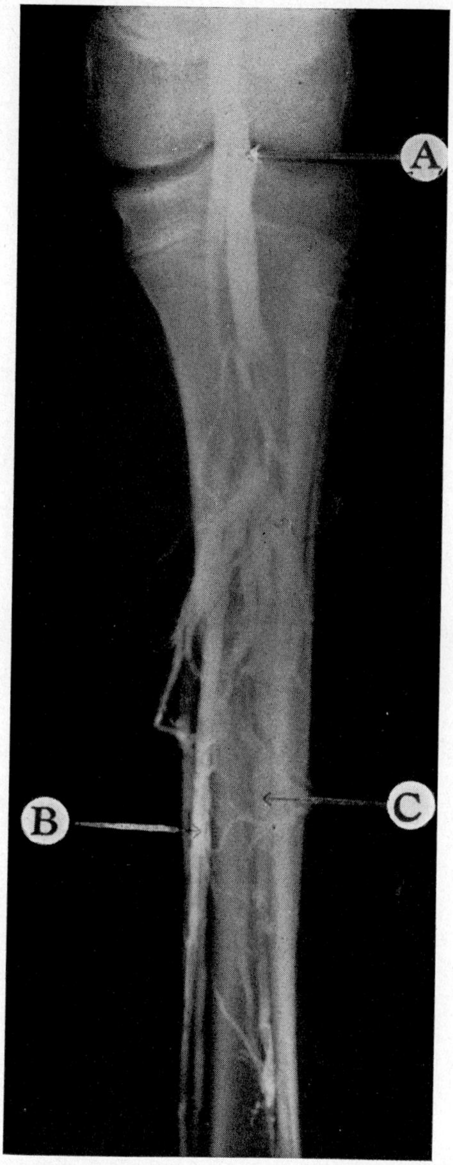

Fig 1.—Anteroposterior view of a normal phlebogram showing: *A*, popliteal vein, *B*, posterior tibial vein, and *C*, peroneal vein. There is almost no dye in the superficial systems.

TABLE 2.—*Clinical Findings*

	Recent Group	Late Group
Symptomless	10	0
Symptoms present	12	6
Pain	8	6
Ankle edema	8	6
Varices since deep venous thrombosis	3	6
Induration	0	3
Ulcer	0	4
Pigmentation and eczema	1	5
Trophic changes	0	3

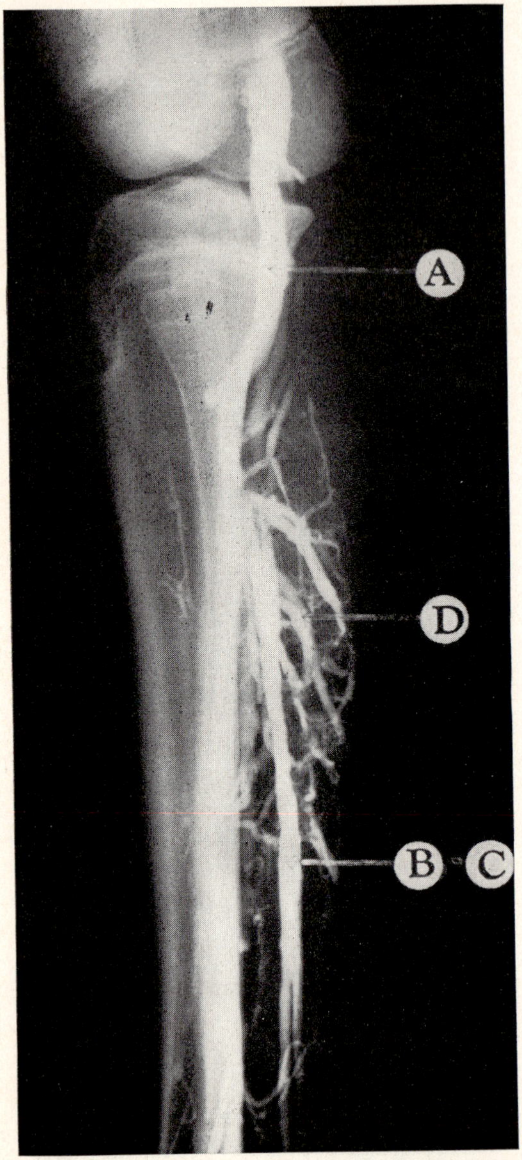

Fig 2.—Lateral view of limb in preceding normal phlebogram showing: *A,* popliteal vein, *B,* posterior tibial vein, *C,* peroneal vein, and *D,* arrows a normal intermuscular vein.

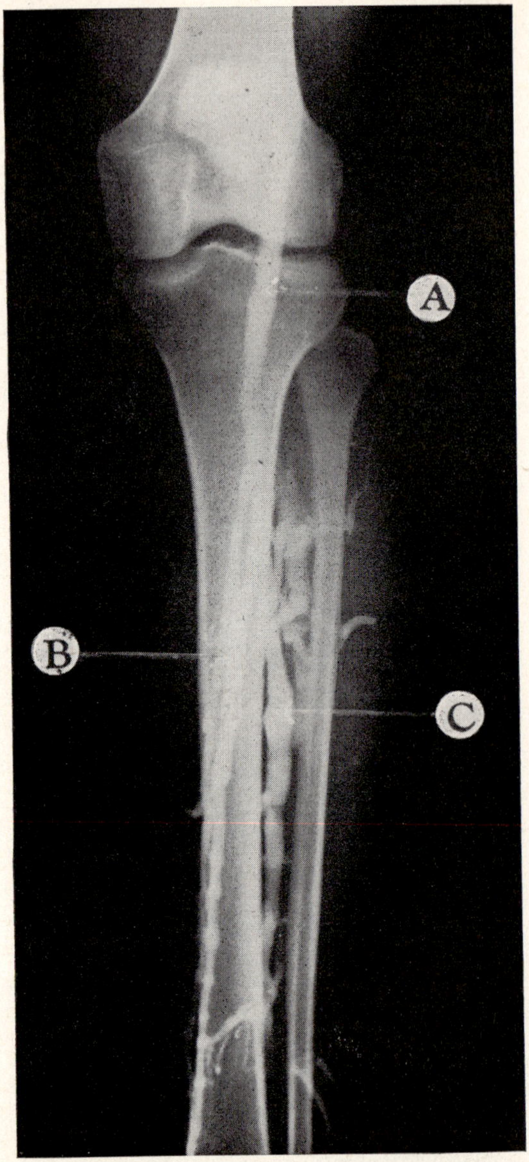

Fig 3.—Anteroposterior view of a normal phlebogram showing: *A,* popliteal, *B,* posterior tibial, and *C,* peroneal veins. There is no dye in the superficial system.

practitioners. It is worthy of note that varices of the superficial system were present in three, but their significance was difficult to assess in that, although having been present for many years, they may have worsened since the thrombotic incident.

The time lapse since the deep venous thrombosis in those with no symptoms was 23.2 months, and in those with symptoms, 29.5 months.

It is well recognized that a deep venous thrombosis need not be accompanied by symptoms or signs. A silent thrombosis may be present in a so-called normal limb, while its opposite counterpart may manifest the typical evidence of thrombosis. Although in the recent group there were no symptoms in the "normal" legs at the time of review, phlebograms were performed to detect the presence of previous damage to deep veins.

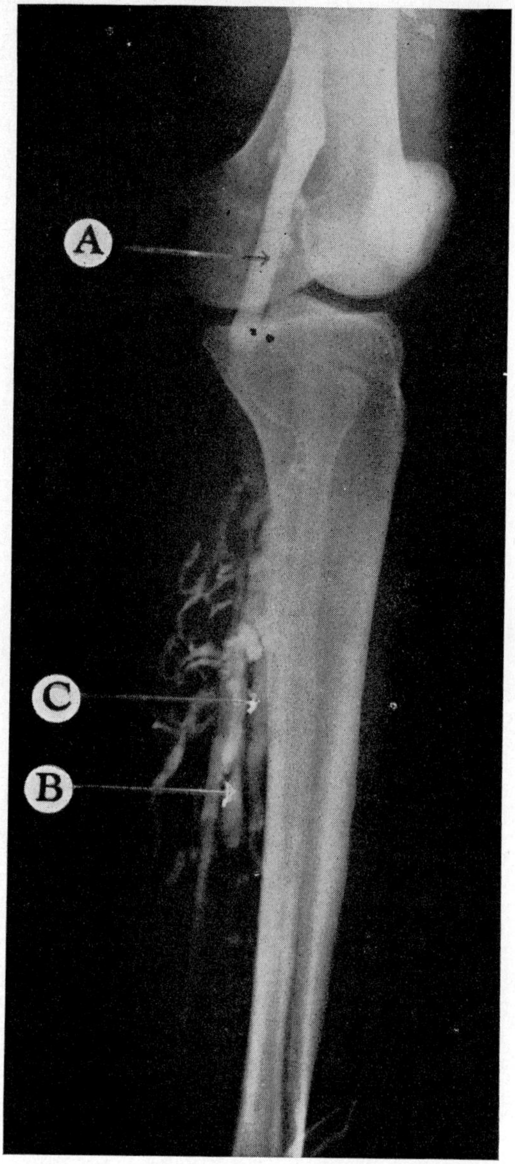

Fig 4.—Lateral view of the previous normal limb showing: *A,* popliteal, *B,* posterior tibial, and *C,* peroneal veins.

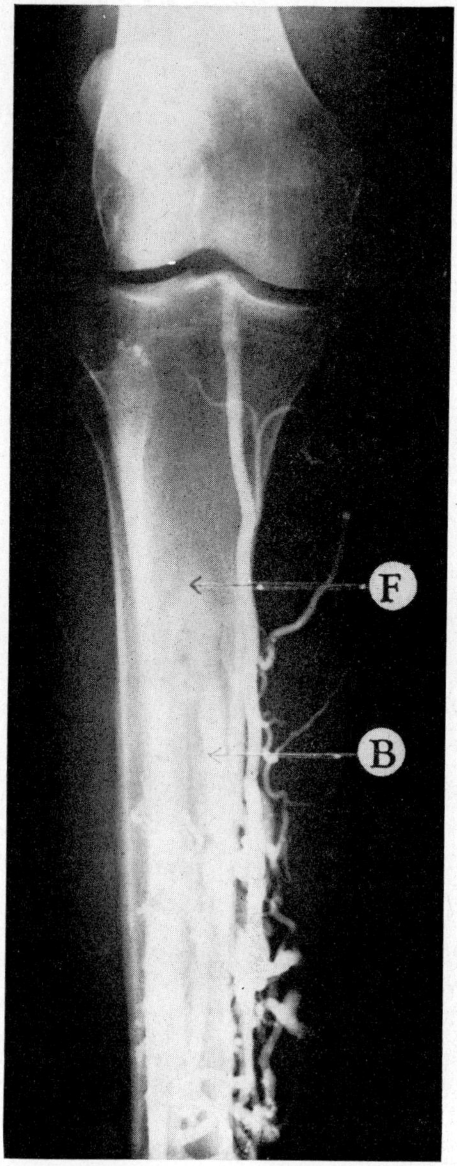

Fig 5.—Anteroposterior phlebogram showing a sudden cessation of filling (*F*) in the posterior tibial vein (*B*). The intermuscular plexus is well filled and spilling over into the saphenous system.

Phlebographic Results

Before embarking upon a description of phlebograms in the groups under study, a brief summary of normal phlebographic findings is presented.

1. The peroneal and posterior tibial veins, single or double trunks, are well filled.
2. The peroneal vein lies deeply in the calf on the interosseous membrane. The posterior tibial lies on the posterior surface of the tibia.
3. Normally, thick walled branches drain to these.
4. The anterior tibial vein is inconstant in its filling.
5. The popliteal vein, large and well filled, is a direct continuation of peroneal and posterior tibial veins, but in its lower part, filling may be poor or absent because the soleus muscle at its fibrous origin from the soleal line of the tibia compresses the dye from the vein.
6. The subcutaneous veins fill poorly.
7. The internal and external saphenous veins are poorly filled or inconstant.

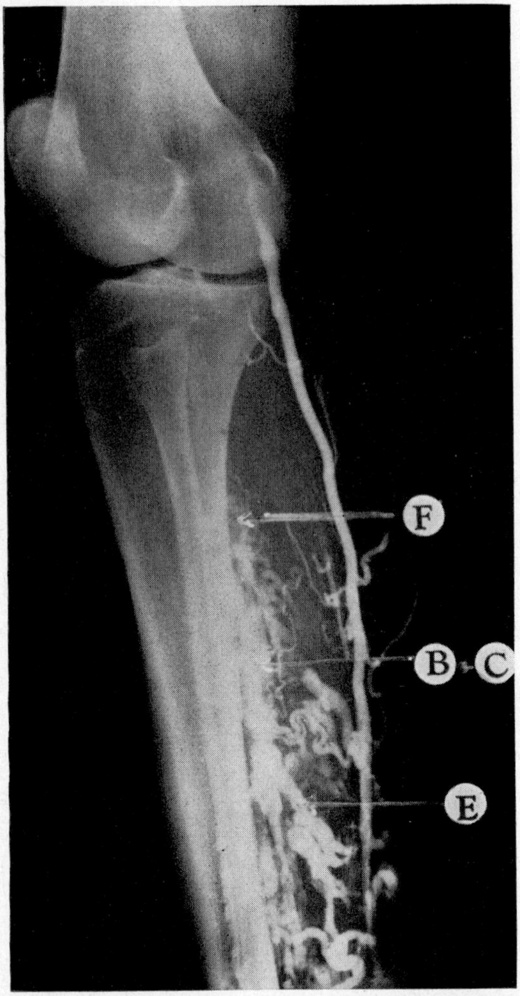

Fig 6.—Lateral view of the previous patient showing a sudden block (*F*) in posterior tibial and peroneal veins (*B* + *C*). *E* marks an incompetent perforator allowing spill over into the superficial systems.

Fig 1-4 demonstrate the normal phlebogram. Fig 5-14 display the findings at phlebography where damage exists in the deep venous systems.

Table 3 presents the phlebographic findings in the two groups. It is of note that all in the late group showed evidence of damage to the deep veins. In ten of the recent group the deep veins were normal, but in two of these there was noted the presence of a solitary medial sural vein, the pathological significance of which is disputed. Bauer [1] states that the sural veins are rarely seen in the healthy limb, but when an obstruction of the deep trunks has occurred, the sural veins generally make their appearance on the phlebogram in a very short time. On the other hand, Mathieson,[12] in discussing the results of tilt phlebography, considers the sural veins to be normal features. It would appear then, in the absence of radiological evidence of deep vein damage, that the presence of a sural vein is of no pathological significance. However, there can be no doubt that deep veins showing a sudden block or a length of vein which fails to fill with radiopaque material signify previous damage in the form of thrombosis. A grossly dilated deep venous channel with no apparent valvular pattern was at first thought to signify recanalization after thrombus organization. In seven limbs this phenomenon was noted, although in four there was an accompanying venous block. Bearing in mind the difficulties of interpretation of phlebograms the dilation was thought to be due to back pressure by the thigh tourniquet rather than an indication of recanalized thrombus.

TABLE 3.—*Phlebogram Results*

	Late Group	Recent Group
Normal deep veins	0	10
Complete block with superficial varicosity	4	9
Local absence of filling in deep veins	2	3

In the recent group, the phlebograms are compared in those patients presenting symptoms and those who were symptomless. This is illustrated in Table 4.

From this table it is noted that those in whom symptoms are present already show a high proportion of abnormal phlebograms. There are, however, four patients as yet symptomless, who show radiological evidence of a blocked deep vein.

It is a fact that venous thrombosis may occur silently, particularly when the opposite limb manifests florid evidence of clot formation. Hence phlebograms were carried out on these "normal" legs, and the findings are presented in Table 5. It is of interest to note

TABLE 4.—*Recent Group*

	Symptoms	No Symptoms
Normal phlebogram	4	6
Deep vein block	5	4
Local absence of filling in a deep vein	3	0

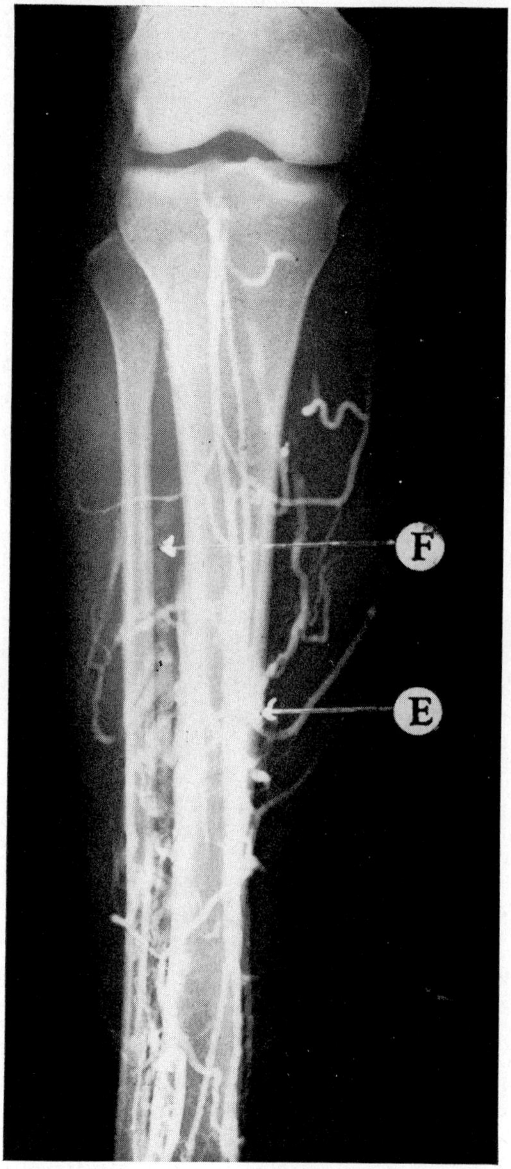

Fig 7.—This is an anteroposterior phlebogram showing (*F*) a sudden block in the posterior tibial and peroneal veins. *E* marks an incompetent perforating vein. There is considerable filling of the superficial system.

that three limbs show radiological evidence of deep vein block.

Superficial varicose veins although commonly a primary disorder may well be secondary to damage in the deep veins. After initial hypertrophy, they become varicose as a result of degeneration when the venous pressure they have to bear becomes excessive. In the late group, with the gravitational ulcer syndrome, four patients displayed clinical evidence of failure of the superficial venous system, whereas in the recent group this was evident in ten patients, five being in those

Fig 8.—Lateral view of the preceding phlebogram. There is a sudden block (*F*) of the posterior tibial and peroneal veins. Through an incompetent perforator (*E*) the superficial system are filling well.

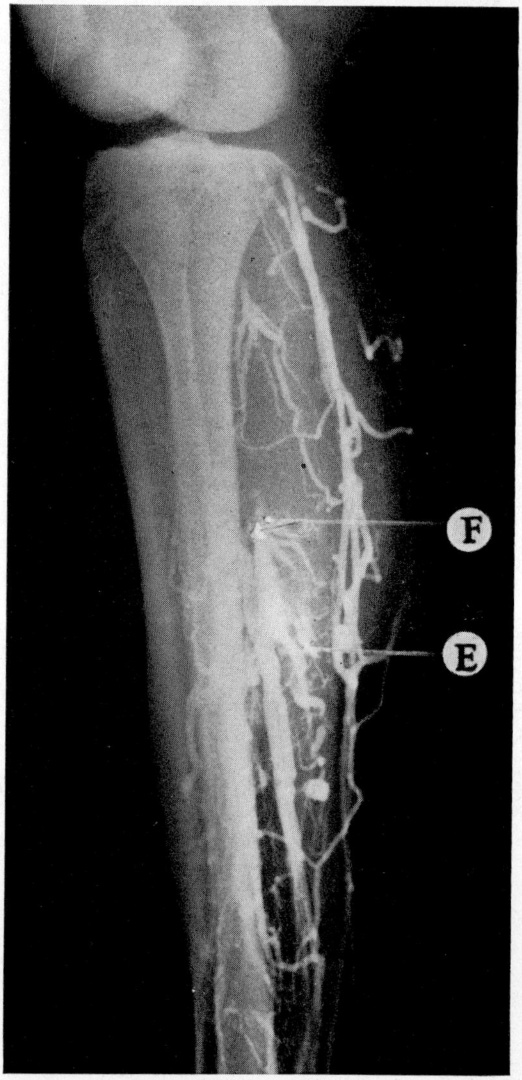

TABLE 5.—*Phlebograms of 24 "Normal" Legs*

Normal phlebogram	21
Complete deep vein block	3

with no symptoms. In these patients in the recent group who had superficial varices, 29.6 months had elapsed since the thrombotic incident, while in those in whom the superficial veins remained intact, 26.2 months had elapsed. The difference is not statistically significant.

Fig 9.—Anteroposterior phlebogram in which a large segment of posterior tibial vein (*S*) fails to fill although the popliteal vein (*A*) is filling well. Dye is spilling over into the superficial systems.

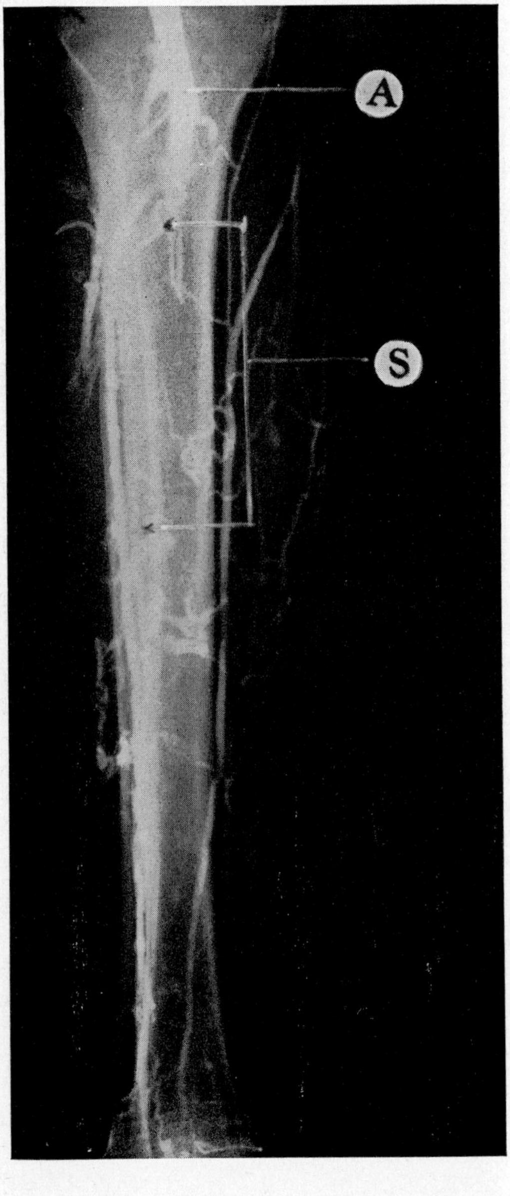

The deep and superficial venous systems in a limb communicate directly or indirectly by means of vessels which perforate the deep fascia. These, in health, permit a unidirectional blood flow, viz, from superficial to deep. A reversal of flow is caused by valvular destruction and incompetence consequent upon thrombosis or, alternatively, when venous pressure becomes excessive, a phenomenon which may occur as a result of valvular destruction in the deep veins. In 54 phlebograms, no less than 37 incompetent perforators could be detected. In legs thought to have been the site of previous thrombosis, 24 showed incompetent perforators, and in the normal limbs, no less than sixteen displayed these. Table 6 is presented to show the occurrence of incompetent perforators in limbs which clinically had and had not varicose veins. One is struck by the high percentage of incompetent perforators in those with no clinical evidence of varicose veins.

Comment

In their text book, Dodd and Cockett [6] (1956) discuss the site and progress of deep venous thrombosis. The process begins in the intramuscular plexus of veins and spreads proximally to popliteal and femoral veins. Consequently, until the main trunks are involved, viz, peroneal or posterior tibial, obstruction to the limb's venous return is minimal, and the long term prognosis remains favorable. According to text books of pathology, in a complete deep vein block, thrombus becomes organized and gradually revascularization leads on to recanalization by the fusion of the newly formed vessels, so that it is possible for such large and continuous lumina to arise with resulting

TABLE 6.—*Occurrence of Incompetent Perforators*

Varicose Veins		Perforators	No Perforators
Present, clinically	18	14	4
Absent, clinically	36	23	13

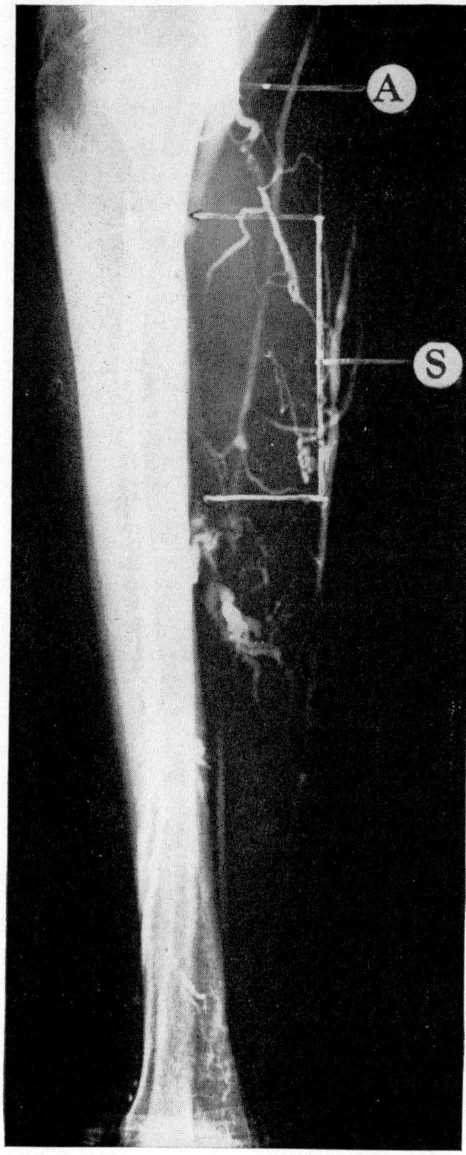

Fig 10.—This is the lateral view of the previous limb again showing the segmental deep vein block (*S*) and the popliteal vein (*A*). The long saphenous is beginning to fill but is not varicose.

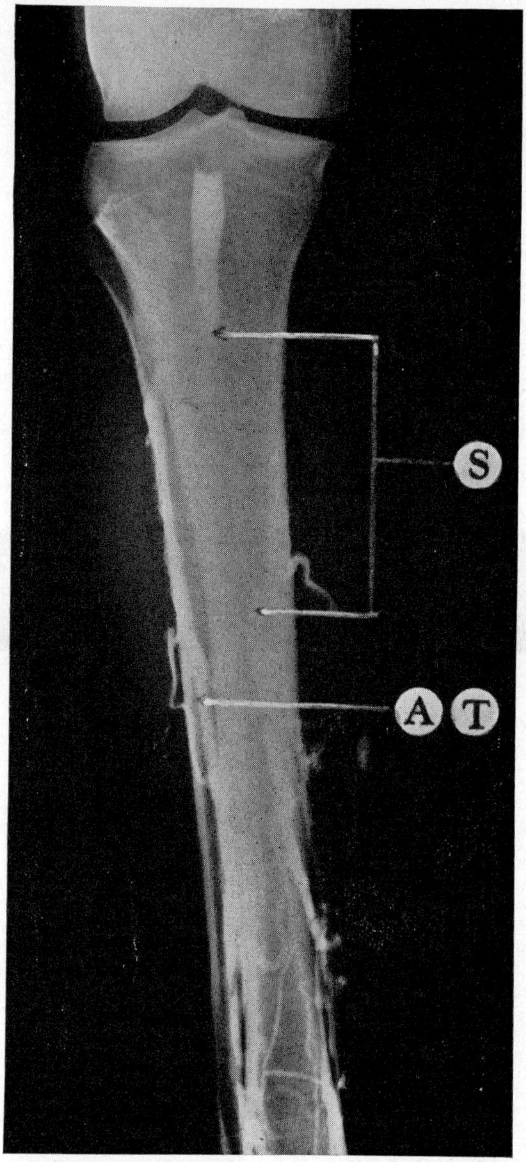

Fig 11.—Anteroposterior phlebogram showing a segmental deep vein block (*S*). The anterior tibial vein (AT) is showing up well. There is visible a varicose superficial vein.

restoration of blood flow. However, Bauer [1] (1942) states:

> My own experience founded on evidence from those cases of chronic thrombosis which I have venographically investigated tends to show, however, that such a recanalization is rare and where it exists, only incomplete and of almost no value to the venous circulation as a whole in the leg. The venous return stands or falls with the subcutaneous accessory system that may have been formed.

When heparin is used in deep venous thrombosis, the thrombotic process can be halted with the result that post-thrombotic symptoms are considerably minimized, although the length of vein involved by the thrombus too is important in prognosis. Bauer's original observation quoted above was made before the introduction of heparin; his work continued into the anticoagulant

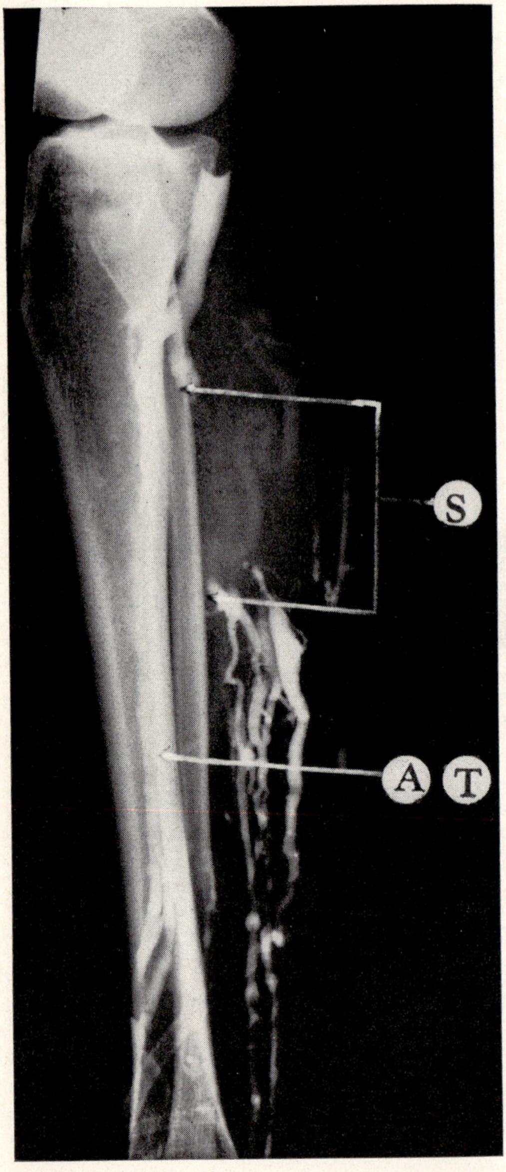

Fig 12.—Lateral view of the preceding limb, again showing a segmental deep vein block (*S*) and the anterior tibial vein (AT).

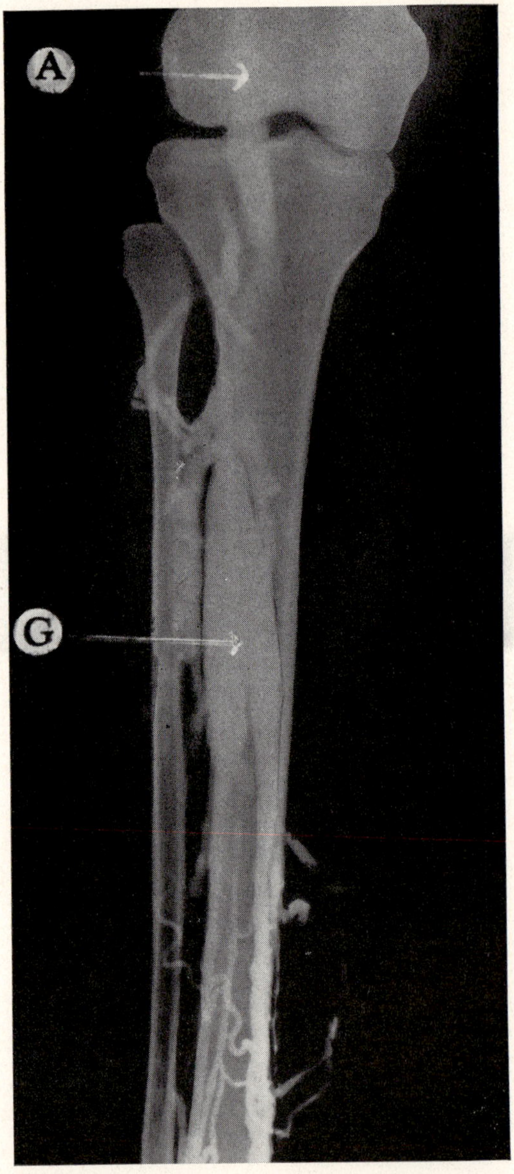

Fig 13.—This anteroposterior phlebogram shows well-filled deep veins. The popliteal vein (*A*) is filling well from the posterior tibial and peroneal veins which are dilated and show no obvious valve pattern (*G*)—believed due to back pressure from the thigh tourniquet.

era so that he concludes that heparin is a very effective prophylactic against post-thrombotic swelling, induration, and ulceration. However, Bauer has not produced a phlebographic follow-up series in patients whose thrombosis had been treated by anticoagulants.

In this present study, both in recent and late groups, the original diagnosis of deep venous thrombosis was made on clinical grounds alone. Of the recent group, 20 had received anticoagulants and 2 supportive therapy only. Yet despite this deterrent to spread of thrombus, 20 of 21 had already developed symptoms of a minimal nature and these within a period of 29.5 months. In the group who had gone on to the gravitational ulcer syndrome, all, on phlebography, confirmed the presence of deep vein damage: four showed a complete block of the deep veins of the calf, and two, a local absence of filling in the deep veins. The original treatment given to these patients was not known, but all could not have received heparin because of the year in which the thrombotic incident occurred. In the recent group, only ten had radiologically normal deep veins. Twelve legs displayed evidence of complete or local block. In these 12 the deep veins were in the same state as those of the late group, and in eight patients symptoms of a minimal nature were present at the time of investigation.

That being so, it is reasonable to conclude that when the accessory superficial systems degenerate under excessive pressure, as they must after a shorter or longer period, these patients will progress to the gravitational syndrome. If there is partial recanalization of a thrombosed segment of vein, and this may have occurred in these patients with dilated deep veins and loss of valve pattern at phlebography who were eventually thought to have normal phlebograms, valves are not reformed. Consequently, the muscle pump, in the absence of venous valves, can only increase the pressure within the pathological vein segment. This will cause incompetence of the valves guarding the perforators and lead on to ulceration and induration (Buchan and Falconer [2]). Twelve patients, 54%, with abnormal deep veins (or 15, 68%, if local dilatation of a venous segment due to recanalization can be diagnosed at phlebography) will progress to the gravitational ulcer syndrome. If this is correct, then prophylaxis or the rapid institution of effective treatment in deep venous thrombosis assumes important proportions.

Crafoord and Jorpes [4] in 1941 had already recognized the importance of heparin in preventing thrombosis. Despite this, anticoagulating all patients admitted to hospitals remains a theoretical possibility only. Surgical operations become hazardous when the prothrombin level is depressed. Postoperative anticoagulation may not always have been instituted in time to prevent thrombosis. A deep venous thrombosis may occasionally occur in the presence of adequate depression of circulating prothrombin (De Bakey, Schroeder, and Oschner [5]).

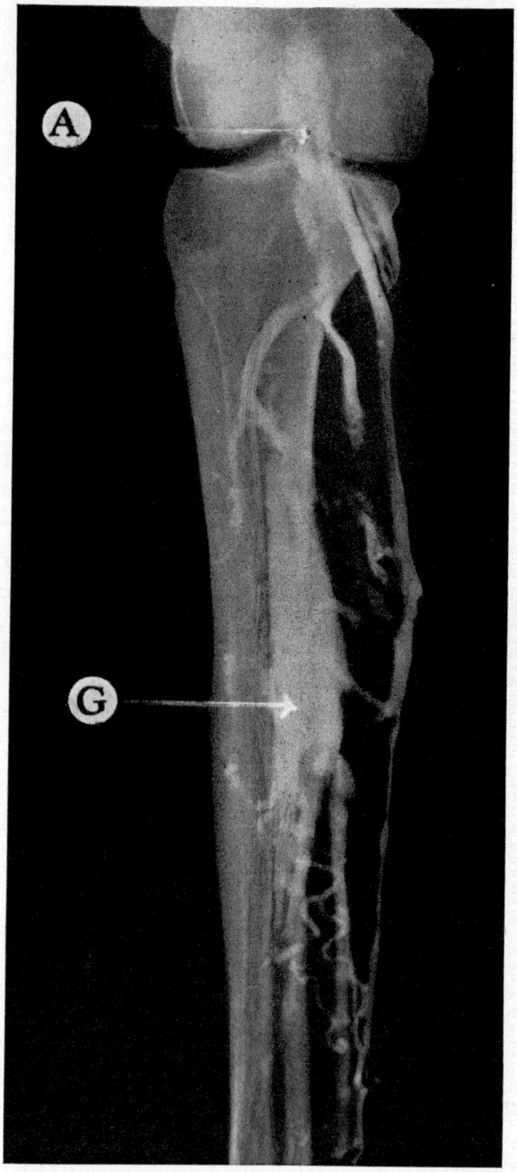

Fig 14—The lateral aspect of the preceding limb again showing well-filled deep veins. *A* marks the popliteal vein. Posterior tibial and peroneal veins (*G*) are dilated with no obvious valve pattern.

It has been shown that extension of thrombosis is prevented by the use of anticoagulants, but the seeds have already been sown for the future development of an edematous, indurated, or ulcerated leg if the thrombus has extended into the principal calf veins. The value of anticoagulants is not disputed, but their effectiveness is limited. A drug capable of lysing thrombus before organization can occur would go far to reduce the total number of patients in danger of progressing to the gravitational ulcer syndrome. Fibrinolysin (plasmin) and trypsin have been shown to have such an action.[3,8-10,13,14]

In the phlebograms done in this study, incompetent perforating veins were detected in 37 legs, yet there would seem to be little corelation with the clinical presence of varicose veins in that in 23 limbs incompetent perforators were present despite the absence of such varices. It would appear reasonable to conclude that this method of phlebography is of little value in determining the significance of such perforators with any accuracy. It is claimed by both Mathiesen[11,12] (1958) and Dohn[7] that tilt phlebography is the method of choice in depicting radiographically incompetent perforators.

Summary

A phlebographic study has been undertaken to discover the state of the deep veins in legs previously the seat of deep venous thrombosis. The findings are compared with those of a group who had already progressed to the development of severe post-thrombotic manifestations. The method of phlebography and the normal phlebographic findings are described.

The conclusion that 12 (54%) of 22 patients with a history of deep venous thrombosis and positive radiographic evidence of deep vein damage will progress in time to the gravitational ulcer syndrome is reached.

It is noted with interest that three of 24 "normal" legs displayed x-ray evidence of vein damage.

The shortcomings of heparin as a prophylactic and therapeutic agent in deep venous thrombosis are discussed.

The inaccuracy of the method of direct ascending phlebography in demonstrating the significance of incompetent perforating veins is admitted.

C. W. A. Falconer, FRCS gave permission to investigate his patients, and special help was given by the staff of the X-Ray Department of the Western General Hospital, Edinburgh, Scotland.

Robert S. Phillips, MB, ChB, FRCSE, Cleveland Metropolitan General Hospital, Cleveland 9, Ohio.

REFERENCES

1. Bauer, G.: A Roentgenological and Clinical Study of the Sequels of Thrombosis, Acta Chir Scand 86, suppl 74, 1942.

2. Buchan, A. C., and Falconer, C. W.: The Management of Chronic Swelling and Ulceration of the Leg, J Roy Coll Surg Edinb 2:279, 1957.

3. Cliffton, E. E.: Early Experience With Fibrinolysin, Angiology 10:244, 1959.

4. Crafoord, C., and Jorpes, J. E.: Heparin as a Prophylactic Against Thrombosis, JAMA 116:2831, 1941.

5. DeBakey, M.; Schroeder, G. F.; and Oschner, A.: Significance of Phlebography in Phlebothrombosis, JAMA 123:738, 1943.

6. Dodd, H., and Cockett, F. B.: Pathology and Surgery of the Veins of the Lower, Limb, Edinburgh: E. & S. Livingstone, Ltd., 1956.

7. Dohn, K.: Tilt Phlebography: Retrograde Phlebography By Ascending Injection, Acta Radiol (Stockholm) 50:293, 1958.

8. Harole, J. P.: The Treatment of Some Problem Cases of Thromboembolic Disease With Fibrinolysin, Angiology 10:283, 1959.

9. Innerfield, I.; Schwartz, A.; and Angrist, A.: Intravenous Trypsin: Its Anticoagulant, Fibrinolytic and Thrombolytic Effects, J Clin Invest 31:1049, 1952.

10. Kryle, L.; Arnoldi, C.; and Kupperman, H.: The Therapeutic Effectiveness of Trypsin in the Treatment of Thrombophlebitis, Ann NY Acad Sci 68:178, 1957.

11. Mathiesen, F. R.: Tilt Phlebography: A Reliable Method of Diagnosing Incompetent Communicating Veins, Acta Radiol (Stockholm) 50:430, 1958.

12. Mathiesen, F. R.: Tilt Phlebography of Normal Legs, Acta Radiol (Stockholm) 50:493, 1958.

13. Moser, K. M.: Thrombolysis with Fibrinolysin (Plasmin): New Therapeutic Approach to Thromboembolism, JAMA 167:1695, 1958.

14. Sokal, J.; Ambrus, J. L.; Ambrus, C. M.: Treatment of Thrombosis With Fibrinolysin, JAMA 168:1314, 1958.

Renal Tubular Necrosis After Oral Cholecystography

RONALD A. MALT, MD
BOSTON
HARRY G. OLKEN, MD
AND
WILLIAM J. GOADE, JR., MD
LYNN, MASS

Recognition of the utility of large and repeated doses of oral cholecystographic compounds to visualize biliary tract disease unrevealed by the conventional amounts carries with it the hazard of also revealing new toxic effects of the contrast agents. Since 1959 four transient and one fatal case of renal insufficiency after ingestion of double doses of these substances have been recorded.[1-3] The case reported below represents a second fatality, with a description of the pathologic findings.

Submitted for publication April 3, 1963.

An Established Investigator of the American Heart Association (Dr. Malt).

From the Department of Surgery, Massachusetts General Hospital and Harvard Medical School and the Departments of Pathology and Radiology, Lynn Hospital and Tufts University Medical School.

Report of a Case

A 69-year-old widow entered Lynn Hospital on April 11, 1960, complaining of upper abdominal pain of one week's duration. Similar, but less severe, attacks had occurred intermittently for 50 years. She was otherwise healthy save for Bell's palsy, eight years of hypertension "over 200," and an evanescent left hemiplegia four years before admission.

Her temperature was 98.6 F (37 C) rectally, pulse 100/min, and blood pressure 212/114 mm Hg. Bilateral basal rales and moderate cardiomegaly were present. There was a grade 3 harsh apical systolic murmur and a grade 2 harsh basal systolic murmur radiating to the neck. Abdominal examination was normal except for a sharp liver edge palpable 4 cm below the costal margin.

The blood hemoglobin was 14.2 gm/100 ml, white blood cell count 8,500/cu mm with 81% polymorphonuclear leukocytes. Specific gravity of the urine was 1.021; no sugar and only a trace of albumin were detected. Five red blood cells and three white blood cells were seen per high-power field.

Parenteral fluids, sedatives, digoxin, and chlorothiazide were administered on the day of admission. Bunamiodyl * 4.5 gm was given orally in preparation for a cholecystogram.

The following morning the fasting level of blood sugar was 204 mg/100 ml, blood urea nitrogen 12 mg/100 ml, and total serum bilirubin 1.2 mg/100 ml. No gall bladder opacification was seen on the x-ray films; examination of the colon and upper gastrointestinal tract with barium was normal. An additional 4.5 gm of bunamiodyl was given that evening.

Roentgenograms on the third hospital day again failed to demonstrate the gall bladder. The levels of electrolytes and proteins in the serum at this time were normal. Several pooled samples of urine on this day had a combined volume of 110 ml and a specific gravity of 1.010. With the completion of digitalization, the pulse rate was 68/min.

The fasting level of blood sugar on the next day was 131 mg/100 ml. Persistent vomiting precluded a glucose tolerance test. An excretory urogram with 30 ml of diatrizoate sodium,† 50%, showed no contrast material in the urinary tract in the 30 minutes following injection. Because of the interest of the Department of Radiology in an abnormal urogram despite a normal blood level of urea nitrogen, the study was repeated later the same day. Twenty-five milliliters of acetrizoate sodium ‡ resulted in prompt bilateral nephrograms persisting for 30 minutes.

Inasmuch as the patient, a probable diabetic, was still vomiting and having increasing epigastric pain, celiotomy was undertaken on her fifth day in the hospital. An acutely and chronically inflamed gall bladder filled with a solid cast of debris was removed. Five hundred milliliters of compatible group A, Rh positive blood was given without incident. The blood pressure was well maintained throughout the operation and recovery period.

After urinating 60 ml in the first few hours after surgery, the patient voided only 10 ml in the next 24 hours. This urine contained many white and red blood cells, but no casts. On the day after surgery, the blood urea nitrogen was 100 mg/100 ml. The lungs became filled with secretions from which *Escherichia coli* was cultured. A program of strict fluid and electrolyte control was instituted.

On the third postoperative day the level of blood urea nitrogen was 125 mg/100 ml and on the fourth 158. Diuresis began on the fourth day, eight days after the first dose of bunamiodyl, and was copious by the fifth day. As there was no urinary catheter and the patient was incontinent, the exact amount of urine was not known.

* Orabilex, E. Fougera & Co., Inc., Hicksville, NY.

† Hypaque, Winthrop Laboratories, New York.

‡ Urokon, 30%, Mallinckrodt Pharmaceuticals, St. Louis, Mo.

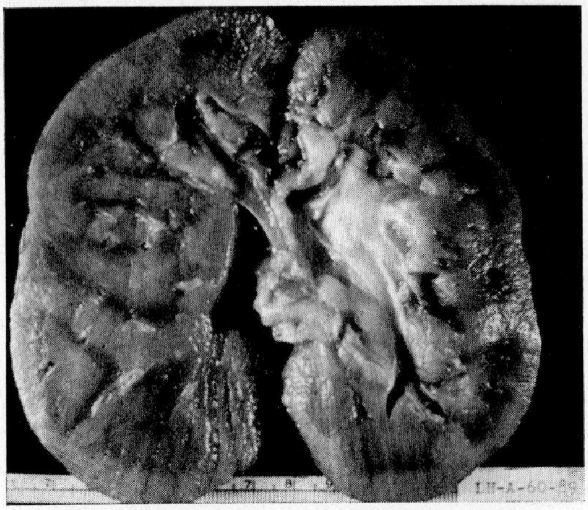

Fig 1.—Gross appearance of the kidneys.

Pulmonary secretions became overwhelming just as the diuresis began. The temperature rose to 104. Antibiotic therapy and a tracheostomy were of no help, and the patient died on the fifth postoperative day. The blood urea nitrogen was 143 mg/100 ml.

Necropsy

There was evidence of hypertensive and arteriosclerotic heart disease. The heart weighed 440 gm; right and left ventricular hypertrophy and pulmonary edema were found. There was bilateral lower lobe bronchopneumonia. The acutely congested liver weighed 2,350 gm.

The kidneys together weighed 310 gm. Their cortices were grossly pale and sharply demarcated from the medulla (Fig 1). Proximal and distal tubules showed histologic changes of swelling and degeneration. Eosinophilic debris, blood, and occasional birefringent crystals were seen within the lumens (Fig 2). Occasional mitotic figures were present in the tubular walls. The parenchyma was infiltrated with lymphocytes and polymorphonuclear leukocytes. Glomeruli were normal.

Comment

The nephrotoxicity of one of the older oral cholecystographic agents § demonstrated by Modell [4] in cats has not commonly had its

§ Iodoalphionic acid; Priodax, Schering Corporation, Bloomfield, NJ.

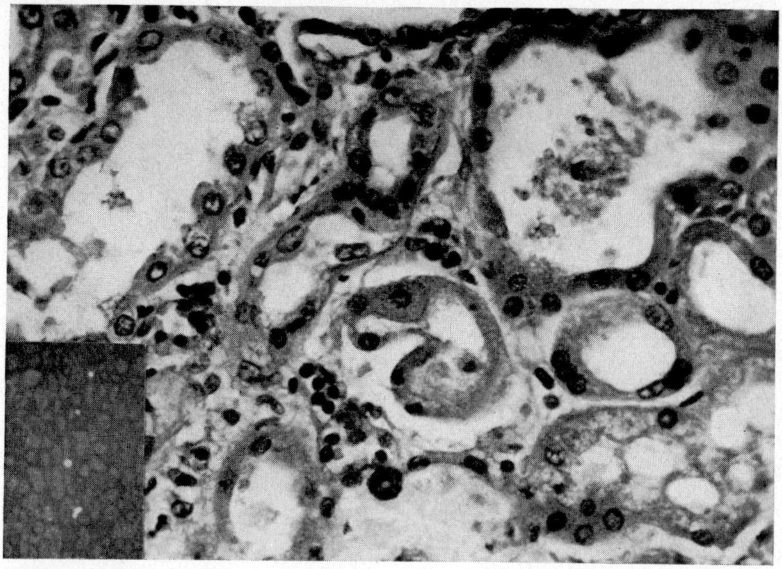

Fig 2.—Microscopic picture of the kidneys. Inset: doubly refractile bodies in the tubules.

counterpart in clinical medicine. Laboratory animals sometimes die with associated renal failure after a single 500 mg oral dose of the contrast medium (equivalent to about 7.5 gm for a 60 kg subject), and albuminuria is frequent with doses as low as 100 mg/kg. Obviously species differences, such as the tendency of cats to excrete urine of pH 1-2,[5] must be considered before transferring to the ward the experience with toxicity in the laboratory; however, as knowledge of the usefulness of repeated administration of contrast materials to detect occult biliary disease becomes more widespread, the population at risk of whatever ill effects are possible must also necessarily increase.

All previously recorded cases of renal insufficiency after cholecystography have followed administration of double doses of the iodinated media within a day. In one instance, the drug was iopanoic acid,# in one iopanoic acid and bunamiodyl, and in all the others bunamiodyl alone. The relationship between ingestion of two 4.5 gm doses of bunamiodyl and the subsequent renal failure in this case reported above is clouded by intervening events. However, circumstantial evidence is strong that renal failure preceded the excretory urograms, operation, and blood transfusion. First, the blood urea nitrogen level (100 mg/100 ml) on the day after surgery is too high to be ascribed to oliguria of only one day's duration. Second, both the scant isosthenuric specimen collected the day after the attempted cholecystograms and the excretory urograms reflect existent renal damage. Prompt appearance of a nephrogram implies that glomerular function, but not tubular, was intact at the time of the test. Third, there is no evidence of a hypotensive episode during x-ray examinations or of hypotension or transfusion reaction during surgery. Finally, the onset of diuresis and the histologic evidence of tubular regeneration are most compatible with an insult at least eight days previous, the approximate time the bunamiodyl was given.

Renal injury following administration of three different cholecystographic drugs suggests that the toxic fraction is the common tri-iodinated aromatic nucleus. The toxicity could be moderated through many influences: among them the well-known fluctuations in gastrointestinal absorption, impairment in hepatic removal of drug from the blood,[3] and perhaps alterations of pH enhancing dissociation of inorganic iodide, to result in the nephrotoxicity and tubular swelling seen in deaths from acute iodism.[2] For example, alkaline environments might readily result in γ-lactone formation and splitting off the 2,6-

Telepaque, Winthrop Laboratories, New York.

iodo groups; an extremely acid medium could conceivably cause dissociation and formation of free HI. Any relationship between the birefringent crystals found within the tubules of our patient and the renal failure is not apparent.

In any event, oliguria following the administration of double doses of oral cholecystographic agents has been reported often enough that a sequential relationship may reasonably be suspected.

Summary

Tubular necrosis of the kidney and death following ingestion of two 4.5 gm doses of a cholecystographic agent, bunamiodyl, is reported. Mechanisms to account for the toxicity of widely used contrast media in this and five similar cases are proposed.

Ronald A. Malt, Department of Surgery, Massachusetts General Hospital, Boston 14, Mass.

Addendum

Additional cases of renal failure after ingestion of large doses of bunamiodyl have recently been reported by Setter, Maher, and Schreiner.[7]

REFERENCES

1. Blythe, W. B., and Woods, J. W.: Acute Renal Insufficiency After Ingestion of a Gall-Bladder Dye: Report of a Case, New Eng J Med 264:1045-1046, 1961.

2. Finkelstein, R., and Jacobi, M.: Fatal Iodine Poisoning: Clinicopathologic and Experimental Study, Ann Intern Med 10:1283-1296, 1936.

3. Gottlieb, A.; Spiera, H.; and Gordis, E.: Fatal Renal Insufficiency After Oral Cholecystography, New Eng J Med 267:389-392, 1962.

4. Modell, W.: Pharmacology of β(3,5 di-iodo-4-hydroxyphenyl)α-phenyl propionic acid, J Lab Clin Med 27:1376-1384, 1942.

5. Miller, S. A., Department of Nutrition, Massachusetts Institute of Technology: Personal communication to the author.

6. Rene, R. M., and Mellinkoff, S. M.: Renal Insufficiency After Oral Administration of Double Dose of Cholecystographic Medium: Report of Two Cases, New Eng J Med 261:589-592, 1959.

7. Setter, J. G.; Maher, J. F.; and Schreiner, G. E.: Acute Renal Failure Following Cholecystography, JAMA 184:102-110, 1963.

Regional Lymph Node Dissection and Malignant Melanoma

Effect on Survival

WILLIAM E. PRICE, MD
AND
MERLIN K. DuVAL, JR., MD
OKLAHOMA CITY

The biological behavior of malignant melanoma is so ubiquitous that the outcome, in any given instance, may bear no predictable relationship to the choice of therapy. This paradox is especially evident when one considers that the primary lesion, when on the skin, is ordinarily readily accessible to inspection and palpation and, therefore, should lend itself to effective eradication at an early stage. Until such time as our knowledge of cellular chemistry permits a chemotherapeutic attack on the disease, the surgeon is obliged to pursue a vigorous course of extirpative therapy that can accomplish no more than physical separation of the disease from the host, in one "region" of the body.

While there is uniform agreement that wide regional excision of melanoma is the basis of primary treatment, there is a considerable divergence of opinion on two points. 1) How "wide" is wide surgical excision, and 2) what is the role of the regional lymph nodes? The review which follows does not concern itself with the first of these controversies, except indirectly, but was done to determine whether or not prognosis was affected by regional lymph node excision.

Many authors have stated that regional lymph node dissection is an essential part of the primary therapy of melanoma [4,8-11] as long as the nodes are in a predictable and accessible location. Others have not been convinced that regional node dissection enhances the prognosis over that which follows adequate radical excision of the melanoma itself, in those instances in which the regional lymph nodes are not clinically involved with tumor.[5,7,12] They emphasize particularly that tumor cells travel slowly through the lymphatics and, therefore, regional dissection of the nodes cannot hope to arrest the spread of the tumor by this route, especially if the dissection is accomplished out of continuity with the primary lesion.

In order to confine our study specifically to this question, we have reviewed all cases of malignant melanoma of the skin of an extremity seen at the University of Oklahoma Hospitals between Jan 1, 1941, and Dec 31, 1957. By confining the study to extremity lesions, the "regional" nodes were both predictable and accessible to examination and removal.

Case Material

The charts and records of all patients seen at the University of Oklahoma Hospitals between Jan 1, 1941, and Dec 31, 1957, with a proven diagnosis of malignant melanoma arising on an extremity, were reviewed. There were 70 cases seen in this period of time. Fig 1 illustrates the age distribution of this series, which was 3 to 84 years with peak incidence in the sixth decade. The single prepubescent lesion is included since it not only recurred locally, after its removal, but also metastasized, thus differentiating itself from the usual juvenile melanoma which has been so well described by Allen and Spitz.[1] There were 27 males (39%) and 43 females (61%). Sixty patients were white, nine were Negroes, and one was Indian. Forty-four of the

Submitted for publication April 15, 1963.

From the Department of Surgery, The University of Oklahoma Medical Center.

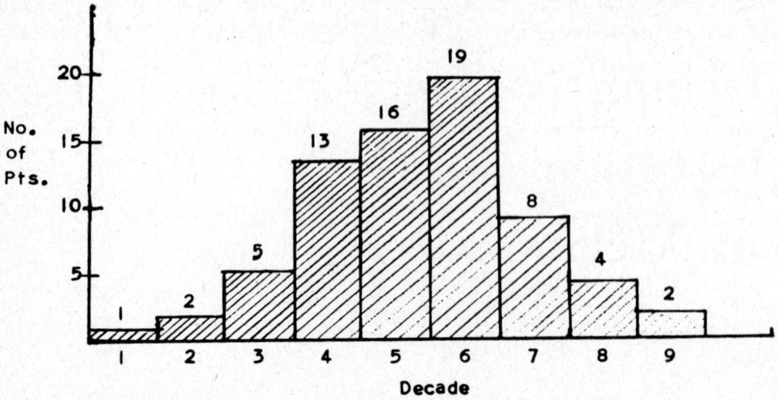

Fig 1.—Age distribution observed among 70 patients with malignant melanoma of an extremity.

melanomas occurred in the lower extremity, and 26 in the upper extremity (Table 1).

Twenty patients were categorically excluded from this study because they had distant metastases (beyond the regional nodes) when first admitted to our hospital. The 50 remaining form the study group. All were categorized according to the presence or absence of clinical evidence of involvement of the regional lymph nodes prior to their undergoing extirpative surgery for this primary tumor. Follow-up data have been secured in all instances.

TABLE 1.—*Correlation of Age, Sex, and Location of Melanoma With Survival* *

	Incidence, 70 Patients	Survival, 18.5%
Age, yr	3-84	3-74
Sex	27 M (38.6%)	5 M (38.5%)
	43 F (61.4%)	8 F (61.5%)
Upper extremities	26 (37.1%)	7 (26.9%)
Lower extremities	44 (62.9%)	6 (13.7%)

* This table includes the 20 patients who were incurable when first seen.

Findings

There have been 13 survivors, without evidence of recurrent melanoma, in this series, ie, 26% for those treated, and 18.5% for all. The mean duration of survival since the institution of treatment in these 13 patients is 7.3 years. Table 1 correlates survival with the location of the primary tumor and age and sex of the patient. Note that eight were female and five male, the same ratio as the incidence of the disease in this series. Similarly, there were eleven whites and two Negroes among the survivors, also the same incidence as the disease itself, in this series. The prognosis seemed somewhat better among those with upper extremity tumors, ie, 26.9% as opposed to 13.7% for the lower extremity, including those cases that were incurable when first seen.

Fig 2 summarizes the data relative to survival, regional lymph node involvement, and

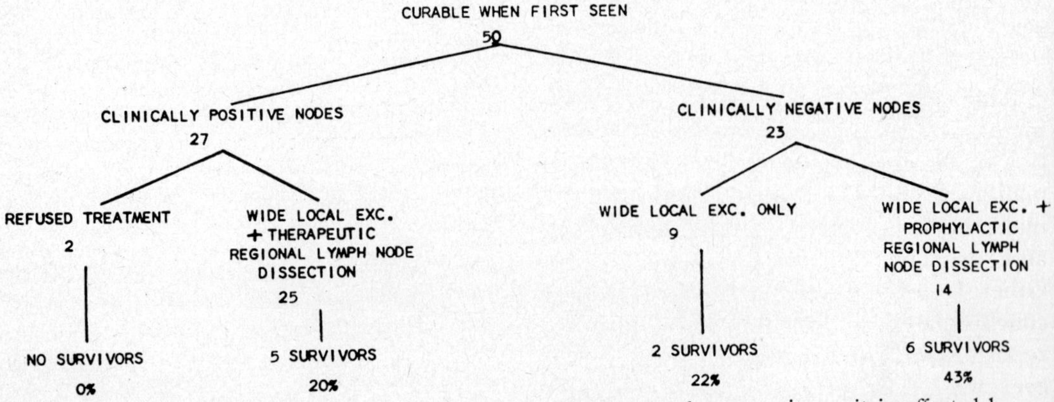

Fig 2.—Summary chart of the prognosis of melanoma on the extremity as it is affected by regional lymph node involvement in the 50 patients, curable when seen, in our study.

surgical dissection among the 50 patients who were not incurable when first seen. These findings may be summarized as follows:

Lymph Nodes Clinically Involved.—Twenty-seven patients (54%) demonstrated clinical evidence of involvement of the lymph nodes draining the extremity when they were first seen. Two of these patients refused any treatment whatsoever, and both died of metastatic melanoma. The other 25 underwent wide, local surgical excision of the primary tumor and radical, "therapeutic" resection of the involved regional lymph nodes. There were no operative deaths. Five of these patients have survived and are living and well, without evidence of recurrent disease (20%). Histologically, the involvement of these regional nodes was confirmed in 24 of the 25 patients.

Lymph Nodes Not Clinically Involved.—There were 23 patients (46%) who had no clinical evidence of involvement of the regional lymph nodes at the time they underwent treatment of their primary tumor. Nine of these underwent wide local excision of the primary tumor only, two of whom have remained well, without evidence of recurrent melanoma (22%). Fourteen were subjected to "prophylactic" dissection of the regional lymph nodes in addition to wide local excision of the primary tumor, six of whom have survived, free of tumor to this follow-up (43%). It is of particular interest that, histologically, none of the lymph nodes examined in these 14 patients showed involvement with tumor.

Comment

Although some reports fail to indicate an increased survival rate after surgical resection of the regional lymph nodes in cases of malignant melanoma, such reports generally make no distinction between "therapeutic" and "prophylactic" lymph node dissection.[3,6] Other reviews merely state that a definite conclusion cannot be drawn.[5,7,12] In those reports that do make this distinction, however, the results seem to be significant. Table 2 summarizes some of them. Note that Da-

TABLE 2.—*Effect of "Prophylactic" Resection of Regional Lymph Nodes on Survival in the Absence of Clinical Involvement, as Reported in the Literature*

Series	Wide Local Excision Only, % Survivors	Wide Local Excision + Prophylactic Regional Lymph Node Dissection, % Survivors
Daland	45	72
Pack	34	40
Block & Hartwell	38	50
University Hospital	22	43

land reports an increase of 27% in the survival rate when prophylactic regional node dissection is added to wide local excision of the tumor.[4] Block and Hartwell recorded a 12% increase in survival,[2] and Pack, 6% among the relatively small portion of his total series studied with respect to this question.[10]

Our observations at the University of Oklahoma Hospitals indicate that for melanoma of the extremity, if there is clinical evidence of regional lymph node involvement, the prognosis will not exceed 20%-25% even if these nodes are surgically extirpated along with the primary tumor. This should not be interpreted as an argument against the surgical removal of regional lymph nodes that are clinically involved, since there are no figures available to indicate that wide local excision of the primary tumor alone will give the same prognosis even if the regionally involved nodes are not treated. Rather, it should be interpreted as an expression of the seriousness of the disease itself.

More important, perhaps, is the question of what to do about the patient who demonstrates no clinical evidence of involvement of the regional lymph nodes in the presence of a melanoma of the extremity. In this group, our experience supports the view that prophylactic removal of these regional lymph nodes increases survival by approximately 20%. Further, in our own series, this appears to be true even though these prophylactically extirpated nodes were not histologically involved with tumor. It is impossible, of course, to present a rational explanation for this observation, although it has been noted by others as well, with the conjecture that regional lymph node dissection has the effect of imposing a fibrous and lymph-stasis "barrier" between the primary site and the rest of the body, thereby trapping the disease in the extremity.

There are other factors involved in the treatment of melanoma that have not been adequately evaluated. Chief among these are the histologic characteristics of melanoma with respect to the degree of local invasion, frequency of mitotic figures, etc, which have been credited with bearing a relationship to the biological nature of the tumor. While further conclusions with regard to the best program of therapy for melanoma will need elucidation of such factors, in the meantime, it would seem that the prognosis may be enhanced by removing uninvolved regional lymph nodes prophylactically.

Summary and Conclusions

The records of 70 patients with malignant melanoma of the extremity seen at the University of Oklahoma Hospitals from 1941 through 1957 have been reviewed.

Twenty of the patients were incurable when first seen.

Twenty-seven patients had clinical evidence of involved regional lymph nodes (54%). The survival rate in this group was 20% after regional lymph node dissection and wide local excision of the primary tumor.

Twenty-three patients had no clinical evidence of involvement of the regional lymph nodes (46%). Survival in this group was 22% after wide, local excision and 43% after wide local excision plus prophylactic removal of the regional lymph nodes.

It is concluded that removal of the regional lymph nodes in patients with malignant melanoma of an extremity enhances the survival by approximately 20%.

Merlin K. DuVal, Jr., MD, Department of Surgery, The University of Oklahoma Medical Center, 800 NE 13th St, Oklahoma City 4, Okla.

REFERENCES

1. Allen, A. C., and Spitz, S.: Malignant Melanoma, Cancer, 6:1, 1953.

2. Block, G. E., and Hartwell, S. W.: Malignant Melanoma: A Study of 217 Cases, Ann Surg 154: 74, 1961.

3. Catlin, D.: Melanomas of the Skin of the Head and Neck, Ann Surg 140:796, 1954.

4. Daland, E. M.: Malignant Melanoma: Personal Experience With 170 Cases, New Eng J Med 260:453, 1959.

5. Johnson, R. E.: Occult Lymphatic Metastases in Malignant Melanoma of the Skin, Ann Surg 146:931, 1957.

6. Kragh, L. V., and Erich, J. B.: Malignant Melanomas of the Head and Neck, Ann Surg 151: 91, 1960.

7. Lund, R. H., and Ihnen, M.: Malignant Melanoma: Clinical and Pathologic Analysis of 93 Cases; Is Prophylactic Lymph Node Dissection Indicated? Surgery 38:652, 1955.

8. McCune, W. S., and Letterman, G. S.: Malignant Melanoma: Ten-Year Results Following Excisonal and Regional Gland Resection, Ann Surg 141:901, 1955.

9. Meyer, H. W., and Gumport, S. L.: Malignant Melanoma: Appraisal of the Disease and Analysis of 105 Cases, Ann Surg 138:643, 1955.

10. Pack, G. T.: End Results in the Treatment of Malignant Melanoma: A Later Report, Surgery 46:447, 1959.

11. Royster, H. P., and Baker, L. M.: The Management of Malignant Melanoma, Ann Surg 145:888, 1957.

12. Vogler, W. R.; Garland, D. P.; and Wilkins, S. A.: A Clinical Evaluation of Malignant Melanoma, Surg Gynec Obstet 108:586, 1958.

Iron Metabolism After Portacaval Shunt in Dogs

CAPT R. C. DOBERNECK, MC, USAR
CAPT DANIEL B. NUNN, MC, USAR
CAPT DALE G. JOHNSON, MC, USAR
AND
B. K. CHUN, MD
MINNEAPOLIS

Recent reports suggest that iron metabolism is altered after surgically induced portacaval shunting in patients with cirrhosis. These reports show that after such shunting extensive parenchymal deposition of stainable iron takes place.[1,4-8] Other reports clearly show that such iron deposition occurs in the absence of surgically induced portacaval shunting in patients with cirrhosis[3] and consequently the exact role played by the shunt remains unknown. This study was made to elucidate the role of the portacaval shunt in the metabolism of iron.

Method

Seventeen healthy adult dogs underwent liver biopsy and construction of an end-to-side portacaval shunt.* All animals were anesthetized with pentobarbital sodium, 25 mg/kg of body weight. The portal vein was divided on the hepatic side of the entry of the cephalic gastroduodenal vein into the portal system so that the entire portal blood flow was diverted into the inferior vena cava. The dogs were followed for the duration of life after portacaval shunting. During that period no medication of any sort was given, and a diet consisting solely of adequate amounts of Ralston Purina dog chow and water was consumed. Autopsy was performed on all dogs after death. At autopsy all shunts were widely patent and portal collaterals

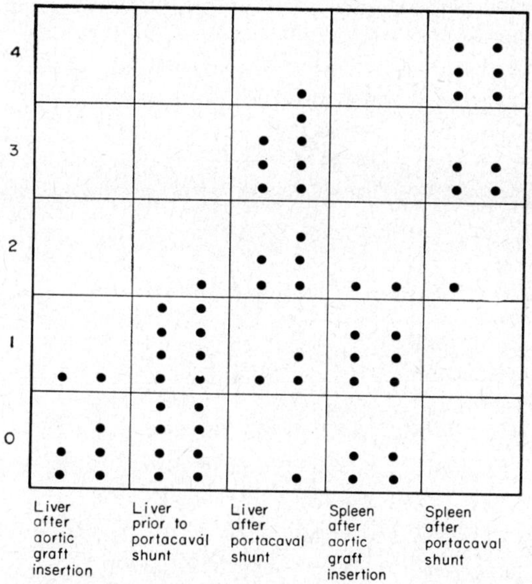

Fig 1.—Scattergram illustrates the grades assigned to sections of liver before and after portacaval shunting and after aortic grafting, and spleen after portacaval shunting and aortic grafting. Each circle represents one dog.

Table 1.—*Amount of Iron in Spleen and Liver at Autopsy in Dogs After Abdominal Aortic Grafting, Graded 0-4*

Dog No.	Survival, Wk	Spleen	Liver
1	2	0	—
2	2	0	0
3	4	1	0
4	4	1	0
5	6	1	0
6	6	1	1
7	13	0	—
8	13	2	1
9	13	2	—
10	13	0	—
11	26	1	—
12	26	1	0
Av	10.8	0.8	0.3

Submitted for publication April 6, 1963.

From the Department of Experimental Surgery, Walter Reed Army Institute of Research, Washington 12, DC.

The illustrations are US Army Photographs (ANWSO).

* The principles of laboratory animal care as promulgated by the National Society for Medical Research were observed.

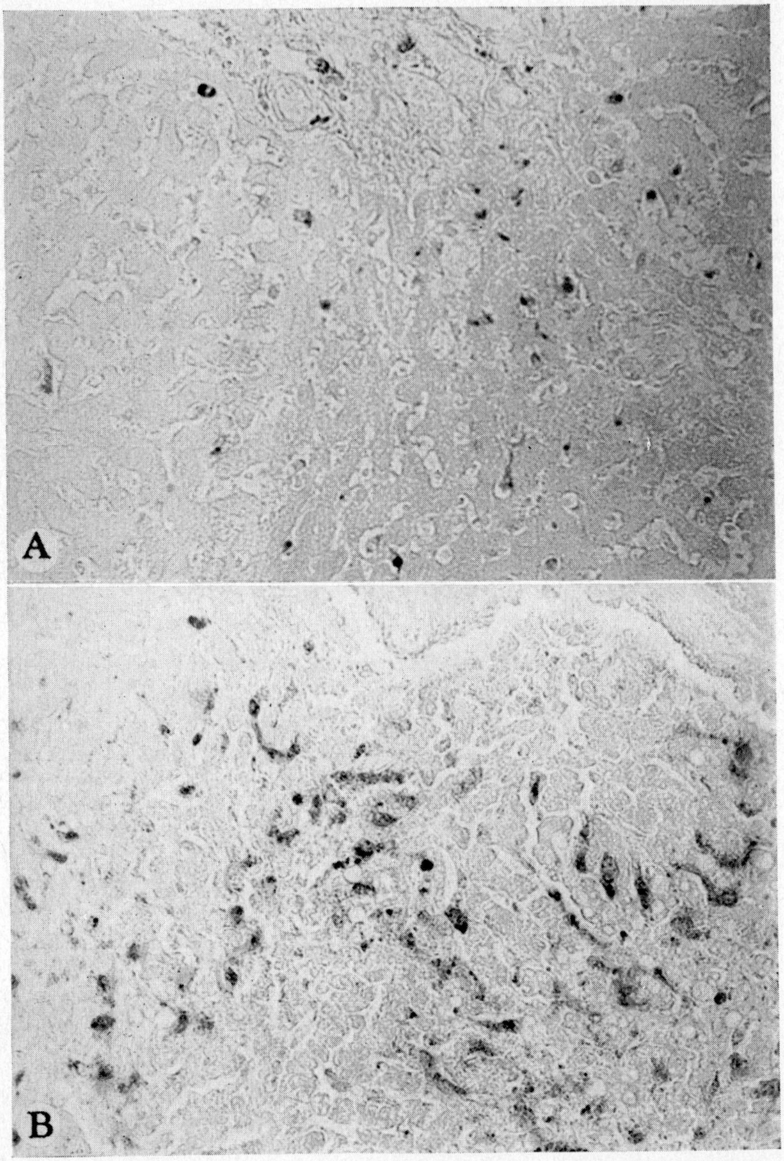

Fig 2.—*A*, photomicrograph of liver obtained prior to portacaval shunting. Note the minimal amount of stainable iron which appears black. Grade 1. Potassium ferrocyanide; reduced 8% from mag × 150; *B*, photomicrograph of liver obtained from the same dog two months after portacaval shunting. Note the increased amount of stainable iron which appears black. Grade 3. Potassium ferrocyanide; reduced 8% from mag × 150.

to the liver were absent. Autopsy specimens for microscopical examination were obtained from spleen, adrenal gland, pancreas, and duodenum in addition to several areas of liver. All specimens were fixed in 10% buffered formalin and stained with both potassium ferrocyanide for iron and hematoxylin and eosin. All sections were graded as to the amount of stainable iron present on a basis of 0 to 4, the higher figure indicating the presence of more stainable iron. The sections of liver obtained at autopsy were then compared to those obtained at operation.

In order to eliminate the nonspecific effects of anesthesia and operative trauma on iron metabolism, specimens of liver and spleen were obtained at autopsy from dogs which had had insertion of abdominal aortic grafts. These specimens were fixed and stained and the sections were graded in the same manner as those from dogs which had had construction of portacaval shunts. The sections obtained at autopsy from both groups of dogs were also compared. The survival after operation was similar in both groups of dogs.

Results

Only two of seven sections obtained at autopsy from the livers of dogs which had had insertion of abdominal aortic grafts were graded 1; the remaining five sections were graded 0. The average grade was 0.3. Only

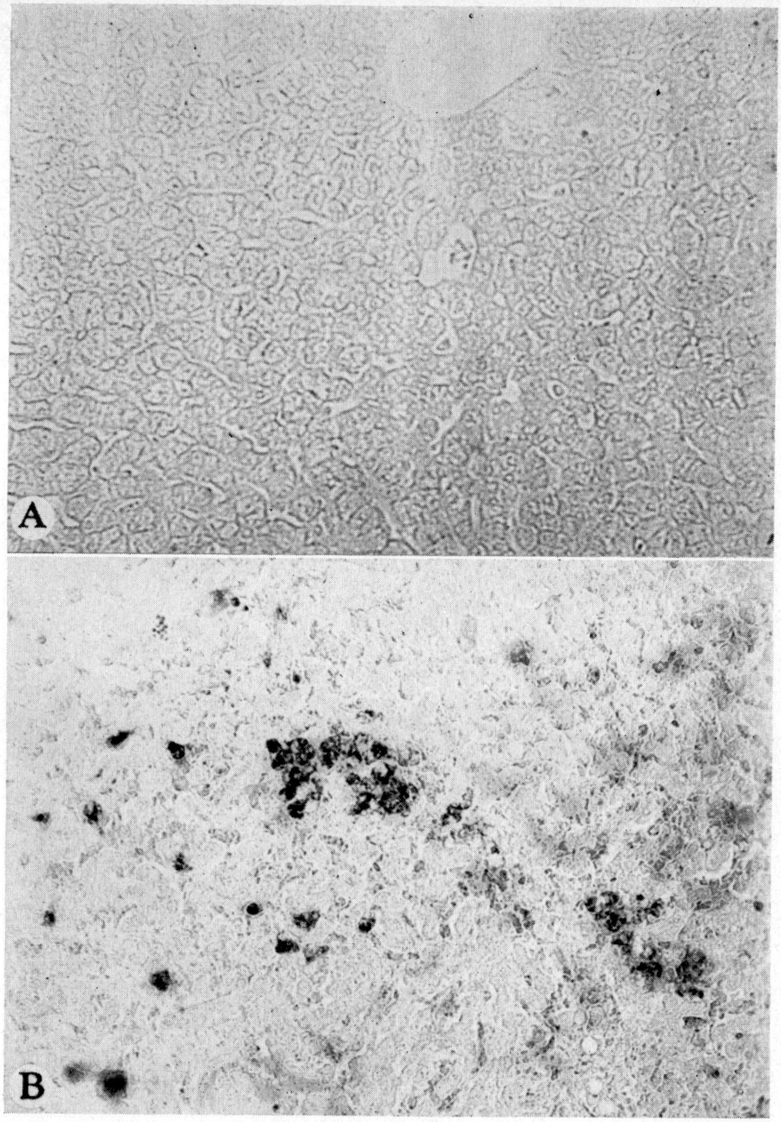

Fig 3.—*A,* photomicrograph of liver obtained prior to portacaval shunting. Note the lack of stainable iron. Grade 0. Potassium ferrocyanide; reduced 8% from mag × 150. *B,* photomicrograph of liver obtained from the same dog two months after portacaval shunting. Note the increased amount of stainable iron which appears black. Grade 3. Potassium ferrocyanide; reduced 8% from mag × 150.

TABLE 2.—*Amount of Iron in Liver and Spleen of Dogs Before and After Portacaval Shunting, Graded 0-4*

Dog No.	Survival, Wk	Liver at Operation	Liver at Autopsy	Spleen at Autopsy
1	5	0	2	3
2	5	1	2	3
3	6	1	2	—
4	6	0	3 *	—
5	7	0	3	4
6	7	0	0 †	3
7	8	1	2	—
8	8	1	4 ‡	—
9	8	1	1 ‡†	—
10	8	1	3 ‡	4
11	8	0	3	—
12	9	0	3 ‡	—
13	10	2	3	4
14	12	0	2 ‡	4
15	13	1	3	3
16	13	1	1 †	4
17	16	0	1 ‡	2
Av	8.5	0.6	2.2	3.5

* Severe fatty change.
† Severe postmortem autolysis.
‡ Minimal fatty change.

two of 12 sections obtained at autopsy from the spleens of these dogs were graded 2; the remaining ten sections were graded 0 or 1. The average grade was 0.8 (Table 1, Fig 1). Only one of 17 control sections of liver obtained at operation at the time of portacaval shunting was graded 2. All remaining sections were graded 0 or 1; the average grade was 0.6 (Table 2, Fig 1).

In contrast to the grades assigned the sections obtained from the aortic graft dogs at autopsy and those obtained from the portacaval shunt dogs at operation, were the grades assigned the sections obtained from the portacaval shunt dogs at autopsy. Thirteen of 17 sections of liver obtained at autopsy from the dogs which had had portacaval shunting were graded 2 or greater. The average grade was 2.2, and the sections

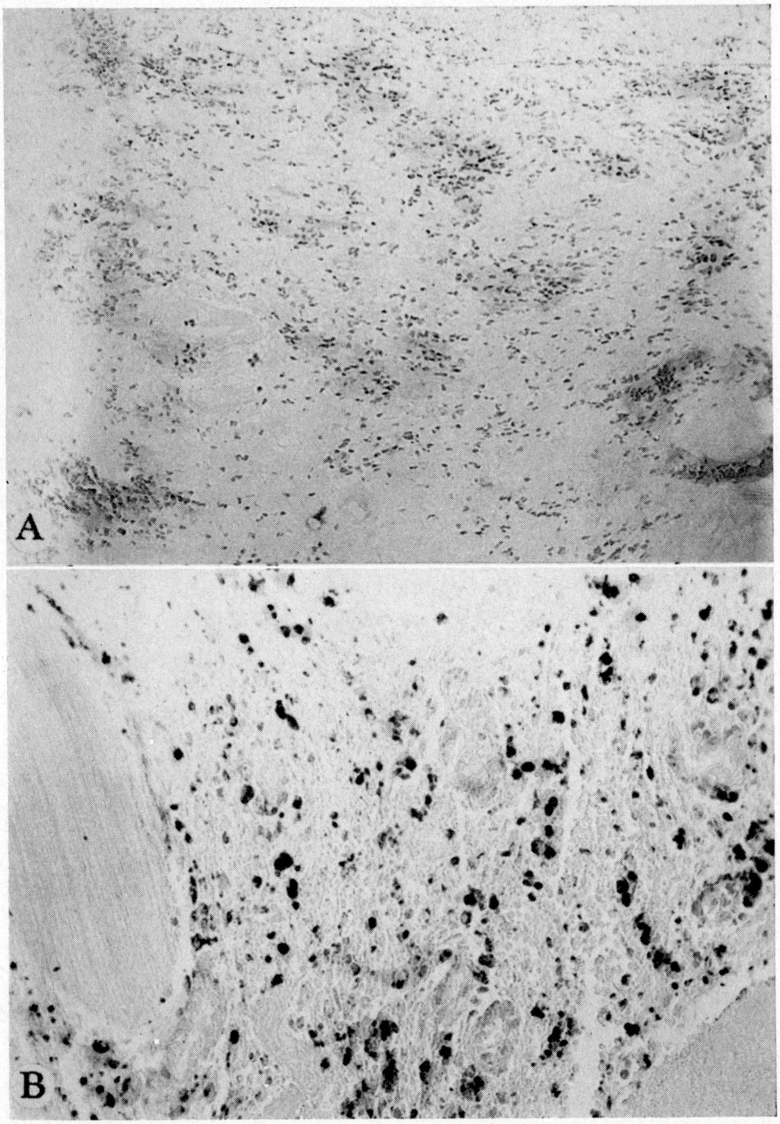

Fig 4.—*A*, photomicrograph of spleen obtained three months after aortic grafting. Note the lack of stainable iron. Grade 0. The small cells which appear darker than the surrounding areas are erythrocytes. Potassium ferrocyanide; reduced 8% from mag × 150. *B*, photomicrograph of spleen obtained three months after portacaval shunting. Note the large amount of stainable iron which appears black. Grade 4. Potassium ferrocyanide; reduced 8% from mag × 150.

of liver from 14 of the 17 dogs were assigned a higher grade at autopsy than at operation. The increases ranged from 1 to 3 grades (Table 2, Fig 1-3). Ten of 11 sections of spleen obtained at autopsy from the dogs which had had portacaval shunting were graded 3 or greater, and the remaining section was graded 2. The average grade was 3.5 (Table 2, Fig 1-4).

In all instances stainable iron was found in both parenchymal and reticuloendothelial cells although the latter contained the greater amount. The amount of stainable iron appeared to have no relation to either the duration of survival or to the presence of fatty hepatic change after portacaval shunting. Fatty change of varying degrees after shunting occurred in only seven of 17 dogs. The three dogs which failed to show an increase in the amount of stainable hepatic iron were the only animals which had severe postmortem autolysis.

Three of 11 sections of adrenal gland and two of 12 sections of pancreas obtained at autopsy from the dogs which had had portacaval shunting were graded 1; all the remaining sections of adrenal and pancreas and all sections of duodenum obtained at autopsy were graded 0.

Comment

The results of this study clearly indicate that the amount of stainable iron in both liver and spleen is increased after portacaval shunting and suggest that iron metabolism is altered after such shunting. The amount of stainable iron in both liver and spleen may be increased by either increased absorption [6] or by a transfer of iron from other sites.[2] This study gives no direct information regarding iron absorption or transfer. Conceivably, a change in the state of the pre-existing unstainable iron in these tissues may occur after shunting so that such iron merely becomes stainable.

The precise mechanism whereby these changes occur after portacaval shunting is unknown, but either the profound metabolic alterations due to the lack of portal blood flow to the liver or the lack of portal blood flow itself after portacaval shunting may be responsible for an increased absorption [6] or a transfer of iron from erythrocytes to the liver and spleen.[2] Future studies of iron absorption and transfer after portacaval shunting are planned.

Since the survival periods of these dogs is not of sufficient duration and since their iron intakes after shunting are not excessive, increased iron absorption cannot be the sole explanation for the presence of increased amounts of stainable iron in the livers and spleens. The transfer of iron to the liver and spleen from erythrocytes is also probably operative after portacaval shunting. Such transfer is known to occur in certain forms of anemia, both hemolytic and nonhemolytic.[2] Hemolysis alone is not responsible since in that condition stainable iron is found almost exclusively in the reticuloendothelial cells,[2] whereas the stainable iron is found in both the hepatic parenchymal and reticuloendothelial cells of dogs after portacaval shunting. This study gives no direct information concerning the presence or absence of a nonhemolytic anemia in dogs after portacaval shunting, and, therefore, a nonhemolytic anemia cannot be excluded.

Finally, whatever may be the mechanism of the presence of increased amounts of stainable iron in the livers of dogs after portacaval shunting, liver damage is not responsible since no relation exists between the amount of stainable iron and the presence or absence of fatty hepatic change. If, in fact, the amount of hepatic iron is increased after portacaval shunting and if iron is toxic to the hepatic parenchymal cell, an additional explanation for the deterioration of liver function occasionally observed after portacaval shunting in the cirrhotic patient is apparent. Similarly, the presence of stainable iron in the livers of cirrhotic patients may be due to spontaneous portacaval shunting, and the lack of stainable iron due to the lack of spontaneous shunting.

Summary

A marked increase in the amount of stainable iron was found in sections of liver obtained at autopsy from 14 of 17 dogs after portacaval shunting when compared to those obtained prior to shunting. Sections of both liver and spleen obtained at autopsy from dogs after portacaval shunting consistently had greater amounts of stainable iron than those obtained at autopsy from dogs after aortic grafting with comparable survival periods. The increased amount of stainable iron was not attributable to anesthesia, nonspecific trauma of operation, hemolysis, excessive iron intake, or liver damage alone. The results suggested that the integrity of the portal blood flow to the liver was essential for the normal metabolism of iron.

Raymond C. Doberneck, MD, University of Minnesota Hospital, Minneapolis 14, Minn.

REFERENCES

1. Hoffbauer, F. W.: Primary Biliary Cirrhosis: Observations on the Natural Course of the Disease in 25 Women, Amer J Dig Dis 5:348, 1960.

2. Kent, G., and Popper, H.: Secondary Hemochromatosis: Its Association With Anemia, Arch Path 70:623, 1960.

3. MacDonald, R. A., and Mallory, G. K.: Hemochromatosis and Hemosiderosis, Arch Intern Med 105:686, 1960.

4. Popper, H., and Schaffner, F.: The Liver and Its Diseases, Gastroenterology 40:536, 1961.

5. Schaefer, J. W.; Amick, J.; Oikawa, Y.; and Schiff, L.: The Development of Hemochromatosis Following Portacaval Anastomosis, Gastroenterology 42:181, 1962.

6. Sherlock, S., and Turner, M. D.: Liver Disease, Gastroenterology 42:612, 1962.

7. Tisdale, W. A.: Parenchymal Siderosis in Patients With Cirrhosis After Portasystemic-Shunt Surgery, New Eng J Med 265:928, 1961.

8. Tuttle, S. G.; Figueroa, W. G.; and Grossman, M. I.: Development of Hemochromatosis in a Patient With Laennec's Cirrhosis, Amer J Med 26:655, 1959.

CALL FOR PAPERS, SCIENTIFIC EXHIBITS, AND MOTION PICTURES FOR THE 113TH ANNUAL MEETING OF THE AMERICAN MEDICAL ASSOCIATION, SAN FRANCISCO, JUNE 21-25, 1964

Those who desire to present scientific papers before the Sections of the Scientific Assembly should communicate with the Secretary of the appropriate Section (see list below) well in advance of the *deadline date, Dec 15, 1963.*

Those who wish to apply for space in the Scientific Exhibit should request application forms from the Representative to the Scientific Exhibit of the appropriate Section (see list below) or from the Director, Scientific Exhibit, Department of Scientific Assembly, American Medical Association, 535 N Dearborn St, Chicago 10, well in advance of the *deadline date for receipt of applications, Jan 10, 1964.*

Those who desire to present motion pictures should request application forms from the Director, Medical Motion Pictures and Television, Department of Scientific Assembly, American Medical Association, 535 N Dearborn St, Chicago 10, well in advance of the *deadline date, Jan 10, 1964.*

Section	Secretary	Representative to the Scientific Exhibit
Anesthesiology	Kenneth K. Keown, MD University of Missouri Medical Center Columbia, Mo.	Donald E. Hale, MD 2020 East 93rd St. Cleveland 6, Ohio
Diseases of the Chest	Howard S. Van Ordstrand, MD 2020 East 93rd St. Cleveland 6, Ohio	Edwin R. Levine, MD 111 N. Wabash Ave. Chicago 2, Ill.
Gastroenterology	Lloyd G. Bartholomew, MD 200 1st St., S.W. Rochester, Minn.	Arthur P. Klotz, MD University of Kansas Medical Center Kansas City, Kansas
Orthopedic Surgery	John C. Wilson, Jr., MD 2010 Wilshire Blvd. Los Angeles 57, Calif.	E. Burke Evans, MD 815 Avenue C Galveston, Texas
Proctology	Norman D. Nigro, MD 7815 E. Jefferson Ave. Detroit, Mich.	Willard H. Bernhoft, MD 2900 Main St. Buffalo, N.Y.
Radiology	Clyde A. Stevenson, MD Sacred Heart Hospital West 101 Eighth Ave. Spokane 4, Wash.	Richard H. Chamberlain, MD 3400 Spruce St. Philadelphia 4, Pa.
General Surgery	Blaise F. Alfano, MD 663 Main St. Melrose 76, Mass.	Charles H. Lupton, MD Suite 515 Wainwright Bldg. 229 W. Bute St. Norfolk 10, Va.
Urology	Myron H. Nourse, MD 1711 N. Capitol Indianapolis 7, Ind.	Charles Rieser, MD Emory University Clinic 1364 Clifton Road, N.E. Atlanta 22, Ga.

Parotid Gland as a Focus of Metastasis

JOHN CONLEY, MD
AND
SEBASTIAN ARENA, MD
NEW YORK

The involvement of the parotid gland by tumors other than those of a primary nature has certain curious and practical considerations. This involvement may result from metastasis into the lymph structures of the parenchyma of the gland, metastasis into the paraglandular lymph nodes, and also by direct invasion of the gland from an adjacent tumor. The histopathology covers a wide range of neoplasms with melanoma and squamous cell cancer predominating. The primary sites contributing to parotid gland involvement are predominantly the scalp and ear, but other regions in the head and neck must be considered as potential foci. The significance of this analysis reflects on the application of surgery to the parotid gland for obvious metastatic disease of the gland, for presumptive metastasis to the gland, or as a perimeter of normal tissue about neoplasms that are proximal to the parotid gland.

Submitted for publication April 6, 1963.

From Head and Neck Department, Pack Medical Group and Department of Otolaryngology, Columbia Presbyterian Medical Center.

Anatomy

The character of the lymph system throughout the parenchyma of the parotid gland and in the immediate paraglandular area is considerably more abundant than has been illustrated (Fig 1). Illustrations showing a few large lymph nodes in the tail of the parotid gland are misrepresentative. The gland contains from 20 to 30 lymph follicles and lymph nodes connected with a rich interlacing network for lymph vessels. Lymph entrance into the gland may be direct without involvement of the paraglandular lymph nodes, may be secondarily deposited from a paraglandular lymph node, or may contami-

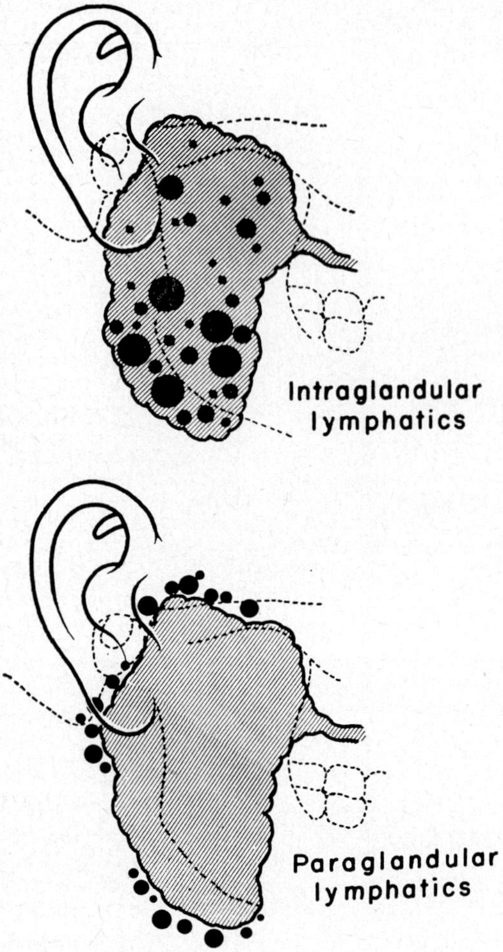

Fig 1.—Distribution of lymph nodes in and about the parotid gland.

nate the system by retrograde extension from massive metastases in the neck.

Paraglandular lymphatics are particularly abundant in the pre- and supratragal area, and this is a favorite depot for spread from the temple, scalp, and ear. Other lymph nodes are in association with the lateral, posterior, deep, and inferior portions of the gland. The anterior portion of the gland is rarely involved as a metastatic focus by either parenchymal or paraglandular lymph nodes.

Clinical Data

Eighty-one cases of parotid gland involvement as a secondary extension of a malignant tumor were found in the files of the Pack Medical Group in the past ten years. It is not felt that this is the total volume, as filing for this particular category did not exist and it was necessary to search these cases from other cross indices. The accumulated data, however, present important criteria in relationship to the parotid gland as a metastatic focus for malignant tumors in the head and neck.

Involvement of the parotid gland by invasion or spread by metastasis from malignant tumors in the head and neck is uncommon, with the exception of melanoma of the temple, scalp, and ear and anaplastic squamous cell cancer of the ear and ear canal. In an analysis of 81 cases, the majority (45.7%) were involved with metastatic melanoma. This rather unusually high statistic derives from a group of 175 cases of melanoma of the head and neck, and unquestionably overbalances the data that would be seen in an average clinical practice. Of these, 37% are associated with squamous cell cancer and 17.3% with other types of malignant tumors.

The other types of malignant tumors that involve the parotid gland include six types of sarcomas originating in structures about the gland and extending into the gland. Three cylindromas of the ear canal invaded the gland. Two adenocarcinomas, one from the cheek and one from the thyroid, and one muco-epidermoid cancer spread into the intraglandular lymph nodes. An esthesioneuroblastoma metastasized to the paraglandular nodes and a basal cell cancer of the brow metastasized to the intraglandular nodes.

The site of involvement of the parotid gland showed a majority (40.7%) in the paraglandular nodes. This figure is influenced by the preponderance of melanoma again which has a predilection for the paraglandular lymph nodes. The intraglandular nodes were involved in 35.8%, and 23.5% invaded the parenchyma directly.

Melanoma

Of 37 cases of melanoma with parotid gland involvement, 70% involved the paraglandular lymph nodes. A review of melanoma of the temple and scalp characteristically revealed metastases to the pre- and supratragal nodes in over 80% of those cases. Intraglandular and parenchymal involvement was uncommon in this instance. Melanoma of the ear and postauricular area involved the paraglandular nodes at a lower level, extending from the tragus inferiorly under the lobule of the ear and along the posterior part of the parotid gland. Melanoma of the face may metastasize to the parotid gland before it is discoverable in the neck. Melanoma of the neck or palate may present bizarre spread to the parotid gland. One in-

TABLE 1.—*81 Cases According to Histologic Diagnosis*

Incidence

Histology	No.	Rate, %
Melanoma	37	45.7
Squamous-cell carcinoma	30	37.0
Other malignant tumors	14	17.3
Total	81	100.0

Determinate Group

Total	Histology	Free of Malignancy: 5 Yr & More	Free of Malignancy: Less Than 5 Yr	Living With Malignancy	Dead of Malignancy	Dead of Other Causes
37	Melanoma	3	8	2	21	3
30	Squamous-cell carcinoma	3	5	3	15	4
14	Other malignant tumors	1	3	3	5	2
	56 determinate cases: 7 + 8 + 41					

End Results

	Total Determinate Cases	5-Yr Cure: No.	5-Yr Cure: Rate, %
Melanoma	26	3	11.5
Squamous-cell carcinoma	21	3	14.3
Other malignant tumors	9	1	11.1
	56	7	

Definitive 5-yr cure rate: 7 of 56 determinate cases = 12.5%

teresting case of metastasis of melanoma to the intraglandular lymph nodes has never revealed a primary focus and is free of clinical disease three years postoperatively. In five instances, the intra- and paraglandular systems were involved by melanoma.

Squamous Cell Cancer

Metastatic squamous cell cancer in the parotid gland occurred in 30 cases (37%) and involved the intraglandular lymph nodes in 47% of the cases. This is in marked contrast to melanoma where metastasis was predominantly in the paraglandular system. The ear and postauricular sites (eight) and oral cavity (eight) were the dominant primary foci. The cheek and lip presented five cases with metastasis to the parotid gland. Only four cases came from the temple and scalp, and again it would appear that squamous cell cancer in this area does not metastasize as readily as melanoma to the lymph drainage bed at the parotid level. Large squamous cell cancers of the oral cavity and sinuses have a significant capacity to spread to the parotid gland. Hypopharyngeal and supralaryngeal cancers rarely involved the parotid gland, and when it did occur it was almost always associated with massive metastasis in the neck with retrograde extension.

Other Types of Cancer

Involvement of the parotid gland by contiguous spread comprises the smallest group of 14 cases, an incidence rate of 17.3%. Sarcomas of adjacent tissues with extension into the parotid region were the most common variety of tumor. The mandible (two), malar area (one), temple (one), submaxillary (one), and pretragal (one) were the specific primary sites in these instances. The cylindroma of the ear canal has a definite predilection to eventually, over a period of years, involve the parotid gland. In a large group of cases certain curiosities of spread will appear in the data. In this category

TABLE 2.—*81 Cases According to Site of Parotid Gland Involvement*

Incidence

Site	No.	Rate, %
Parotid parenchyma (by invasion or infiltration)	19	23.5
Intraglandular lymphatics (by metastasis)	29	35.8
Paraglandular lymph nodes (by metastasis)	33	40.7
Total	81	100.0

Determinate Group

Total	Site	Free of Malignancy: 5 Yr or More	Free of Malignancy: Less Than 5 Yr	Living With Malignancy	Dead of Malignancy	Dead of Other Causes
19	Parotid parenchyma	2	2	2	10	3
29	Intraglandular lymphatics	2	5	3	16	3
33	Paraglandular lymph nodes	3	9	3	15	3
	56 determinate cases: 7 + 8 + 41					

End Results

	Total Determinate Cases	5-Yr Cure: No.	5-Yr Cure: Rate, %
Parenchymal invasion	14	2	14.3
Intraglandular metastasis	21	2	9.5
Paraglandular metastasis	21	3	14.3
	56	7	

Definitive 5-year cure rate: 7 of 56 determinate cases = 12.5%

metastatic basal cell cancer of the brow and metastasis from a papillary cancer of the thyroid emphasize the unpredictable nature of tumor behavior in a small percentage of cases. The predominant type of involvement in this group was parenchymal.

TABLE 3.—*Melanoma Metastatic to Parotid Gland*

Site of Primary	No. Cases	Area of Parotid Involvement: Parenchyma	Area of Parotid Involvement: Intraglandular Lymphatics	Area of Parotid Involvement: Paraglandular Lymph Nodes
Skin of neck:				
Anterior	2	—	2	—
Posterior	1	—	—	1
Postauricular and upper posterior neck	2	1*	1*	—
Ear:				
External	5	1*	—	4
Canal	1	—	1	—
Skin of face:				
Pretragal	2	—	—	2
Brow	1	—	—	1
Cheek	1	—	1	—
Temple	16	—	2*	14
Scalp	4	—	1	3
Palate (hard & soft)	1	1	—	—
Occult	1	—	1	—
Totals	37	3	9	25

* Also metastasized to paraglandular lymph nodes.

TABLE 4.—*Squamous Cell Carcinoma Metastatic to Parotid Gland*

Site of Primary	No. Cases	Area of Parotid Involvement: Parenchyma	Intraglandular Lymphatics	Paraglandular Lymph Nodes
Ear:				
External	1	1	—	—
Canal	4	3 *	1 †	—
Middle	1	—	1 †	—
Postauricular	2	1	1	—
Scalp	1	—	1	—
Temple ‡	3	1	2	—
Cheek	3	1	1	1
Lip §	2	1	1	—
Tongue	1	—	—	1
Alveolus & mandible	2	—	—	2 ‖
Buccal mucosa	2	—	—	2 ‖
Floor of mouth	1	—	1	—
Tonsil & palate	2	—	1	1
Supralaryngeal	3	—	3	—
Maxilla	2	—	1	1
Totals	30	8	14	8

* One of this group also metastasized to intraglandular lymphatics.
† Also metastasized to paraglandular nodes.
‡ In one instance, primary lesion also involved tragus and ear.
§ In one case, primary lesion also involved nose, cheek, etc.
‖ Also infiltrated into parenchyma of gland.

Frequency of Sites

The primary focus and specific histopathology revealed general patterns of clinical and biological behavior (Fig 2.) Twenty-five cases originated in the temple and scalp, and 20 of these were melanoma. This highlights the relative frequency of melanoma at this site and its proclivity for paraglandular metastasis by rapid and diffuse spread throughout the lymph channels of the scalp to this first filtering depot.

Nineteen cases began in the ear, ear canal, and postauricular area and were divided between melanoma (eight), squamous cell cancer (eight), and other types (three). Malignant tumors about the ear readily involved the parotid system.

TABLE 5.—*Metastasis to Parotid Gland From Malignant Tumors of Various Histologic Pathology*

Histology Site of Primary	No. Cases	Area of Parotid Involvement: Parenchyma	Intraglandular Lymphatics	Paraglandular Lymph Nodes
Embryonic rhabdomyosarcoma, temple	1	1	—	—
Fibrochondromyxosarcoma, mandible	1	1	—	—
Spindle-cell sarcoma, submaxillary area	1	1	—	—
Fibrosarcoma,				
Cheek: pretragal	1	—	—	1
malar	1	—	1	—
Mandible	1	1	—	—
Adenocarcinoma,				
Thyroid (Anaplastic Adenocarcinoma)	1	1	—	—
Buccal mucosa	1	—	1	—
Cylindroma, ear canal	3	3	—	—
Basal-cell carcinoma, brow	1	—	1	—
Mucoepidermoid carcinoma, submaxillary gland	1	—	1	—
Esthesioneuroblastoma, nasal cavity	1	—	—	1
Totals	14	8	4	2

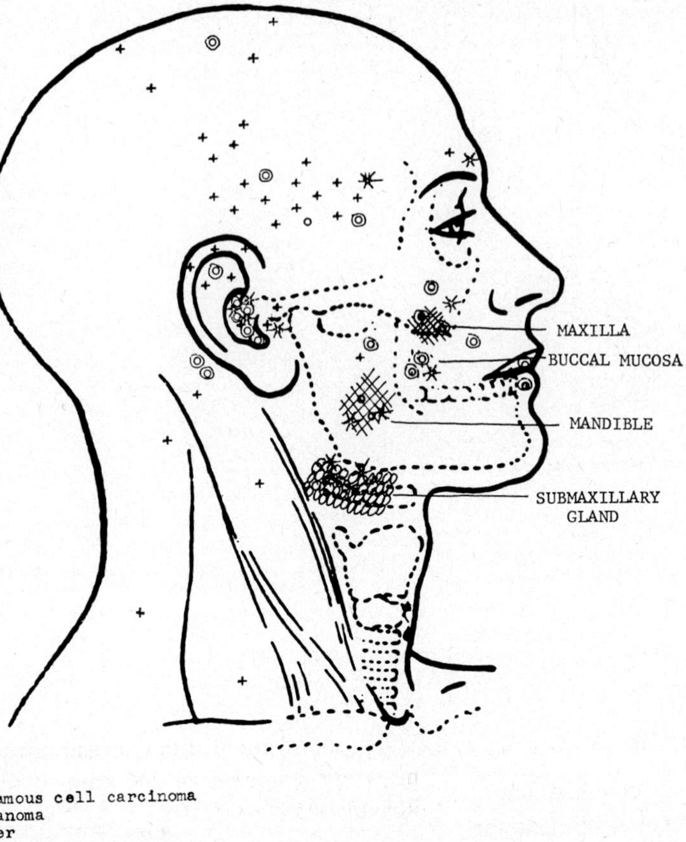

Fig 2.—Sites of primary neoplasms contributing to parotid gland involvement.

Tumors of the mucous membrane comprised 16 cases with a heavy preponderance of squamous cell cancer (13) (Fig 3). This emphasizes the phenomenon of direct or retrograde metastatic spread from the predominant variety of neoplasm of these sites. It also points out the relative infrequency of parotid involvement by squamous cell cancer originating in the head and neck in comparison with its proclivity for metastasis to the lateral neck.

The face and neck contributed 15 cases with spread to the parotid by direct metastasis. Melanoma occurred seven times and squamous cell cancer five times. The noninvasive melanoma of the face in females does not tend to metastasize, but the invasive type metastasizes to both parotid gland and neck. Squamous cell cancer of the face has a higher incidence of metastasis to the neck, but occasionally involves the parotid gland.

Treatment

The management of metastasis to the parotid gland is based on the adequate removal of the primary neoplasm, the parotid gland, and the lateral neck contents (Fig 1). In the majority of cases this can be carried out as an incontinuity operation, but there are obviously situations where incontinuity dissections are not applicable (eg, esthesioneuroblastoma, occult primary, etc) and where its application has limited biological significance (eg, brow, occiput, etc). In paraglandular metastasis the facial nerve is almost always preserved, unless the metastatic disease is massive in size. In intraglandular metastasis in the lateral lobe the facial nerve may be salvaged. Metastasis to the deep lobe of the parotid gland, massive involvement of the gland, and invasion of the gland require radical resection of the facial nerve system as part of the extirpative technique.

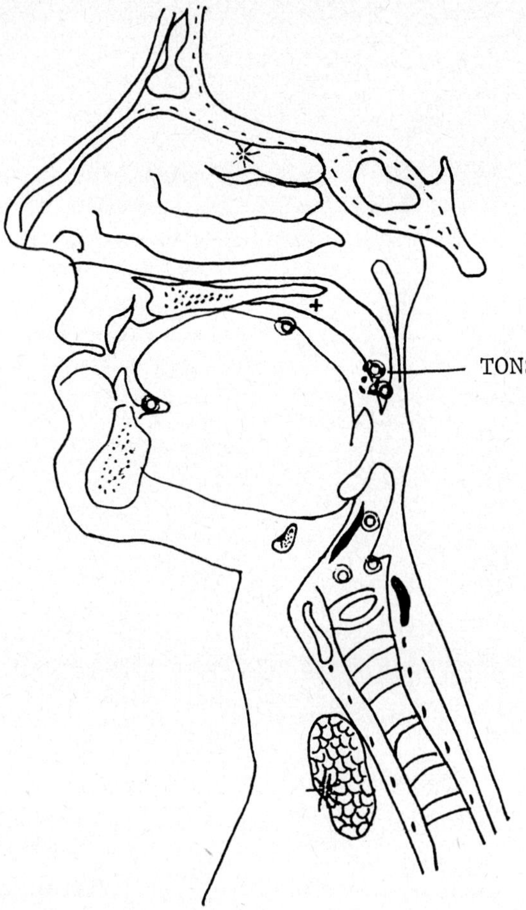

Fig 3.—Sites of primary neoplasms contributing to parotid gland involvement.

o = Squamous cell carcinoma
+ = Melanoma
✻ = Other

If the primary neoplasm has been treated previously, a decision must be made regarding the adequacy of the prior operation or irradiation administered. When there is doubt of cure or control of the primary neoplasm, its resection should be included with the parotid gland and neck dissection.

Inclusion of the tail of the parotid gland in radical neck dissection is rarely a therapeutic technique for the removal of possible metastatic lymph nodes at this site, but should be considered more as establishing an adequate cuff of normal tissue at this particular margin of the specimen. This extra cuff of parotid tissue is particularly desirable when there is massive metastasis in the neck with retrograde extension or when the subdigastric area is heavily involved. If there is a question of parotid involvement under these circumstances, it is preferable to do a total parotidectomy. The advisability of removing the tail of the parotid gland as a routine measure in all neck dissections is open to question.

Prognosis

Once the parotid gland has become a focus of metastasis in malignant tumors of the head and neck, the prognosis is grave. This is partially explained on the vicious nature of melanoma of the scalp that metastasizes to this area, the extensiveness and inaccessibility of some of the primary squamous cell

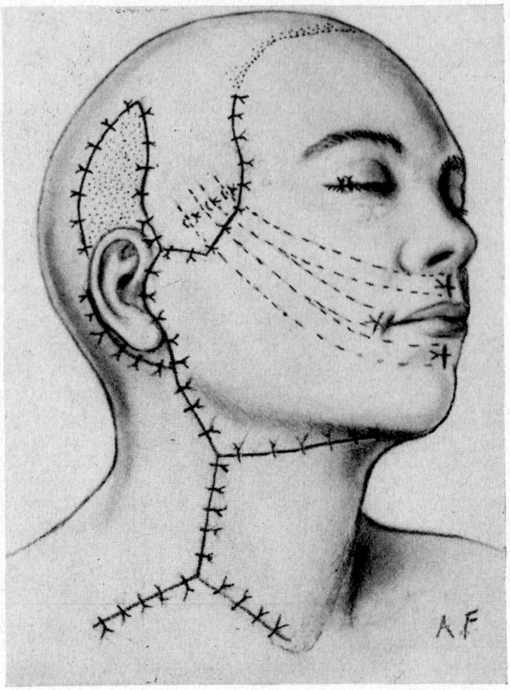

Fig 4.—Wound rehabilitation with transposed hair-bearing flap to the temple, free skin graft posteriorly, autogenosus facial nerve grafting, fascial stripping for face suspension, and tarsorrhaphy for eyelids.

cancers that contribute to this condition, the retrograde lymph spread associated with massive metastasis in the neck, and the technical difficulties and biological aggressiveness of many of the infiltrative somatic and epithelial tumors involving the parotid region. In some clinical respects metastasis to the parotid gland is an unpredictable behavior pattern and is often associated with other bizarre metastases.

The five year determinate cure rate was 11.5% for melanoma, 14.3% for squamous cell cancer, and 11.1% for other malignant tumors.

The five year determinate cure rate was 14.3% for parenchymal invasion, 9.4% for intraglandular metastasis, and 14.3% for paraglandular metastasis.

Histologically, squamous cell cancer enjoys a slightly better prognosis than other types of neoplasms. Anatomically intraglandular metastasis presents the most serious type of metastasis. The over-all cure rate was 12.5%.

Conclusions

The paraglandular lymph nodes are the frequent and common repository for metastasis of melanoma of the temple, scalp, and ear, 80%.

The intraglandular lymph nodes are the most frequent repository for metastasis of squamous cell cancer of the mucosal lining of the oral, sinus, and pharyngeal cavities and of epithelial tumors of the ear.

The involvement of the parotid gland by metastatic squamous cell cancer in the head and neck is, however, not a common occurrence in comparison with its incidence of metastasis to the neck.

Metastasis reaches the parotid gland by direct drainage from the scalp, face, ear, oral, nasal, and pharyngeal cavities. It may also appear from retrograde spread, in bizarre routing and direct invasion.

In the majority of instances metastasis to the parotid gland is associated with metastasis to the neck or disseminated disease.

All varieties of involvement by any type of neoplasm have a grave prognosis.

The treatment is composite reaction of the primary neoplasm, the parotid gland, and the neck.

The over-all five year determinate rate was 12.5%.

John Conley, MD, 139 E 36th St New York, NY.

Histological Changes After Regional Chemotherapy

Brain and Face Tumors

M. S. MAHALEY, JR., MD; GUY L. ODOM, MD; AND BARNES WOODHALL, MD, DURHAM, NC

Introduction

When regional chemotherapeutic perfusions of neoplasms of the brain and face were begun, histological examination of specimens following perfusion was undertaken in order to evaluate the effect of the anticancer drug used. Sixty patients have undergone carotid perfusions, and half of these have had postperfusion histological sections on one or more occasions. This paper reports local histological changes following regional chemotherapy and the relationship between this histopathology and the therapeutic response.

Method

Regional Perfusion Technique.—The extracorporeal perfusion circuit consisted of a dual channel pump, a bubble oxygenator, a heat exchanger, a venous reservoir bottle, and a bubble trap, interconnected with plastic tubing.[1] Donor blood was the perfusate for all internal carotid and some external carotid perfusions. Dextran was used in place of blood in some external carotid perfusions. One hundred per cent oxygen was used in the oxygenator, and the heat exchanger was maintained at 45 C in all except the first four brain perfusions which were hypothermic. Each chemotherapeutic drug was dissolved in Ringer's solution just prior to perfusion and was mixed in the perfusate. The inflow catheter was inserted into the carotid artery, and the outflow catheter in the corresponding jugular vein. Perfusions lasted from 20 to 30 minutes.

Clinical Material.—All patients had primary or metastatic brain tumors or primary face neoplasms. In all brain lesions and some of the face tumors perfusion was considered palliative therapy, performed after incomplete surgical resection. In some patients with face tumors regional perfusion was performed as an adjunct to definitive surgery in an effort to improve the therapeutic result over and above what one would expect from surgery alone. Preperfusion histological sections were available in all cases. Postperfusion sections were obtained at subsequent resections, excisions, biopsies, or autopsy. Histological sections of primary brain tumors were examined with hematoxylin and eosin, phosphotungstic acid, Masson's, and gold and silver impregnate stains; other tumors had routine hematoxylin and eosin stains. The peripheral nerves present in some sections of perfused face tumors were treated with special nerve stains: Bodian and Luxol-fast blue and periodic acid-Schiff (LFB-PAS).

Submitted for publication April 8, 1963.

From the Division of Neurosurgery, Duke University Medical Center.

Supported by USPHS grants CA-04751-04 and H-3582 (Center for Study of Aging).

Results

Table 1 lists the postperfusion histological changes resulting from each drug. As regards mechlorethamine hydrochloride (a nitrogen mustard [HN2*]), two internal carotid perfusions caused changes in both tumor and brain tissue, with cellular as well as axis cylinder injury (Fig 1). In external carotid perfusions, no change was noted in the one basal cell carcinoma, where a relatively low dosage was used. One of the five squamous cell carcinomas showed no histological changes four months later. In the remainder, there was severe damage to the cytoplasm and nuclei of tumor cells during the first month. In one case with serial histological sections over a period of 15 months, a return of tumor growth was evident five months after perfusion, at which time definitive radical surgery was carried out (Fig 2).

A139† was used in a variety of tumors. The glioblastoma multiforme sections showed evidence of drug effect upon the

* HN2: methyl-bis (β-chloroethyl) amine hydrochloride.

† A139: 2, 5-diethylenimino-3, 6-bis-(2-methoxyethoxy)-1, 4-benzoquinone.

TABLE 1.—*Histological Changes Following Regional Chemotherapeutic Perfusions*

Drug	Tumor	Patient	Dosage, Mg/Kg	Postperfusion Therapy	Postperfusion Histological Changes	Survival †
Mechlorethamine hydrochloride	Glioblastoma multiforme	1	2		10 days: microcystic areas, swollen astrocytes, demyelinization, perivascular deposition of granular material	D, 10 days
	Ependymoblastoma	2	1.5	Partial resection, 10 mo	10 mo: rare groups of tumor cells, with vesiculated nuclei and no mitoses; encephalomalacia and demyelinization of white matter	D, 12 mo
	Basal cell carcinoma	3	0.5	Cobalt therapy, 2 wk	2 wk: no change; 2 mo: no change	D, 4 mo
	Squamous cell carcinoma	4	2	Local excision and hemimandibulectomy, 3 mo	4 mo: no change	D, 11 mo
	Squamous cell carcinoma	5	2.5		1 mo: no tumor present	D, 6 mo
	Squamous cell carcinoma	6	1.5	Radical neck, hemimandibulectomy, and hemiglossectomy, 13 days	13 days: swollen tumor cells, loss of nuclei, pale cytoplasm	L, 36 mo
	Squamous cell carcinoma	7	2	Radical neck and hemimandibulectomy, 5 mo	17 days: ghosts of tumor cells, rare groups with indistinct cytoplasm and nuclei; 5 mo: islands of normal tumor cells, with necrotic centers; 15 mo.: leukoplakia	L, 39 mo
	Squamous cell carcinoma	8	0.75	Radical dissection, 2 wk; infusion, 2 mo; irradiation, 6 mo; partial glossectomy, 10 mo	9 days: inflam. tissue, no tumor 20 days: swollen tumor cells hyperchromatic nuclei, no mitoses; 5 wk: nests of cells with necrotic centers, swollen cells, pale cytoplasm, no mitoses; 10 mo: few mitoses, pale cytoplasm, swollen cells, necrotic areas	L, 12 mo
A139	Glioblastoma multiforme	9	1.5		17 days: loss of tumor cells, shrunken cells with hyperchromatic nuclei and disruption of nuclear membrane, abnormal mitoses, increase in multinucleated cells	D, 17 days
	Breast carcinoma, brain metastases	10 *	3.6	Partial resection, 2 days	2 days: no change	D, 13 mo
	Adenocystic carcinoma	11	1	Common carotid perfusion, 1 yr	2 days: no tumor present 10 mo: no tumor present	L, 30 mo
	Adenocystic carcinoma	12	0.8		9 mo: no change	D, 14 mo
	Adamantinoma	13	1	Cyclophosphamide, 1 yr	4 mo: no change 8 mo: no change	L, 24 mo
	Adenoacanthoma	14	1.5		3 mo: no change	D, 3 mo
	Ependymoblastoma	15	2		2 mo: no change	D, 2 mo
Thio-tepa	Breast carcinoma, brain metastasis	16	5		11 days: no change	D, 11 days
Thienylalanine & ethionine	Ependymoblastoma	17 *	1,257 gm & 15 gm		2 mo: small nodule of residual tumor surrounded by gliosis; encephalomalacia of white matter	D, 2 mo
Methionine sulfoxide	Glioblastoma multiforme	18 *	90	Partial resection, 1 mo	1 mo: no change 3 mo: no change	D, 3 mo

Cyclophosphamide	Squamous cell carcinoma	19	40	Radical neck, hemimandibulectomy, and glossectomy, 8 days	8 days: no change 2 mo: no change	D, 3 mo
	Squamous cell carcinoma	20	40	Radical excision, 13 days; radical excision, 19 days	10 days: no change 13 days: no change 19 days: no change	L, 24 mo
	Squamous cell carcinoma	21	40	Local excision, 14 days; local excision, 15 mo	3 days: no mitoses beyond metaphase; 7 days: no mitoses beyond metaphase; 14 days: no change; 23 days: no change; 14 mo: no change; 15 mo: no change	D, 21 mo
	Squamous cell carcinoma	22	40		6 days: necrosis of centers of nests of cells	D, 6 days
	Squamous cell carcinoma	23	40	Radical excision, 6 mo; local excision, 9 mo	7 days: no tumor present 6 mo: nests of tumor cells, some with vacuolated cytoplasm; 9 mo: normal tumor cells; 16 mo: parakeratosis	L, 36 mo
	Squamous cell carcinoma	24	40	Radical neck and hemimandibulectomy, 8 days	8 days: rare, atypical tumor cells	L, 40 mo
	Squamous cell carcinoma	25	40	Radical neck and hemimandibulectomy, 9 days	9 days: necrosis of centers of nests of tumor cells	D, 6 mo
	Squamous cell carcinoma	26	40	Radical neck and hemimandibulectomy, stat. Maxillectomy, 5 mo	11 days: vacuolated cytoplasm, nuclear destruction, bizarre mitoses; 4 mo: same as above; 5 mo: normal tumor cells; 7 mo: no change	D, 14 mo
	Squamous cell carcinoma	27	40		5 mo: no tumor present; 7 mo: no tumor present; 15 mo: no tumor present	L, 15 mo
	Squamous cell carcinoma	28	40	Cobalt therapy, 6 mo	11 mo: pale cytoplasm and vesiculated nuclei	D, 28 mo
	Lymphoepithelioma	29	40		4 mo: necrosis of centers of nests of tumor cells	D, 4 mo
	Parotid carcinoma	30	40	Radical excision, 7 days; irradiation, 5 mo	7 days: degeneration of some cells	D, 11 mo
	Spongioblastoma	31	40	Partial resection, 14 mo	14 mo: no change; 19 mo: no change	D, 19 mo

* Hypothermic perfusion.
† D: died; L: living.

79 *Mahaley et al*

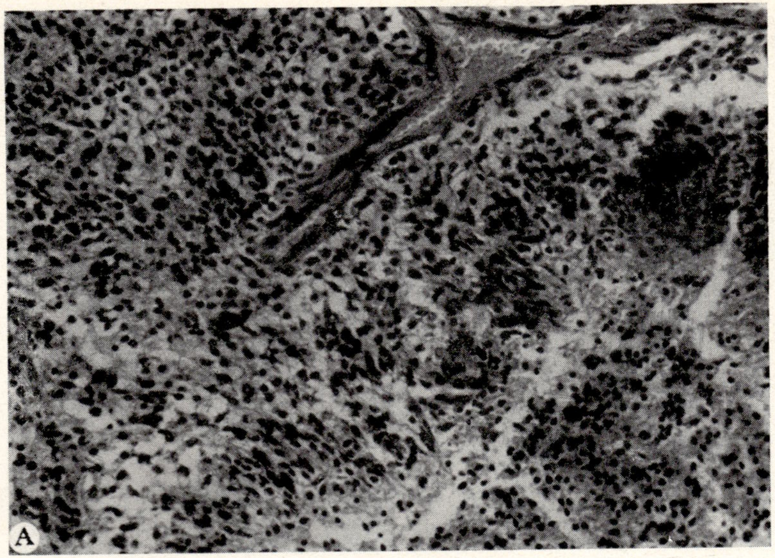

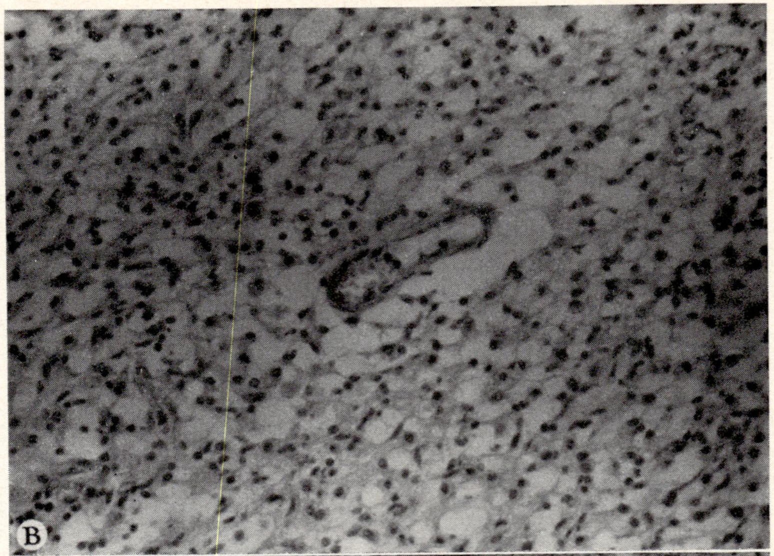

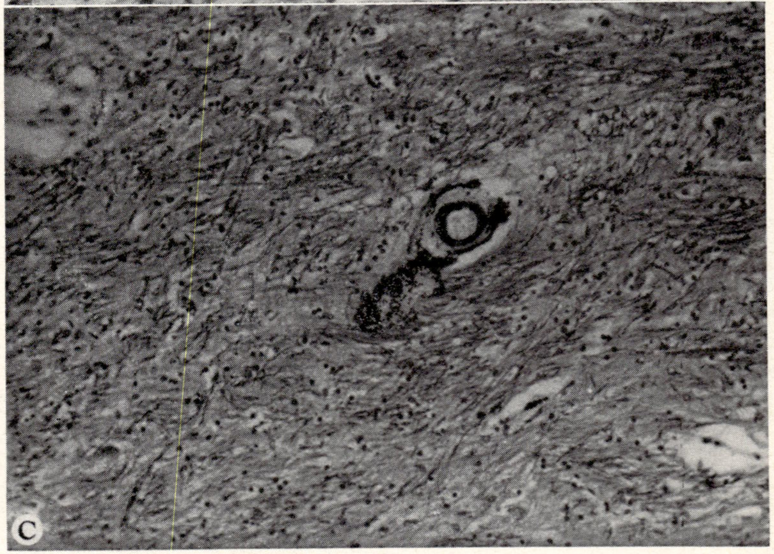

Fig 1*A*.—Glioblastoma multiforme, patient 1, 28 days preperfusion. Hematoxylin and eosin; reduced 37% from mag × 64.

Fig 1 (*B* and *C*).—Glioblastoma multiforme: *B*, Ten days postperfusion. This section demonstrates the predominance of astrocytes with swollen cytoplasm of poor staining quality, as well as "microcystic" areas. Hematoxylin and eosin; reduced 37% from mag × 64. *C*, Ten days postperfusion. Breakdown of normal myelin structure and perivascular deposition of dark, granular material was present in the white matter. Luxol-fast blue and periodic acid-Schiff; reduced 37% from mag × 51.

Fig 2.—Squamous cell carcinoma, patient 7: *A*, preperfusion. Hematoxylin and eosin; reduced 37% from mag × 64. *B*, 17 days postperfusion, mechlorethamine hydrochloride. Several pale-staining tumor cells are present among predominantly inflammatory cells and fibroblasts. Hematoxylin and eosin; reduced 37% from mag × 64. *C*, five months postperfusion. Rare tumor cells are scattered among chronic inflammatory tissue in this specimen from a radical neck dissection and hemimandibulectomy. Hematoxylin and eosin; reduced 37% from mag × 64. *D*, 15 months postperfusion, five months postradical surgery. Leukoplakia, with no evidence of recurrence. Hematoxylin and eosin; reduced 37% from mag × 64. For this Figure, see facing page.

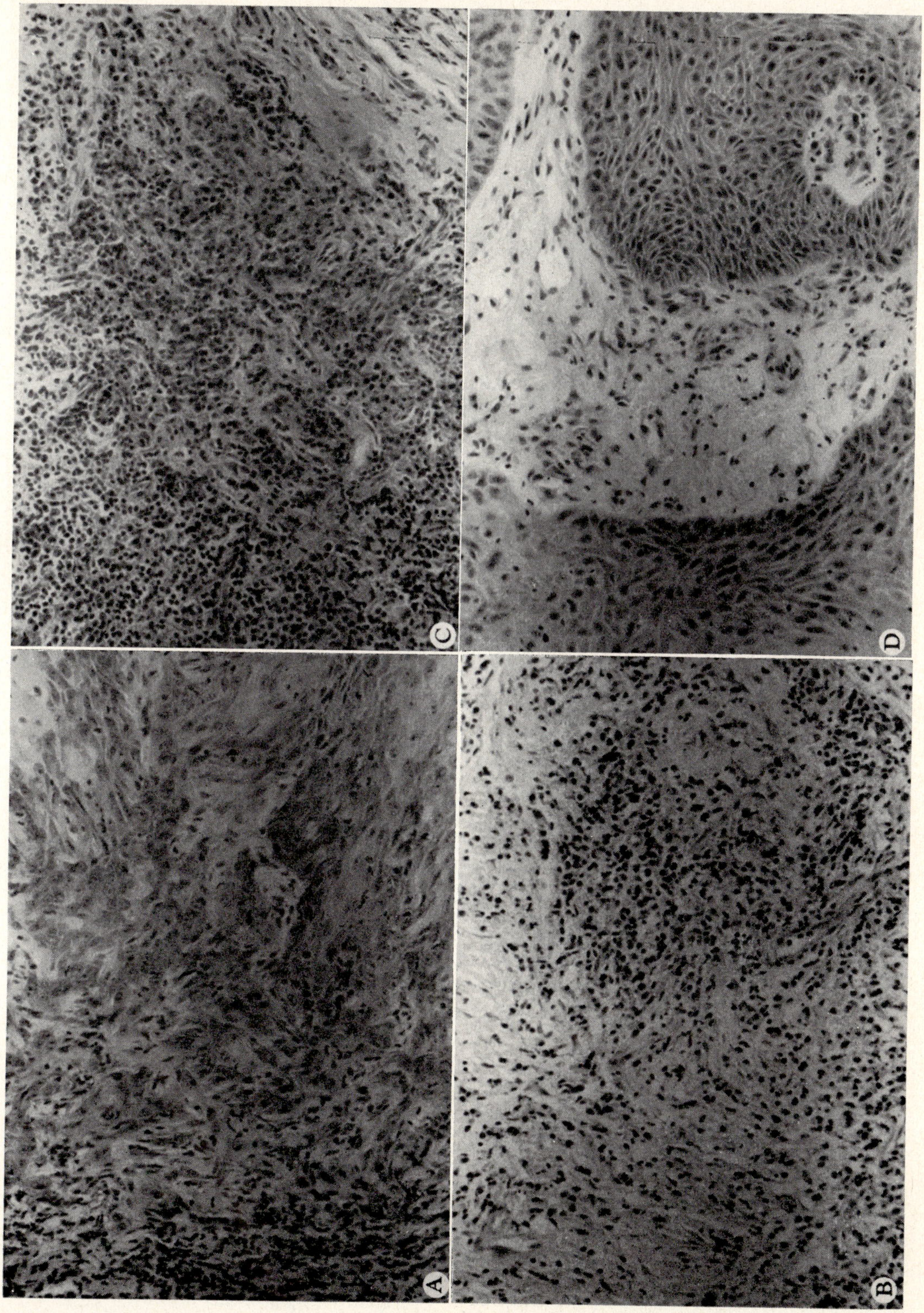
C
D
A
B

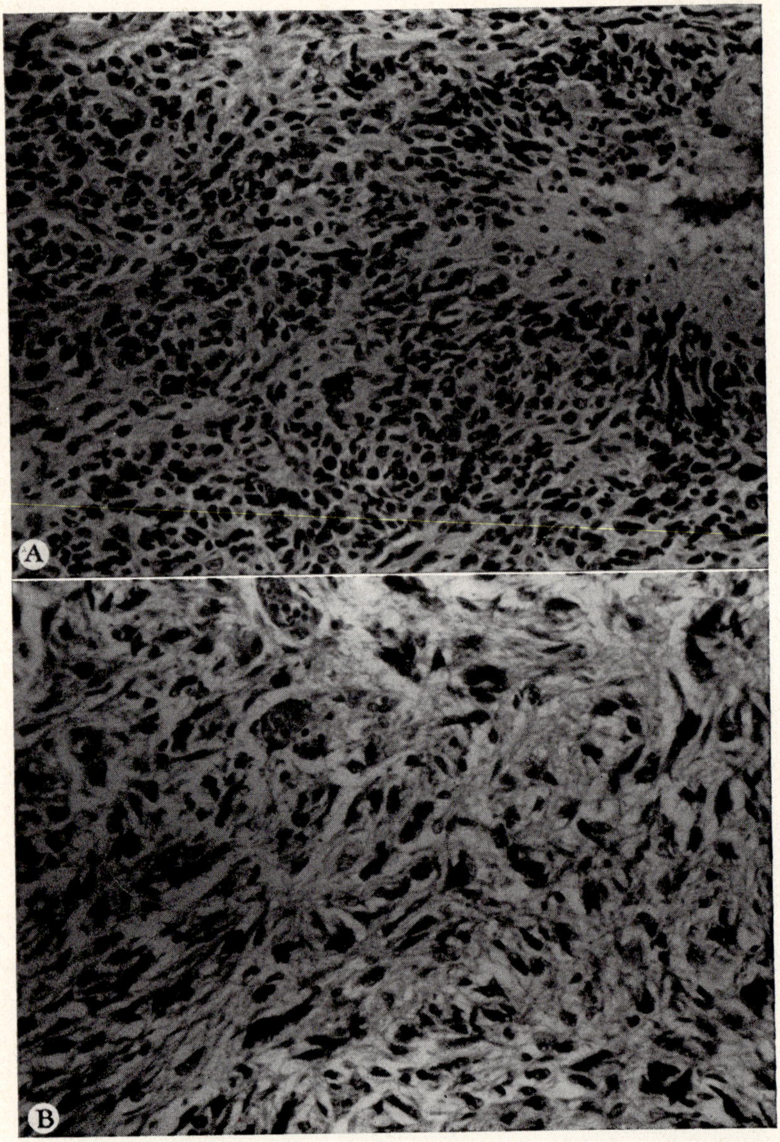

Fig 3. — Glioblastoma multiforme, patient 9: *A*, preperfusion. Hematoxylin and eosin; reduced 37% from mag × 64. *B*, 17 days postperfusion, A139. There are shrunken tumor cells with hyperchromatic nuclei and abnormal mitoses. Hematoxylin and eosin; reduced 37% from mag × 64.

nuclei of tumor cells in 17 days after perfusion, with no drug-induced changes in the surrounding brain tissue (Fig 3). One adenocystic carcinoma has shown no evidence of recurrence over a 30 month period. No histological changes were noted in postperfusion sections from metastatic breast carcinoma, adamantinoma, adenoacanthoma, ependymoblastoma, and one of the two adenocystic carcinomas.

The single perfusions with thio-tepa ‡ and methionine sulfoxide caused no histological tumor changes. The perfusion with thienylalanine and ethionine resulted in a small nodule of residual tumor two months later with considerable gliosis and encephalomalacia.

The drug used in the majority of carotid perfusion was cyclophosphamide (Cytoxan).§ Of the ten squamous cell carcinomas, two showed no histological evidence of drug effect eight days to two months later. The earliest postperfusion sections in the other eight

‡ Thio-tepa: Triethylenethiophosphoramide.

§ Cytoxan: 2H-1, 3, 2-oxazaphosphorine, 2-bis (chloroethyl) amino-tetra-hydro-2-oxide.

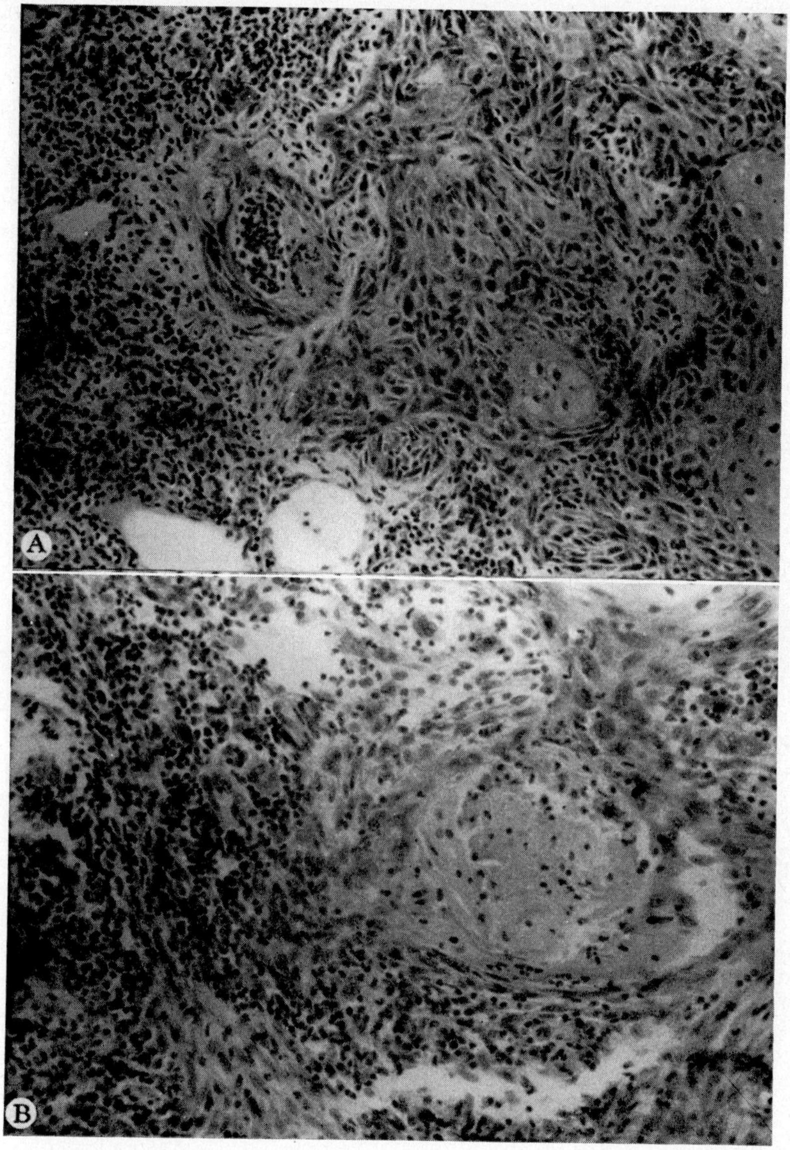

Fig 4.—Squamous cell carcinoma, patient 24: *A,* preperfusion. Hematoxylin and eosin; reduced 37% from mag × 64. *B,* eight days postperfusion, cyclophosphamide. This small group of possible tumor cells, with very poor staining qualities and no mitoses, was the only area of viable tumor tissue present at the time of radical neck dissection and hemimandibulectomy. Hematoxylin and eosin; reduced 37% from mag × 64.

showed mitotic arrest, destruction of tumor cells (Fig 4), and resulting necrosis of perivascular areas in the centers of tumor cell nests (Fig 5) during the first two weeks. Evidence of cellular damage was present for up to five months. Sections from the lymphoepithelioma showed histological evidence suggestive of perivascular tumor necrosis but continued peripheral cellular growth around these necrotic areas four months after perfusion. The parotid carcinoma had some evidence of cellular damage seven days postperfusion. No histological change was noted in the single spongioblastoma 14 and 19 months postperfusion.

In the postperfusion histological sections of eight patients, peripheral nerve tissue was present (Table 2). A139 perfusions resulted in myelin but no axis cylinder changes four months later. Mechlorethamine hydrochloride perfusion caused both myelin and axis cylinder changes four months later (Fig 6). Pathological nerve changes were present after one of the cyclophosphamide perfusions.

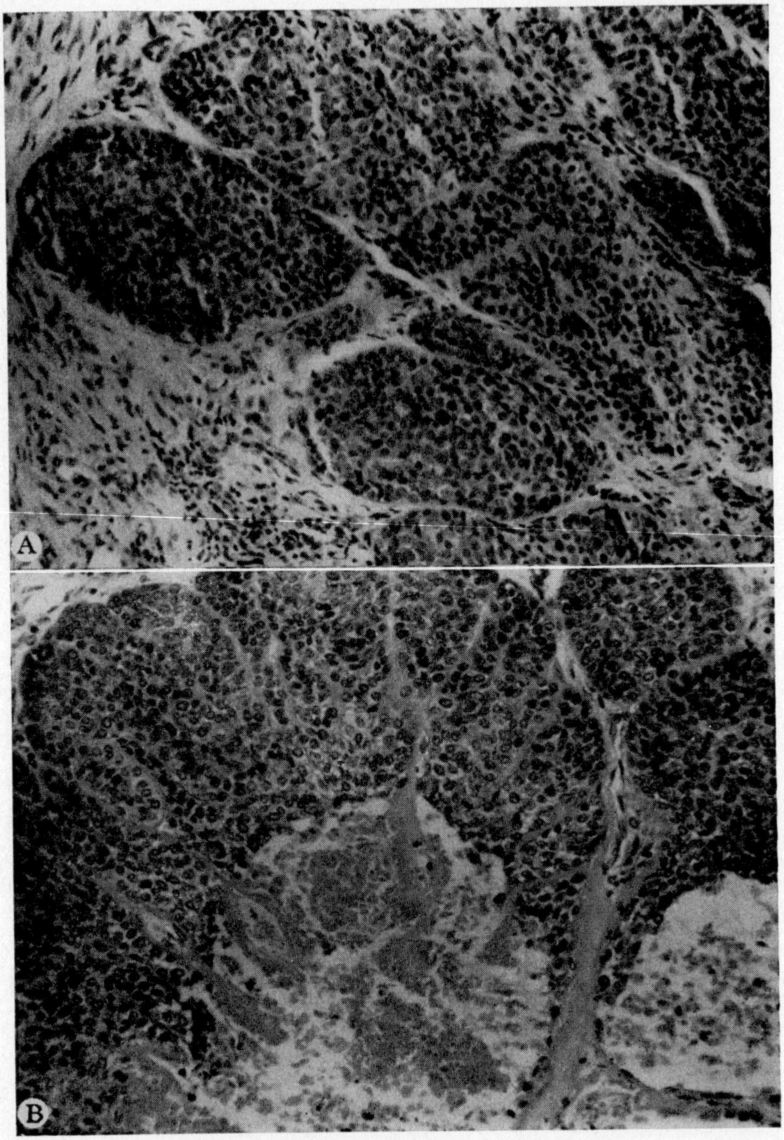

Fig 5.—Squamous cell carcinoma, patient 25: *A*, preperfusion. Hematoxylin eosin; reduced 37% from mag × 64. *B*, nine days postperfusion, cyclophosphamide. There was necrosis in the centers of nests of tumor cells. Hematoxylin and eosin; reduced 37% from mag × 64.

Table 2.—*Histological Changes in Peripheral Nerves Following Perfusion*

Drug	Patient	Dosage, Mg/Kg	Postperfusion Histological Changes in Peripheral Nerve Tissue
A139	13	1	4 mo: myelin vacuolization, displacement away from Schwann sheath and disappearance
Mechlorethamine hydrochloride	4	2	4 mo: myelin displacement away from Schwann sheath, pale staining, and disappearance; shrunken, displaced axis cylinders
Cyclophosphamide	30	40	7 days: myelin vacuolization, displacement away from Schwann sheath, and disappearance; loss of axis cylinders
Cyclophosphamide	21	40	23 days: normal
Cyclophosphamide	20	40	10 days: normal
			13 days: normal
Cyclophosphamide	25	40	9 days: normal
Cyclophosphamide	19	40	8 days: normal
Cyclophosphamide	24	40	8 days: normal

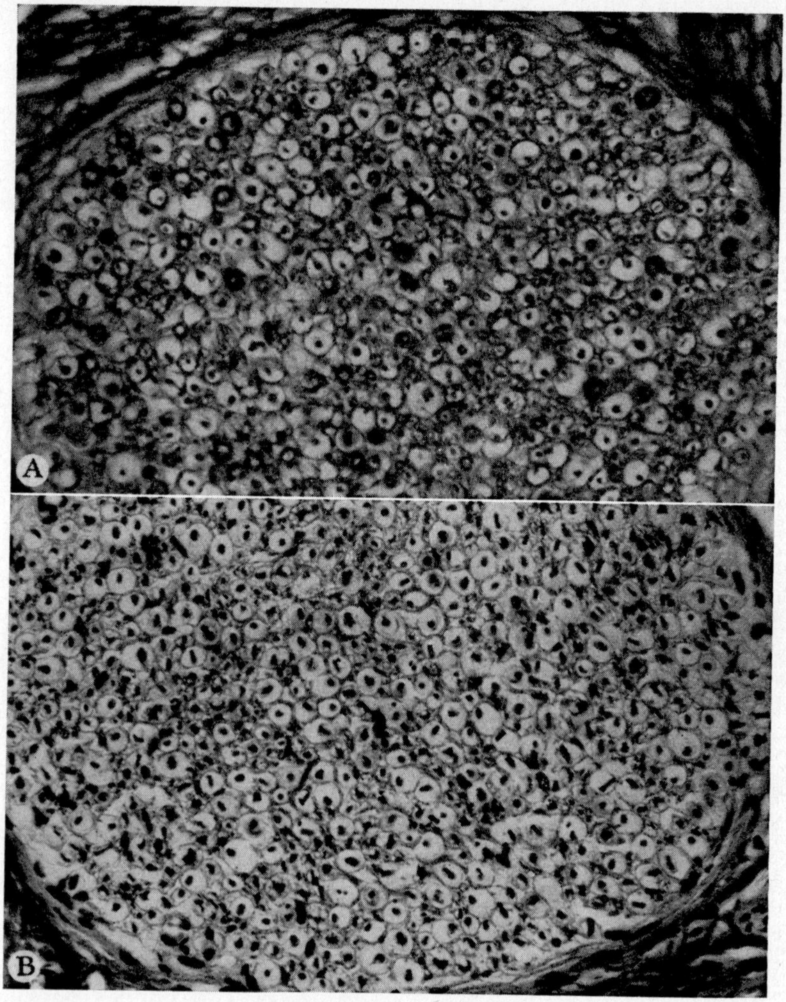

Fig 6. — Peripheral nerve, cross section, patient 4: *A*, four months postperfusion, mechlorethamine hydrochloride. The normally dark-stained myelin about each nerve fiber here shows loss of the normal rosette appearance, pale staining, displacement away from the Schwann sheath, and absence in a larger number of fibers. Luxol-fast blue and periodic acid-Schiff; reduced 33⅓% from mag × 100. *B*, four months postperfusion, mechlorethamine hydrochloride. This is the same section shown in *A*. Here the axis cylinders, which are normally stained dark and are located in the centers of fibers, are absent in some cases and displaced to the side, toward the Schwann sheath, in others. Bodian; reduced 33⅓% from mag × 100.

Comment

The systematic study of the effect of regional chemotherapeutic perfusion upon the morphology of perfused tissues is handicapped because of several factors. Frequent postperfusion serial biopsies on each individual patient were not possible in the case of intracranial tumors and were restricted to a limited number of face tumors. Thus, more than one postperfusion section was available in 13 of the 31 patients in this series. Several variables must be considered as possible influences upon the appearance of postperfusion sections: other subsequent therapy, such as irradiation; individual tumor variation in response to perfusion with a given drug; and selection of biopsy site, when entire lesions are not available for histological sectioning.

Nevertheless, histological evidence of tissue damage, not present in preperfusion sections, has been present in a number of postperfusion sections. Mechlorethamine hydrochloride, as a rule, caused cytoplasmic and nuclear damage, with changes for several months. Abnormal mitoses in carcinomas of the cervix have been reported as early as four hours after regional perfusion with mechlorethamine hydrochloride, with necrosis occurring primarily about arterioles, and histological changes occurred for up to 46 days.[2] A139 caused histological changes in only a few cases; most of the changes were within the nuclear structure. Cyclophosphamide, in some cases produced toxic changes throughout the tumor cells, with evidence of drug effect for at least six months in the squamous cell carcinoma group. Histological changes in peripheral nerves occurred after mechlorethamine hydrochloride and A139 perfusions but not after most of the cyclophosphamide perfusions, the changes being similar to those reported in dogs.[3] As previously described in animals, [4] no destructive changes were present in normal surrounding tissues within the area of perfusion, with the exception of the central nervous system and the peripheral nerves.

As regards prognostication on the basis of postperfusion histological appearance, all patients who are presently living and show no gross or histological evidence of recurrence had definite evidence of drug-induced morphological changes in postperfusion sections. On the other hand, all patients who showed no morphological changes in the postperfusion histological sections have either died from further tumor growth or are living with gross evidence of continued tumor growth. Although no prolongation of survival time occurred in the brain tumor cases, the use of regional chemotherapeutic perfusion as an adjunct to definitive surgery in carcinomas of the face has produced long-term survival without recurrence in a significant number of cases. The largest single group of tumors perfused are the squamous cell carcinomas. If one analyzes this entire group of 21 patients, 15 of which have had postperfusion histological sections and are included in Table 1, two patients are found to have died of postoperative complications and could not be considered in a long-term survival study. Of the other 19 patients, 7 are living 15 to 40 months postperfusion with no evidence of recurrence (37%), 1 is living with recurrence, and 11 have died (Table 3).

TABLE 3.—*Survival of Patients With Squamous Cell Carcinomas Following Perfusion*

	Living		
	No Recurrence	Recurrence	Dead
With definitive surgery	5	1	6
No definitive surgery	2	0	5 *

* Two additional patients died of postoperative complications.

Summary

Histological changes in tumors of the head and neck following regional chemotherapeutic perfusion with several anticancer drugs occur early after therapy and, in some cases, are present some months later after further growth of surviving tumor cells is evident. Although histological changes were present in the postperfusion sections of some brain tumors, no prolongation of survival time occurred in this group of patients. The largest group of tumors studied was the squamous cell carcinomas of the face. All patients in this group who are presently living and have shown no gross or histological evidence of recurrence had definite evidence of drug-induced morphological changes in the postperfusion sections, and most of these patients had regional chemotherapy performed as an adjunct to definitive surgery. Even in a relatively specific type of tumor such as the squamous cell carcinoma occurring in the face area, there were some postperfusion sections which showed no anticancer drug effect, just as the postperfusion course of some patients seemed unaltered by chemotherapy. The need for an accurate means of selecting individual tumors for perfusion with specific drugs is emphasized.

M. S. Mahaley, Jr., MD, Department of Surgery, Division of Neurosurgery, Duke University Medical Center, Durham, NC.

REFERENCES

1. Woodhall B.; Reynolds, D. H.; Mahaley, S., Jr.; and Sanders, A. P.: The Physiologic and Pathologic Effects of Localized Cerebral Hypothermia, Ann Surg 147:673, 1958.

2. Malm, J. R.; Herter, F. P.; Frick, H. C.; Long, M. E.; and Demetz, A.: Evaluation of Isolated Perfusion Chemotherapy in the Treatment of Advanced Malignant Disease, Surg Forum 10:743, 1960.

3. Woodhall, B.; Mahaley, S., Jr.; Boone, S.; and Huneycutt, H.: The Effect of Chemotherapeutic Agents Upon Peripheral Nerves, J Surg Res 2:373, 1962.

4. Mahaley, M. S., Jr.; Woodhall, B.; and Knisely, W. H.: Selection of Anti-Cancer Agents for Regional Brain Cancer Perfusion, Surg Forum 10:774, 1960.

Anatomy of Duodenal Papilla and Genesis of Pancreatic Reflux

Z. MESTER, MD
G. CSANAKY, MD
L. MOCSAY, MD
AND
O. EPSTEIN, MD
SALGOTARJAN, HUNGARY

The sphincter of Oddi occupies a central position in the function of the biliary ducts. It closes not only the common bile duct but the pancreatic duct as well. It regulates the discharge of the bile into the duodenum and the pressure in the biliary ducts. Since Oddi's time a large number of authors have discussed its functions, but many problems still remain unsolved. Not until recent times has the motor function of the sphincter of Oddi received proper attention, and its mechanism, as well as its importance, just begins to be understood (Foti, Mester, and Juhasz; Stalport, Nicholas, and Demelenne). Our present investigation shall be devoted, in the first place, to a closer study of its motor function.

In the cholangiograms we found that the sphincter of Oddi has not only a simple mechanic function, but that it has a contracting and relaxing activity of its own as well. Already Mirizzi, Mallet-Guy, and other authors have made mention of the peristalsis of the biliary ducts. We also tried to demonstrate the peristalsis of the common bile duct, attributing to it the active function. Since that time several papers took the stand that no peristalsis can be demonstrated in the biliary ducts. The cholangiographic part of this study, published elsewhere, confirms this opinion. No peristalsis can be demonstrated in the common bile duct. The active motor function is limited to the sphincter, and it consists of periodical contractions and relaxations (Mester, Csanaky, and Mocsay).

A number of detailed studies have been published about the anatomy of the sphincter of Oddi (Schoen; Boyden; Kreilkamp and Boyden; Schwegler and Boyden; Leger and Lataste), but none of the authors have ever studied the relation of the muscle fibers to the opening of the Wirsungian duct, nor the problem of projecting it on the cholangiographic pictures, which are often so difficult to evaluate anyway. The anatomy of the sphincter of Oddi shows many varieties which do not fit into the classic pattern, but which still cannot be overlooked or neglected when we study their pathological function. We, therefore, decided to dissect 100 sphincters of Oddi and to study them, in the first place, from the point of view of their function. This paper will report on the results of this anatomic investigation.

Material and Method

For the purposes of our study we dissected from 100 random bodies of full-grown persons those parts of the duodenum which contained Vater's papilla, together with their surrounding tissues within a circle of 3 to 4 cm, without having cut open either the common bile duct or the Wirsungian duct. We placed the material into a 20% nitric acid solution for 12 to 18 hours and, after elapsing of this time, into a 3% to 4% formol solution. After this preparatory treatment the muscles became visible in the form of massive puffy fibers, while the connective tissue was macerated, so that it was easy to prepare the muscular parts.

Submitted for publication April 10, 1963.

Chief of the Surgical Service, Candidatus of the Hungarian Academy of Sciences (Dr. Mester).

From the Surgical Department of the Hospital of the County of Nograd, Salgotarjan, Hungary.

This method was originally worked out by Marcacci who treated the material in a mixture of 20% nitric acid solution and glycerin, after which he proceeded with the preparation immediately (Hendrickson). We started by following the same method; however, it soon turned out that whenever we removed the specimen we would not have time to make the examination and the measurements forthwith. The material can be just as well prepared after fixing it in formol as before, and the material fixed in this way will keep indefinitely. This means that, after the work is done, the material can be taken out again at any later time and supplementary measurements can be made. We also eliminated glycerin from our nitric acid mixture, because, in some instances, the mixture began boiling under the formation of nitrous gases. From the point of view of specimens, admixing of glycerin did not bring about any advantages. When the preparations were ready we measured the sizes by the span of a pair of compasses and checked the span on a ½ mm graduated ruler. Decimals of millimeters have been established by estimation. The measurements were made consistently by the same person, in order to keep the subjective errors at the same uniform level.

Results

1. *Relation of the Sphincter to the Duodenal Mucosa.*—At the dissection, Vater's papilla looks like a small plica of the mucous membrane—often hard to find among the number of similar plicae. The orifice itself is, as a rule, only of pinpoint size. When the bile does not empty, this papilla is hardly discernible. Of the 100 preparations we made, the orifice of Vater's papilla was found to be pinpoint in 88 cases, while in another 12 cases it was larger by a measurable difference. With these larger papillae we found the diameter to be 0.5 to 4.5 mm. The distribution of the values taken for the diameters of the orifices is shown on Fig 1.

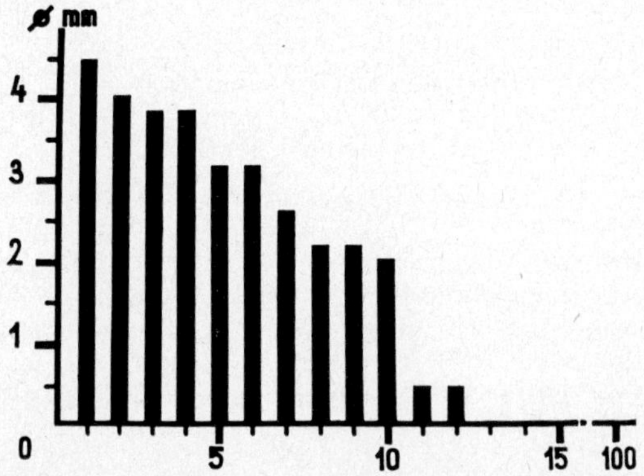

Fig 1.—Distribution of the diameters of the papillar orifices. Abscissa: number of cases. Ordinate: diameter of the papillar orifice in millimeters. Beginning with case 13, the diameter of the papilla was only of pinpoint size.

In two cases, larger lobules of mucous membrane were found to be bending over the Vater's papilla, but these lobules were not actually connected with the papilla proper, so that they did not make a proper diverticulum. In fresh cadaverous material it is possible in almost every instance to pull a similar lobule over the papilla, because the mucous membrane is movable above the duodenum muscles; however, the plica that can be produced in this way may not be confused with a true diverticulum, nor can it be mistaken for the mucous membrane pouch located in front of the muscles, the so-called ampulla Vateri.

The mucous membrane of the duodenum adheres to the base tightly at the orifice of Vater's papilla, and adheres somewhat more loosely to the intraduodenal portion of the sphincter. During preparation, this adhesion can be easily felt. We examined especially fresh cadaverous material of five corpses and found that the adhesion could still be noticed; this adhesion is firm enough in fresh cadaverous material to prevent the mucous membrane that covers the sphincter of Oddi from turning inside out, like a glove, thereby forming a pseudodiverticulum in front of the opening, or, in other words, to prevent the formation of a pseudoampulla Vateri.

In fresh cadaverous material the cylindrical shape of the duodenal portion of the sphincter of Oddi can be palpated with ease through the mucous membrane; this portion is capable of moving a few millimeters over its muscular base, for the sphincter is fixed at its base only. The apex of the intraduodenal section, will move together with the mucous membrane.

If, after the preliminary treatment described above, we remove the mucous membrane from the duodenal muscle, the preparation will go forth easily until it reaches the Vater's papilla. At the base of the Vater's papilla we hit tougher fascicules

TABLE 1.—*Orifices of the Diverticula Located Beside the Vater's Papilla*

Diameter, Orifice of Diverticulum, Mm	No. Cases
18 by 8.5	1
11-10 by 6-5	2
9-6 by 5-4	5
3 by 3 or smaller	6
Total	14

of the connective tissue; after having these dissected gradually, we have greater difficulties in removing the section of the mucous membrane immediately covering the Oddi's musculature. Finally, the thus removed mucous membrane will adhere to the preparation at the apex of the Vater's papilla only—where it continues in the mucous membrane of the ampulla.

During the preparation work of the 100 cases we had 14 where diverticula were found in the immediate vicinity of the Vater's papilla; in 11 cases we had one diverticulum, and in 3 cases two diverticula (Table 1). The orifice on the intestine side was 18 by 8.5 mm in the largest of these, whereas in the smallest diverticula the orifice was less than 3 by 3 mm. In depth the diverticula varied from 16 to 6.5 mm. In every case the diverticulum extended into an opening in the musculature, so that after removing the mucous membrane a hiatus of adequate size remained in the muscle of the duodenum wall, right beside the sphincter of Oddi.

2. *External Appearance of the Sphincter Mechanism.*—After the removal of the mucous membrane the sphincter of Oddi emerges slantwise from the duodenal musculature (Fig 2). The intraduodenal portion of the sphincter of Oddi has an average length of 10.6 mm on the mucous membrane side, and 6.6 mm on the intestinal wall side. The cylinder formed by the sphincter is 5.9 mm in diameter. Table 2 shows the extent of the dispersion of the cases, the standard deviation, as well as their highest and lowest values. Fig 3 presents diagrammatically the measurements of the largest, smallest, as well as the average duodenal parts in natural size.

If we prepare the muscles on the outer surface of the duodenum wall also, and remove the pancreas and the connective tissue that adheres to the muscles, then we have before us the entry of the common bile duct

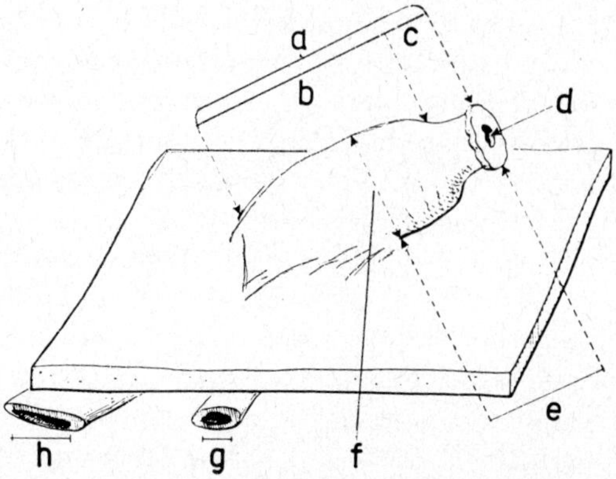

Fig 2.—Diagrammatic drawing of the sphincter of Oddi, after removal of the mucous membrane as seen from the side of the intestinal lumen: *a* indicates length of intraduodenal portion of Vater's papilla on the mucous membrane side, *b* indicates length of the sphincter muscle within the duodenum, *c* indicates length of the mucous membrane in front of the musculature, *d* indicates diameter of the orifice of the Vater's papilla, *e* indicates length of the intraduodenal portion on the side of the intestinal wall, *f* indicates diameter of the sphincter of Oddi, *g* indicates diameter of the pancreatic duct, *h* indicates diameter of the common bile duct.

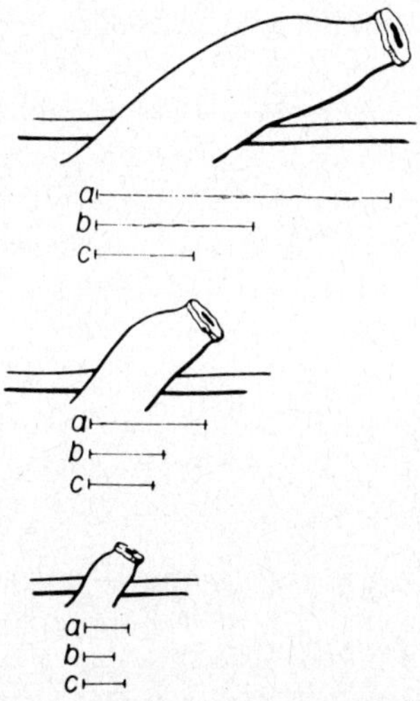

Fig 3.—Diagrammatic drawing of the largest (top), average (middle), and smallest (bottom) sphincter of Oddi in natural scale. The respective measurements are quoted below the figures: *a* indicates length of intraduodenal portion of Vater's papilla as seen from the mucous membrane, *b* indicates length of intraduodenal portion as seen from the duodenal wall, *c* indicates diameter of the intraduodenal portion.

TABLE 2.—*Measurements of the Vater's Papilla*

Data (No.)	Mean Value, Mm	SD	Value, Mm Greatest	Smallest	No. Cases
1. Length of intraduodenal section on the aspect toward the mucous membrane (*a*) *	10.6	3.5	27.4	3.5	100
2. Length of intraduodenal section on the aspect toward the muscle layer of the duodenum (*l*) *	6.6	2.2	14.2	2.5	100
3. Diameter of intraduodenal section (*f*) *	5.9	1.0	8.9	3.8	98
4. Length of common bile duct within the sphincter (*i*) *	11.2	5.0	27.9	4.8	100
5. Percentage of Vater's papilla within duodenum on the aspect toward the:					
mucous membrane	94	—	98 †	72 †	
musculature	58	—	50 †	52 †	

* Letters in parentheses refer to symbols used in Fig 2 and 6.
† Calculated from the data measured on the largest and smallest Vater's papilla.

into the musculature; and it can be distinctly seen how the Wirsungian duct branches off, quite close to the entry, at right angles (Fig 4). The orifices of many small ducts can be easily observed on the Wirsungian duct, but we also found cases where this duct bifurcated at just a few millimeters distance from the sphincter.

On our specimens, the relation of the sphincter of Oddi and the duodenal musculature can be well observed; the duodenal muscles are usually sharply separated from the sphincter, from which they can be removed without exerting any force. Usually no muscle bundles of any importance connect the duodenum with the sphincter. Perhaps the fibers which have been described by a number of authors are delicate and thin, and in our preparations they were rarely discernible. In Table 3 we can see the degree of adhesion between the duodenal musculature and the sphincter in the cases examined by us. As can be seen, only in 22 cases out of 100 a strong adhesion was found, while in 29 cases hardly any adhesion could be evidenced.

TABLE 3.—*Grade of Adhesion Between the Sphincter of Oddi and the Musculature of the Duodenum*

None	2
Very weak	2
Poor	25
Medium	49
Strong	20
Very strong	2
Total	100

The musculature of Oddi's penetrates the wall of the duodenum obliquely, so that the rear one-third muscle is attached to the duodenum musculature. On the mucous membrane side the duodenal muscle is connected to the sphincter farther back than on the intestine wall side. From Table 2 it appears that the difference between these locations is 4 mm on the average. (This is the difference between Data 1 and 2.) In the largest sphincter this value was as high as 13.2 mm, and even with the smallest of the sphincters, this difference was 1 mm. At the mucous membrane side, 94% of the length of the sphincter of Oddi lay within the duodenum, while, at the intestine wall side, 58% of the sphincter was found to be inside.

In consideration of these findings it is hard to believe that any contraction of the duodenal muscle would completely close the lumen of the biliary duct; it is not capable even of exerting any important pressure upon the sphincter, because the muscle fibers separate at a rather obtuse angle when they enfold the sphincter.

Since in the duodenal muscle there is no holding force that would act vertically to the direction of the fibers, this muscle cannot exert a relatively powerful force in a lateral direction, nor can this bond be supplemented by the concentric muscle fibers which easily separate from each other. If the duodenal muscle plays any part at all in the closing of the common bile duct this can occur only in the case of the small, short sphincters of Oddi, where the fulcrums of the muscle are comparatively less apart from each other on the frontal and rear walls. When the sphincter of Oddi is longer, then the distance between the two fulcrums is substantially greater, so that the muscle is less likely to exert pressure. The frequency of cases of hiatuses also seems to prove that the sphincter would rather tend to push the fibers apart. All in all, it seems that the role of the duodenal musculature in closing the common bile duct is rather doubtful.

However, intraduodenal pressure may have a very strong effect on the intraduodenal part traversing obliquely under the mucous membrane. This may have been the reason why Greenfield, Siegel, and Francis' experiment—to fill up the common bile duct and the pancreatic duct by introducing contrast material under heavy pressure between two inflatable balls—was doomed to failure. Their experiment was unsuccessful, among other things, because pressure inside the intestine—acting like a valve—closes the said duodenal portion fully. This is probably the mechanism through which the peristaltic motion of the duodenum can be demonstrated in a continuous common bile duct debimetric graph (Stalport).

Fuchsig and associates demonstrated that the resistance of the sphincter of Oddi will diminish under the influence of intraduodenal suction. This phenomenon was observed incidentally on an operated patient and was later verified by animal experiment. In knowledge of the anatomical layout described above, the phenomenon can be properly explained. If, in the duodenum, pressure decreases, then the said valve-like closing effect will stop, and the flow will be free. In the case of an active suction one may suppose that the suction effect, exerted upon the surface of the closing muscle at the duodenal side, tends to pull apart the fibers of the sphincter and that in this way results a more relaxed discharge in the biliary duct. It follows from its anatomic location that this suction effect is more energetic when the intraduodenal portion of the sphincter is fairly long than in cases of short stubby sphincters.

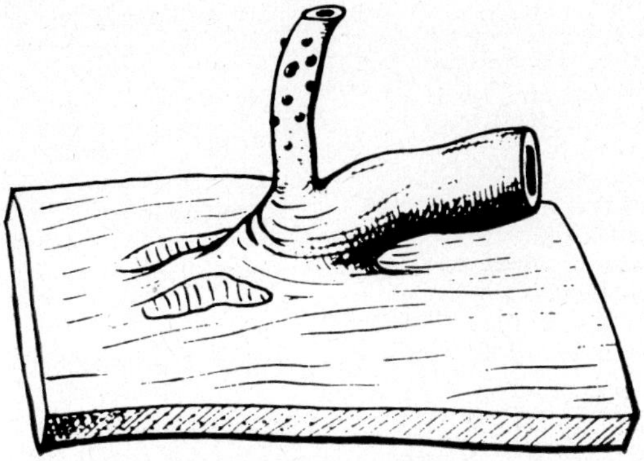

Fig 4.—Diagram of the sphincter of Oddi as seen from the outer surface of the duodenum. It can be clearly seen that the pancreatic duct enters the sphincter at a sharp angle outside of the duodenum.

3. *The Musculature of the Sphincter of Oddi.*—When studying the intraduodenal portions of our specimens the massive sphincter musculature can be, in general, clearly seen. This musculature has a rather compact, slightly protruding outline (Fig 2 and 5). However, towards the apex of Vater's papilla the sphincter musculature usually ends in a sharp edge, and, in front of it, up to the apex of the papilla, another mucous membrane pouch, generally of 3.5 mm, is left. In histological investigation we can observe massive muscle bundles at the portion corresponding to the sphincter of Oddi; these bundles come to an end at a certain point while progressing towards the apex of Vater's papilla, whereas in the rest of the mucous membrane one can find only a few dispersed and usually single muscle fibers. This portion corresponds to Vater's ampulla.

We could not discover any macroscopically appreciable fibers surrounding the Wirsungian duct separately; these merge into the homogenous sphincter mass. As we mentioned before, the Wirsungian duct enters the mass of the constrictor muscle outside the duodenum, at its remotest part; and, from the outside, it looks as if it originated from the common bile duct at an acute angle. When the sphincter is dissected it can be distinctly seen that the two ducts follow a parallel course, inside the homogenous muscle, as far as the orifice. The musculature closes around both ducts uniformly.

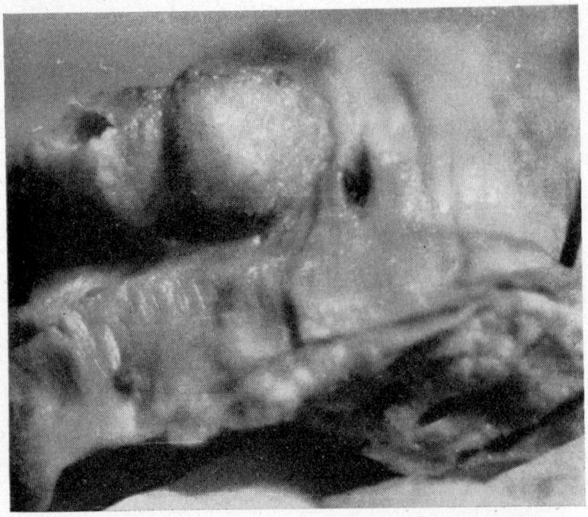

Fig 5.—Photograph of the intraduodenal portion after removal of the mucous membrane. The muscular part and, in front of it, the mucous membrane can be well observed.

The full length of the constrictor muscle is 8.1 mm, its thickness being 5.9 mm on the average (Table 4). Its volume could be computed by considering it as a cylinder and finding its cubic content—(the total length of sphincter muscle by the square of the diameter of the muscle by $\pi/4$).

The cubic content of the sphincter, when calculated by this method gives an average value of 275 cu mm, its greatest value having been 873 cu mm and the smallest 58.3 cu mm. From this value, the volume of the intrasphincteric sections of the bile and the pancreatic canals should be deducted. Anyway, the resulting value has been found suitable for the comparison of the volumes of the single sphincters.

When performing sphincterectomy we cut through the sphincter from the duodenal side. It is of importance that we make a cut also through a certain part of the muscle itself—beside the mucous membrane pouch, in front of the sphincter. This cut, however, must not extend over the muscular layer of the duodenum, or else the bilious and duodenal contents may reach the loose fatty tissue around the duodenum, and this may cause an expanding bilious infiltration or bilious phlegmon, or, even, duodenal fistula. For these reasons Doubilet proposes a 10 mm cut.

Our investigations enabled us to check this problem. Fig 12 shows the cases studied for this purpose. The upper curve refers to the lengths of the intraduodenal portion of Vater's papilla, measured on its duodenal lumen side. We classified the cases according to size and stated their frequency in percentages. In the same manner, the lower curve refers to the length of the mucous membrane pouch from the apex of Vater's papilla to the first sturdy muscle fibers, which is equivalent to the length of the ampulla, comparing their values in percentages. The graph proves that had we made a sphincterectomy with a cut of only 1 cm in each of these cases, we would not have reached the sphincter muscle and would have incised the ampulla in not more than 1% of the cases. On the other hand, in 40% of the cases we would have damaged the duodenum muscle (see section of the upper curve, corresponding to the 60% to 100%). Had we made a 1.5 or 2 cm cut the result would have been even worse, for, with the shorter cut we would have touched the duodenal muscles in 90% of the cases, whereas with the 2 cm cuts, in 99% of the cases, the duodenal muscles would have been cut also.

In practice we drew the conclusion that the surgeon should in every case establish the length of the cut according to the size of the Vater's papilla. If the latter is large,

Table 4.—*Measurements of the Musculature*

Data (No.)	Mean Value, Mm	SD	Value, Mm Greatest	Smallest	No. Cases
1. Length of the intraduodenal portion of sphincter (*b*) *	6.6	2.3	16.0	1.1	100
2. Total length of sphincter (i−c)*	8.1	3.6	24.4	3.2	88
3. Volume of sphincter in cu mm	275.7	175.9	873.0	58.5	99
4. Length of mucous membrane in front of the sphincter (c) *	3.5	1.8	12.5	0	88

* Letter in parentheses refers to symbols used in Fig 2 and 6.

Table 5.—*Data of the Wirsungian Duct*

	Mean Value, Mm	SD	Value, Mm: Greatest	Value, Mm: Smallest	No. Cases
Length of the Wirsungian duct within the sphincter from entrance to orifice (*l*) *	6.5	5.6	4.5	3.6	96
Location of the exit from the sphincter, measured from the rear portion of the musculature (i-j-l) *	0.6	3.1	+7.1	—4.9	96
Possibility of backflow, length of fibers closing the way of both ducts, measured from first fiber of the sphincter of Oddi to the orifice (*k*) *	0.7	2.3	+5.5	—4.0	88
Length from orifice to apex of Vater's papilla (*j*) *	4.3	2.7	16.0	0	100
Diameter of common bile duct (*h*) *	5.8	1.8	14.0	2.5	100
Diameter of Wirsungian duct (*g*) *	2.5	1.0	6.5	1.0	100

* Letters in parentheses refer to symbols used with Fig 2 and 6.

the cut might even be longer than 10 mm, whereas if the Vater's papilla is small, it is more appropriate that we make a somewhat shorter cut.

4. *The Intrasphincteric Bile Duct and Wirsungian Duct.*—When we make a cut through the whole length of the common bile duct—right to the apex of Vater's papilla—we can clearly see that the lumen of the common bile duct narrows quite sharply at the point of start of the sphincter musculature. In the cases studied by us the average width of the common bile duct was found to be 5.8 mm, and that of the Wirsungian duct 2.6 mm. The greatest and smallest values, as well as the standard deviation, can be taken from Table 5. This diameter narrows down at a distance of 11.2 mm, on the average, from the apex of Vater's papilla (see Table 2, data 4) and becomes a virtual duct, which will have an actual lumen only when the sphincter opens (Fig 6). This can be observed very clearly on the cholangiographs on which the column of contrast material is visible to this very point, namely, the upper edge of the sphincter. When the sphincter opens, the shadow of the common bile duct suddenly narrows at this point, and the contrast material gives a distinct outline of the canal, or duct, within the sphincter.

In the intrasphincteric portion of the common bile duct, two parts are distinguishable (Fig 6). The mucous membrane of the rear portion (that is the part closer to the biliary pathways) is smooth, sometimes with tiny longitudinal plicae, with some hardly visible, pinpoint-size openings of a few glands. On the front part, that is the portion closer to the intestine, well-distinguishable transverse plicae can be seen. The orifice of the Wirsungian duct is located in the hindmost cross plica. Behind the orifice of the Wirsungian duct no cross plica has ever occurred. Cross plicae were present, however, in every case, even when the Wirsungian duct emptying took place right at the apex of Vater's papilla

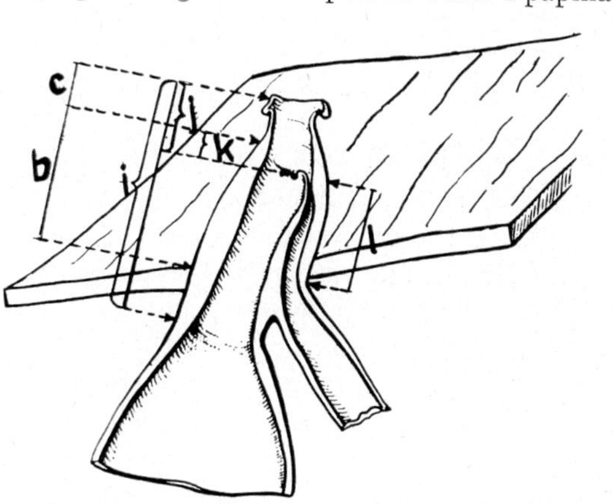

Fig 6.—Diagramatic view of the Vater's papilla after cutting of the common bile duct and the pancreatic duct: *b* indicates length of the intraduodenal portion of the sphincter muscle, *c* indicates mucous membrane section located in front of it, *i* indicates total length of Vater's papilla between the orifice in the intestine and the hindmost sphincter fiber (at this last point, a narrowing of the lumen of the common bile duct can be observed), *j* indicates distance from the papillar pore to the orifice of the pancreatic duct, *k* indicates distance from the frontmost fibers of the sphincter to the opening of the pancreatic duct (where the pancreatic duct empties behind the frontal muscle fibers, we use a [positive] + sign; where it empties in front of them, we use a [negative] — sign), *l* indicates distance between the pancreatic orifice and the entry in the sphincter muscle. At the point of entry into the sphincter muscle the lumen of the pancreatic duct narrows.

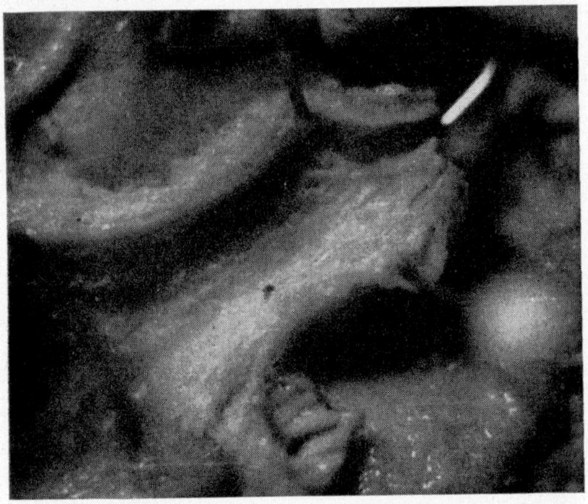

Fig 7.—Photograph of the bile duct cut open. Below, on the left side, we see the common bile duct narrowing at the point of entry into the sphincter. In the center of the photograph the canal of the common bile duct within the sphincter is held in position by pins. At the location of the orifice into the intestine, the probe introduced into the pancreatic duct is shining. It can also be seen that the orifice of the common bile duct is very close to the papillar orifice.

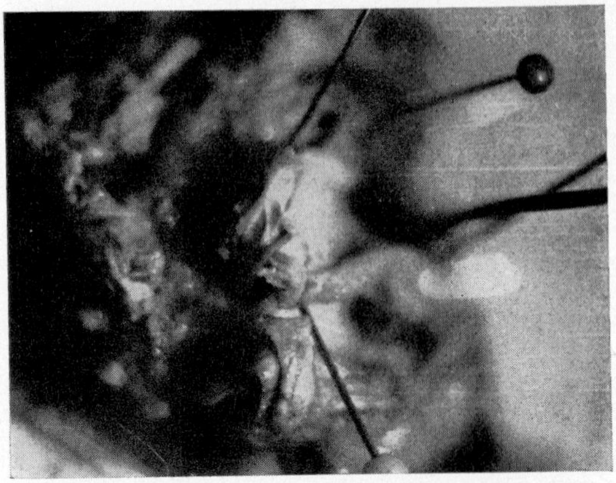

Fig 8.—The Vater's papilla, shown on the previous figure, as photographed from the papillar pore. In the center, one can well observe the probe projecting from the pancreatic duct, and, right above the same, the transverse plicae crammed together in a semicircle.

(Fig 7 and 8). Nevertheless, these plicae converge upon the apex of Vater's papilla, resembling the form of a rose.

The portion provided with cross plicae, which, as we have mentioned before, extends to the orifice of the Wirsungian duct, is of an average length of 4.3 mm. This portion is called Vater's ampulla and, actually, is the section without musculature we discussed above. These mucous membrane plicae have been described in full detail in the thesis of Holle and Giermann.

As we have mentioned before, the front orifice of Vater's ampulla is very narrow, so that it makes it possible that a stone, pressed through the shpincter, is caught in the portion which, actually, does not have any muscle elements.

In our material we found only one case of such a phenomenon. In this case we noticed a stone of pea size in the ampulla. A somewhat larger stone was discovered in an earlier case during the dissection of a patient who died of acute pancreatitis. In both cases, the stone—borne through the sphincter—was embedded in the mucous membrane pouch and thus closed the orifices of both ducts. The stone was held firmly against the orifice by the elasticity of the mucous membrane. In case of a more vigorous bile secretion the mixing of the two secreted fluids is assisted by this mechanism.

The Wirsungian duct empties at the bottom of the hindmost plica. In six instances this plica ended aslant in an upper fissure and the Wirsungian duct opened into the hindmost corner of this fissure.

After having made a cut into the Wirsungian duct we could see distinctly that the portion within the sphincter was running parallel to the common bile duct. The musculature closes around both uniformly, but some muscle fibers lie between the two. This can well be seen in histological sections. When we reach the upper portion of the sphincter, the Wirsungian duct changes its direction at angles from 45 degrees to 90 degrees and proceeds straight into the pancreas. This point of exit of the Wirsungian duct, when the dissection was made from the pancreas side, can be seen (Fig 4). For this reason it is very difficult to probe into the Wirsungian duct—either from the side of the orifice or of the pancreas—after the material is fixed. In both cases the probe gets stuck in the curve. On a living patient or in a fresh body, when the tissues are much softer and pliable, this bend can be followed much easier, and the probing will encounter difficulties only when the sphincter is spasmodically constricted.

The average length of the Wirsungian duct, measured from the entrance in the sphincter to the orifice, is 6.5 mm. It runs parallel to the common bile duct. Its mucous membrane is smooth and shiny, no plicae can be found on it. The diameter of the Wirsungian duct, similar to the common bile duct, narrows sharply at its entrance into the sphincter, and from that point on it is a virtual canal only. The Wirsungian duct itself joins the sphincter farther forward than the hindmost fibers, this distance being 0.6 mm on the average.

5. *The Emptying of the Wirsungian Duct From the Point of View of the Possibility of Mixing the Pancreatic Fluid With the Bile.*—According to the classical description, which originates from Opie, there are three varieties of emptying of the Wirsungian duct. There are cases when the Wirsungian duct empties at a considerable distance from the orifice of the common bile duct, independently from the latter; in other instances the Wirsungian duct empties beside the common bile duct at the apex of the papilla; and, it is also possible that the Wirsungian duct empties within the sphincter of Oddi (Hegge Eivind; Mekmen; Hjorth; Cameron and Noble). In the first two instances there is no possibility of mixing the pancreatic fluid with the bile, whereas in the last case the possibility exists.

Fig 9.—A pancreatic duct emptying at the bottom of long fissure. To the left from the fissure a few transverse plicae can be seen. In the center of the picture the unfolded common bile duct can be observed.

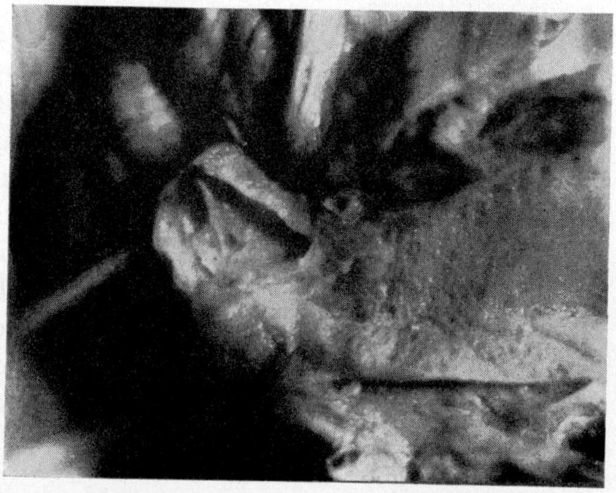

In the 100 cases studied by us there was only one in which the common bile duct emptied at the apex of Vater's papilla, whereas the Wirsungian duct emptied at a distance of 16 mm, through a small separate papilla. There was no orifice of any pancreatic duct through Vater's papilla which served the common bile duct. Both of the papillae were poorly developed; the one serving the common bile duct had the following measurements: 5.8 mm at the front, 4.0 mm at the back, the diameter 4.5 mm. The papilla for the pancreatic duct measured 4.2 mm at the front, 4 mm at the back, and its diameter was 5.1 mm.

Holle described yet another anomaly in the area of Vater's papilla, where the front wall of Vater's papilla was entirely missing and appeared as a deep fissure on the duodenum side. We could not find any anomaly of this kind in our work.

In our material we found nine cases (Fig 10) where the Wirsungian duct emptied exactly on the apex of Vater's papilla, that is at 0 mm distance from the apex. In the other 90 cases the Wirsungian duct emptied slightly farther inside from the apex of Vater's papilla, and this distance varied from 0.5 mm to 15 mm. The distribution of our material from this point of view is shown on Fig 10. It can be seen that, in most cases, the duct empties at about 2 to 8 mm behind the apex of Vater's papilla. The average dis-

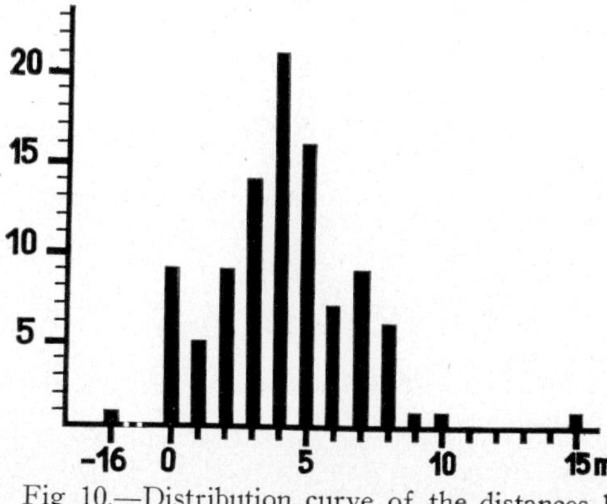

Fig 10.—Distribution curve of the distances between the apex of Vater's papilla and the orifice of the pancreatic duct. Abscissa: distance in millimeters. Value —16 means that in a given case the pancreatic duct emptied through a separate papilla located 16 mm from the papilla that closes the common bile duct. Ordinata: number of cases.

tance from the apex of the papilla to the orifice proved to be 4.3 mm.

In the foregoing we have just demonstrated that the Vater's ampulla is in front of the orifice of the Wirsungian duct, and that its wall is rather thin and does not contain muscle fibers. Consequently this portion plays little role in closing Vater's papilla ahead of the orifice; it is more important to know whether the Wirsungian duct empties in front of or behind the frontal fibers of the sphincter. When we scrutinize our material from this viewpoint we find that the Wirsungian duct's orifice, generally, is located close to the front edge of the bulkier sphincter musculature. However, the actual location of the orifice is not absolutely identical with the location of the frontal fibers, but, in the majority of the cases, is slightly in front or behind this point. The distribution of our cases from this point of view is indicated on Fig 11. On the abscissa we marked, in millimeters, the distance between the location of the front fibers of the Wirsungian duct and its orifice. Those cases where the Wirsungian duct empties in front of the frontal sphincter fibers are indicated by a negative sign (−) on the graph. The cumulative percentage is shown by the curve above the graph originating from the greatest positive values as a basis.

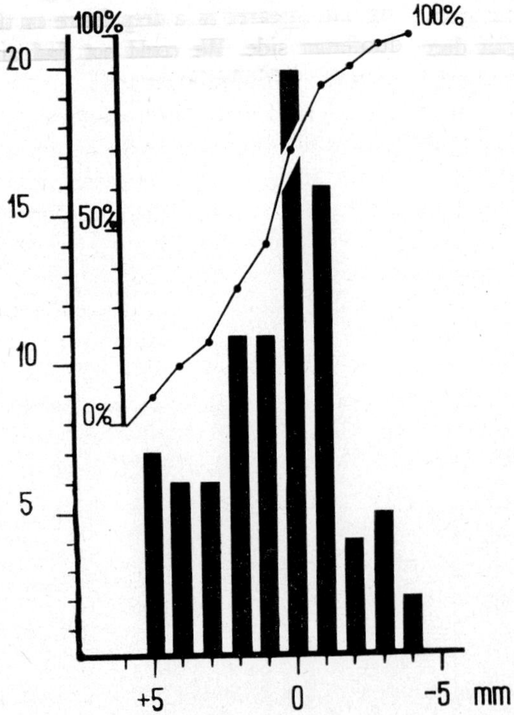

Fig 11.—Relationship between the location of the orifice of the Wirsungian duct and the frontal fibers of the sphincter. Abscissa: distance of the pancreatic duct from the frontmost fiber of the sphincter muscle. When the orifice is located behind the frontmost fibers, we indicated it with a positive number, when it was in front of these fibers we marked it with a negative number. Distances are given in millimeters. Ordinata: the number of cases. On the upper curve the cumulative percentile ratio of the cases in the column below is shown as against the total number of cases; that is, in other words, the values indicated in the columns on the left side of the column in question were added.

From this curve it is easy to read the location of the orifice of the Wirsungian duct which corresponds to the frequency of filling up the Wirsungian duct in the cholangiograms, with the double condition that, in cholangiography, the filling of the Wirsungian duct will depend exclusively on this one factor and the series of cases with cholangiography is comparable with that of this series.

In the cholangiographs in our material the Wirsungian duct filled in 25.6% of the cases. It can be seen from the graph that in those cases the Wirsungian emptied at a location 2 mm minimum behind the frontal muscle fibers.

If we consider that the above two conditions are far from being absolutely sure, then it would seem likely that in those cases in which the x-ray picture reveals a backflow of the contrast material we can expect rather higher values. This follows from the fact that in the cholangiographical series we always dealt with patients suffering from illness of the biliary duct, whereas our anatomical preparations were taken mostly from bodies of patients whose biliary ducts had not been attacked. It is probable that especially those persons would have a stronger inclination to biliary conditions whose anatomical build would make it more probable that their pancreatic fluid would flow back. Concerning the first condition, we should assume that, in addition to anatomical facts, certain functional or pathological factors may also affect the filling of the Wirsungian duct.

TABLE 6.—*Data of the Sphincter of Oddi in Various Pathological Cases*

Case No.	Diagnosis	Possible Role of Digestion	Diameter of Papillary Pore (*d*),* Mm†	Length: From Orifice to Apex of Vater's Papilla (*j*),* Mm	Length: Between Orifice and Behind the Frontal Fiber of Musculature (*k*) * Mm	Volume of Musculature, Cu Mm	Length of Vater's Papilla (*i*),* Mm	Diameter of Wirsung's Duct (*g*), * Mm
1	Gangrenous cholecystitis	+?		3.5	+0.4	154	13.1	1.5
2	Acute pancreatitis	+		7.5	+3.7	207	11.2	2.5
3	Acute pancreatitis	+		4.6	+2.5	146	9.6	1.5
4	Acute pancreatitis	+		7.6	+4.0	128	15.0	4.0
5	Acute pancreatitis	+	3.2	4.1	+3.1	728	19.6	2.0
6	Choledocholithiasis; fistula cholecystoduodenalis	+?	2.6	4.9	+0.6	563	15.0	2.0
Av (M)	—	—	—	5.35	2.4	326	13.5	2.25
SD	—	—	—	1.6	1.5	232	2.2	0.85

* Letters in parentheses refer to symbols used in Fig 2 and 6.
† Calculated from the data measured on the largest and smallest Vater's papilla.

However these may act in the opposite sense because they would increase the percentage of the frequency of the backflow of the contrast material.

We wish to point out here that in some of the cases, as we have already described above, the orifice was located at the bottom of a long, slanting fissure sticking far out; from the point of view of backflow this is particularly fortunate because this canal directs the contrast material towards the Wirsungian duct. Being familiar with this type of anatomical structure the question arises how it is possible for a muscle section, only 2 or 3 mm long, to close the emptying towards the duodenum and, at the same time, to permit the flow towards the Wirsungian duct. We shall try to answer this question studying the x-ray pictures.

6. *The Emptying of the Wirsungian Duct in Bodies of Patients Who Had Died of Acute Pancreatitis and Cholecystitis.*—For the purpose of complementing our material we also prepared Vater's papilla from the bodies of six patients who had presumably died from illnesses caused by autodigestion of biliary ducts and pancreas. These cases are compiled in Table 6. We had four cases of pancreatitis, one acute gangrenous cholecystitis, and one lithiasis of the common duct. In the two latter cases (1 and 6) the destructive effect of the pancreatic fluid may have played some role, but this was not clearly evidenced.

We can see in this Table that in these six cases the Wirsungian duct emptied, on the average, at 5.3 mm from the apex of Vater's papilla, which is 1 mm greater than that of the average. Also the dispersion data are far narrower than in the healthy cases. (Standard deviation is $\sigma = 1.6$, as contrasted with 2.8 in the healthy series.) This indicates that the distance between the apex of Vater's papilla and the orifice of the Wirsungian duct was comparatively large. Extremely great and extremely small values were not found in the series. In the four cases of pancreatitis the Wirsungian duct emptied at a location 2.5 to 4 mm behind the frontal fibers of the musculature, whereas in both of the cholecystitic cases this distance was only 0.5 and 0.6 mm. Here again we found definitely higher values than in the general series.

Similar investigations were conducted by Hegge Eivind. In his material, two out of three pancreas necrosis cases and 14 of the 17 other cases described in the literature were such that the pancreatic duct emptied high; according to him this is a prerequisite for the development of the illness.

The volume of the sphincter was found lower than average in four cases and decidely high in one case. The length of the papilla was generally greater than the average. These

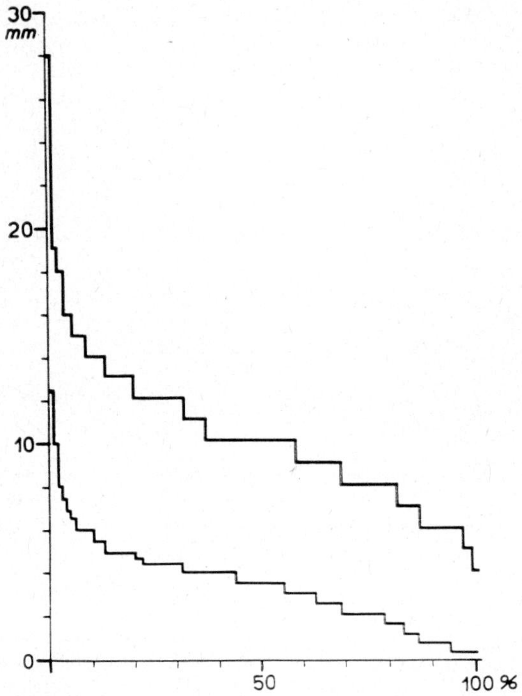

Fig 12.—Length of the intraduodenal section as seen from the side of the mucous membrane (line *a* in Fig 2) and the length of the amuscular mucous membrane portion in front of the sphincter muscle (line *c* in Fig 2) presented in ratios of percentages. Abscissa: number of cases expressed in percentages. Ordinata: values in millimeters.

data indicate that pancreatitis or pathological syndromes of autodigestion occur more often when the orifice is located in a raised position, and, also, mostly in such cases when the Wirsungian duct empties behind the frontal fiber of the musculature.

Summary

The authors studied the musculature of Vater's papillae taken from 100 bodies by maceration technique. They found that the orifice of Vater's papilla towards the intestine was a narrow, pinpoint-like one in 88 instances out of 100 and that it was slightly larger in size, namely 0.5 to 4.5 mm, in 12 cases only. The intraduodenal portion of the sphincter of Oddi was found, on the side of the intestinal lumen, to be 10.6 mm long on the average and, on the side of the intestinal wall, 6.6 mm long on the average. The diameter of the sphincter cylinder was 5.9 mm on the average. Certain values, as compared with the above averages, showed substantial deviations. The sphincter mechanism is placed, in the shape of a slanting cylinder, below the mucous membrane, and, thus, there exists a possibility that it becomes compressed by the pressure developing inside the duodenum, or rather this pressure exerts an influence upon the flow through the sphincter. This mechanism might serve as an explanation of those reports which state that the common bile duct and the Wirsungian duct, when exposed to intraduodenal pressure, fail to fill and that, under suction, they empty more readily. The duodenal musculature is only loosely connected with the musculature of the sphincter of Oddi, and the contraction of the duodenal muscle probably does not affect the emptying through the sphincter. In front of the sphincter of Oddi there exists, in most of the cases, a mucous membrane pouch provided with hardly any muscles; in this pouch a stone borne through the musculature may get caught and thereby may close the orifices both of the Wirsungian duct and the common bile duct. When performing sphincterotomy it is important to make a cut of a length proportional to the dimensions of the Vater's papilla—so as not to damage the muscular layer of the duodenum yet to reach the initial fibers of the sphincter of Oddi. Making a standard cut of 10 mm will be satisfactory in the majority of the cases, nevertheless there are a few cases when this will not be satisfactory. In all cases the emptying of the Wirsungian duct takes place in front of the main bulk of the sphincter musculature—close to the frontal fibers—whereas in half of the cases the orifice is located behind the frontal fibers, at a distance of 1 to 5 mm. This arrangement is significant chiefly from the point of view of filling of the Wirsungian duct at cholangiography. The orifice of the Wirsungian duct is generally located at 4.3 mm from the apex of Vater's papilla. The section between the top of the Vater's papilla and the orifice of the Wirsungian duct is provided with transverse plicae and is known as Vater's ampulla; the Wirsungian duct empties at the bottom of the hindmost cross plica. The Wirsungian duct joins the common bile duct at the rear end of the sphincter musculature; within the sphincter muscle they run parallel. Finally, the authors also investigated the position of the orifice of the Wirsungian duct in six pathological cases and found that the orifice was located, in the instances, slightly higher than the average, behind the frontal muscle fibers of the sphincter. This arrangement may have had also some role in the development of the condition.

Z. Mester, MD, 41 Claxton Blvd, Toronto 10, Ontario, Canada.

REFERENCES

1. Bergkvist, A., and Seldinger, S. I.: Pancreatic Reflux in Operative Cholangiography in Relation to Pre- and Postoperative Pancreatic Affection, Acta Chir Scand 114:191, 1957.

2. Boyden, E. A.: The Anatomy of the Choledochoduodenal Junction in Man, Surg Gynec Obstet 104:641, 1957.

3. Boyden, E. A.: The Sphincter of Oddi in Man and Representative Mammals, Surgery 1:25, 1937.

4. Cameron, A. L., and Noble, J. F.: Reflux of Bile up the Duct of Wirsung Caused by an Impacted Biliary Calculus, JAMA 8:1410, 1924.

5. Doubilet, H.: Treatment of Pancreatitis by Sphincterotomy, Amer J Surg 24:205, 1958.

6. Doubilet, H.: Indications and Precautions in Choledochal Sphincterotomy, Surg Clin N Amer 38:1279, 1958.

7. Eichhorn, E. P., and Boyden, E. A.: The Choledochoduodenal Junction in the Dog: A Restudy of Oddi's Sphincter, Amer J Anat 97:431, 1955.

8. Greenfield, H.; Siegel, H.; and De Francis, N.: Attempted Visualization of the Pancreatic Ducts by Ampullary Reflux, Gastroenterology 29:280, 1955.

9. Foti, M.; Mester, Z.; and Juhasz, B.: Oddi-Sphincter und Choledochusperistaltic, Arch Exper Path Pharmakol 224:95, 1955.

10. Hendrickson, W. F.: On the Musculature of the Duodenal Portion of the Common Bile Duct and of the Sphincter, Anat Anz 17:197, 1900.

11. Holle, G.: Die Bauprinzipien der Vaterschen Papille und ihre funktionelle Bedeutung unter normalen und krankhaften Bedingungen, Deutsch Med Wschr 85:648, 1960.

12. Ivy, A. C.: Motor Dysfunction of the Biliary Tract, Amer J Roentgen 57:1, 1947.

13. Kreilkamp, B. L., and Boyden, E. A.: Variability in Composition of Sphincter of Oddi, Anat Rec 76:485, 1940.

14. Lan, H. C.: An Evaluation of Sphincterotomy of Oddi, Chin J Surg 7:60, 1959.

15. Leger, L., and Lataste, J.: Le sphincter du canal de Wirsung joue-t-il un rôle dans la pathologie du pancréas? Presse Med 62:289, 1954.

16. Mester, Z.: Über die Innervation der Gallenwege aus dem Gesichtspunkt des Chirurgen, Zbl Chir 78:1128, 1953.

17. Foti, M., and Mester, Z.: Durch Cholangiographie nachgewiesene Entwicklungsanomalien, Fortschr Roentgenstr 76:212, 1952.

18. Mester, Z.; Csanaky, G.; and Mocsay, L.: The Motor Function of the Sphincter of Oddi and Its Role in the Pancreatic Reflux, J Int Coll Surg to be published.

19. Nemours-Auguste, S., and Barag, N.: Cholangio-Cholécystographie: Considérations préliminaries sur 100 observations, Presse Med 62:300, 1954.

20. Roux, M.; Rettori, R.; Debray, Ch.; and Le Canuet, R.: Diverticules duodenaux juxtaoddiens et maladie du choledoque terminale, J Chir (Paris) 78:337, 1959.

21. Schoen, H.: Zur funktionellen Morphologie der Gallen und Pancreasgangpapille bei Mensch und Rind, Z Zellforsch 35:194, 1950.

22. Schwegler, R. A., Jr., and Boyden, E. A.: The Development of the Pars Intestinalis of the Common Bile Duct in the Human Fetus With Special Reference to the Origin of the Ampulla of Vater and the Sphincter of Oddi, Anat Rec 68:17 and 193, 1937.

23. Stalport, J.; Nicholas, E.; and Demelenne, A.: Evaluation fonctionelle du sphincter d'Oddi: La debitmetrie peroperatoire, J Int Coll Surg 30:591, 1958.

Partial Hepatectomy in the Dog

A Revised Technique Based on Anatomic Considerations

BERNARD SIGEL, MD
PHILADELPHIA

Partial hepatectomy has served as a valuable experimental tool with which to study liver regeneration and function. The presence of rather complete fissures between the hepatic lobes of laboratory animals has greatly facilitated resection and has provided a means of estimating the amount of tissue which has been removed. The techniques of partial excision in the rat [2] and the dog [1] are well standardized. Both methods are designed to resect about two-thirds of the liver and consist of ligating the base of the lobes to be removed with amputation of liver tissue distal to the ligature. Although this procedure is simple and rapid, it is associated with a high mortality where other surgical maneuvers are needed concomitantly (eg, partial hepatectomy and Eck fistula in dogs). This situation could be due to 1) excessive trauma of operation associated with retention of devitalized liver tissue, 2) production of a severe physiologic deficit resulting from resection, or 3) a combination of these two factors. If an operation could be devised to provide safe closure of blood vessels without excessive crushing of liver tissue, the mortality of partial hepatectomy might be reduced and even permit the performance of simultaneous procedures upon the liver. These considerations have prompted the use of a revised technique of partial hepatectomy in the dog. This method consists of isolating the structures in the hepatic bed with individual closure and division of bile ducts and blood vessels. The liver tissue actually strangulated by ligatures after such a dissection is minimal.

Submitted for publication April 16, 1963.

Recipient of Research Career Development Award from the National Institute of Arthritis and Metabolic Diseases, Public Health Service, No. AM-K3-16,679; Assistant Professor of Surgery, Woman's Medical College of Pennsylvania.

From the Department of Surgery, Woman's Medical College of Pennsylvania.

Supported by Research grant No. A-4255-C1 from the National Institute of Arthritis and Metabolic Diseases, Public Health Service.

Method

Anesthesia in dogs is induced with thiopental (Pentothal) and maintained by ether insufflation through a cuffed endotracheal tube. The peritoneal cavity is entered through a vertical midline incision and a self-retaining retractor is inserted. The gastrohepatic ligament is incised to the left of the vascular and ductular structures at its free edge (Figure, *A*). The operator then loops a finger about the pedicle in the hepatoduodenal ligament consisting of the bile duct, portal vein, and hepatic artery. By pulling down on the duodenum and elevating the overhanging lobes of the liver with a retractor, the porta hepatis is clearly visualized. The liver of the dog consists of six lobes which have rather complete fissures down to the hilum. These lobes appear to radiate about an axis which is defined by the position of the portal vein at the liver hilum. For practical and anatomic reasons, the six lobes with an exception to be described may be considered as grouped into three divisions. The left division consists of the left lateral lobe (usually the largest lobe in the dog) and the left central lobe. The central division sometimes called "the gallbladder lobes" is formed by the quadrate and right central lobes. These lobes on their contiguous undersurfaces form a fossa which contains the gall-

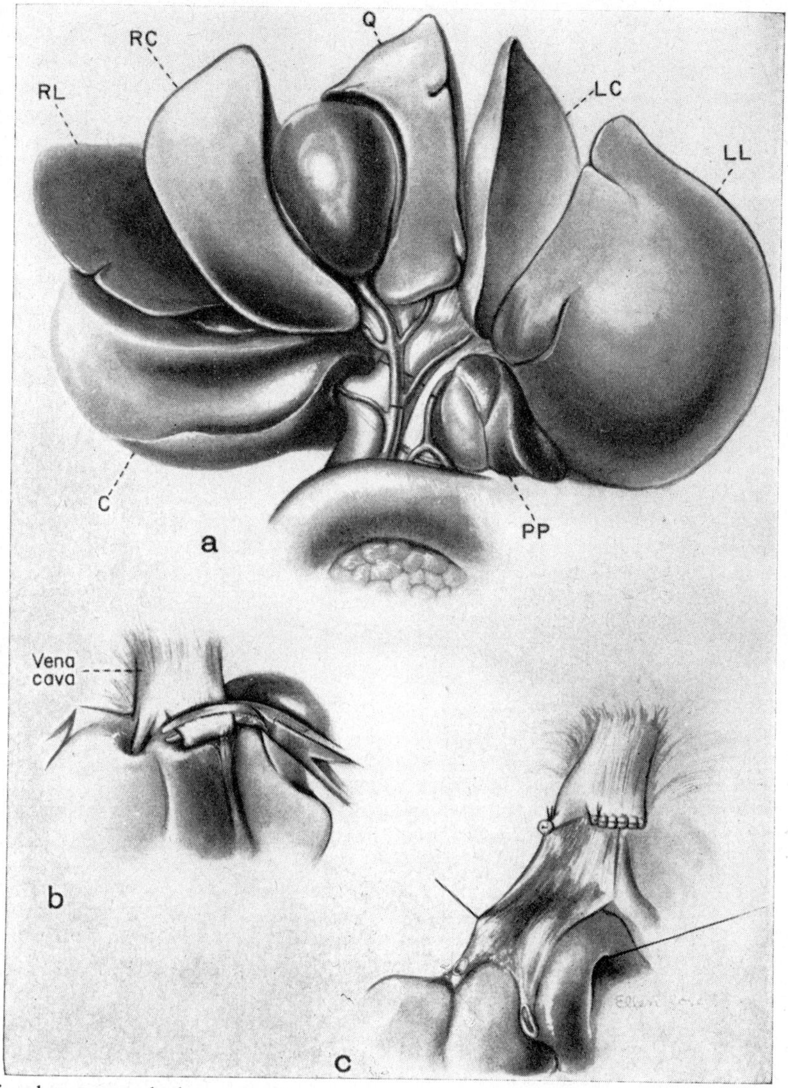

Technique of 70% hepatectomy in the dog. (*a*) Subhepatic area. The gastrohepatic and hepatoduodenal ligaments have been removed except for the attachment to the liver and porta hepatis structures. The lobes of the liver are the left lateral, *LL;* left central, *LC;* quadrate, *Q;* right central, *RC;* right lateral, *RL;* and caudate, *C.* The papillary process, *PP,* of the caudate lobe emerges medial to the porta hepatis and is ordinarily covered by the gastrohepatic ligament. The heavy transverse lines indicate the sites where the porta hepatis structures are divided. The lines of transection for the hepatic duct and portal vein are above the branches of the right lateral and caudate lobes. The arterial branch to the right division usually emanates from the common hepatic artery before its bifurcation into the hepatic proper and gastroduodenal arteries and enters the lobes along the dorsal surface of the portal vein branch. (*b*) Suprahepatic area. The liver is retracted downward, and the left triangular and gastrohepatic ligaments have been incised. A vascular clamp is applied to the large hepatic vein draining the left division lobes. A smaller hepatic vein from the central division lobes is lateral. The cut edge of the gastrohepatic ligament is shown attached to the liver. (*c*) Suprahepatic area. The hepatic veins have been closed. That portion of liver to be removed (left lateral, left central, quadrate, right central lobes, and gallbladder, and the papillary process of the caudate lobe) is retracted out of the operative incision. A ligature has been placed about the bridge of liver tissue between the caudate lobe and its papillary process.

bladder. The right division consists of the right lateral and caudate lobes. A projection of the caudate lobe passes ventrally to the vena cava and dorsally to the portal vein to emerge as the papillary process of that lobe on the left side of the portal vein. The left and central divisions and the papillary process of the caudate lobe comprise about 70% of the liver and constitute the tissue to be removed. The position of the papillary process is the exception to the arbitrary description of lobes arranged in divisions because, while a part of the caudate lobe, it is in close relation to the lobes of the left and central divisions. There is a tissue connection between the process and the bases of the lobes of the left and central divisions. The tissue link provided by the papillary process serves as the main parenchymal union between the lobes of the right division and the remainder of the liver. This isthmus of tissue between the caudate lobe proper and the papillary process is quite narrow, measuring 2 to 3 cm in diameter. It constitutes, therefore, an ideal location for transecting the liver during excision. This rather discrete separation between the left and central division lobes from the right division lobes was clearly described in the older literature where the left and central divisions were called the "main liver mass" and the right division lobes, "lateral mass."[3] The afferent blood supply, hepatic veins, and bile ducts of the left and central divisions and papillary process are arranged to permit ligation and division while preserving the structures of the right division.

Bile ducts from the various lobes converge to form the hepatic duct along the ventral portion of the porta hepatis in the hepatoduodenal ligament. The ducts from each lobe in the central division join with the cystic duct to form the most proximal portion of the hepatic duct. There is usually a single duct from the left division which enters the hepatic duct 1 to 3 cm from its origin. The duct from the right division also is usually a solitary structure and joins the hepatic duct ½ to 1 cm distal to the entry of the duct from the left division. The hepatic duct is dissected from its bed immediately above the entry of the duct from the right division and is ligated and divided. The hepatic artery is then identified medial and slightly dorsal to the hepatic duct. Some areolar and lymphatic tissue obscures the artery and must be cleared first. The hepatic artery proper is then isolated proximal to the level where the hepatic duct is sectioned. When the artery is gently retracted to expose the dorsal aspect of the hepatoduodenal ligament, the arterial branch or branches to the right division can be seen in most instances to arise from the common hepatic artery before it bifurcates into the hepatic proper and gastroduodenal arteries. Thus, ligation and division of the hepatic artery above the level of hepatic duct transection usually preserves the arterial supply to the right division. The hepatic artery proper may branch immediately distal to its origin, but these branches can usually be regarded as a single trunk and managed by one set of ligatures. After the bile duct and hepatic artery are divided, the portal vein, located dorsal to the hepatic duct, becomes visible. The portal vein at the liver hilum provides a large branch to the right division and then arches to the left to supply the remainder of the liver. Careful dissection with a right angle clamp frees the portal vein above its first major branch, after which the vein is ligated in continuity and divided. At this time, the lobes of the right division appear red and are turgid in consistency, while the lobes of the left and central divisions and the papillary process are dark and flaccid.

Attention is next directed to the area between the dome of the liver and the diaphragm. By downward traction on the liver, the falciform and coronary ligaments are exposed. The falciform ligament is divided. The medial extension of the coronary ligament, the left triangular ligament, is usually well formed, while the right triangular is not. The left triangular ligament is incised taking care to avoid the left phrenic vein and to secure a small vessel usually located in the free edge of the ligament. Two rather constant hepatic veins are now seen entering the vena cava (Figure, *B*). The larger of the two veins is the hepatic vein from the left division. The visible portion of this vessel is about 1 to 2 cm wide and only 1 or 1½ cm in length. The medial most portion of the gastrohepatic ligament obscures the medial edge of the vein and is best incised to clearly define the vessel. The smaller hepatic vein is lateral to the larger hepatic vein and drains the central division lobes. The hepatic vein from the left division is too short and too wide to be safely ligated. After dissection with a right angle clamp behind the vessel, a vascular clamp is applied; the vein is divided; and the stump is closed with a continuous 4-0 arterial silk suture. The hepatic vein from the central division can usually be secured by simple ligation. Whatever remains of the gastrohepatic ligament is now incised. The liver tissue to be resected is elevated out through the operative incision (Figure, *C*). A slim bridge of liver tissue about 2 to 3 cm in diameter is the only attachment remaining. Before placing a heavy silk ligature around this tissue bridge, the operator defines the level of color change between the papillary process and the remainder of the caudate lobe and determines the position of the preserved bile duct to the right division. The ligature is then applied in an area of viable liver tissue on the caudate lobe below the area of discoloration of the papillary process and above the location of the bile duct of the right division. The tissue bridge is then sectioned and the specimen removed. The reason for ligating the tissue bridge is to secure small interlobar blood vessels and bile ducts. No drains are inserted, and the abdomen is closed in two layers. When no other procedure is performed at the same operation, antibiotics and blood transfusions are not administered.

Results

The animals react from anesthesia rapidly and are usually standing in their cages within an hour of operation. When mortality occurs, it is almost always immediate and has resulted in nearly all instances from an error in technique, particularly related to the dissection and closure of the hepatic veins. Very occasionally an animal becomes jaundiced and pursues a declining course as a result either of accidental occlusion of the bile duct to the hepatic remnant or absence of a direct bile duct between the remnant and the hepatic duct (instances where the right division drains into an interlobar duct). Mortality has been higher when another procedure is performed simultaneously or if extensive adhesions have resulted from previous surgery. The described procedure has been employed in 95 animals. When performed alone (25 animals), the total mortality, including preliminary developmental procedures and anesthesia deaths, has been 20%. When performed in conjunction with other liver operations at the same or at subsequent times, the mortality has been higher (41% to 76%) but still less than in reported instances employing conventional partial hepatectomy. Most of the mortality was encountered in the earlier phases of the study and has been reduced with accumulated experience. After the operation, the animals appear healthy and resume their normal diets in a day or two. The morbidity is greater where concomitant procedures produce various degrees of hepatic insufficiency.

In 76 normal dogs, the percent of body weight comprised by the liver and the proportion each lobe represents of the whole liver has been determined. The liver is 2.7%±0.6% * of the body weight (gallbladder removed). The relative proportion which each lobe constitutes of the whole liver is as follows: left lateral 28.7%±3.3%; left central 13.7%±2.1%; quadrate 6.9% ±1.6%; right central 17.1%±2.5%; right lateral 17.5%±2.8%; and caudate 16.1%± 2.7%. In 20 animals, a partial hepatectomy has been performed, the animal immediately sacrificed, and the remnant of liver removed to determine the actual extent of resection using the described technique. The resected specimen has comprised 71.0%±5.0% of the whole liver.

Comment

The anatomy of the canine liver readily permits the dissection and individual closure of bile ducts and blood vessels supplying that portion of the liver to be removed. The technique described may seem more intricate than the mass ligature method. However, once mastered it may be performed in from 30 to 60 minutes with an acceptable mortality. The main positive features of the procedure are: 1) a minimal amount of devitalized liver tissue is left behind, and 2) a secure closure of major blood vessels and bile duct is attained. The practical advantage of this is that other operations upon the liver or its blood supply may be combined with this operation.

*All figures preceded by a ± sign represent one standard deviation.

Summary

A method for resecting about 70% of the liver in the dog is presented. This technique is based on anatomic dissection and individual closure of the blood vessels and bile ducts supplying the portion of liver to be resected while preserving these structures to the remnant. The procedure is associated with minimal necrosis of hepatic tissue and safe closure of blood vessels. It appears to be helpful in reducing mortality in instances where partial hepatectomy is combined with other experimental procedures of the liver.

Bernard Sigel, MD, Department of Surgery, Woman's Medical College of Pennsylvania, Philadelphia 29, Pa.

REFERENCES

1. Fishback, F. C.: A Morphologic Study of Regeneration of the Liver After Partial Removal, Arch Path 7:955-977, 1929.

2. Higgins, G. M., and Anderson, R. M.: Experimental Pathology of the Liver: Restoration of the Liver of the White Rat Following Partial Surgical Removal, Arch Path 12:186-202, 1931.

3. McMaster, P. D., and Rous, P.: The Biliary Obstruction Required to Produce Jaundice, J Exp Med 33:731-750, 1921.

Blood Transfusion Hepatitis in Open-Heart Surgery

EUGENE P. ADASHEK, MD
AND
WILLIAM H. ADASHEK, MD
LOS ANGELES

One of the major problems confronting blood banks is the occurrence of hepatitis following blood transfusions. It has always been difficult to obtain valid statistics because the incubation period of hepatitis may be relatively long. Hence some cases are unrelated and unreported.

With the use of many blood transfusions for open-heart surgery to prime the pump oxygenator and to replace blood loss, and because of the close contact established with these patients by our Regional Blood Center, we felt that this group of surgical cases presented an ideal opportunity for the investigation of hepatitis possibly due to massive blood transfusions.

By the end of 1962, the Los Angeles-Orange Counties Red Cross Regional Blood Center had collected 2,173,156 units of blood since its inception as a civilian blood program in 1946. Table 1 depicts the yearly blood collections at the Regional Blood Center since 1954 and the number of cases of hepatitis reported to us each year. In this past year we have uncovered additional cases of hepatitis through the cooperation of the local health departments which have sent in reports on some cases not known to the hospitals where the blood was administered.

The Regional Blood Center supplies almost 100% of the blood used in Orange County

TABLE 1.—*Yearly Collections: Usage of Whole Blood—Reported Cases of Post-Transfusion Hepatitis, 1954-1961*

Year	Pints Collected	Hospital Usage Whole Blood	Reported Cases Hepatitis
1954	167,154	111,213	15
1955	144,291	122,671	34
1956	144,247	129,584	21
1957	147,201	117,629	38
1958	160,100	139,321	37
1959	154,957	127,363	36
1960	153,730	129,471	41
1961	165,524	136,533	47

Submitted for publication April 15, 1963.

Associate Clinical Professor of Surgery, University of California Medical Center (Dr. E. P. Adashek).

Medical Directors, Los Angeles-Orange Counties Red Cross Regional Blood Center.

TABLE 2.—*Special Collections of Blood for Open-Heart Surgery at the Los-Angeles-Orange Counties Regional Blood Center*

Year	No. Collections	No. Units Blood *
1957	3	48
1958	166	3,331
1959	400	7,266
1960	588	10,901
1961	655	13,016

* Includes units collected in both heparin and acid citrate dextrose (ACD) solutions.

and approximately 65% of the blood used in Los Angeles County, distributed to 219 hospitals approved by its medical advisory committees (appointed by the two county medical associations).

The Regional Blood Center started special collections for open-heart surgery in 1957. Table 2 lists the number of such collections. The over-all average collected for the individual patient in 1961 was 19.9 units and varied from 12 units for a child to a maximum of 35 for an adult.

In order to determine the incidence of hepatitis following open-heart surgery, it was decided to conduct the survey beginning with the first scheduled cases in 1957 and to cut off the survey as of Dec 31, 1961. This permitted the lapse of at least six months before the follow-up was conducted, since the analysis was not begun until August, 1962.

A questionnaire with a covering letter was sent to each patient known to have survived the surgical procedure in order to determine the possibility of a post-transfusion hepatitis. A second questionnaire was sent to the patient's attending physician. With the contact established with both the patient and his physician, as well as the excellent cooperation of the cardiac surgeons, we have been able to obtain accurate follow-up information.

Questionnaires were sent to 1,229 patients. A total of 494 patients have not replied, and 91 questionnaires were returned by the post office. We have received replies from 644 patients who received a total of 11,597 units of blood, or an over-all average of 18.01 units per patient. Of the 644 patients there were 12 cases of hepatitis reported to us. This represents a case incidence of 1.86%, or an infectivity incidence of 0.1032%. The individual cases reported are reviewed in Table 3. It should be noted that three patients received additional blood postoperatively from proprietary blood banks; one patient received fibrinogen; and two patients received commercial lyophilized pooled plasma ("Anti-Hemophilic Plasma"). Some patients received medications which in rare instances have been known to cause jaundice. One patient gave a history of infectious hepatitis in 1954. All of these patients had many venipunctures for blood tests, cardiac catheterizations, and numerous intravenous medications. There is always a possibility that one of these factors might have been the cause of the hepatitis. For the purposes of our study, however, the hepatitis reported was always presumed to have been transmitted by the blood from the Regional Center. In the entire group of cases surveyed thus far, there were fortunately no deaths attributable to hepatitis.

When a case of post-transfusion hepatitis is reported to the Regional Blood Center, an attempt is made to learn whether the donor involved actually understood the questions relating to the possible history of jaundice. In acceptance of donors, a person who has had infectious hepatitis within two years is automatically rejected; if the hepatitis occurred more than two years before, he may be accepted for blood to be used for fractiona-

TABLE 3.—*Reported Cases of Hepatitis After Open-Heart Surgery, 1957-1961*

Sex, Age (Yr)	No. Units Hep & ACD ARC * Blood	Other Transf Not ARC *	Days Approx Incubat
F, 22	21	0	28
M, 41	22	0	22
F, 16	16	2	135
M, 59	21	0	84
F, 35	22	2 Fibrinogen	145
M, 45	17	0	38
F, 45	20	0	70
M, 36	22	3 "Anti-Hemo. Plasma"	66
M, 23	27	6	76
M, 18	23	0	140
F, 40	13	4	18
F, 55	23	1 "Anti-Hemo. Plasma"	40

* Symbol used locally to designate units from Regional Center.

tion only. A donor who has had "contact" within the past six months with a case of infectious hepatitis is also rejected, as is a donor with a history of transfusion of blood or blood derivatives within six months. All donors whose blood is involved with a case of post-transfusion hepatitis are removed from the donor panel.

In the years that we have followed up on such donors, the number of persons responding with an amended medical history has been so insignificant that it is obvious that our chief problem is with the silent carrier who may harbor the virus of hepatitis in his blood and yet have no knowledge of any illness to account for it.

Hoxworth [1] reported 19 cases of hepatitis, or an infectivity incidence of 0.259%, in a study of 3,349 patients who had received blood transfusions (7,315 units) from carefully screened donors (family plus 4% paid donors) at the Cincinnati General Hospital in 1958. He stated that he deplored the use of blood from professional donors since many of these are unfortunates who, in order to receive their pay, would be disinclined to give an adequate medical history. Blood from persons such as narcotic addicts, alcoholics, etc, would be much more likely to harbor the virus of hepatitis. Hoxworth estimated that if only professional donors were used, there would be over 39,000 cases of serum hepatitis annually in the United States; with a limited use of the professional donor, there might be an estimated 12,900 cases.

In a recent and most careful study, Allen and Sayman [2] stated that it has been demonstrated that the chances of a professional donor's being a carrier of hepatitis are essentially six times greater than those of a volunteer or family donor. In this report, Allen and Sayman found the over-all attack rate for all patients (2,547) transfused with blood only was 3%, there being 77 cases of hepatitis in this group. The average patient received 3.4 units of blood. They found a direct relationship between the number of units of blood received and the susceptibility to hepatitis. Thus, in cases where 7 to 9 units of blood were given, the attack rate was 5.4%; where 10 to 20 units were given, the rate was 6.8%; and where more than 20 units were given the rate went up to 7.8%.

In a paper presented at the IXth Congress of the International Society of Blood Transfusion, Norris [3] pointed out that Potter and associates [4] found the incidence of abnormal hepatic function tests as 75% in imprisoned narcotic addicts, whereas only 16% of nonaddicted prisoners in the same institution had abnormal tests.

In his studies, Norris [3,5] reported an investigation of blood donors suspected of having transmitted viral hepatitis where only a single blood transfusion had been given each patient. Tests performed on sera of these donors, mailed to his laboratory from Red Cross centers and community and hospital blood banks, showed abnormal liver function tests in four of 25 such samples. In contrast, 16 of 33 donors in his own group of donors had abnormal liver function tests. It became apparent to Norris, in a closer study of the donors in his own group who are paid a fee for their blood, that there were addicts who had escaped detection by the usual manner of examination and others were alcoholics in whom there was evidence of a chronic form of hepatitis. When his single donor group was subdivided further into those who were in a low economic group and who were paid for donation, and those who were contributing their blood on behalf of friends or relatives, it was found that the incidence of abnormal hepatic function tests in the paid group was identical with the incidence in the known narcotic addicts. In other words, three fourths of this paid group had abnormal liver function tests.

In spite of numerous studies as to the value of thymol turbidity,[6] serum glutamic oxaloacetic acid transaminase,[7] and bilirubin tests in an attempt to screen out hepatitis carriers, it would appear that these tests would result in the loss of too many donors whose blood would not transmit viral hepatitis. Jennings [6] concluded in his study on the thymol turbidity test in screening blood donors that although the incidence of serum hepatitis might be reduced, it could not be claimed that the use of this test would eliminate the danger.

For a number of years, as indicated in Table 1, our experience at the Regional Blood Center has been a low incidence of post-transfusion hepatitis reported to us. We felt that this was because of our healthy, voluntary blood donor who receives no payment for his donation. Since we also felt that many cases of hepatitis may not be diagnosed and not reported, we wondered if this same low incidence would be duplicated in the present series where it was possible to follow accurately the recipients of the blood.

It is theoretically possible that some of the factors peculiar to open-heart surgery might have significance in the low incidence of hepatitis reported. The blood for the most part is collected in heparin and is circulated through the pump oxygenator. Stokes [8] has recommended the giving of γ-globulin with each unit of blood followed by a second injection a month later, in order to lower the incidence of transfusion hepatitis. Perhaps the γ-globulin accumulated in the patient through the many blood transfusions given within a short space of time may have a deterrent effect on the subsequent development of hepatitis.

Regardless of other factors that might influence the low incidence of hepatitis in this series, the use of the voluntary blood donor at the Regional Blood Center has proved a most satisfactory way of obtaining blood.

Summary and Conclusion

1. A survey was conducted at the Los Angeles-Orange Counties Red Cross Regional Blood Center of patients who had open-heart surgery, in order to determine the incidence of hepatitis where massive blood transfusions are used.

2. In all, 644 patients who received a total of 11,597 units of blood participated in this survey. A total of 12 cases of hepatitis allegedly due to blood transfusions was reported, a case incidence of 1.86% or an infectivity rate of 0.1032%.

3. In view of the low incidence of hepatitis in this series of open-heart surgery patients, we believe the use of the voluntary blood donor to be most satisfactory.

Eugene P. Adashek, MD, Los Angeles and Orange Counties Regional Blood Center, 1130 S Vermont Ave, Los Angeles 6, Calif.

REFERENCES

1. Hoxworth, P. I., et al: The Risk of Hepatitis From Whole Blood and Pooled Plasma, Surg Gynec Obstet 109:38-42 (July) 1959.

2. Allen, J. G., and Sayman, W. A.: Serum Hepatitis From Transfusions of Blood, JAMA 180:1079-1085 (June 30) 1962.

3. Norris, R. F.: Present Status of Hepatic Function Tests in the Detection of Carriers of Viral Hepatitis, paper presented at IXth International Congress of Society of Blood Transfusion, Mexico City, September, 1962.

4. Potter, H. P., Jr., et al: Chronic Hepatic Dysfunction in Heroin Addicts, JAMA 174:2049-2051 (Dec 17) 1960.

5. Norris, R. F.: "The Carrier of Viral Hepatitis as a Blood Donor," in Proceedings of the VIIIth Congress of the International Society of Blood Transfusion, 1960, White Plains, NY: Albert J. Phiebig, Books, 1962, pp 37-44.

6. Jennings, E. R., et al: The Thymol Turbidity Test in Screening of Blood Donors, Amer J Clin Path 27:489-502 (May) 1957.

7. Bang, N. U., et al: Detection of Hepatitis Carriers by Serum Glutamic Oxalacetic Transaminase Activity, JAMA 171:2303-2306 (Dec. 26) 1959.

8. Gamma Globulin Can Eliminate Serum Hepatitis, Medical News, JAMA 180:29 (May 5) 1962.

A Comparison of Three Mechanical Ventilators

Effects on Pulmonary Blood Flow

KHLAR E. McDONALD, MD; CAPT FRANK A. CAMP, USAF (MC); AND
WORTHINGTON G. SCHENK, JR., MD, BUFFALO

The effect of mechanical ventilation on pulmonary blood flow has both experimental and clinical implications. Most major surgical procedures are currently being done while using mechanical ventilation. Experimental plans often require thoracotomy and, hence, mechanical ventilation.

This study was aimed at evaluating alterations in pulmonary blood flow resulting from ventilation with three commonly used mechanical ventilators.

Methods

Eleven mongrel dogs weighing from 10.9 to 21.31 kg were studied under light intravenous sodium pentobarbital (12 mg/kg) anesthesia. Each animal was intubated with a cuffed endotracheal tube, and mechanical ventilation with room air was accomplished by one of three ventilators: *a*) intermittent positive-negative piston type (Jefferson*), *b*) continuous positive pressure operated diaphragm (pneophore†), or *c*) positive-negative pressure operated diaphragm (anesthetizer-vaporizer-resuscitator, [A-V-R] ‡). Polyethylene catheters of identical dimensions were placed in a peripheral artery, the pulmonary artery, and the left atrial appendage. From these, arterial pressure and pulmonary artery less atrial differential pressure (ΔP) were recorded using Sanborn pressure transducers. The differential transducer was stabilized at the level of the left atrium.

A noncannulating electromagnetic probe § was then placed about the main pulmonary artery for the purpose of measuring pulmonary artery blood flow by the square wave electromagnetic flowmeter.‖ Endotracheal pressure was recorded by means of an 18-gauge needle inserted into the endotracheal tube and attached to a Sanborn pressure transducer (No. 267A).

With this preparation it was then possible to make simultaneous recordings of:

1. pulmonary artery blood flow
2. differential pulmonary pressure (ΔP)
3. peripheral arterial pressure
4. endotracheal pressure

All studies were performed with the thorax open.

Results

The type of intratracheal pressure variation produced by the ventilators is seen in Fig 1 recorded at a paper speed of 50 mm/sec. The Jefferson ventilator wave-form is more or less a rectangular wave except at rates of 40/min or higher. At rates of 40/min or more it becomes sawtoothed in shape. With each stroke the wave returns to or passes through zero pressure. As previously demonstrated by Dameron and Green,[1] the pneophore produces a sawtooth shaped respiratory wave. It never returns to zero pressure but bottoms at +4 to +5 mm Hg. The A-V-R produces a pattern similar to the pneophore except that it has a negative spike of −9 to −12 mm Hg at

Submitted for publication April 15, 1963.

Buswell Fellow in Surgical Research (Dr. Schenk).

From the Department of Surgery, School of Medicine of the State University of New York at Buffalo and the Edward J. Meyer Memorial Hospital.

Supported by grants-in-aid from the United States Public Health Service H-3181 and the Heart Association of Erie County.

The contents reflect the opinions of the author and are not to be construed as official Air Force Policy.

Animals used in these experiments were treated in accordance with the rules regarding animal care established by the American Medical Association.

* Made by Air Shields, Inc., Hatboro, Pa.

† Made by Mine Safety Appliances Co., Pittsburgh.

‡ Made by National Cylinder Gas Division of Chemation Corporation, Chicago.

§ Electromagnetic Probe Co., Winston-Salem, NC.

‖ Carolina Medical Electronics, Winston-Salem, NC.

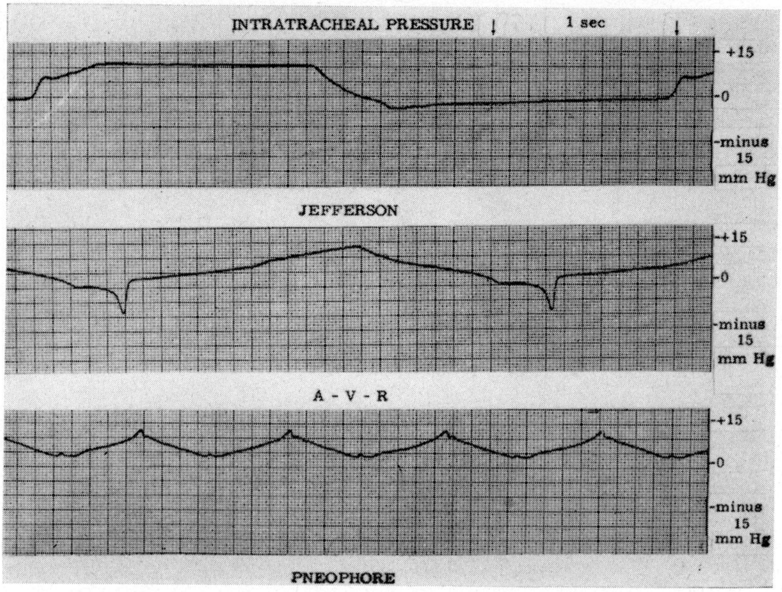

Fig 1.—Intratracheal pressure variation produced by three ventilators. Paper speed 50 mm/sec.

the termination of expiration. As seen in Fig 1 this negative spike is of short duration. The wave forms of the A-V-R and the pneophore remained essentially unchanged throughout the range of operation studied.

Instantaneous pressure-flow relationships resulting from the use of these three ventilators are shown in Fig 2, 3, and 4. In each instance it will be noted that there are phasic alterations in both pressure and flow recordings, synchronous with phase of ventilation.

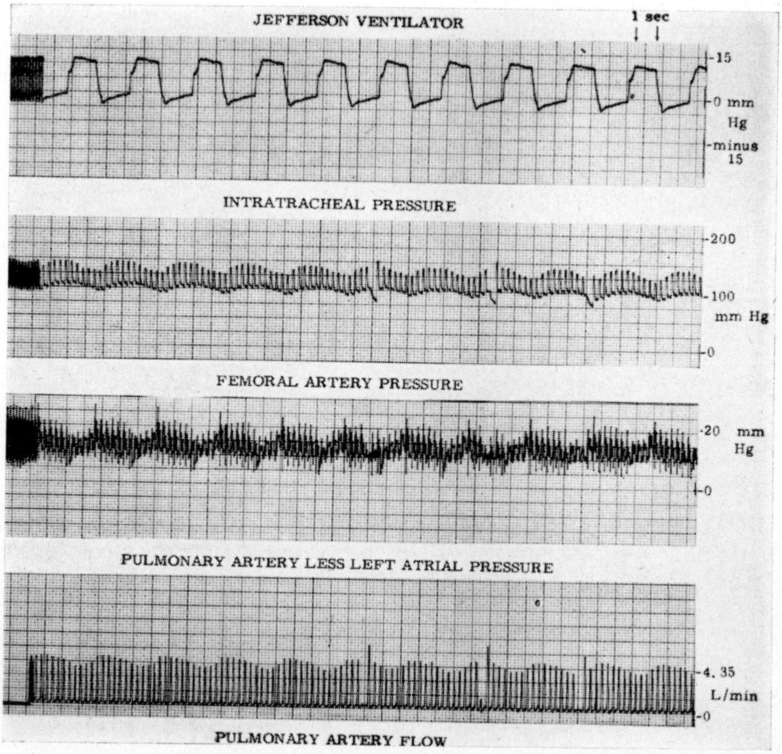

Fig 2.—Simultaneous recording of alterations in intratracheal pressure, femoral artery pressure, pulmonary differential pressure, and pulmonary artery flow as produced by Jefferson Ventilator.

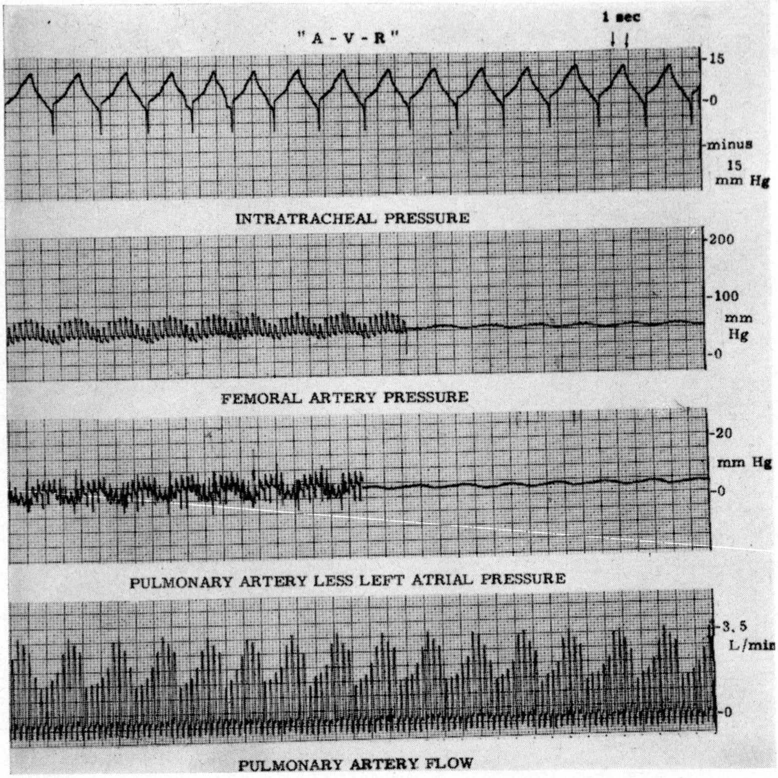

Fig 3.—Simultaneous recording of alterations in intratracheal pressure, femoral artery pressure, pulmonary differential pressure, and pulmonary artery flow as produced by A-V-R ventilator.

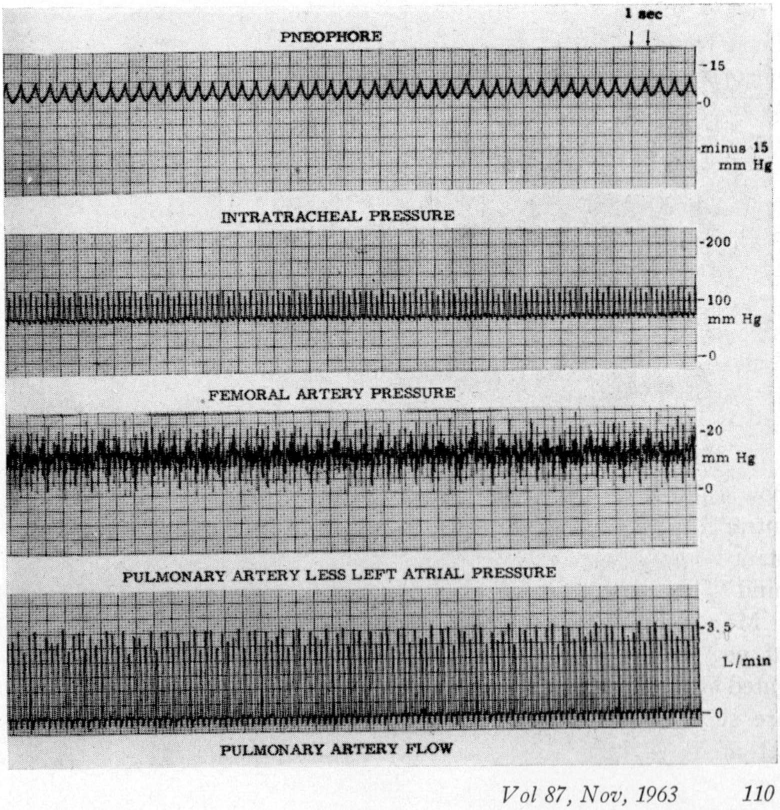

Fig 4.—Simultaneous recording of alterations in intratracheal pressure, femoral artery pressure, pulmonary differential pressure, and pulmonary artery flow as produced by Pneophore.

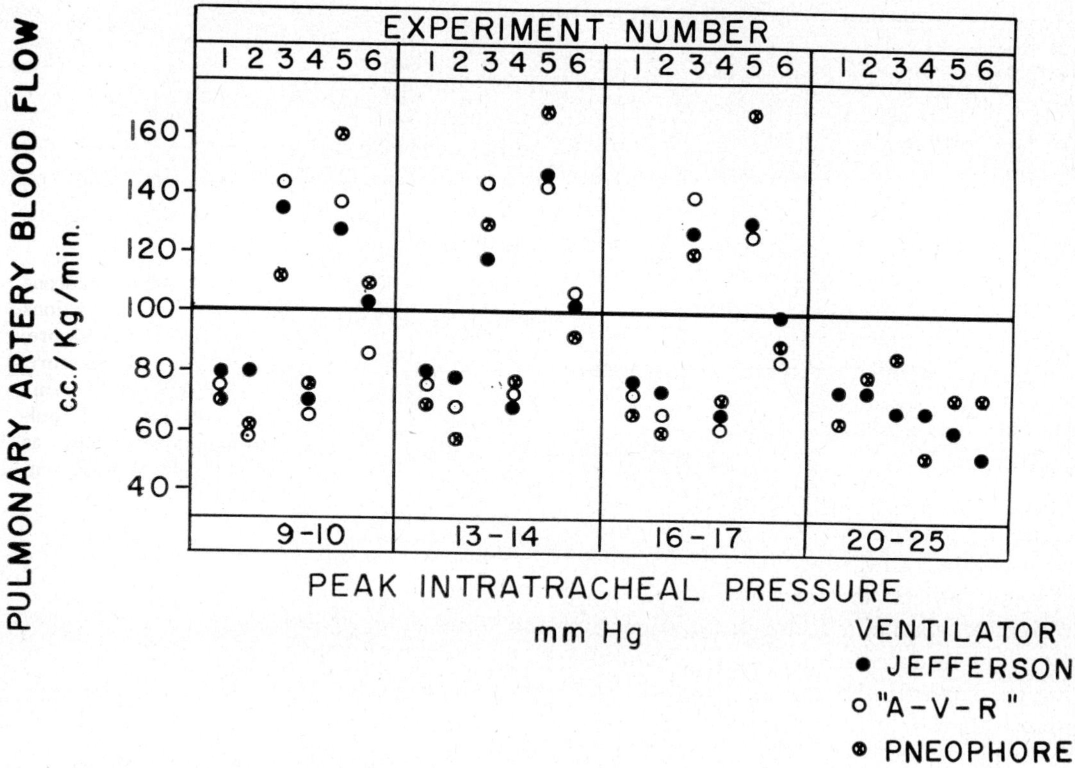

Fig 5.—Scattergram showing mean pulmonary blood flow observed during use of three different ventilators at varying pressure ranges. Each value plotted is a mean of two to four observations.

Such changes are minimized using the pneophore due to the rapid ventilatory rate. With both the Jefferson and the A-V-R the slower rates make the phase relationships easier to identify. It will be seen that the pulmonary artery flow and systemic arterial pressure vary reciprocally with intratracheal pressure while ΔP varies directly. The magnitude of this instantaneous change in pulmonary blood flow with alteration in ventilatory pressure is best illustrated in Fig 3. It can be noted that maximum flow peaks of 3.5 liters/min occur almost synchronously with the negative pressure "spikes." This flow value is reduced 50% by the positive intratracheal pressure peaks. In both instances the flow alteration lags slightly behind the intratracheal pressure change.

Mean pulmonary blood flow as a function of peak intratracheal pressure was investigated at five pressure ranges, and the results are shown in Fig 5. Respiratory rate was set at 18-20/min using the Jefferson and A-V-R ventilators but could not be controlled on the pneophore in which the rate is a function of the maximum inflation pressure. Values are not shown in Fig 5 below 9 mm Hg since inflation pressure below this level resulted in a clinical picture of hypoxia, including cyanosis, respiratory efforts, and struggling. The values shown represent means of two to four pulmonary blood flow measurements per point plotted. All six animals used in this portion of the study were changed in random fashion from one pressure range to another and from one ventilator to another. At least ten minutes were allowed after each change of pressure or ventilator for accommodation. It is apparent that throughout the 9-17 mm Hg peak intratracheal pressure range there is no essential difference in mean flow related to either pressure or type of ventilator. When the pressure exceeded 20 mm Hg a sharp drop in mean pulmonary blood flow occurred with both the Jefferson and the pneophore.

The A-V-R will not operate in this pressure range.

Comment

It has been established by Cournand and his group[2] that a fall in cardiac output caused by excessive intratracheal pressure is first reflected in the right ventricular output. In our observations, a consistent change in right ventricular output in the dog was first seen at intratracheal pressure above 20 mm Hg. This closely approximates Cournand's recommendation that mask pressure should not exceed 25 cm water (18.45 mm Hg). Excessive intratracheal pressure was also reflected in our study by a rise in differential pulmonary pressure suggesting increased pulmonary resistance. Observations reported by Edwards[3] and by Ankeney[4] strongly indicate that increase in pulmonary resistance is a major factor in fall of cardiac output with excessive intratracheal ventilating pressure. In the dog we found the optimum range of ventilating positive pressure to be quite narrow (+9 to +17 mm Hg). The variation in shape of the endotracheal pressure curves produced by these machines had no apparent effect on pulmonary artery blood flow when optimum ventilating pressures were used. However, the ratio of the duration of inspiration to the duration of expiration is within the recommended limits,

Negative pressure during the expiratory phase had no apparent effect on right ventricular output as studied here. However, the effect of this negative component on pulmonary exchange of blood gases was not investigated in this study but may be important.

Investigators have repeatedly emphasized the clinical importance of the detrimental effect of excessive positive intratracheal pressure in the open chest. Of equal importance is the careful control of ventilating intratracheal pressures in investigative work. It is easy to understand how lack of adequate control of ventilating pressure may give erroneous results in hemodynamic studies with the chest open.

Summary and Conclusions

Alterations in main pulmonary artery flow and pulmonary differential pressure produced by three different mechanical ventilators were studied in open-chest dogs.

Wide variations in instantaneous pulmonary artery flow occurred in reciprocal relationship to intratracheal pressure.

Pulmonary differential pressure varied synchronously with intratracheal pressure.

Mean pulmonary blood flow remained in accepted normal ranges with peak positive ventilatory pressure ranging from +9 to +17 mm Hg, while inflating pressures exceeding 20 mm Hg consistently diminished mean pulmonary blood flow.

Presence or absence of a negative phase in the ventilatory cycle did not affect mean pulmonary blood flow; blood gas exchange was not investigated in this study.

In two of the ventilators studied, (Jefferson, pneophore) it was possible to produce extremes of pressure which interfered with pulmonary blood flow, while the third (A-V-R) allowed such a narrow range of adjustment as to never interfere with pulmonary blood flow.

Worthington G. Schenk, Jr., MD, 462 Grider St, Buffalo 15, NY.

REFERENCES

1. Dameron, J. T., and Greene, D. G.: Use of the Burns Valve as a Simple Respirator for Intrathoracic Surgery in the Dog, J Thorac Surg 20:706, 1950.

2. Cournand, A.; Motley, H. L.; Werko, L.; and Richards, D. W., Jr.: Physiological Studies of the Effects of Intermittent Positive Pressure Breathing on Cardiac Output in Man, Amer J Physiol 152:162, 1948.

3. Edwards, W. S.: The Effects of Lung Inflation and Epinephrine on Pulmonary Vascular Resistance, Amer J Physiol 167:756, 1951.

4. Ankeney, J. L.; Hubay, C. A.; Hackett, P. R.; and Hingson, R. A.: The Effect of Positive and Negative Pressure Respiration on Unilateral Pulmonary Blood Flow in the Open Chest, Surg Gynec Obstet 98:600, 1954.

Postfracture Vascular Changes and Healing Process

JAMES B. WRAY, MD, AND H. O. GOODMAN, PhD, WINSTON-SALEM, NC

Introduction

Recent investigations have documented the sequence of vascular changes in the postfracture period. Fracture of a long bone leads to acute vasodilation throughout the traumatized limb.[6] Acute vasodilation is followed by chronic enlargement of the potential vascular space of the limb. With the passage of time, the enlarged vascular space gradually shrinks to prefracture size.[5,7,8]

While the relationship of these vascular changes to the healing process is unknown, two chief possibilities come to mind. Vascular alterations may be accompanied by metabolic adjustments that may or may not be essential to the fracture healing process. Second, vascular changes, or more specifically, the gradual return of the enlarged vascular bed to prefracture levels, may be related to the consolidation of bony union at the fracture site.

It is this latter possibility, a possible relationship of vascular bed recession to bony union, that is the concern of this investigation. The strength of the bony union at the fracture site was measured with an especially constructed apparatus. Vascular bed size was estimated by a technique of plastic injection that has been reported elsewhere.[5] The accumulated data have been subjected to statistical evaluation and are presented in the following report.

Submitted for publication April 17, 1963.

Professor of Surgery, Chairman of Division of Orthopedic Surgery, State University of New York, Upstate Medical Center (Dr. Wray); Assistant Professor of Preventative Medicine and Medical Genetics, Bowman Gray School of Medicine (Dr. Goodman).

From The Bowman Gray School of Medicine.

Materials and Methods

A total of 393 four-month-old male rats of the C. F. Nelson strain was used in this study which extended over a period of 80 days. Each rat was randomly assigned to one of several experimental groups. All animals were maintained on a diet of Purina Rat Chow and water *ad libitum* and were housed in metal cages in groups of six or seven rats.

Twenty-six of the animals were not operated upon and were utilized as controls. The remaining 367 rats were operated upon in the following manner. After each animal had been anesthetized with ether, one hind limb was painted with a 10% tincture of iodine. A small incision was made over the subcutaneous surface of the tibia in the mid portion of the bone just above the point of union of the fibula to the tibia. The tibia was then sectioned at this level with a small dental rongeur, and the skin wound was closed with a single small skin clip. No effort was made to immobilize the fractures, and, in the great majority of cases, spontaneous fracture occurred in the fibula.

Of the animals so operated upon, 156 were used to estimate the strength of the fracture site (Table 1). At selected days after fracture each animal was sacrificed with an overdose of ether. Both hind limbs were amputated. The fractured limb was x-rayed, and both fractured and nonfractured tibias were dissected free of soft tissues.

The cleaned tibia was then placed in an apparatus (Fig 1) constructed to measure the amount of force necessary to break the bone at the fracture site (or the corresponding area of the opposite nonfractured bone). The disrupting force was recorded in arbitrary units on a maximum reading dial. The difference in breaking strength between paired fractured and nonfractured limbs was then calculated.

The tibias of the 26 control animals were cleaned, and the breaking force necessary to disrupt each tibia at the experimental level was determined.

The remaining 211 animals were utilized to estimate changes in the potential vascular space of the limb on the side of the fracture (Table 2).

The technique of vascular space measurement has been published elsewhere but will be briefly described.[5] Immediately after death the thoracic

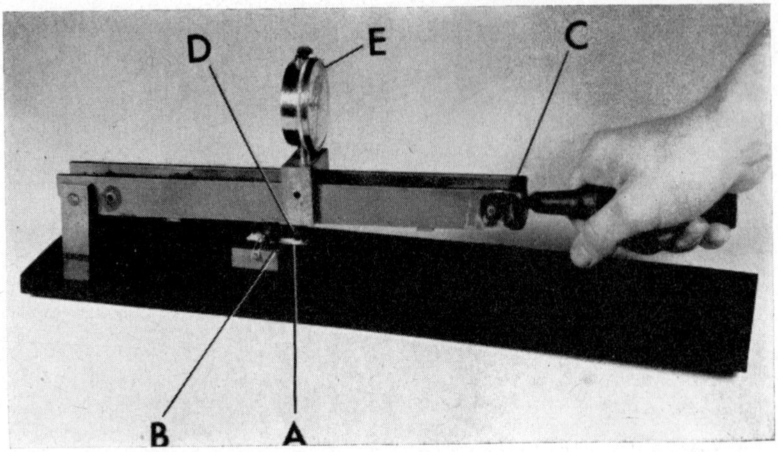

Fig 1.—Apparatus used to determine the breaking strength of the fracture callus. The test bone (*A*) is secured to the block (*B*) with the fracture site (or corresponding area of a nonfractured bone) directly over the sharpened end of the block. Depression of the lever (*C*) applies strain to the bone through two metallic arms. Pressure transmitted by the metallic arm (*D*) closest to the operator's hand is measured by the gauge (*E*). Breaking strength is registered as revolutions of the needle at the time of bone disruption.

aorta of each animal was cannulated with an injection system of polyethylene tubing, three-way stopcock, and 10 cc syringe. After a thorough flush of the vascular system with isotonic sodium chloride, 10 cc of methyl methacrylate, with promoter and catalyst added, was injected. After the plastic hardened, the carcass was skinned and both hind limbs were disarticulated at the hip. Paired limbs were then macerated in alternate solutions of KOH and HCl. At the completion of treatment, a plastic mold of the vascular space of each limb remained. The weight of each mold was compared to its paired counterpart.

Results

Analyses of relative strengths of tibias after fracture were based on paired comparisons, the unfractured tibia on the contralateral side serving as the control for each fractured tibia. All computations employed formulas from either Walker and Lev[4] or Snedecor.[3] Support for the use of paired rather than group comparisons was provided by the high correlation between breaking strengths of right and left tibias in the group of 26 controls ($r_{xy}=0.90$, $P<0.001$), and the wide variability between these animals.

The results of analyses of relative fracture strengths are presented in Table 1. The breaking strength of fractured tibias at the fracture site was unequivocally less than that of the unfractured controls through the 36th postfracture day. On day 42, the fractured

TABLE 1.—*Analyses of Mean Differences in Breaking Strength of Fractured Tibias Compared to Contralateral Unfractured Tibias*

Postfracture Day	N	$\bar{D}$ *	$SE_{\bar{D}}$ †	*t* ‡	*P* §
6	13	−2.04	0.10	−20.40	0.001
12	12	−1.39	0.15	− 9.27	0.001
18	12	−1.39	0.18	− 7.72	0.001
21	12	−1.30	0.19	− 6.84	0.001
24	13	−1.07	0.20	− 5.35	0.001
27	13	−1.15	0.18	− 6.39	0.001
30	12	−1.11	0.27	− 4.11	0.005
36	13	−1.17	0.18	− 6.50	0.001
42	12	−0.23	0.36	− 0.64	0.50
50	12	−0.62	0.22	− 2.82	0.05
65	12	−0.41	0.28	1.46	0.10
80	10	1.14	0.26	4.38	0.005

* Mean difference (fractured minus nonfractured tibias).
† Standard error of the mean difference.
‡ "Student" *t*-test.
§ Probability that a mean difference as large or larger could have arisen by chance if true mean difference = 0.

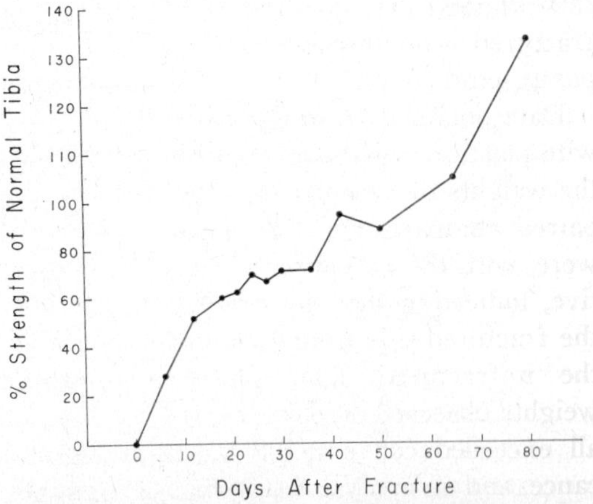

Fig 2.—Graph of the healing process in the fractured rat tibia expressed as resistance of breaking strain. Breaking strength of the fracture is expressed as a per cent of the breaking strength of the normal paired tibia and is plotted against time in days after fracture.

TABLE 2.—*Analyses of Mean Differences in Weights of Plastic Molds (Fractured Minus Unfractured) According to Postfracture Day*

Post-fracture Day	N	$\overline{D}$ *	$SE_{\overline{D}}$ †	t ‡	P §
3	17	0.128	0.027	4.74	<0.001
6	18	0.013	0.021	0.62	>0.50
9	18	0.015	0.031	3.39	<0.005
12	18	0.088	0.026	3.38	<0.005
15	16	0.014	0.027	0.52	>0.50
18	17	0.034	0.040	0.85	>0.40
21	18	−0.078	0.017	4.59	<0.001
24	18	0.020	0.032	0.62	>0.50
27	18	−0.038	0.034	−1.12	>0.20
30	18	0.023	0.020	1.15	>0.20
36	18	0.023	0.036	0.64	>0.50
42	17	0.056	0.026	2.15	<0.05

* Mean difference in mg.
† Standard error of mean difference in mg.
‡ "Student" *t*-test.
§ Probability that mean difference as large or larger could have arisen by chance if true $\overline{D} = 0$.

tibia values were still less than those of their paired counterparts, but the differences between the two were not statistically significant.

By the 65th day the fractured tibia was stronger than its paired nonfractured member. On the 80th postfracture day this strength differential had increased to a statistically significant level.

Fig 2 presents the average strengths of fractured tibias expressed in per cent of the strengths of the unfractured tibias. As shown in Table 1 the fractured tibias of these rats attained the same strength as their unfractured counterparts around the 60th postfracture day.

Data obtained from the 211 rats perfused with plastic are given in Table 2. Analyses of the weights of vascular casts are based upon paired comparisons. The mean differences were, with the exception of day 27, all positive, indicating that the weights of casts on the fractured side were greater than those on the unfractured side. The difference in weights observed on days 3, 9, 12, 21, and 42 all exceeded conventional levels of significance, and an analysis including all days also indicated a significant difference ($t=5.22$, $P<0.001$). It seems likely that failure of some samples to reach conventional significance levels resulted from sampling error.

The correlation between the mean differences in breaking strength and the mean differences in vascular volumes was computed to study the possibility of a relationship between breaking strength and vascular volume as measured by the plastic injection technique. The over-all correlation was 0.26 which cannot be shown to differ significantly from zero ($P>0.40$). Examination of Table 2 indicates a decrease in the mean difference of the plastic casts over the days 6, 12, 18, and 21. The correlation coefficient computed for these days alone was negative ($r_{xy}=-0.11$). Though again it cannot be shown to be different from zero ($P>0.50$). For days 24, 27, 30, 36, and 42 there appears a gradual, if erratic, increase in the differences of the plastic casts ($r_{xy}=0.69$, $P<0.20$). Though this coefficient is not significantly different from zero, it should be mentioned that it was based on only three degrees of freedom since only five pairs of means were used. This limitation was imposed in all of these correlations by the fact that the same animal could not be used for both fracture strength and vascular volume estimates.

Review of the x-rays of the fractures evaluated for their resistance to breaking was of interest but allowed no critical comment. In general, x-ray evidence of fracture healing roughly paralleled the gain in strength at the fracture site. On the other hand, the relationship between evidence of ossification as shown by x-ray and the breaking point of the fracture did not appear close enough to permit a critical estimate of the healing process.

Comment

A postfracture increase in total vascular space of the injured limb has been observed in earlier work which demonstrated a rise to maximum values at 9 to 12 days which was followed by a rapid return to prefracture levels. In this study, however, significantly larger plastic casts were noted on the fracture side as late as 21 and 42 days after fracture. While these observations might be attributed to sampling error, the authors are inclined to the view that the more persistant vascular reaction is due, at least in part, to the relatively slower fracture healing that follows the technique of open fracture employed in this study.

A reasonably clear picture of the fracture healing process is offered by Fig 2 in spite of the fact that overriding and angulation of a fracture occasionally occurred. The over-all pattern is similar to that observed in the two comparable studies of healing of the rat fibula that have been reported in the literature.[1,2] In brief, the most rapid increase in fracture breaking strength was observed in the first 12 days after fracture.

This initial gain in strength was followed by a slightly less rapid increase in strength that continued throughout the experiment. By 65 days the fractured tibia offered greater resistance to breaking than the opposite normal tibia, an observation that may be in part the consequence of excessive callus formation due to overriding of the fracture. It is noteworthy that this study and the two others that might be compared to it offer suggestive, if inconclusive, evidence that a period of relatively limited healing activity occurs around the 24th to 30th day after fracture.[1,2] The significance of this observation is unclear at this time.

The repeatedly demonstrated initial increase in vascular volume, the observed regular increase in fracture strength, and the hypothesis that vascular volume does not remain permanently altered all lead one to expect an association between the two variables in appropriate data. However, the data and computations derived in this study indicate that no simple linear relationship exists between the two. Indeed, failure to demonstrate a significant degree of association over the 42-day period during which the vascular volume was estimated suggests that the increasing bone strength and decreasing vascular volume are manifestations of separate and nondependent physiological mechanisms.

Conclusions

1. A surgically produced fracture of the tibia of the rat leads to enlargement of the vascular space of the entire limb.

2. Healing of surgically produced fractures, as measured by the breaking strength of the callus, occurs at a rapid and surprisingly constant rate. Eighty days after fracture the callus is stronger than a comparable area in the opposite normal tibia.

3. There is no apparent relationship between the postfracture vascular volume increase and the progressive attainment of union at the fracture site. It is likely that the two processes are due to entirely different physiologic mechanisms.

James B. Wray, MD, Division of Orthopedics, Department of Surgery, State University of New York, Upstate Medical Center, Syracuse, NY.

REFERENCES

1. Copp, D. H., and Greenberg, D. M.: Studies on Bone Fracture Healing: I. Effect of Vitamins A and D, J Nutr 29:261-267, 1945.

2. Lindsay, M. K., and Howes, E. L.: The Breaking Strength of Healing Fractures, J Bone Joint Surg (Amer) 13:491-501, 1931.

3. Snedecor, G. W.: Statistical Methods Applied to Experiments in Agriculture and Biology, Ames, Iowa: The Iowa State College Press, 1956.

4. Walker, H. M., and Lev, J.: Statistical Inference, New York: Henry Holt and Company, Inc., 1953.

5. Wray, J. B., and Lynch, C. J.: The Vascular Response to Fracture of the Tibia of the Rat, J Bone Joint Surg (Amer) 41:1143-1148, 1959.

6. Wray, J. B., and Spencer, M. P.: The Vasodilatory Response to Skeletal Trauma, Surg Forum 11:444-445, 1960.

7. Wray, J. B.: The Effect of Refracture on the Vascular Response to Fracture, Surg Gynec Obstet 112:421-424, 1961.

8. Wray, J. B.: The Effect of Age on the Vascular Response to Fracture, J Trauma 1:576-582, 1961.

Coronary Artery Pressure in the Perfused Heart

EDWIN G. MEYER, MD
AND
WILLIAM H. FALOR, MD
AKRON, OHIO

During extracorporeal perfusion multiple factors effect the coronary arterial pressure. Two of the most significant factors are controllable because they are functions of the bypass, viz, (1) the rate of flow and (2) the temperature of the perfusate. A third important factor, controllable by the surgeon during the operative procedure, is left heart decompression. Finally a fourth factor, only in part controllable, is ventricular fibrillation. The following report is an assay of the effect of these four factors on coronary arterial pressure.

Coronary arterial blood flow is approximately 5% of total cardiac output.[3,12] In the dog, the right coronary, carrying 20% of the total coronary flow, supplies the right auricle, interauricular septum, and a small portion of the right ventricle.[3,12] In this experiment the left coronary artery, carrying 80% of the total coronary flow to the remaining portions of the heart, was chosen for cannulation and perfusion. Left coronary perfusion rates of normal estimated flow to six times normal estimated flow were chosen

Submitted for publication April 18, 1963.
Supported in part by a grant from the Akron District Heart Association.

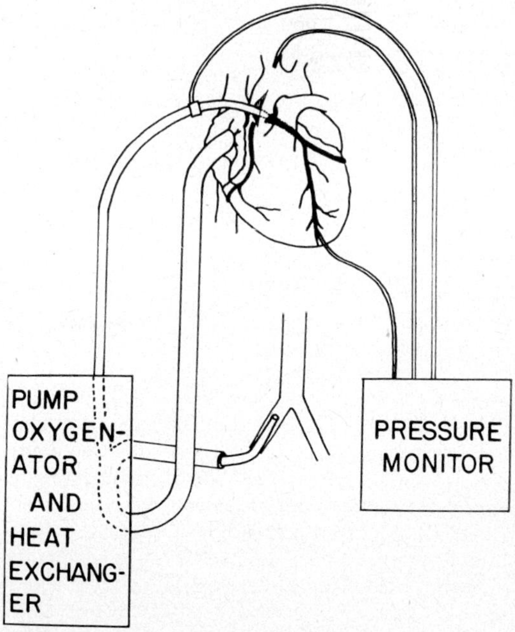

Fig 1.—Extracorporeal perfusion and arterial pressure monitoring system.

Table 1.—*Systemic and Left Coronary Artery Pressure and Flow Rates Before and During Extracorporeal Perfusion*

		Arterial Pressures, Mm Hg					
		Before Bypass		Complete Bypass *			
Dog	Weight, Kg	Internal Mammary	Left Coronary	Internal Mammary	Left Coronary	Total Body Perfusion, Cc/Min	Total Body Perfusion, Cc/Kg/Min
1	22.7	150/135	135/125	140	130	1,300	57.2
2	20.0	140/125	130/125	135	130	1,100	55.0
3	22.7	130/120	125/120	130	125	1,300	57.2
4	18.6	135/125	125/120	130	125	1,200	64.0
5	13.6	120/100	100/95	120	110	900	66.0
6	17.3	140/120	130/120	120	115	1,200	69.0
7	20.1	160/140	150/140	130	125	1,300	65.0
8	17.3	150/135	140/135	125	125	1,100	64.0
9	20.0	150/135	140/135	130	130	1,200	60.0
10	13.5	160/140	150/140	130	130	900	66.0

* During complete bypass the occlusive pump produces a constant pressure.

for each experiment. Arbitrary temperatures of 37 C, 28 C, and 18 C were used to represent normothermia, moderate hypothermia, and profound hypothermia, respectively.

Materials and Methods

Ten adult mongrel dogs, weighing 13 to 23 kg, anesthetized with thiopental sodium (Pentothal Sodium), were intubated and placed on an automatic respirator. Through a median sternotomy incision the pericardial sac was opened vertically. A bulb-tipped 23-gauge scalp vein needle was carefully inserted in the lumen of the most distal portion of the ramus descendens of the left coronary artery (Fig 1). The needle, held in place by sutures in the adjacent myocardium, was connected to a strain gauge for continuous arterial pressure recordings. A portion of the distal left coronary arterial flow was obstructed by this technique. The needle was kept patent with saline until heparinization was effected with the dose of 2 mg/kg animal weight. Systemic pressures (Fig 1) were electronically recorded from a cannula inserted into one of the internal mammary arteries. Having established baseline coronary and systemic arterial pressures, routine cannulation and cardiopulmonary bypass was effected with an occlusive pump (Pemco) and a Kay-Cross disc oxygenator. Total body perfusion flows were adjusted to restore systemic and coronary arterial pressure as near as possible to prebypass level (Table 1). Total body perfusion remained at this flow throughout the experiment. Blood was cooled by a Pemco heat exchanger; myocardial temperatures were registered on a telethermometer attached to a thermocouple placed next to the left ventricle.

The ascending aorta was clamped just proximal to the brachiocephalic artery; the proximal aorta was then opened in its long axis, and a No. 12 polyethylene cannula with a flanged end[10] was inserted in the left coronary os and immobilized with a purse-string suture. The left coronary artery was perfused by a separate pump calibrated for a flow rate of 4% of total perfusion flow.

Results

During bypass, perfusion flows necessary for maintenance of prebypass systemic arterial pressures ranged from 900 cc/min to 1,300 cc/min, or from 55 cc/kg/min to 69 cc/kg/min. Clamping of the aorta, aortotomy, and decompression of the heart reduced the pressure in the left coronary artery system to zero as expected. However, subsequent cannulation of the left coronary ostia and perfusion with the estimated normal left coronary arterial flow (Table 2) raised the

Table 2.—*Left Coronary Artery Pressure During Closed and Open Perfusion of the Heart*

		Left Coronary Arterial Pressure, Mm Hg	
Dog	Estimated Normal Left Coronary Flow, Cc/Min	Closed Perfused Heart	Open Decompressed Heart Perfused at Estimated Left Coronary Flow
1	52	130	50
2	44	130	35
3	52	125	35
4	48	125	40
5	36	110	40
6	48	115	50
7	52	125	40
8	44	125	50
9	48	130	40
10	36	130	30

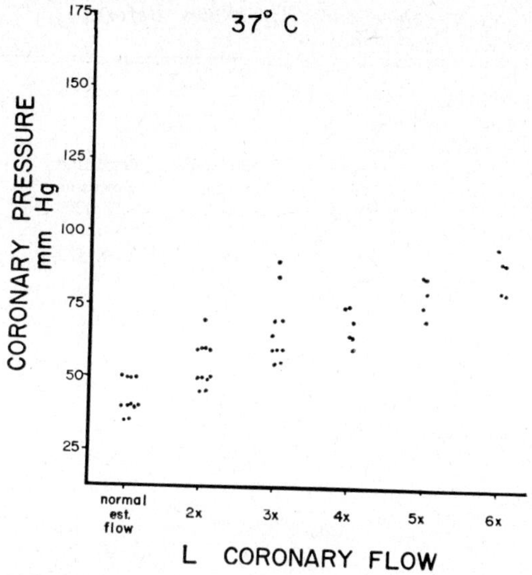

Fig 2.—Response to left coronary artery perfusion in the 37 C decompressed heart.

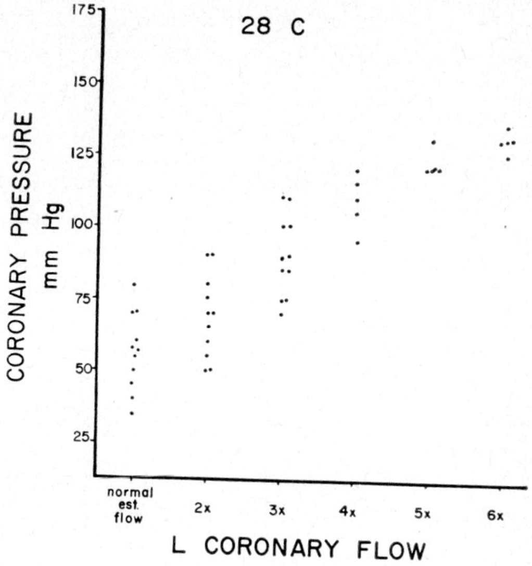

Fig 3.—Response to left coronary artery perfusion in the 28 C decompressed heart.

coronary arterial pressure to less than one half the coronary pressure of the closed perfused heart. Flow rates through the left coronary artery of the normothermic heart were then increased arbitrarily as multiples of the estimated normal left coronary arterial flow. As the flow increased the pressure increased to a very limited degree (Fig 2). At 37 C, flows of six times estimated normal did not produce a left coronary pressure equal to the predecompressed perfused heart.

After the cooling of the perfusate and heart muscle to 28 C (moderate hypothermia), the left coronary artery again was perfused at multiples of the normal estimated left coronary arterial flow. Coronary arterial pressures (Fig 3) are noted to be slightly higher than during normothermic perfusion. Finally with the perfusate and heart muscle cooled to 18 C (profound hypothermia), coronary arterial pressures (Fig 4) are noted to be higher than at either normothermia or at moderate hypothermia. Many of the 18 C

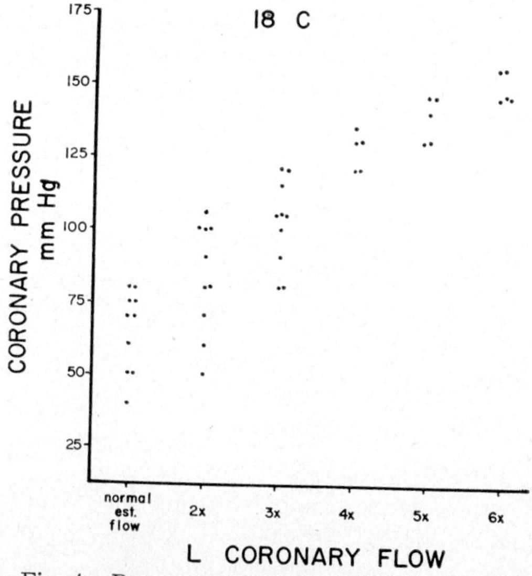

Fig 4.—Response to left coronary artery perfusion in the 18 C decompressed heart.

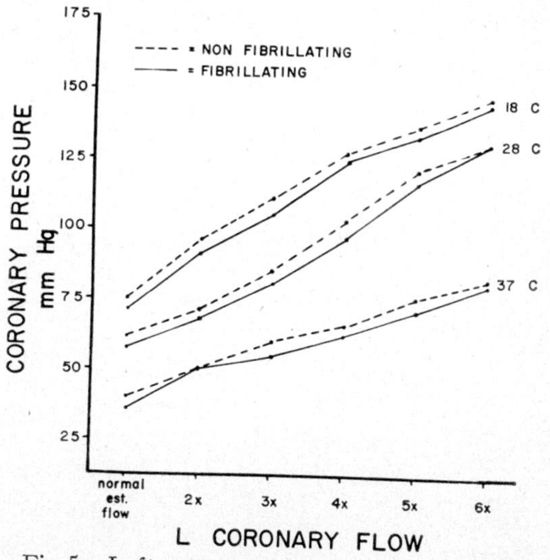

Fig 5.—Left coronary artery pressure in the perfused fibrillating and nonfibrillating decompressed heart.

hearts developed petechiae as the perfusion rate of the left coronary artery approached five to six times normal estimated arterial flow.

In four perfused hearts, coronary arterial pressures were recorded at alternate periods of normal beating and ventricular fibrillation. Myocardial fibrillation was initiated at 37 C, 28 C, and 18 C either by anoxia and by mechanical myocardial stimulation or by hypothermia alone at low temperature levels (Fig 5). Of significance, however, in normothermic and even in profoundly hypothermic hearts was the defibrillation that frequently followed left coronary arterial perfusion with flows of five or six times the estimated normal.

Comment

Arterial pressure is a product of flow times resistance (P=FR). In this study of left coronary arterial pressures, the blood flow was carefully controlled. Resistance, however, is a function of several factors: (1) the hydrostatic pressure of the full ventricles, especially of the left, (2) the viscosity of the blood, (3) the tone of the coronary arteries, and (4) the tissue tension of the myocardium.

From these experiments one cannot assay the importance of each of these factors in the determination of the ultimate left coronary arterial pressure. It is evident, however (Table 2), that the hydrostatic pressure of a bolus of blood in the left ventricle is a major force. Normally 40% of the coronary venous return is by thebesian flow into the ventricles.[3] It seems likely that with the reduction in ventricular resistance in the opened heart, thebesian flows may increase and thus contribute to the coronary arterial pressure drop.[12]

Cardiac output in the normothermic dog has been estimated at about 100 cc/kg/min.[4,6,9] In our experiments systemic perfusion flow required to restore each dog's systemic pressure to prebypass level averaged 64 cc/kg/min. This may have led to a moderately false low in estimated left coronary flow. However, estimated left coronary flow was increased by multiples, and this created only slight to moderate changes in the left coronary system pressure in the open perfused heart.

By comparing Fig 1, 2, and 3 it can be seen that as the perfusate and myocardial temperature is progressively lowered from 37 C to 28 C to 18 C, the coronary arterial pressure increases moderately. It is concluded that sludging and increased blood viscosity accounts for much of this increase. Hegnaur et al [6] demonstrated a two- to threefold increase in blood viscosity as the temperature was lowered to 20 C. On the other hand, it was concluded by Berne [2] that in the experimental animal with normal cardiac innervation a lowering of coronary arterial temperature resulted in a decrease in arterial tone and thus in a decrease in coronary pressure. Regardless, in the present experiments where flow rate and myocardial muscle tension have been constant and where hypothermia has tended to lower pressure by virtue of decrease in arterial tone, the ultimate progressive coronary arterial hypertension of hypothermia is felt to reflect an increasing resistance to flow by the remaining determinant of pressure, viz, blood viscosity.

Coronary arterial perfusion flow rates two, three, and four times normal, commonly at even deep hypothermia, reverted ventricular fibrillation to a normal beat. The mechanism for this phenomena is not known, however, adequate oxygenation is inferred. The constancy of the response suggests the use of increased coronary perfusion in the clinical case of refractory ventricular fibrillation. Nevertheless, in the dog's heart at 18 C, left coronary artery perfusion flow greater than three times normal produces coronary arterial hypertension and is associated with petechiae.

Conclusion

During normothermic extracorporeal circulation, left coronary arterial pressure is reduced by at least 50% by the decompression of the left ventricle and is only moderately raised by increasing the coronary flow rate even to six times normal. Progressive hypothermia down to 18 C is associated with a progressive slight elevation of left coronary arterial pressure, presumably secondary to increasing viscosity of the perfusate.

The onset of fibrillation in the open perfused heart does not significantly change the coronary arterial pressure. Increasing the flow rate of coronary perfusion will commonly lead to defibrillation regardless of the cardiac temperature but during profound hypothermia will tend to produce myocardial petechiae.

Edwin G. Meyer, MD, Akron City Hospital, 525 E Market St, Akron 9, Ohio.

REFERENCES

1. Anrep, G. V.; Blalock, A.; and Hammouda, M.: The Distribution of the Blood in the Coronary Blood Vessels, J Physiol (London) 67:87, 1929.

2. Berne, R. M.: Coronary Flow in Immersion Hypothermia, Circ Res 2:236, 1954.

3. Best, C. H., and Taylor, N. B.: The Physiological Basis of Medical Practice, ed 5, Baltimore: The Williams and Wilkins Company, 1950, pp 322-325.

4. Edwards, W. S.; Tuluy, S.; Reber, W. E.; Siegel, A.; and Bing, R. J.: Coronary Blood Flow and Myocardial Metabolism in Hypothermia, Ann Surg 139:275, 1954.

5. Hegnaur, A. H., and D'Amato, H. E.: Oxygen Consumption and Cardiac Output in the Hypothermic Dog, Amer J Physiol 178:138, 1954.

6. Hegnaur, A. H.; Shuler, W. J.; and Haterius, H. O.: Cardiovascular Response of the Dog to Immersion and Hypothermia, Amer J Physiol 161: 455, 1950.

7. Littlefield, J. B.; Lowiedi, E. M.; and Muller, W. H.: Experimental Left Coronary Perfusion Through an Aortotomy During Cardiopulmonary Bypass, J Thorac Cardiov Surg 40:685, 1960.

8. McGoon, D. C., in discussion of Gordon, A. S.; Meyer, B. W.; and Jones, J. C.: Open-Heart Surgery Using Deep Hypothermia Without an Oxygenator, J Thorac Cardiov Surg 40:801-802, 1960.

9. Sabiston, D. C.; Theden, E. O.; and Gregg, D. E.: The Relationship of Coronary Blood Flow and Cardiac Output and Other Parameters in Hypothermia, Surgery 38:498, 1955.

10. Sharp, W. V.: Personal communication.

11. Shumway, N. E.; Gliedman, M. L.; and Lewis, F. J.: Coronary Perfusion for Longer Periods of Cardiac Occlusion Under Hypothermia, J Thorac Surg 30:598, 1953.

12. Wiggers, C. J.: Physiology in Health and Disease, ed 3, Philadelphia: Lea & Febiger, 1939, p 701.

Gastric Cancer: A Midcentury Look

M. MICHAEL EISENBERG
AND
EDWARD R. WOODWARD
GAINESVILLE, FLA

There has been recent editorial emphasis on the long-standing observation that gastric malignancy in the United States has been on the steady decrease for the past 2½ decades and very probably longer (Fig 1).[64] During the years 1930 to 1955 the age-adjusted mortality rates have fallen approximately 23%.[45,64] From a clinical aspect the decline has become so striking, in fact, that a number of medical centers have recorded a drop in admissions for this disease in excess of 50% since 1952.[64] By way of contrast, death from carcinoma of all types has increased during the same interval, and, while the mortality rate from carcinoma of the stomach has fallen from 19.8 to 11.2 per 100,000 population, that from carcinoma of the colon and rectum has remained stable (Fig 2).[45] The trend has not been confined to the United States alone; comparably reduced death rates have been recorded for Holland, Norway, and Great Britain.[100]

Submitted for publication April 22, 1963.

From the Department of Surgery, University of Florida College of Medicine.

At various times during the last half century students of the disease have implicated dietary and hereditary factors, infectious organisms, chronic and specific irritations, endogenous or internal inciting factors such as hormones, and premalignant conditions such as gastric ulcer, chronic gastritis, gastric polyps, and hypochlorhydria or achlorhydria.[33,45,96,61] While under certain circumstances one or more of these factors can be incriminated, present evidence is insufficient to single out any one influence as the prime mover.

Attempts to clarify this dramatic decline by epidemiologic means have not met with notable success. There has been a great deal of recent evidence presented, largely from European clinics but supported as well by American studies, which has suggested that there is an increased incidence of gastric cancer in patients with blood group type A. Hogg and Pack,[42] in a review of 5,678 cases of gastric carcinoma presented in the international literature, noted an increased rate

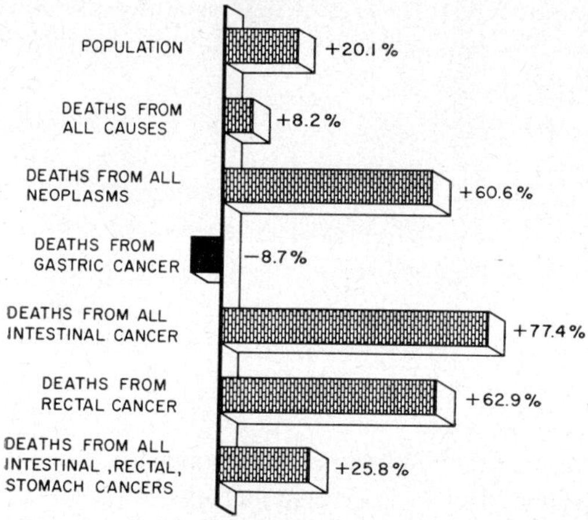

Fig 1.—Percentage change during the years 1933 to 1950. During this era of marked population increase, mortality rates per 100,000 people for all causes combined and for all neoplasms have risen sharply. During the same interval deaths from carcinoma of the stomach have declined. (Based on data from Ivy.[45])

of 7.12% over that which may be expected in the normal population in the five countries studied. They have concluded that either blood type O protects against gastric cancer or blood type A imposes an increased predilection. On the other hand in a review of 237 cases of their own, no statistically significant increase was noted among type A patients. Billington[13] in a review of 483 British patients with gastric carcinoma also found no real association with the type A blood grouping. Aird, Bentall, and Fraser Roberts[1] in Britain, Hollander[43] in Switzerland, and Køster, Sindrup, and Seele[52] in Denmark have shown a higher relationship with type A blood, and these studies have been corroborated on American patients by Buckwalter and co-workers.[20,21] The latter were not able, however, to demonstrate any relationship between age, sex, social and economic status, past or familial history, gastric acid secretion, or degree of malignant spread and the blood type. While no firm conclusions can be drawn from these studies, there appears to be a small but significantly increased risk of gastric carcinoma among blood type A patients.[42,61]

These observations, even if valid, do not appear to appreciably enlighten our understanding of either the etiology of the disease or the observed decrease in incidence during recent times. Although important genetic and hereditary factors cannot be completely excluded, the marked variation of over-all incidence of stomach cancer in different countries, the higher incidence in higher latitudes,[61] and the inverse correlation with economic status[61] may all represent clues to an environmental basis.[64] For example, while England, Wales, and United States have recorded a drop in gastric carcinoma, Finland, Japan, and Iceland continue to sustain the highest rates in the world.[61,64,100]

Despite the apparent and genuine decline in the incidence of this disease, it continues to remain secondary only to cancer of the

Fig 2.—Death from gastrointestinal malignancy in terms of percentages of all deaths from neoplasms. While deaths from carcinoma of the rectum and colon have remained stable, mortality from cancer of the stomach has declined. (Based on data presented by Ivy.[45])

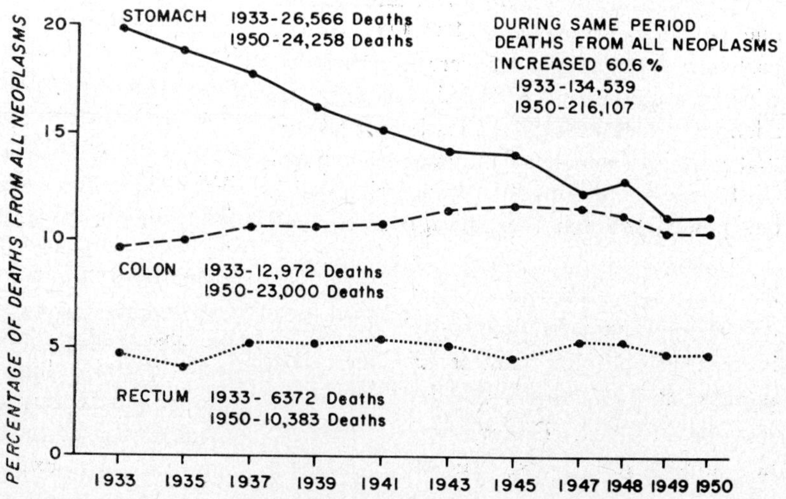

colorectal area in frequency of malignant neoplasms of the gastrointestinal tract. Cancer of the stomach was said, in 1939, to be responsible for more deaths than all malignant tumors of the lip, tongue, cheek, tonsil, pharynx, larynx, salivary glands, thyroid, male and female breasts, ovary, cervix, and uterus combined.[54,110] Cancer in the gastrointestinal tract accounts for approximately one third of all malignancies of the body, and it has been likewise estimated that one third of these can be cured. Texter and Barborka [106] have pointed out that in the mouth there is a 30%-70% cure rate, in the colon and rectum a 30%-50% cure rate, but in the stomach an over-all cure rate of only 5%-14%. The Connecticut Registry figures have shown the five-year-survival rate in carcinoma of the stomach for the years 1935 to 1951 to vary between 4% and 7%.[14] Numerous other series have corroborated these findings. While intensive efforts have been made on a number of fronts to clarify the etiology and to effect a respectable salvage rate, and despite improvements in diagnostic techniques and education of the public, cure rate in diagnosed carcinoma of the stomach continues relatively static. For these reasons the disease remains one of the more compelling challenges to both the researcher and the clinician.

Experimental Work

Spontaneous gastric carcinoma is extremely uncommon among lower animals. In one postmortem study of 100,000 rats, no gastrointestinal neoplasms were found. Likewise, in an autopsy of 381 baboons only one adenoma was located.[55] It has been reported that gastric carcinoma has never been noted in the enormous amount of material which has passed through the Chicago stockyards over the years.[110] Morson [68] and others [45] have expressed the opinion that this species difference cannot be due entirely to an inherent susceptibility, and it has been proposed that living and environmental habits may be involved. Dietary factors such as hot liquids and foods, seasoning, coloring, medicinals, alcohol and tobacco, and the general increased level of anxiety among men are examples.

For many years experimental efforts directed toward the production of gastric carcinoma in lower forms by the use of carcinogenic hydrocarbons, deficient diets, endocrines, parasites, bacteria, and viruses met with little success.[45,110] It has become apparent, therefore, that additional cocarcinogens or a suitable tissue environment is a necessary accompaniment for the success of experimental production of such lesions. It has been widely substantiated, for example, that trauma enhances the effect of chemical carcinogens on skin.[32,45,99] It appears likely that the same holds true for all epithelia including that of the gastrointestinal tract, and experimental gastric tumors have been elicited by similar techniques. The rate of malignant transformation, on this basis, is noted to be considerably higher in those instances in which the carcinogen is applied to areas of epithelial discontinuity.

Stein-Werblowsky [99] has stated that the decisive factor in malignant transformation appears to be intimate contact of the carcinogen and young regenerating elements of tissue as is occasioned in areas of ulceration, abrasion, or wound repair. Moreover, the intramural introduction of carcinogens has produced malignancy in experimental animals,[101] whereas simple per oral feeding of comparable materials has not. Similarly, the addition of hydrophilic or lipophilic agents to carcinogens appears to potentiate their effect and has greatly facilitated the production of experimental tumors.[3,9,45,92] It has been postulated that human gastric malignancy may have a similar genesis, that is, exposure of basal or regenerating cells such as may occur under conditions of atrophic gastritis or ulceration, to exogenous dietary carcinogens. It is significant that comparable observations have been made on colonic lesions, and a high incidence of malignant change has been noted in long-standing cases of ulcerative colitis.[6,61] There is no evidence, however, that experimental carcinomas are

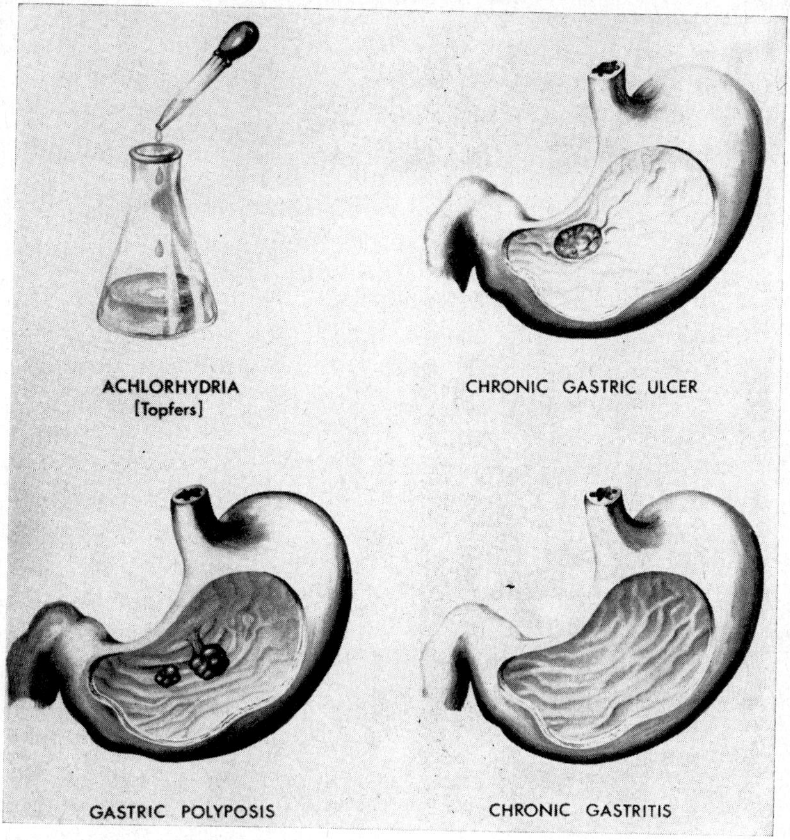

Fig 3.—Four benign conditions which have been implicated as possible precursors of gastric malignant degeneration in man.

preceded in animals by any of the so-called precancerous conditions.

Premalignant Conditions

In general there are four benign conditions of the stomach which have been implicated as precursors of gastric malignancy. These are achlorhydria, chronic atrophic gastritis, chronic gastric ulcer, and adenomatous gastric polyps (Fig 3).

1. *Achlorhydria and Chronic Gastritis.*—Von den Velden [108] in 1879 and Konjetzny [50] in 1938 were among the first to recognize a relationship between achlorhydria and carcinoma of the stomach.[40,61] Corroborating evidence for this observation is abundant. Comfort, Kelsey, and Berkson [26] have stated that achlorhydria probably precedes development of carcinoma in a large percentage of cases. They have noted a three times higher incidence in the absence of acid. Surveys at the University of Minnesota have demonstrated that 70%-75% of patients with gastric carcinoma are achlorhydric, and an additional 10%-15% are hypochlorhydric with less than 30 degrees free acid.[40] Sommers has also noted a high frequency of achlorhydria in 204 cases of carcinoma of the stomach.[96]

Observations concerning the high incidence of achlorhydria and subsequent development of gastric cancer in patients with pernicious anemia have also been widely reported.* Zamcheck and co-workers [113] have shown that 10% of patients with pernicious anemia have carcinoma of the stomach by the time of death. Jenner [46] has found cancer of the stomach in 4% of 180 pernicious anemia patients. Mosbech and Videbaek [69,70,71] have noted a three times higher incidence of cancer in pernicious anemia in the populations studied in several Scandinavian countries. Hitchcock, Sullivan, and Wangensteen,[40] in a study of 3,439 patients 50 years or older with hypochlorhydria but

* References 26, 41, 50, 81, 93, 103, 61.

without the diagnosis of pernicious anemia, followed their group for up to 9½ years. Hydrochloric acid secretion was tested by intubation with three injections of 0.5 mg of histamine phosphate used as the gastric stimulant. Patients were classified as achlorhydric or hypochlorhydric (free hydrochloric acid below 30 degrees). Thirty-eight carcinomas, or 4.5 times the incidence of gastric cancer in the general population, were turned up in this study. In the presence of pernicious anemia, on the other hand, an 18.3 times incidence of malignancy was noted.

While the coincidental association of achlorhydria, atrophic gastritis, and gastric carcinoma is well established,[26] a sequential relationship has not been proved, and it is postulated by many that gastric secretion may simply be a reflection of epithelial integrity rather than a cause of subsequently observed pathology.[61] Barrett [7] has pointed out that the incidence of achlorhydria in the normal population approaches 20%-25% and in patients with gastric carcinoma 50%. Eklöf and co-workers [29] have reported a 19%-35% achlorhydric rate in normal patients. Meadows and Lefeber [60] in a 14-year survey of over 1,000 consecutive gastroscopic examinations found chronic atrophic gastritis to be a common finding irrespective of the reason of the examination, and its significance was seriously questioned. Guiss and Stewart [34] were unable to demonstrate any direct relationship between atrophic gastritis, achlorhydria, and gastric carcinoma, and they noted an increased frequency of atrophy with longevity. Hebbel,[38] in a study of almost 200 specimens resected for malignancy, noted gastritis of all degrees and extent, independent of the size of the carcinoma. He was also able to correlate the degree of atrophy with achlorhydria to histamine but could make no firm conclusions as to whether or not gastritis antedated carcinoma in a significant percentage of cases.

Mider [61] has raised the question, based in part on observations similar to these, as to whether achlorhydria and chronic gastritis are not simply coincidental and concurrent processes with no etiologic relationship to malignant degeneration. If chronic atrophic gastritis leads to the development of malignant change, do the factors responsible for the production of the atrophy lead to neoplastic transformation or do they simply permit other noxious agents to act on an area of increased susceptibility? Fairley and coworkers,[30] in a five-year survey of 32 cases of atrophic gastritis proven by gastric biopsy (12 male and 20 female), found that no gastric carcinoma developed. It is apparent, therefore, that no clear-cut conclusions on this point may be drawn at this time, and the question of a direct etiologic relationship between achlorhydria, atrophic gastritis, and malignancy remains unsettled.

2. *Adenomatous Polyps.*—It has been frequently stated and generally accepted that benign adenomatous polyps of the stomach *may* undergo malignant degeneration.† Eklöf, Engstedt, and Reizenstein,[29] in an extensive survey of polyps of the stomach and duodenum, found that 32 out of 176 patients with polyposis had proven malignancy, and two additional patients had "pre-malignant polyps." They demonstrated that 80% or more of patients with gastric polyposis are achlorhydric; similarly in patients with cancer of the stomach 50%-85% are achlorhydric. The problem of the relationship of gastric polyps to malignancy is also interrelated with achlorhydria and gastric atrophy since there is similarly increased incidence of polyps with achlorhydria.[10,19,31,35,41,44,49] Moreover there is an associated gastric atrophy in most instances. The predominant type of gastric malignant growth occurring in pernicious anemia is polypoid, and this, too, has suggested to some a possible relationship between adenocarcinoma and adenoma.[31,90,112] Atrophic gastritis has been reported by biopsy in almost every case of pernicious anemia and is widely reported to be associated with gastric carcinoma and with polyps.[10,29,31,44] Eklöf and co-workers,[29] however, while conceding that the link between intrinsic factor deficiency, idiopathic pernicious anemia, achlorhydria, gas-

† References 10, 16, 44, 48, 50, 66, 67, 102, 103.

tric polyps, and carcinoma *may* be atrophic gastritis, stress the observation that causal relationship is not yet completely understood. They further point out that polyps may simply be a manifestation of a generally increased susceptibility to tumor although with an indubitable tendency to malignant degeneration.

Plachta and Speer,[80] Breslaw,[18] and others [63] have maintained that malignant polyps are *primarily* malignant and have indicated that there is no conclusive proof of a single polyp undergoing malignant degeneration. While Southwick and Cole [97] have reported a 16.3% malignant rate in gastric polyps, gastroscopic studies have not supported this thesis. Carey and Hay,[23] in a long-term gastroscopic study in a series of patients with gastric polyps, were unable to find a single instance of malignant degeneration. While others favor the view of polyps undergoing malignant degeneration with a reported incidence of between 6.7% and 27%, this question too remains unsettled.[10] Moreover, Monaco, Roth, Castleman, and Welch [63] have made careful histologic and pathologic studies of 153 consecutive patients with gastric polyps. They found no evidence that adenomatous polyps progress to the usual type of invasive, infiltrating carcinoma or that residual stomachs after polypectomy are more prone to the development of cancer. Despite occasional areas microscopically suggestive of cancer in situ, it is believed that if these tumors are removed while benign adenomatous tissue is identifiable histologically, they act in a biologically benign manner. Ten per cent of polyps in their study had carcinoma in situ though only in small foci. There was only one case of actual invasive carcinoma, and in no cases were metastases noted; nor was there any evidence of progression of the lesion. A number of authors have noted an increased incidence of malignant change in polyps greater than 2 cm.[10,29,109] In the study by Monaco and his co-workers,[63] 10% of polyps were 2 cm or greater in diameter. In none was there any evidence of metastases except in those with a separate invasive carcinoma.

The frequently cited analogous relationship between benign colonic polyps and carcinoma of the colon bears close scrutiny. A recent rash of evidence has been presented to refute any direct association between the benign adenomatous polyp of the large bowel and adenocarcinoma. Castleman and Krickstein [25] and Spratt, Ackerman and Moyer,[98] on re-examination of previous reports of malignant degeneration of polypoid lesions, have concluded that the overwhelming majority of cancers of the colon arise as carcinoma *de novo* or in villus adenomas and not in adenomatous polyps. They have stated that the adenomatous polyp is a lesion of negligible malignant potential.

It is entirely possible if not probable that the relationship between gastric polyposis and malignancy may require similar, more extensive re-evaluation. It should also be noted, that, since gastric carcinoma has a 5.5 times greater frequency than gastric polyposis, polyps do not, in any event, occur in a sufficient number of instances to account for more than a very small number of malignant cases.[45] Such observations are consistent with the theory that while carcinoma is more prone to occur in the presence of chronic inflammatory or degenerative processes, this does not necessarily imply a direct etiologic relationship.

3. *Chronic Gastric Ulcer.*—The long standing controversy surrounding the etiologic relationship between carcinoma of the stomach and chronic gastric ulcer has never been satisfactorily settled. The incidence of benign gastric ulcer undergoing malignant degeneration has been variously reported as having an incidence of from 0% to 100%.[100] Flood [31] has pointed out that, based on histopathologic studies, 5%-15% of gastric ulcers are associated with malignancy. Orator,[74] in a review of 700 cases of gastric ulcer and 150 cases of gastric carcinoma, reported that 80% of carcinoma arose from a precancerous gastritis and 20% from gastric ulcer. A direct causal relationship between benign gastric ulcer and cancer, however, is not consistent with the prevailing point of view, and, in general, wide-

spread clinical experience has not supported this concept. Rienhoff and Baker [83] have stated that either an ulcer is malignant from the beginning or never undergoes malignant degeneration.

It has been suggested that ulcers which appear to be benign by all standard diagnostic criteria but which ultimately prove to be malignant may simply represent examples of slow growing carcinoma.[106] Notkin,[73] Palmer and Humphreys [76] and Bone and Broome [15] have demonstrated that healing may occur in an ulcerated cancer as well as in a benign lesion. Mallory [57] has stated that carcinoma in situ may be almost completely digested leaving only a tiny area of the original lesion intact and may, therefore, present as an example of an apparent gastric ulcer with a small focus of carcinoma in its edge. Review of pathologic data [45] concerning the location of the lesion has demonstrated that in 66% of the cases benign ulcers are found on the lesser curvature between 1 to 3 cm from the cardia and 3 to 5 cm from the pylorus (Fig 4). In 20% of the cases the ulcers are in the pyloric canal and the antrum within 3 to 4 cm of the pyloric orifice. *Roughly speaking the opposite is true of carcinoma.* Forty to 71% of cancers are found in the antrum in postmortem studies and 26%-83% in clinical data.

While it is probable that a small number of localized malignancies may develop at the margin of an otherwise benign peptic ulcer,[27] it appears unlikely that more than 2% or 3% of gastric carcinomas ever develop on this basis. The statement made by Ewing in 1919 that the relationship of gastric ulcer to gastric cancer is "rather close, quite obscure, and as yet incompletely explained," has retained its validity.[100]

Physicians are aware, however, that the etiologic relationship between chronic gastric ulcer and carcinoma is at present academic. To the physician confronted by a patient with roentgenologic evidence of an ulcerated gastric lesion, the important question which must be answered is: Does the lesion represent a benign ulcer or is it malignant at the time of diagnosis? This continues to be one of the most challenging and absorbing problems in clinical medicine. Since the benign gastric ulcer can be sometimes successfully managed by medical means alone and since the only known cure for gastric carcinoma depends upon adequate surgical treatment, the question of when to hesitate and when to operate is of paramount importance. Moreover, the surgical approach to the treatment of the two diseases should be entirely different. Boles [14] has expressed serious concern for the 80%-90% of patients with truly benign gastric ulcer who undergo unneces-

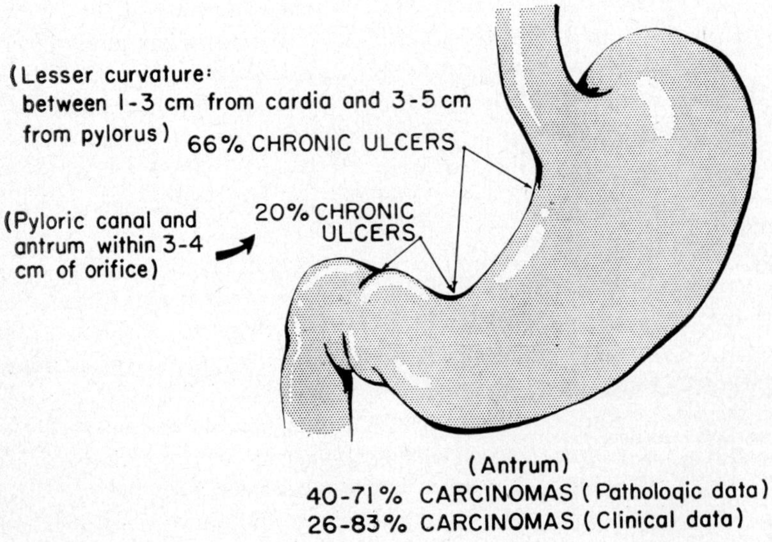

Fig 4.—Distribution of carcinoma and chronic ulcer of the stomach. In general, clinical and pathologic data support the contention that benign gastric ulcer and gastric carcinoma have different anatomic locations. (Based on data presented by Ivy.[45])

sarily extensive gastric resection. Fortunately, diagnostic acumen has developed to the point where the difference between benign and malignant disease of the stomach imposes little difficulty in the modern clinic.[4,104] Ill advised radical surgery for the benign lesion can, on this basis, be minimized.

Diagnosis of Carcinoma of the Stomach

Symptomatology is the commonest and most often the earliest clue to an underlying malignancy. In carcinoma of the stomach the symptoms may be absent or minimal, may resemble peptic ulcer, or may be vague and misleading.[106] In review of 1,708 patients with gastric carcinoma Marshall[59] found epigastric pain and discomfort, anorexia and vomiting, and weight loss to be among the earliest symptoms. Great weight loss, severe anemia, vomiting, hematemesis, and melena are all evidence of *advanced* carcinoma. Jonas and Stauffer[47] report that anorexia, distaste for meat, postprandial fullness, and long-standing indigestion are present in 25% of cases. As an early symptom, pain is unreliable, and only about half of the patients with carcinoma of the stomach have this complaint when first seen.[106] Occult blood in the stool is common but may be a later sign.[47,91] Symptoms referable to

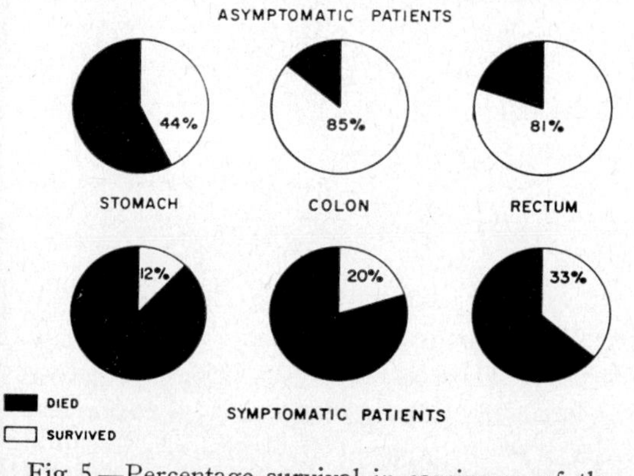

Fig 5.—Percentage survival in carcinoma of the stomach, colon, and rectum; University of Minnesota study.[28] Survival rate after treatment for cancer of the gastrointestinal tract is markedly reduced in those patients in whom symptomatology has played a role in diagnosis. Patients in whom treatment is instituted prior to the onset of symptoms are far more amenable to cure.

iron deficiency anemia from blood loss are also noted frequently and consist of weakness, dizziness, dyspnea on exertion, and, in the late stages, cardiac failure and syncope. Since only late lesions may be diagnosed on the basis of physical examination, in general this aspect of diagnosis contributes little or nothing to the early treatment of gastric carcinoma.[73]

In a cancer detection clinic such as is found at the University of Minnesota,[28] the survival percentage of patients with carcinoma of the stomach was 44% in those patients in which there was no symptomatology. In colon carcinoma the cure rate was 85% and in carcinoma of the rectum 81%. In a similar group studied which, however, were *symptomatic,* only 12% of carcinomas of the stomach were curable, 20% of carcinomas of the colon, and 33% of carcinomas of the rectum (Fig 5). While symptomatology is, therefore, the most important clue to the existence of underlying malignant disease, it is apparent that once symptoms have occurred the vast majority of patients have already been lost in terms of potential cure. Indeed, one out of two patients are said to be *inoperable* by the time they seek hospital care.[22] A great deal of energy has been expended in an effort to educate the public in the value of early reporting of symptomatology and the importance of immediately seeking competent medical care. For carcinoma of the stomach, at least, there appears to have been little gained by this approach. A logistically feasible mass screening test for the detection of *presymptomatic* gastric carcinoma is not yet a reality.

Diagnostic Techniques

While available material reviewed thus far has revealed a discouraging picture as far as the etiology and early detection of the malignant gastric lesion is concerned, accurate diagnosis is none the less important from the point of view of palliation. Moreover, it is obligatory to separate the benign gastric lesion from the malignant one in order that unnecessarily extensive radical procedures not be applied where they are not needed.[14]

Of the diagnostic tools available for differentiating between benign and malignant lesions of the stomach, exfoliative cytology, endoscopy, radiography, and gastric analysis are the most helpful and most important.

1. *Exfoliative Cytology.*—Although not available in every institution, this approach has been felt by some to represent the most useful technique for the early detection of carcinoma.[14,86] A variety of procedures has been devised whereby carcinomatous cells are obtained by means of gastric lavage. Antral abrasive balloons,[79,87] brushes,[5,111] high pressure fluid streams,[89] lavage with papain,[85] chymotrypsin in a buffered acetate solution,[88] and simple lavage with saline have all been used.[86] Many clinics have abandoned the brush techniques because they have found them to be cumbersome and unreliable, largely due to difficulty in positioning of the tube. The chymotrypsin method has also been abandoned by some in favor of a simple saline wash because of the difficulty in preparation and maintenance of the lytic solutions. Saline alone has been found to offer the same degree of yield and accuracy as any of the more complex lavage solutions.[86]

While there is not general agreement as to the over-all value of the cytologic techniques when compared to x-ray and gastroscopic examination, the reports have been for the most part encouraging. Schade,[89] by using a simple lavage technique, disclosed 25 cases of carcinoma in which radiographic and gastroscopic studies were negative. Ross, McGrath, Crozier, and Rohart,[86] in a study of 252 patients with gastric disease, found 56 proven carcinomas. In five cases in which the roentgen diagnosis was equivocal and in two in which it was benign although carcinomas were actually proven, cancer cells were found by cytologic examination. There were 27 out of 40 correct x-ray diagnoses for an accuracy rate of 67.5% and 29 out of 41 correct cytological diagnoses, a rate of 71%. In only six cases were both the x-ray and the cytologic diagnoses incorrect. The combined accuracy of the two methods was 85%. Cytology has been shown to have its highest degree of accuracy in that group of patients in whom x-ray is also definitive. In cases wherein the radiologist misses the diagnosis the cytologic error may be as high as 38%. In a study of 2,500 patients it was found that the best diagnostic material came from small gastric lesions or those confined to the mucosa.[89]

2. *Radiology.*—In an evaluation of the radiological diagnosis alone, Strandjord and co-workers[104] reviewed 283 cases of gastric carcinoma. A correct diagnosis of cancer was made in 78% of the cases. In 6% an undecided diagnosis was made, and in 16% the wrong diagnosis was made. The position of the lesion in the stomach apparently influenced the degree of failure. Of the lesions of the corpus 47% were failures, while in only 24% of the antral lesions was the diagnosis missed. The proximal stomach is, therefore, a particularly difficult area to evaluate by roentgenographic means alone. Amberg,[2] in a review of 35,396 x-ray reports on 21,738 patients, found 861 cases of carcinoma of the stomach. Sixty-seven cases were diagnosed as carcinoma incorrectly; 72 cases were diagnosed as benign or equivocal and were, in fact, carcinomas. Twenty-seven benign ulcers were called malignant. On the other hand 30 carcinomas were diagnosed as benign or probably benign disease. In summary, false-positive diagnoses were present in 7.8% and false-negative diagnoses in 8.4%. Mitty and co-workers[62] reported a 91% accuracy rate in 155 patients with abdominal complaints. Hennig and Harvey,[39] in a review of 1,250 gastric lesions, found that 19 out of 150 resectable cancers were not correctly diagnosed preoperatively, for an accuracy rate of 88%.

3. *Gastroscopy.*—The use of gastroscopy in the diagnosis of various lesions of the stomach has met with a considerable degree of success and enthusiasm since the first practical design of a flexible gastroscope in 1932 by Schindler.[17] Benedict[8] has pointed out that lesions high on the greater curvature are frequently difficult to palpate and study by radiographic means alone but are usually well seen through the gastroscope. On the

other hand, small pyloric lesions, particularly on the lesser curvature of the antrum, high on the lesser curvature of the body, and high on the fundus are much better seen by the radiologist. The anterior and posterior walls of the stomach, often difficult to interpret by x-ray, are easily viewed by gastroscopic means.[17] Berry [12] has stated that if the lesion can actually be seen at gastroscopy, in most cases it can be diagnosed with a greater degree of accuracy than by roentgenologic means.

Within the past few years improvements in technique, more sophisticated instruments, and a greater number of trained observers have all contributed to making gastroscopy an acceptable and desirable part of the diagnostic work-up in patients with gastric disease. While there are several important absolute contraindications to the use of gastroscopy and a few relative contraindications, in general, accidents and complications are rare.[17] Smith and Tanner,[94] in a review of 7,200 gastroscopies and 605 esophagoscopies performed since 1943, noted 35 esophageal perforations. No instances of gastric perforation were incurred. Palmer,[75] in a review of 25,000 endoscopies by several operators, noted 27 perforations for a rate of 0.108% and eight deaths for a rate of 0.032%. Eleven of the 27 perforations were esophageal.

The relative value of the gastroscopic examination in the diagnosis of carcinoma of the stomach has been described by Villako.[107] Forty-three patients with gastric neoplasms were investigated with the gastroscope and x-ray. All were subsequently operated upon, and the diagnosis was confirmed in all but one case. X-ray alone could not make the diagnosis in six cases in which gastroscopic examination was conclusive. There were seven cases in which the diagnosis was made by x-ray but which were missed by the endoscopist. In all other cases the diagnosis was confirmed by both gastroscope and x-ray. In another series a positive diagnosis was made by gastroscopy in 38% of the 64 cases reported wherein a positive diagnosis could not be accomplished by x-ray alone.[107]

TABLE 1.—*Gastric Carcinoma Diagnostic Accuracy According to Technique*

Isolated Techniques		
Gastroscopy alone:	Arnold, et al (4)	95.3%
	Villako (107)	83.7%
Cytology alone:	Arnold, et al (4)	97.7%
	Nieburgs, et al (72)	80.0%
	Ross, et al (86)	71.0%
X-ray alone:	Amberg (2)	83.8%
	Arnold, et al (4)	92.7%
	Ross, et al (86)	67.5%
	Strandjord, et al (104)	78.0%
	Villako (107)	86.0%
Combined Techniques		
Cytology and x-ray	Ross, et al (86)	85.0%
Gastroscopy and x-ray	Villako (107)	100. %
X-ray, cytology, and gastroscopy	Arnold, et al (4)	99.3%
	Strandjord, et al (104)	94.0%

It is readily apparent, therefore, that while gastroscopy alone may not have a significantly higher percentage of correct diagnoses, it offers a valuable adjunct to the other available diagnostic methods. By using the three techniques of gastroscopy, x-ray, and cytology, correct diagnosis may be made in from 94% [104] to 99.3% [4] of the cases preoperatively, leaving an over-all error in the range of from less than 1% to 6%. The low rate of diagnostic error has been confirmed by other studies in which two or three of the investigative modalities have been used in conjunction with one another (Table 1).[86,107] It is also of considerable interest to note that direct vision of the lesion at the operating table may not offer as high a diagnostic yield as the indirect methods. Hennig and Harvey,[39] in reporting on 42 cases of penetrating or superficially spreading gastric carcinoma, pointed out that the surgeon handling the lesion was able to make the correct diagnosis only 19 times. It may be concluded, therefore, that while individual techniques for detecting and differentiating carcinoma from benign disease of the stomach may have an accuracy in the range of 60%-80%, by combining all the available modalities of x-ray, gastroscopy, cytology, gastric analysis, and history and physical examination, an accuracy approaching the absolute may be achieved.

Treatment of Gastric Carcinoma

While the prevailing concept is that complete surgical extirpation represents the only truly effective management of gastric malignancy, this does not imply that surgery has been found to be a satisfactory method of treatment.[14,53,78] Despite improved techniques, more radical attacks on the lesion, and a better understanding of the natural history of gastric cancer, the cure rate remains discouragingly low. Smyth[95] has pointed out that operability and favorable prognosis are in general related to the duration of history. The most frequently encountered lesions are the rapidly growing lethal ones, and, on this basis, he feels there is little virtue in early diagnosis and urgent treatment after diagnosis. Others have corroborated this point of view.[78] He has concluded that data suggest that partial or total gastrectomy is not curative under these circumstances, and he feels that the disease is either curable or does not require extensive surgery for cure or successful palliation. Radiation and tumor chemotherapy are at present inadequate for absolute control of the disease and have been reserved for palliative attempts only.[64,100]

Although there remains considerable disagreement among surgeons as to which lesions deserve what operative approach, in general, surgery consists of radical subtotal or radical total gastrectomy.[58,59,100] While the over-all cure rate has stagnated in the range of 5%-10% over the last two decades, somewhat better and more encouraging statistics may be obtained by examining those patients in whom earlier diagnosis has been achieved (Table 2).

In 155 patients with carcinoma of the stomach reviewed by Mitty and co-workers,[62] 15% were not operated upon because of obvious extension of their disease. Twenty-eight per cent were operated upon, but only exploratory laparotomy and histologic diagnosis were carried out. An additional 25% were treated by palliative bypass or resection. Only 32% underwent a curative resection, and in this group a 38% survival rate was noted *if there were no metastases present.* The over-all five-year-survival rate for this group of 155 patients was a disappointing 7.7%.

Hennig and Harvey[39] reported a five-year-survival rate of 18% in *resectable* lesions and a 32% five-year-survival rate for a group of 44 *resectable* carcinomas of the ulcerating, nonfungating variety which appeared to be benign at the time of operation. Marshall,[58] in reporting a follow-up of 1,701 out of 1,708 patients treated for carcinoma of the stomach, reported an operative mortality rate of 3.2% for subtotal gastrectomy and 7% for total gastrectomy. He reported a curability rate of 39.5% for five years and 16.6% for ten years in *resectable* lesions.

Operability, resectability, and curability have all increased to some small extent over the past 50 years: operability from 60% (1902-1916) to 90.8% (1951-1955), resectability from a low of 12.3% (1931-1940)

TABLE 2.—*Amenability to Surgical Treatment Among Patients With Carcinoma of the Stomach*

Author	Operability, %	Resectability, %	Curability, % (Resectable Lesions Only)
Berkson, Walters, Gray, & Priestley, 1952 (11)	80.0	44.0	—
Ransom, 1953 (82)	64.4	36.3	—
Moore & Morton, 1955 (65)	81.7	38.2	37.5
Shahon, Horowitz, & Kelly, 1956 (91)	85.4	73.3	54.8
McNeer, Lawrence, Ashley, & Pack, 1958 (56)	90.8	74.3	41.6
Marshall, 1958 (58)	97.5	38-41	39.5 (5 yr) 16.6 (10 yr)
Hennig & Harvey, 1959 (39)	—	46.3	18.0
Mitty, Rousselot, & Grace, 1960 (62)	85.0	32.0	38.0

to a high of 74.3% (1951-1955), and curability from a low of 15.5% to a high of 54.8% (in *resectable* lesions). While these figures are culled from the reports of a number of different clinics and are not necessarily comparable, they do suggest a slight trend to an over-all improvement in the surgical treatment of gastric malignancy. Still, no one could be satisfied with the treatment of a disease from which nine out of ten people die despite the most heroic methods of attack. Lipp [53] reviewed 18 series comprising 12,728 cases with 9,177 followed for five years. Only 466 patients were alive at the end of five years for an over-all survival rate of 5.7%. Smyth [95] has pointed out that the average survival in inoperable, palliative, and nonresective cases is six months. In patients in whom palliative resection is a feasible approach the average survival time is 15 months, and in patients in which a curative resection is attempted the average survival is 4.3 years.

In view of the fact that approximately a quarter of a million people die of carcinoma of the stomach in each decade, the disease continues to represent one of the most perplexing, frustrating, and important challenges to the contemporary physician. It has been pointed out by a number of authors that the death rate for this disease may increase as the average age of the population is elevated unless a fresh approach to diagnosis and treatment is instituted.[45]

The primary function of the physician in society is, after all, the prevention of disease, and, only in failing that, the treatment, and, if possible, the cure. Disease in itself represents a failure of our art; inadequate treatment doubly so. In view of the tantalizing observation that gastric carcinoma is on the decrease, and that this decline is probably on a spontaneous environmental basis, it would appear that our efforts need to be turned in another direction. We have gone about as far as we can insofar as bigger and better operations are concerned,[78] and, since our diagnostic acumen is approaching perfection,[4,104,107] there appears little more to be gained on that front. Moore [64] has advocated additional epidemiological studies of a radical nature to further our understanding of the basics of this disease. He has suggested, irrespective of the practical difficulties, controlled studies on large groups of school children in those countries in which the rate of gastric malignancy is highest, with variations in vitamin intake and dietary factors and with special emphasis on determination of gastritis, alteration of gastric function, dietary habits, and infection.

To quote directly: "The striking decrease that has occurred in the frequency and incidence of gastric cancer is adequate proof that gastric cancer is not inevitable and must be associated with environmental factors. These *must* be identified." [64]

M. Michael Eisenberg, MD, Department of Surgery, University of Florida College of Medicine, Gainesville, Fla.

REFERENCES

1. Aird, I.; Bentall, H. H.; and Fraser Roberts, J. A.: A Relationship Between Cancer of Stomach and the ABO Blood Groups, Brit Med J 1:799, 1953.

2. Amberg, J. R.: Accuracy of Roentgen Diagnosis in Carcinoma of the Stomach, Amer J Dig Dis 5:259, 1960.

3. Arffmann, E.: Heated Fats and Allied Compounds as Carcinogens: A Critical Review of Experimental Results, J Nat Cancer Inst 25:893, 1960.

4. Arnold, W. T.; Hampton, J.; Olin, W.; Glass, H.; and Carruth, C.: Gastrict Lesions, Including Exfoliative Cytology, JAMA 173:1117, 1960.

5. Ayre, J. E., and Oren, B. G.: A New Rapid Method for Stomach-Cancer Diagnosis: The Gastric Brush, Cancer 6:1177, 1953.

6. Bargen, J. A., and Gage, R. P.: Carcinoma and Ulcerative Colitis: Prognosis, Gastroenterology 39:385, 1960.

7. Barrett, M. K.: Avenues of Approach to the Gastrict Cancer Problem, J Nat Cancer Inst 7:127, 1946.

8. Benedict, E. B.: Correlation of Gastroscopic, Roentgenologic and Pathologic Findings in Diseases of the Stomach, Amer J Roentgen 55:251, 1946.

9. Berenblum, I., and Haran, N.: The Influence of Croton Oil and of Polyethylene Glycol-400 on Carcinogenesis in the Forestomach of the Mouse, Cancer Res 15:510, 1955.

10. Berg, J. W.: Histological Aspects of the Relation Between Gastric Adenomatous Polyps and Gastric Cancer, Cancer 11:1149, 1958.

11. Berkson, J.; Walters, W., Gray, H. K.; and Priestley, J. T.: Mortality and Survival in Cancer

of the Stomach: A Statistical Summary of the Experience of the Mayo Clinic, Proc Mayo Clin 27:137, 1952.

12. Berry, L. H.: Newer Trends and Technics in Gastroscopy, Rev Gastroent 18:791, 1951.

13. Billington, B. P.: Gastric Cancer: Relationships Between ABO Blood-Groups, Site, and Epidemiology, Lancet 2:859, 1956.

14. Boles, R. S.: In discussion on Marshall, S. F.[58]

15. Bone, F. C., and Broome, R. A., Jr.: Temporary Healing of a Cancerous Gastric Ulcer, J Florida Med Ass 49:129, 1962.

16. Bowden, L.: Adenocarcinoma in a Small Gastric Polyp, Cancer 15:468, 1962.

17. Brandborg, L. L.: "Upper Gastrointestinal Endoscopy," in H. N. Harkins and L. M. Nyhus: Surgery of the Stomach and Duodenum, Boston: Little, Brown & Company, 1962.

18. Breslaw, L.: Malignant Disease and Gastric Polyps, Calif Med 92:430, 1960.

19. Brunn, H., and Pearl, F.: Diffuse Gastric Polyps—Adenopapillomatosis Gastrica, Surg Gynec Obstet 43:559, 1926.

20. Buckwalter, J. A.; Wohlwend, C. B.; Colter, D. C.; and Tidrick, R. T.: Natural Selection Associated With the ABO Blood Group, Science 123:840, 1956.

21. Buckwalter, J. A.; Wohlwend, C. B.; Colter, D. C.; Tidrick, R. T.; and Knowler, L. A.: The Association of the ABO Blood Groups to Gastric Carcinoma, Surg Gynec Obstet 104:176, 1957.

22. Burnett, W.; MacFarlane, P. S.; Park, S. D. S.; and Kay, A. W.: Cancer of the Stomach: An Evaluation of Diagnostic Methods Including Exfoliative Cytology, Brit Med J 1:753, 1960.

23. Carey, J. B., and Hay, L. J.: Gastric Polyps, Gastroenterology 14:280, 1950.

24. Carlson, E., and Ward, J. G.: Surgical Considerations in Gastric Polyps, Gastric Polyposis, and Giant Hypertrophic Gastritis in 74 Cases, Surg Gynec Obstet 107:727, 1958.

25. Castleman, B., and Krickstein, H. I.: Do Adenomatous Polyps of the Colon Become Malignant? New Eng J Med 267:469, 1962.

26. Comfort, M. W.; Kelsey, M. P.; and Berkson, J.: Gastric Acidity Before and After the Development of Carcinoma of the Stomach, J Nat Cancer Inst 7:367, 1947.

27. Comfort, M. W.; Gray, H. K.; Dockerty, M. B.; Gage, R. P.; Dornberger, G. R.; Solis, J.; Epperson, D. P.; and McNaughton, R. A.: Small Gastric Cancer, AMA Arch Intern Med 94:513, 1954.

28. Editorial: Neoplasms in Medical Practice, GP 19:167, 1959.

29. Eklöf, O.; Engstedt, L.; and Reizenstein, P.: Intrinsic Factor Deficiency, Achlorhydria, and Malignancy in Polyps of the Stomach and Duodenum, Acta Med Scand 171:601, 1962.

30. Fairley, K. F.; Turner, C. N.; Mackay, M. A.; and Joske, R. A.: Atrophic Gastritis: A Five Year Survey of 32 Cases Proven by Gastric Biopsy, Med J Aust 2:1085, 1955.

31. Flood, C. A.: Precancerous Disease of the Gastrointestinal Tract, Amer J Dig Dis 6:555, 1961.

32. Gottfried, B.: Molomut, N.; and Patti, J.: Effect of Repeated Surgical Trauma on Chemical Carcinogenesis, Cancer Res 21:658, 1961.

33. Graham, S., and Lilienfeld, A. M.: Genetic Studies of Gastric Cancer in Humans: An Appraisal, Cancer 11:945, 1958.

34. Guiss, L. W., and Stewart, F. W.: Chronic Atrophic Gastritis and Cancer of the Stomach, Arch Surg 46:823, 1943.

35. Gutmann, R. A.; Bertrand, I.; and Péristiany, T. J.: Le Cancer de l'estomac au début: Étude clinique, radiologique et anatomo-pathologique, Paris: Gaston Doin & Cie, 1939.

36. Harkins, H. N., and Nyhus, L. M.: Surgery of the Stomach and Duodenum, London: Little, Brown & Company, 1962.

37. Hay, L. J.: Gastric Polyps, Minnesota Med 34:362, 1951.

38. Hebbel, R.: The Topography of Chronic Gastritis in Cancer-Bearing Stomachs, J Nat Cancer Inst 10:505, 1949.

39. Hennig, G. C., and Harvey, H. D.: The Problem of the Diagnosis of Gastric Lesions, Ann Intern Med 50:43, 1959.

40. Hitchcock, C. R.; Sullivan, W. A.; and Wangensteen, O. H.: The Value of Achlorhydria as a Screening Test for Gastric Cancer, Gastroenterology 29:621, 1955.

41. Hitchcock, C. R.; MacLean, L. D.; and Sullivan, W. A.: The Secretory and Clinical Aspects of Achlorhydria and Gastric Atrophy as Precursors of Gastric Cancer, J Nat Cancer Inst 18:795, 1957.

42. Hogg, L., Jr., and Pack, G. T.: The Controversial Relationship Between Blood Group A and Gastric Cancer, Gastroenterology 32:797, 1957.

43. Hollander: Cited by Aird, I.; Bentall, H. H.; and Fraser Roberts, J. A.[1]

44. Hurst, A. F.: Precursors of Carcinoma of the Stomach, Lancet 2:1023, 1929.

45. Ivy, A. C.: Experimental Observations on the Etiology of Gastric Carcinoma, Gastroenterology 28:325, 1955.

46. Jenner, A. W. F.: Perniziöse Anämie und Magenkarzinom (Pernicious Anemia and Gastric Cancer), Acta Med Scand 102:529, 1939.

47. Jonas, K. C., and Stauffer, H. M.: "Stomach and Duodenum," in Jonas, K. C., editor: Babcock's Principles and Practice of Surgery, ed 2, Philadelphia: Lea & Febiger, 1954, p 1254.

48. Kaplan, H. S., and Rigler, L. G.: Pernicious Anemia and Carcinoma of the Stomach: Autopsy Studies Concerning Their Interrelationship, Amer J Med Sci 209:339, 1945.

49. Konjetzny, G. E., in Anschütz, W., and Konjetzny, G. E.: Die Geschwülste des Magens, Stuttgart: Ferdinand Enke, 1921.

50. Konjetzny, G. E.: Der Magenkrebs, Stuttgart: Ferdinand Enke, 1938.

51. Konjetzny, G. E.: Die Beziehungen zwischen Gastritis und Magenkrebsentwicklung, Arch Klin Chir 204:4, 1943.

52. Køster, K. H.; Sindrup, E.; and Seele, V.: ABO Blood Groups and Gastric Acidity, Lancet 2:52, 1955.

53. Lipp, W. F.: In discussion on Marshall, S. F.[58]

54. Livingston and Pack: Cited by Webster, D. R.[110]

55. McCoy: Cited by Webster, D. R.[110]

56. McNeer, G.; Lawrence. W; Ashley, M. P.; and Pack, G. T.: End Results in the Treatment of Gastric Cancer, Surgery 43:879, 1958.

57. Mallory, T. B.: Carcinoma in Situ of the Stomach and Its Bearing on the Histogenesis of Malignant Ulcers, Arch Path 30:348, 1940.

58. Marshall, S. F.: Treatment of Cancer of the Stomach: End Result, Gastroenterology 34:34, 1958.

59. Marshall, S. F.: "Tumors of the Stomach," in L. Davis: Christopher's Textbook of Surgery, Philadelphia: W. B. Saunders Company, 1960.

60. Meadows, J. C., and Lefeber, E. J.: Gastroscopy: A 14 Year Survey of Over 1,000 Consecutive Examinations, Ann Intern Med 42:69, 1955.

61. Mider, G. B.: Causative Factors in Gastrointestinal Cancer, Gastroenterology 39:271, 1960.

62. Mitty, W. F., Jr.; Rousselot, L. M.; and Grace, W. J.: Carcinoma of the Stomach, Amer J Dig Dis 5:249, 1960.

63. Monaco, A. P.; Roth, S. I.; Castleman, B.; and Welch, C. E.: Adenomatous Polyps of the Stomach: A Clinical and Pathological Study of 153 Cases, Cancer 15:456, 1962.

64. Moore, G. E.: The Decrease in Incidence of Cancer of the Stomach, Editorial, Surg Gynec Obstet 114:209, 1962.

65. Moore, J. R., and Morton, H. S.: Gastric Carcinoma, Ann Surg 141:185, 1955.

66. Morson, B. C.: Gastric Polyps Composed of Intestinal Epithelium, Brit J Cancer 9:550, 1955.

67. Morson, B. C.: Intestinal Metaplasia of the Gastric Mucosa, Gastroenterologia 85:181, 1956.

68. Morson, B. C.: Precancerous Lesions of the Upper Gastrointestinal Tract, JAMA 179:311, 1960.

69. Mosbech, J., and Videbaek, A.: Mortality From and Risk of Gastric Carcinoma Among Patients With Pernicious Anemia, Brit Med J 2:390, 1950.

70. Mosbech, J.: Heredity in Pernicious Anemia: A Probe and Study of the Heredity and the Relationship to Cancer of the Stomach, Copenhagen: Ejnar Munksgaards, Forlag, 1953.

71. Mosbech, J.: Genetic Considerations in Polyps and Cancer of the Gastrointestinal Tract, Acta Int Un Cancr 17:302, 1961.

72. Nieburgs, H. E.; Werther, J. L.; Hollander, F.; and Janowitz, H. D.: The Cytologic Diagnosis of Gastric Cancer and Evaluation of the Abrasive Brush Technic in 125 Cases, Amer J Dig Dis 5:63, 1960.

73. Notkin, L. J.: Carcinoma Occurring on the Basis of Pre-Existing Gastric Ulcer, Canad Med Ass J 72:288, 1955.

74. Orator, V.: Virchow Arch Path Anat 256:292, 1925.

75. Palmer, E. D.: The Risks of Peroral Endoscopy, US Armed Forces Med J 5:974, 1954.

76. Palmer, W. L., and Humphreys, E. M.: Gastric Carcinoma: Observations on Peptic Ulceration and Healing, Gastroenterology 3:257, 1944.

77. Palmer, W. L.: Certain Aspects of Benign and Malignant Gastric Ulcer, Bull NY Acad Med 26:527, 1950.

78. Palmer, W. L.: In discussion on Marshall, S. F.[58]

79. Panico, F. G.; Papanicolaou, G. N.; and Cooper, W. A.: Abrasive Balloon for Exfoliation of Gastric Cancer Cells, JAMA 143:1308, 1950.

80. Plachta, A., and Speer, F. D.: Gastric Polyps and Their Relationship to Carcinoma of the Stomach, Amer J Gastroent 28:160, 1957.

81. Pollard, H. M.: Precancerous Gastric Disease, Amer J Dig Dis 4:1039, 1959.

82. Ransom, H. K.: Cancer of the Stomach, Surg Gynec Obstet 96:275, 1953.

83. Rienhoff, W. F., Jr., and Baker, B. M., Jr.: The Medical and Surgical Aspects of Peptic Ulcer, Int Clin 2:167, 1934.

84. Rieniets, J. H., and Broders, A. C.: Gastric Adenomas: A Pathologic Study, Western J Surg 54:21, 1946.

85. Rosenthal, M., and Traut, H. F.: The Mucolytic Action of Papain for Cell Concentration in the Diagnosis of Gastric Cancer, Cancer 4:147, 1951.

86. Ross, J. R.; McGrath, J. M.; Crozier, R. E.; and Rohart, R. R.: Exfoliative Cytology: Its Practical Application in Diagnosis of Gastric Neoplasms, Gastroenterology 34:24, 1958.

87. Rubin, C. E.; Massey, B. W.; Kirsner, J. B.; Palmer, W. L.; and Stonecypher, D. D.: The Clinical Value of Gastrointestinal Cytologic Diagnosis, Gastroenterology 25:119, 1953.

88. Rubin, C. E., and Benditt, E. P.: A Simplified Technique Using Chymotrypsin Lavage for the Cytological Diagnosis of Gastric Cancer, Cancer 8:1137, 1955.

89. Schade, R. O. K.: Exfoliative Cytology of Gastric Carcinoma, Brit Med J 1:743, 1958.

90. Schell, R. F.; Dockerty, M. B.; and Comfort, M. W.: Carcinoma of the Stomach Associated

With Pernicious Anemia, Surg Gynec Obstet 98:710, 1954.

91. Shahon, D. B.; Horowitz, S.; and Kelly, W. D.: Cancer of the Stomach, Surgery 39:204, 1956.

92. Shemiakina, T. V.: The Importance of the Solvent and Mode of Administration of a Carcinogenic Substance in Inducing Experimental Cancer of the Preventriculus in Mice, Vop Onkol (Eng) 5:333, 1959.

93. Siurala, M., and Seppälä, K.: Atrophic Gastritis as a Possible Precursor of Gastric Carcinoma and Pernicious Anemia, Acta Med Scand 166:455, 1960.

94. Smith, C. C. K., and Tanner, N. C.: The Complications of Gastroscopy and Oesophagoscopy, Brit J Surg 43:396, 1956.

95. Smyth, J.: Carcinoma of the Stomach: A Critical Review, Med J Australia 2:15, 1955.

96. Sommers, S. C.: Constitutional Aspects of Gastric Carcinoma, AMA Arch Path 66:487, 1958.

97. Southwick, H. W., and Cole, W. H.: Cancer of Gastrointestinal Tract, Amer J Dig Dis 4:491, 1959.

98. Spratt, J. S.; Ackerman, L. V.; and Moyer, C. A.: Relationship of Polyps of the Colon to Colonic Cancer, Ann Surg 148:682, 1958.

99. Stein-Werblowsky, R.: An Experimental Study of Gastric Cancer in Relation to Gastric Ulcer, Gut 3:129, 1962.

100. Stevenson, J. K.: "Gastric Carcinoma" in Harkins, H. N., and Nyhus, L. M.: Surgery of the Stomach and Duodenum, London: Little, Brown and Company, 1962.

101. Stewart, H. L., and Lorenz, E.: Adenocarcinoma of the Pyloric Stomach and Other Gastric Neoplasms in Mice Included With Carcinogenic Hydrocarbons, J Nat Cancer Inst 3:175, 1942.

102. Stewart, M. J.: Precancerous Lesions of the Alimentary Tract, Lancet 2:669, 1931.

103. Stout, A. P.: New York J Med 45:973, 1945.

104. Strandjord, N. M.; Moseley, R. D., Jr.; and Schweinefus, R. L.: Gastric Carcinoma: Accuracy of Radiologic Diagnosis, Radiology 74:442, 1960.

105. Tanner, N. C.: A Critique of Gastroscopy, Brit Med J 2:849, 1944.

106. Texter, E. C., Jr., and Barborka, C. J.: Diagnosis of Gastrointestinal Cancer, Med Clin N Amer 44:151, 1960.

107. Villako, K. P.: Gastroscopy in the Diagnosis of Gastric Cancer, Klin Med (Wien) 37:69, 1959.

108. Von den Velden, R.: Über Vorkommen und Mangel der freien Salzsäure im Magensaft bei Gastrektasie, Deutsch Arch Klin Med 23:369, 1879.

109. Wangensteen, O. H.: Cancer of the Esophagus and the Stomach, New York: American Cancer Society, Inc., 1951.

110. Webster, D. R.: "The Stomach, Duodenum and Small Intestine," in Moseley, H. F.: Textbook of Surgery, St. Louis: C. V. Mosby Company, 1955, p 575.

111. Welch, G. E.: In discussion on Marshall, S. F.[58]

112. Woolf, C. M.: A Genetic Study of Carcinoma of the Large Intestine, Amer J Hum Genet 10:42, 1947.

113. Zamcheck, N.; Grable, E.; Ley, A.; and Norman, L.: Occurrence of Gastric Cancer Among Patients With Pernicious Anemia at the Boston City Hospital, New Eng J Med 252:1103, 1955.

Metastatic Epidural Tumor of the Spine

A Study of 45 Cases

WILLIAM O. WILD, MD
AND
ROBERT W. PORTER, MD
LONG BEACH, CALIF

The attitude of physicians toward metastatic epidural tumor of the spine has changed somewhat during the past two decades from one of pessimism and therapeutic nihilism [8,16] to one which is more therapeutically aggressive.* Our experience, however, reveals that many physicians are still unaware of the benefits to be derived from the surgical therapy of this disease and the need for prompt action in such cases with neurological involvement. In an attempt to evaluate this subject further and obtain additional information useful in the selection and treatment of these patients, 45 cases of metastatic epidural tumor of the spine with neurological involvement were reviewed. These cases were analyzed with respect to the duration of symptoms, degree of paresis, tumor level, tumor type, postoperative irradiation, and their relation to the postoperative return of function. All of the patients in this series were seen at the Long Beach Veterans Administration Hospital during the period from 1953 to 1962, and all received a decompressive laminectomy with removal of as much of the tumor as advisable.

Duration of Symptoms

The symptoms of neurological involvement fell into three main groups (Table 1): sensory impairment, motor weakness, and sphincter disturbances. Sensory symptoms usually consisted of numbness, tingling, or coldness, singly or in combination. Motor symptoms presented as weakness in the lower extremities. Sphincter symptoms consisted of bowel and bladder disturbances as manifested by constipation progressing to obstipation, and urinary hesitancy or frequency progressing to urinary retention or incontinence.

The most common complaint which resulted in the patients' referral to the neurosurgical department was muscle weakness in the lower extremities. The history revealed, however, that sensory symptoms were usually the first to appear. Sphincter symptoms were the last to appear in 87% of the cases, this late appearance indicating that this modality is the most resistant of the three to compression. Table 2 gives the average duration of symptoms in each of the three symptom categories as related to the degree of postoperative return of motor function. As shown, the average duration of sensory and motor symptoms was shorter and the average duration of sphincter symptoms was longer in those patients who experienced no post-

TABLE 1.—*Duration of Symptoms for the Three Main Symptom Categories*

	Extremes	Av
Sensory	24 hr-6 mo	23 da
Motor	24 hr-5 mo	18 da
Sphincter	0 hr-1.5 mo	5 da

Presented at the annual meeting of the Western Neurosurgical Society, Phoenix, Ariz, Oct 28, 1962.

Surgical Service, Veterans Administration Hospital, Long Beach, Calif, and the departments of anatomy and surgery, University of California School of Medicine, Los Angeles.

* References 1-3, 5, 9, 10, 13, 15, 19, 20.

TABLE 2.—*Average Duration of Symptoms for the Three Main Symptom Categories as Related to Postoperative Return of Motor Function*

	Duration of Preop Symptoms, Av Da		
Postop Motor Return	Sensory	Motor	Sphincter
Good	29	23	4
Moderate	10	6	4
None	22	16	10

TABLE 3.—*Postoperative Relief of Paresis as Related to Degree of Preoperative Paresis*

Degree of Preop Paresis	Postop Relief of Paresis
None, 2%	Became paraplegic
Mild, 4%	1 returned to normal; 1 remained ambulatory 12 da
Moderate, 16%	71% good; 14% no change; 14% worse
Marked, 78%	31% good; 26% improved; 43% none

operative return of motor function than in those who became ambulatory. Since the sphincter modality is the most resistant of the three to compression, it would appear to be an indicator of the severity of spinal cord dysfunction. Hence, the length of time between the onset of motor symptoms and that of sphincter symptoms may serve as an index of the rapidity of progression of neurological deficit. Table 2 illustrates that this length of time was significantly shorter in the group of patients that experienced no postoperative return of function than it was in the group that experienced good recovery of function.

Degree of Paresis

Muscle weakness in the lower extremities was classified as mild, moderate, or marked. Mild refers to those patients who exhibited clinically demonstrable weakness, but were still able to ambulate unassisted. Moderate is used to indicate those patients who required assistance in order to ambulate. Marked refers to those with complete paralysis, or paresis to such a degree that they were unable to support their body weight. The majority of the patients in this series presented with marked paresis as shown in Table 3. Analysis of the degree of postoperative relief of paresis in relation to the degree of preoperative paresis revealed the following (Table 3): 31% of those patients whose paresis was marked at the time of surgery became ambulatory postoperatively, whereas 71% of those whose preoperative paresis was only moderate regained their ability to walk.

Tumor Level

The level of the epidural tumor was at T-1–T-4 in 38% of the cases in this series. The cauda equina was the site of tumor involvement in 13% of these cases and there was one case of involvement above C-7. The remaining segment of the cord, T-5–L-1, was involved in 47% of the cases. The least favorable postoperative results occurred in those patients with tumor involvement at T-1–T-4. Only 24% of these became ambulatory whereas 83% of those with cauda equina and 43% of those with involvement of T-5–L-1 became ambulatory postoperatively.

Routine x-rays of the spine revealed vertebral involvement at the tumor level in 67% of the cases. Lumbar puncture study was recorded in 38 patients, and a complete manometric block was demonstrated in 34, or 89%, of these. The cerebrospinal fluid protein levels ranged from 34 mg% to 1,623 mg%. There was no apparent correlation of tumor type or level with the protein level.

Tumor Type

Seventeen different histologic cell types were represented by the tumors encountered in this predominantly male population, which excludes tumors usually limited to the female. Tumors of the lung, kidney, and prostate gland comprised 48% of the group (Table 4). Based on the postoperative return of function and longevity, tumors of the prostate gland, multiple myeloma, and malignant lymphomas were the most favorable tumors of this group. Bronchogenic, renal, and testicular tumors were the least favorable.

Postoperative Irradiation

Of the patients, 51% received postoperative x-ray irradiation to the appropriate level of the spine ranging from a palliative dose of 400 r in air to 5,600 r in air. Of those pa-

TABLE 4.—*Postoperative Results by Tumor Type*

Tumor Type	No. Patients	Postop Longevity	Results
Bronchogenic	11, 24%	Av 2.4 mo	3 patients ambulatory and 3 catheter free
Prostatic	6, 13%	Av 24 mo (1 patient living at 1 yr and 1 at 8 yr)	4 patients ambulatory and 2 catheter free (1 obstructed)
Renal	5, 11%	Av 3.3 mo	None ambulatory or catheter free
Testicular	4, 9%	Av 30 mo (1 patient living at 8½ years)	1 patient ambulatory and catheter free
Hodgkins	3, 7%	Av 6 mo	1 patient ambulatory and catheter free
Malignant melanoma	2, 4%	Av 4 mo	2 patients ambulatory, none catheter free
Multiple myeloma	2, 4%	Still living at 1 yr	2 patients ambulatory and catheter free
Bladder	2, 4%	Av 1.9 mo	None ambulatory or catheter free
Leukemia	2, 4%	Av 1.5 mo	None ambulatory or catheter free
Thyroid	1, 2%	Still living at 1 yr	Ambulatory and catheter free
Liposarcoma	1, 2%	Still living at 2 yr	Ambulatory and catheter free
Angiosarcoma	1, 2%	Died at 3 yr	Ambulatory and catheter free
Pancreatic	1, 2%	Died at 2 mo	Not ambulatory or catheter free
Gastric	1, 2%	Died at 3.5 wk	Not ambulatory or catheter free
Lymphosarcoma	1, 2%	Died at 6.5 mo	Ambulatory and catheter free
Hypopharyngeal	1, 2%	Died at 1 wk	Not ambulatory or catheter free
Reticulum cell	1, 2%	Still living at 6 yr	Ambulatory and catheter free

tients who received irradiation, 44% became ambulatory whereas only 26% of those who did not receive irradiation regained their ability to walk. Further analysis from a different aspect revealed that of those patients who experienced good postoperative return of function, 61% had received postoperative irradiation, whereas of these patients who experienced no postoperative return of function only 39% had received postoperative irradiation.

Postoperative longevity averaged 14.5 months for those patients who received irradiation and 8 months for those who did not.

Comment

This series again demonstrates the tendency of metastatic epidural tumors of the spine to develop neurological deficit fairly rapidly and to be characterized by a steadily progressive course. This is in contrast to benign tumors which may take months to develop paraplegia and may be characterized by a remissive course.[6] The rate of progression of the neurological deficit and its duration were related to the postoperative return of function in the cases included in this study. The more rapid the progression and the longer a severe deficit remained present, the less favorable the prognosis in this regard. These findings are in agreement with those of Tarlov [19] in his study of return of function following relief of spinal cord compression.

The degree of paresis prior to surgery was related to the postoperative return of function in these cases: the more severe the paresis the less likelihood of a good recovery. Mullan and Evans [12] obtained similar results. Botterell and Fitzgerald [5] found "Recovery from paraplegia rare once the latter is fully established." The importance of early diagnosis and treatment in cases of metastatic epidural tumor of the spine is stressed by others [3,5,12,13,19] and by the above findings. Immediate surgical decompression is indicated in cases with progressing paresis and even in cases where sphincter symptoms have already developed. The presence of sphincter symptoms was found to be a useful and practical clinical indication of the severity of the disruption of spinal cord function in this series.

The relative role of direct pressure as compared to the interference with vascular supply in the development of neurological deficit has been studied by McAlhany and Netsky [11] and by Tarlov [18] who concluded that the major effect is a mechanical one at the site of the tumor. The thoracic cord segments T-1–T-4 ventrally and dorsally are considered to be most susceptible to vascular insult [21] by virtue of the anatomical arrangement of the vascular supply to the spinal cord. The cases in this series were studied with this concept in mind, and as mentioned earlier the least favorable prognosis for return of function occurred in those patients with epidural tumor in the T-1–T-4 segment of the spinal cord.

Roentgenography of the spine is helpful in localization of the level of the lesion in a high percentage of cases of metastatic epidural tumor. The abnormalities noted on x-ray consisted of osteolytic changes in the pedicles and bodies, collapse or complete destruction of the vertebral bodies, scoliosis, and in some cases a paraspinal mass. Increased density of the involved vertebrae occurred in cases of osteoblastic metastasis, eg, prostatic carcinoma. Scirrhus carcinoma of the breast has also been observed to produce osteoblastic metastasis,[3] as has renal carcinoma.[22] These changes are characteristic of metastatic tumor and can be distinguished from those of primary tumors which produce erosion of the pedicles and widening of the interpedicular space.

Lumbar puncture combined with myelography is an important guide in the management of these cases. The danger of increasing the patient's disability by these procedures is a recognized complication,[8,12,19] but the advantages to be gained outweigh the risks involved. The technique of performing one lumbar puncture for cerebrospinal fluid study and for injection of the radiopaque dye helps to minimize the complication of subdural dye injection [17] which could completely frustrate any attempted myelographic study. Myelography not only serves to localize the exact site of the lesion but also indicates the character of the offending lesion, eg, whether it is extradural or intradural.

The need for caution in manipulating patients during evaluation is illustrated by the case of a man, not included in this series, who was undergoing investigation for multiple myeloma with possible epidural involvement. During the positioning on the x-ray table he experienced mid-dorsal pain and 20 minutes later was markedly paraparetic. After being transferred to the Long Beach Veterans Administration Hospital, the patient received a decompressive laminectomy which revealed epidural extension of multiple myeloma with an extensive hematoma within the tumor itself. This is thought to have occurred during the x-ray examination and resulted in a marked change in the expected clinical course for his illness.

The results obtained in this series in relation to the various tumor types are comparable to those of other series.[3,5,13] The influence on postoperative longevity of various tumors is related to the inherent characteristics of growth and spread of the particular cell type. The relation of postoperative return of function to tumor type is more obscure. Analysis of the duration of symptoms for specific tumor type reveals that the least favorable tumors listed above either had an acute onset and rapid progression of motor symptoms or had sphincter symptoms of relatively long standing. The most favorable tumors as listed above on the other hand, underwent slow progression of motor symptoms and developed sphincter symptoms quite late in this progression, with a notable exception of the malignant lymphoma group in which the onset of motor and sphincter disturbances was closely related and rapidly progressive. The duration of all symptoms in this latter group was quite short, however, indicating early diagnosis and treatment. The postoperative return of function as related to tumor cell type would appear to follow the generalization made at the beginning under the discussion of the duration of symptoms, namely, a less favorable prognosis in those cases with rapid progression of neurological involvement and/or in those where sphincter disturbances have developed.

The figures in this series which favor x-ray irradiation as a part of the therapeutic regimen in the cases under discussion are biased, for in this series postoperative irradiation was given selectively to those patients with known radiosensitive tumors whose general condition was otherwise satisfactory. Nevertheless, postoperative x-ray irradiation appears to have been efficacious and is recommended for those patients with radiosensitive tumors whose general condition is satisfactory.

The curious predilection of metastatic tumor for the epidural space as well as the protective barrier which the dura forms between even the most extensive and highly malignant tumor and the intrathecal contents has been commented upon by Rogers.[15] Batson [4] added to our knowledge and understanding of this subject by his study and description of the valveless, vertebral veins. The dura was not opened routinely in the cases in this series because of a reluctance to break down this protective barrier but was opened in those cases where the surgeon was not satisfied with its pulsation following decompression and in those cases where a satisfactory explanation for the clinical picture was not found.

Of additional interest is the rarity of metastatic intradural tumor of the spine [6,14] as compared to cerebral and cerebellar metastases. No cases of intradural or intramedullary metastasis of the spine were encountered in this series.

Symptoms or signs of spinal cord compression were the first evidence of malignant disease in 53% of this series. Botterell and Fitzgerald [5] reported this phenomenon in 77% of their series. Of this series, 47% were known to have a malignancy at the time of surgery, and in 24% the presence of a malignancy was suspected after the preoperative evaluation.

It has been possible from an analysis of the cases included in this study to arrive at certain generalizations in regard to the prognosis in various cases of metastatic epidural tumor of the spine. It has not been possible to establish consistently reliable criteria for the selection or exclusion of those cases that would be amenable to surgical treatment. For this reason it is our opinion that the treatment of choice in cases of metastatic epidural tumor of the spine with evidence of progressive spinal cord or cauda equina impairment is decompressive laminectomy, provided the patient's general condition is otherwise satisfactory. The purpose of decompressive laminectomy in these cases is not necessarily to restore full activity although this was the gratifying result in a significant percentage of this series. The relief of pain, the prevention of decubiti, the restoration of sphincter control, the relief of painful flexor spasms, the partial return of muscle control are worthwhile benefits of surgery and all help to lighten the nursing burden and make the patient's remaining life more comfortable. That this treatment is effective even after repeated application to the same patient is illustrated by one of the cases in this series. This patient originally presented with marked paraparesis and bladder involvement due to metastatic epidural liposarcoma of T-12 to L-1. This was decompressed and subtotally excised on Jan 25, 1960, and subsequently irradiated with 4,800 r in air. The patient made an excellent recovery, became ambulatory, regained sphincter control, and was discharged. The paraparesis returned in the fall of 1961, and on Oct 1, 1961, additional liposarcoma was subtotally excised from T-1–T-4 and T-9–L-1. It was interesting to note the recurrence of a myelographic block at the site of the original laminectomy since this phenomenon was thought to be quite unlikely. The reason became obvious at surgery and was found to be due to the formation of dense scar tissue in the previously irradiated area. This formed nearly as firm an encasing to the spinal cord as the vertebral arches did prior to their removal. Consequently, the recurring tumor once again was firmly encased and its pressure was directed to the spinal cord. The patient again made an excellent recovery with return of motor and sphincter function. His recovery was short-lived this time, however, and he returned in December of 1961 with marked paraparesis, this time accompanied by painful flexor spasms. Decompression of T-4–T-8 on December 28, 1961, failed to result in the return of the patient's ambulation, but the painful flexor spasms were relieved. No apparent disability occurred that could be attributed to his extensive laminectomy from C-7 to L-2.

Summary

Forty-five cases of metastatic epidural tumor of the spine with neurological involvement representing 17 different histologic cell types were reviewed. These cases were analyzed with respect to the duration of symptoms, degree of paresis, tumor level, tumor type, postoperative irradiation, and their relation to the postoperative return of function. In general, the more rapid the rate of progression, the longer the duration, and the more severe the degree of neurological deficit the less favorable was the prognosis with regard to postoperative return of function. The importance of early diagnosis and surgical treatment in order to prevent irreversible neurological deficit is stressed.

William O. Wild, MD, Department of Neurosurgery, Veterans Administration Hospital, 5901 E Seventh St, Long Beach 4, Calif.

REFERENCES

1. Alexander, E., Jr.; Davis, C. H., Jr.; and Field, C. H.: Metastatic Lesions of Vertebral Column Causing Cord Compression, Neurology (Minneap) 6:103-109, 1956.

2. Arseni, C. N.; Simionescu, M. D.; and Horwath, L.: Tumors of the Spine, Acta Psychiat Scand 34:398-410, 1959.

3. Barron, K. D.; Hirano, A.; Araki, S.; and Terry, R. D.: Experiences With Metastatic Neoplasms Involving the Spinal Cord, Neurology (Minneap) 9:91-106, 1959.

4. Batson, O. V.: Role of Vertebral Veins in Metastatic Processes, Ann Intern Med 16:38-45, 1942.

5. Botterell, E. H., and Fitzgerald, G. W.: Spinal Cord Compression Produced by Extradural Malignant Tumors: Early Recognition, Treatment and Results, Canad Med Ass J 80:791-794, 1959.

6. Cantor, M. B., and Stein, J. M.: Intramedullary Spinal Cord Metastasis, J Nerv Ment Dis 115: 351-355, 1952.

7. Chambers, W. R.: Intraspinal Tumor: A Difficult Diagnosis, Amer J Surg 87:824-829, 1954.

8. Elsberg, C. A.: Surgical Diseases of the Spinal Cord, Membranes and Nerve Roots, New York: Paul B. Hoeber, Inc., Medical Book Department of Harper & Bros., 1941, p 501.

9. Kennedy, J. C., and Stern, W. E.: Metastatic Neoplasms of the Vertebral Column Producing Compression of the Spinal Cord, Amer J Surg 104:155-168, 1962.

10. Love, J. G.; Miller, R. H.; and Kernohan, J. W.: Lymphomas of the Spinal Epidural Space, AMA Arch Surg 69:66-76, 1954.

11. McAlhany, H. J., and Netsky, M. G.: Compression of the Spinal Cord by Extramedullary Neoplasms: A Clinical and Pathologic Study, J Neuropath Exp Neurol 14:276-287, 1955.

12. Mullan, J., and Evans, J. P.: Neoplastic Disease of the Spinal Extradural Space: A Review of 50 Cases, AMA Arch Surg 74:900-909, 1957.

13. Perese, D. M.: Treatment of Metastatic Extradural Spinal Cord Tumors, Cancer 11:214-231, 1958.

14. Rasch, G. C.; Rosenbaum, D.; and Heimburger, R. F.: Intramedullary Spinal Cord Metastases From Lung Carcinoma Simulating Primary Cervice Cord Tumor, Neurology (Minneap) 3:311-315, 1953.

15. Rogers, L.: Malignant Spinal Tumors and the Epidural Space, Brit J Surg 45:416-422, 1958.

16. Shenkin, H. A.; Horn, R. C., Jr.; and Grant, F. C.: Lesions of Spinal Epidural Space Producing Cord Compression, Arch Surg 51:125-146, 1945.

17. Spurling, R. G.: Lesions of the Cervical Intervertebral Disc, Springfield, Ill: Charles C Thomas, Publisher, 1956.

18. Tarlov, I. M.: Spinal Cord Compression Studies: III. Time Limits for Recovery After Gradual Compression in Dogs, AMA Arch Neurol Psychiat 71:588-597, 1954.

19. Tarlov, I. M., and Herz, E.: Spinal Cord Compression Studies: IV. Outlook With Complete Paralysis in Man, AMA Arch Neurol Psychiat 72: 43-59, 1954.

20. Törmä, T.: Malignant Tumors of the Spine and the Extradural Space, Acta Chir Scand suppl 225, pp 1-176, 1957.

21. Truex, R. C., editor: Strong and Elwyn's Human Neuroanatomy, ed 4, Baltimore: Williams & Wilkins Company, 1959, p 74.

22. Wohl, G. T.: Vertebral Metastasis in Renal Carcinoma: An Anatomic Correlation, Amer J Roentgenol 75:930-937, 1956.

Studies on Portal Venous Oxygen Saturation

ROBERT A. HARDIN, MD
HARRIS B. SHUMACKER, JR., MD
AND
CHIEN SHENG SU, MD
INDIANAPOLIS

Oxygen saturation of the portal venous blood has been found to be higher than that of the systemic venous blood of anesthetized and unanesthetized dogs [1,2] and human subjects.[2-4] This has been observed in patients with and without liver disease. Regardless of the role of arteriovenous shunting in bringing about an elevated portal venous oxygen saturation, a number of other factors might conceivably have a part. This study was initiated in order to investigate several of them. It was our aim to learn the effect of the anesthetic state, of active body exercise, of digestion, and of hypoxia.

Materials and Methods

Adult mongrel dogs weighing from 11 to 18 kg were used. Anesthesia was induced by the intravenous administration of sodium thiopental. Tracheal intubation was carried out, and the lungs were inflated rhythmically with 100% oxygen by means of a mechanical respirator. The animals had received nothing by mouth for at least 15 hours prior to the study. Using aseptic technique, a midline abdominal incision was made, and a small plastic catheter was passed into the portal vein through a mesenteric vein and secured in place with a ligature. The wound was closed, and the end of the plastic tube was exteriorized. A sample of blood was drawn, and the catheter was filled with a heparin solution.

Approximately 18 hours later, fasting blood samples were withdrawn from the portal and femoral veins. Some animals were then fed an ordinary meal of kennel rations, and portal blood was drawn for study one hour later. Other dogs were exercised by walking for one-half hour. Samples of portal venous blood were obtained from them immediately thereafter and again 30 minutes later. In still other animals, samples were removed after one-half hour of exercise, and then, after a period of rest, the animals were fed. One hour later, portal venous blood was again drawn for analysis.

After a control period during which they were breathing pure oxygen, six dogs anesthetized intravenously and intubated were made to rebreathe into an anesthetic bag containing 100% oxygen. Five minutes later blood was withdrawn at the same time from the portal vein and from the femoral artery

Submitted for publication May 7, 1963.

From the Department of Surgery and the Heart Research Center, Indiana University School of Medicine.

This investigation was supported in part by Public Health Research grant H-207 from the National Institutes of Health and in part by a grant from the James Whitcomb Riley Memorial Association.

TABLE 1.—*Observations of Oxygen Saturation in Dogs* *

Dog	Portal Vein: At Operation	Portal Vein: Fasting, Resting State	Femoral Vein: Fasting, Resting State	Portal Vein: After 30 Min of Exercise	Portal Vein: 30 Min After Completion of Exercise	Portal Vein: 1 Hr After Eating
1		72		56		60
2		92		83		73
3	40	76	34	64		76
4	84	74	17	45		64
5	71	70 } 76	48	45 } 64		64 } 69
6	89	82	63	77		88
7	81	74		63		69
8	68	77	61	83		75
9	78	73 } 75	23	59 } 66		59
10	91	73	34	64		63
11	76	69	56	63	68	
12	79	78	34	59	72	
13	43	71	30	64	64	
14	59	56 } 73	38	62 } 70	73 } 73	
15	54	83	81	77	80	
16	86	82	63	80	83	
17	92	71	33	70	69	
18	99	93	92			93
19	87	83				84
20	90	82 } 78	55			78 } 81
21	74	64	63			82
22	92	81	48			83
23	81	64	54			75
24	94					
25	87					
26	91					
27	99					
28	84					
29	82					
30	92					
31	85					
32	89					
33	86					
34	88					
Mean	81	76	49	66	73	

* All values expressed in per cent.

for gas analysis. Again five minutes later, after a ten-minute period of rebreathing into the bag, portal and femoral arterial blood was withdrawn simultaneously for study. Each animal then breathed 100% oxygen once again for 15 minutes before final blood samples were removed.

Oxygen saturation was determined by the Roughton-Scholander technique.

Results

The results are tabulated in Tables 1 and 2. Portal venous oxygen saturation was determined at the time of operation in 32 animals. The mean value was 81%.* It should be pointed out, however, that a high saturation was not found in every animal. In five of them the value was actually less than 70%. No explanation is available for these exceptionally low values.

In 21 of these dogs and in 2 additional ones, portal venous oxygen saturations were determined in the resting and fasting state approximately 18 hours after operation. The mean value was 76, the range from 56% to 93%. Fifteen of the 21 dogs studied during operation and also during the wake state the following day had higher values during anesthesia and operation. In 17 animals simultaneous femoral venous oxygen saturations were determined. These varied rather widely but averaged 49%.† The femoral venous

* This is precisely the same value that was found by Womack and Peters [2] whose anesthetized dogs had an average portal venous oxygen saturation of 80.9%.

† This again is almost precisely the same value obtained by Womack and Peters for vena caval blood, 46.4%.

TABLE 2.—*Influence of Rebreathing Into a Bag on Oxygen Saturation of Portal Venous and Arterial Blood* *

	Control		5 Min Rebreathing		10 Min Rebreathing		15 Min Rebreathing O_2	
Dog	Portal	Femoral	Portal	Femoral	Portal	Femoral	Portal	Femoral
	92.8	103.8					92.8	104.3
1	95.3	106.3					95.3	106.8
	97.8	108.8	97.4	104.4	85.2	78.3	97.8	109.3
	71.5	90.4					73.6	85.8
2	73.9	92.8					75.9	88.2
	76.3	95.2	86.9	88.4	40.8	35.7	78.4	90.6
	79.4	102.1					84.9	101.5
3	81.9	104.7					87.3	103.8
	84.5	107.3	86.1	98.7	83.6	91.3	89.6	106.2
	56.2	97.6					57.0	96.9
4	59.5	100.9					60.2	100.2
	62.8	104.2	88.9	101.6	95.4	112.2	63.2	103.4
	81.0	91.2					80.0	95.0
5	83.0	93.3					82.0	97.1
	85.0	95.5	82.2	94.1	68.0	68.0	84.0	99.2
	77.2	89.0					85.3	91.0
6	80.2	91.5					88.3	94.0
	83.2	94.4	83.3	91.0	63.1	66.0	91.3	97.0
Mean	81.5	101.0	87.0	96.0	73.0	75.0	84.0	101

* All values are expressed in percentages.

blood was, in general, less well saturated than the portal. In three exceptional animals, however, the oxygen saturation was approximately the same in portal and systemic venous blood.

In 17 dogs portal venous oxygen saturation immediately after 30 minutes of exercise was found to average 66%. Values in these same 17 dogs before exercise averaged 75%. In seven of the same animals additional determinations were made 30 minutes after the exercise had been terminated. In five of them the portal oxygen saturation had risen (slightly in two, more so in three) from that found immediately after exercise, while in two it remained essentially unchanged. On the average the saturation rose from 68% to 73%.

A meal was given to ten animals after they had been exercised and had then been given a short period of rest. One hour later, portal samples were obtained. The average value was 69% as compared with an average control value of 76% in the same animals earlier in the morning while they were fasting and resting. A decrease was observed in eight of the ten animals, while in one exceptional animal no change was observed and in the other the postprandial value was actually higher. A meal was given to six other dogs which had had no previous exercise. The average value was 81% as compared with an average preprandial value of 78%.

Observations made in the six animals studied while rebreathing into a bag initially filled with 100% oxygen suggested a relationship between the oxygen saturation of both portal venous blood and systemic arterial blood and the adequacy of ventilation. The average control values with the animals breathing 100% oxygen were 81.5% for portal venous blood and 101% for systemic arterial blood. Curiously enough, five minutes after the animals had rebreathed into a bag originally filled with 100% oxygen, the average values rose slightly for portal and fell slightly for arterial blood. Ten minutes after the animals had rebreathed into the bag, however, both values had fallen sharply (73% and 75% saturation, respectively). Finally, when the dogs had breathed 100% oxygen once again for 15 minutes, the values returned essentially to those observed initially under the same circumstances. In five of the six animals studied, the trend was essentially the same. In one, the observations were at variance and could not be explained.

Comment

These studies tend to confirm the general impression that portal venous blood at the time of operation is relatively well saturated. In 84% of our animals studied under anesthesia at the time of operation there was a high oxygen saturation, the average value being 86.5%. In nine of them the saturation was 90% or more. At the same time the values were rather low in four animals.

Our investigations indicate that the adequacy of ventilation may be a factor which influences the portal venous oxygen saturation. The high values noted when the animals breathed 100% oxygen fell sharply after they had been rebreathing for ten minutes into a bag originally filled with oxygen.

When the portal venous blood was studied in the postoperative state in the unanesthetized animal, the saturation was found to be somewhat less than that observed under anesthesia and mechanical ventilation with oxygen. The average value the morning after operation in 23 dogs was 76% (in contrast to 81%). All the dogs with high oxygen saturation at the time of operation had somewhat lower values the following day, but in two of them the change was of doubtful magnitude. In those showing a definite change, the average value was 86% at operation and 76% the day afterward. The mean femoral venous oxygen saturation of the unanesthetized dogs the day after operation was 49%.

Our studies seem to indicate that active body exercise brings about a decrease in the saturation of portal venous blood, just as it is known to do with respect to systemic venous blood. Immediately after dogs had walked for 30 minutes the average saturation of the portal venous blood was 66%, significantly less than that of the control resting samples (75%). After one-half hour of rest, recovery towards normal tended to occur. In those animals in which all three studies were made, the control resting portal venous oxygen saturation averaged 73%, that immediately after exercise 68%, that one-half hour later 73%.

The mechanism for the decreased saturation of portal venous blood following physical activity is not evident from our experiments. One possible factor may be a redistribution of blood flow during physical activity. One might assume that with greater blood flow into the extremities there is a correspondingly decreased portal flow and consequently greater oxygen extraction. It is also possible that some of the arteriovenous shunts may be closed during active exercise.

Equivocal results were obtained after the ingestion of food. The average values were somewhat lower than the control resting values, 69% as compared with 76%. In these studies, however, the meal was given rather soon after a period of active exercise which itself reduced the portal venous oxygen saturation. In six other animals, a meal was given after resting values were determined. They were studied an hour later. The average portal venous oxygen saturation in them was 81% after eating as compared with 78% prior to the ingestion of food. These studies, therefore, do not permit us to conclude that eating alone has any relatively constant effect upon portal oxygen saturation.

In two patients during convalescence from portacaval anastomosis, Smythe, Fitzpatrick, and Blakemore [4] observed an augmentation of arterioportal venous oxygen difference following the ingestion of a small meal. On one occasion the difference increased from 3.2 to 5 vol% and on another from 3.4 to 5.1. Peters and Womack felt that their studies indicated that gastric secretory activity brought about a closure of arteriovenous shunts which tended to be open in the resting state. This conclusion was based upon injection studies after gastric perfusion with histamine and after gastric perfusion with epinephrine. These observations are quite convincing. Their conclusions are also based in part upon observations of portal venous oxygen saturation and pressure which led them to generalize that histamine increases portal pressure and does not change oxygen saturation. They did not, however, observe a constant change in their oxygen saturation values. The saturation rose in three, fell in three, and remained unchanged in one animal. It is also not clear that there was any significant change in portal pressure since the pressure remained the same in three of seven animals studied, rose only 1 mm of mercury in one, and only 2 mm in another.

It is apparent that further investigations are needed in order to clarify the possible role of active digestion upon portal venous oxygen saturation. It might prove worthwhile to perform animal studies similar to those we carried out but with a longer period between the operative insertion of the portal venous catheter and the study itself. It also might be worthwhile to measure the portal venous oxygen saturation at varying time intervals after the ingestion of food. Further observations in man might prove enlightening.

Summary

Experimental observations on portal venous oxygen saturation in dogs are reported. A relatively high saturation of portal venous blood at the time of operation performed with adequate ventilation was noted in over 80% of the dogs. Arterial hypoxia induced by rebreathing into a bag reduced portal venous oxygen saturation. The saturation of the portal venous blood tended to be somewhat less in the unanesthetized resting state than at the time of operation. Physical activity resulted in a significant fall in the saturation of portal blood. The response to the ingestion of food was variable and inconstant.

Harris B. Shumacker, Jr., MD, Department of Surgery, Indiana University Medical Center, 1100 W. Michigan St, Indianapolis 7, Ind.

REFERENCES

1. Blalock, A., and Mason, M. F.: Observations on the Blood Flow and Gaseous Methabolism of the Liver of Unanesthetized Dogs, Amer J Physiol 117:328, 1936.

2. Womack, N. A., and Peters, R. M.: An Investigation of the Relationship Between Portal Venous Pressure and Inferior Vena Caval and Portal Venous Oxygen Saturations, Ann Surg 146:691, 1957.

3. Bradley, S. E.; Smythe, C. M.; Fitzpatrick, H. F.; and Blakemore, A. H.: The Effect of Portacaval Shunt on Estimated Hepatic Blood Flow and Oxygen Uptake in Cirrhosis, J Clin Invest 32:526, 1953.

4. Smythe, C. M.; Fitzpatrick, H. F.; and Blakemore, A. H.: Studies of Portal Venous O_2 Content in Unanesthetized Man, J Clin Invest 30:674, 1951.

5. Peters, R. M., and Womack, N. A.: Hemodynamics of Gastric Secretion, Ann Surg 148:537, 1958.

Carcinoma of Cecum Associated With Intussusception

FRANK G. MOODY, MD
AND
JOHN M. BEAL, MD
NEW YORK

Intussusception in adults is uncommon and, in contrast to children, is usually caused by an intrinsic lesion of the intestine. The diagnosis of intussusception is seldom made in adults before operation which is probably related to its infrequency and to the unusual manifestations. Carcinoma of the cecum has been encountered as a cause of intussusception in three patients on the pavilion surgical service of The New York Hospital-Cornell Medical Center over a six-year period. The diagnostic and therapeutic considerations which have been suggested by these patients stimulated this report.

Report of Cases

CASE 1.—A 78-year-old white woman first noted intermittent right lower quadrant pain approximately one year prior to admission. The pain increased in severity two months before admission and during the last four weeks was associated with one or two loose stools daily. The patient had not suffered from nausea, vomiting, or melena. She reported a 70-pound weight loss during the year.

Examination.—Blood pressure was 160/100, pulse 88, respirations 14, and temperature 37 C (98.6 F).

Abdomen: A diffusely tender mass occupied the entire right lower quadrant of the abdomen and did not seem to be movable. There was moderate guarding and muscle spasm; bowel sounds were normal.

Laboratory Findings.—Urinalysis was normal; hematocrit 35% on admission, increased to 43% after 1,000 cc whole blood transfusion. White cell count was 20,000.

An intravenous pyelogram demonstrated promptly functioning upper urinary tracts. A barium enema was reported to show an obstructing lesion of the transverse colon, presumably carcinoma.

Operation was performed on Oct 4, 1957. The entire right colon was intussuscepted into the transverse colon. The leading point was fixed and could not be reduced. A right hemicolectomy was performed.

The surgical pathologist reported a mass 28 cm in length. The mass that had produced the intussusception was an ulcerating neoplasm of the cecum that lay close to the ileocecal valve. A portion of the intussusceptum was markedly hemorrhagic. The diagnosis was carcinoma, cecum; intussusception, colon; infarct, colon.

The patient made a satisfactory recovery and was able to leave the hospital ten days after opera-

Submitted for publication May 13, 1963.

The Department of Surgery, The New York Hospital-Cornell Medical Center.

tion. She is now confined to a nursing home five years after operation without evidence of recurrence of carcinoma.

CASE 2.—A 38-year-old white man was admitted March 4, 1963, with complaints of abdominal pain and postprandial vomiting for three months.

The patient had a history of excessive ingestion of alcoholic beverages for many years which he discontinued upon medical advice five months before admission. At this time he developed mild cramping lower abdominal pain which was relieved by belching, vomiting, or defecation. Loss of approximately 25 pounds of body weight had been noted during the past three months. Pain in the right lower portion of the abdomen had been frequent for two weeks, and he had vomited frequently. His family and past history was otherwise unremarkable.

Physical findings were as follows: Blood pressure was 120/75, pulse 100, temperature 38 C (100.4 F), respirations 20. The patient was thin and appeared chronically ill. In the abdominal examination, the liver was felt 2 cm below the costal margin and the liver edge was smooth and not tender. A slightly tender, 8 cm × 10 cm firm movable mass was present in the right lower quadrant of the abdomen. Bowel sounds were active.

Laboratory Findings.—Hematocrit was 30%; white cell count 12,300. Urinalysis was unremarkable; stools were negative for occult blood on three examinations; chest roentgenogram was unremarkable. A barium enema was reported to demonstrate carcinoma of the right colon with associated intussusception (Fig 1).

Course.—Proctoscopic examination was performed, and the rectal mucosa was normal in appearance for a distance of six inches above the anus. After suitable preparation laparotomy was performed on March 11, 1963.

When the peritoneal cavity was entered, a large mass which represented the colon was found in the upper abdomen. It became apparent that the terminal ileum and ascending colon had intussuscepted into the transverse colon. A right hemicolectomy was performed.

The surgical pathologic report recorded that an 8 × 12 cm fungating polypoid mass was present in the cecum just distal to the ileocecal valve. The ileum and proximal ascending colon had invaginated into the proximal transverse colon for a distance of 7 cm. The intussusceptum was hemorrhagic and edematous. Microscopically, nests of anaplastic cells penetrated the full thickness of the bowel wall. However, the regional lymph nodes did not contain metastatic carcinoma. The diagnosis was carcinoma of cecum.

His postoperative course was satisfactory and he was discharged 11 days after operation.

CASE 3.—A 62-year-old white man developed fever, anorexia, and generalized cramping abdominal pain one month before admission to the hospital. These symptoms persisted for approximately one week and then subsided spontaneously. Two weeks before his entry into the hospital, epigastric cramping pain recurred and was associated with five to seven loose stools each day. Nausea and vomiting occurred one week later. The pain became increasingly severe. He reported 15 to 20 pounds' weight loss during the month. Stools had been brown without gross evidence of blood.

Examination.—Blood pressure was 140/90, temperature 37 C (98.6 F), pulse 90, and respirations 16. In the abdomen a large mass in the right upper quadrant extended to the left of the umbilicus. It was slightly tender and did not seem to be movable. Bowel sounds were hypoactive but present.

Laboratory.—Hematocrit was 43%; white cell count 15,500 with shift to left. Urinalysis was unremarkable. One stool was guaiac negative. BUN was 27 mg%. Serum sodium, potassium, and CO_2 combining power were within normal limits.

Barium enema examination demonstrated obstruction in the midtransverse colon, the margins of which were smooth. On the postevacuation film, the barium was noted to outline a large mass, approximately the size of a small football, which appeared to be continuous with the transverse colon (Fig 2).

Laparotomy was performed March 21, 1963. A large edematous fluid-filled mass occupied the right side of the abdomen. The mass lay within the

Fig 1.—Barium enema examination in case 2 demonstrates the "coiled spring" sign, typical of intussusception of the colon.

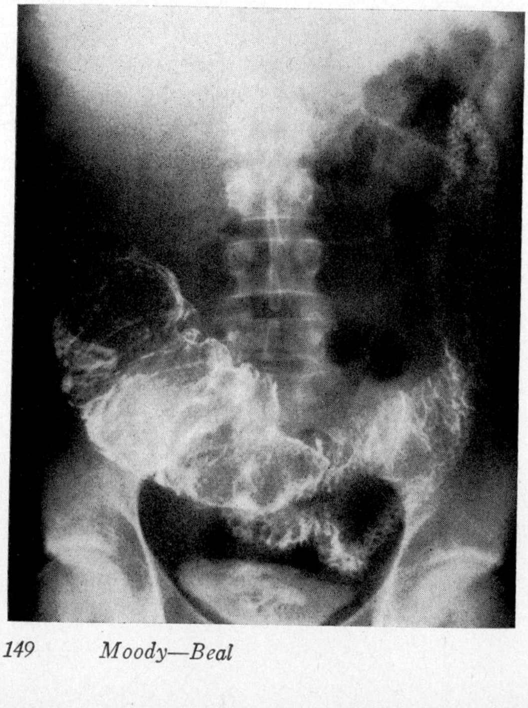

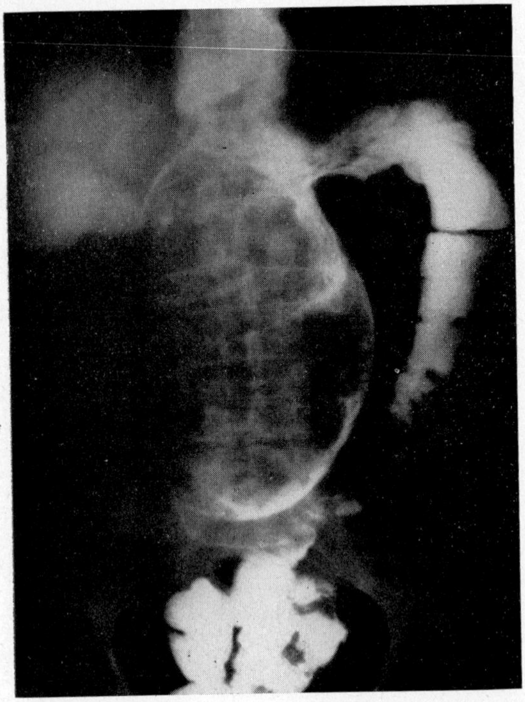

Fig 2.—Barium enema examination in case 3 demonstrates a large barium-coated mass in the postevacuation film which resembles a football in shape. The contour of the mass resulted from torsion of the intussuscepted colon.

transverse colon and extended to the midline. The terminal ileum had intussuscepted within the mass, and an inflamed appendix protruded from the proximal portion adjacent to the ileum. The entire mass was rotated 180° on the hepatocolic ligament. Approximately 100 cc of serosanguineous fluid was present. A right hemicolectomy was performed with end-to-end ileotransverse colostomy.

The surgical pathologic findings noted 30 cm of bowel, some areas of which were edematous, others hemorrhagic. The lesion that had produced the intussusception was a flattened polypoid lesion 4 cm in diameter, surrounding the ileocecal valve. When reduced, 50 cm of colon were measured from the cecum to the transected transverse colon, and 14 cm of ileum were present proximal to the ileocecal valve. The appendix was infarcted. The microscopic diagnosis was carcinoma of the cecum. Metastases were not found in the regional lymph nodes.

The patient made a satisfactory recovery and was discharged from the hospital 12 days after operation.

Comment

Intussusception in adults accounts for 5% to 10% of all cases of intussusception.[6] In contrast to this condition in children, intussusception in adults is usually caused by a definite lesion of the intestine.[7] The majority of the lesions that have produced intussusception in adults have been benign, although approximately 60% of the cases from the Mayo Clinic series were caused by malignant neoplasms.[3] Carcinoma of the cecum appears to be a relatively infrequent cause of intussusception. Donhauser and Kelly reviewed the literature from 1901 to 1947 and collected 665 cases, including 12 of their own. They were able to find 25 instances in which carcinoma of the cecum had produced intussusception.[4] Roper analyzed 410 cases from the British and American literature for the years 1947 to 1952 and found 42 cases of carcinoma of the cecum as cause of intussusception. Carcinoma of the cecum, however, was not implicated as a cause of intussusception in series reported more recently by Briggs and associates [1] and by Cotlar and Cohn.[2]

The symptoms associated with colonic intussusception are not specific and suggest partial obstruction of the large intestine. Intermittent cramping abdominal pain is usually described. The wide variation in duration of symptoms, one month to one year, in the present group of patients is comparable to that recorded in other reports. Dean and associates commented on the relative infrequency with which acute intestinal obstruction occurs in adult intussusception.[3] The three patients in this report had lost significant amounts of body weight, 20 to 70 pounds, during the course of their illness.

An abdominal mass was palpated in each patient in the present report. They did not, however, exhibit the contractile or "disappearing" tumor which Roper described as a key physical sign. This sign implies a reducible intussusception which was not present in these three patients.

Barium enema has been the most reliable diagnostic method. This examination may reveal only the site of obstruction, as illustrated in case 1. However, three signs have been reported which are considered diagnostic of intussusception when visualized by barium enema: (1) the "coiled spring" or "spiral sheath," (2) the crescentic edge, and (3) the "pitchfork" sign. The last is applicable to an unreduced ileoileal intussusception. The "coiled spring" sign was exemplified by the roentgenographic appearance in case 2 (Fig 1). The third case presented a radiologic finding that was not properly interpreted before operation. The postevacuation film demonstrated a large ovoid cavity, coated with barium, which was described by the radiologist as resembling a small football and might thus be labeled the "football" sign (Fig 2). This cavity apparently represented the dilated intussusception which was distended as a result of the obstruction produced by the intussusception and the torsion on the mesentery.

There is general agreement that adult intussusception should be treated by laparotomy and resection. However, several reports state that an effort at reduction should be made and that resection of the intussuscepted mass should be carried out if reduction fails.[1,6] Attempts at reduction of the intussusception may be justified in ileoileal intussusception because many of these are caused by Meckel's diverticula or other benign lesions. However, manipulation of ileocolic or colocolic invaginations in adults seems unwise. The majority of these are due to malignant neoplasms and most cannot be reduced. The frequency with which vascular change has been observed in the bowel wall suggests the likelihood of spread of tumor cells by injudicious handling. Primary resection was undertaken in the three cases in this report with good immediate results.

The prognosis after surgical treatment of intussusception of the colon associated with carcinoma of the cecum is uncertain. Roper [7] has stated, "malignant tumors occurring in this location are rare . . . highly malignant and . . . carry a bad prognosis. . . ." This conclusion was based on his analysis of the literature and upon his own experience. The first patient (case 1) in the current study has survived five years and is free of evidence of recurrent neoplasm. The other two patients have been operated upon too recently for any observations of survival. However, spread of carcinoma to the regional lymph nodes was not detected in any of this group. Thus, it is possible that the prognosis may not be as ominous if primary resection is performed without manipulation of the intussusception.

Summary

Three cases of intussusception of the colon due to carcinoma of the cecum have been reported. The treatment consisted of resection of the intussusception and primary anastomosis of the ileum and transverse colon. One patient has survived more than five years. The other patients have been operated upon recently.

Barium enema is the most important aid in diagnosis of this uncommon problem. An unusual radiologic picture was presented by one of the patients in this series.

John M. Beal, MD, Department of Surgery, New York Hospital-Cornell Medical Center, 525 E 68th St, New York 21, NY.

REFERENCES

1. Briggs, D. F.; Carpathios, J.; and Zollinger, R. W.: Intussusception in Adults, Amer J Surg 101:109, 1961.

2. Cotlar, A. M., and Cohn, I., Jr.: Intussusception in Adults, Amer J Surg 101:114, 1961.

3. Dean, D. L.; Ellis, F. H., Jr.; and Sauer, W. G.: Intussusception in Adults, AMA Arch Surg 73:6, 1956.

4. Donhauser, J. L., and Kelly, E. C.: Intussusception in the Adult, Amer J Surg 79:673, 1950.

5. Keeley, J. L.: Intussusception Associated With Aberrant Pancreatic Tissue, Arch Surg 60:691, 1950.

6. Orloff, M. J.: Intussusception in Children and Adults, Int Abstr Surg 102:313, 1956.

7. Roper, A.: Intussusception in Adults, Surg Gynec Obstet 103:267, 1956.

Drug Effects on Survival of Homografts of Skins

WARREN T. SUTTON, MD
FORD VAN HAGEN, MD
B. HEROLD GRIFFITH, MD
AND
FREDERICK W. PRESTON, MD
CHICAGO

Many attempts have been made to prolong the survival of homografts by suppressing the reticuloendothelial system of the host with drugs and other agents. A study of the Bagg lymphosarcoma in our laboratory showed that the growth of homografts of this tumor in rats was enhanced when the recipient animals were preconditioned with certain cytotoxic drugs and antimetabolites.[4] This study has been extended to determine if these agents affect the survival of homograft of normal skin. The transparent chamber technique was used because it provides an accurate criteria of survival of homografts. Skin is an organ which is very sensitive to the homograft rejection mechanism. Drugs which affect the survival of homografts of skin might have a similar effect upon homografts of other tissues. It is hoped that the simple technique described in this paper might be useful in the selection of drugs for the conditioning of animals for homotransplantation of other organs.

Method

Adult female mice of the AKR/J and C57BL/6J strains were used. Prior to grafting the mice were housed eight to a cage measuring 25.3×16.5×13.2 cm and fed water and a balanced formula. Treated animals received intraperitoneal injections of one or more drugs prior to, or prior to and after the grafting of the skin. The drugs used were selected from drugs currently undergoing clinical and laboratory trials as cancer chemotherapeutic agents. There were four antimetabolites, three alkylating agents, three antibiotics, and one miscellaneous drug, methylglyoxal-bis(guanylhydrazone).

Various dosage schedules were used in an attempt to determine specific suppression of the homograft rejection mechanism apart from the nonspecific debilitating effects of the drugs. An attempt was made to keep the doses of drugs within the sublethal range.

In order to have a clear-cut end-point for survival of the skin homografts, we utilized the transparent chamber technique devised by Algire[1] and subsequently modified by Edgerton and associates[3] and by Conway and associates.[2] The skin of the back of the mouse was suspended on a copper wire splint so that grafting and subsequent observation could be accomplished easily. A full-thickness defect of skin was created on one side of the dorsal fold exposing the vessels that lie between the panniculus adiposus and the panniculus carnosus. A homograft of full-thickness skin of the ear was removed from a donor mouse and applied to the defect. A similar defect was created on the opposite side of the skin fold to receive an autograft of ear skin from the recipient mouse. All grafting was done under a dissecting microscope in order to avoid injury to the delicate blood vessels in the grafts and in the recipient sites. Sterile technique was used. Care was taken to place the vessels of the graft at right angles to the vessels of the host in each recipient area. The autograft was thinner than the skin it replaced and was exactly opposite the homograft. This facilitated the transmission of light through the preparation when it was viewed under the dissecting microscope. After grafting, animals were caged separately, and grafts were observed daily. When a take of the

Submitted for publication May 21, 1963.

From the Department of Surgery, Veterans Administration Research Hospital and Northwestern University Medical School.

Aided by grants from the United Fund of Northfield Illinois, Inc., and from the Illinois Division of the American Cancer Society.

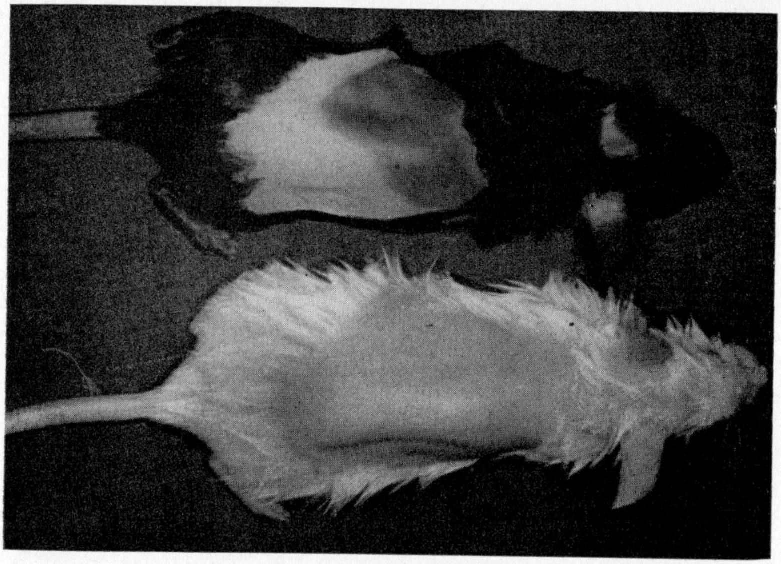

Fig 1.—Mice prepared for skin grafting.

graft occurred, blood could be seen to flow through the vessels of the graft within four to six days of grafting. Fig 1 shows a mouse prepared for grafting and Fig 2 shows a mouse with splint in place. The end-point of survival was considered to be the dilation of the vessels of the homograft and the slowing of the blood flow within them. When blood no longer flowed from the host animal into the vessels of the graft, necrosis and sloughing of the graft soon followed. The characteristics of a viable skin graft and the changes which occur when the graft is rejected have been described in detail by Edgerton and associates.[3] Their criteria for the determination of viability and for determining the rejection end-point were followed by us.

Results

Many grafts failed to "take" initially. Most of these failures occurred while we were developing our skill with the technique. Some mice died preoperatively from lethal amounts of the drugs or from the anesthetic. Mice in the hair growth cycle were not used because changes in the skin which occur at this period might alter the survival of the homografts. Autografts in which initial takes occurred remained permanently viable. Successful homografts in untreated animals had a mean survival time of approximately seven days. Animals which died prior to rejection of homografts were not included in the tabulation of results. A comparison is made between the mean survival times of the homografts in the treated animals and those in the control group. The results are given in tables 1-4.

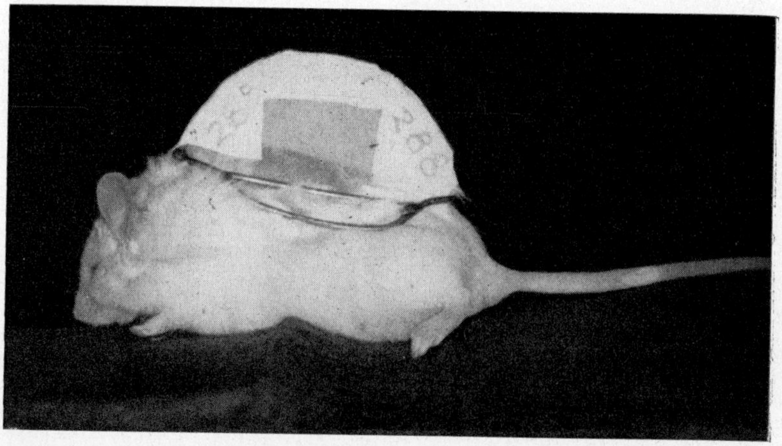

Fig 2.—Mouse with splint in place.

TABLE 1.—*Effect of Alkylating Agents on Skin Homograft Survival in Mice*

Drug	Dose: Amt. Injected, Mg/Kg	Dose: No. Injections	No. Mice	Mortality, %	Successful Grafts: No. Mice	Successful Grafts: Survival, Days Mean ± SD	Successful Grafts: *P* Value
None (control)	—	—	52	0	34	6.9±0.14	—
Sarcolysin	1/48 hr	12	26	4	8	7.5±0.42	<0.30
	2/48 hr	12	4	0	4	7.5±0.50	>0.50
	2/24 hr	12	4	0	2	8.0±0.00	<0.02
	2.5/24 hr	12	19	16	9	7.6±0.44	>0.20
	5/48 hr	12	41	10	18	8.4±0.59	>0.02
	5/24 hr	12	20	55	4	8.0±0.71	>0.20
	10/48 hr	12	7	29	0	—	—
	7.5/24 hr	12	4	75	0	—	—
Cyclophosphamide	20/24 hr	12	106	5	51	8.3±0.24	< <0.001
	25/24 hr	12	118	17	24	10.2±0.57	< <0.001
	50/24 hr	6	12	42	6	9.3±1.78	>0.20
	30/24 hr	12	42	19	7	11.7±1.53	<0.02
	35/24 hr	12	66	39	9	8.6±0.76	<0.10
	70/24 hr	6	12	25	0	—	—
	50/24 hr	12	51	59	9	14.0±0.71	< < <0.001
2-chloroethyl-methane-sulfonate	50/24 hr	12	26	8	17	6.8±0.19	>0.20
	60/24 hr	12	30	0	26	6.9±0.15	>0.60

TABLE 2.—*Effect of Antimetabolites on Skin Homograft Survival in Mice*

Drug	Dose: Amt Injected, Mg/Kg/24 Hr	Dose: No. Injections	No. Mice	Mortality, %	Successful Grafts: No. Mice	Successful Grafts: Survival, Days Mean ± SD	Successful Grafts: *P* Value
None (control)			52	0	34	6.9±0.14	—
6-mercaptopurine	20	6	11	9	8	9.1±0.64	>0.01
	50	6	29	21	8	7.9±0.23	<0.01
	50	12	37	27	11	7.8±0.33	<0.05
5-fluorouracil	15	12	22	5	15	9.0±0.44	<0.001
	20	12	13	54	5	8.0±0.32	>0.02
Methotrexate	3	12	38	13	19	9.4±0.44	< <0.001
	4	12	53	23	22	9.7±0.44	< <0.001
	5	12	41	20	15	8.3±0.41	<0.05
6-azauridine	7	12	18	0	7	7.4±0.58	<0.50
	8	12	22	0	20	7.4±0.44	>0.40
	10	12	22	0	17	6.8±0.19	<0.60

TABLE 3.—*Effect of Antibiotics on Skin Homograft Survival in Mice*

Drug	Dose: Amt Injected, Mg/Kg/24 Hr	Dose: No. Injections	No. Mice	Mortality, %	Successful Grafts: No. Mice	Successful Grafts: Survival, Days Mean ± SD	Successful Grafts: *P* Value
None (control)	—	—	61	0	39	7.2±0.70	—
Cycloheximide	50	12	40	15	9	6.7±0.44	>0.30
	100	12	6	50	0	—	—
Mitomycin C	1	12	54	9	31	7.1±0.24	>0.70
	1.5	12	21	14	7	7.1±0.41	>0.90
Actinomycin D	25	12	18	6	9	6.7±0.24	>0.10
	50	12	30	17	20	8.0±0.26	>0.02
	60	12	22	5	14	8.1±0.47	>0.10
	75	12	12	0	3	8.3±0.41	<0.10

TABLE 4.—*Effect of Methylglyoxal Bis(Guanylhydrazone) on Skin Homograft Survival in Mice*

Drug	Dose: Amt Injected, Mg/Kg/24 Hr	Dose: No. Injections	No. Mice	Mortality, %	Successful Grafts: No. Mice	Successful Grafts: Survival, Days Mean ± SD	*P* Value
None (control)	—	—	52	0	34	6.9±0.14	—
Methylglyoxal	30	12	24	0	11	6.2±0.23	>0.01
	40	12	18	0	13	5.8±0.91	>0.001

Comment

Others authors have investigated the effect of drugs on the homograft rejection mechanism with particular reference to homografts of skin. Schwartz and Dameshek [7] and Meeker and associates [6] have found significant prolongation of survival of skin homografts in rabbits conditioned with 6-mercaptopurine but not with mechlorethamine hydrochloride (a nitrogen mustard) or thio-tepa (triethylenethiophosphoramide). Meeker and associates point out that the results of experiments concerned with prolongation of skin homograft survival are related to the species of animal used. Studies in which mice were used by these authors failed to show any prolongation of skin homograft survival in a large number of experiments using a wide range of doses of drugs. It is perhaps noteworthy that cyclophosphamide, the drug which produced the most effect in our test system, was not included among the drugs studied by these investigators. Furthermore these authors used as an end-point the slough of the graft as observed grossly, a technique which does not provide as sharp an end-point as the transparent chamber method.

Summary

Adult female mice of AKR/J and C57BL/6J strains were prepared with skin autografts and homografts to study the effect of suppression of immune mechanisms on homograft survival.

Four antimetabolites, three alkylating agents, three antibiotics, and a miscellaneous drug, methylglyoxal-bis(guanylhydrazone) were investigated.

Results show statistically significant prologation of homograft survival with 6-mercaptopurine, 5-fluorouracil, methotrexate, and cyclophosphamide. Of these, cyclophosphamide had the greatest effect.

The authors are indebted to Miss Judith Brandly for technical assistance.

Frederick W. Preston, MD, Chief, Surgical Service, Veterans Administration Research Hospital, 333 E Huron St, Chicago, Ill.

REFERENCES

1. Algire, G. H.: Microscopic Studies of the Early Growth of a Transplantable Melanoma of the Mouse, Using the Transparent-Chamber Technique, J Nat Cancer Inst 4:13, 1943.

2. Conway, H.; Griffith, B. H.; Shannon, J. E., Jr.; and Findley, A.: Re-Examination of the Transparent Chamber Technique as Applied to the Study of Circulation in Autografts and Homografts of Skin, Plast Reconstr Surg 20:103, 1957.

3. Edgerton, M. T.; Peterson, H. A.; and Edgerton, P. J.: The Homograft Rejection Mechanism, AMA Arch Surg 74:238, 1957.

4. Henegar, G. C.; Jackson, E. J.; and Preston, F. W.: Host Conditioning for Homologous Tumor Transplants, Surg Forum 12:165, 1961 .

5. Levinson, M. E., and Necheles, H.: Successful Prolongation of Survival of Skin Homografts, Plast Reconstr Surg 17:218, 1956.

6. Meeker, W. R., Jr.; Condie, R. M.; Good, R. A.; and Varco, R. L.: Alteration of the Homograft Response by Antimetabolites, Ann NY Acad Sci 87:203, 1960.

7. Schwartz, R., and Dameshek, W.: Drug-Induced Immunological Tolerance, Nature (London) 183:1682, 1959.

Interrelationship of Diabetes Mellitus and Pancreatitis

HERMAN T. BLUMENTHAL, MD
J. G. PROBSTEIN, MD
AND
A. W. BERNS, BS
ST. LOUIS

Several types of relationships between pancreatitis and diabetes mellitus have been studied: (1) A transitory hyperglycemia and glycosuria have been observed during acute attacks of pancreatitis which have been attributed to secondary, temporary effects of the acute inflammatory process on the islets of Langerhans. After recovery from the acute episode, the defect in carbohydrate metabolism usually disappears.[1] However, the damage appears to be permanent in some cases since Shumacker [2] has reported that 3%-10% of patients with acute pancreatitis develop permanent diabetes. (2) The development of acidosis and coma during an attack of acute pancreatitis in an already established diabetes has been particularly stressed by Root [3] and more recently by Hughes.[4] It appears that in such cases the diabetes antedates the onset of acute pancreatitis. But it remains uncertain whether or not the presence of diabetic coma renders the patient more susceptible to attacks of acute pancreatitis. Evidently Tully and Lowenthal [5] believe that this is the case since they suggest that the relationship should be stated as the acute pancreatitis of diabetic coma rather than the diabetic coma of acute pancreatitis. (3) Comfort [6] has reported that diabetes mellitus is one of the more common complications of chronic relapsing pancreatitis, and presumably this is attributed to progressive, permanent destruction of the islets of Langerhans with recurrent acute episodes. On the other hand Bell [7] has found that among 2,217 diabetic subjects there were only eight cases (0.36%) which could be attributed to chronic pancreatitis. However, he also noted that nearly one half of the subjects with

Submitted for publication May 22, 1963.

From the Laboratories of the Clinical Research Program on Aging, Veterans Hospital, Jefferson Barracks, and the Departments of Surgery, The Jewish Hospital and Washington University of Medicine.

This study was supported in part by the Louis Monheimer-Clara K. London Memorial Research Fund and in part by Grant No. AM-07116, National Institute of Arthritis and Metabolic Disease, National Institutes of Health.

pancreatic lithiasis developed permanent diabetes.

That the acute proteolytic processes which are peculiar to necrosis of the pancreas can destroy islets as well as acinar tissue would appear to be supported by a number of older reports by Lattes,[8] Levin,[9] Wells,[10] and Katz and Winkler[11] of permanent diabetes after traumatic injury to the pancreas. While occasionally permanent diabetes has also been observed after severe attacks of acute pancreatitis by Bernhard [12] and by Gambill et al,[13] this would appear to be a relatively infrequent complication. Warren and LeCompte [14] have pointed out that this complication would probably be more frequent were it not that the lesions which destroy enough of the pancreas to produce an insulin insufficiency are generally also sufficiently severe to cause death from the pancreatitis itself before there has been opportunity for diabetes to become manifest. Presumably, in chronic relapsing pancreatitis sufficient time does elapse for an islet insufficiency to occur, since according to Comfort [6] only about one third of the patients die as a result of the pancreatitis.

It may be significant, however, that in the study by Comfort [6] another third of the patients died of vascular disease. Until recently the vascular phenomena associated with diabetes have been considered a complication of the metabolic disease. However, the reports of Freedman,[15] Arnold et al [16] and Ellenberg [17] emphasize that diabetes must be suspected in the differential diagnosis of any renal lesion of uncertain etiology. Such suspicion may be enhanced by the presence of a family history of diabetes, retinopathy,[18] neuropathy as manifested by absent deep reflexes,[19] or peripheral gangrene or severe peripheral vascular disease.[20] Certain of these reports[15-19] indicate that various of these phenomena may sometimes even antedate the onset of hyperglycemia and glycosuria. During the past several years studies by Blumenthal et al [21-28] further support the concept that the special angiopathies associated with diabetes may actually be an integral part of the total disease process rather than a complication in the ordinary sense.

TABLE 1.—*Frequency of Pancreatitis at Autopsy in Diabetic and Nondiabetic Subjects*

	Diabetic	Nondiabetic
Total cases	281	3,540
Cases up to 20 yr	4	649
Pancreatitis up to 20 yr	0	6 (0.9%)
Cases over 20 yr	277	2,891
Pancreatitis over 20 yr	31 (11.2%) *	152 (5.3%) *
Males over 20 yr	131	1,614
Pancreatitis in males over 20 yr	17 (13.0%)	92 (5.7%)
Females over 20 yr	146	1,277
Pancreatitis in females over 20 yr	14 (9.6%)	60 (4.6%)

* $P < 0.001$ by the χ^2 test.

It is therefore possible that, in some cases of acute pancreatitis in which diabetes appears to occur as a complication, an abnormal state of glucose metabolism may have been present but undetected prior to the onset of pancreatitis or that angiopathies of diabetes were present without manifest hyperglycemia or glycosuria. These possibilities deserve exploration since, as we have previously pointed out,[29] vascular disease may play an important role in the genesis of pancreatitis. In the latter concept, the existence of a diabetic angiopathy in the pancreas might actually constitute a significant mechanism which would render the patient more susceptible to attacks of acute pancreatitis. The present report therefore, deals with a search for evidence which would support such a concept regarding the interrelationship of diabetes and pancreatitis.

Materials and Methods

There were two phases to this study, the first a statistical one and the second, histopathological. In the first phase the records of 3,821 autopsy cases performed at the Jewish Hospital over a period of approximately 35 years were examined for the presence of diabetes and/or pancreatitis. A comparison was then made of the frequency of pancreatitis between the diabetic and nondiabetic groups as shown in Table 1. The frequency of pancreatitis in diabetic subjects was then compared with the frequency of other complications in diabetes-associated angiopathies in the same autopsy population, as shown in Table 2.

TABLE 2.—*Comparison of Frequency of Infarcts in Diabetics and Nondiabetics*

Infarction	Diabetic, % *	Nondiabetic, % *	Ratio D/ND †
Myocardial	49.6	19.2	2.6/1
Cerebral	30.2	19.4	1.6/1
Renal	6.2	3.0	2.1/1
Pancreatitis	11.2	5.3	2.1/1
Gangrene, lower extremity	7.3	0.9	8.1/1

* $P < 0.001$ by the χ^2 test with the exception of renal infarction which was $0.05 > P > 0.01$.
† D/ND designates diabetic/nondiabetic ratio.

In the second phase of this study, sections of the pancreas in the 184 cases of pancreatitis were studied for the presence of various lesions of small intraparenchymal vessels. Successive sections in each case were stained with hematoxylin and eosin, the Verhoeff-Van Gieson stain, and by the periodic acid-Schiff and colloidal iron techniques as in previous studies dealing with the vasculopathies encountered in diabetes.[21-18] The vascular lesions encountered were then tabulated, as shown in Table 3, and a comparison made as to the frequency of each between diabetic and nondiabetic subjects with pancreatitis. The characteristics of these various types of vascular lesions have also been described in previous studies.[21-18]

Results

The Frequency of Pancreatitis in Diabetes Mellitus.—Because of the small number of cases of diabetes under age 20 (only four) and also the small number of cases of pancreatitis in this age group (only six, previously reported),[30] the comparison of the frequency of pancreatitis in diabetic and nondiabetic subjects was limited to the cases over 20 years of age. There was a total of 3,168 cases over this age, including 183 cases of pancreatitis. Thus, the frequency of pancreatitis in this autopsy population was 5.8%. The frequency of such pancreatitis in the diabetic group was 11.2% as compared with only 5.3% in the nondiabetic autopsy population, or well over a two-fold increase, and statistically significant. In both groups the frequency in males was higher than in females, although the sex difference was greater in the diabetic than in the nondiabetic group.

In Table 2 a comparison is shown of the frequency of various complications of vascular disease in the diabetic and nondiabetic groups in this autopsy population. There is a considerable difference in the frequency of infarction in various organs between the two groups, with a striking and significant increase in the frequency of infarction in diabetes. In the case of infarction of the heart, brain, or kidney, the ratio of diabetic to nondiabetic patients is about 1.5 to 2.5:1. This ratio is considerably higher only with respect to gangrene of the lower extremity. It is noteworthy that the ratio between the two groups in respect to the frequency of pancreatitis is about the same as with infarction of the heart, brain, or kidney.

The Vascular Lesions.—The frequency of the various types of vascular lesions within the pancreas is shown in Table 3. This tabulation refers to lesions in intralobular vessels and smaller, down to arteriolar size. The data refer primarily to lesions on the

TABLE 3.—*Frequency of Various Vascular Lesions in Diabetic and Nondiabetic Subjects With Pancreatitis*

Group	Vascular Lesions: Inflammatory (%)	Thrombotic (%)	Atheromatous *(%)	Hemodynamic (%)	Proliferative (%)
Diabetic males	17/17 (100)	4/17 (23.5)	4/17 (23.5)	13/17 (76.5)	11/17 (64.7)
Diabetic females	14/14 (100)	4/14 (28.6)	4/14 (28.6)	14/14 (100)	12/14 (85.7)
Combined	31/31 (100)	8/31 (25.9)	8/31 (25.9)	27/31 (87.1)	23/31 (74.2) †
Nondiabetic males	92/92 (100)	10/92 (10.9)	10/92 (10.9)	86/92 (93.5)	14/92 (15.2)
Nondiabetic females	60/60 (100)	5/60 (8.3)	7/60 (11.7)	43/60 (71.7)	7/60 (11.7)
Combined	152/152 (100)	16/152 (9.9)	17/152 (11.2)	129/152 (84.9)	21/152 (13.8) †

* This includes ten cases of atheromatous embolization: two each in diabetic males and diabetic females, four in nondiabetic males, and two in nondiabetic females.
† $P < 0.001$ by the χ^2 test.

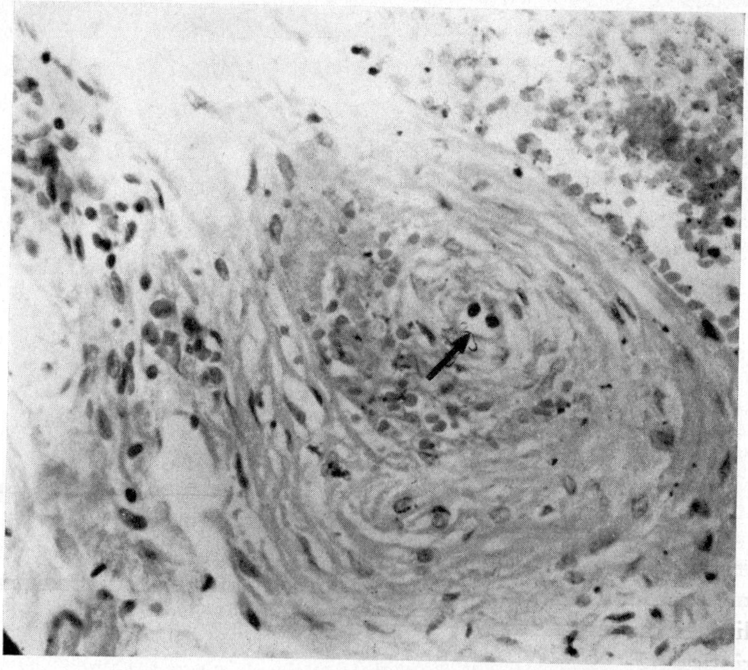

Fig 1.—Section of an interlobular artery of a diabetic patient with acute pancreatitis. The lumen is almost completely occluded by a mass of endothelial cells. Arrow indicates the tiny residual lumen. Hematoxylin and eosin stain; reduced 61% from mag approximately × 450.

arterial side of the circulation, although occasional lesions of some types, eg., inflammatory, thrombotic, and proliferative, were occasionally seen in veins. Since all of the specimens had evidence of pancreatitis, the presence of inflammatory vascular lesions in all cases in both groups is as would be expected. Thrombotic and atheromatous lesions show a slightly over two-fold increase in the diabetic group. On the other hand, the frequence of hemodynamic lesions is about the same in the two groups. The most striking difference is found in the frequency of proliferative lesions; the latter were present in about three fourths of the cases of pancreatitis in the diabetic group, and this repre-

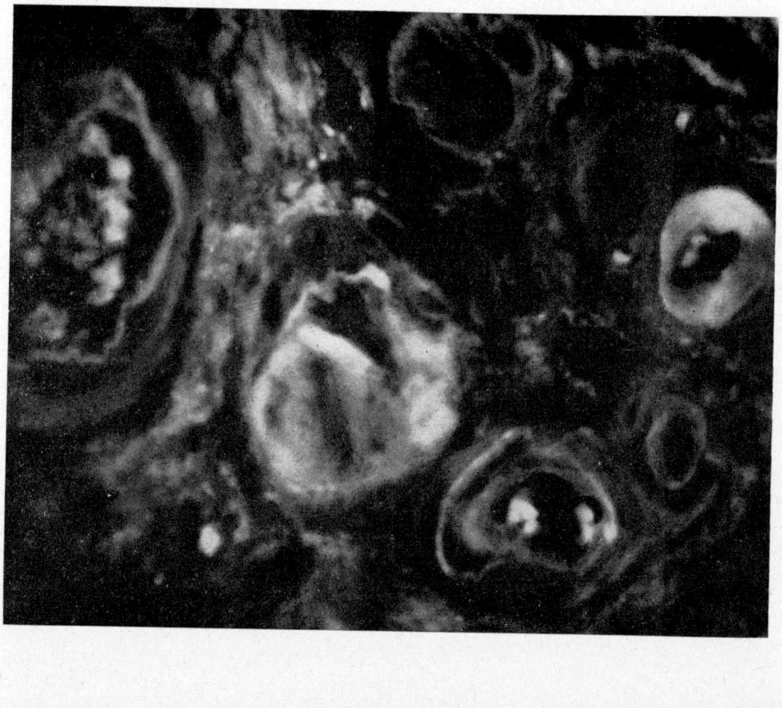

Fig 2.—Section showing a cluster of interlobular arteries of a diabetic patient with acute pancreatitis. Section has been stained with fluorescein conjugated insulin and photographed with ultraviolet light. In the center is a markedly hyalinized artery showing brilliant fluorescence, and a somewhat smaller artery, also hyalinized, is seen along the right margin. Several other arteries in the right half of the figure show autofluorescence of the internal elastic lamella. The same is the case with the large artery along the left margin, but here even more brilliant staining of endothelial cells is seen.

sents over a five-fold increase in frequency over that in the nondiabetic group. This is a statistically significant difference.

These proliferative lesions are characterized by an ingrowth of endothelial cells into the lumen, with narrowing and eventually occlusion of the latter (Fig 1). This process is accompanied by the deposition of fine fibrils between endothelial cells which give a positive periodic acid-Schiff reaction and a negative one with the colloidal iron technique. They differ from the atheromatous lesion in that they do not contain lipid in significant amounts [24] and from the hemodynamic one in that the latter consists of thickening of the intima by acellular hyaline material and reduplicated or degenerated elastic fiber. In later stages the periodic acid-Schiff positive material may coalesce, giving the appearance of a hyalinized arterial wall similar to that characteristic of the hemodynamic lesion, and at this point a distinction between the two types may not be possible by conventional stains.

However, both the proliferative lesions and some of the hyalinizing ones characteristically bind fluorescein conjugated insulin (Fig 2). Whereas such a binding reaction was found in all of the pancreatitis cases with diabetes, it was found in less than 1% of the nondiabetic subjects with comparable vascular lesions. The techniques involved in such fluorescence microscopy studies have been detailed previously.[26,27] The specificity of the reaction is indicated further by the fact that if such sections are first immersed in nonfluorescent insulin to saturate the hormone-binding sites, the binding of fluorescent insulin can be inhibited. Unstained sections show only blue auto-fluorescence as contrasted with the green fluorescence of the conjugated hormone. Fluorescein conjugated snake venom protein used as a control for nonspecific protein binding gives a negative reaction.

Comment

It is evident from the foregoing results that this report addresses itself primarily to the relationship between an already established diabetes and the occurrence of pancreatitis. A striking feature of these data is that they show that pancreatitis occurs more frequently among diabetic than among nondiabetic patients in our autopsy population and that this increase in frequency is of about the same order of magnitude as that which occurs in respect to myocardial, cerebral, and renal infarction.

Such data therefore suggest that the initiating mechanism may be an infarction of the pancreas. As we have pointed out previously [29] there is a considerable body of evidence suggesting such an initiating event, but the anatomic features of infarction may be soon lost because of the superimposed proteolytic activity of enzymes peculiar to the pancreas. Hranilovich and Baggenstoss [31] have pointed out that occlusion of a large artery does not inevitably lead to infarction, particularly since the pancreas is richly endowed with potential collateral channels. It therefore becomes important to evaluate the state of small collaterals in the pancreas in diabetes if the infarction hypothesis is to have a valid basis.

The principal difference in the present study as regards the state of the vascular supply in diabetic and nondiabetic subjects with pancreatitis is the finding of about a five-fold increase in the frequency of proliferative lesions of small vessels, principally arteries and arterioles, in the diabetic group. This, then, could account for differences in the competency of collateral channels as between diabetic and nondiabetic subjects. Another possibility has been offered by Tourtellotte and Tyler [32] who have pointed out that diabetes may be associated with hyperlipemia and fat emboli to the pancreas. This mechanism has also been stressed by Klatskin and Gordon.[33] While this may have applicability in some cases, it should be pointed out that such hyperlipemia is infrequent in the adequately controlled diabetic patient. Moreover, it has been shown [24] that the proliferative lesion associated with diabetes does not contain a significant quantity of lipid demonstrable by conventional fat stains.

The occurrence of such vascular phenomena might also constitute an important factor in chronic relapsing pancreatitis. As has already been pointed out, the diabetes often associated with the latter disease is considered to be a complication resulting from the progressive destruction of islets of Langerhans by recurrent inflammatory processes. It is equally possible that, at least in some instances, the vascular lesions and pre- or inapparent diabetes may be present. With repeated episodes of infarction and subsequent healing, as well as with progressive fibrosis resulting from a diminished blood supply, the same end-picture could result in the pancreas.

As we have pointed out in past studies,[21-28] these proliferative lesions have characteristics similar to those obtained with experimentally induced immune states and can also be found in nondiabetics with disease states considered to occur on a hyperimmune basis. Among the latter are rheumatoid arthritis, chronic glomerulonephritis, lupus, and others. The demonstration of insulin binding by vascular lesions in diabetics suggests that this hormone may be the responsible antigenic agent. In recent studies[34] it has been possible to reproduce such lesions by producing an immunity to insulin in rabbits.

One clinical observation which has perhaps obscured the relationship between these two diseases is the discovery of the diabetic state for the first time during or shortly after an acute attack of pancreatitis. As pointed out in the introduction, this has led to the conclusion that the acute inflammatory process destroys islet as well as acinar tissues, thus leading to an insulin insufficiency diabetes. An alternative possibility is that the vascular manifestations may antedate the clinical manifestations of both diabetes and pancreatitis. Support for such a thesis derives from the observations already noted[15-19] of the occurrence of the various angiopathies associated with diabetes prior to the onset of hyperglycemia and glycosuria. Furthermore, Bell[7] has suggested that hyalinization of the islets of Langerhans of nondiabetic patients may similarly represent pre- or potential diabetes, and our recent study on the pancreas[28] suggests a link between such islet lesions and the proliferative vascular ones when the latter involve the islets of Langerhans. Thus the association of pancreatitis and diabetic acidosis[3-5] may represent a concomitant onset of both diseases linked with the presence of an associated vascular phenomenon.

Herman T. Blumenthal, MD, Director, Clinical Research Program on Aging, Veterans Administration Hospital, Jefferson Barracks, St. Louis 25, Mo.

REFERENCES

1. Paxton, J. R., and Payne, J. H.: Acute Pancreatitis: Statistical Review of 308 Established Cases of Acute Pancreatitis, Surg Gynec Obstet 86:69, 1948.

2. Shumacker, H. B., Jr.: Acute Pancreatitis and Diabetes, Ann Surg 112:177, 1940.

3. Root, H. F.: Diabetic Coma and Acute Pancreatitis With Fatty Liver, JAMA 108:777, 1937.

4. Hughes, P. D.: Diabetic Acidosis With Acute Pancreatitis, Brit J Surg 49:90, 1961.

5. Tully, G. T., and Lowenthal, J. J.: The Diabetic Coma of Acute Pancreatitis, Ann Intern Med 48:310, 1958.

6. Comfort, W. W.: Chronic Relapsing Pancreatitis: Its Clinical Course, Sequelae, Diagnosis, and Medical Treatment in Cases in Which Disease of Biliary or Gastrointestinal Tract Did Not Exist, Proc Mayo Clin 22:548, 1947.

7. Bell, E. T.: Diabetes Mellitus: A Clinical and Pathological Study of 2,529 Cases, Springfield, Ill: Charles C. Thomas, Publishers, 1960.

8. Lattes, L.: Über Pancreasvergiftung, Virchow Arch Path Anat 211:1, 1913.

9. Levin, I.: Effects of Experimental Injuries of the Pancreas, J Med Res 16:419, 1907-08.

10. Wells, H. G.: Post-Traumatic Calcification of the Pancreas With Diabetes, Amer J Med Sci 164:476, 1922.

11. Katz, A., and Winkler, F.: Experimentelle Studien über die Fettgewebsnekrose des Pancreas, Arch Verdauungskr 4:289, 1898.

12. Bernhard, F.: Das Auftreten des Diabetes mellitus nach akuten Pankreaserkrankungen (Untersucht an 50 operativ gehellten (Fällen), Klin Wschr 10:632, 1931.

13. Gambill, E. E.; Baggenstoss, A. H.; Van Patter, W. C.; and Power, M. H.: Acute Hemorrhagic Pancreatitis: Study of a Patient Having Disseminated Fat Necrosis, Hypocalcemia, Hypopotassemia, Uremia, Diabetes Mellitus, Ascites, and

Bilateral Hydrothorax, Gastroenterology 11:371, 1948.

14. Warren, S., and LeCompte, P. M.: The Pathology of Diabetes Mellitus, ed 3, Philadelphia: Lea and Febiger, 1952.

15. Freedman, L. R.: Inapparent Diabetes Mellitus as a Cause of Renal Insufficiency Due to Kimmelstiel-Wilson Lesions, Bull Hopkins Hosp 100:132, 1957.

16. Arnold, J. D.; Tarlov, A. R.; Spargo, B.; and Brewer, G. J.: Subclinical Diabetes Mellitus in Patients Presenting With Clinical Chronic "Glomerulonephritis", Trans Ass Amer Physicians 71:186, 1958.

17. Ellenberg, M.: Diabetic Nephropathy Without Manifest Diabetes, Diabetes 11:197, 1962.

18. Becker, B.: Diabetic Retinopathy, Ann Intern Med 37:273, 1952.

19. Ellenberg, M.: Absent Deep Reflexes: A Diagnostic Clue in Unsuspected Diabetes, Amer J Med Sci 242:183, 1961.

20. Dry, T. J., and Hines, E. H., Jr.: The Role of Diabetes in the Development of Degenerative Vascular Disease, Ann Intern Med 14:1893, 1941.

21. Burstein, R.; Blumenthal, H. T.; and Soule, S. D.: Histogenesis of Pathological Processes in Placentas of Metabolic Disease in Pregnancy: II. The Diabetic State, Amer J Obstet Gynec 74:96, 1957.

22. Goldenberg, S.; Alex, M.; and Blumenthal, H. T.: A Non-Atheromatous Peripheral Vascular Disease of the Lower Extremity in Diabetes Mellitus, Diabetes 8:261, 1959.

23. Blumenthal, H. T.; Alex, M.; and Goldenberg, S.: A Study of Lesions of the Intramural Coronary Artery Branches in Diabetes Mellitus, Arch Path 70:13, 1960.

24. Blumenthal, H. T.; Alex, M.; and Goldenberg, S.: A Nonatheromatous Proliferative Vascular Lesion of the Retina in Diabetes Mellitus: Role in the Etiology of Diabetic Retinopathy, Amer J Med 31:382, 1961.

25. Alex, M.; Baron, E. C.; Goldenberg, S.; and Blumenthal, H. T.: An Autopsy Study of Cerebrovascular Accident in Diabetes Mellitus, Circulation 25:663, 1962.

26. Berns, A. W.; Owens, C. T.; Hirata, Y.; and Blumenthal, H. T.: The Pathogenesis of Diabetic Glomerulosclerosis: I. The Significance of Various Histopathological Components of the Disease, and II. A Demonstration of the Insulin Binding Capacity of the Various Histopathological Components of the Disease by Fluorescence Microscopy, Diabetes 11:296, 308, 1962.

27. Berns, A. W.; Hirata, Y.; and Blumenthal, H. T.: Application of Fluorescence Microscopy to the Study of Possible Insulin-Binding Reactions in Formalin-Fixed Material, J Lab Clin Med 60:535, 1962.

28. Berns, A. W., and Blumenthal, H. T.: A Histo- and Immunopathological Study of the Vascular and Islet Lesions of the Pancreas in Diabetes Mellitus, to be published.

29. Blumenthal, H. T., and Probstein, J. G.: Pancreatitis: A Clinical Pathologic Correlation, Springfield, Ill: Charles C. Thomas, Publishers, 1959.

30. Blumenthal, H. T., and Probstein, J. G.: Acute Pancreatitis in the Newborn, in Infancy and in Childhood, Amer Surg 27:533, 1961.

31. Hranilovich, G. T., and Baggenstoss, A. H.: Lesions of the Pancreas and Malignant Hypertension, Arch Path 55:443, 1953.

32. Tourtellotte, C. R., and Tyler, R. D.: Hyperlipemia Associated With Diabetes Mellitus and Pancreatitis: A Case Report With Autopsy, Ann Intern Med 45:691, 1956.

33. Klatskin, G., and Gordon, M.: Relationship Between Relapsing Pancreatitis and Essential Hypertension, Amer J Med 12:3, 1952.

34. Hirata, Y.; Berns, A.; and Blumenthal, H. T.: The Experimental Production of a Disseminated Vasculopathy Similar to Diabetic Vasculopathy in Man, presented at the 22nd Annual Meeting of the American Diabetic Association, June, 1962.

Bile Ascites

DON R. SANTSCHI, MD
KENNETH A. HUIZENGA, MD
HAROLD H. SCUDAMORE, MD
WILLIAM H. DEARING, MD
AND
JOHN M. WAUGH, MD†
ROCHESTER, MINN

Free escape of bile into the peritoneal cavity in adults generally is considered to be an acute and serious situation with a high mortality rate. In a review of more than 7,000 cases of perforation of the gallbladder, collected from six authors, Eliason and McLaughlin [1] reported a mortality rate in adults of 10% to 85%. In a series reported by Butler and Harkins,[2] all patients with untreated acute perforation of the gallbladder died. Mentzer [3] stated that infected bile spreading diffusely throughout the peritoneal cavity produces an acute peritonitis that would be fatal unless treated surgically. Morse and associates [4] wrote that the mortality rate in all untreated cases of acute perforation of the gallbladder is 100%.

Our interest in this subject was stimulated by experience with four adults during the past eight years who, clinically, did not present with the usual acute picture associated with peritoneal contamination with bile. Three of these patients had massive ascites instead of acute peritonitis, and the ascites did not recur after surgical repair of a leak in the biliary tract. In the fourth patient, only paracentesis was necessary. This paper reports these cases and reviews briefly the recent literature on this subject.

Report of Cases

CASE 1.—A 30-year-old white married woman registered at the Mayo Clinic in September, 1961, with the chief complaint of progressive abdominal distention of one month's duration. During the previous two years, she had experienced three episodes of pain in the right upper quadrant of the abdomen which required meperidine (Demerol) for relief. In April, 1961, cholecystectomy had been performed, but the common bile duct was not explored. Two days after this operation she had noted the onset of progressive jaundice without fever, dark urine, light-colored stools, and steatorrhea; she then was treated with methylprednisolone (Medrol). Because of progressive jaundice and pruritus, the abdomen had beeen re-explored two weeks later, and the surgeon's report stated that the only positive finding was a dilated and mucus-filled common bile duct. A T-tube had been inserted, but it subsequently had been displaced. At dismissal one week later, the patient still had had jaundice, anorexia, nausea, and vomiting, but had had no external drainage from the wound. During the following two months, she had noticed a gradual abatement of the jaundice and an increase in appetite. However, in August, 1961, anorexia, nausea, and malaise had recurred, associated with constipation, increase of weight, and abdominal distention; but there was no increase in jaundice. She then had been treated with diuretics without benefit, and was referred to the Mayo Clinic.

On admission, she complained of abdominal distention, vague generalized abdominal distress, dyspnea, orthopnea, and "heartburn." Positive physical findings consisted of massive abdominal distention, shifting abdominal dullness, and mild jaundice.

Laboratory studies of blood provided the following values: hemoglobin, 13.4 gm/100 ml; leukocyte count, 8,600 per cubic millimeter; and erythrocyte

Submitted for publication May 25, 1963.

Fellow in Medicine, Mayo Foundation (Dr. Santschi), Section of Medicine (Dr. Huizenga, Dr. Scudamore, Dr. Dearing) Section of Surgery (Dr. Waugh), Mayo Clinic and Mayo Foundation, Rochester, Minn.

† Dr. Waugh died Aug 12, 1962.

sedimentation rate, 75 mm in one hour (Westergren method). The serum bilirubin was 4.2 mg/100 ml by the direct method and 0.9 mg by the indirect method. Other analytical results were: total cholesterol, 175 mg/100 ml of plasma; alkaline phosphatase, 85.2 King and Armstrong units per 100 ml of serum; blood urea, 36 mg/100 ml of blood; thymol turbidity, 2+; and prothrombin time, 20 seconds. Three days later electrolyte concentrations were: sodium, 120 mEq, and potassium, 2.9 mEq per liter of serum; and chloride, 70.4 mEq per liter of plasma. Carbon dioxide combining power was 27 mEq per liter of plasma.

Four days after admission an abdominal paracentesis was performed, with the removal of 12,400 ml of dark-green ascitic fluid which had the color and fluidity of crankcase oil and which contained large amounts of bile salts. After this procedure, her abdomen was flat with minimal abdominal tenderness, and her dyspnea and orthopnea disappeared. No abdominal organs were palpable. Nine days later, an additional 11,500 ml of fluid, identical to that removed before, was removed from the abdominal cavity, and on the following day exploratory laparotomy was performed. On the morning of operation the values of the serum electrolytes were essentially normal.

At operation the peritoneal surfaces were found to be thickened, rather fibrous, injected, and bile stained. The liver was normal on gross examination. Bile was found flowing freely from an opening in the proximal part of the common bile duct. An end-to-end hepaticocholedochostomy was performed, and a T-tube was used as a splint for the anastomosis. The patient's postoperative recovery was uneventful. She remained afebrile and alert throughout her hospital course and abdominal pain and tenderness was never more than minimal. The jaundice had completely cleared before she was dismissed from the hospital.

Case 2.—This 45-year-old white married woman first registered at the Mayo Clinic in September, 1955, with the chief complaints of jaundice and abdominal distention. She had a 20-year history of recurrent abdominal pain in the right upper quadrant, but no fever, jaundice, or change in the stool. In 1954 a cholecystogram had revealed a nonfunctioning gallbladder. In August, 1955, cholecystectomy had been done because of acute cholecystitis. Two days later she had noticed the onset of jaundice, dark urine, and light-colored stools. One week postoperatively, progressive abdominal distention had begun with dyspnea and abdominal pain in the right upper quadrant.

Positive physical findings on admission were jaundice, abdominal distention, shifting abdominal dullness, and moderate pedal edema. The liver extended 6 cm below the right costal margin. The spleen was not palpable.

The results of laboratory studies on blood were: hemoglobin, 10.8 gm; leukocyte count, 9,200; sedimentation rate, 115 mm in one hour; direct serum bilirubin, 2.96 mg; indirect bilirubin, 0.18 mg; and alkaline phosphatase, 91.2 King and Armstrong units. Prothrombin time was 27 seconds, but decreased to 19 seconds after the oral administration of menadiol sodium diphosphate (Vitamin K Analogue).

Abdominal paracentesis yielded 8,000 ml of greenish-yellow fluid. Five days later an exploration was performed; an additional 3,000 ml of the same fluid was removed from the abdominal cavity. The upper end of the common bile duct was found to be open, and bile was flowing freely from it. The distal end of the common duct was located 1.5 cm away, and reanastomosis of the two free ends over a T-tube as a splint was followed by an uneventful recovery. The jaundice disappeared, and intra-abdominal fluid has never reaccumulated.

Case 3.—A 42-year-old woman registered at the Mayo Clinic in June, 1960, 50 days after cholecystectomy had been performed elsewhere. At that operation, hydrops of the gallbladder and many stones had been found. It was not known whether the common bile duct had been explored, but an abdominal tube had drained black fluid until it had been removed, three days postoperatively. Jaundice first had been noted four days later, and the patient had been rehospitalized two weeks later because of jaundice, anorexia, and progressive abdominal distention. Three paracenteses had yielded a total of 12,000 ml of fluid. There had beeen no response to treatment with vitamins, low sodium diet, and various diuretics including spironolactone (Aldactone). On transfer to the Mayo Clinic, she also complained of six to ten loose stools per day since the cholecystectomy, but denied having had chills or fever.

Physical examination revealed a thin woman with no acute abdominal distress. No icterus was observed. Marked abdominal distention with a prominent fluid wave and minimal generalized abdominal tenderness were noted, but no abnormal intra-abdominal organs or masses were palpable.

The results of laboratory studies on blood were: hemoglobin, 12.3 gm; leukocyte count, 16,800; and sedimentation rate, 105 mm in 1 hour. Direct serum bilirubin was 1.2 mg and indirect bilirubin, 0.2 mg.

Five days after admission, abdominal paracentesis yielded 5,500 ml of yellow-olive ascitic fluid. Three days later an abdominal exploration was performed; an additional 4,000 to 5,000 ml of ascitic fluid was removed from the abdominal cavity. A stricture was found in the common bile duct; the proximal ends of both hepatic ducts were open, and bile was flowing from them. Repair was effected through a double hepaticoduodenostomy over two Mayo-Sullivan tubes. The patient was dismissed from the hospital on the 34th postoperative day.

An examination 2½ years later revealed symptoms and findings compatible with a mild degree of secondary biliary cirrhosis, but the patient was feeling well and working full time. Icterus or ascites had not recurred. The direct serum bilirbuin was 0.9 mg/100 ml and indirect, 0.5. The sulfobromophthalein test showed 22% retention at the end of one hour. The serum alkaline phosphatase was 66 King and Armstrong units, and total lipids were 733 mg/100 ml of plasma.

CASE 4.—A 51-year-old woman had been operated on at another institution in February, 1958, because of an episode of severe pain in the upper part of the abdomen with fever, jaundice, and dark urine. At operation a third of the gallbladder had been removed because of a single large gallstone and acute cholecystitis, and a catheter had been sewn into the gallbladder. Jaundice and progressive abdominal distention had begun within the next five days. The degree of icterus had abated somewhat when the catheter in the gallbladder first had started to drain copious amounts of bile (seventh postoperative day), but had increased again one week later. Abdominal distention, jaundice, and the passage of dark urine and six to seven light-colored, loose stools daily persisted until she was transferred to the Mayo Clinic on the 28th postoperative day.

Initial examination revealed a temperature of 101.4 F (rectal), marked abdominal distention with a prominent fluid wave, minimal abdominal tenderness, and mild scleral icterus. Hemoglobin concentration was 11.7 gm, leukocyte count was 14,900, and a thoracic roentgenogram showed effusion in the left pleural space. Paracentesis of the left lower quadrant yielded 2,400 ml of bile-stained fluid, on which both cytologic and bacteriologic studies gave negative results. Thoracentesis on the left side yielded 1,100 ml of bile-stained fluid. Culture of this fluid revealed *Staphylococcus aureus,* and appropriate antibiotic therapy was begun. A cholangiogram, made after injection of contrast medium via the catheter in the gallbladder, was considered normal with no evidence of fistula of the biliary tree.

Eleven days after admission here, her temperature increased to 102.8 F (oral), and a tender mass in the left upper quadrant of the abdomen became palpable. Four days later, 1,000 ml of odorless, creamy pus was removed from an abscess in the left subdiaphragmatic region; culture of this pus revealed *S aureus.* Two days later, no fluid was obtained on thoracentesis. Antibiotic therapy was continued to the 25th day of hospitalization, and the patient was dismissed on the 35th hospital day. She had not been examined again, but an answer to inquiry indicated that she is feeling relatively well five years later with no abdominal symptoms or recurrence of jaundice or ascites.

Comment.—Two differences in the clinical course of this patient, as compared to that of the first three patients, are apparent. First, an acute febrile complication occurred that necessitated drainage of a purulent subdiaphragmatic abscess. Second, a second operation on the biliary tract was neither performed nor deemed necessary, since the cholangiogram was normal and also since reaccumulation of intrapleural or intra-abdominal fluid could not be demonstrated during the period of observation. It is assumed, however, that this patient had generalized bile ascites because of the site at which the abdominal paracentesis was performed and the quantity of bile-tinged fluid obtained.

Two other similar cases have been observed at the Mayo Clinic.* In each of these cases, abdominal distention due to bile ascites developed a few days after the patient had been dismissed from the hospital after cholecystectomy. There was no icterus or fever in either case. Paracentesis was performed on three occasions in each patient, and each time produced large but decreasing amounts of bile-colored ascitic fluid. After the third procedure, no further ascites accumulated, and the remainder of the convalescence was uneventful. It was thought that the bile ascites developed from a slow leakage from the operative site in the common bile duct. This leakage stopped when healing was complete.

Comment

The presenting complaints in the four cases reported and the two cases mentioned briefly differed markedly from the usual clinical picture of generalized bile peritonitis in the adult. In each, the presenting complaint was abdominal distention, with dyspnea in one case and jaundice in another. In none was abdominal pain, abdominal tenderness, fever, or leukocytosis prominent. In the first three cases, surgical exploration established that the bile ascites was general-

* These cases were brought to our attention by Dr. D. O. Ferris of a section of surgery of the Mayo Clinic.

ized in the abdominal cavity. In the other three cases, the bile ascites was either generalized or localized but did not recur after repeated paracentesis. The exact location of bile leakage was not ascertained in these cases, but it was thought to have occurred at the operative site. All cases were postoperative complications of surgical procedures on the biliary tract.

McKenzie,[5] in 1955, listed the possible causes of leakage of bile after cholecystectomy as: 1) slippage of the cystic duct ligature; 2) operative damage to the bile ducts; 3) leakage from unrecognized accessory ducts; 4) dislodgment of the drainage tube in the common bile duct; and 5) seepage from the common bile duct at the suture line. In his presentation, 13 of 20 patients were classified as having had a subacute or insidious onset and course. None had a course limited only to the development of ascites without peritonitis.

No other cases similar to the six presented or mentioned herein could be found in the literature since 1955 or in the files of the Mayo Clinic for the period from Jan 1, 1952, through Dec 3, 1961. Among the Mayo Clinic cases, 18 were found in which there was generalized leakage of bile, but all of these patients were acutely ill with peritonitis and the majority of them were considered to be surgical emergencies.

In the adult, the most common cause of leakage of bile is perforation of the acutely or chronically inflamed gallbladder. The incidence of such perforation in three large series (6,217 cases) of consecutive operations on the gallbladder or biliary tree for all reasons varied from 0.9% to 2.6%.[2,6,7] The most common disease of the biliary tract leading to perforation of the gallbladder was acute cholecystitis. The reported incidence of perforation or rupture in acute cholecystitis has varied from 2.5% to 25% and is about 8% to 13% in most large series.[4,6,8,9]

Although infrequent, trauma that results in leakage from extrahepatic bile ducts is the second most common cause of generalized bile peritonitis. Only 102 cases of injury to the gallbladder were noted among a combined total of 5,305 cases of abdominal trauma in two large series.[10,11] Only 66 cases of traumatic rupture of the common bile duct have been reported in the literature.[12,13]

Spontaneous perforation of the biliary tract is uncommon in the adult.[14] Hart[15] reported that perforation rarely occurs unless there has been an operation, trauma, or obstructing calculi, and mentioned increased intraductal pressure, duct infection, cysts, diverticula, and calculi as possible contributory causes. Hills and associates[16] stated that about 90% of cases of spontaneous rupture of the common bile duct are caused by a stone impacted in that duct, but the cause is obscure in the remainder.

Torsion of the gallbladder rarely causes perforation. The first case associated with cholelithiasis and perforation was reported by Wendel[17] in 1898. In 1957, Rais and Thulin[18] collected reports of 112 such cases, only two of which were diagnosed correctly preoperatively.

Perforation of the gallbladder has been reported in a number of other circumstances, including: steroid therapy,[19,20] typhoid fever,[21] acute pancreatitis,[22] biliary opisthorchiasis,[23] and ruptured hepatic hydatid cyst.[24]

In adults, the typical clinical picture associated with free escape of bile into the peritoneal cavity is acute and progressive peritonitis, with a high mortality rate. When extravasation of bile follows inflammation and perforation of the gallbladder, there invariably is abrupt worsening in the patient's condition. In Butler and Harkin's[2] series, the mortality rate was 12% for all types of perforation, and 100% in all untreated cases of free perforation. In 433 cases from the literature collected by Cowley and Harkins,[6] the mortality rate was 20.8%, and in their own 25 cases, it was 24%. Other authors have reported mortality rates varying from 10% to 100%.[1,4]

On the other hand, in infants and children the causes and the usual clinical picture of intra-abdominal bile leakage seem to be different. Spontaneous rupture without operation, trauma, or infection is the most common cause of leakage. Ericsson and Rudhe[25] collected reports of 14 such cases and added one of their own. In only three was there an acute onset of symptoms. In the other 11, the most common presenting signs were jaundice, nausea, emesis, acholic stools, and, especially, abdominal distention due to ascites. Fever, abdominal tenderness, and rebound tenderness were minimal. Davies and Elliot-Smith[26] described two cases of bile peritonitis in infants and mentioned other reported cases in which the patients showed only a chronic, mild illness without acute peritonitis. They suggested that the slow leakage of bile is the basis for this difference. Pettersson[27] described four cases, in three of which the presenting symptom was abdominal distention due to ascites. Gertz[28] discussed 11 patients who were between 2 weeks and 22 months of age; eight of them had subacute courses. All 11 showed abdominal distention; and in five, shifting dullness could be elicited.

Oates[29] has reviewed the problem of acute cholecystitis in childhood and found it to be rare. He described an eight-week-old female infant with congenital obstruction of the common bile duct, who presented with acute cholecystitis (empyema) and perforation of the gallbladder. Downie[30] has reported a case of acute cholecystitis in a 15-month-old infant, and acute cholecystitis also has been reported in childhood as a complication of scarlet fever[31] and typhoid fever.[32] In the latter,[32] perforation of the gallbladder was found at operation in nine of the 18 patients with acute cholecystitis, and each of these nine had had the typical clinical picture of acute peritonitis.

Perhaps the slow rate of bile leakage[26] and, especially, the absence of major bacterial contamination of the bile[3] might account for the clinical condition of chronic benign bile ascites commonly seen in children and occasionally observed in adults. Therapy consists of abdominal exploration with repair of the leakage site in cases with rapid ascites formation and, in those with slow accumulation of ascites, of paracentesis performed one to four times.

Summary

Four nonfatal cases of chronic bile ascites in adults, which developed after cholecystectomy and choledochostomy, are reported and two others are mentioned briefly. The clinical picture was characterized by bile ascites with abdominal distention and sometimes jaundice, anorexia, nausea, acholic stools, or diarrhea, but without the overt evidence of acute peritonitis that usually accompanies leakage of significant amounts of bile into the peritoneal cavity. In three patients, the bile ascites was caused by unintentional severance of the bile ducts at operation and required surgical repair. The cause was undetermined in the other three but probably was due to slow leakage at the operative site in the biliary tract; only repeated paracentesis was required in treatment.

The recent literature on bile ascites and bile peritonitis was reviewed, and the different types of clinical syndromes in adults and children were analyzed.

Mayo Clinic, Rochester, Minn.

REFERENCES

1. Eliason, E. L., and McLaughlin, C. W.: Perforation of the Gall-Bladder, Ann Surg 99:914-921 (June) 1934.

2. Butler, R. M., and Harkins, H. N.: Perforation of the Gallbladder With Special Reference to Cholecystenteric Fistulas, Amer J Surg 101:717-726 (June) 1961.

3. Mentzer, S. H.: Bile Peritonitis, Arch Surg 29:227-241 (Aug) 1934.

4. Morse, L.; Krynski, B.; and Wright, A. R.: Acute Perforation of the Gallbladder, Amer J Surg 94:772-775 (Nov) 1957.

5. McKenzie, G.: Extravasation of Bile After Operations on the Biliary Tract, Aust New Zeal J Surg 24:181-191 (Feb) 1955.

6. Cowley, L. L., and Harkins, H. N.: Perforation of the Gall Bladder: A Study of 25 Consecutive Cases, Surg Gynec Obstet 77:661-668 (Dec) 1943.

7. Fletcher, A. G., Jr., and Ravdin, I. S.: Perforation of the Gallbladder, Amer J Surg 81:178-185 (Feb) 1951.

8. Diffenbaugh, W. G.; Sarver, F. E.; and Strohl, E. L.: Gangrenous Perforation of the Gallbladder: Analysis of 19 Cases, Arch Surg 59:742-749 (Sept) 1949.

9. Becker, W. F.: Perforation of the Gallbladder (Editorial) Surg Gynec Obstet 105:636 (Nov) 1957.

10. Gordon-Taylor, G.: Second Thoughts on the Abdominal Surgery of "Total" War: A Review of Over 1,300 Cases, Brit J Surg 32:247-258 (Oct) 1944.

11. Hall, E. R., Jr.; Howard, J. M.; Jordan, G. L., Jr.; and Mikesky, W. E.: Traumatic Injuries of the Gall Bladder, AMA Arch Surg 72:520-524 (Mar) 1956.

12. Fletcher, W. S.; Mahnke, D. E.; and Dunphy, J. E.: Complete Division of the Common Bile Duct Due to Blunt Trauma: Report of a Case and Review of the Literature, J Trauma 1:87-95 (Mar) 1961.

13. Stewart, R., and Silen, W.: Traumatic Rupture of the Common Bile Duct: Review of the Literature and Report of a Case of Rupture Following Cholecystectomy and Choledochotomy, Arch Surg 82:387-390 (Mar) 1961.

14. Gans, H. M., and Reydman, M.: Non-Traumatic Perforation of the Common Bile Duct, Amer J Surg 74:811-814 (Dec) 1947.

15. Hart, D. E.: Spontaneous Perforation of the Common Bile Duct, Ann Surg 133:280-282 (Feb) 1951.

16. Hills, W. J.; Gregory, E. J., Jr.; and Wright, R. M.: Spontaneous Perforation of the Common Bile Duct: Report of Two Cases With Recovery, Amer Surg 21:1211-1213 (Dec) 1955.

17. Wendel, A. V.: A Case of Floating Gall-Bladder and Kidney Complicated by Cholelithiasis With Perforation of the Gall-Bladder, Ann Surg 27:199-202, 1898.

18. Rais, O., and Thulin, C. A.: Torsion of the Gallbladder: Report of One Case and Review of the Literature, Acta Chir Scand 113:289-293 (Oct 31) 1957.

19. Kolisch, P. deR.: Rupture of Gall Bladder Associated With Steroid Therapy: Report of a Case, J Med Soc New Jersey 57:81-83 (Feb) 1960.

20. Mouzas, G. L., and Briggs, J. H.: Perforation of Gall-Bladder During Prednisone Treatment, Brit Med J 2:450-451 (Aug 24) 1957.

21. Protić, M. F., and Goldberger, A.: Gallbladder Perforation as a Complication of Typhoid Fever, Med Arh 10:81-85 (Sept-Oct) 1956.

22. Butler, D. E., and Eichhorn, R.: Acute Pancreatitis With Necrosis and Perforation of Common Bile Duct: Case Report, Amer Surg 22: 512-516 (May) 1956.

23. Kraft, I. A.: Zhelchyne peritonity pri opistorkhoze, Med Parazit (Moskva) 25:291-294 (Oct-Dec) 1956.

24. Hiddlestone, H. J. H.: Bile Peritonitis From Ruptured Hepatic Hydatid Cyst, New Zeal Med J 55:320-322 (Aug) 1956.

25. Ericsson, N. O., and Rudhe, U.: Spontaneous Perforation of the Bile Ducts in Infants: Presentation of a Case and Review of the Literature, Acta Chir Scand 118:439-445 (April 14) 1960.

26. Davies, P. A., and Elliot-Smith, A.: Bile Peritonitis in Infancy, Arch Dis Child 30:174-176 (April) 1955.

27. Pettersson, G.: Spontaneous Perforation of the Common Bile Duct in Infants, Acta Chir Scand 110:192-201 (Dec 31) 1955.

28. Gertz, T. C.: Spontaneous Perforation of the Common Bile Duct: Report of a Case, AMA Arch Surg 78:7-11 (Jan) 1959.

29. Oates, G. D.: Perforated Empyema of the Gall-Bladder in an Infant, Brit J Surg 48:686-688 (May) 1961.

30. Downie, V. J.: A Case of Acute Cholecystitis Occurring in an Infant, Brit J Surg 25:914-915 (Dec) 1938.

31. Swing, A. T., and Bullowa, J. G. M.: Acute Cholecystitis Complicating Scarlet Fever: Report of Two Cases and Review of the Literature, Amer J Dis Child 55:521-525 (Mar) 1938.

32. Reid, M. R., and Montgomery, J. C.: Acute Cholecystitis in Children as a Complication of Typhoid Fever, Bull Hopkins Hosp 31:7-11 (Jan) 1920.

An Iodophor for Preoperative Skin Preparation

ALVIN M. COTLAR, MD, AND ISIDORE COHN, JR., MD, NEW ORLEANS

The recently introduced "iodophor" compounds are reported to retain the germicidal effects of iodine but lack the undesirable properties of alcoholic iodine solutions. Miller [10] and Mannix and Dineen [9] reported effective antibacterial action without allergic reactions, irritating effects, or prolonged staining after skin preparation with an iodophor, Ioprep.* Ioprep consists of a complex compound of iodine and two nonionic surface active agents. The solution contains a 1% concentration of free or available iodine for antibacterial activity.

The present study was designed to evaluate Ioprep clinically and compare its effects with a skin preparation of ether followed by tincture of thimerosal (Merthiolate). In the course of the study, observations were made concerning the general incidence of wound infection and the effects of various factors including type of operative procedure and the influence of prophylactic antibiotics.

Clinical Study

Four hundred patients subjected to surgical procedures on the Louisiana State University Surgical Service at Charity Hospital were evaluated. The types of operations (Table 1) were predominantly "clean" surgical procedures. Two hundred patients had preoperative skin preparation with solvent ether cleansing followed by tincture of thimerosal. Another 200 patients received a three-minute scrub with Ioprep. Patients were randomly assigned to ether-thimerosal or Ioprep groups by a flip of a coin at the time of operation. There were approximately the same number of a specific type of operation in each group. The two groups consist essentially of paired cases.

No special effort was directed toward preparing the patient's skin until after induction of anesthesia. Some patients in each group bathed with an antiseptic soap on the night prior to operation. The use of skin towels, wound irrigations, prophylactic antibiotics, and other special techniques was left to the discretion of the operator. The method of random assignment distributed these patients equally between the two groups.

Patients were observed for evidence of wound infection, skin sensitivity reactions, and other complications. All wounds were followed for a minimum of six weeks postoperatively. There were 220 females and 180 males ranging in age from newborn to 88 years. Two thirds of the patients were Negroes. All except 14 of the 400 operations were elective procedures.

Results

Seventeen of the 400 patients developed postoperative wound infection (4.3%). There were nine wound infections in the ether-thimerosal group and eight in the Ioprep group. No significant difference occurred between the two groups with regard to the types of procedures in which wound infection developed. Table 1 lists the infection rates according to the type of operation for the entire series. The hernioplasty group in which there was a 2.4% incidence of infection is comprised of all types of hernias including incisional hernias. The enbloc dissections had the highest infection rate (26.6%) in the series. This high figure may be correlated with intra-oral resections (tongue, floor of the mouth, mandible) in four of the eight radical neck dissections.

Submitted for publication May 28, 1963.

Chief Resident in Surgery (Dr. Cotlar), Professor and Chairman, Department of Surgery (Dr. Cohn).

Department of Surgery, Louisiana State University School of Medicine and the Louisiana State University Surgical Service, Charity Hospital of Louisiana.

* Johnson & Johnson.

Table 1.—*Types of Operations and Incidence of Wound Infections in Each Category*

Operation	No. Performed	No. Infections	Infection Rate, %
Hernioplasty	115	3	2.4
Cholecystectomy	51	2	3.9
Thyroidectomy	40	1	2.5
Exploratory laparotomy	32	0	0.0
Extremity operations	29	0	0.0
Thoracotomy	29	0	0.0
Gastrectomy	26	1	3.8
Minor neck operations	26	0	0.0
Breast biopsy	22	3	13.6
Colectomy	15	3	20.0
Radical neck operation	8	3	37.0
Radical mastectomy	7	1	14.0
Total	400	17	4.3

The preoperative nutritional status was classified as good in 314 patients, fair in 54, and poor in 19. There was no significant difference in the incidence of wound infection in these three groups. The age of the patient did, however, influence the incidence of wound infection. Although only 25% of all patients were over 60, 53% of the wound infections occurred in this older age group.

There were no allergic reactions attributed to either type of skin preparation. Occasionally vesicles appeared at the site of hernioplasty incisions in young children when collodion was used instead of a gauze dressing to cover the wound. The "collodion blisters" occurred in both groups and were attributed to the use of the collodion rather than either of the materials used to prepare the skin.

The influence of postoperative prophylactic antibiotics is shown in Table 2. Although this study was not designed to specifically evaluate this factor, the available evidence suggests that prophylactic antibiotics did not reduce the incidence of postoperative wound infection. The highest infection rate occurred after colectomy and radical neck dissection despite the routine use of antibiotics in these cases.

Comment

The importance of preoperative skin sterilization as a factor in reducing the incidence of wound infection has not been definitely established. Black et al[3] demonstrated that although the double application of an antiseptic to the operative area significantly reduced the amount of bacterial growth, the wound infection rate was the same as when a single application was used. There was a seven-fold increase in pathogenic organisms on the skin at the end of the operation, but there was no increase in nonpathogenic organisms. These findings were consistent with contamination during the procedure, and bacteria present on the skin before operation were not considered important causes of postoperative wound infections. By contrast, Jarvis and Wigley[7] showed a significant relationship between the preoperative presence of staphylococci on the patient's skin at the operative site and the development of operating-room-acquired infections. There was also a high

Table 2.—*Influence of Prophylactic Postoperative Antibiotics on the Incidence of Wound Infection*

Operation	Prophylactic Antibiotics	No. Infected	No Antibiotics	No. Infected
Hernioplasty	9	0	106	3
Cholecystectomy	15	0	36	2
Thyroidectomy	1	0	39	1
Exploratory laparotomy	15	0	17	0
Extremity operation	5	0	24	0
Thoracotomy	20	0	9	0
Gastrectomy	11	0	15	1
Minor neck operation	3	0	23	0
Breast biopsy	1	0	21	3
Colectomy	15	3	0	0
Radical neck operation	8	3	0	0
Radical mastectomy	4	0	3	1
Total	107	6	293	11

correlation between staphylococci in the patient's nose and in the operative area. Shepherd and Kinmonth [13] demonstrated a reduction in postoperative wound infection after more thorough preparation of the skin and isolation of the wound from the surrounding skin by the use of plastic, waterproof drapes.

Studies of a large variety of materials for skin sterilization indicate the widespread interest in this problem. Even in concentrations less than 1%, iodine in alcoholic solution is more effective than other antiseptics.[5,8,14] The irritating properties of tincture of iodine have limited its use, however. The iodophor used in the present study appears to be a safe iodine antiseptic. There were no adverse local or systemic effects in 200 patients in this study. Although Ioprep was no more effective than ether-thimerosal skin preparation in controlling infection in this study, Ioprep has some advantages. Only one solution is needed when Ioprep is used. The surfactants are contained in solution with the iodine, thereby making mechanical cleansing with ether unnecessary.

Goldenberg et al [6] noted that a four-minute scrub with Ioprep was three times more effective in sterilizing the skin than a ten-minute scrub with a liquid hexachlorophene detergent. They found Ioprep to be highly effective against the skin flora and to be nonirritating. Miller et al [10] studied Ioprep in 150 patients and concluded that the skin could be sterilized by a one-minute scrub but recommended a three-minute scrub for additional safety. No skin irritation occurred among their 150 patients. Mannix and Dineen [9] reported that immediately after the application of Ioprep ("J" iodine) there was a 96% reduction in skin flora which was maintained up to four hours. Mannix and Dineen reported no allergic reactions, irritating effects, or prolonged staining of the skin. On the basis of in vitro studies, Blatt and Maloney [2] concluded that the iodophor compounds were germicidal and that their effectiveness was due to the free iodine. They found no advantage in the addition of the surfactants.

Although the present study demonstrated no difference between two types of skin preparations in preventing wound infections, useful information regarding the over-all incidence of postoperative infection on the surgical service was obtained.

The infection rates (Table 1) are based upon wound infections which required incision and drainage. Stitch abscesses are not included since they are of minimal significance, are not always recorded, and are classified by some as foreign-body reactions rather than true wound infections.[15]

The over-all major wound infection rate (4.3%) in the present study compares favorably with other reports. All of the infections in the present series responded readily to incision and drainage and specific antibiotic therapy. Shepherd and Kinmonth [13] noted a 16.7% wound infection rate in "block" dissections. This is the highest incidence in their series, but it is less than the 26.6% in the present group. Caswell et al [4] whose low incidence of postoperative wound infection is not duplicated by most authors [1,12,13,15] found an average 6.6% incidence of infection after radical neck dissection and radical mastectomy and only 2.1% after colectomy.

Moreland et al [11] reviewed 261 surgical cases on this same service in 1961 and found a 3.5% incidence of major wound infection. That series varied somewhat from the present in types of cases reported, and the differences are not thought to represent a true increase in wound infection rates.

Infections occurred more commonly in the older age groups in Moreland's series also. Of the infected wounds in that series, 65% occurred in patients over 50 years of age. Moreland noted an infection rate (including minor infections) of 28.6% in patients of poor nutritional status as compared to a rate of 8.8% for the entire series. This is in contrast to the present study in which the infection rate was not affected by nutritional status. Of Moreland's 261 patients, 21 were classified as poorly nourished, while only 19 of the 400 patients in the present series were placed in this catagory. Unfortunately the small number of cases in some operative categories makes the wound infection rate meaningless for that particular operation.

The failure to find significant benefit from prophylactic antibiotics is consistent with the work of others. Barnes et al [1] found that prophylactic antibiotics did not reduce the incidence of postoperative infection, and further resistant strains of bacteria developed in the infected wounds of those patients that received these antibiotics. Rocha [12] found no difference between control and antibiotic-treated groups in regard to infection rate or hospital stay. He noted that the *Staphylococcus* was the most common organism involved, and that this organism was usually resistant to the prophylactic antibiotic administered. The use of antibiotics was limited to 25% of the cases in the present series, and this represents a progressive improvement over the past few years. There has been a gradual realization among surgeons that the availability of new antibacterial agents does not preclude the necessity for adequate preparation of the skin of the patient and hands of the surgeon as well as aseptic technique in the operating room.

Summary and Conclusions

An iodophor, Ioprep, was used for preoperative skin sterilization in 200 patients. An additional 200 patients received an ether-thimerosal (Merthiolate) preparation.

There was no significant difference in wound infection rate between the Ioprep and ether-thimerosal groups.

There was no skin irritation or other adverse effect with either Ioprep or the ether-thimerosal preparation.

The over-all incidence of major wound infection was 4.3%. The highest incidence of infection occurred after colectomy and en bloc operations.

Nutrition did not significantly affect the rate of wound infection. Patients over 60 years of age had a higher infection rate than the younger age groups.

Prophylactic antibiotics were not of value in preventing postoperative wound infection.

The iodophor preparations have eliminated the undesirable effects of alcoholic solutions of iodine but retain their germicidal activity.

Isidore Cohn, Jr., MD, Department of Surgery, Louisiana State University School of Medicine, 1542 Tulane Ave, New Orleans 12, La.

REFERENCES

1. Barnes, J.; Pace, W. G.; Trump, D. S.; and Ellison, E. H.: Prophylactic Postoperative Antibiotics: A Controlled Study of 1,007 Cases, AMA Arch Surg 79:190, 1959.

2. Blatt, R., and Maloney, J. V.: An Evaluation of the Iodophor Compounds as Surgical Germicides, Surg Gynec Obstet 113:699, 1961.

3. Black, T.; Lynch, P. F.; and Summers, M. M.: Preoperative Skin Preparation, Lancet 1:612, 1962.

4. Caswell, H. T.; Schreck, K. M.; and Burnett, W. E.: Staphylococcal Wound Infection in Selected Surgical Procedures: An Analysis of 7,691 Operations, Surg Clin N Amer 40:1469, 1960.

5. Gardner, A. D.: Rapid Disinfection of Clean Unwashed Skin, Lancet 2:760, 1948.

6. Goldenberg, I. S.; Haley, L. D.; and Higaski, G. I.: An Evaluation of an Iodine Preoperative Scrub Detergent, Surg Gynec Obstet 114:329, 1962.

7. Jarvis, A. W., and Wigley, R. D.: Staphylococcal Surgical Wound Infections, With Particular Reference to Skin Flora, and a Comparison of Two Preoperative Skin Preparations, Med J Aust 2:542, 1961.

8. Lowbury, E. J. L.; Lilly, H. A.; and Bull, J. P.: Disinfection of the Skin of Operation Sites, Brit Med J 2:1039, 1960.

9. Mannix, H., Jr., and Dineen, P.: "Germicides" for Skin Preparation Before Surgery, Arch Surg 83:752, 1961.

10. Miller, J. M.; Jackson, D. A.; Collier, C. S.; and Johnson, H. R.: The Microbial Property of a New Iodophor Antiseptic Solution, Milit Med 126:441, 1961.

11. Moreland, J. A.; Hunter, P. R.; and Cohn, I., Jr.: A Plastic Spray for Preoperative Skin Preparation, Surgery 51:461, 1962.

12. Rocha, H.: Postoperative Wound Infection, Arch Surg 85:456, 1962.

13. Shepherd, R. C., and Kinmonth, J. B.: Skin Preparation and Towelling in Prevention of Wound Infection, Brit Med J 2:151, 1962.

14. Story, P.: Testing of Skin Disinfectants, Brit Med J 2:1128, 1952.

15. Walker, P. E.: Surgical Infection Rates: What Should They Be?, Bull Amer Coll Surg 46:7, 1961.

Antitoxic Effect of Aldosterone on Cats in Endotoxic Shock

Further Studies

HIROSHI HAYASAKA, MD
JOSEPH F. O'MALLEY, MD
AND
JOHN M. HOWARD, MD
PHILADELPHIA

Within recent years, several investigators have utilized corticosteroids in the treatment of shock due to Gram-negative organisms. Bein and Jaques [1] reported a lifesaving effect in cats when aldosterone was given intravenously in a single injection after an otherwise fatal injection of the endotoxin of *Proteus*.

Previous work [2] in this laboratory showed that 46% of 46 cats survived when given a single intravenous injection of aldosterone (0.1 mg/kg), 30 minutes after receiving intravenously an otherwise fatal dose of the endotoxin of *E scherichia coli.* The purpose of the current investigation has been to further explore this antitoxic effect and if possible to extend its sphere of potential usefulness.

Submitted for publication May 28, 1963.

From the Department of Surgery, Hahnemann Medical College.

Supported by a grant (A1-04064) from the Institute of Allergy and Infectious Diseases, National Institutes of Health.

Methods

Healthy cats of either sex weighing 1.5-4.5 kg were used. A femoral cut down exposed the artery for recording blood pressure and the vein for intravenous injections. The cats were anesthetized with diallybarbituric acid (Dial)-urethane (1.1 ml/kg) intravenously. The temperature of the cats was measured using a telethermometer with a 401 probe inserted in the rectum. The physiological observations were made for five hours, after which time the animals were kept under observation for four days. Survival rates were determined on the basis of survival for four days after receiving the endotoxin. Autopsy of selected animals was performed in each study group.

Control Studies.—A. The rectal temperature, blood pressure, and survival rates were measured in 19 cats, after the intravenous administration to each of 2.5 mg/kg of the lipopolysaccharide of *E coli.** Because the temperature of the cat fell sharply after the administration of the endotoxin, the studies were repeated except that the temperature was maintained at normothermic levels by means of an electrical blanket.

B. Since the maintenance of normothermia was found to increase the cats' tolerance to endotoxin, all other studies were carried out with normothermia being maintained until the cats regained activity.

*Difco Co.

Animals in series were then given endotoxin in varying amounts as a single intravenous injection to establish the minimal quantity which would result in a 100% fatality rate in normothermic animals.

C. In the third group, 33 cats were studied to standardize the dosage of *d*-aldosterone. All animals were kept at normal body temperature. The criterion used for the standardization of aldosterone was to select the largest dose which did not in itself cause death in any of the animals and which did not appear to cause other toxic manifestations.

Therapeutic Effectiveness of Aldosterone. In the experiments described below each cat was given 3.5 mg of endotoxin as a single intravenous injection.

A. In the first group the aldosterone was diluted in 100 ml of 5% dextrose. This was administered as an intravenous drip, starting 30 minutes after the endotoxin had been injected and continuing over a four-hour period.

B. In the second group two injections of aldosterone were given; the first, (0.09 mg/kg), 30 minutes after the endotoxin and the second, (0.04 mg/kg), 90 minutes after the endotoxin.

C. In the third group aldosterone (0.09 mg/kg) was administered as a single intravenous injection 30 minutes after the endotoxin.

Effectiveness of Aldosterone With Hydrocortisone.—Control studies: Standardization of a dosage of hydrocortisone was carried out as with aldosterone. Various single doses were injected intravenously, and survival and toxic manifestations were recorded. The highest apparently nontoxic dose was selected.

B. Effect of hydrocortisone: A single intravenous injection of hydrocortisone (50 mg/kg) was given 30 minutes after the intravenous injection of endotoxin (3.5 mg/kg).

C. Effect of aldosterone and hydrocortisone: Aldosterone (0.09 mg/kg) and hydrocortisone (50 mg/kg) were mixed and injected intravenously 30 minutes after the endotoxin which had been given intravenously in the same dose as in the preceding group.

Control Studies.—The changes in the rectal temperature and in the systolic blood pressure of an anesthetized cat after the injection of endotoxin is shown in Figure. Under anesthesia, the cat's rectal temperature was found normally to be 100-102 F. The temperature dropped during the first hour after anesthesia; at first quite rapidly and then more gradually. After administration of the endotoxin of *E coli,* the temperature of the anesthetized cat would fall faster, beginning within a few minutes after hypotension developed. The drop in temperature was as much as 10 F. With the cat on the electric blanket, a normal temperature was maintained.

Immediately after the endotoxin the blood pressure would fall rapidly, but within 15 minutes it would rise almost back to normal levels. Subsequently another fall in pressure would occur and hypotension would then persist, the pressure falling until the animal died.

Autopsy of the cats dying in endotoxic shock revealed pulmonary atelectasis with edema, congestion, and hemorrhage. The liver and spleen were congested and had small hemorrhagic areas. The renal tubules showed cloudy swelling. The adrenal glands and the gastrointestinal tract revealed minimal changes.

In the absence of control of temperature, 2½ mg of endotoxin per kilogram of body weight proved fatal to each of the 19 cats. If the cats were maintained at normothermic levels, two of nine cats survived after this dose of endotoxin (Table 1). With nor-

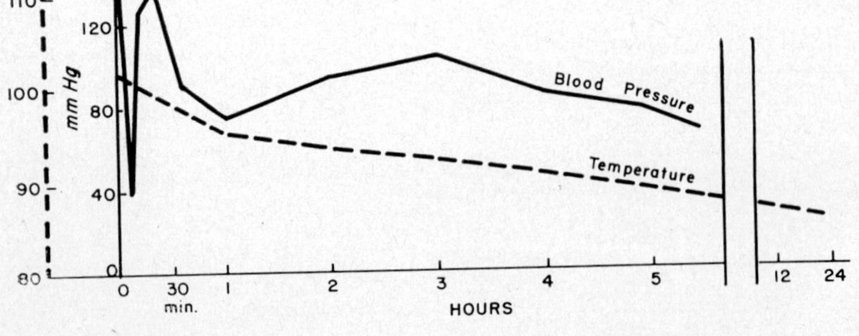

Temperature changes and blood pressure responses demonstrating the hypotensive and hypothermic course of anesthetized cats after the intravenous administration of *E coli* endotoxin (2.5 mg/kg). The above measurements in a single animal reflect the general pattern which was observed unless the temperature of the animals was maintained by an electrical blanket.

TABLE 1.—*Survival of Cats Receiving 2.5 Mg/Kg of Endotoxin of E Coli: The Effect of Temperature*

	No. Cats	No. Dying	Time of Death, Hr
No external heat applied	19	19	16-20
Normothermia maintained by electrical blanket	9	7	8-24

mothermia maintained, all animals died, however, after a dose of endotoxin of 3.5 mg/kg (Table 2).

Under normothermia each of five cats receiving only anesthesia survived.

In studying the toxicity of aldosterone, single intravenous doses ranged from 0.09-0.2 mg/kg in respective experiments. Although with both 0.09 mg/kg and 0.1 mg/kg, no adverse effects were definitely detected (Table 3); 0.09 mg/kg was selected for use in the present experiment because it appeared to be better tolerated.

Doses of hydrocortisone in excess of 50 mg/kg were associated with fatalities (Table 4), so this dosage was selected for therapeutic trial.

The Effect of Aldosterone and Hydrocortisone.—In the first group, which received 0.09 mg/kg of aldosterone as an intravenous drip, one of 19 cats (5%) survived (Table 5). In the second group, receiving two doses of aldosterone (0.09 mg/kg and 0.04 mg/kg), two of ten cats (20%) survived. In the third group, receiving 0.09 mg/kg aldosterone as a single intravenous injection 30 minutes after the endotoxin, 16 of 26 (62%) survived. When aldosterone was given 30 minutes after the endotoxin, a gradual and progressive restoration in blood

TABLE 3.—*Standardization of Dosage of Aldosterone*

Dose of Aldosterone, Mg/Kg	No. Cats	No. Dying	Time of Death, Hr
0.20	7	4	20-72
0.15	10	4	27-72
0.10	8	0	—
0.09	8	0	—

TABLE 2.—*Studies of the Toxicity of Endotoxin of E Coli: Survival of Cats Maintained Normothermic*

Dosage of Endotoxin, Mg/Kg	No. Cats	No. Dying	Time of Death, Hr
2.5	9	7	8-24
3.0	6	5	10-24
3.5	8	8	6-20
5.0	11	11	6-20
10.0	5	5	6-20

pressure to near normal levels took place during the late hypotensive phase.

A single intravenous injection of hydrocortisone (50 mg/kg), administered 30 minutes after the endotoxin, was followed by the survival of five of 12 (42%) cats (Table 6). However, 0.09 mg/kg aldosterone and 50 mg/kg hydrocortisone, mixed and injected intravenously, resulted in the survival of nine of 12 (75%) cats.

Comment

In an earlier study[2] reported from this laboratory, cats were given endotoxin in a dose of 2.5 mg/kg. In the current study the dose was increased to 3.5 mg/kg. Compared to the previous investigation (46% survival), the reasons for the increase in survival rate (62%) in the current study may be due to several factors. First, the cats were currently protected from a drop in temperature due to the anesthesia and endotoxin. Second, the dosage of 0.09 mg/kg aldosterone appeared to be better tolerated than 0.1 mg/kg, even though the difference in dosage is quite small. The cats were maintained in a lighter plane of anesthesia in the current study.

TABLE 4.—*Standardization of Dosage of Hydrocortisone*

Dose of Hydrocortisone, Mg/Kg	No. Cats	No. Dying	Time of Death, Hr
150	2	1	48
100	5	2	24-48
50	6	0	—
30	2	0	—
15	2	0	—
10	3	0	—

TABLE 5.—*Effect of Aldosterone on Cats Given Endotoxin of E Coli*

Treated Group	No. Cats	No. Dying	Survival Rate, %
Previous study (2*): endotoxin (2.5 mg/kg) followed by aldosterone (0.1 mg/kg) 30 min later	46	25	46
Endotoxin (3.5 mg/kg) followed by aldosterone (0.1 mg/kg) started 30 min after endotoxin as an IV drip over 4 hr	19	18	5
Endotoxin (3.5 mg/kg) followed by aldosterone (0.09 mg/kg) 30 min later, (0.04 mg/kg) 90 min later	10	8	20
Endotoxin (3.5 mg/kg) followed by aldosterone (0.09 mg/kg) 30 min later	26	10	62

* Reference number.

Cats given aldosterone 30 minutes before the administration of the endotoxin of *E coli* failed to receive any protection.[2] The drip type of injection of aldosterone, over a four-hour period, resulted in little if any protection. Both of these methods presumably resulted in low levels of aldosterone in the blood during the period when the endotoxin was present in a high concentration. The time relationship between endotoxin and aldosterone may be important in determining the survival rate. This could not, however, explain the failure of a supplementary injection of aldosterone. The latter result may reflect in part the toxicity of too much aldosterone.

Spink [3] recently reported that a small dose of aldosterone and of angiotension II, administered to the monkey after an otherwise fatal dose of endotoxin, resulted in survival in each of five experiments. The monkeys which received only the endotoxin died.

An increase in temperature has been reported in dogs and in patients after injection of endotoxin. By contrast the temperature of the cat drops after endotoxin. Other species differences in the responses to endotoxin have been described.[4]

TABLE 6.—*Effect of Aldosterone and Hydrocortisone on Cats Given Endotoxin of E Coli*

Treated Group	No. Cats	No. Dying	Survival Rate, %
Hydrocortisone (50 mg/kg) 30 min after endotoxin	12	7	42
Aldosterone (0.09 mg/kg) + hydrocortisone (50 mg/kg), both 30 min after endotoxin	12	3	75

Cortisone,[5] prednisolone,[6] and hydrocortisone [7] have been shown earlier to have a protective effect against endotoxin when given, respectively, to the mouse, rat, or dog. Under the specific conditions of the current study, aldosterone provided added protection. Certainly, aldosterone provides far more protection on a weight basis.

The mechanism of the action of aldosterone against endotoxin is not known, but it exhibits an unquestionable antitoxic effect against the lethal dose of the endotoxin of *E coli* which has been studied.Acting either directly or indirectly, aldosterone significantly restores the blood pressure in the late phase of endotoxic shock. Earlier, Kuida and associates [8] demonstrated that after administration of the endotoxin of *E coli* to cats, pooling of blood occurred in the vascular bed of the lungs. This is believed to be a significant cause of the hypotension in cats, resulting in a decreased venous return and a fall in cardiac output. The pooling was still present in the shocked cats in this study which failed to respond to steroid therapy. Lillehei [7] demonstrated the ability of hydrocortisone to prevent the plasma loss which followed the administration of endotoxin to dogs. Weil [9] found that the protective action of prednisolone against endotoxin in the dog did not exert its effect by prevention of acidosis, at least within the two-hour period of his observations. Spink [10] postulated that the pharmacological doses of adrenocorticosteroids utilized in these studies prevent an increase in vascular permeability after administration of the endotoxin.

After the administration of the endotoxin of *Proteus* to the cat, Bein and Jaques[1] demonstrated that levarterenol (Norepinephrine) may fail to produce a rise in arterial blood pressure. Epinephrine, after endotoxin, was found to cause a fall in blood pressure. Under these circumstances, aldosterone resulted in a restoration of the pressor response to each of the catecholamines. Neither prednisolone nor hydrocortisone, however, exhibited this property of restoring responsiveness. Aldosterone has not been considered to have any anti-inflammatory function but does have a salt-retaining function. Bein[11] quoted Desaulles that another steroid, 19-oxyprogesterone, has no anti-inflammatory nor salt-retaining activity but does protect the cat against endotoxin.

Recently in this laboratory the endotoxin of *E coli* and *d*-aldosterone, mixed and incubated at 37 C for 30 minutes prior to injection into the cat, resulted in a lower mortality rate than did the simultaneous injection of comparable unmixed preparations.[12] This result suggests that aldosterone may have a direct effect on endotoxin itself.

Conclusions

Aldosterone, in pharmacological doses, protects the cat against death from the endotoxin of *Escherichia coli.* The timing of the aldosterone injection in respect to the administration of the endotoxin appears to be important. The best results occurred when aldosterone was given rapidly 30 minutes after the endotoxin had been injected.

Hydrocortisone provides moderate protection against endotoxin if used in pharmacological doses. Greater protection was afforded in this study when both hydrocortisone and aldosterone were given simultaneously.

John M. Howard, MD, Professor of Surgery, Hahnemann Medical College & Hospital, 230 N. Broad St, Philadelphia 2, Pa.

REFERENCES

1. Bein, H. J., and Jaques, R.: The Antitoxic Effect of Aldosterone, Experientia 16:24, 1960.

2. Bondoc, C. C.; Beskid, G.; Wolferth, C. C.; Howard, J. M.; and O'Malley, J. F.: Cardiovascular and Antitoxic Effects of Aldosterone on Cats in Endotoxin Shock, Surg Gynec Obstet 114:43, 1962.

3. Spink, W. W.: Reversal of Endotoxin in Monkeys May Keep More Humans Alive: Report to the American College of Physicians JAMA 180:27, 1962.

4. Gilbert, R. P.: Mechanisms of the Hemodynamic Effects of Endotoxin, Physiol Rev 40:245, 1960.

5. Abernathy, R. S., and Spink, W. W.: Resistance to Endotoxin After Protection Against Initial Lethal Challenge With Adrenocorticoids or Chlorpromazine, Proc Soc Exp Biol Med 95:580, 1957.

6. Weil, M. H.; Bradley, G. M.; and Spink, W. W.: Unpublished observation quoted by Weil, M. H.: Adrenocortical Steroid for Therapy of Acute Hypotension, Amer Practit 12:162, 1961.

7. Lillehei, R. C., and MacLean, L. D.: The Intestinal Factor in Irreversible Endotoxin Shock, Ann Surg 148:513, 1958.

8. Kuida, H.; Hinshaw, L. B.; Gilbert, R. P.; and Visscher, M. B.: Effect of Gram-Negative Endotoxin on Pulmonary Circulation, Amer J Physiol 192:335, 1958.

9. Weil, M. H.: Adrenocortical Steroid Therapy of Acute Hypotension, Amer Practit 12:162, 1961.

10. Spink, W. W.: "Brucellosis as a Model for Metabolic Studies on Bacterial Shock and Inflammation," in Council for International Organizations of Medical Sciences: Biochemical Reponse to Injury; A Symposium, Springfield, Ill: Charles C Thomas, Publishers, 1960.

11. Bein, H. J.: "Aldosterone and Alteration in Circulatory Reactivity Following Endotoxins," Symposium on Shock, Stockholm, 1961, in Pathogenesis and Therapy; Berlin Springer-Verlag, 1962.

12. Hayasaka, H., and Howard, J. M.: Studies of the Mechanisms of Action of D-Aldosterone in Endotoxic Shock, Surgery, to be published.

Surgical Wire Welding

IRVING FELLER, MD
AND
CHARLES C. HILL, PE
ANN ARBOR

The incorporation of technological improvements from the physical into the biological sciences has led to rapid advances in medicine. One such accomplishment was the introduction of stainless steel wire as a suture material. This material affords greater strength than the organic sutures and also has the advantage of eliciting a lesser foreign-body reaction. However, there are problems accompanying the use of wire sutures, such as breaking at the knot and difficulty of tying, due to the rigidity of the metal. To resolve these problems and at the same time improve the use of wire sutures, the authors have investigated another engineering technique, wire welding.

The project to develop welded wire sutures began six years ago with bench tests to determine and confirm the parameters controlling welded sutures. The parameters investigated included wire composition, size, and tension; weld current pulse; electrode contact pressure; and effect of body fluid. The most sensitive variable is weld current pulse.

With a relatively simple power supply, developed concurrently with the bench test, the current pulse can be adjusted and controlled to give consistant weld quality over the range of wire sizes commonly encountered in surgery. When the bench test and the equipment development was completed, animal experimentation was begun.

Commonly used surgical incisions were made in a series of dogs. The wire sutures were inserted in the usual manner, and the joints were welded rather than knot tied (Fig 1). The wire closures were used in the deep fascia layers as well as on the surface. The wound healing was observed for periods up to one year, and tissue sections were submitted to the pathology laboratory for examination. At the completion of the animal experimentation, it was evident that the wire could be welded without tissue damage. Wound healing was normal, and tissue studies revealed that there were no differences in tissue reaction between the conventionally knotted wires and those that were welded. Welding sutures was faster than tying, with less discomfort to the surgeon and with less wire remaining at the joint.

Clinical applications to date include umbilical and inguinal herniorrhaphies, and fascial closure of transverse abdominal incisions. More recently the surgical wire welder has been used to repair broken electric conducting wires in cardiac pacemakers previously inserted into patients. In one case, the electrical lead broke at the costal margin within the subcutaneous tissues ten months after the system was installed (Fig 2). In a second case the wires broke where they entered the heart. Local anesthesia was used in the first

Submitted for publication June 1, 1963.

Department of Surgery, University of Michigan Medical Center, St. Joseph Mercy Hospital, Ann Arbor; Michigan Research Corporation, Troy.

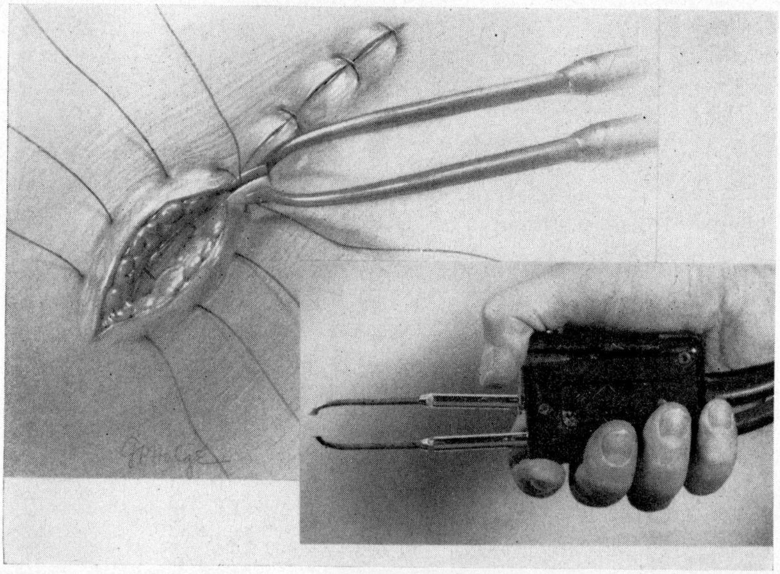

Fig 1.—The photographic inset illustrates the size of the hand piece of the surgical welding instrument. The drawing demonstrates the technique of welding stainless steel wires.

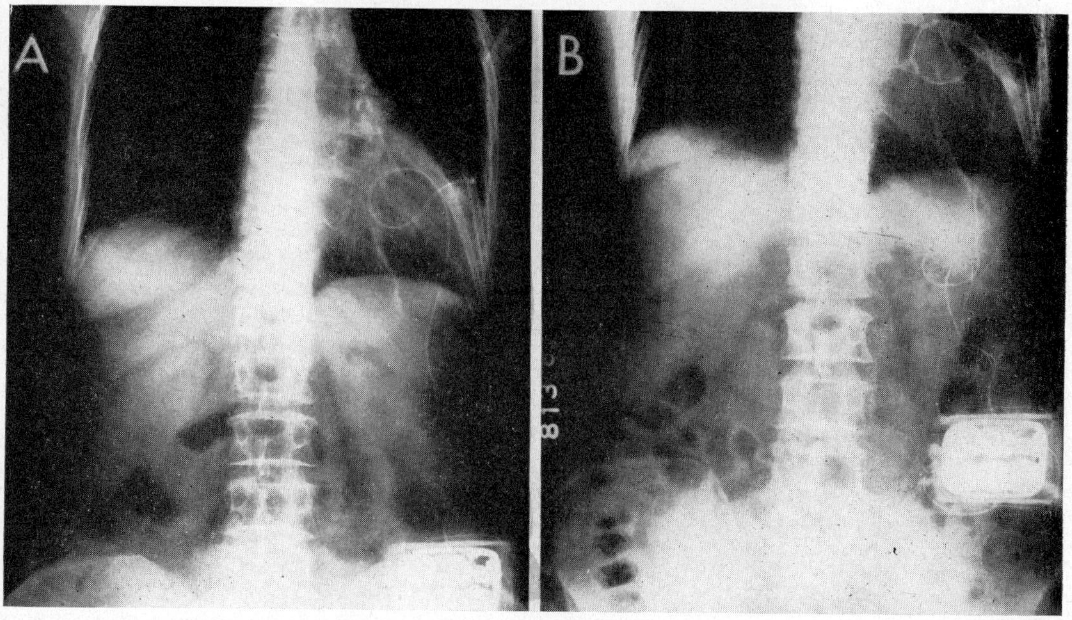

Fig 2.—The location of the cardiac pacemaker and wires can be seen in roentgenogram. *A,* the break in the wires can be seen above the pacemaker. *B,* the method of repair is illustrated. A loop of wire was inserted between the broken ends and welded into place. Parallel horizontal incisions were used to repair the wires.

repair and nonexplosive general anesthesia in the second case. In both cases the wires were welded within the body, obviating the need for the more complicated operation that would be necessary to replace the entire system.

Summary

A technique for surgical wire welding has been devised, tested in animals, and successfully applied clinically.

Irving Feller, MD, Department of Surgery, University of Michigan Medical Center, Ann Arbor, Mich.

Mandibular Fractures Treated With Plastic Polymers

IRWIN LIGHTERMAN, MD, DDS
AND
JOHN J. FARRELL, MD
MIAMI, FLA

Injuries to the maxillofacial area have been on the increase primarily as a result of increased numbers of automobile accidents. A substantial number of maxillofacial injuries also occur in industry. Of all the injuries, fractures of the facial skeleton produced the greatest morbidity.

Present methods of treating jaw fractures have satisfactorily restored cosmetic and functional deformities resulting from these injuries. However, prolonged fixation, the necessity of hairline reduction, and the multitude of complications which are associated with these fractures have prompted a review of our present treatment methods and a possible new approach to therapy.

Plastic polymers,[2] such as polyvinyl sponge,[4,11] have been successfully used to bridge osseous defects in the maxillofacial region. Even plaster of Paris had been used in bone defects with satisfactory results.[9] Ballen [1] has used methyl methacrylate in orbital defects but stated that its employment in stress situations has not been evaluated. Each of these materials, while creating a "bridge" to induce healing, is not strong enough nor sufficiently adherent to be useful as a "bone glue." Successful "bone gluing" with plastic polymers was first reported by Mandarino.[5-8,10] His treatment of human and experimental fractures has been almost exclusively limited to the long bones. Canty [3] was reported having success with polyester resin as a bone glue. However this work has not been subsequently confirmed. It was the concept of bone gluing

Presented to the meeting of the American College of Surgeons, Atlantic City, NJ, Oct 16, 1962.

Research Instructor, Department of Surgery (Dr. Lighterman); Clinical Professor of Surgery (Dr. Farrell).

From the Department of Surgery, University of Miami School of Medicine, Jackson Memorial Hospital.

This investigation was supported by Research grant D-1415 from the National Institute of Dental Research of the National Institutes of Health, United States Public Health Service. Aided by a Fellowship from the Dazian Foundation for Medical Research.

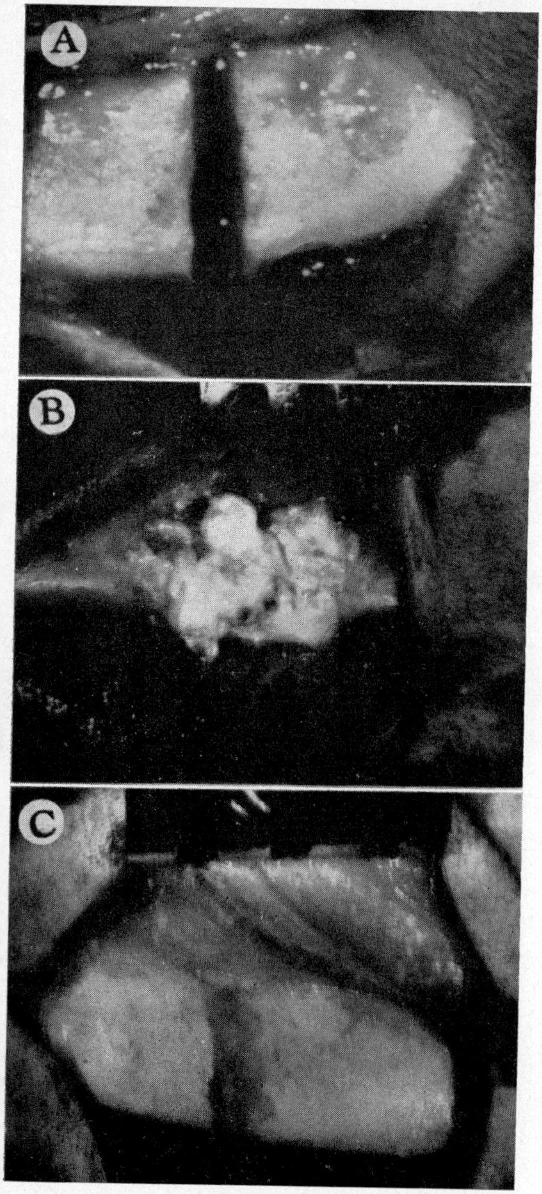

Fig 1.—*A,* a surgically induced linear fracture of the mandible is made in the bicuspid or molar area. *B,* polyurethane foam at the fracture site after polymerization. *C,* the excess polyurethane foam is removed just before the periosteum is approximated.

and immediate use of the fractured bone which prompted our studies in the treatment of mandibular fractures with plastic polymers.

Method and Materials

Dogs were selected as the ideal experimental animal because of their large mandibles.

Sixty-one adult dogs were divided into control group A and experimental group B. The mandible was surgically exposed in all cases, and a controlled fracture was made under aseptic conditions (Fig 1*A*). All fractures were induced in an interproximal space of the bicuspid or molar area.

Control Group A.—Eleven dogs served as controls. After fracture, no other surgery was performed except closure of the wound. Particular attention was given to the approximation of the previously retracted periosteum.

No attempt was made to fix the fracture. Instead, the unfixed mandible was considered a parallel study to the unwired "glued" mandible in experimental group B. Roentgenograms were taken every two weeks to determine the degree of osseous healing, and the dogs were sacrificed in pairs at two-week intervals. Gross and microscopic postmortem studies were carried out in all cases for comparison with material obtained from experimental group B.

Experimental Group B.—The 50 dogs used in experimental group B were divided into two groups of 24 and 26 dogs, respectively, to test polyurethane polymer and methyl cyanoacrylate monomer in parallel studies with each other.

Polyurethane polymer is a rigid porous foam supplied by the manufacturer in special kits. Each kit contains two sterilized viscous liquids; one a prepolymer and the other a catalyst. The liquids are accurately measured and then mixed at a temperature of 100 F. Sterile wire beaters must be machine driven and allowed to agitate the two liquids rapidly for exactly seven seconds. Failure to mix the liquids for this prescribed period of time results in poor polymer formation, while mixing too long will cause the polymer to set too rapidly. The mixture is then poured into the fracture defect. Polyurethane polymer liberates heat and carbon dioxide as it is setting, causing the plastic to foam (Fig 1*B*). It becomes hard in seven minutes, but it is recommended that the excess material not be removed for 20 minutes (Fig 1*C*). The polymer at this point will be found hard and adherent to the bone so that the fractured segments are immobile.

Methyl cyanoacrylate monomer, the second "glue" is modified with a thickening agent and a plasticizer. Polymerization occurs readily when the monomer is pressed into a thin film between two surfaces. No heat or catalysts are necessary for the reaction, and polymerization occurs with no appreciable change in volume.

After the surgically induced fracture, and after bleeding and salivary flow (if present) were controlled, the plastic polymer being tested was placed subperiosteally around the surgically created defect. The wounds were closed in layers, and the dogs permitted to chew a soft ration after recovery from anesthesia.

Roentgenograms were taken every two weeks to demonstrate replacement of plastic by osseous tissue, bone resorption, gross pathological changes, and distraction of the fractured segments. The dogs were also weighed and examined weekly to delineate changes in the nutritional status, determine the stability of the fracture, and note the presence of inflammation and/or infection.

The dogs were sacrificed in pairs 1, 2, 3, 4, 5, 10, 20, 30, 60, 90, 135, and 180 days after surgery.

Histological studies were carried out in all phases of the project to demonstrate the manner in which bone tissue replaces implanted plastic, osteoblastic and/or osteoclastic activity, inflammatory reactions, the induction of abnormal cells by the plastics, etc.

Results

Species differences in bone consistency between dog and man presented us with a significant variable when applying the results of these experiments to human values. The mandibular bone of man is relatively weak, and the incidence of dental fracture, along with jaw fracture, is relatively insignificant. The canine mandible, on the other hand, is very durable, and teeth fracture readily when the trauma is sufficient to effect fracture. The high incidence of dental fracture in our studies is thought to be the prime factor in the great number of infections which occurred.

Group A Control Dogs

Eleven dogs were periodically sacrificed in pairs and followed for a period of ten weeks. All dogs showed signs of infection at some period of their convalescence. However, only three dogs had evidence of infection or inflammation at the time of sacrifice. One of the three, which was sacrificed after ten weeks, showed evidence of osseous union (Fig 2, *A* and *B*). A second presented with bone necrosis at the fracture line as well as osseous hyperplasia 7 mm away from the fracture line due to a low grade infection. The third dog showed bone necrosis with gingival inflammation and sloughing at the fracture line. The eight dogs without inflammation had an intact periosteum even though a nonunion may have been present.

Three of the 11 dogs persistently lost weight. It is interesting that these dogs did not have signs of infection or inflammation at the time of sacrifice.

Only two dogs showed any evidence of union; there was one case of bony union and one of fibrous union (Fig 2*C*). Fracture of two root apices occurred in the first case at the time of surgery. One of the apices later sequestrated into the soft tissues, while the other formed an abscess cavity at the inferior border of the mandible. The defect was found to contain granulation tissue and greenish-yellow pus on postmortem examination (Fig 2*A*). The remaining portion of the fracture line was in good position and

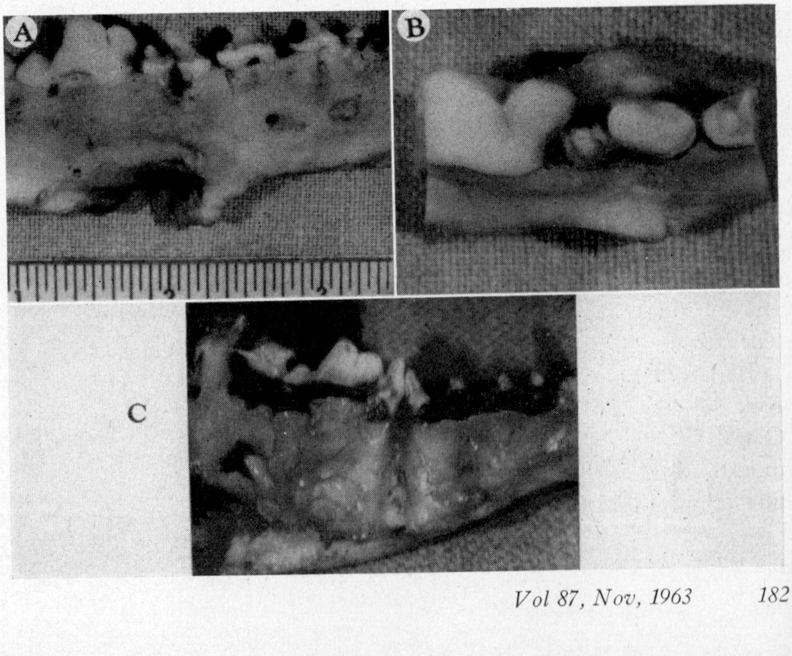

Fig 2.—*A*, osseous union in a control dog ten weeks after surgery showing excellent dental occlusion. Note the fracture of the fourth bicuspid tooth. There is an abscess cavity at the inferior border of the mandible where a root apex remained as a nidus of chronic infection. *B*, the same specimen presented in 2*A* showing an increased buccolingual diameter of the mandible due to exuberant callus formation. *C*, fibrous union in a control dog ten weeks after surgery showing excellent dental occlusion. Note the fracture of the fourth bicuspid tooth. A thin layer of bone was deposited across the fracture line at the lingual plate.

formed a firm bony union. The case of fibrous union was associated with thickening and expansion of the lingual plate. The fracture line was completely bridged by strong bands of fibrous tissue except at the lingual plate where a thin layer of bone had developed (Fig 2*C*). The occlusion was good, and there was no evidence of soft tissue inflammation.

Group B Experimental Dogs

Group I. Polyurethane Polymer Series.—The 24 polyurethane polymer animals had immediately good results in all but five cases. Of these, three were poorly stable because of improper mixing or excessive trimming of the polyurethane foam. Three dogs were fixed by the reverse inlay technique described by Mandarino.[8] However, this did not provide any special advantage and was discontinued. The long-term results of this group were generally poor.

Only seven animals had a stable mandible at the time of death or sacrifice. Of these, two died within the first 24 hours because of surgical shock; one died of an upper respiratory infection; two were sacrificed after refracture which occurred while forcibly opening the mouth under light anesthesia; and one was sacrificed after refracture when jumping off an examining table. Two dogs having a stable mandible showed evidence of inflammation, and a third, while clinically asymptomatic, demonstrated inflammatory changes on postmortem examination.

Seventeen fractures were unstable at the time of sacrifice or death. These include five of the unstable cases reported at the time of surgery. The remaining twelve cases were all clinically stable at surgery but became unstable in a period of 20 to 40 days. Instability coincided with pus formation in ten cases.

In an attempt to get increased stability, four cases were studied in which excess Ostamer * was placed in the floor of the mouth. In two, the polyurethane foam ulcerated into the mouth. In the other two cases, sacrificed at two and four days, respectively, early color changes were present which indicated ischemia and impending pressure necrosis.

Inflammation was clinically absent in eight dogs at postmortem examination. Of these, only one was followed longer than ten days, and this was the one edentulous case in our series. The remaining 16 animals demonstrated some evidence of inflammation. This included a serous, seropurulent, serosanguineous, or purulent exudate draining into the mouth through a fistula in the suture line or through a partial or complete dehiscence of the suture line.

There were three typical cases of mandibular osteomyelitis. Two of the dogs had giant gingival ulcerations and necrosis; one ulcer exposed the underlying bone from the fourth bicuspid to the second molar tooth. Miscellaneous reactions include two cases of ecchymosis and one of noma (Fig 3). The latter began as a "moist gangrene" of the cheek. After sloughing, the wound edges epithelialized in response to daily penicillin-streptomycin injections. Despite meticulous care, the dog ran a downhill course and, presumably, died from electrolyte imbalances associated with uncontrolled drooling.

Group II. *The Methyl Cyanoacrylate Monomer Series.*—The operative technique used in the methyl cyanoacrylate monomer study differed somewhat from the polyurethane polymer series. In the latter group,

Fig 3.—Noma (gangrenous stomatitis) in a polyurethane polymer dog. The wound edges have epithelized forming a mucocutaneous junction along the entire border of the cheek.

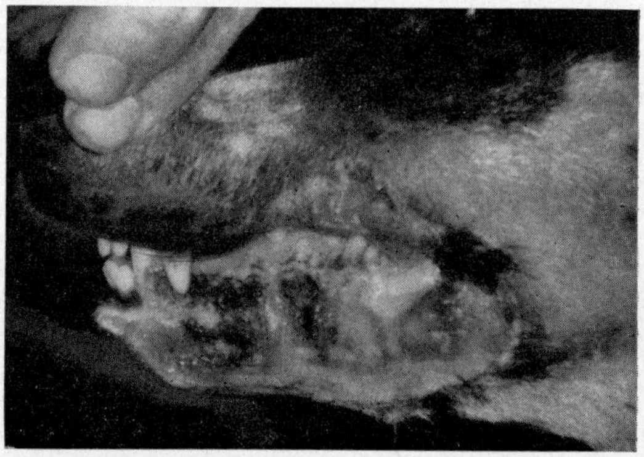

* Ostamer was supplied through the courtesy of the William S. Merrell Company, Cincinnati, Ohio.

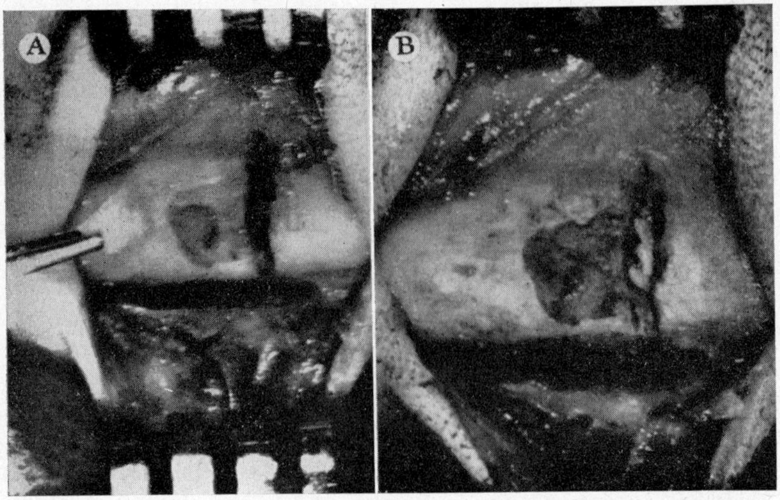

Fig 4.—*A*, autogenous cortical bone taken from the distal segment of the fractured mandible. *B*, bone graft placed in the fracture defect prior to methyl cyanoacrylate "gluing."

bone loss at the fracture site (caused by the bur) permitted replacement by a greater bulk of Ostamer.

The strength of the bond was increased by a bulk of polyurethane foam across the fracture line. On the other hand isovolumetric methyl cyanoacrylate required replacement of the lost bone with a graft; autogenous cortical bone from the proximal and/or distal segment of the fractured mandible was obtained for this purpose (Fig 4, *A* and *B*). Separate records were kept for our experiences with AD/here † and Eastman 910 adhesive.‡ Although chemically identical cyanoacrylate monomers, a review of our cases indicated definite superiority of the Eastman 910 adhesive series.

AD/here: Sixteen AD/here cases were followed for a period of 1 to 136 days. Of these, seven showed good stability, eight showed fair stability, and one showed poor stability at surgery. It appeared that the presence of moisture (blood, saliva, etc) and the use of old stock AD/here (or Eastman 910 adhesive) were the greatest factors leading to instability of the "glued" bone.

† AD/here was supplied through the courtesy of the Borden Company, Chemical Division, Philadelphia.

‡ Eastman 910 adhesive was supplied through the courtesy of Ethicon, Inc., Somerville, NJ. It is manufactured by Eastman Chemical Products, Inc., Kingsport, Tenn.

Of the five fractures which were stable at the time of death or sacrifice, only two were studied for a period of longer than five days (20 and 90 days, respectively). The 90 day dog had a fibrous union (Fig 5), while the 20 day animal appeared to have only a physical union. One of the remaining three cases had a 20 cc collection of bloody, seropurulent fluid at the operative site.

Of the 11 dogs which had unstable mandibular fractures at the time of sacrifice or death, seven were unstable in ten or less days. The remaining four maintained their stability for 20 to 67 days. Discontinuity of the fracture line coincided with the appearance of a purulent or seropurulent exudate in all cases.

With the exception of one dog, all animals initially lost weight. Of these, eight were

Fig 5.—Fibrous union in a methyl cyanoacrylate dog 90 days after surgery. Note the dental occlusion.

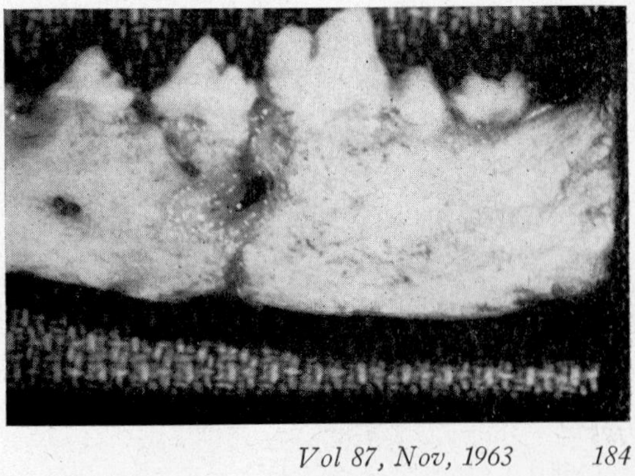

able to adjust to their new environment and were later able to maintain or gain weight. The remaining seven either continued to lose weight and finally died from inanition or were sacrificed in short-term studies before adjusting to their fracture.

All but three dogs had partial or total separation of the suture line or a gingival fistula at some time of their convalescence. These dehiscences were associated with a serous, purulent, or seropurulent discharge. The remaining three were sacrificed at three days, three days, and one day, respectively, and most likely did not survive long enough for inflammatory changes to develop.

All dogs of both the AD/here and Eastman 910 adhesive series developed mild to severe postoperative edema. This was attributed to chemical irritation by the cyanoacrylate monomer. However, the tissues appeared to tolerate the material well, after regression of the edema.

There was stripping of the periosteum and denudation of bone in three cases. One of these occurred in a case where there was extensive dehiscence of the suture line and exposure of the mandible. A second occurred where the AD/here had "tented" on the surface of the bone and was not removed before closing the soft tissues.

Other findings include two cases with sequestrum formation. Radiolucence developed at the fracture line in one of these dogs due to chronic infection. Another animal showed radiographic evidence of osteomyelitis, but sequestrum formation never occurred.

Two dogs had gingival ulceration and necrosis spanning one and three teeth away from the fracture line, respectively. A third animal developed gingival ulceration where the AD/here had "tented" subgingivally.

Eastman 910 Adhesive: Ten Eastman 910 adhesive cases were followed for a period of 1 to 180 days. The presence of blood appeared to have less of an adverse effect on the Eastman 910 Adhesive than on AD/here, but saliva affected polymerization equally in both series.

The postsurgical complications occurring with Eastman 910 adhesive were comparable to the AD/here series. Eight of ten dogs initially lost weight. Of these, five were later able to maintain or gain weight, while the remaining three ran a downhill course and died or were sacrificed before adjusting to their fracture. In general, the Eastman 910 adhesive series of animals were able to maintain their weight better than the AD/here series, and both did considerably better than the Ostamer group.

All but three dogs had partial or total separation of the suture line or a gingival fistula at some time during their convalescence. As in the AD/here series, the dehiscences were usually associated with a serous, purulent, or seropurulent exudate. One wound separation did not go on to suppuration and began to heal by secondary intention shortly thereafter. Of the three dogs which did not dehisce, one had no postsurgical complication, and another was sacrificed at surgery because of failure to effect a physical union.

The two dogs which had an intact fracture line throughout their postoperative course were followed 138 and 180 days, respectively. The former had no complications throughout its entire postsurgical course, and callus was readily observed in radiographs. The dog died of unexplained weight loss with osseous union across the fracture line, good occlusion, and no evidence of inflammation. The other dog had mandibular continuity for 180 days, although presenting with radiographic signs of osteomyelitis (Fig 6*A*), incomplete healing of the fracture at the inferior border of the mandible (Fig 6*B*), and some necrotic soft tissue on postmortem examination (Fig 6*C*). Sequestrum formation occurred three times during the six-month period. It is interesting that the only other dog with sequestra was the other 180-day dog which developed an infection and refractured early in the postsurgical period.

Only one case presented with periosteal stripping and exposure of bone. In this instance the bone appeared grossly necrotic.

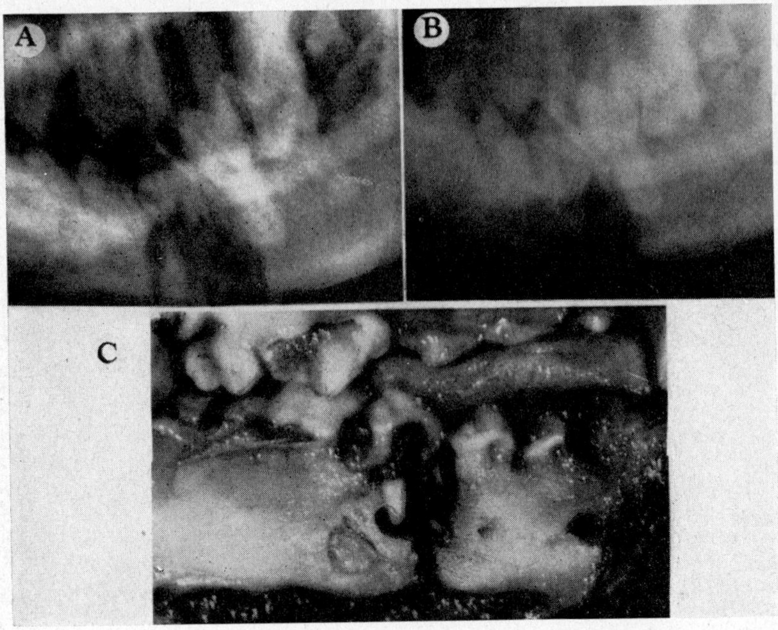

Fig 6.—*A,* acute osteomyelitis with sequestrum formation in a dog "glued" with methyl cyanoacrylate monomer. Note the fracture of the fourth bicuspid root. *B,* 36 days later a large osseous defect is present at the inferior border of the mandible. The radiograph is consistent with chronic osteomyelitis. *C,* mandibular continuity is still present at 180 days. Necrotic soft tissue and the mesial root of the fourth bicuspid tooth are contained in the fracture line.

Pathology §

Control Group A.—The control series followed the usual healing pattern reported by others in experimentally induced fractures. However, inflammatory changes were more pronounced in all phases of this study because of the absence of fixation and the oral flora which frequently contaminated the fracture site.

The early specimens primarily showed inflammatory changes. Callus and new bone formation both continued to increase during the succeeding weeks, and, by the tenth week, fibrosis and new bone were present between the fragments. A persisting chronic inflammatory exudate was also present in the last specimens.

Experimental Group B.—The most noteworthy observation in the experimental group of animals was the poor correlation between clinical inflammation and the histopathological findings, which were much less severe.

Polyurethane Polymer: The polyurethane polymer series showed hemorrhage, inflammatory changes, some fibrosis or granulation tissue, and the presence of the plastic in the first five days. Osteoplastic and osteoclastic activity were first noted on the fourth and fifth days.

Fibrosis and callus began to develop in the period between five and ten days. Irregular partially calcified trabeculae then formed, and repair of the traumatized bone continued during the succeeding weeks. A persisting inflammatory exudate and the polyurethane foam were noted in many of the specimens. Atypical bone cells were present in sections taken at 28 and 30 days.

Beginning at 46 days there was noted ulceration, infection, an inflammatory exudate, and granulation tissue formation. Fibrosis, epithelial inclusions, and cyst formation were found at 59 days. Bone healing progressed during this period, but the new bone was poorly and irregularly calcified.

Healing continued until the end of the study when the bone trabeculae appeared dense and well calcified.

Methyl Cyanoacrylate Monomer: The cyanoacrylate monomer series did not show any tissue reaction until the fourth day, when sections indicated inflammatory changes and areas of osteoclastic activity around some of the bone spicules. Bone healing continued in the later specimens but the inflammatory exudate also persisted.

§ W. A. D. Anderson, MD.

Fibrosis and new bone formation were observed at 13 days. Some large cells were present in the bone, but it could not be determined if these represented osteoblastic activity or degenerative changes. Similar findings were later found along with a more pronounced inflammatory reaction and some atypical bone fragments. The latter was believed to be a degenerative process.

Fibrosis and callus formation were consistently present in most of the histologic sections. An inflammatory exudate was frequently found between the newly forming bone trabeculae. One series of slides showed irregular staining properties and variable calcification densities in the cellular stroma at the apex of a tooth adjacent to the fracture line.

Fibrous tissue and remnants of the cyanoacrylate polymer continued to be present in the later studies. The fibrous tissue merged into areas of irregular bone trabeculae having variable amounts of calcification. Minimal to moderate inflammation persisted in most sections with both osteoblastic and osteoclastic activity present.

Comment and Conclusions

It is well known that failure to fix mandibular fractures may result in inflammation, infection, nonunion, fibrous union, or bony union with malocclusion. On the other hand, it has been demonstrated that untreated cases occasionally go on to complete healing with restoration of function. All of these changes were recorded in our control series. The high incidence of infection reported in the control dogs must be attributed to exposure of bone to the oral flora and unavoidable dental trauma during surgery.

Polyurethane polymer requires bone adhesion over a relatively wide area in order to have it fix the fracture and remain undisturbed during the period of healing. Conditions in the fractured mandible differ from those in long bones where the plastic has been successfully deposited within the medullary cavity. "Gluing" of the mandible is anatomically limited by the adjacent teeth and the absence of a marrow cavity. Attempts to broaden the area of bone contact by extending the polyurethane foam into the floor of the mouth resulted in soft tissue damage.

Stability of the bone fragments with Ostamer for a period of 20 to 40 days suggests a physical union which is interrupted when osteogenesis again becomes active. Whether loss of stability can be attributed to some enzyme system, presumably liberated by the bone cells or the persisting inflammatory exudate, cannot be determined from our histological specimens. It appears, though, that Ostamer does not fulfill the necessary requirements of a bone glue in the dentulous mandible.

Methyl cyanoacrylate monomer has properties more consistent with a successful "bone glue." It polymerizes without dimensional changes or the liberation of heat, is strong, and is well tolerated by the tissues. The methyl cyanoacrylate polymer forms a physical union between the bone fragments for 20 to 50 days, at which time refracture occurs. This relatively impervious plastic film, like polyurethane polymer, appears to be partially removed by enzymatic action, and refracture occurs because of the masticatory stresses placed upon the weakened mandible. Whether the enzymes originate from the bone cells or the inflammatory cells again is not known. Experience has shown that Eastman 910 adhesive is clinically superior to AD/here even though they are chemically identical plastics.

Eastman 910 adhesive "glued" a mandibular fracture for 138 days without incident. We believe that avoidance of dental trauma during surgery was the greatest factor in this success. (Two other dogs maintained bone continuity for 90 and 180 days, respectively, but were not free of infection or inflammatory changes during their convalescence.)

From these studies it is concluded that polyurethane polymer and methyl cyanoacrylate monomer are not adequate substitutes for presently used methods of treating dentulous mandibular fractures.

Summary

Mandibular fractures were surgically induced in 61 dogs. Fifty of these had the continuity of their jaw restored with either polyurethane polymer (Ostamer) or methyl cyanoacrylate monomer (Eastman 910 adhesive or AD/here).

The great number of infections in both the experimental and control groups was attributed to the high incidence of inadvertent tooth fracture during surgery. Enzymes produced by this infection or the cells engaged in osteogenesis later remove enough of the bone glue to disturb the physical union and cause refracture.

It is concluded that polyurethane polymer and methyl cyanoacrylate monomer are not adequate substitutes for presently used methods of treating dentulous mandibular fractures.

Irwin Lighterman, MD, DDS, Department of Surgery, University of Miami School of Medicine, Jackson Memorial Hospital, Miami, 36, Fla.

Addendum

Limited studies have been carried out in edentulous dogs to evaluate Eastman 910 adhesive in the absence of dental infection. Excellent results have been obtained when the monomer was used within two weeks of receipt from the manufacturer. Our experience indicates that there is sufficient promise from Eastman 910 adhesive as a bone glue to warrant further animal studies in the edentulous mandible. Modifications are also being sought to increase the shelf life of this plastic.

REFERENCES

1. Ballen, I.: Personal communication.
2. Blum, G.: Experimental Observations of Use of Absorbable and Nonabsorbable Plastics in Bone Surgery, Proc Roy Soc Med 38:169, 1944.
3. Canty, T.: Personal communication.
4. Grindlay, J. H., and Waugh, J. M.: Plastic Sponge Which Acts as a Framework for Living Tissue: Experimental Studies and Preliminary Report of Use to Reinforce Abdominal Aneurysms, AMA Arch Surg 63:288, 1951.
5. Mandarino, M. P., and Salvatore, J. E.: Polyurethane Polymer (Ostamer): Its Use in Fractured and Diseased Bones: Experimental Results, Surg Forum 9:762, 1958.
6. Mandarino, M. P., and Salvatore, J. E.: The Use of Polyurethane Polymer: Its Use in Fractured and Diseased Bones, Amer J Surg 97:442, 1959.
7. Mandarino, M. P.: The Use of Polyurethane Polymer (Ostamer) in Fractured and Diseased Bones, Surg Clin N Amer 40:243 (Feb) 1960.
8. Mandarino, M. P., and Salvatore, J. E.: A Polyurethane Polymer (Ostamer): Its Use in Fractured and Diseased Bones; Report of 35 Cases, AMA Arch Surg 80:623, 1960.
9. Peltier, L. F.; Bickel, E. Y.; Lillo, R.; and Maung, S. T.: The Use of Plaster of Paris to Fill Defects in Bone, Ann Surg 146:61, 1957.
10. Salvatore, J. E., and Mandarino, M. P.: Polyurethane Polymer, Its Use in Osseous Lesions: An Experimental Study, Ann Surg 149:107, 1959.
11. Struthers, A. M.; Grindlay, J. H.; and Figi, F. A.: An Experimental Study of Formation of Autogenous Bone Within Polyvinyl Sponge, Plast Reconstr Surg 15:274, 1955.

Chemical Irrigation of Wounds Inoculated With Cancer Cells

BRIAN McKIBBIN, FRCS
JOHN GAZET, FRCS
EVERETT HOPPE
AND
CONSTANCE SCHWAB, MD
CHICAGO

The recurrence of malignant tumors in surgical wounds continues to be a problem. Although there is no doubt that in some cases this is the result of incomplete primary excision, there is a great deal of evidence that in many instances the growth originated from free cancer cells contaminating the wound of an otherwise adequate operation.

The idea that these cells might be destroyed by chemical means is not at all new, and as long ago as 1896, Lack,[1] appreciating the parallel with bacterial contamination, recommended the use of Lister's carbolic solution for this purpose. Since then a variety of alternative solutions have been suggested, although in most cases the expectation of their efficacy was based on theoretical argument rather than experimental evidence.

Submitted for publication June 3, 1963.

From the Department of Surgery, University of Illinois College of Medicine.

Supported in part by a grant from the United States Public Health Service, No. 3482.

Of recent years there have been several attempts to select a suitable compound on the basis of experimentation with animal tumors.[2-4,7,10] In particular McDonald, Gines, and Cole [5] in this laboratory screened 50 or more compounds as wound irrigants using the Walker 256 carcinosarcoma in wounds in the abdominal wall of the rat. They concluded that, taking toxicity factors into account, the most suitable were mechlorethamine hydrochloride (a nitrogen mustard) in a strength of 1 mg% and sodium hypochlorite 0.5% buffered to pH 9.

From the clinical and practical standpoint both these drugs have some disadvantages. In the case of mechlorethamine the systemic effects of the drug constitute a major obstacle, since this precludes the simultaneous use of any other systemic agent which might also depress the marrow. Sodium hypochlorite is an unstable compound in solution and must be freshly prepared. It is effective only within a narrow pH range and therefore requires careful buffering. These are not insurmountable obstacles, but nevertheless they constitute a grave disadvantage in a drug which is intended for regular and frequent clinical use.

In the continuing search for the ideal drug several other agents have been investigated here. All have been tested against the already evaluated hypochlorite solution to provide a yardstick of their effectiveness. As shown below several other groups throughout the country have been working on this problem.

ACL 60, or sodium dichloro-isocyanurate, is a new compound marketed by the Monsanto Chemical Company as a bleaching and disinfecting agent. In aqueous solution it releases hyperchlorous acid and has a pH of around 6. It was hoped that by virtue of its chlorine content it would have an anticancer action equal to that of hypochlorite but would have greater stability and convenience in use. Chloramine-T is another commercial chlorine releasing drug which was found to be effective as a wound irrigant in mice by Thomas and associates.[2] Quinacrine (Atabrine) has been used in a 2% solution by Gellhorn and associates [6] in the control of neoplastic effusion, and these same authors found that when given intraperitoneally it prolonged the survival time of mice with the Ehrlich ascites tumor. Proflavine hemisulfate 0.1% was found by Nash [7] to be 90% to 96% effective in preventing tumor growth in wounds seeded with Cloudman 5-91 melanoma.

Material and Methods

The agents used in this experiment were sodium hypochlorite 0.25%, ACL 60 in a 0.5%, 0.25%, 0.1%, and 0.05% solution, chloramine-T 1%, quinacrine 1% and 2%, and proflavine hemisulfate 0.1%. Isotonic saline was used as a control. All the solutions were freshly prepared in one liter of sterile pryrogen-free distilled water. The hypochlorite solution was buffered to pH 9 by the method described by McDonald et al.[5]

Female albino rats of the Sprague-Dawley strain weighing from 150 to 220 gm were anesthetized with intraperitoneal pentobarbital sodium (Nembutal) 32 mg/kg and immobilized supine in groups of 15. After skin preparation an identical surgical wound was created in each one. Two types of defect were employed, the one a pouch in the subcutaneous tissues of the abdominal wall and the other a wound involving muscle in the pectoral region. Only one type of defect was used in any particular experiment.

Subcutaneous Pouch.—This is a modification of the wound described by McDonald et al.[5] A transverse incision 1.5 cm long was made in the skin and subcutaneous tissues of the abdominal wall 2 cm caudal to the xiphisternum. The lower flap of the wound was mobilized with a hemostat, creating a subcutaneous pouch measuring approximately 1.5 × 2.5 cm.

Muscle Wound.—Here a skin incision was made starting at the manubriosternal junction and extending downward and laterally at 45 degrees. This exposed the origin of the sternal head of the pectoralis major, and that muscle belly was divided completely in the line of the skin incision. This produced a deep wound whose walls were formed by divided muscle and whose apex was the axilla. The defect could be accurately reproduced in successive animals.

A tumor suspension was prepared from the Walker 256 carcinosarcoma according to the method described by McDonald et al.[5] The cells were suspended in Hanks solution and after the addition of eosin 1:1,000 in Tyrode's solution to a sample, the cells were counted in a blood counting chamber. The suspension was then adjusted so that there were 40,000 unstained cells in 1 ml of suspension.

After creation of the surgical wound it was inoculated (under the skin flap) with 0.25 ml of the tumor suspension containing 10,000 cells. In exactly one hour irrigation was begun with the test solution. The bottles containing the test fluid were suspended above the table at such a height that 100 ml of solution took approximately one minute to flow out through the nozzle of the standard plastic venoclysis set which was used for the irrigation. Each wound was irrigated with 100 ml of solution after which closure was effected with a continuous cotton suture. The animals were observed every other day, at first for evidence of delay in wound healing, and later for the appearance of tumor. Observations were continued for 80 days.

Results

It is evident from Table 1 that all of the drugs tested were extremely effective in preventing tumor growth. Certainly none of them appear to be inferior to the hypochlorite in this respect. It was notable that the few tumors which did appear in the treated group were located in the extreme depths of the pouch, indicating that the growth may have been caused by a mechanical rather than a chemical failure. Dilution

TABLE 1.—*Walker Tumor in Subcutaneous Pouch*

Solution Tested	Total No. of Rats	% Tumor Growth
Saline	120	92
Sodium hypochlorite 0.25 %	55	16
ACL 60, 0.5 %	73	4
ACL 60, 0.25 %	57	3
ACL 60, 0.1 %	29	7
ACL 60, 0.05 %	28	4
Chloramine-T 1 %	41	2
Quinacrine 2 %	29	3
Quinacrine 1 %	30	3
Proflavine 0.1 %	30	3

TABLE 2.—*Walker Tumor in Muscle Wound*

Solution Tested	Total No. of Rats	% Tumor Growth
Saline	30	94
ACL 60, 0.5 %	30	7

of ACL 60 ten times did not appear to weaken its action, and Table 2 shows that it is equally effective in a wound involving muscle.

All the wounds in the rats irrigated with ACL 60 healed by first intention, although in a few animals slight induration was noted in the animals irrigated with the 0.5% solution. This normal healing was not the case with quinacrine, for with both the 1% and 2% solutions there was sloughing of the entire skin over the pouch with the formation of a large ulcer. Neither the proflavine nor the chloramine-T produced significant delay in wound healing. Proflavine provided a special problem because of the coloration it caused. All the drapes became deeply stained and had to be either laundered separately or discarded. The fur of the animals remained bright yellow throughout the period of observation.

Comment

With the compounds tested herein the beneficial action appears not to be related to a systemic action of the drug. Rather is it likely that the inoculated tumor cells are killed primarily because they lack stromal support and, being unprotected, are destroyed by a drug which has general cytotoxic properties. It has been established that should tumor cells escape the action of a chemotherapeutic agent, their chance of growth may actually be enhanced as the result of the toxic effect on normal cells.[4,8-10] In other words the distinction between a destructive effect and an enhancing effect is a very thin one. For this reason caution must be utilized in the selection of a wound irrigant. Numerous compounds capable of killing cancer cells in a wound are available; the problem is to select the one with the greatest safety factor from the standpoint of the enhancing factor and the toxicity on normal cells. Failure to observe these principles may result not only in failure to control the growth of implanted cells but in actual exacerbation of the tumor growth.

The newly acquired drug ACL 60 appears to fulfill these requirements. It has been shown to be effective down to a concentration of 0.05%, while a 0.5% solution had no obvious local toxic effects. There is, therefore, a safety factor of at least 10:1. From the practical standpoint the drug has many advantages. It is remarkably stable in the dry form, so that no special storage is required.[11] It is readily soluble in water, the 0.05% solution having a pH of 6.2. After standing for 24 hours at room temperature the pH of the solution had fallen only to 6.05.

The tumor which has been used for these experiments is an animal explant. Accordingly, it is premature to assume that the same effects will be seen with human tumors and its full evaluation must await clinical trial. The drug is being introduced in our hospital for the irrigation of neck and breast wounds after cancer surgery, and although it is too early to make any statement about its anticancer properties, no untoward effects on wound healing have been seen in any of our patients up to date. A concentration of 0.25% was selected for clinical use since this lies well within the range of proven effectiveness without ever having shown signs of local toxicity.

It is necessary to emphasize that the action of the drug depends on the differential action on normal and tumor cells; although the anticancer effect has been established in the subcutaneous tissue of the rat it does not follow that the toxicity ratio will be the same for all tissues. Indeed further experiments with the drug in the peritoneal cavity[12] indicate that its local toxicity on the tissues here is greatly increased, and tumor growth may actually be enhanced under certain circumstances. We are continuing work on this observation which suggests that the action of certain anticancer compounds may differ in various tissues.

The other drugs tested in this series of experiments were effective but possessed some notable disadvantages. Quinacrine produced such severe local tissue toxicity that we consider it unacceptable for irrigation of a wound. Chloramine-T and proflavine have not been fully evaluated although both drugs are very much more expensive than ACL 60. The coloration produced by the proflavine constitutes a minor objection.

Summary

Several compounds (sodium hypochlorite, ACL 60 [sodium dichloro-isocyanurate], chloramine-T, quinacrine hydrochloride [Atabrine], and proflavine) have been tested for their efficiency as wound irrigants in preventing the development of tumors in artificially seeded wounds in the rat, using the Walker 256 tumor. All were highly successful in preventing tumor, but the local effect on the wound was too severe with quinacrine to allow its consideration for wound irrigations.

A new compound, sodium isocyanurate (ACL 60), was found to combine effectiveness against cancer cells with a remarkably low toxicity and chemical stability. Of the five chemicals tested, ACL 60 appears to be the most desirable because of its lack of tissue toxicity, chemical stability, and an anticancer effect equal to that of the others. We have observed no untoward reactions in its use to irrigate wounds of the neck and breast after radical resection for cancer, but it is too early to determine what the clinical results might be. However, we strongly advise it *not* be used for irrigation purposes in the peritoneal cavity.

Brian McKibbin, FRCS, c/o Warren H. Cole, MD, Department of Surgery, University of Illinois College of Medicine, 840 S Wood St, Chicago 12, Ill.

REFERENCES

1. Lack, H. L.: Contribution to Operative Treatment of Malignant Disease of the Larynx, With Special Reference to Danger of Cancerous Wound Infection, Lancet 1:1638-1641, 1896.

2. Thomas, C. G.; Weeds, P. M.; and Brown, B. C.: Control of Tree Tumor Cell Growth by Topical Chemotherapeutic Agents, Surgical Forum 9:598-603, 1958.

3. Hatiboglu, I.; Moore, G. E.; Wilkins, H. J.; and Hoffmeister, F.: Effects of Chemotherapeutic Agents on Wounds Contaminated With Tumor Cells, Ann Surg 152:559-567, 1960.

4. Ship, A. G.; Eck, R. V.; and Smith, R. R.: Local Chemotherapy of Experimentally Tumor-Seeded Wounds, Cancer 11:687-695, 1958.

5. McDonald, G. O.; Gines, S. M.; and Cole, W. H.: Wound Irrigation in Cancer Surgery, Arch Surg 80:920-927, 1960.

6. Gellhorn, A.; Zaidenweber, J.; Ultmann, J.; and Hirchberg, E.: The Use of Atabrine (Quinacrine) in the Control of Recurrent Neoplastic Effusions, Dis Chest 39:165-176, 1961.

7. Nash, S. C.; Ketcham, A. S.; and Smith, R. R.: Effect of Local Irrigation With Proflavine Hemisulfate on Wounds Seeded With Tumor Cells, Ann Surg 155:465-471, 1962.

8. Laszlo, J.; Burk, D.; and Wight, K.: Inhibition and Enhancement Effects of Hypochlorite in Ascites Tumor Cell Metabolism and Growth, J Nat Cancer Inst 23:351-364, 1959.

9. Kondo, T., and Moore, G. E.: The Limitations and Adverse Effects of Cancer Chemotherapy, Surg Forum 9:607-611, 1958.

10. Ketcham, A. S.: The Use of a Hyperchlorous Acid Derivative in the Control of Cancer, Cancer 13:20-24, 1960.

11. Monsanto Chemical Company: Monsanto Technical Bulletin I-177, Chicago: the Company, 1962, p 6.

12. Unpublished data.

Lymphatic Pressures in Extremities of Dogs

STUART MILLER, AB
JOHN B. LAINE, MB, FRCS
AND
JOHN M. HOWARD, MD
PHILADELPHIA

In reviewing the literature concerning the peripheral lymphatic system, one discovers a relative lack of information with regard to its basic physiology, in terms of accurate measurements of peripheral intralymphatic pressure.

In 1933, Drinker and Field[1] reported tying a glass T-tube into a lymphatic lying below the popliteal lymph node of the dog, attaching the tube to a manometer and measuring pressure in centimeters of water. The dog's foot was attached to a rotator which flexed and extended the limb at a rate of 73 times/minute. The pressures which were measured under these conditions were as follows: 41 cm of water after ten minutes and 68 cm of water after 40 minutes of exercise. They recorded no intralymphatic pressure with the animal at rest. In 1932, McMaster and Hudack[2] measured the pressure indirectly in the lymphatics of the mouse's ear as 2-4 cm of water. They rendered the vessels visible by subcutaneous injections of vital red dye and measured the pressure which, when applied to the ear, was sufficient to occlude them. In 1947, McMaster[3] recorded the pressure manometrically in the cutaneous lymphatics of the mouse's ear as ranging between 0.0 and 2.7 cm of water. These earlier investigators did not have the advantage of modern scientific apparatus, and the reliability of their subsequent measurements is, perhaps, open to doubt. Measurements were not taken frequently and thus did not show whether or not there was fluctuation of pressure.

With the availability of sensitive pressure transducers and fine polyethelene tubing for cannulation purposes, a limited study was undertaken to obtain accurate and more complete peripheral intralymphatic pressures in the extremity of the dog.

Submitted for publication June 4, 1963.

From the Department of Surgery, Hahnemann Medical College.

Supported by grants from the American Heart Association and from the National Heart Institute (HE 04182).

Technique

Fourteen mongrel dogs of either sex, weighing between 32 and 41 lb, were anesthetized with pentobarbital sodium, 50 mg/kg body weight. To render the lymphatics of the extremity visible, 5 ml of Evans blue dye was injected subcutaneously into the paw. Operative exposure of the femoral triangle was developed until the femoral sheath was seen, meticulous regard being paid to hemostasis. Careful dissection of the sheath usually revealed several dye-filled lymphatic vessels of approximately 0.5-1.0 mm in diameter, lying beneath loose fascia, either placed superficially between the femoral artery and vein, or deep to the femoral vein. Utilizing the dissecting microscope, one of these lymphatics was cleared of its surrounding fascia for approximately 2 cm. After this, the vessel was seen to distend, as though previously restrained by the fascial coat. The utmost care had to be exercised, as the lymphatic wall, although tolerant to a fair degree of handling, was relatively easily torn. The lymphatic was opened with a transverse incision. Polyethelene tubing (No. 10 or No. 20) was inserted into the lymphatic, being directed toward the paw for approximately 5-10 cm. Successful cannulation was evidenced by the flowing of blue lymph through the polyethelene tubing, with no extravasation from the lymphatic at the point of insertion. A No. 30 or No. 27 needle was used to connect the free end of the polyethelene tubing to a Statham pressure transducer which was placed at the same level as the cannulated lymphatic. The transducer was connected to an electronic recorder and balanced to atmospheric pressure with isotonic saline in the transducer. The observed pressures were regarded as end pressures. It is to be noted here that lateral pressures were also recorded in four of the dogs.

Since it was difficult to construct a single T-tube of such fine dimensions as would be necessary for these lymphatics, a modified T-assembly was arranged in the following way. After inserting a cannula against the direction of lymph flow as described above, another segment of polyethelene tubing was inserted into the same lymphatic in the direction of lymph flow, approximately 1 cm cephalad from the point of initial cannulation. The two polyethelene tubes were joined by a 2 cm segment of rubber tubing. Lymph was observed to flow through the first tubing, into the rubber connection, through the second tubing, and back into the proximal lymphatic. A No. 20 polyethelene tubing was then inserted into the side of the rubber connection to complete the T. The latter limb was connected to the pressure transducer for the recording of lateral pressures.

Serial pressure recordings at one-minute intervals were made under the following conditions:

1. Limb at rest
2. Temporary occlusion of femoral vein
3. Temporary occlusion of femoral artery
4. Temporary occlusion of both femoral artery and vein
5. Intramuscular injection of 0.4 ml epinephrine (1:1,000)
6. Uniform massage of paw
7. Intra-arterial injection of 2.0 ml tolazoline HCl (25 mg/ml)
8. Subcutaneous injection of 10.0 ml physiological saline into the paw of the extremity under study

Pressures were taken at 1 minute intervals for at least 15 minutes for each procedure, and continued until the pressure stabilized.

The substitution of an injection of 10 ml. physiological saline subcutaneously into the paw, instead of the Evans Blue Dye, showed the lymphatics to be distended at least twice their normal size, and this method was sometimes utilized as an aid in cannulation. With practice the lymphatics could be readily seen without the aid of dye. The initial drop of lymph at the orifice of the transected lymphatic acted as a magnifying medium, and allowed the stoma to be viewed quite clearly.

Findings and Significance

Limb at Rest.—With the dog at rest, no significant difference between end and lateral pressures was observed. The average pressures were very close to 5 mm Hg throughout the period of observation provided the animal remained at rest (Fig 1). In each dog, there was a fluctuation of pressure with the limb at rest of not more than 2 mm Hg per minute. The mean intralymphatic pressures of individual dogs ranged from 1.0 mm to 13.7 mm of mercury. This variation

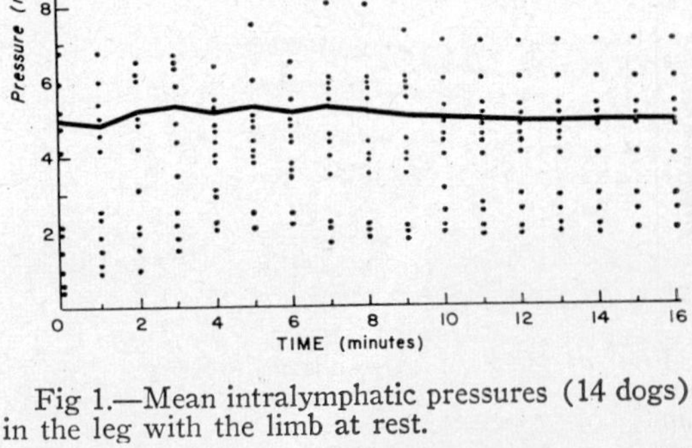

Fig 1.—Mean intralymphatic pressures (14 dogs) in the leg with the limb at rest.

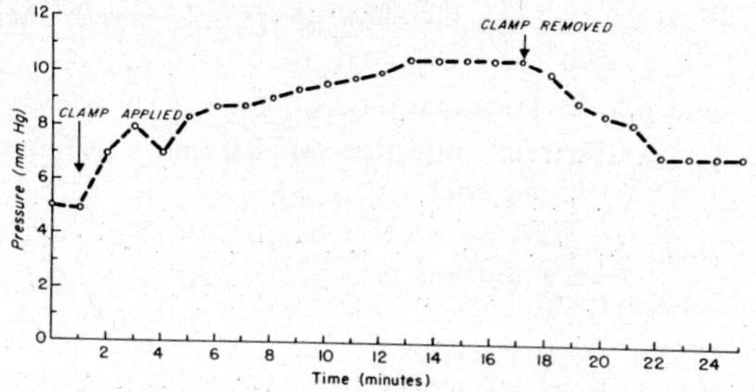

Fig 2.—Mean intralymphatic pressures (ten dogs) before and after occlusion of femoral vein. Limb at rest.

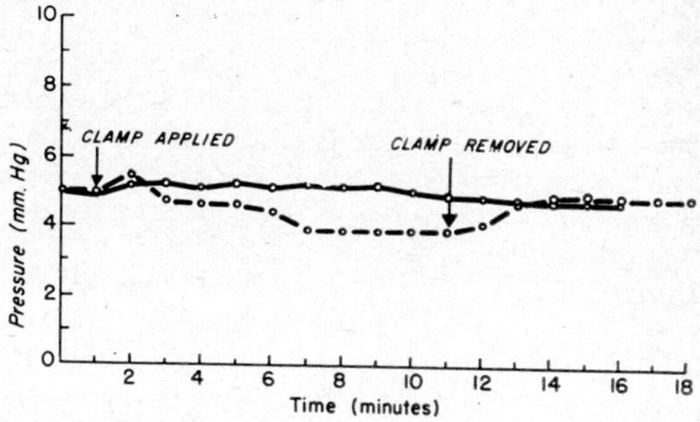

Fig 3.—Mean intralymphatic pressures (broken line) before and after occlusion of the femoral artery. The solid line from Fig 1 represents the mean pressures without manipulation.

in pressure between animals does not support the observations of Drinker and Field.[1]

Vascular Occlusion.—As might be expected from the dependency of the lymphatic system upon arteriolar—capillary—venular pressure and permeability relationships, temporary venous occlusion caused a rise (Fig 2) whereas temporary arterial occlusion produced a fall (Fig 3) in intralymphatic pressure. However, a greater influence of the venous system is shown by a comparison of Fig 2 to Fig 3. This is again illustrated in Fig 4, as complete occlusion of the main blood vessels of the limb still produced a significant rise in intralymphatic pressure. The increment may have been due in part to an increased capillary permeability secondary to ischemia and stasis. The modest ischemia, believed to have occurred as a result of temporary arterial occlusion alone, did not result in an increment in lymphatic pressure.

Vasoactive Drugs.—Injection of epinephrine, 0.4 ml (1:1,000) intramuscularly, caused a delayed but perceptible rise in intralymphatic pressure that coincided with an increase in the rate and force of the cardiac beat. Whether this increase was due to any resultant contraction of the lymphatic or to a general adrenergic effect which would increase muscular blood flow of the limb, and hence perhaps to increased lymphatic flow, is a questionable point that cannot be proved by this study. Injections of 4 ml of tolazoline hydrochloride (Priscoline), with its adrenergic blocking action, failed in each instance to produce a change in intralymphatic pressure.

Massage.—Uniform massage of the related paw resulted in an increase in pressure in every animal. Although Fig 6 shows this fairly well, it fails to indicate that in two dogs end pressures were recorded as high as 700 mm of mercury, a truly remarkable pressure for a lymphatic to withstand without rupture. One can only postulate that these high pressures were not achieved in every instance because most of the dogs possessed more extensive collateral lymphatic circulation and were thus better able to dissipate

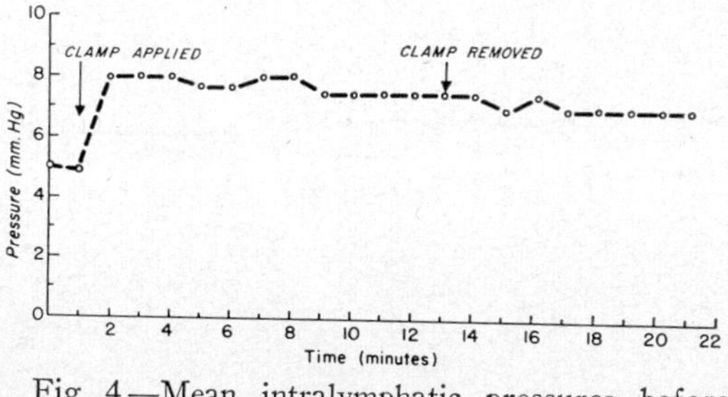

Fig 4.—Mean intralymphatic pressures before and after occlusion of both femoral artery and vein. Limb at rest (ten dogs).

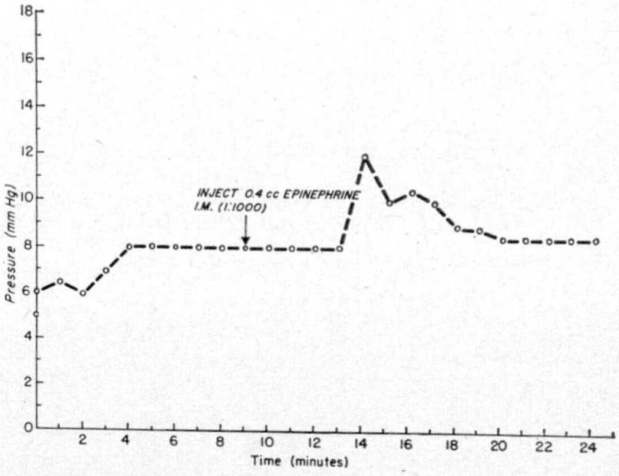

Fig 5.—Mean intralymphatic pressures after epinephrine injection (five dogs). Limb at rest.

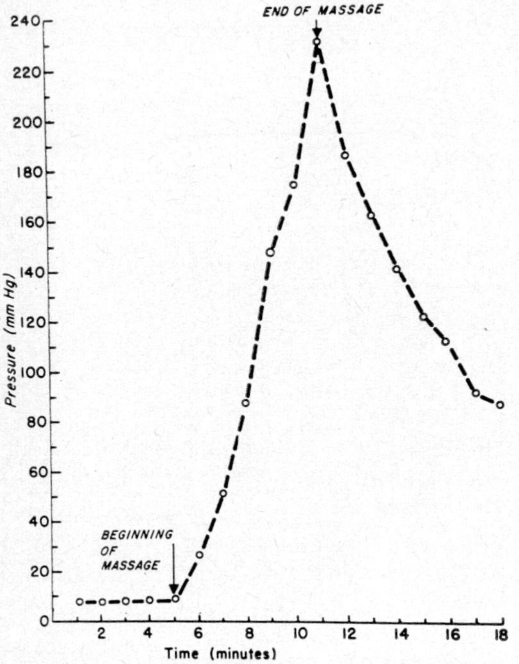

Fig 6.—Mean intralymphatic end pressures (14 dogs) with uniform massage of paw. These pressures, well above arterial pressures, reflect the forcing of fluid by massage into a system in which egress by collaterals or through possible nodal-venous anastomoses was obviously inadequate to maintain a normal pressure.

the increased flow that was caused by the massage. These high pressures are not considered physiologic, since they reflect the response to external pressures (massage) to a system which in these specific instances must have reflected a system closed at the outflow end.

Isotonic Saline.—A significant negative finding was that the injection of small volumes (10-20 ml) of isotonic saline subcutaneously into the involved paw produced no apparent alteration in intralymphatic pressure. This is especially noteworthy as the lymphatics of the limb can be observed to be dilated after injection.

Comments

A recent study by Blocker and associates [4] stresses the importance of the need for accurate studies of lymphodynamics. Although he recorded negative intralymphatic pressures in the extremity of the dog which is obviously not in agreement with our results, he has demonstrated the application of a knowledge of normal lymphodynamics to clinical medicine.

The measurements in the current study were made at internodal points, between the popliteal node and the iliac nodes. The significance of the node and any abnormality of its function to the peripheral pressure has not been studied.

Summary

Studies of the intralymphatic pressure of the extremity of the dog at rest consistently reveals it to be positive. Massage of the related paw increases the lymphatic pressure and can raise the end pressure within the lymphatic well above arterial pressure. Temporary occlusion of the ipsilateral femoral vein or the systemic administration of epinephrine resulted in a modest rise in lymphatic pressure.

John M. Howard, MD, Professor of Surgery, Hahnemann Medical College and Hospital, 230 N Broad St, Philadelphia 2, Pa.

REFERENCES

1. Drinker, C. K., and Field, M. E.: Lymphatics, Lymph, and Tissue Fluid, Baltimore: The Williams & Wilkins Company, 1933.

2. Hudack, S., and McMaster, P. D.: The Permeability of the Wall of the Lymphatic Capillary, J Exp Med 56:223, 1932.

3. McMaster, P. D.: The Relative Pressures Within Cutaneous Lymphatic Capillaries and the Tissues, J Exp Med 86:293, 1947.

4. Blocker, T. G.; Lewis, S. R.; Smith, J. R.; Dunton, E. F.; Kirby, E. J.; and Meyer, J. V.: Lymphodynamics, Plast Reconstr Surg 25:337, 1960.

Vertebral Artery Insufficiency

MARVIN WAGNER, MD

EARL KITZEROW, MD

AND

ARTHUR TAITEL

MILWAUKEE

The postoperative complications peculiar to thyroidectomy are crisis, bleeding, inadequate airway, and tetany. The one being reported is another consideration, namely, vertebral artery insufficiency.

Powers [1] records four principal complexes that characterize the clinical features of vertebral artery insufficiency. These are (1) cochlear-vestibular symptoms, including vertigo, tinnitus, and nerve deafness; (2) vascular headache, usually unilateral and pounding in character with or without an aura and frequently associated with blackout spells; (3) visual symptoms of the perceptive type including diplopia, visual claudication, and transient bilateral field defects; and, finally, (4) numbness and paresthesia of the arms. The case being presented fits into Power's second category.

Submitted for publication April 8, 1963.

Attending Staff (Dr. Wagner) and Surgical Resident (Dr. Kitzerow), Milwaukee County General Hospital; Junior Student, Marquette University School of Medicine (Mr. Taitel).

From the Department of Surgery, Marquette University School of Medicine.

Report of Case

The patient was a 54-year-old white male, admitted to the Milwaukee County General Hospital in June, 1962, because of an episode of transient headache, lightheadedness, and near syncope occurring spontaneously while sitting. Similar episodes had occurred in the past, associated principally with turning his head to the right. The patient dated these symptoms back to 1958 after which time he underwent a right subtotal thyroidectomy for a nodular nontoxic goiter.

In reviewing the patient's hospital record at the time of his thyroidectomy, it was noted that the patient had a hemorrhage postoperatively and was returned to the operating room for control of bleeding from the right inferior thyroid artery.

Physical Examination.—This showed a blood pressure 114/80 right, 104/70 left; pulse 80. The neck was free of masses or bruits. Compression of the left carotid artery produced lightheadedness. The rest of the examination was essentially unremarkable. The patient had a neurological work-up including bilateral carotid angiograms, which showed no abnormalities.

On July 16, 1962, the patient was readmitted because of persistence of symptoms. Aortic arch studies were performed employing retrograde

Fig 1.—Retrograde brachial angiography with the head in normal forward position. No apparent occlusion of the right vertebral artery.

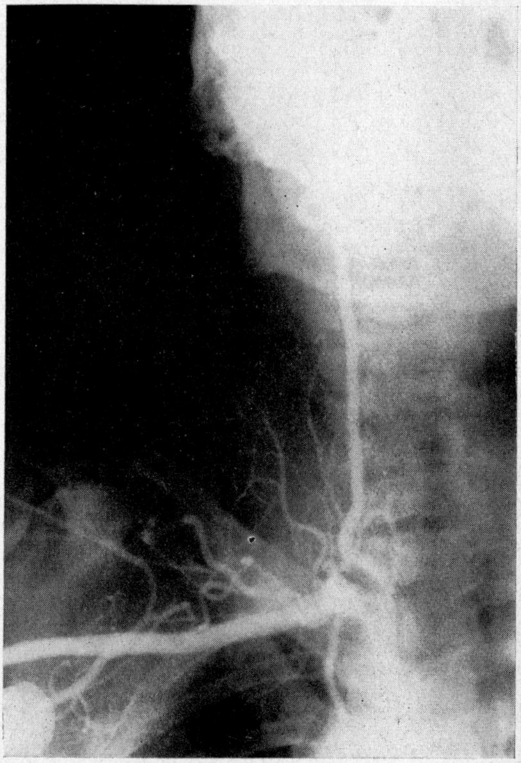

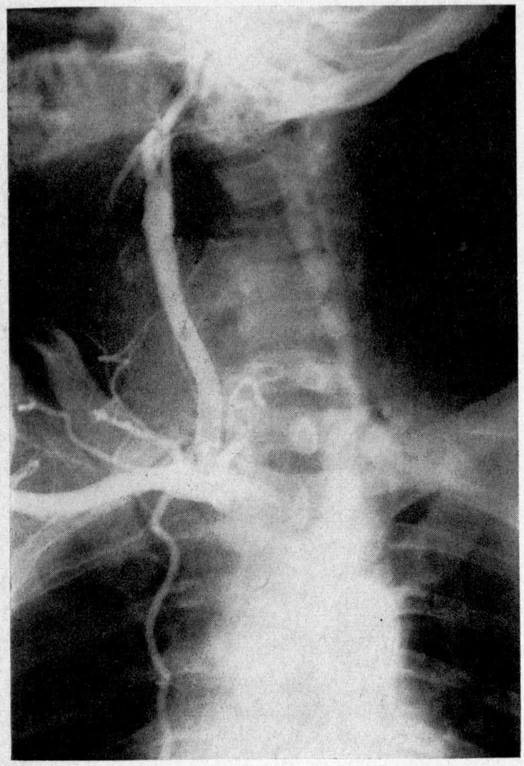

Fig 2.—Retrograde brachial angiography with the head rotated to the right shows occlusion of the right vertebral artery in its proximal segment.

brachial angiography, and an occlusion of the right vertebral artery was noted. This occlusion was visualized only when the patient turned his head to the right (Fig 1 and 2).

On Aug 6, 1962, the patient underwent a neck exploration. Cicatricial bands were noted about the right vertebral artery, which twisted and occluded the artery at the point of fixation when the head was turned to the right. These cicatrices were lysed. The postoperative course was uneventful. The patient has been followed in the outpatient department for seven months and has had no recurrence of symptoms.

Comment

In Cole's book, *Operative Technic in General Surgery,* the following is stressed in the procedure of thyroidectomy: "In this region, the blood supply to the thyroid, the lymphatic drainage, the position of the recurrent laryngeal nerves and the location of the parathyroid glands are of particular importance." However, if one scrutinizes the "anatomical abode" of the thyroid gland, the contiguous structures of the carotid sheath and its contents, the vertebral artery and its close proximity to the thyrocervical trunk are also of importance. In the case presented, bleeding was encountered postoperatively involving the inferior thyroid artery on the right side, and it required a second exploration and control. Operative findings at the time of vertebral artery exploration showed cicatrices involving the thyrocervical trunk and the proximal segment of the vertebral artery. When the head was turned to the right it twisted the vessel at its point of fixation, cutting off its flow into the head.

Evidently the complication of bleeding with secondary cicatricial formation and fixation of the proximal segment of the vertebral artery was this man's difficulty. What was an important consideration in this man's case is that he had bilateral carotid angiograms and yet his pathology was not determined. In patients who manifest cerebral symptoms, and where angiography is indicated, one is remiss in working up a patient completely if only the carotid systems are visualized, for visualization of the entire brachiocephalic axis which includes the vertebral artery and the proximal segment of the carotid must be demonstrated. The technique of retrograde brachial angiography as described by Kuhn has served as an ideal approach for complete visualization of the brachiocephalic run-off, as was illustrated in this case.

Summary

A case of vertebral artery insufficiency is presented. The causative factor was cicatrices about the vertebral artery due to hemorrhage after a thyroidectomy. Of prime concern is the importance of visualizing the entire brachiocephalic run-off in patients suspected of having cerebral symptoms due to extracranial vascular disease, and how retrograde brachial angiography is an excellent procedure in one's armamentarium for such study.

Marvin Wagner, MD, 1212 W Wisconsin Ave, Milwaukee 3, Wis.

REFERENCES

1. Powers, S. R.; Drislane, T. M.; and Iandoli, E. W.: The Surgical Treatment of Vertebral Insufficiency, Arch Surg 86:60-64, 1963.

2. Cole, W. H., editor: Operative Technic in General Surgery, ed 2, New York: Appleton-Century-Croft, Inc., 1955, pp 834-854.

Control of Bleeding in Suprapubic Prostatectomy

Use of Bilateral Ligation of the Hypogastric Arteries

L. M. KINMAN, MD
AND
E. M. JENNINGS, MD
ROSWELL, NM

The control of bleeding during and after suprapubic prostatic surgery is often difficult to accomplish. The methods currently used to control bleeding present many problems and add greatly to postoperative discomfort. Bilateral ligation of the hypogastric arteries during surgery has resulted in a marked decrease in bleeding during and following suprapubic prostatectomy. Patient discomfort has been greatly reduced.

Reich and Nechtow [1] reported nine cases of alarming gynecologic and obstetrical hemorrhage which were controlled by ligation of one or both hypogastric arteries. They noticed no ill effects from this procedure.

Technique

Extraperitoneal Approach.—A low midline incision is made from pubis to umbilicus. The rectus muscle is retracted laterally. The posterior rectus sheath is carefully incised just above its lower border, thus entering the preperitoneal space (Fig 1). The incision is carried upward the length of the wound. It is then extended inferiorly, dividing the thin ill-defined transversalis fascia below the lower border of the posterior rectus sheath. The peritoneum is then swept off the undersurface of the left rectus muscle and the lateral pelvic wall. This is started just above the lower border of the posterior rectus sheath, because this is about the level of the pelvic brim. The peritoneum is also more loosely attached to the pelvic wall at this level than below. The brim of the pelvis is exposed. The first structure encountered is the external iliac artery. As the peritoneum is further retracted medially, the ureter will be encountered, attached to the peritoneum (Fig 2). The peritoneum is then retracted slightly further medially and the hypogastric artery can be identified coursing inferiorly and medially. It is noted that as the ureter is released it will lie over and run parallel to the artery for a short distance (Fig 3). A convenient site on the artery is selected for ligation. This is usually just distal to its origin, and the dissection is

Submitted for publication April 13, 1963.

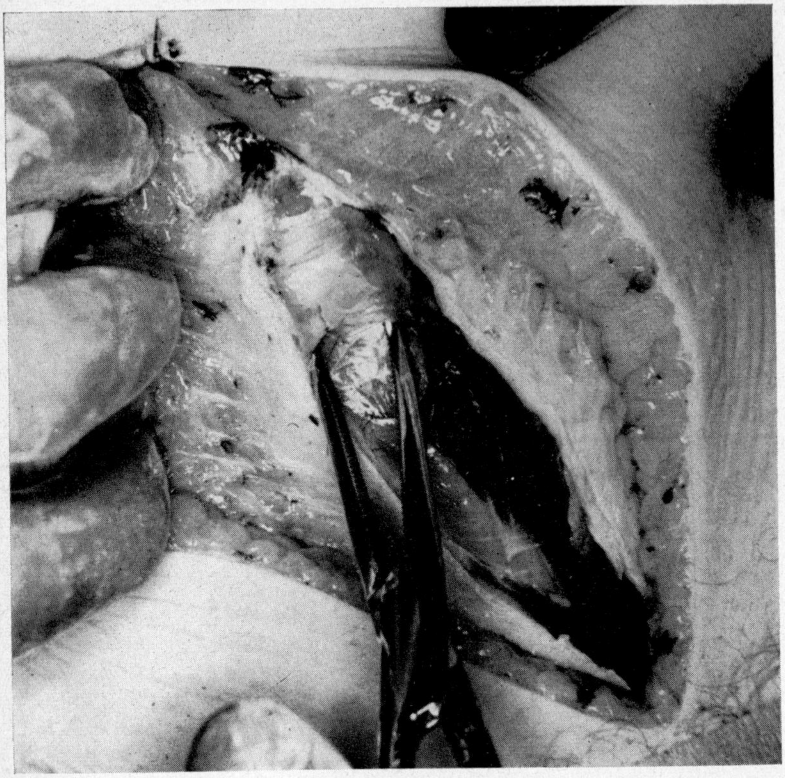

Fig 1.—The forceps are under the posterior rectus sheath.

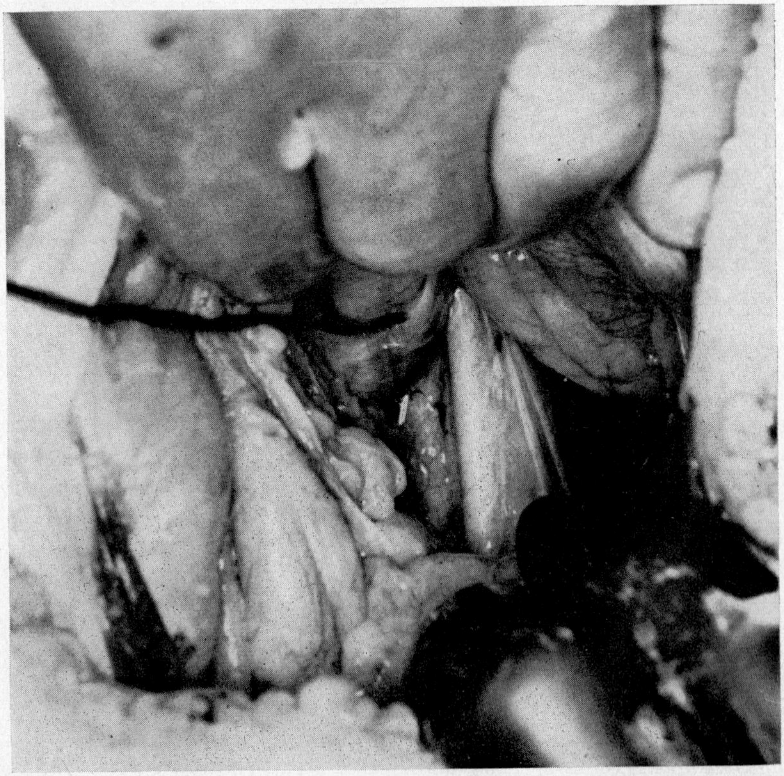

Fig 2.—The end of the probe surrounds the left ureter attached to the peritoneum at the left pelvic brim. The external iliac artery covered by areolar tissue is shown laterally.

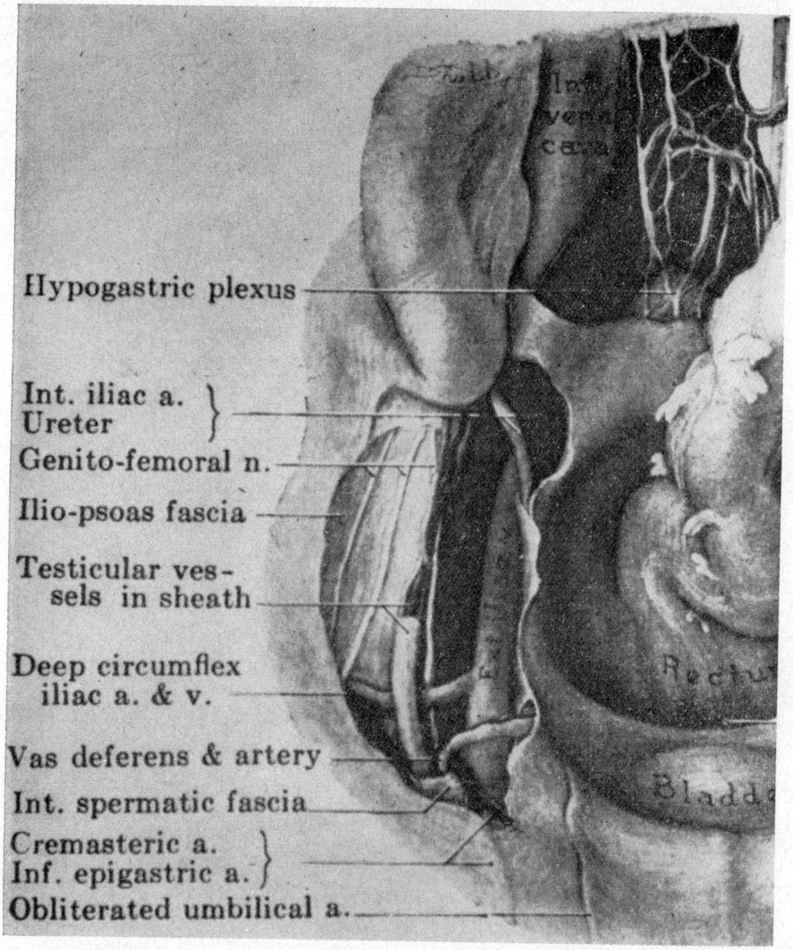

Fig 3.—The relationship of the ureter to the hypogastric artery is illustrated.

usually carried out in the crotch formed by the division of the common iliac into the external iliac and hypogastric arteries. The sheath of loose connective tissue on the anterior aspect of the artery is dissected free and the artery is dissected away from the vein with a right-angle gallbladder clamp (Fig 4). This should be done with care, as the vein lies immediately posterior to the artery. After a 1 cm segment of the artery has been dissected, it is either singly or doubly tied with No. 2 chromic suture. The artery is not cut. The peritoneum is then swept off of the right pelvic wall and the same procedure carried out on the right side. No drainage to the areas of ligation is instituted.

Transabdominal Approach.—The abdomen is opened through a low midline incision. The abdomen is explored. A self-retaining retractor is inserted and the small bowel is packed superiorly. The rectosigmoid is then retracted to the left. The posterior peritoneum is incised on the right side. The right hypogastric artery is identified, dissected free, and ligated. The artery is not cut. The sigmoid colon is then retracted to the right and its attachment to the peritoneum at the left brim of the pelvis is cut. The sigmoid is then retracted further medially and the left hypogastric artery is ligated. The incisions in the posterior peritoneum are not sutured since, when the sigmoid is allowed to fall in place, the edges of the incisions fall together. The peritoneum is then closed tight with 0-chromic suture without drainage.

After the hypogastric arteries have been ligated by either method, the bladder is opened and the hyperplastic prostatic tissue

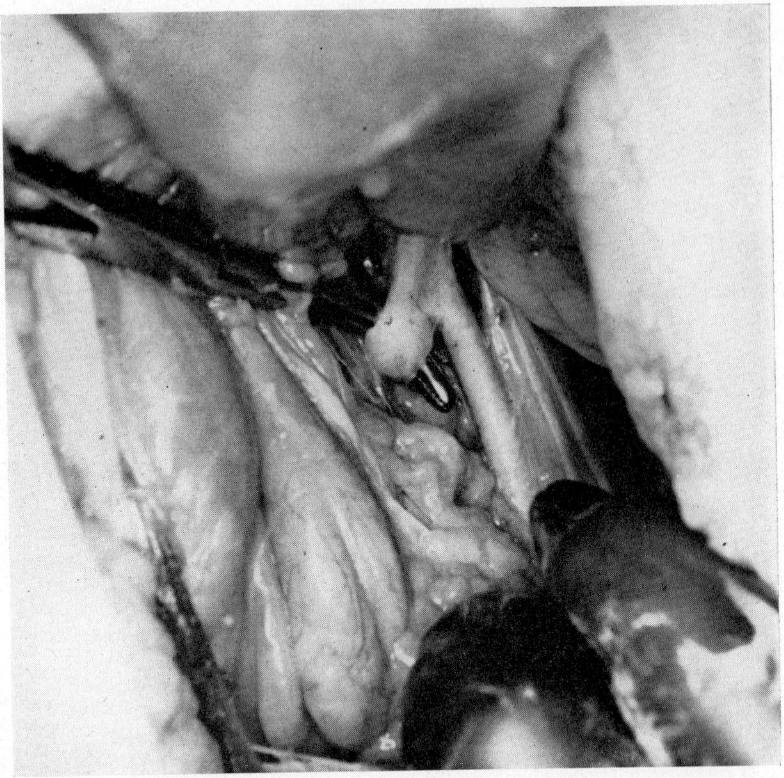

Fig 4.—Retroperitoneal area at the left brim of the pelvis. The bifurcation of the common iliac is shown. The forceps are behind the left hypogastric artery.

is enucleated bimanually. A No. 24 continuous irrigating urethral catheter is inserted, and the bag is filled with enough water to keep it out of the prostatic fossa. The catheter is placed so that the bag is against the neck of the bladder, but no traction is placed on the catheter. The bladder is closed tight with two layers of 0-chromic suture. Immediately after the first layer has been completed, continuous irrigation with isotonic saline is begun to prevent clot formation. The wound is closed in layers around a Penrose drain, which is placed in the space of Retzius and brought out through the lower end of the incision.

Comment

Twenty-five suprapubic prostatectomies with bilateral ligation of the hypogastric arteries have been performed by us. In the first three cases the hypogastrics were ligated through a transabdominal approach. One of these developed a wound disruption involving all layers which necessitated a return to surgery for secondary closure. The last 22 cases were ligated through an extraperitoneal approach. Although the transabdominal approach allows for an intra-abdominal exploration in an elderly patient, the danger of wound dihiscence and postoperative intestinal obstruction offers a serious objection. For this reason the extraperitoneal approach is preferred unless there is some good reason for abdominal exploration.

The reduction in bleeding following prostatic enucleation has been striking in every case, especially in the first half-hour. Usually in about 30 minutes after removal of the prostate the drainage is highly colored and the irrigation system is opened wider. The drainage usually lessens in color in about three hours and the irrigation is slowed. In 24 hours only a slow drip is required. It is not implied that the postoperative course is completely bloodless, for if it was, the procedure of bilateral ligation of the hypogastrics could not be done. The catheter has not been plugged up with clots a single time. Formerly blood transfusions were almost a routine procedure during or after surgery, whereas now only an occasional case requires blood during surgery and no cases have required blood after leaving the operating room. Surprisingly enough the hypogastric arteries have been large, pliable, pulsating vessels in most cases.

The most rewarding feature of this procedure to the patient has been the decrease in postoperative discomfort. With elimination of the suprapubic tube and bag tube traction, bladder spasm has been no more of a problem than that encountered in transurethral prostatic surgery. The patient is gotten out of bed on the second postoperative day. The irrigation by this time is cut down to a very slow drip. The irrigation bottle is attached to a mobile intravenous stand and the patient's catheter is attached to a plastic leg bag. The patient then pushes the intravenous stand up and down the hospital hall. The drip may be discontinued whenever it seems desirable. The catheter is removed when the wound appears healed.

There have been no ill effects from ligation of the hypogastric arteries other than the wound dehiscence in one of the early cases that was done through a transabdominal approach. The penis and buttocks have not changed color or temperature, and there have been no decubitus ulcers after a follow-up period of 14 months. No cases had to be returned to surgery because of bleeding. The length of the stay in the hospital has been less than that for the usual suprapubic prostatectomy. The shortest was seven days and the longest three weeks. This has depended largely upon the general condition of the patient before surgery.

After the patient leaves the hospital, the course has been much the same as in the usual suprapubic prostatectomy. The urine clears up in 8 to 12 weeks. No case has developed a urethral stricture. There has been no urinary incontinence. In this series only two patients were under 69 years of age. Postoperatively they are able to have satisfactory sexual intercourse. One patient who complained of preoperative severe intermittent claudication stated that he no longer has pain in his legs upon walking since surgery.

Summary

Control of operative and postoperative bleeding by bilateral ligation of the hypogastric arteries is presented and discussed. Two techniques are described. The hypogastric arteries are routinely ligated in open prostatic surgery. Ligation has also been found useful in cystectomy.

L. M. Kinman, MD, 111 N Union Ave, Roswell, NM.

REFERENCE

1. Reich, W. J., and Nechtow, M. J.: J Int Coll Surg 36:157, 1961.

Scalenotomy in Patients With and Without Cervical Ribs

Analysis of Surgical Results

HENRY A. SHENKIN, MD, AND FREDRIC M. SOMACH, MD, PHILADELPHIA

The syndrome of cervical rib causing pain in an upper extremity was described early in this century.[1] Adson and Coffey[2] in 1927 first pointed out that section of the scalene muscle alone could relieve a patient of pain due to the presence of a cervical rib. Thereafter it was reported that in some instances the scalene muscle of itself could cause compression of the brachial plexus and/or the subclavian artery in the absence of a cervical rib.[3,4] Many confirmatory reports appeared, and some suggested that the scalene syndrome could be divided into primary and secondary varieties, depending on whether altered anatomical relationships would lead the scalene muscle to compress the neurovascular structures beneath it or whether a reflex spasm of the muscle due to pathological changes in adjacent areas was the etiological factor. However, other reports[5-10] in the last 20 years question the efficacy of sectioning the scalene muscle in the absence of a cervical rib, and even the existence of such an entity as a scalene syndrome is doubted.[6]

We have reviewed our experience in this area in order to give added testimony in this controversy and, if possible, delineate further criteria in the selection of patients who will benefit from scalenotomy. Sixty-four patients in whom the scalene muscle was sectioned between 1950 and 1960 have been evaluated. This provided a follow-up period of 3 to 13 years, and information was obtained on all patients. For this purpose the patients were divided into diagnostic categories depending on whether a cervical rib was present or not and whether, in the absence of a rib, the scalene syndrome accompanied significant changes in the cervical spine.

Submitted for publication April 15, 1963.

Director (Dr. Shenkin) and Resident (Dr. Somach), Department of Neurosurgery, Episcopal Hospital.

From the Department of Neurosurgery, Episcopal Hospital.

Primary Scalene Syndrome

There were 17 patients with upper extremity pain who had no restriction of movements of the neck and normal x-rays of the cervical spine, and were tender to palpation over the appropriate scalene muscle. Four of this group had cervical myelograms, all proving to be normal. There were 15 females and only two males and their ages averaged 35, ranging from 25 to 51. The duration of symptoms averaged 1½ years, ranging from four weeks to five years. Over-all, there were nine worthwhile results and eight patients who were unimproved by the operative procedure.

This group was evaluated as to the presence of an overt emotional problem, and such was found to be the case in ten. The emotional stability of the patient was judged from the full history available on each patient by two independent evaluations of these records. In 14 of the 17 patients, a neuropsychiatric evaluation had been recorded prior to surgery. A good result was obtained in only four of this group as opposed to five good results in the remaining seven patients judged to be emotionally undisturbed.

The value of evidence of vascular compression (Adson's sign, abduction effects on radical pulse, etc) was evaluated. In the ten patients with some sign of vascular involvement, six obtained good results as opposed to three good results out of the seven patients operated upon without evidences of vascular compression. In six patients the symptoms definitely were referred to the ulnar distribution, and in this group only two patients obtained worthwhile results. Four other patients had symptoms referred to the thumb and first two fingers, and three of these four had a good result. When the factors of vascular signs, median or ulnar distribution, and sex were related to the presence or absence of an emotional problem, the only apparent correlation with results obtained was the finding that of the six females without an emotional problem five obtained a good result. All four patients with a median distribution of pain were judged to be uninvolved emotionally and three had good results.

Primary Scalene Syndromes With X-Ray Abnormalities of the Cervical Spine

All patients in this category had upper extremity pain with tenderness over the scalene muscle but without limitation or discomfort of movements of the head upon the neck. They all had changes in the x-ray of the cervical spine consisting of evidences of arthritis and/or loss of cervical lordosis. All had cervical myelograms that were normal and had had symptoms, on the average, over two years before being operated upon.

There were 11 patients in this group and again the results were evenly divided, being worthwhile in five and without benefit in six. The ages averaged 43 years, ranging from 24 to 62. There were eight females in this group with only three worthwhile operative results, but two of the three males did well postoperatively. There was an emotional disturbance judged to be present in five of this group, and of these only one obtained relief through surgery. Four out of six patients judged to be stable personalities did well after scalenotomy. None of this group had evidence of vascular compression. In only one of this group did symptoms clearly radiate to the ulnar side of the hand, and no result was obtained in this individual. Four patients had a median distribution of pain, two had a good result, and two failed to improve after surgery.

Secondary Scalene Syndrome With Positive Myelograms

There were 14 patients with upper extremity pain, all of whom had distinct abnormalities on x-ray of the cervical spine (arthritis with spurring, narrowed interspaces, foraminal encroachment) and all had myelograms that were positive (multiple filling defects; ridging). The relationship of the myelographic defects to the patient's symptoms was often not specific. The patients all were markedly tender over the appropriate scalene muscle. They had not responded satisfactorily to conservative treatment, and scalenotomy was offered for the following reasons. (1) The diagnosis of cervical spine changes as the cause of upper extremity pain was not clear. Scalenotomy was done because of distinct tenderness over the scalene muscle often with palpable muscle spasm, and it seemed, at the time, to be the lesser of the two available surgical procedures (11 cases). A poor cardiac status in two patients of this group gave an additional reason to avoid laminectomy. (2) Laminectomy had already been done, but pain persisted and there were tenderness and palpable spasm in the scalene area (three cases).

There were, over-all, 11 good results and three patients without postoperative improvement. Of the three patients who had previous cervical spine surgery, two obtained good results following scalenotomy in relieving residual upper extremity pain. Scalenotomy was done one to two years after the original cervical laminectomy. The reason for persisting symptoms in the third patient after laminectomy and scalenotomy is not entirely clear, but the patient did have an emotionally disturbed background. Of the 11 patients in whom scalenotomy was done as a lesser of two operative procedures, nine had excellent results and two were unimproved and subsequently underwent cervical hemilaminectomy and foraminotomy and were relieved of their pain.

These 14 patients had had symptoms on the average of two years before coming to surgery, with a range of one month to 15 years. There were 11 males and three females, and the average age was 45 ranging from 31 to 62 years. Only three of the 14 were judged to have an overt emotional problem, and eventually two of these three did well. Two patients had pain radiating to the ulnar side, and one belonged to the small group with poor results in this category. There were four patients with pain or paresthesias radiating to the thumb and/or the first two fingers, and all of these were relieved of pain by scalenotomy.

Cervical Rib Series

There were 22 patients in this category and all obtained good results. Bilateral scalenotomy alone was done in three patients. Unilateral scalenotomy was carried out in 11 patients, and scalenotomy with partial removal of a cervical rib was done in seven. One patient had a bilateral scalenotomy and partial removal of one rib. Criterion for removal of a rib was the slightest suggestion at the operating table that pressure was still being exerted on the brachial plexus by the cervical rib after the scalene muscle had been sectioned. The syndromes were equally divided as to sidedness, but for some reason the ribs removed were predominantly left (7:1).

The ages averaged 37 years with a range of 14 to 68; there were 18 females and four males. A distinct emotional disturbance was present in four, but, nevertheless, they all obtained a good result. Three patients had a distinct ulnar distribution of their symptoms, and four had radiation of pain or paresthesias to the medial distribution. Seventeen of the 22 patients had had evidences of vascular compression by the various maneuvers, and in three instances actual thrombosis of the subclavian artery had occurred.

Comment

The diagnosis of a scalene syndrome in the absence of a cervical rib was arrived at in any individual patient who complained of upper extremity pain and had distinct tenderness over the scalene muscle and in whom the possibilities of a cervical disc syndrome, shoulder bursitis or tendonitis, a sympathetic shoulder-arm dystrophy, or neoplasm of the lung has been eliminated. This diagnosis obviously was inadequate, for the results of scalenotomy in our 28 primary scalene syndrome patients were only 50% worthwhile. The majority of our patients had preliminary injection of the scalene muscle for diagnostic purposes, and this certainly added nothing to the definitiveness of the syndrome. There were as many patients obtaining a good result from surgery with no relief of pain following preliminary injection of the scalene muscle as those who failed to improve after scalenotomy and had had immediate improvement in their complaints following injection. The inadequacy of injection of the scalene muscle as a diagnostic criterion has been pointed out by others.[6] Analysis of results in relation to presence of evidence of vascular compression failed to yield a criterion for improving these results. It has been stated the scalene syndrome primarily caused pain radiating to the ulnar side of the hand and fingers, but again analysis of our results correlated to this type of pain failed to yield an improved criterion for surgery. Only two of the seven patients with this distribution of pain obtained relief from scalenotomy. Indeed, patients with distinct median distribution of pain, if anything, got better results from surgery (five of eight).

An effort to correlate results with overt evidences of emotional disturbance in the primary scalene syndrome group was more fruitful. Only five of 15 patients with obvious emotional disturbances in the primary scalene categories obtained relief of symptoms from scalenotomy, whereas nine of 13 similar patients but without apparent emotional disturbance did well postoperatively. A more careful psychiatric evaluation of these patients indeed might yield better results and should be part of the evaluation for each patient in whom this type of surgery is contemplated. The vast preponderance of females in the primary scalene category (23:5) has been previously noted and felt to be due to the greater tendency of the shoulder to sag in this sex. It is to be noted that the females predominated also in the cervical rib group (18:4), and all in this group had excellent results.

The primary scalene syndrome category was subdivided in two groups depending on whether or not abnormalities were noted in the cervical spine x-rays. This was done in the hope a distinction would be found in the two groups in regard to results obtained from surgery. Such was not the case. There was a difference of significance in the average age of the two groups; as might be anticipated the primary scalene group with cervical arthritic change was older (43 versus 35 years).

While a 50% effectiveness of operation in this primary scalene group may be construed as evidence that the results are only those which would occur by chance, our retrospective opinion is different. Many patients had pain that appeared obvious, were disabled, and had failed to respond to a variety of treatments extending over years only to have immediate and dramatic relief of pain from scalenotomy and termination of their disability. If operative intervention is confined to individuals whose pain appears obvious over a prolonged period of time and who have been carefully evaluated from a psychiatric point of view, then we believe the percentages of poor results will be reduced. It must be assumed that the treatment of a syndrome whose diagnosis rests on so little objective criteria will always comprehend a large percentage of failures. This should not be used as evidence that the syndrome does not exist at all. It is worth pointing out that no morbidity was encountered in this entire series of cases.

The number of satisfactory results in the secondary scalene syndrome group was particularly surprising. These patients were operated upon, for the most part, early in the series. It should be pointed out that the choice between attacking the primary lesion in the cervical spine and the possible secondary scalene syndrome was offered the patient most often a decade ago when operation on the cervical spine seemed more formidable to us than it is felt to be at present. Nonetheless, that a secondary scalene syndrome may be the cause of persisting complaints following cervical laminectomy for a radicular syndrome is emphasized by the fact that two of three patients who had previous laminectomies and foraminotomies were relieved of residual pain by scalenotomy done one and two years, respectively, after cervical laminectomy, and they have remained free of pain 3 and 11 years after scalenotomy.

The results reported by our cervical rib group of patients are truly gratifying. Others, too, have reported excellent relief of pain in these cases following surgery, but not as consistently. We can confirm Adson's observation that in many instances scalenotomy alone is effective in relief of symptoms. Indeed, in only eight of the 22 patients with cervical rib was the rib removed in addition to scalenotomy. Our technique of scalenotomy comprehends dissecting out and full visualization of the subclavian artery after the muscle is cut to be certain all compression of it has been relieved. While the brachial plexus is not always isolated, it is carefully inspected and palpated to be certain it, too, is decompressed. It is of interest that five of this group did not manifest evidences of vascular compression prior to surgery and, therefore, the etiology of the upper extremity pain must have been primary brachial plexus compression. Undoubtedly the neurosurgeon would be most apt to see patients with pain syndromes due to scalene or cervical rib compression in the absence of evidence of vascular compression.

It would seem the efficacy of scalene section alone in relieving a cervical rib syndrome so consistently points up the possible role of this muscle in causing compression on neurovascular structures in this area, in the absence of a cervical rib, despite the opinion of some to the contrary.[6,10]

To sum up, scalenotomy with occasional partial removal of the cervical rib has been entirely satisfactory in relieving patients with a cervical rib who have upper extremity pain. We have previously emphasized [11] that even minimal symptoms with evidences of vascular compression in the presence of a cervical rib are sufficient indication for surgical decompression of the subclavian artery. We have reported subclavian thrombosis occurring in such circumstances without prior severe pain or disability.

Summary

Sixty-four patients subjected to scalenotomy from 1950 to 1960 have been reviewed. They were divided into categories consisting of 28 patients with a primary scalene syndrome, 14 patients with what was judged to be a secondary scalene syndrome, and 22 patients with a cervical rib syndrome.

Of the primary scalene syndrome patients, 50% obtained a lasting good result. Separating out the factors of evidences of vascular compression, ulnar or median distribution of pain, and the presence or absence of x-ray abnormalities of the cervical spine failed to yield improved criteria for surgery. An evaluation of the emotional background of each patient in this category did reveal that the number of poor results could be reduced by avoiding operation on patients suspected of a primary scalene syndrome and harboring an overt emotional disturbance.

Eleven patients of 14 operated upon with demonstratable cervical spine disease and presenting evidence of a scalene syndrome did well. Three of this category of patients were operated upon after cervical laminectomy, and two did well. Two patients of this total of three with poor results in this group were subsequently relieved of their symptoms by cervical laminectomy and foraminotomy.

Pain in all patients with evidence of a cervical rib was overcome by surgery. In the majority of patients scalenotomy alone was sufficient to give lasting relief from pain. Only in one third of the patients was a part of the offending cervical rib removed.

Henry A Shenkin, MD, Department of Neurosurgery, Episcopal Hospital, Front St and Lehigh Ave, Philadelphia 25, Pa.

REFERENCES

1. Murphy, J. B.: Case of Cervical Rib With Symptoms Resembling Subclavian Aneurism, Ann Surg 41:399-406, 1905.

2. Adson, A. W., and Coffey, J. R.: Cervical Rib: A Method of Anterior Approach for Relief of Symptoms by Division of the Scalenus Anticus, Ann Surg 85:839-857, 1927.

3. Ochsner, A.; Gage, M.; and DeBakey, M.: Scalenus Anticus (Naffziger) Syndrome, Amer J Surg 28:669-695, 1935.

4. Naffziger, H. C., and Grant, W. T.: Neuritis of the Brachial Plexus Mechanical in Origin: The Scalenus Syndrome, Surg Gynec Obstet 67:722-730, 1938.

5. Kirgis, H. D., and Reed, A. F.: Significant Anatomic Relations in the Syndrome of the Scalene Muscles, Ann Surg 127:1182-1201, 1948.

6. Telford, E. D., and Mottershead, S.: Pressure at the Cervico-Brachial Junction: An Operative and Anatomical Study, J Bone Joint Surg (Brit) 30:249-265, 1948.

7. Stammers, F. A. R.: Pain in Upper Limb From Mechanisms in Costoclavicular Space, Lancet 1:603-607, 1950.

8. Raaf, J.: Surgery for Cervical Rib and Scalenus Anticus Syndrome, JAMA 157:219-223, 1955.

9. Clagett, O. T.: Research and Prosearch, J Thorac Cardiov Surg 44:153-166, 1962.

10. Bucy, P. C., and Oberhill, H. R.: Pain in the Shoulder and Arm From Neurological Involvement, JAMA 169:798-803, 1959.

11. Shenkin, H. A.: Cervical Rib and Thrombosis of the Subclavian Artery, JAMA 165:335-338, 1957.

Chemodectoma

A Review With Two New Cases

JAMES P. CAREY, MD
AND
ROBERT L. BRADLEY, MD
HUNTINGTON, W VA

Since Von Haller[1] described the carotid body in 1743, nonchromaffin paragangliomas have been discussed frequently in the surgical literature. The term chemodectoma derives from the Greek words χημεία, an infusion, and δέχεσθαι, to receive, and -ωμα, tumor, and was so named by Mulligan[2] in 1950. Synonyms for this interesting tumor which arises in the chemoreceptor system in various locations of the body are: receptoma, nonchromaffin paraganglioma, and carotid body-like tumor. These tumors may be found anywhere the scattered structures of neural, epithelial, and vascular components known as the chemoreceptor system are located but most frequently are encountered in the neck arising from the carotid body, over 400 tumors in this region having been reported. Over 100 have been reported to arise in the glomerula jugulare located in the adventitia of the jugular bulb. They have been encountered along the auricular branch of the vagus nerve, the tympanic branch of the glossopharyngeal nerve, and within the glomus intravagale of the vagus nerve. At least five chemodectomas of the aortic body have been reported arising within the mediastinum.

These lesions have also been described as arising in the ciliary body near the ciliary ganglion within the orbit, and at least five have been reported from the femoral region.[3] Recently Korn and associates[4] have described multiple lung lesions histologically resembling chemodectomas.

The exact origin of the chemoreceptor system is not known nor are its complete anatomy and function delineated. These bodies differ from true paraganglia such as the adrenal medulla in that they do not secrete endocrine substance and do not give the true chromaffin reaction. Only the carotid and aortic bodies have yet been shown to have physiologic function. When stimulated by lowered oxygen tension, increased carbon dioxide tension, lowering of the pH, or increase in the body temperature, they act to increase the rate and depth of respiration and

Submitted for publication May 13, 1963.

also the activity of the sympathetic nervous system.

Muratori, in Italy, found chemoreceptors in the ganglion nodosum of birds in 1932. White, in 1935, found chemoreceptor cells in the perineurium of the vagus nerve of man just below the ganglion nodosum. This has been termed "the vagal body" by Birrell and may actually be in multiple small foci in the vagus nerve at the level of the ganglion nodosum in the upper neck. The term "vagal body tumor" was given to chemodectomas in this area by Birrell [5] in 1953. Perez, Harrison, and ReMine [6] reviewed the literature and added two cases to make a total of 20 reported cases of chemodectoma of the vagal body in December of 1960. Johnson, Beahrs, and Harrison [7] have recently added four new cases to make a total of 24 reported cases of vagal body origin arising high in the neck. Chamberlin,[8] in 1956, reported a chemodectoma located 5 cm below the carotid bifurcation arising in association with the vagus nerve. Jernstrom and Fry [9] reported a second incidence of a nonchromaffin paraganglioma of the cervical portion of the vagus nerve; and the present case reported represents the third known reported chemodectoma of the vagus nerve located in this more inferior cervical portion. Watzka, in Berlin, reported finding parasympathetic paraganglions along the course of the vagus nerve at a distance from the ganglion nodosa in 1943. With this in mind chemodectoma may be found low in the cervical region as reported here.

These lesions are frequently multicentric and generally behave in an essentially benign manner, but several cases have been reported with lymph node metastases. Burman [10] in 1955 described a case which metastasized to lungs, skull, pelvis, and vertebra and probably was of vagal body origin.

The most common variety of this tumor is located in the carotid body and is usually asymptomatic. Lesions which form in the region of the glomerula jugulare, however, may cause a variety of symptoms most common of which are increasing deafness, aural discharge, and cranial nerve involvement. There may be a polypoid mass present in the ear canal. In the cervical region some reported cases have been asymptomatic; other patients have complained of hoarseness and blacking-out spells, dizziness, nausea and sweating postprandially, and palpitations. The principal symptom in this reported cervical case was a dry hacking type of cough which has been noted in one case previously in the reported literature. No general symptoms attended the femoral lesion reported here.

Complete surgical excision has been most often successful in the treatment of these tumors, although radiation has been of some palliative value in those superiorly located and larger lesions which have not been amenable to surgery. Of the 20 cases collected by Perez, Harrison, and ReMine [6] in 1960, surgical excision was successful in 15 over a 3- to 17-year follow-up period. Sixteen patients had total resection, one of whom died 17 years later of brain involvement. Radiation was of symptomatic value in one of two cases in which it was given.

Grossly the chemodectoma of the cervical region of the vagus nerve presents as an ovoid or a nodular, firm, rubber, encapsulated mass contiguous to or arising from the vagus nerve most commonly above or involving and replacing the ganglion nodosum. Small vessels may be seen on the external surface of the tumor and grossly the fibers of the vagus nerve seem to contribute to the capsule. On cut section the appearance is meaty and rather pinkish with yellowish bands of fibrosis running throughout. Microscopically the clusters of cells termed *Zellballen* are most characteristic. These are nests of rather uniform cells which have small dark central nuclei and abundant pale eosinophilic cytoplasm with indistinct borders. Various degrees of fibrosis and angiomatous appearance of spindle cells in a vascular type of framework have been reported as well as giant cells which may give the appearance of cancer on some occasions.

Report of Cases

Case 1.—This 51-year-old rather nervous and anxious-appearing male patient complained of

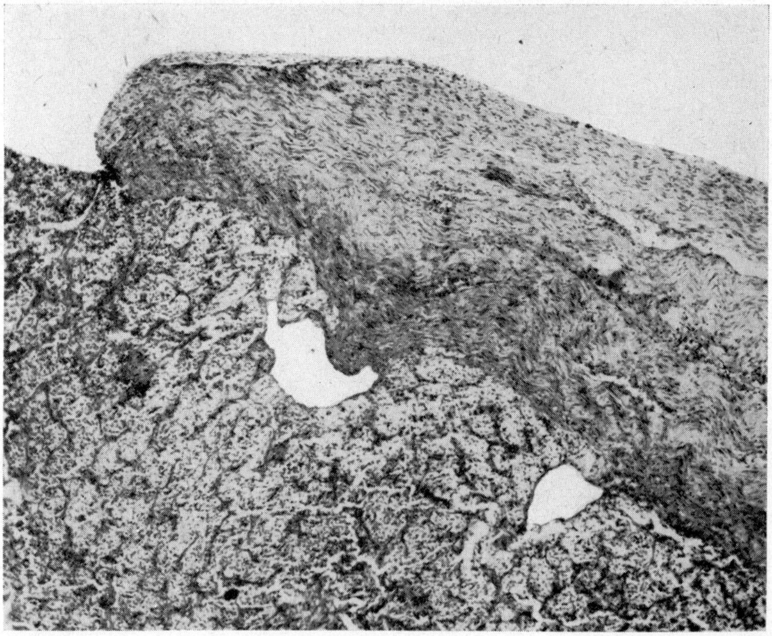

Fig 1.—Low-power view of vagal body tumor showing vagus nerve origin of the tumor.

paroxysms of coughing usually terminating in vomiting for about one year. He had come to realize that these episodes of coughing could be stimulated by pressure on the right side of the neck and that it had become impossible to tolerate a tight collar or necktie for this reason. Also, merely turning the neck, particularly to the right side and if done quickly, initiated these attacks of coughing. He had been treated for stomach trouble without relief. He also believed that the right side of his neck had become more prominent gradually over this period of time. Physical examination revealed a firm mass at the anterior border of the right sternocleidomastoid muscle about its midportion. This tumor could not be palpated satisfactorily because it produced severe paroxysms of coughing which were thought to be accentuated or overemphasized by the patient's anxiety and nervousness. It was definitely posterior to the carotid bifurcation, however, and on a level somewhat inferior to it. No lymphadenopathy was noted in the neck, and general physical examination otherwise was essen-

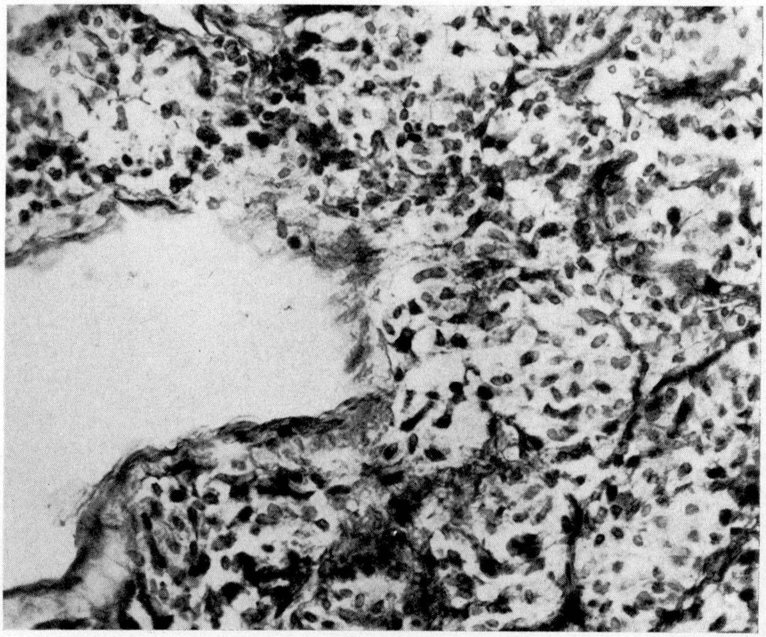

Fig 2.—View showing the nerve contribution to the capsule of the tumor.

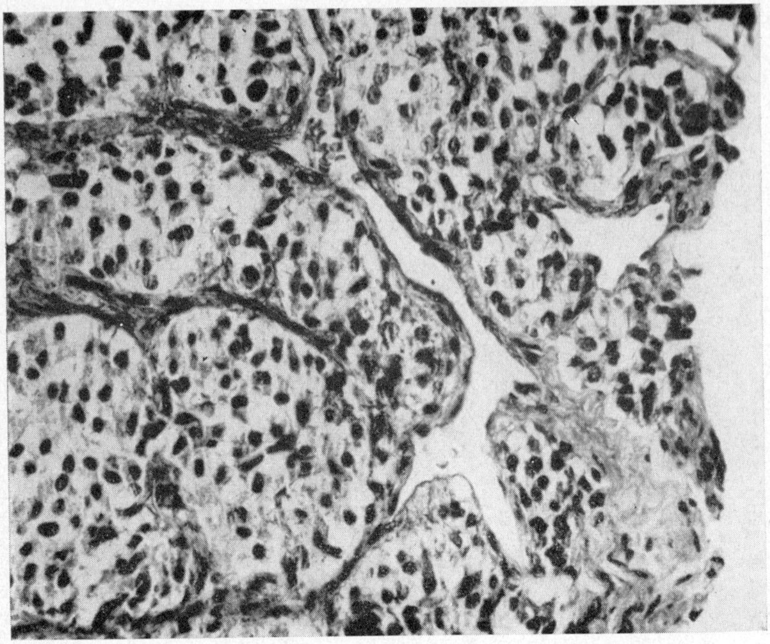

Fig 3.—Typical *Zellballen* arrangement of uniform cells with small dark central nuclei of tumor in Fig 1.

tially negative. X-rays of the chest, upper gastrointestinal series, and routine laboratory work were all within normal limits. The patient stated that he had lost 14 lb (6.3 kg) of weight over the last year, because of his frequent vomiting. On Nov 9, 1961, the tumor was explored surgically and found to lie within the posterior portion of the carotid sheath behind the internal jugular vein and to originate from the vagus nerve. The tumor was removed with a segment of the vagus nerve on either side along with several small normal-appearing lymph nodes of the jugular chain. Frozen section diagnosis was probable nerve tumor, probably benign.

Grossly the tumor consisted of a firm, rubbery, grayish mass of an ovoid shape measuring about 3×2 cm in size. Projecting from either end of the tumor were stumps of nerve-like tissue (Fig 1). These stumps of tissue could not be dissected from the tumor proper. On cut section it had a pinkish homogeneous appearance. Microscopically the nerve did not appear to be an essential part of the tumor

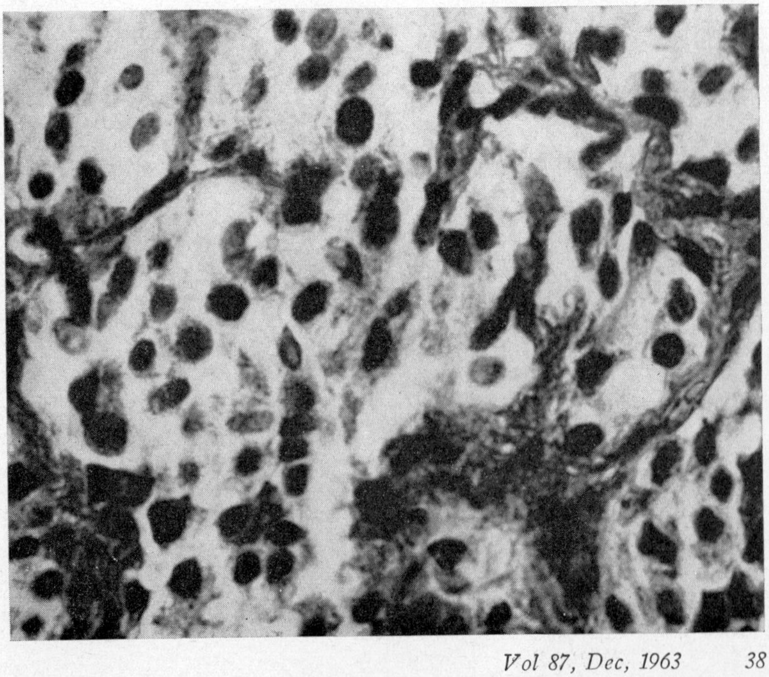

Fig 4.—Higher magnification of the vagal body tumor demonstrating the fine reticulum separating the nests of cells.

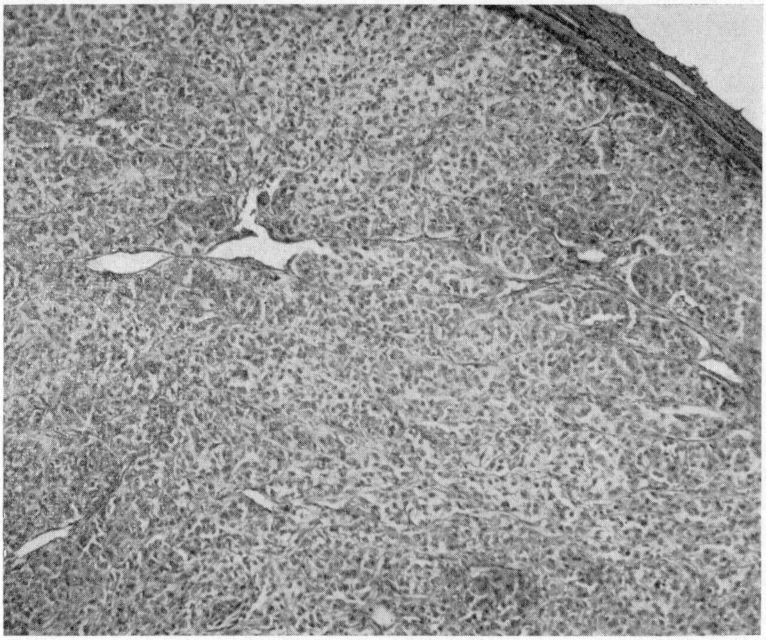

Fig 5.—Femoral body tumor showing homogeneous pattern of cell nests with a definite capsule.

but to contribute to its capsule (Fig 2). The typical *Zellballen* of rather uniform cells with small dark central nuclei and pale eosinophilic cytoplasm were noted (Fig 3 and 4). No malignant features were apparent. The lymph nodes removed were normal.

Postoperatively the patient noted the complete disappearance of his tendency to cough and to vomit. He noted hoarseness also which was due to right vocal cord paralysis, of course incident to excision of the vagus nerve. On follow-up examinations to 16 months postoperatively the patient has had no recurrence of his symptoms, and the operated region can be palpated and pressed without producing any coughing or vomiting. There has also been no evidence of recurrence or other foci of tumor.

Case 2.—A 42-year-old white male was admitted Oct 15, 1951. He first noticed a 2 cm painless mass in the anterior aspect of the left thigh five months prior to admission, after a minor injury to the area. Three weeks prior to admission the mass rapidly enlarged with some associated pain and overlying redness of the skin.

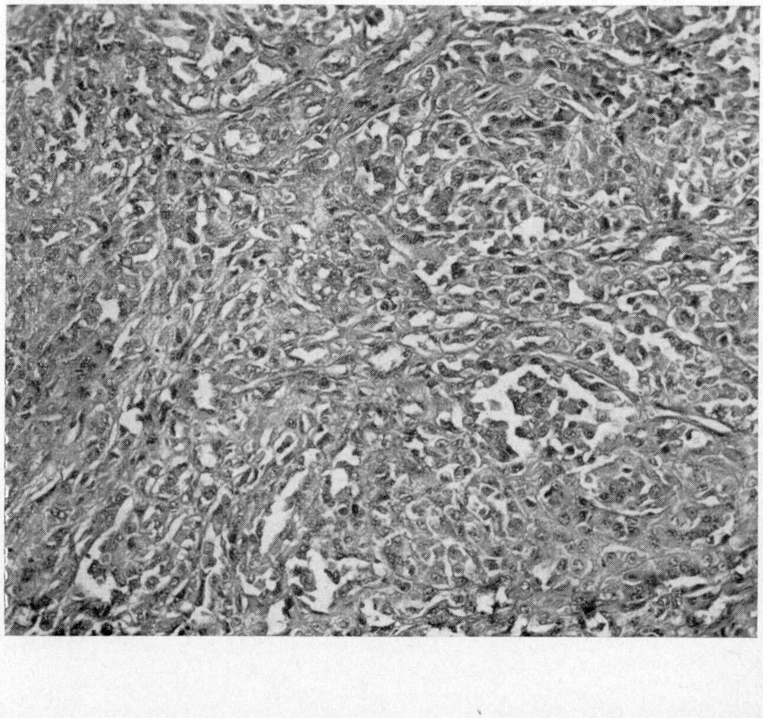

Fig 6.—Another view of tumor shown in Fig 5 with bizarre sizes and shapes of cells and irregular disposition.

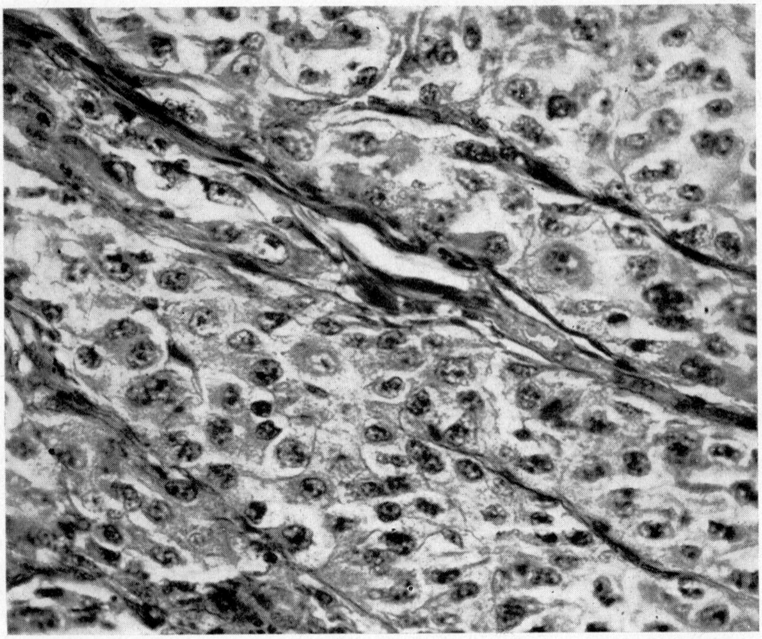

Fig 7. — High-power view of the same femoral body tumor with cords of cells and stroma well seen.

Physical examination was negative except for a firm 7×10 cm mass situated on the anterior aspect of the left thigh at the apex of Scarpa's triangle. It was tender to palpation and had the suggestion of fluctuation in the center. There were no enlarged inguinal nodes or lymphangitis, and examination otherwise was essentially negative.

The mass was removed by wide local excision on Oct 23, 1951, and diagnosis by the Armed Forces Institute of Pathology was malignant paraganglioma, nonchromaffin in type (Fig 5, 6, and 7). A wide excision of the operative site and radical groin dissection in continuity were carried out on Nov 28, 1951. Two recurrent nodules in the skin at the site of the primary excision were removed on Sept 5, 1952. After this, on Oct 8, 1952, re-excision of the primary site was carried out on this patient with skin grafting. Follow-up examinations revealed no further local recurrence, but on Nov 9, 1953, multiple metastases to the lungs and the skull were seen. The patient died at home Nov 23, 1953, of his metastases.

Summary

The literature has been briefly reviewed in regard to chemodectoma, especially of the vagus nerve, and two new cases have been added: one in which the tumor originated in the cervical portion of the vagus nerve, probably at the lowest level yet reported, and the other in the femoral region. The two lesions are strikingly similar in appearance but differ vastly in clinical behavior, the neck lesion being essentially benign and the femoral lesion causing death by metastases.

Robert L. Bradley, MD, Chief, Surgical Service, Veterans Administration Hospital, 1540 Spring Valley Dr, Huntington 1, W Va.

REFERENCES

1. Von Haller, A.: Icones Anatomicae, Gottingen: A. Vandenhoeck, 1743-1756.

2. Mulligan, R. M.: Chemodectoma in the Dog, Amer J Path 26:680, 1950.

3. Byrne, J. J.: Carotid Body and Allied Tumors, Amer J Surg 95:371, 1958.

4. Korn, D.; Bensch, K.; Liebow, A. A.; and Castleman, B.: Multiple Minute Pulmonary Tumors Resembling Chemodectomas, Amer J Path 37:641-672, 1960.

5. Birrell, J. H. W.: Vagal Body and Its Tumour, Aust New Zeal J Surg 23:48-54 (Aug) 1953.

6. Perez, P. E.; Harrison, E. G.; and ReMine, W. H.: Vagal-Body Tumor (Chemodectoma of the Glomus Intravagale), New Eng J Med 263:116-1121 (Dec) 1960.

7. Johnson, W. S.; Beahrs, O. H.; and Harrison, E. G., Jr.: Chemodectoma of the Glomus Intravagale (Vagal-Body Tumor), Amer J Surg 104:812 (Dec) 1962.

8. Marcuse, P. M., and Chamberlin, J. A.: Multicentric Paragangliomas: Case Report With Demonstration of Intravagal Paraganglionic Tissue at Previously Undescribed Level, Cancer 9:288-292 (March-April) 1956.

9. Jernstrom, P., and Fry, K.: Nonchromaffin Paraganglioma of the Cervical Portion of the Vagus Nerve: An Unusual Case, Amer J Clin Path 28:393-399 (Oct) 1957.

10. Burman, S. O.: Vagal Body Tumor (Paraganglioma), Ann Surg 141:488-489 (April) 1955.

Chemodectoma of the Mediastinum

GENE W. SPECTOR, MD; CHARLES L. ROPER, MD; AND JOHN S. SPRATT, JR., MD, COLUMBIA, MO

In 1950, the term "chemodectoma" was proposed as the generic name for tumors arising from the nonchromaffin neuroepithelial cells located in the adventitia of blood vessels derived from the branchial arches. The ganglia of the glossopharyngeal and vagus nerves are also sites of the neoplasms.[1-3]

These cell aggregates have neither endocrine nor motor function. They have the propensity for perceiving chemical changes in the circulatory system and thus act as a sensory component in a reflex arc which allows transmission of impulses centrally over afferent parasympathetic nerve fibers. In this way, blood flow and respiratory rate may be controlled.[4,5]

Although these neuroepithelial cells are found in many sites, by far the most common location of neoplasm is the carotid body at the main carotid bifurcation. This entity was first described by Marchand in 1891.[6] Chemodectomas arising from aortic bodies situated in the mediastinum are rarely seen.[7] To date, 13 cases have been reported in the literature. It is the purpose of this paper to present the 14th reported case of mediastinal chemodectoma and the first which permitted calculation of growth rate.

Report of Case

A 67-year-old white female entered Ellis Fischel State Cancer Hospital on May 9, 1962, with the chief complaint of a "lump" in the abdomen.

Submitted for publication May 17, 1963.

Chief Resident, Department of Radiology, The Jewish Hospital of St. Louis, formerly Resident in Radiotherapy at Ellis Fischel State Cancer Hospital (Dr. Spector); Assistant Professor in Surgery (Thoracic), Washington University School of Medicine, St. Louis, Consultant in Thoracic Surgery at Ellis Fischel State Cancer Hospital (Dr. Roper); Chief Surgeon, Ellis Fischel State Cancer Hospital (Dr. Spratt).

From the Ellis Fischel State Cancer Hospital.

Present Illness.—In 1946, the patient had a left radical mastectomy performed for adenocarcinoma of the breast. At the time of her operation no lymph node metastasis was found. In the interval, the patient had done well until approximately one year prior to her present admission. At that time, she had noted recurrent episodes of vague upper abdominal pain, and upon one occasion an episode of syncope had occurred. Her physician, who had been treating her for hypertension for years, noted a questionable abdominal mass.

The patient's past history was unremarkable except for the previously mentioned radical mastectomy.

Review of systems was essentially negative.

Physical examination revealed a blood pressure of 170/70, a pulse of 80, and respiratory rate of 20. The head and neck were within normal limits with no adenopathy being noted. Examination of thorax revealed a left radical mastectomy scar which was well healed without evidence of local or regional recurrence. The lungs were clear to auscultation and percussion. There was a grade 2 apical systolic murmur, and no abnormality of heart rhythm was noted. Upon examination of the abdomen there was a suggestion of a mass in the midepigastric region. Pelvic examination revealed only a small cervical polyp.

Laboratory Data.—The patient's hemoglobin was 13 gm with hematocrit of 39%. The WBC was 6,120 with adequate platelets and a normal differential. The BUN was 11 mg%, and her postprandial blood sugar was 14 mg%. VDRL was nonreactive. The urinalysis revealed a specific gravity of 1.010 with no sugar or albumin. The ECG showed left axis deviation.

Hospital Course.—During the patient's hospitalization, both intravenous pyelograms and barium studies were performed to rule out the presence of an abdominal mass. A chest roentgenogram was taken, which revealed the presence of a large midmediastinal mass. An esophagogram showed rather marked deviation of both the trachea and the esophagus. In reviewing past chest roentgenograms of this patient, it was found that a small mediastinal mass could be seen at the time of her surgery in 1946. Subsequent x-rays had revealed the mass to be progressively enlarging (Fig 1). On May 23, 1962, a scalene node biopsy was performed, and histological examination of the fat pad

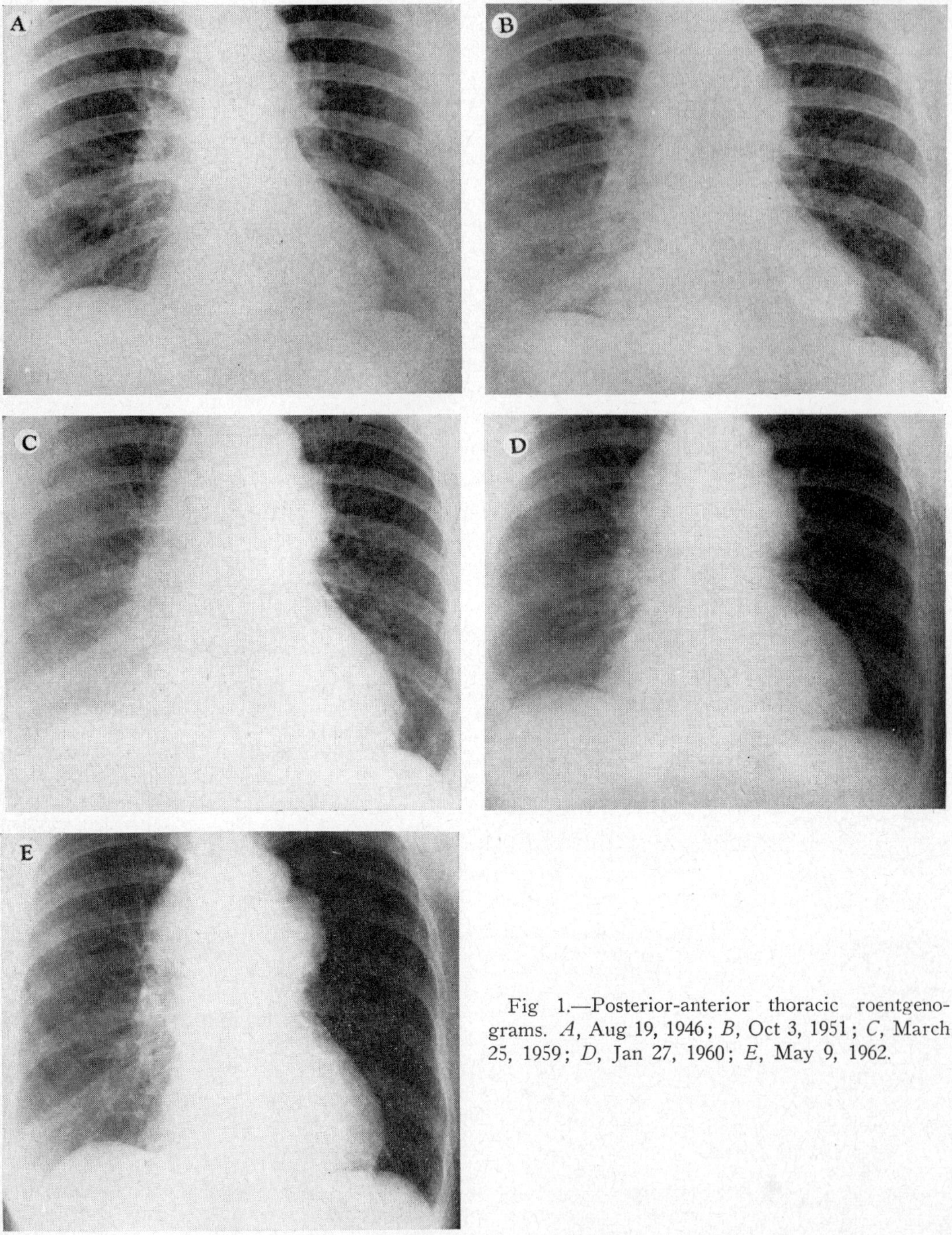

Fig 1.—Posterior-anterior thoracic roentgenograms. *A*, Aug 19, 1946; *B*, Oct 3, 1951; *C*, March 25, 1959; *D*, Jan 27, 1960; *E*, May 9, 1962.

revealed no evidence of metastatic adenopathy. On May 28, 1962, left thoracotomy was performed. A highly vascular 9 by 7 cm mass was found lying adherent to the inferior aspect of the aortic arch (Fig 2). By means of careful dissection, the tumor was grossly completely excised. Profuse oozing of blood from the adventitia of the aortic wall was noted throughout the procedure, and this was controlled by laparotomy sponges and Gelfoam. Postoperatively, the patient did well and was discharged on June 6, 1962. The patient was last seen in October, 1962, and a roentgenogram was taken at that time which revealed no evidence of recurrent tumor.

The photomicrograph of the resected tumor showed the typical aggregates of multishaped and

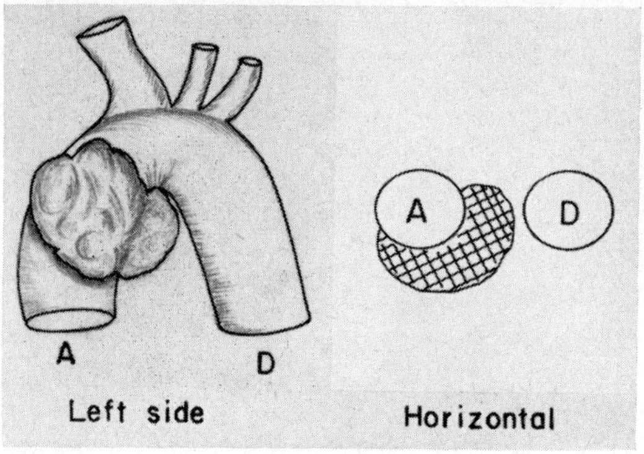

Fig 2.—Location of mediastinal chemodectoma with respect to the aortic arch.

sized epithelial cells embedded in an extremely vascular stroma (Fig 3). The cells are arranged in *Zellballen* or "cell balls" which are characteristic of chemodectoma.[8] No mitoses were seen.

Comment

Nathan, Collins, and Adams have shown that pulmonary lesions with doubling times of over 500 days are virtually always benign.[9] We have confirmed this observation with our own data.[10,11] The film observations on this chemodectoma span a period of approximately 6,000 days. During this time the diameter of the tumor doubled. Therefore, the volume of the tumor increased by a factor of eight. Assuming an exponential growth pattern, there were three doublings of the tumor volume requiring 2,000 days each. In Nathan's studies, tumors with equally long doubling times were usually benign hamartomas.

The nonaggressive nature and slow growth of this tumor point out the typical charac-

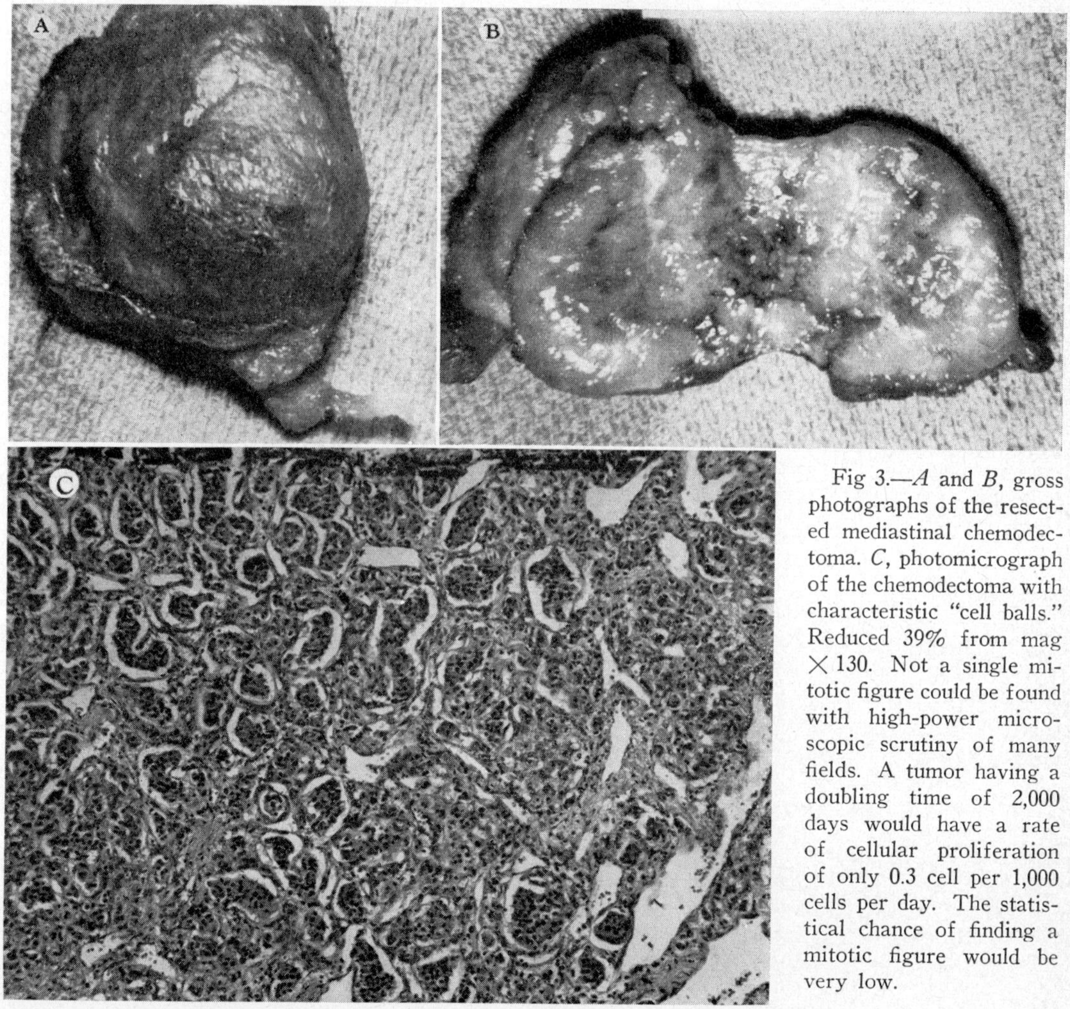

Fig 3.—*A* and *B*, gross photographs of the resected mediastinal chemodectoma. *C*, photomicrograph of the chemodectoma with characteristic "cell balls." Reduced 39% from mag × 130. Not a single mitotic figure could be found with high-power microscopic scrutiny of many fields. A tumor having a doubling time of 2,000 days would have a rate of cellular proliferation of only 0.3 cell per 1,000 cells per day. The statistical chance of finding a mitotic figure would be very low.

teristic of chemodectomas. Of the previously reported 13 cases, six were in the anterior mediastinum.[7,12-16] Nine were asymptomatic and were discovered incidentally.[7,13-15,17-20] One patient had chest pain and one had superior venacaval obstruction.[16] There is some tendency for these tumors to be multiple.[7]

Treatment has included total and partial excision and irradiation. Prognosis is good.[16] Only one chemodectoma has been proved to metastasize.[12]

Summary

A 14th case of chemodectoma of the mediastinum is reported. The growth rate as determined from serial roentgenograms confirms the histologic picture of benignancy.

Consultation was made with Drs. R. E. Johnson and C. M. Waggoner, the respective chiefs of Pathology and Diagnostic Radiology at the Ellis Fischel State Cancer Hospital.

John S. Spratt, Jr., MD, the Ellis Fischel State Cancer Hospital, Columbia, Mo.

REFERENCES

1. Boyd, J. D.: "The Development of the Human Carotid Body," in Contributions to Embryology, publication No. 479, Washington, DC: Carnegie Institute, 1937.

2. Nonidez, J. F.: The Aortic (Depressor) Nerve and Its Associated Epitheliod Body, the Glomus Aorticum, Amer J Anat 57:259-293, 1935.

3. Smetana, H. F., and Scott, W. R., Jr.: Malignant Tumors of Non-Chromaffin Paraganglia, Milit Surg 109:330-341, 1951.

4. Schmidt, C. F., and Comroe, J. H., Jr.: Functions of Carotid and Aortic Bodies, Physiol Rev 20:115-157, 1940.

5. Dripps, R. D., Jr., and Comroe, J. H.: The Clinical Significance of the Cartoid and Aortic Bodies, Amer J Med Sci 208:681-694, 1944.

6. Marchand, F.: Beitrage sur Kenntniss der normalen und pathologischen Anatomie der Glandula Carotica und der Nebennieren, Virchow Arch Path Anat 1:535-581, 1891.

7. Lottes, R.: Non-Chromaffin Paraganglioma of Ganglion Nodosum, Carotid Body and Aortic Arch Bodies, Cancer 3:667-694, 1950.

8. LeCompte, P. M.: Tumors of the Carotid Body and Related Structures (Chemoreceptor System), sect IV, fasc 16, Atlas of Tumor Pathology, US Armed Forces Institute of Pathology, 1951.

9. Nathan, M. H.; Collins, V. P.; and Adams, R. A.: Differentiation of Benign and Malignant Pulmonary Nodules by Growth Rate, Radiology 79:221-232, 1962.

10. Spratt, J. S., Jr.; Roper, C. L.; and Spjut, H. J.: The Frequency Distribution of the Rates of Growth and the Estimated Duration of Primary Pulmonary Carcinomas, Cancer 16:687-693, 1963.

11. Spratt, J. S., Jr., and Spratt, T. L.: The Rates of Growth of Pulmonary Metastases and Host Survival, Ann Surg, to be published.

12. Monro, R. S.: The Morphology of the Branchial Glomera and Their Tumours: With a Report of a Case of Aortico-Pulmonary Glomus Tumour, Brit J Surg 38:105-109, 1950.

13. McDonald, O. G.; Aufderheide, A. C.; and Fuller, J.: Chemodectoma (Non-Chromaffin Paraganglioma) of the Mediastinum, Ann Surg 140:254-256, 1954.

14. Mendelow, H., and Slobodkin, M.: Aortic-Body Tumor (Chemodectoma) of the Mediastinum: Report of a Case and Review of the Literature, Cancer 10:1008-1014, 1957.

15. Madden, T. J.: Mediastinal Chemodectoma, Ann Surg 148:943-950, 1958.

16. Tama, L.; Ellis, F. J., Jr.; Hodgson, C. H.; and Dockerty, M. B.: Chemodectoma of the Mediastinum: Report on a Patient With Superior Vena Caval Obstruction Treated by a Shunt from the Right Innominate Vein to the Right Atrium, J Thorac Cardiov Surg 43:585-594, 1962.

17. Duncan, D. K., and McDonald, J. R.: Chemodectoma ("Non-Chromaffin Paraganglioma") of the Mediastinum: Report of Two Cases, Amer J Clin Path 21:515-520, 1951.

18. Davies, J. R., and Randall, K. J.: Benign Aortic-Body Tumour, J Path Bact 68:247-250, 1954.

19. MacDonald, R. A.: A Carotid-Body-Like Tumor on the Left Subclavian Artery, AMA Arch Path 62:107-111, 1956.

20. Taylor, M. J., and Evans, P. V.: Non-Chromaffin Paraganglioma (Chemodectoma) of Mediastinum: Report of Case and Review of Literature, AMA Arch Surg 77:242-247, 1958.

Alterations in Vascular Volume After Long Bone Fracture

H. ZEIDMAN, MD
J. B. WRAY, MD
AND
A. J. SCHNEIDER, MD
SYRACUSE, NY

Introduction

Fracture of a long bone in the dog produces dramatic alterations in the hemodynamics of the injured region. Widespread vasodilation with accompanying increase in blood flow occurs in the fractured limb.[4] Associated changes in the general circulation have not been clearly demonstrated.

Textbooks of surgery and orthopedic surgery imply that extensive blood loss follows fracture of a long bone.[1,2] On the other hand, we have been unable to find documented proof that significant hemorrhage accompanies the usual uncomplicated fracture. The present study was carried out in an effort to estimate, in a reasonably critical fashion, the amount of hemorrhage that accompanies a closed fracture of a long bone. Fracture sites were restricted to areas with relatively little paraskeletal soft tissue, in an effort to separate the effects of skeletal trauma from those of soft tissue injury. The dog rather than the human was employed in this investigation due to the fact that baseline blood volume measurements, made in the prefracture period, are not available in the human but are easily obtained in the animal.

Submitted for publication May 19, 1963.

Division of Orthopedic Surgery (Drs. Zeidman and Wray); Department of Pediatrics (Dr. Schneider).

State University of New York, Upstate Medical Center.

Supported by grant No. AM-04868 of the National Institutes of Health.

Direct measurements of red cell mass were made with Cr^{51}-tagged red cells. Each fracture was exposed for the estimation of local blood loss. The data strongly support rather surprising conclusions and are the subject of the following report.

Material and Methods

Twenty-three adult mongrel dogs ranging from 10 to 15 kg in weight were used in this study. Nineteen of the animals were splenectomized four weeks or longer before experimentation. The remaining four animals were not splenectomized and were employed as "intact" animals.

All volume determinations were carried out with the animals under intravenous pentobarbital anesthesia. In the experiments when fracture was to be performed, one carotid artery was cannulated to permit continuous blood pressure monitoring (Fig 1). A fracture was produced in each animal by manipulation with padded monkey wrenches. At the completion of the experiment, each animal was sacrificed with an overdose of pentobarbital. The fracture was then exposed and free blood at the fracture site measured by absorption into weighed sponges.

Circulating red cell mass was measured directly with radioactive chromium. An amount of ten ml of blood was drawn from each animal into a heparinized syringe. The sample was centrifuged and the cells suspended in acid citrate dextrose solution. Ten microcuries of radiochromate were added, and the mixture was allowed to stand for 45 minutes. The cells were then separated from the mixture, washed three times with saline, and resuspended in their own plasma. One aliquot of the prepared sample was used for injection into the test animal, and one aliquot was used for the preparation of standards by dilution.

Thirty minutes were allowed for mixing after injection of the radioactive cell mass. Samples were

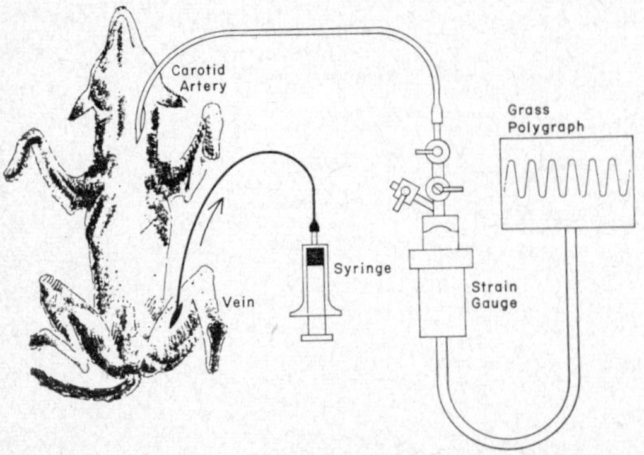

Fig 1.—Experimental setup for single extremity fractures. The animal is maintained in the supine position during the entire experiment. A large vein was cannulated in an unfractured extremity to permit sample withdrawal. A carotid artery was cannulated for continuous blood pressure monitoring. Another cannula, not shown here, was inserted into a second vein, remote from the fracture site, to permit the injection of tagged cells. In fractures of all four limbs, one jugular vein was cannulated for sample withdrawal.

then drawn at designated intervals before and after fracture. Duplicate aliquots of each sample were counted in a NaI crystal deep well counter.* A portion of each sample was used for hematocrit determinations which were performed in duplicate by the capillary tube method. Circulating red cell mass was then calculated by the formula:

$$\text{Red Cell Volume} = \frac{\text{Hct} \times \text{Vol Tagged Cells Injected} \times 200 \times \text{c/m Std}}{\text{c/m Whole Blood Sample}}$$

where 200=dilution, and c/m=counts per minute per milliliter counted.

This injection technique was employed in three different situations.

In the first instance, repeated red cell mass determinations were performed at two-week intervals in the same unfractured dog.

In the second instance, a single injection was made. Red cell mass estimations were made before fracture and at intervals of ten minutes over a 90-minute period after fracture.

* Counter—Nancy Wood Counter Laboratory Model SC-2L, Scaler-Baird Atomic Model 1030.

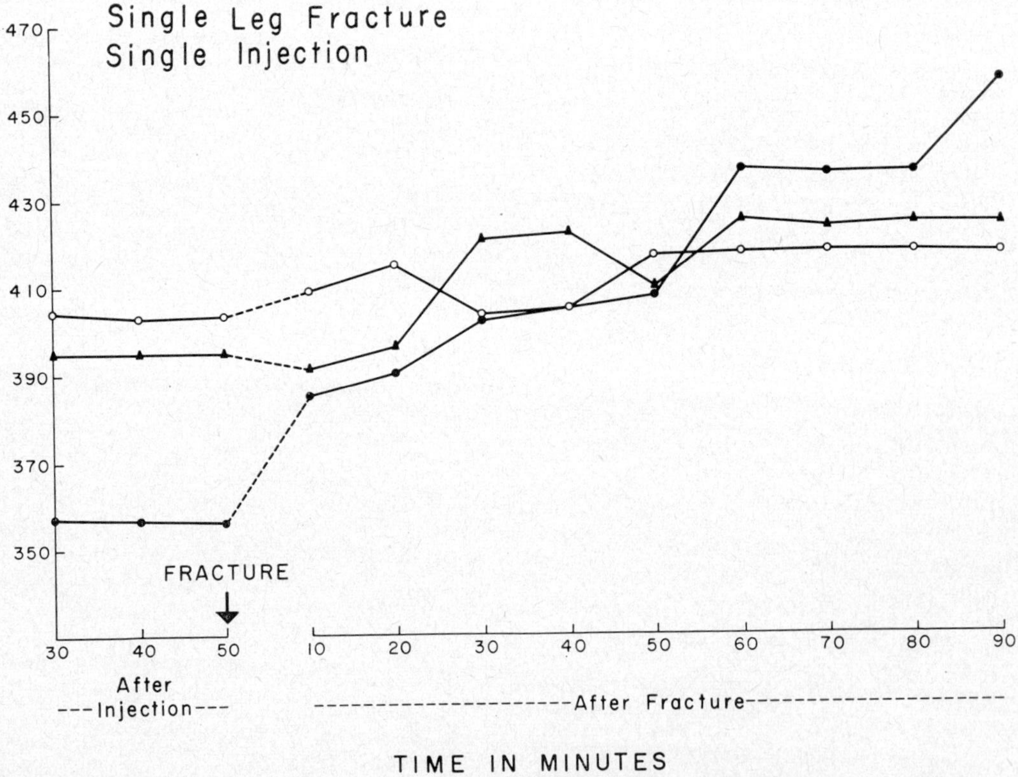

A

Fig 2A.—Fig 2A-2D show volume changes estimated by the single injection of tagged red cells. The red cell volume in cubic centimeters is plotted on the vertical axis in each instance, while the time in minutes before and after fracture is plotted on the horizontal axis. Graph 2A-2C represents data obtained in splenectomized animals. Red cell volume showed minimal variation during the prefracture period. After fracture, however, the calculated red cell mass was found to increase in all instances. This increase was greatest in the nonsplenectomized animals. Such increases in calculated red cell mass could be caused by the dilution of tagged cells, the loss of tagged cells into the tissues, or by a combination of both.

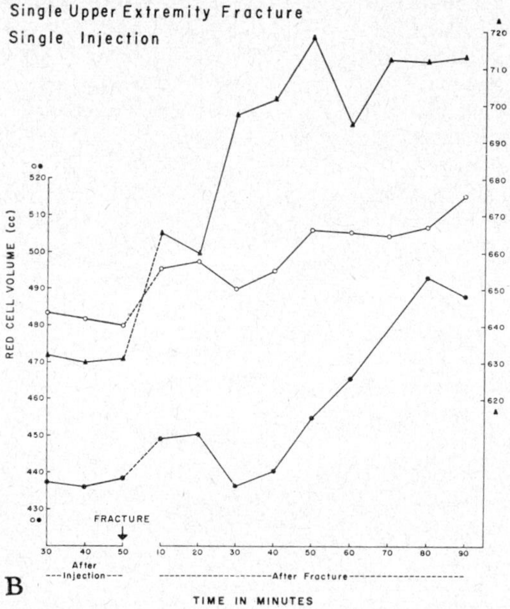

B

Fig 2B.—Splenectomized animal (see Fig 2A).

Finally, four animals were studied with a double injection of tagged cells. Baseline samples were drawn after one injection; one tibia in each animal was then fractured, samples were drawn, and a second injection of tagged red cells was carried out. After 30 minutes were allowed to elapse for mixing, further samples were drawn.

Results

Five splenectomized animals were used to estimate red cell mass at two-week intervals. Considerable variation was noted in red cell mass for any given animal over a two-week period, and this method was not employed further.

Animals studied with a single injection of radioactive cells showed definite changes in the postfracture period.

The results obtained in a series of three splenectomized animals following a fracture of one tibia are shown in Fig 2A. The increase in calculated red cell mass volume has occurred by ten minutes and persists during the entire sampling period. A similar response is noted with fracture of a single upper extremity (Fig 2B).

When all four limbs were fractured in three splenectomized animals (Fig 2C), there was an initial decrease in calculated cell volume followed by a persistent rise beyond baseline values.

When four intact dogs, ie, nonsplenectomized, were subjected to fracture of a single tibia (Fig 2D), there was an increase

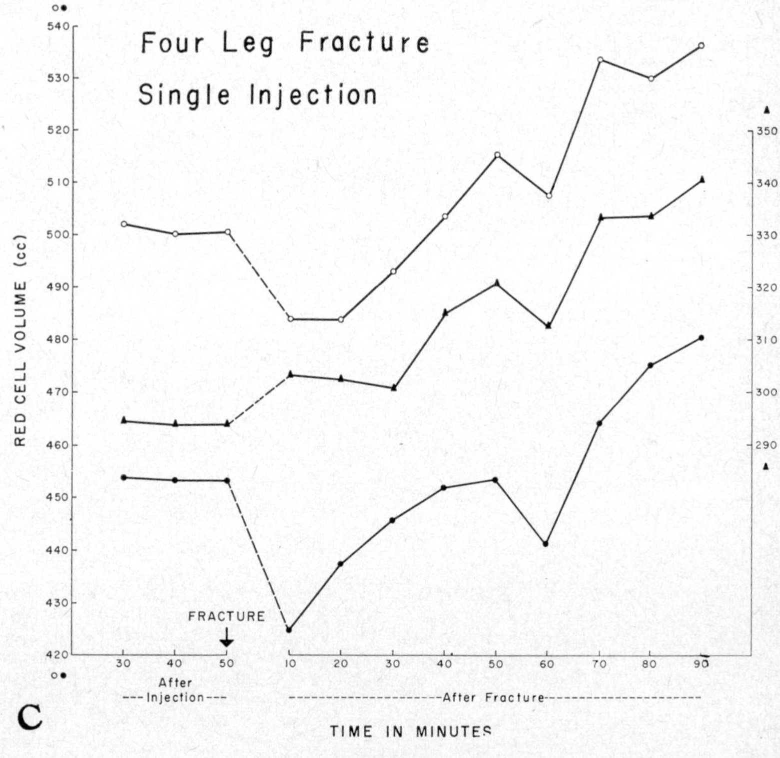

C

Fig 2C.—Splenectomized animal (see Fig 2A).

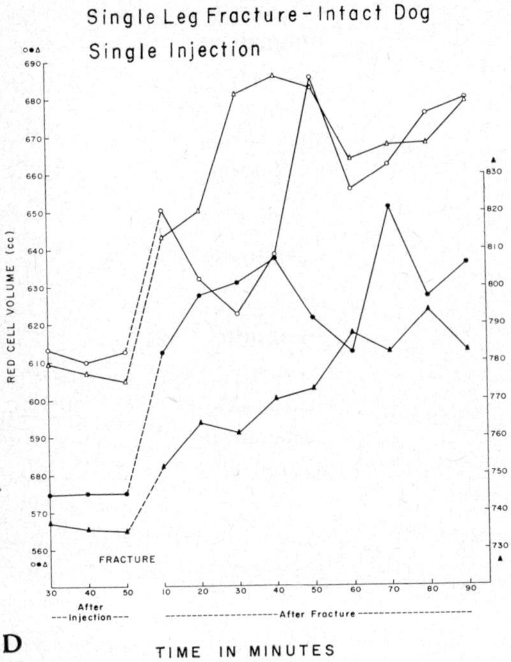

Fig 2D.—Data obtained from nonsplenectomized animals (see Fig 2A).

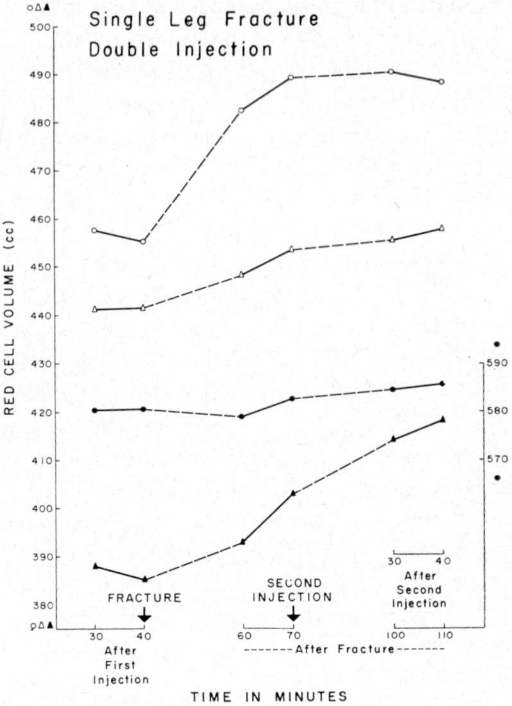

Fig 3.—Volume changes estimated by double injections of tagged cells. The red cell volume is plotted on the vertical axis in cubic centimeters and time on the horizontal axis in minutes. An increase in calculated red cell mass was again noted. A second injection of tagged cells 70 minutes after fracture demonstrates that the increase in circulating red cell mass is real and is the result of an influx of untagged cells into the active circulation.

in calculated red cell volume at ten minutes. This increase persisted throughout the entire sampling period and appeared to be of greater degree than was noted in any of the previous groups.

A final group of four splenectomized animals was studied with double injections of tagged cells (Fig 3). After a single injection of tagged cells, samples were drawn and one tibia was fractured. One hour was allowed to elapse, and two postfracture samples were drawn. A second injection of tagged cells was then carried out. After 30 minutes two more samples were obtained. Red cell increases greater than prefracture levels were noted in both initial postfracture and reinjection estimations.

There were no significant changes in hematocrit or blood pressure noted in any of the above series except for the nonsplenectomized dogs which showed a persistent increase of three to five hematocrit units following fracture.

All fractures were exposed to estimate local blood loss. In no case did free blood at a fracture exceed 5 cc. An equal amount was estimated to be present in the surrounding soft tissue.

Comment

The increase in calculated red cell volume following fracture is evidence only of dilution of the original red cells by new, untagged cells. Of itself, it is not sufficient to demonstrate an increase in the total red cell mass. Indeed, it is conceivable that an actual decrease, or no change, in red cell mass could have occurred in spite of the dilution curves observed with a single injection. The increased postfracture volumes found after the use of the reinjection technique show, however, that an actual increase in circulating red cell mass follows long bone fracture.

It has been shown that major hemorrhage followed by reinfusion of the shed blood produces an increase in calculated circulating red cell volumes as measured by dilution techniques.[3] On the other hand, the increases in red cell volume observed in this study were associated not with major hemorrhage but rather with limited blood loss. Further, blood loss due to sampling during the control period is of a similar magnitude to that at the fracture site (10 cc), and no increase in red cell mass is observed.

The red cells added to the circulation after fracture would appear to be derived from a relatively inactive vascular bed which is not fully participating in the general circulation prior to fracture. Of interest in this regard is the finding that red cell mass measurements repeated after a two-week interval were less reproducible than those that were repeated immediately. While this may be due, in part, to the variable replacement of lost red cells by newly formed cells, it also suggests that the size of the actively circulating red cell mass is inconstant.

Although the more marked response of the nonsplenectomized animals to fracture suggests that the splenic circulation may contribute, it seems likely that the fractured limb itself is the major donor to the increased circulating red cell mass. It is now known that vasodilation occurs throughout the involved limb in the immediate postfracture period.[4] The resultant opening of additional channels in the involved limb would facilitate a liberation of relatively inactive red cells into the general circulation.

It is important to bear in mind that the observations that were made in this study were drawn from fractures that were accompanied by minimal soft tissue damage. Certain fractures, such as fracture of the femoral shaft, however, may be associated with much greater soft tissue injury and may result in considerable blood volume depletion.

Conclusions

1. Closed fracture of one tibia in the dog is accompanied by minimal local blood loss.

2. Fracture of one or more long bones in the nonsplenectomized or splenectomized dog leads to an increase in the circulating red cell mass as measured with Cr^{51}-tagged red cells.

3. Severe associated soft tissue damage might reasonably be expected to alter these findings.

J. B. Wray, MD, Division of Orthopedics, Department of Surgery, State University of New York, Upstate Medical Center, Syracuse 10, NY.

REFERENCES

1. Watson-Jones, R.: Fractures and Joint Injuries, ed 4, Baltimore: The Williams & Wilkins Company, 1957, p 227.

2. Committee on Trauma, American College of Surgeons: An Outline of the Treatment of Fractures, ed 7, Philadelphia: W. B. Saunders Company, 1960, p 5.

3. Shoemaker, W. C.: Measurement of Rapidly and Slowly Circulating Red Cell Volumes in Hemorrhagic Shock, Amer J Physiol 202:1179-1182, 1962.

4. Wray, J. B., and Spencer, M. P.: The Vasodilatory Response to Skeletal Trauma, Surg Forum 11:444, 1960.

Are Postoperative Narcotics Necessary?

BENSON B. ROE, MD
SAN FRANCISCO

The routine liberal administration of narcotics to the postoperative patient is a deeply rooted surgical tradition based on the erroneous impression that devastating pain is the inevitable consequence of a major surgical procedure. It is the purpose of this paper to assess the factors relating to pain in the postoperative period and to report an experience with a large consecutive series of surgical patients who have received (and required) either very small doses of narcotics or none at all.

From observations on laboratory animals and human infants (whose pain threshold has been demonstrated to be lower than that of adults [1]), it is notable that major pain and discomfort are rarely evident after surgical procedures. It is also well known that a person can sustain major tissue damage in war combat or in an athletic contest and yet continue in active motion with minimal discomfort, sometimes being completely unaware of the injury. Beecher [2] noted a marked difference in response to pain of war wounds compared to that of surgical incisions: less than one third of seriously wounded soldiers requested medication for pain, whereas four fifths of postoperative patients demanded narcotics.

Bishop [3] has recognized the problem of measuring pain: "This unpleasant sensation will vary with emotional state, anxiety, anticipation of disaster, etc., and is almost impossible to deal with quantitatively since it has such a large component of what is referred to as a reaction to sensation." Hardy, Wolff, and Goodell [4] state: "Pain of high intensity resulting from noxious stimulant is seldom of more than brief duration because such intense stimulation either (1) destroys the neural equipment implicated, or (2) so damages the tissue . . . so as to prevent the stimuli from reaching the nerve ending." Since these and many other observations

Submitted for publication May 28, 1963.

Associate Professor of Surgery and Chief, Cardiac Surgery.

From the Department of Surgery, University of California Medical Center.

have emphasized the large psychological element in postoperative pain, our program was undertaken to parallel the objectives in the management of surgical patients that Read[5] proposed for "natural childbirth."

The physical well-being and rapid convalescence of the patient who makes light of his operation is in striking contrast to the course of the frightened patient who requires heavy sedation. Thus, in an effort to promote better ventilation, early mobility, and greater confidence, it has been the policy on our service since 1958 to restrict the use of narcotics in the postoperative period, both in the frequency of administration and in the size of the dose.

For successful execution of this policy it is necessary preoperatively to devote time and effort to each patient in order to obtain his cooperation after the procedure, since a patient already in pain and fear is poorly receptive to assurances. The patient is carefully told (1) that his incision will be securely closed and cannot be disrupted by his moving or coughing, (2) that his pain is the expected consequence of the operation and is not in any way abnormal, (3) that early mobility and ventilation are essential for his safe and rapid convalescence, and (4) that "limbering up" the operative area despite the initial pain will reduce his over-all discomfort and disability. Each patient is taught deep breathing and coughing, and the positive pressure breathing apparatus routinely used after operation is demonstrated to him. He is given the opportunity to converse with patients on the ward who have recently undergone similar procedures and whose healthy appearance provides effective confidence. Complete understanding and cooperation by the patient are essential if a restrictive narcotic policy is to be accepted.

Our policy of narcotic administration has stressed the following considerations: (1) restlessness alone is considered an indication for narcotics only when it can be ruled out as a sign of hypoxia; (2) genuine pain which cannot be assuaged by reassurance or other supportive measures is treated with narcotics as needed; (3) evaluation of the need for narcotics is made by an experienced member of the staff and not by a nurse; and (4) on the basis of personal preference, morphine sulfate has been used almost exclusively in doses of 0.25 to 1 mg in children and 1 to 2 mg in adults administered intravenously at intervals of 10 to 30 minutes until the desired effect is obtained. No routine narcotic order is written. "Titration" of the narcotic against pain is carried only to the point of relieving the discomfort and never to the level of somnolence. Early full mobilization of the painful areas is encouraged and is further emphasized during the period of analgesia when narcotics are given. Under this regimen it has been observed that once the pain has been relieved it seldom recurs to the same degree of severity and often a repeat dose of narcotic is not necessary.

While it has not been our primary intent to see how small an amount of drug we can successfully use, it has been useful to evaluate the efficacy of the program on a quantitative basis. As a result of this policy, in the past five years the actual consumption of narcotics has been reduced from the traditional 50 to 100 mg of morphine (or its equivalent) per surgical case to a documented average of less than 4 mg morphine per case; many patients have received no narcotics.

More than 600 patients have been treated with this regimen, nearly all of whom have had a thoracotomy. In many of these operations sternal splitting or sternal transecting incisions were made, and the procedures often involved extensive mediastinal and pleural dissection. Lateral thoracotomies have involved resected or transected ribs; pericostal or peristernal sutures were used in closure. Large (No. 40 French) chest tubes have been used routinely, and postoperative management has included vigorous measures to maintain the patency of the tracheobronchial airway and chest tubes, both of which necessarily involve considerable manipulation of the patient and potential discomfort.

Since this postoperative narcotic policy is a significant departure from traditional practices, it understandably has been criticized and its effect on the patient has been questioned. Visitors and personnel on the service who were initially unaware of the regimen consistently expressed surprise when they learned how little narcotic the patients were receiving. Indeed, I myself unknowingly observed a series of my own patients under the management of an overly enthusiastic resident who gave no narcotics at all to 26 consecutive patients, none of whom appeared to have unusual discomfort.

In recognition of the large subjective element in postoperative pain we considered the various methods of evaluating subjective responses as reviewed by Beecher [2] in his comprehensive monograph and were unable to find one that would apply to this project. The basic departure from "routine" management was not only that of drug dosage or any single controllable factor, but rather a program consisting of psychological preparation and personal attention which introduces a number of variables. For this reason, it is impossible to present objective evidence to support the method, and evaluation must be made on the necessarily crude basis of subjective comparisons. The total experience is sufficiently large and covered a long enough period that it could be assessed by a number of professional personnel whose clinical experience provided adequate basis for evaluation. A questionnaire was submitted to all members of the attending staff, resident staff, and nursing personnel who have extended contact with 25 or more of these patients. Their unsigned responses (Table) may be summarized as follows: only six of 36 observers believed that these patients suffered more discomfort than patients getting routine narcotic dosages. The postoperative course was thought to be improved by 26 observers and unchanged by 11; no one thought the regimen was detrimental to recovery. Only five observers supported the suggestion that somewhat less restrictive use of narcotics might be preferred. Paradoxically, two of the four nurses who said that there was more early suffering voted that the policy was not too severe. Recovery from major discomfort was thought to occur sooner by 22 observers and to be unchanged by 11; only one observer thought the period of pain was extended.

Patients who had undergone other major surgical procedures (or the same procedure in the case of mitral reoperations) elsewhere were asked to compare their suffering and postoperative courses. These patients were pleased with their management, and only one complained of insufficient pain medication.

Distribution of Responses to Questionnaire Submitted to Staff Members

Question	Choice of Answer	Visiting Staff	Resident Staff	Nurses *	Total
Do deprived patients suffer more than routine patients?	(a) No	3	19	3	25
	(b) Uncertain	0	3	3	6
	(c) Yes	1	1	4	6
Do you think the postoperative course of the deprived patient compared to the routine patient is generally	(a) Better	2	18	6	26
	(b) No different	2	5	4	11
	(c) Worse	0	0	0	0
Do you believe that the policy (as outlined) is too restrictive and that somewhat more liberal use of narcotics is desirable?	(a) No	3	21	8	32
	(b) Yes	1	2	2	5
Do the deprived patients get over major discomfort?	(a) Sooner	2	14	6	22
	(b) No difference	2	9	3	14
	(c) Later	0	0	1	1

* Intensive care unit nursing staff and private duty nurses with large experience.

Deviations from this policy were necessary in surprisingly few patients under our management. In most instances where the frequency or dosage of narcotic administration was more than minimal the patient was either particularly apprehensive or had not been psychologically prepared for the regimen. Variations in the pattern of narcotic administration occurred as new residents interpreted the policy more or less liberally than others; however, none of the patients received narcotics on a scale approaching that which has been considered routine on other services. Most of these patients had assisted respiration postoperatively which aided in maintaining adequate respiratory exchange; however, when restricted ventilatory excursion could not be corrected by pursuasion it was found valuable to "break" the restriction with small doses of morphine which seldom needed repeating.

The type of surgical incision may be a factor in postoperative pain. Some observers have the clinical impression that sternal splitting and trans-sternal anterior incisions are less painful than posterolateral thoracotomy or laparotomy incisions; however, the wide range of individual variation and other factors such as surgical retraction make this generality unreliable. While a majority of the patients in our series had anterior thoracotomy incisions, approximately one third were subjected to posterolateral thoracotomy; the latter group did not require significantly more narcotics postoperatively although their discomfort was somewhat greater.

Summary

In more than 600 patients seen during a five-year period, postoperative administration of narcotics was sharply reduced from the usual dosage of 50 to 100 mg to 4 mg or less. Improved ventilation, earlier mobility, and less postoperative fear were noted by the attending staff, residents, and nurses who cared for these patients.

The success of this regimen depends upon the cooperation of the patient which is obtained by the careful preoperative instruction in techniques of deep breathing and coughing. The positive pressure breathing apparatus is demonstrated to the patient and it is explained to him that his incision will be securely closed and cannot be disrupted by coughing or movement. He is told that early mobility and ventilatory motion are essential for his safe and rapid convalescence. The amount of postoperative pain was not noticeably increased by this restrictive regimen. Larger doses of morphine were necessary in only a few cases.

Benson B. Roe, MD, Department of Surgery, University of California Medical Center, San Francisco, Calif.

REFERENCES

1. Chapman, W. P., and Jones, C. M.: Variations in Cutaneous and Visceral Pain Sensitivity in Normal Subjects, J Clin Invest 23:81-91, 1944.

2. Beecher, H. K.: Measurement of Subjective Responses: Quantitative Effects of Drugs, New York: Oxford University Press, 1959.

3. Bishop, G. H.: quoted by Beecher,[2] p 6, from a personal communication.

4. Hardy, J. D.; Wolff, H. G.; and Goodell, H.: Pain Sensations and Reactions, Baltimore: The Williams & Wilkins Company, 1952.

5. Read, G. D.: Childbirth Without Fear: The Principles and Practice of Natural Childbirth, New York: Harper & Brothers, 1944.

Laboratory Findings in Massively Bleeding Gastroduodenal Ulcers

A Review of 2,008 Cases

DONALD D. KOZOLL, MD
AND
KARL A. MEYER, MD
CHICAGO

We have previously reported on general factors influencing the incidence and mortality of 1,904 patients admitted to the Cook County Hospital with a proved acute perforation of a gastroduodenal ulcer [1] and of 2,008 ulcer patients admitted to the same hospital for massively bleeding gastroduodenal ulcer.[2] In other publications [3,4] we commented on the signs and symptoms which influenced the prognosis of both of these two groups of patients and upon the laboratory findings in acute perforated gastroduodenal ulcer.[5] In this paper, we wish to report the laboratory findings of the 2,008 ulcer patients treated for massive bleeding between 1936 and 1955.

Only those cases were accepted whose history gave overt evidence of copious intestinal bleeding and which showed radiologic, gastroscopic, operative, or necropsy evidence of a peptic lesion of the stomach or duodenum. We defined massive hemorrhage as: (1) a reduction of blood volume by one third or more (ie, a hemoglobin of less than 60% or 9 gm per 100 ml, erythrocyte counts of less than 3,000,000/cu mm, or a hematocrit of less than 30%); (2) the presence of clinical shock; (3) the need for multiple blood transfusions to forestall or correct the reduced blood volume or shock. Besides the 2,008 cases qualifying under this definition, 541 additional cases could be classified as "moder-

Submitted for publication June 1, 1963.

From the Departments of Surgery of the Cook County Hospital, Northwestern University Medical School, and the Cook County Graduate School of Medicine.

Supported by a grant-in-aid from the Jerome D. Solomon Memorial Research Foundation and the Hektoen Institute for Medical Research of the Cook County Hospital.

TABLE 1.—*Laboratory Procedures Performed in the Stated Number of Cases of a Possible 2,008*

Test	No. Cases	Test	No. Cases
Erythrocyte count	1,826	γ-Globulin	469
Hemoglobin	1,899	Icteric index	475
Hematocrit	452	Cephalin flocculation	103
Leukocyte count	1,818	Cholesterol	333
Sedimentation rate	81	Thymol turbidity	354
Kahn serology test	1,492	Alkaline phosphatase	444
Blood grouping	576	Serum amylase	59
Fasting blood sugar	110	Urinalysis	1,396
Nonprotein nitrogen	1,426	Stool benzidine	1,553
Creatinine	569	Gastric analysis	667
CO_2 combining power	327	Chest x-ray	851
Serum chloride	627	Gastrointestinal x-ray	1,496
Serum potassium	361	Gallbladder x-ray	131
Serum sodium	389	Colon x-ray	483
Phosphorus	304	Gastroscopy	285
Serum total protein	1,022	Proctoscopy	119
Serum albumin	434	Electrocardiograph	445

ate bleeders" because their blood loss was of lesser degree: these were referred to for comparison.

The survey method has been described before.[1] The laboratory data included here are the results of procedures performed by interns on the ward, in the routine biochemical laboratory, or in the x-ray department. They were standard procedures and consisted of the determinations made in the stated number of cases out of a possible 2,008 cases, as shown in Table 1. All results were evaluated as "below normal values," "normal," and "above normal values," depending upon the test in question.

Present Study

Erythrocyte Count.—The incidence of anemia in patients with active gastroduodenal bleeding from peptic ulcer is indicated in Table 2. Using our arbitrary criteria of 3,000,000 red blood cells per cubic millimeter as the level of significant blood loss, the incidence of anemia occurred slightly more often with bleeding gastric ulcers than with duodenal. The incidence of red cell counts of less than 3,000,000/cu mm was 71.61% in gastric cases and 63.40% in duodenal cases. Those with erythrocyte counts less than 3,000,000/cu mm did not have significantly greater mortality rates than those above this level. Even patients with less than 2,000,000 cells per cubic millimeter did not have significantly higher mortality rates. In contrast to this, patients with bleeding duodenal ulcers with more than 4,500,000 cells per cubic millimeter showed a higher mortality rate; hemoconcentration was noted less often with gastric lesions. Mitty et al [6] were unable to correlate the mortality rate of 421 cases of bleeding ulcer with the degree of anemia or the presence or absence of shock. They explain their unexpected finding with the ready use of blood transfusions. Levy et al [7] found a greater mortality as the red blood cell count decreased and that the mortality rate was almost twice as high among patients with gastric bleeding. Gilchrist and Chun [8] in reporting a study of 140 cases of peptic ulcer found that mortality could not be correlated to changes in the erythrocyte count.

Hemoglobin.—The incidence of anemia was higher by this test than with the erythrocyte count: 78.69% of gastric and 75.34% of duodenal cases had hemoglobin levels of less than 60% (9.0 gm per 100 cc). Mortality rates at this abnormal hemoglobin level were not significantly different from those at normal hemoglobin levels, but cases with hemoglobin values in excess of 80% (on the basis of 100% being 15 mg per 100 ml) had significantly higher mortality rates (Fig 1).

Hematocrit.—Hematocrit data presented in Table 2 was collected in the last eight years

TABLE 2.—*Hematologic and Serologic Tests*

	Gastric				Duodenal			
	No. Cases Determined	% Cases Determined	No. Deaths	% Mortality	No. Cases Determined	% Cases Determined	No. Deaths	% Mortality
Erythrocytes (per cu mm)	553	100.0	146	26.4	1,273	100.0	151	11.8
<3 million	396	71.61	110	27.8	807	63.40	104	12.9
3-4.5 "	151	27.31	35	23.1	435	34.17	39	8.95
>4.5 "	6	1.08	1	16.6	31	2.43	8	25.9
Hemoglobin (100 % = 15 mg/100 ml)	577	100.0	157	27.2	1,322	100.0	166	12.5
<60 %	454	78.69	115	25.4	996	75.34	116	11.6
60 %-100 %	119	20.62	40	33.6	319	24.12	46	14.4
>100 %	4	0.69	2	50.0	7	0.54	5	71.5
Hematocrit (%)	134	100.0	51	38.1	318	100.0	43	13.6
<30	96	71.64	36	37.5	219	68.91	33	15.0
30-45	33	24.63	12	36.4	94	29.54	9	9.55
>45	5	3.73	3	60.0	5	1.55	1	20.0
Leukocytes (thousands per cu mm)	556	100.0	146	36.2	1,262	100.0	157	12.4
<5.0	24	4.32	3	12.5	61	4.86	6	9.84
5.0-15.0	449	80.75	108	24.10	1,079	85.48	116	10.75
>15.0	83	14.93	35	42.10	122	9.66	35	28.7
Sedimentation rate (mm/hr)	28	100.0	9	32.10	53	100.0	7	13.2
<15	10	35.72	2	20.0	23	43.39	1	4.35
15-30	13	46.43	3	23.2	18	33.96	3	16.6
>30	5	17.85	4	80.0	12	22.65	3	25.0
Kahn test	439	100.0	121	27.7	1,053	100.0	112	10.7
Neg	407	92.71	107	26.29	997	94.68	106	10.63
+ to +++	17	3.87	8	47.2	39	3.70	4	10.3
++++	15	3.42	6	40.0	17	1.62	2	11.76
Blood group	70	100.0	17	24.3	506	100.0	56	11.1
O	38	54.28	9	24.8	315	62.25	26	8.25
A	26	37.15	7	26.9	121	23.90	24	19.7
B	6	8.57	1	16.66	55	10.88	6	10.9
AB	0	0	0	0	15	2.97	0	0

Fig 1.—Influence of hemoglobin upon prognosis of massively bleeding gastroduodenal ulcer. Approximately three fourths of the cases showed some evidence of anemia; ie, a hemoglobin level 60% or less. There was no correlation between the degree of anemia and the mortality rate; this may have been influenced by early transfusion. Patients with hemoglobin levels in excess of 80% had a far less favorable prognosis.

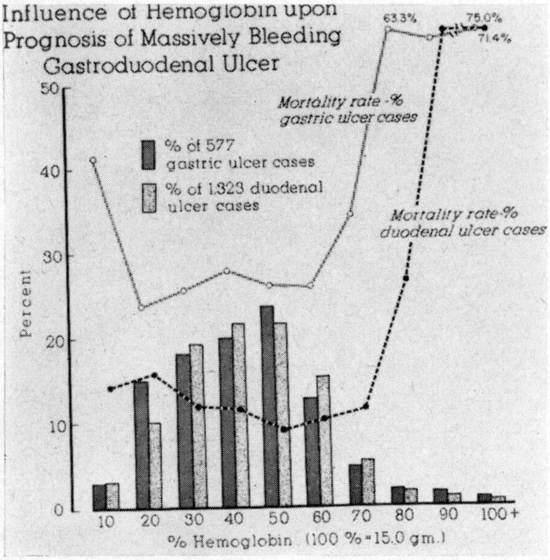

of the study because these determinations were not done routinely in this hospital until 1948. The results were much the same as with erythrocyte or hemoglobin determinations: The majority had hematocrits below 30%, but their mortality rates were not significantly different from those with hematocrits between 30% and 45%. Those patients with hematocrits above 45% showed an increased mortality, especially gastric cases.

From and Shapiro [10] and Saltzstein et al [11] indicated that a hematocrit taken on admission or shortly after hematemesis may be normal or an unreliable indication of the extent of the bleeding in an ulcer patient, because hemodilution is not apparent.

The fact that patients with anemia showed a mortality rate as low as those with normal hematologic data, and better than those with evidence of hemoconcentration, provokes some speculation. These determinations were all performed upon capillary or venous blood, both admittedly having the ability to show the compensatory signs of peripheral vasoconstriction. Dye or isotope techniques were not routinely available for these patients, and would probably not be too reliable in patients in shock.[11] The other possibility exists that these admitting values were not as low as they might have dropped to had hemodilution been allowed to occur before treatment. In an earlier report from this institution by Sullens et al,[12] a grave prognosis was always reported in proportion to the degree of anemia. This report referred to clinical cases having less access to blood transfusions. It is highly probable that the patients with laboratory confirmation of anemia were treated more vigorously with transfusions than those without it, and particularly those with hemoconcentration. The surgical experience reported from Western Reserve University 20 years ago indicated that "normal" may represent hemoconcentration in an acutely bleeding subject. Their patients who were overtly bleeding and were given at least 2,000 cc of blood during gastric resection had a lower operative mortality than those who had "normal" admitting erythrocyte counts and were transfused less.

The determination of the hemoglobin (or erythrocyte count) is of limited prognostic value during the first 48 or 72 hours after hemorrhage because of the phenomenon of hemodilution. This may take anywhere from three hours to several days with an average of 32 hours (Ivy [9]). Thus a declining hemoglobin during this time may mean continued hemorrhage or movement of fluid into the extracellular vascular compartment to maintain an effective circulatory volume. Rate of hemodilution is further influenced by preexisting anemia, dehydration, and recurrence of bleeding. Red cell regeneration does not reach maximal efficiency for approximately 30 days. The same is true of hematocrit or blood volume determinations.

Leukocyte Count.—Most patients had normal leukocyte counts. The incidence of leukocytosis (in excess of 15,000/cu mm) was 14.93% in gastric cases and 9.66% in duodenal cases, and both had significantly higher mortality rates (Table 2). In fact, the relationship of the leukocyte count to the mortality rate appears to be almost a linear one (Fig 2). Leukocytosis was not as great

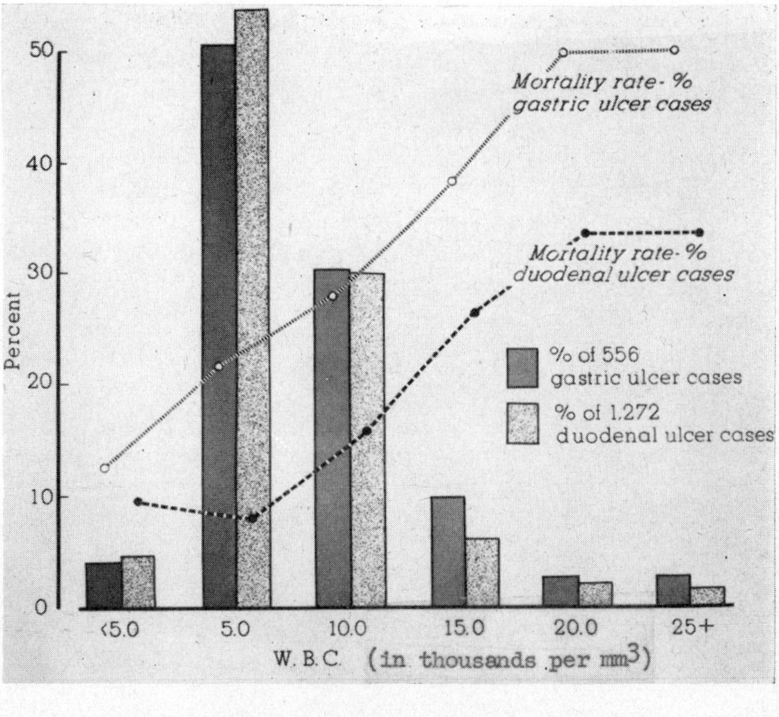

Fig 2.—Influence of WBC on prognosis of massively bleeding gastroduodenal ulcer. A direct relationship existed between the leukocyte count and the mortality rate. The incidence of white blood cell counts in excess of 15,000 per cubic millimeter was 14.9% for cases of gastric hemorrhage and 9.6% for cases of duodenal hemorrhage; this is lower than the incidence of shock noted for the same group of patients, which is the usual explanation for the occurrence of the leukocytosis.

in cases of moderately bleeding gastroduodenal ulcer, but the effect upon the mortality rate was equally unfavorable.

Hoffman[13] reports that an elevated white blood cell count is characteristic of massively bleeding peptic ulcer. From and Shapiro[10] add that this cell count rises early (to about 12,000) and shifts to the left. Harrell and Wilson[14] report that in a series of eight patients, the white blood cell count rose in seven, with a correspondingly high polymorphonuclear leukocytosis. The incidence of leukocytosis after hemorrhage is the same when bleeding is due to ulcer or other causes than ulcer. Schiff et al[15] showed that 65% of 145 patients had leukocyte counts greater than 10,000, some rising to 25,000. The oral administration of citrated blood was not followed by a leukocytosis. The white blood cell count returns to normal in three or four days. This supports the concept that the leukocytosis in patients with hemorrhage is due to the associated shock. Leukocytosis has been identified with other forms of shock as well. However, the incidence of shock in these patients was higher than the incidence of leukocytosis.

Sedimentation Rate.—Though this test was performed in a rather limited series of patients with gastroduodenal bleeding ulcer, it is interesting that those with increased sedimentation rates in excess of normal (30 mm per hour) did show an increased mortality rate. The sedimentation rate increase here is undoubtedly related to the anemia. Hoffman[13] notes that an elevated sedimentation rate is another of the characteristics of a massively bleeding peptic ulcer patient's clinical picture, but he makes no comparisons.

Kahn Serology Test.—Although from 5% to 7% of patients having this test had a positive serology report, the exact significance of the increased mortality rate of the gastric cases with 1+ to 4+ serology reports is not apparent. Rothman[16] reports a nonfatal case of duodenal ulcer of syphilitic origin.

Blood Groups.—Record of the patient's blood group did not appear in the chart of the clinical record; however, through the cooperation of the hospital's blood bank records, the blood group of 576 patients were tallied (Table 2). There is an abnormally high percentage of patients in group O and an abnormally low percentage of patients in group A and AB; the difference is even more striking with duodenal ulcer patients. Our values are similar to those of Aird et al.[17] Snyder and Berne,[18] in a study of 232 peptic ulcer patients from Los Angeles County General Hospital, noted that there was a disproportionately high percentage of patients with duodenal ulcer who had blood type O. In patients with gastric carcinoma, atrophic gastritis, and pernicious anemia the predominance was in group A. Shay and Sun[19] state that an association between group O and duodenal ulcer has received confirmation in every country in which it has been studied. In the case of gastric ulcers, there are conflicting reports. Clarke et al[20] found higher amounts of ABH substances in patients with duodenal ulcer than with controls; they also observed the same high incidence of group O in nonaffected siblings.[21] Evans[22] reported the incidence of group O to be even higher in stomal ulcer than it is in duodenal ulcer.

The Rh factor was determined in 394 patients with massively bleeding duodenal ulcers. It was positive in 89.5% and negative in 10.5%. There were too few gastric cases with such data to evaluate.

Fasting Blood Sugar.—Hyperglycemia (Table 3) was seen in more than half of the 110 patients studied but can be explained when one realizes that the request is often made for patients showing glycosuria or having diabetes. Both Ingegno[23] and Christiansen[24] report hyperglycemia with massive hemorrhage.

Nonprotein Nitrogen.—Azotemia (nonprotein nitrogen in excess of 40mg%) was found in 60.3% of gastric and 52.5% of duodenal cases tested, with moderate increases in the mortality rate. Increases in the NPN up to 60 mg% occurred as often in 335 cases of moderate hemorrhage as in the cases of massive hemorrhage. However, NPN in excess of 60 mg% occurred twice as often with

TABLE 3.—*Blood Chemistry Tests*

	Gastric				Duodenal			
	No. Cases Determined	% Cases Determined	No. Deaths	% Mortality	No. Cases Determined	% Cases Determined	No. Deaths	% Mortality
Fasting blood sugar (mg %)	38	100.0	19	50.0	72	100.0	13	18.1
<80	7	18.42	3	42.86	2	2.78	0	0
80-120	12	31.58	9	75.0	31	43.05	5	16.13
>120	19	50.0	7	36.84	39	54.17	8	20.51
Nonprotein nitrogen (mg %)	445	100.0	133	29.8	981	100.0	126	12.8
<40	177	39.7	35	19.7	467	47.5	28	6.0
>40	268	60.3	98	36.6	514	52.5	98	19.1
Creatinine (mg %)	201	100.0	76	37.7	368	100.0	73	19.8
<2	131	65.1	41	31.3	225	62.4	23	10.0
>2	70	34.9	35	50.0	143	37.6	50	36.2
CO_2 combining power (vol %)	113	100.0	44	39.0	214	100.0	48	22.4
<49	60	53.10	25	41.7	112	52.34	27	24.1
50-70	48	42.47	16	33.3	88	41.12	16	18.1
>70	5	4.43	3	60.0	14	6.54	5	35.7
Serum chloride (mEq/liter)	215	100.0	69	32.1	412	100.0	69	16.7
<100	106	49.31	30	29.8	173	41.99	28	15.6
100-109	86	40.0	29	33.7	189	45.87	28	14.8
>110	23	10.69	10	43.5	50	12.14	13	26.0
Serum sodium (mEq/liter)	126	100.0	49	38.8	263	100.0	41	15.6
<130	11	8.73	4	36.36	29	11.03	9	32.2
130-140	79	62.7	24	30.38	177	67.30	17	9.6
>140	36	28.57	21	58.3	57	21.67	15	26.3
Potassium (mEq/liter)	118	100.0	45	38.1	243	100.0	36	14.7
<3.5	22	18.6	10	45.5	33	13.58	9	27.4
3.5-5.9	91	77.17	31	34.1	206	84.78	26	12.6
>6	5	4.23	4	80.0	4	1.64	1	25.0
Phosphorus (mg %)	94	100.0	39	41.4	210	100.0	34	16.5
<3	12	12.76	8	66.6	28	13.33	6	21.2
3-5.0	67	71.28	24	35.8	158	75.24	21	13.3
>5.0	15	15.96	7	46.6	24	11.43	7	29.1

massive hemorrhage as with moderate hemorrhage with a most adverse effect upon the mortality rate (Table 4). The mortality rate rose progressively with increasing azotemia and was usually higher for gastric than for duodenal ulcer (Fig 3).

Bockus[25] identified the easy digestion and absorption of globin as the source of the alimentary hyperazotemia; several experimenters produced the syndrome by intragastric administration of whole blood. This produced a greater rise in urea nitrogen than introducing whole blood directly into the ileum or colon but less than in clinical subjects.[26-30] Both Bockus[25] and Schiff and Stevens[31] attributed great reliability to the degree of azotemia as a measure of the degree of hemorrhage, particularly in the absence of vomiting, dehydration, shock, renal or hepatic disease; in fact, if the

TABLE 4.—*Comparison of Incidence and Mortality of Azotemia in Massive and Moderate Gastroduodenal Ulcer Hemorrhage*

	Gastric				Duodenal			
	No. Cases Determined	% Cases Determined	No. Deaths	% Mortality	No. Cases Determined	% Cases Determined	No. Deaths	% Mortality
Massive hemorrhage								
NPN <30	177	39.7	35	19.1	467	47.5	28	6.0
" 40-60	175	39.3	51	29.1	248	35.4	37	10.6
" >60	93	21.0	47	50.5	166	17.1	61	36.7
Moderate hemorrhage								
NPN <30	37	49.3	2	5.4	138	53.0	3	2.7
" 40-60	30	40.0	3	10.0	96	36.9	8	8.3
" >60	8	10.7	3	37.8	26	10.1	4	15.3

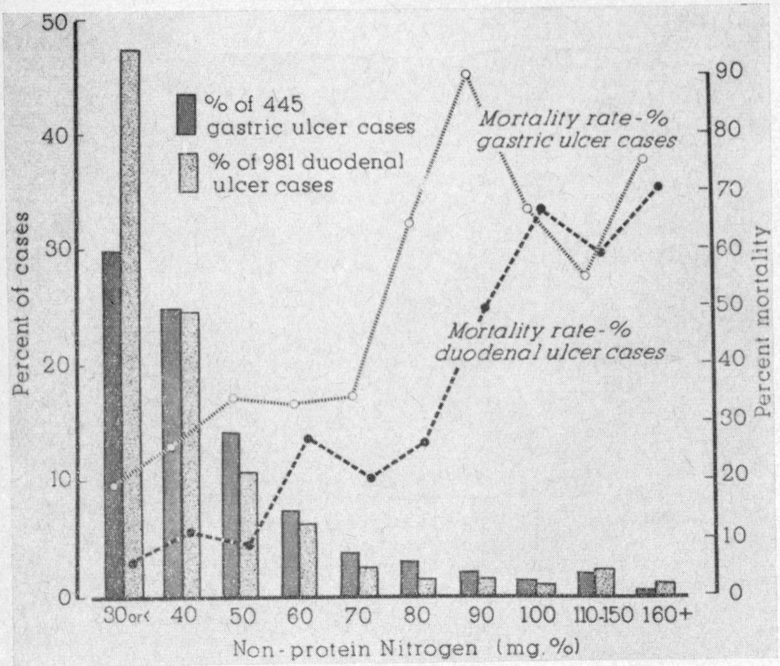

Fig 3.—Influence of NPN upon prognosis of massively bleeding gastroduodenal ulcer. The occurrence of azotemia bore a direct relationship to the mortality rate. This rate did not exceed the average until the nonprotein nitrogen rose to levels in excess of 70 mg per 100 cc. The incidence of abnormally elevated creatinine levels in the blood was less but the effect upon mortality rates more grave.

azotemia persisted more than three or four days after cessation of hemorrhage, they suspected renal disease. This extrarenal hyperazotemia produces no renal parenchymal lesion nor is it necessarily associated with disturbances in electrolyte or acid-base balance. Schiff et al[31] cited two cases in which an elevation in blood urea manifested itself before melena.

The value of urea retention as a measure of degree and activity of bleeding has been seriously challenged.[32] Our experience has been that it indicated extreme degrees of hemorrhage, that it occurred more often in aged patients, and that it usually took more than 72 or 96 hours for the nitrogen levels to return to normal.

Schiff et al[31] noted a 64% mortality rate in patients with urea nitrogen above 100 mg%, 33% died with urea nitrogen between 50 and 70 mg per 100 cc, and 3.7% died with urea nitrogen less than 50 mg%.

Sullens et al[12] found a 100% mortality rate in bleeding ulcer cases with nonprotein nitrogen greater than 100 mg%, 12.5% for NPN between 50 and 100 mg%, and 2.6% for NPN less than 50 mg%.

According to Borst,[33] hemorrhage which is severe enough to produce shock will always be associated with decreased urine output, decreased excretion of urea in the urine, urea elevation in the blood, and decreased urea clearance. Dehydration, by production of oliguria and anuria, predisposes to azotemia. Bogoch[34] states that a urea nitrogen greater than 50 mg% usually indicated a prerenal or actual renal involvement.

Creatinine.—The incidence of abnormally elevated creatinine (above 2.0 mg%) was significantly less than the incidence of azotemia, but it carried with it a higher mortality rate than did azotemia in bleeding patients (Table 3). This is to be expected in patients with extrarenal azotemia, for the creatinine rises only with the more extreme degrees of nitrogen retention. Patients with moderate hemorrhage had almost as high an incidence of creatinemia with comparable effects upon the mortality rate. Creatinemia in patients with perforated ulcer was not quite as frequent but produced an even worse prognosis.

CO_2 Combining Power.—Acidosis occurred more often than alkalosis (Table 3), about half as frequently with moderate hemorrhage. Alkalosis occurred just as often with moderate hemorrhage with just as un-

favorable prognosis as with massive hemorrhage.

Serum Chloride.—Hypochloremia occurred less frequently with hemorrhaging ulcers than with perforating ulcers [5]; however, the effect upon mortality rate was more serious in the case of perforation. Hyperchloremia occurred significantly more often with hemorrhage than with perforation, although the mortality rate with this complication was higher with perforation. Bockus [25] considered the occurrence of hypochloremia in massive hemorrhage, in the absence or presence of azotemia, to be due to emesis associated with gastric retention.

Borst [33] concluded that the renal threshold for chloride excretion was increased in massive hemorrhage, rather than a renal lesion. This explains the decreased urinary excretion of chloride whereas the blood chloride remains undisturbed. If acute renal failure should ensue to the point of oliguria or anuria, then a hyponatremia, hypochloremia, and lowered CO_2 together with a hyperkalemia and increased azotemia may be anticipated.

Serum Sodium.—The test for this component has not been available as long as the test for serum chloride. The incidence of hyponatremia was less than hypernatremia (Table 3). In the case of gastric hemorrhage, hyponatremia was tolerated better; with duodenal hemorrhage both sodium derangements were equally unfavorable. The experience with perforated ulcer was much the same.

Serum Potassium.—Hypokalemia occurred much more frequently than hyperkalemia; the effect of hyperkalemia with gastric bleeding was worse than the effect of hypokalemia. Potassium derangements occurred less often with duodenal hemorrhage and led to smaller increases in mortality rate (Table 3). The experience with perforated ulcer was similar. Borst [33] found increased excretion of potassium in urine with normal or somewhat reduced blood values.

Serum Phosphorus.—Disturbances in serum phosphorus appear more frequently in ulcer patients than is generally understood. Although the series of phosphorus determinations is greater in this series of bleeding patients than in an earlier series of patients who were undergoing perforation, the percentile incidence of phosphorus derangements was higher in the perforation series

TABLE 5.—*Liver Function Tests*

	Gastric				Duodenal			
	No. Cases Determined	% Cases Determined	No. Deaths	% Mortality	No. Cases Determined	% Cases Determined	No. Deaths	% Mortality
Total protein (gm %)	318	100.0	95	29.8	704	100.0	94	13.4
<6	156	49.0	49	31.4	310	44.0	46	14.8
6-7.5	150	47.3	44	29.3	370	52.6	47	12.7
>7.5	12	3.7	2	16.6	24	3.4	1	4.1
Serum albumin (gm %)	167	100.0	51	30.3	367	100.0	54	14.7
<3	33	19.76	15	45.5	65	17.72	19	29.3
3-4	105	62.88	30	28.7	202	55.04	26	12.9
>4	29	17.36	6	20.7	100	27.24	9	9.0
γ-globulin (gm %)	135	100.0	45	33.3	334	100.0	35	10.5
<1.0	40	29.63	12	30.0	89	26.65	8	8.08
1-2	74	55.96	24	34.0	155	46.41	20	12.9
>2	21	14.41	9	43.1	90	26.94	7	7.8
Cephalin	40	100.0	17	42.5	63	100.0	20	31.7
0	9	22.5	1	11.11	—	—	—	—
1+	13	32.5	4	30.77	15	23.81	3	20.0
2+	9	22.5	4	44.44	25	39.68	12	48.0
3+	4	10.0	3	75.0	14	22.22	1	7.14
4+	5	12.5	5	100.0	9	14.29	4	44.44
Cholesterol (mg %)	100	100.0	37	37.0	223	100.0	31	13.9
<150	28	28.0	10	35.7	35	15.02	5	14.8
150-250	60	60.0	22	36.7	141	64.80	18	12.7
>250	12	12.0	5	41.7	47	20.18	8	17.1

and the effect upon mortality rate more deleterious. Wight et al[35] observed phosphorus depletion in postperforation patients and phosphorus elevation in patients with pyloric obstruction.

Serum Protein.—Serum total proteins were abnormally low (less than 6.0 gm%) in 49.0% of gastric cases and 44.0% of duodenal cases (Table 5). Although this would appear to be a remarkable incidence, the influence upon mortality rate was not manifest until the level of total protein fell below 4.0 gm% (Fig 4). This phenomenon may represent hemodilution rather than protein deficiency; early transfusions could easily restore these levels to normal. This incidence was considerably less in ulcer patients who bled moderately. Patients with serum total proteins in excess of 7.5 gm% showed mortality rates considerably lower than average. The incidence of hyperproteinemia was higher in patients with perforated ulcer. The favorable influence of hyperproteinemia would appear to be related to dehydration as its cause and to the ability of the patient to respond to appropriate treatment.

Hypoalbuminemia (serum albumin less than 3.0 gm%) was seen less often than hypoproteinemia and exercised a less deleterious effect than in the case of perforation. Patients with serum albumin more than 3.0 gm% experienced average or lower than average mortality rates. Bockus[25] stressed this biochemical complication as a therapeutic indication for blood plasma infusions. Bogoch[34] describes a transitory rise in plasma proteins as the result of the liver's effort to rid itself of the increased ammonia from the breakdown of blood. He found the determination of blood proteins of no value in estimating the degree of hemorrhage. The determination of serum albumin may reveal an undetected cirrhosis or state of malnutrition preceding the bleeding.

Hypoglobulinemia was seen in slightly less than 10% of patients with average or lower than average mortality rates. Hyperglobulinemia (more than 2.5 mg%) was seen in almost one fourth of those determined, and in these there was a moderate increase in mortality. Borst[33] found that plasma globulin concentration fell soon after hemorrhage, with a rise to levels even above normal a few days later.

γ-Globulin determinations in this series were made in patients with gastric bleeding, who showed some increased mortality, regardless of the level of γ-globulin. The patients with duodenal ulcer bleeding showed a lower than average mortality rate, regardless of the level of γ-globulin.

Icteric Index.—As is indicated in Fig 5, somewhat more than three fourths of the 475

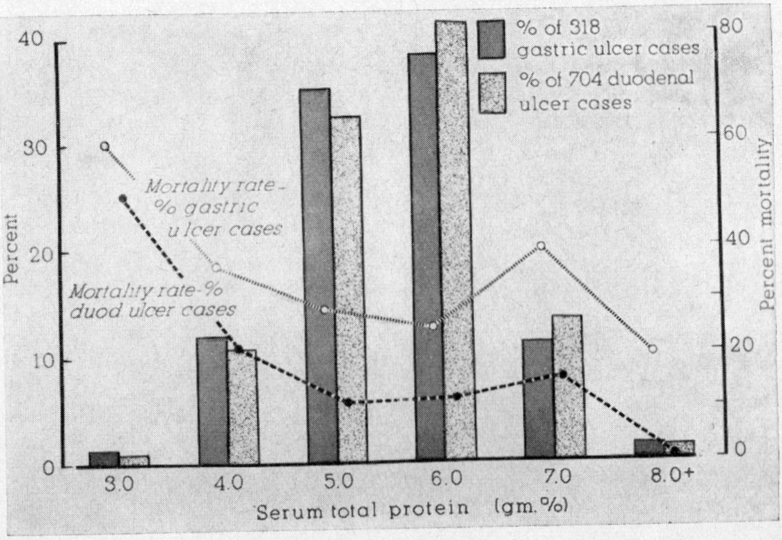

Fig 4.—Influence of serum total protein upon prognosis of massively bleeding gastroduodenal ulcer. Forty-nine per cent of patients with gastric ulcer hemorrhage and 44.0% of those with duodenal ulcer hemorrhage showed serum protein levels of less than 6.0 gm% (hypoproteinemia). This exercised remarkably little effect upon the mortality rate until the level of total protein fell below 4.0 gm%. This phenomenon may well represent hemodilution rather than actual protein deficiency and hence a dramatic response with blood transfusions.

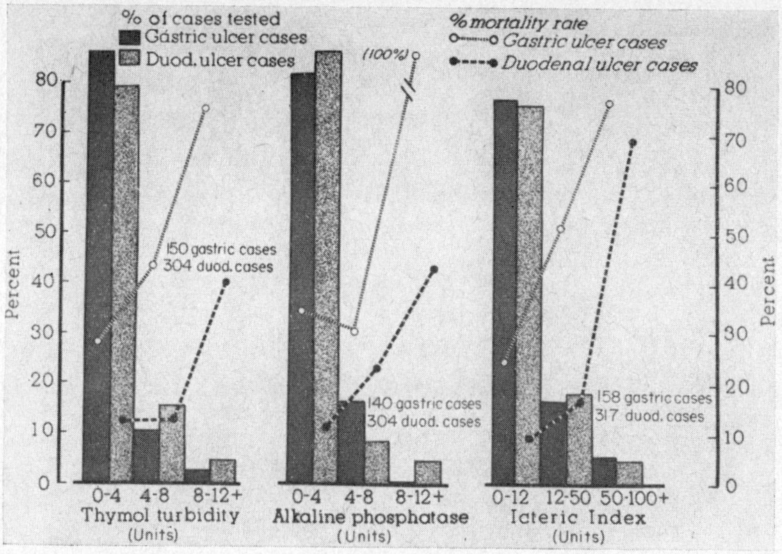

Fig 5.—Influence of liver function upon prognosis of massively bleeding gastroduodenal ulcer. Approximately 25% of patients with massive hemorrhage had an elevation of the icteric index above 12 clinical units; this was associated with an increased mortality rate. Approximately 20% of patients in whom thymol turbidity or alkaline phosphatase tests were done showed abnormal elevations with similar effect upon mortality rates.

patients tested had icteric indices below 12 units, with mortality rates that were average or lower. The remaining patients with elevated indices showed marked increases in mortality rate, which was higher in cases of gastric ulcer. The same trend of the icteric indices was seen in the case of perforated ulcer. Bockus [25] acknowledges the occurrence of slight icterus and, more frequently, slight hyperbilirubinemia as the result of increased reticuloendothelial breakdown of absorbed blood pigment.

Cephalin Flocculation.—Patients with gastric ulcer bleeding showed a close correlation between the degree of flocculation and the mortality rate (Table 5). Patients with duodenal ulcer bleeding showed increased mortality rates which were not as closely correlated with the degree of flocculation.

Cholesterol.—Twelve per cent of patients with gastric ulcer bleeding and 20% of patients with duodenal ulcer bleeding had serum total cholesterols above 250 mg%. Although there was some elevation of mortality rate above that for the entire series, it probably is not significant (Table 5).

Thymol Turbidity.—More than 80% of 454 patients with gastroduodenal bleeding tested had thymol turbidity levels of less than 4 units (normal). The mortality rate at this level was average. Patients with gastric ulcer bleeding showed striking increases in mortality with increases in thymol turbidity (Fig 5). Patients with duodenal ulcer bleeding did not show such increases in mortality rate until the thymol turbidity exceeded 8 units.

Alkaline Phosphatase.—The results were almost identical to thymol turbidity (Fig 5) except that at the level of 4 to 8 Bodansky units, the mortality rate of the patients with duodenal ulcer bleeding rose and that of the gastric cases did not.

Serum and Urine Amylase.—The presence of this pancreatic enzyme has been noted in increased amounts in the serum and urine of patients with perforated ulcer. In 59 patients with gastroduodenal ulcer bleeding tested, there was not a single instance of elevation of this enzyme in the serum. In 12 such patients, having urine amylase determinations, one patient had 256 units; this one case did not have clinical evidence of pancreatitis or perforation. In all other cases, it was considered normal.

Urinalysis.—The range of specific gravity of the urine of patients bleeding from peptic ulcers was quite normal; this is in contrast to patients with perforation who demonstrated a greater frequency of urinary concentration. The gastric bleeding cases with urine specific gravities in excess of 1.025 showed significant increases in mortality rate, whereas comparable duodenal cases did not

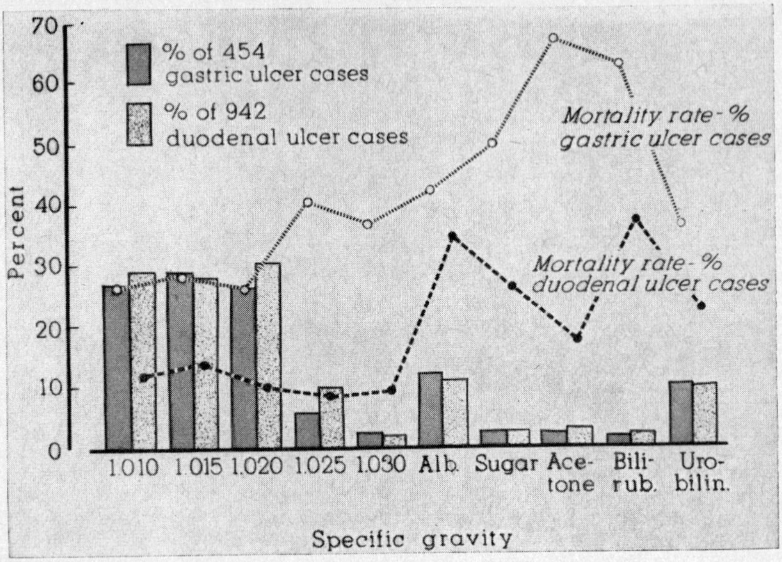

Fig 6.—Urinalysis in 1,396 patients with massively bleeding gastroduodenal ulcer. Except for the cases of gastric hemorrhage, urine specific gravity offered little prognostic value. All patients showing albumin, sugar, acetone, or bile pigments in the urine were associated with increased risk of a fatality.

TABLE 6.—*Stool, X-Ray, and Electrocardiographic Tests*

	Gastric				Duodenal			
	No. Cases Determined	% Cases Determined	No. Deaths	% Mortality	No. Cases Determined	% Cases Determined	No. Deaths	% Mortality
Stool benzidine	452	100.0	120	26.5	1,101	100.0	128	11.6
1+	20	4.43	2	10.0	51	4.63	5	9.8
2+	23	5.09	3	13.04	50	4.55	6	12.0
3+	19	4.2	2	10.53	38	3.44	6	15.79
4+	390	86.28	113	28.97	962	87.38	111	11.54
Chest x-ray	265	100.0	62	23.4	586	100.0	55	9.4
Normal	175	66.1	29	16.5	427	72.6	24	5.6
Pulmonary path.	59	22.1	23	38.9	94	16.0	17	18.1
Cardiac "	31	11.8	10	32.3	65	11.4	14	21.5
Gastrointestinal x-rays *	411	100.0	53	12.9	1,085	100.0	67	6.17
Normal	47	11.43	6	12.8	125	11.52	17	13.6
Gastric ulcer	327	79.5	42	12.9	72	6.63	7	9.7
Gastric deformity	21	5.11	2	9.5	4	0.36	0	0
Gastric niche & incisura	218	52.55	22	9.65	18	1.66	2	11.1
Retention	31	6.7	3	9.7	38	3.60	2	5.3
Additional gastric ulcers	19	4.6	2	10.5	3	0.28	0	0
Ca	66	16.06	10	15.2	14	1.29	2	14.2
Duod. deformity	57	13.86	7	12.3	808	74.47	37	4.6
Duod. crater	5	1.22	0	0	103	9.49	2	1.94
Duod. niche &/or incisura	12	2.92	3	25.0	198	18.26	8	4.02
Duod. diverticulum	12	2.92	2	16.66	49	4.52	5	10.2
Duod. obstruction	1	0.24	0	0	13	1.20	0	0
Colon x-rays	139	100.0	18	13.1	344	100.0	18	5.25
Normal	111	79.86	12	10.81	281	81.69	13	4.63
Diverticuli	16	11.51	3	18.9	36	10.46	3	8.35
Miscellaneous	12	8.68	3	25.0	27	7.85	2	7.4
Gallbladder x-ray	26	100.0	1	3.84	106	100.0	9	8.4
Normal	17	65.4	0	0	75	71.43	6	8.0
Nonvisualization	9	34.6	1	11.1	23	21.95	4	17.4
Calculi	—	—	—	—	8	7.62	1	12.5
EKG	146	100.0	47	32.2	299	100.0	44	14.7
Normal	40	27.39	8	20.0	97	32.4	10	10.31
Arrhythmias	17	11.64	8	47.0	43	15.05	8	18.6
Myocardial disease	31	21.23	9	29.03	41	13.71	8	19.51
Coronary disease	3	2.05	2	66.66	10	3.34	5	50.0
Cardiac enlargement	18	12.32	6	33.33	35	11.69	8	22.9
Abnormal tracing	46	31.51	16	34.8	97	32.34	10	10.31
Low voltage	5	3.42	1	20.0	5	1.67	1	20.0

* Many cases have multiple x-ray findings, which will, therefore, exceed the total number.

(Fig 6). Patients with moderate hemorrhage showed a higher incidence of urinary specific gravities in excess of 1.025, without concomitant increases in mortality rates.

The incidence of albuminuria in bleeding patients was less than in perforating patients; this was also true of glycosuria and acetonuria. However, their mortality rates were of comparable magnitude (Fig 6). The incidence of bilirubin and urobilinogen in the urine is noted in Fig 6; the latter is higher in incidence but exercised less of an effect upon the mortality rate. Hematuria and pyuria were present in a small percentage of cases but demonstrated a more serious prognosis in the gastric than in the duodenal cases.

Stool Examination.—The results of gross examination of the stool of these patients was described in a report preceding this one [4]; 85.5% of gastric and 96.9% of duodenal bleeders show overt evidence of tarry stools. Bright red blood was seen in 10.0% and 15.1%, respectively, of gastric and duodenal cases. The results of the chemical examination of the stool of the majority of these patients are listed in Table 6. More than 85% were 4+ in a grading of 0 to 4+, the latter being maximal. The incidence of 4+ benzidene-positive stools ran 70% in those classified as moderate hemorrhage. There was no correlation between the degree of positive response and the mortality rates.

Gastric Analysis.—This was determined in approximately one third of patients upon cessation of active bleeding according to the methods listed in Fig 7. Achlorhydria was present in 18.0% of gastric and 10.7% of duodenal cases; in patients with moderate hemorrhage achlorhydria occurred less frequently. Hypochlorhydria (up to 20 units of free acid) occurred in 22.3% and 19.5%, respectively, of gastric and duodenal cases; free acid values between 20 and 40 units were found in an almost identical percentage of patients. In 21.8% of gastric and 27.8% of duodenal cases the free acidity varied from 40 to 70 units; 30.7% and 33.3%, respectively, of patients with moderate bleeding from gastric and duodenal ulcer had this same range of acidity. Free acid in excess of 70 units was detected in 12.8% and 22.2% of gastric and duodenal cases, respectively; this degree of acidity was detected in 15.3% and 22.4%, respectively, of moderate gastric and moderate duodenal bleeders. Thus, the incidence of achlorhydria and hypochlorhydria was lower in patients with both

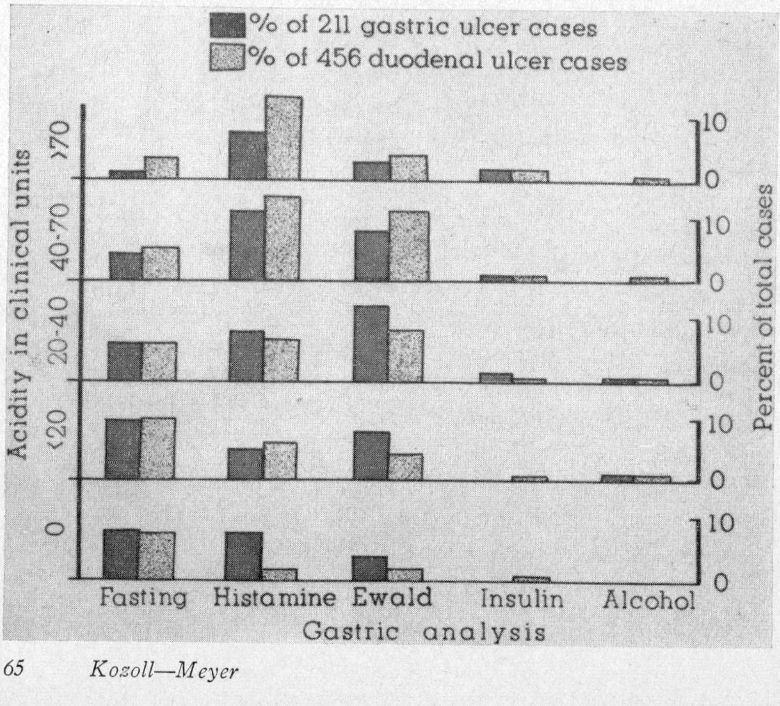

Fig 7.—Gastric analysis in patients with massively bleeding gastroduodenal ulcer. The incidence of achlorhydria and hypochlorhydria was greater in patients with gastric ulcer hemorrhage. The incidence of hyperchlorhydria was greater in patients with duodenal ulcer hemorrhage.

massive and moderate hemorrhage due to gastric rather than duodenal ulcer. Conversely, the incidence of hyperacidity was greater in patients with duodenal lesions. Patients with moderate hemorrhage showed a relatively higher frequency of hyperacidity. The response to histamine stimulation was the best indicator of hypersecretory tendencies.

Chandler and Watkinson (quoted by Bogoch[34]) carried out hourly aspirations of gastric content in patients with acute or chronically bleeding ulcer. They found that 57 of 68 such patients bleeding from duodenal ulcers had nocturnal hyperacidity; 26 of 33 patients with bleeding gastric ulcer had a normal nocturnal acidity; 69 of 78 patients bleeding from acute peptic ulcers (site unspecified) had a hypochlorhydria.

Chest X-Ray.—Routine chest films were taken in approximately 42% of these patients with massive bleeding. In the group of 265 gastric cases, 66.1% of the films were read as normal, 22.1% showed pulmonary pathology, and 11.8% reported cardiac pathology. The mortality rate of those patients with cardiopulmonary pathology was significantly greater (Table 6). In the group of 586 duodenal cases, 72.6% were considered normal, 16.0% were reported to show pulmonary pathology, and 11.4% showed cardiac pathology. Again, the patients with cardiopulmonary findings experienced significantly higher mortality rates (Table 6).

Gastrointestinal X-Ray.—Such studies were taken upon cessation of hemorrhage in approximately three fourths of all patients. In 79.5% of gastric cases studied, a gastric ulcer was diagnosed by x-ray; a second gastric ulcer was found in 4.6%, and a duodenal deformity or crater in addition to a gastric ulcer was found in 15.0%. Other roentgen findings are listed in Table 6.

Of the 1,085 cases of duodenal ulcer hemorrhage, a duodenal deformity was recognized in 74.4% and a crater in 9.49%. A gastric ulcer in addition to the bleeding duodenal ulcer was reported in 6.6%. In duodenal cases, as well as gastric, the roentgen findings bore no relationship to the mortality rate; in fact, the lower than average rates indicated that these studies were carried out principally in the better risk patients.

Gallbladder X-Ray.—These studies were carried out in a very small percentage of cases. The incidence of pathological gallbladders indicated in Table 6 is possibly not out of proportion to the age group studied.

Colon X-Ray.—These studies were available in one fourth of the patients. Approximately 80% of barium enemas were reported as normal, and slightly over 10% had diverticuli (Table 6).

Gastroscopy.—This was carried out in 144 cases of gastric ulcer bleeding of massive amount and a gastric ulcer identified in 67.5%, gastritis in 25.8%, and malignancy misdiagnosed in 13.5%. Of 141 similar duodenal cases gastroscoped, gastritis was the principal finding in 46.8%, an additional gastric ulcer in 14.9%, an erroneous diagnosis of neoplasm in 2.1%.

Proctoscopy.—This examination was done in 38 of the cases of gastric and 81 of the cases of duodenal bleeding. In more than half, the examination was normal. External and internal hemorrhoids were the next most frequent report. Adenocarcinoma (as an incidental finding) was found in one case each of gastric and duodenal ulcer, and polyps in two cases of each group. An ulcerative colitis was recognized in a case of gastric bleeding and an amebic colitis in one case of duodenal bleeding.

Electrocardiograph.—Tracings were taken more frequently than in an earlier series of perforated peptic ulcer patients,[5] and as a result the incidence of abnormal tracings and the resultant mortality rates were not as great as that reported for perforating ulcer patients. The data for the bleeding patients is listed in Table 6.

Craver and Glenn[36] cite an earlier study by Rasmussen and Foss, who noted T wave depression and even lowered ST segments, but others[7,8] do not mention this. Various other authors have mentioned cardiac complications among ulcer patients.

Summary

Approximately three fourths of 2,008 patients with massive bleeding peptic ulcer showed laboratory evidence of anemia; hemoglobin determinations were more sensitive than erythrocyte counts. Hemoconcentration had an even more unfavorable prognosis upon mortality rate than anemia, although occurring much less frequently.

In patients with bleeding gastric and duodenal ulcer, respectively, 14.9% and 9.6% showed evidence of leukocytosis in excess of 15,000 WBC per cubic millimeter. This was associated with a significantly higher mortality rate. This phenomenon is supposed to be related to the occurrence of shock; however, the incidence of shock in this group of patients was greater than the incidence of leukocytosis.

A significantly higher incidence of group O blood type was found in our records of 576 patients with massive gastroduodenal hemorrhage due to ulcer, with a proportionate decrease in groups A and AB; the difference is even more striking with duodenal ulcer than gastric. The Rh factor was positive in 89.5% and negative in 10.5%.

Hyperglycemia was noted in more than half of 110 patients with massive hemorrhage tested.

More than half of cases tested proved to have azotemia; its effect upon mortality was related to its degree. The incidence of excess creatinemia was less, but the effect upon mortality rate was more grave.

Derangements of serum electrolytes occurred less often in this group of patients with massively bleeding ulcers than in a comparable group of patients with acute perforating ulcers. Acidosis occurred more frequently in this group of patients than alkalosis; the effect of the latter was more adverse. A significant incidence of phosphorus depletion was seen.

Serum total proteins less than 6 gm% were found in 49% and 44% of gastric and duodenal ulcer patients, respectively, but had no significant effect upon mortality rate until the level declined below 5.0 gm%. Hypoalbuminemia occurred less often and affected the mortality rates less. A significant percentage of these bleeding patients had derangements of standard liver function tests with unfavorable effects upon mortality rates.

The incidence of achlorhydria and hypochlorhydria was greater in patients with bleeding due to gastric ulcer; the incidence of hyperchlorhydria was greater in patients with bleeding due to duodenal ulcer.

Radiologic studies taken upon cessation of hemorrhage revealed the bleeding ulcer site in more than 75% of cases so studied. Other incidental roentgenographic studies were not particularly rewarding.

A significant incidence of abnormal electrocardiograms was found in patients of this series and is probably related to the degree of anemia and shock.

Donald D. Kozoll, MD, Cook County Hospital, 1825 W Harrison St, Chicago 12, Ill.

REFERENCES

1. Kozoll, D. D., and Meyer, K. A.: General Factors Influencing the Incidence and Mortality of Acute Perforated Gastroduodenal Ulcers, Surg Gynec Obstet 111:607-625, 1960.
2. Kozoll, D. D., and Meyer, K. A.: General Factors Influencing the Incidence and Mortality of Massively Bleeding Gastroduodenal Ulcers, Arch Surg 86:445, 1963.
3. Kozoll, D. D., and Meyer, K. A.: Symptoms and Signs in the Prognosis of Gastroduodenal Ulcers: An Analysis of 1,904 Cases of Acute Perforated Gastroduodenal Ulcer, Arch Surg 82:528-544, 1961.
4. Kozoll, D. D., and Meyer, K. A.: Symptoms and Signs in the Prognosis of Massively Bleeding Gastroduodenal Ulcer, Amer J Surg, accepted for publication, November, 1962.
5. Kozoll, D. D., and Meyer, K. A.: Laboratory Findings in Acute Perforated Gastroduodenal Ulcers, Arch Surg 84:646, 1962.
6. Mitty, W. F.; Breen, W. F. J.; Wallace, R.; and Grace, W. J.: Factors Influencing Mortality in Bleeding Peptic Ulcer: II. The Occurrence of Massive Hemorrhage, Amer J Dig Dis 6:395, 1961.
7. Levy, J. S.; Hardin, J. H.; Juniper, K., Jr.; and Thomas, P. O.: Problems in the Management of Bleeding Peptic Ulcer, Southern Med J 50:759-763, 1957.
8. Gilchrist, R. K., and Chun, N.: Severe Hemorrhage in Presumed Peptic Ulcer, AMA Arch Surg 69:366-377, 1954.

9. Ivy, A. C.; Grossman, M. I.; and Bachrach, W. H.: Peptic Ulcer, Philadelphia: The Blakiston Company, 1950.

10. From, P., and Shapiro, S. W.: Current Concepts in the Management of Bleeding Peptic Ulcer, J Iowa Med Soc 47:367-371 (July) 1957.

11. Saltzstein, H. C.; Mahlin, M. S.; and Scheinberg, S. R.: Bleeding Peptic Ulcer, AMA Arch Surg 67:29-42, 1953.

12. Sullens, W. E.; Steigmann, F.; and Meyer, K. A.: Surgical Considerations in Hemorrhage of the Upper Part of the Gastrointestinal Tract, Arch Surg 59:1244, 1949.

13. Hoffman, E.: Peptic Ulcer With Massive Hemorrhage in the Upper Age Groups, J Amer Geriat Soc 6:324-335, 1958.

14. Harrell, W. B., and Wilson, R. O.: Ruptured Peptic Ulcer Among US Troops in Panama, Milit Surg 96:336-342, 1945.

15. Schiff, L.; Shapiro, N.; and Stevens, R. J.: Observations on the Oral Administration of Citrated Blood in Man: III. The Effect on Temperature and the White Blood Cell Count, Amer J Med Sci 207:465, 1944.

16. Rothman, J.: Massive Hemorrhage From Apparent Syphilitic Gastritis, Med Bull Veterans Admin 18:92-94, 1941.

17. Aird, I.; Bentall, H. H.; Mehigan, I. A.; and Roberts, J. A. F.: The Blood Groups in Relation to Peptic Ulceration and Carcinoma of Colon, Rectum, Breast and Bronchus: Association Between ABO Groups and Peptic Ulceration, Brit Med J 2:315, 1934.

18. Snyder, E. N., Jr., and Berne, C. J.: Management of Massive Hemorrhage From Peptic Ulcer, Amer J Surg 94:368-376, 1957.

19. Shay, H., and Sun, D. C. H.: Chap 24 in Bockus, H. L.: Gastroenterology, ed 2, Philadelphia: W. B. Saunders Company, 1963, vol 1.

20. Clarke, C. A.; Cowan, W. K.; Edwards, J. W.; Howel-Evans, A. W.; McConnell, R. B.; Woodrow, J. C.; and Sheppard, P. M.: The Relationship of the ABO Blood Groups to Duodenal and Gastric Ulceration, Brit Med J 2:643, 1955.

21. Clarke, C. A.; Edwards, J. W.; Haddock, D. R. W.; Howel-Evans, A. W.; McConnell, R. B.; and Sheppard, P. M.: ABO Blood Groups and Secretor Character in Duodenal Ulcer: Population and Sibship Studies, Brit Med J 2:725, 1956.

22. Evans, D. A. P.: Genetic Factors in the Etiology of Duodenal Ulcer, Gastroenterology 40: 371, 1961.

23. Ingegno, A. P.: The Elevated Blood Urea of Acute Gastrointestinal Hemorrhage and Its Significance, Amer J Med Sci 190:770, 1935.

24. Christiansen, T.: The Biochemical Changes in the Organism Produced by Massive Intraintestinal Hemorrhage, Rev Gastroenterol 4:166, 1937.

25. Bockus, H. L.: Gastroenterology, Philadelphia: W. B. Saunders Company, 1943, vol 1.

26. Chunn, C. F., and Harkins, H. N.: Experimental Studies on Alimentary Azotemia: I. The Role of Blood Absorption From the Gastrointestinal Tract, Surgery 9:695, 1941.

27. Schiff, L.; Stevens, R. J.; Goodman, S.; and Garber, E.: Observations on the Oral Administration of Citrated Blood in Man, Amer J Dig Dis 6:597, 1939.

28. Harkins, H. N., and Chunn, C. F.: Experimental Studies on Alimentary Azotemia: II. The Relative Importance of the Plasma and Erythrocyte Fractions of Absorbed Blood, Surgery 10:991, 1941.

29. Greenblatt, I. J., and Cohn, T. D.: Azotemia in Gastrointestinal Bleeding, Amer J Med Sci 221: 565, 1946.

30. Chunn, C. F.; Harkins, H. N.; and Boals, R. T.: Experimental Studies in Alimentary Azotemia: III. Site of Blood Absorption, Surgery 11:56, 1942.

31. Schiff, L.; Stevens, R. J.; Moss, H. K.; and Garber, E. S.: The Prognostic Significance of the Blood Urea Nitrogen Following Hematemesis or Melena, Amer J Dig Dis 9:110, 1942.

32. Murphy, R. T., and Marshall, E. A.: Bleeding Peptic Ulcer: A Review of 200 Consecutive Cases, Amer J Gastroent 37:283-294, 1962.

33. Borst, J. G. G.: The Cause of Hyperchloremia and Hyperazotemia in Patients With Recurrent Massive Hemorrhage From Peptic Ulcer, Acta Med Scand 97:68, 1938.

34. Bogoch, A.: Hematemesis and Melena, chap 28 in Bockus, H. L.: Gastroenterology, ed 2, Philadelphia: W. B. Saunders Company, 1963, vol 1.

35. Wight, A.; Hopkirk, J. F.; Demuydler, E.; and Cope, O.: Metabolic Derangements Imperiling the Perforated Ulcer Patient: II. Derangements and Shifts of Intracellular Electrolytes; The Need for Potassium, Arch Surg 71:839, 1955.

36. Craver, W. C., and Glenn, F.: Massive Hemorrhage From Peptic Ulcer: A Cause of Myocardial Infarction in the Aged, J Amer Geriat Soc 5:969-981, 1957.

Prognosis of Aortic Stenosis

Special Reference to Indications for Operative Treatment

JUN TAKEDA, MD; RICHARD WARREN, MD; AND DANIEL HOLZMAN, MD, WEST ROXBURY, MASS

Introduction

The growth of heart surgery has imposed on surgeons the responsibility of defining the indications for operation in the various disease entities that are being considered for surgical relief. Since the operations for acquired heart disease are as yet seldom without risk or known to be permanently curative, indications for operation in individual cases must be set against the background of the natural history of the particular disease.

Review of the Literature

In aortic stenosis, much study has been concentrated on the clinical course of the disease under nonsurgical treatment. In reviewing articles dealing with the subject, it is important to divide the cases reported into two groups: (1) those with pure aortic stenosis in which all complicating cardiac lesions except an insignificant degree of aortic insufficiency are excluded, and (2) aortic stenosis complicated with significant degrees of aortic insufficiency or with other heart lesions.

Table 1 summarizes the average age at death of patients with aortic stenosis as collected from a few selected reports. According to these reports and a few others,[1,5,13] death in pure aortic stenosis seems to occur on the average in the early part of the seventh decade. If the stenosis is complicated by significant insufficiency, it falls in the sixth decade. If associated with mitral valve disease, death tends to occur in the fifth decade. Furthermore, the prognosis of aortic stenosis seems to relate roughly to symptoms in the following way. On analyzing and combining the same reports for more information, it was found that the average interval from onset of symptoms to death was 4.7 years (range 1 month to 20 years); that angina pectoris (a symptom present in 50% to 80% of patients) carried a prognosis 3.5 to 6 years from onset to death, dyspnea on exertion (present in 50% to 80%) a prognosis of 2 to 3.5 years until death, and syncope (present in less than 50%) a prognosis that, though short, was less well defined (nine months to three years). Heart failure as evidenced by pulmonary edema or orthopnea carried a prognosis of less than two years from onset to death. Kennedy[12] noticed that some patients lived a long time even when they had severe angina or effort syncope, but once signs of left heart failure occurred, the prognosis was extremely poor.

Anderson[1] states that the natural history of calcific aortic stenosis is the insidious undermining of left ventricular functional reserve until symptoms of circulatory failure developed. The course may be relatively benign when the obstruction is less than critical, but at a certain point it becomes malignant, leading to irreversible congestive heart failure or sudden death unless relief of the obstruction can be accomplished.

An attempt has been made by a few authors to measure prognosis against such factors as the intensity of the murmur or the transvalvular pressure gradient. Cosby et al[7] and Mitchell et al[13] both showed that no correlation could be developed. They tried to establish some relationship between the hemodynamic severity of aortic stenosis and the prognosis but failed because of the lack of a clinical or pathological yardstick other than cardiac catheterization for measuring

Submitted for publication June 3, 1963.

West Roxbury Veterans Administration Hospital and Boston Veterans Administration Hospital.

This study was supported in part by training grant HTS-5291 from the National Institutes of Health.

TABLE 1.—*Aortic Stenosis: Mean Age at Death in Years*

	Anderson (1) *	Clawson (4)	Clawson (5)	Contratto (6)	Mitchell (13)
Pure aortic stenosis	63.5	55.8	60-69		65.3
Aortic stenosis with insufficiency				50-59	52.3
Aortic stenosis with mitral valve disease					48.4

* Parentheses indicate reference numbers.

severity. Left heart catheterization has not been done widely enough in this disease for a sufficient length of time to have produced the needed sequential information on gradients or measured valve areas.

Purpose of Study

This study was undertaken to examine the prognosis of aortic stenosis in our institutions in the hope that a review of these patients would give us firsthand information which, when combined with that from the literature, would enable us to make the best possible decisions when asked to consider patients for operation. Although the patients in VA hospitals, being all adult male, are affected more often with aortic stenosis than a group where the sexes are mixed, the disease itself was not expected to have a prognosis that differs greatly from the accepted one.

Materials and Method

Between 1948 and 1959, sixty-five patients were admitted to the Boston and West Roxbury Veterans Administration Hospitals with the diagnosis of pure aortic stenosis. It has already been mentioned that "pure" aortic stenosis means stenosis without additional cardiac lesions other than insignificant aortic insufficiency. For this series, the above definition has, for convenience, been further amplified by including patients with coronary disease, as indicated by electrocardiographic findings of myocardial ischemia or by coronary artery stenosis on coronary angiogram. This was done because when the cases were first studied there seemed little difference in prognosis between those with and those without coronary disease, with a few prominent exceptions that will be mentioned. Because angina pectoris is such a common symptom in aortic stenosis without abnormalities of the coronary arteries, its presence without the above evidence was not sufficient to place a patient in the coronary disease group. During the period, 17 additional patients who would otherwise have fallen under the criteria for study were operated upon for correction of aortic stenosis and have been excluded. In only one of the 65 patients was the aortic lesion suspected of being congenital in origin. In 64 the lesion was acquired.

The medical records of the patients were studied and appropriate data tabulated. Particular attention was paid to the symptoms of chest pain, syncope, dyspnea, and signs of heart failure. Criteria for diagnosis of heart failure were a history of paroxysmal nocturnal dyspnea, orthopnea, peripheral edema, or pulmonary edema, or, in the rare case that underwent cardiac catheterization, an elevated end-diastolic pressure in the left ventricle. All patients who could be traced were followed for at least three years or until death. The longest follow-up was 20 years from the onset of symptoms. Follow-up information was obtained on 60 (92.3%) of the 65 patients. The living patients were personally examined. Of the deaths, the cause was identified in 90%. It could not be determined in 10%.

Results

A. *Total Group (60 Patients)*.—1. Age Distribution (Table 2): The average age of patients on the first admission to the hospital was 57.4 years (range 29-88 years). The average age at time of diagnosis of heart dis-

TABLE 2.—*Aortic Stenosis: Age Distribution According to Diagnosis, First Symptom, and First Hospital Admission*

Age	1st Admission	1st Diagnosis of Heart Disease	1st Symptom
10-19	0	0	1
20-29	1	9	2
30-39	7	7	6
40-49	4	8	5
50-59	19	19	24
60-69	26	14	19
70-79	2	2	2
80-89	1	1	1
Total	60	60	60
Mean age, yr	57.4	48.8	54.4

TABLE 3.—*Aortic Stenosis: Mortality*

Total patients	60
Living	10
Dead	50
Age at death (mean)	62.5 yr

ease was 48.8 years (range 20-86 years), and the age at onset of symptoms was 54.5 years (range 17-90 years).

2. Mortality (Table 3): Fifty (82.3%) of the 60 patients had died by the time of follow-up. The average age at death was 62.5 years.

3. Symptoms (Table 4): Thirty-seven (61.6%) of the 60 patients suffered from angina pectoris. Seven of them are living and 30 are dead. Sixteen (26.6%) of the 60 suffered from attacks of syncope. Four of them are living and 12 are dead. Syncope here is defined as a sudden episode of "blackout" or "grayout" unrelated to posture or known cause other than aortic stenosis. Forty-five (75.6%) of the 60 suffered from dyspnea on exertion. Forty-two (70%) of the 60 patients had a history of cardiac failure. Four of these are still living, 38 are dead.

4. Age at Onset of Symptoms: As has been stated, the average age at onset of any symptoms was 54.5 years. The average age at onset of angina was 53.8 years, of syncope

TABLE 4.—*Aortic Stenosis: Incidence of Symptoms*

Symptom	Total Series (60 Patients) No.	%
Angina	37	61.6
Syncope	16	26.6
Dyspnea on exertion	45	75.0
Heart failure	42	70.0

53.5 years, of dyspnea on exertion 57.4 years, and of heart failure 59.2 years. In 37 (61.7%) of the patients, dyspnea on exertion was the first symptom. In 18 (30%) it was angina, in 3 (5%) it was syncope, and in 2 (3.3%) it was peripheral edema.

5. Durations of Symptoms Prior to Death (Table 5): The average duration of life from the onset of anginal pain to death was 4.4 years, of syncope attack 3.8 years, of dyspnea on exertion 3.7 years, and of heart failure 2.8 years. The average duration of life from the onset of symptoms of any kind was 4.7 years.

6. Cause of Death (Table 6): In 30 of 50 cases death took place in the hospital. Sixteen had autopsies performed. Of the remaining 20, the cause of death was determined by medical clinical diagnosis or reports from laymen in 15; in five it was undetermined. Heart failure was the most common cause of death (46%). Cerebral vascular accident comprised 14% and myocardial infarction 12%. It is of interest that death was "sudden" in only three (6%).

TABLE 5.—*Aortic Stenosis: Prognosis in Relation to Symptoms*

	No. of Patients	Interval From Onset to Death or Follow-Up, Yr: Mean	Range
Angina			
Dead	29	4.4	1-9
Living	8	13.0	6-22
Syncope			
Dead	11	3.8	½-7
Living	5	12.0	9-15
Dyspnea on exertion			
Dead	41	3.7	1 mo-20
Living	4	11.5	4-16
Heart failure			
Dead	38	2.8	2 wk-7
Living	4	11.7	3-13
Symptoms of any kind			
Dead	50	4.7	1 mo-20
Living	10	13.1	4-12

TABLE 6.—*Aortic Stenosis: Cause of Death*

	Total Deaths (%)	Hospital Deaths Diagnosis Clear
Heart failure	23 (46)	17
Cerebral vascular accident	7 (14)	6
Myocardial infarction	6 (12)	2
Postoperative death *	2 (4)	2
Sudden death	3 (6)	
Subacute bacterial endocarditis	2 (4)	2
Pulmonary disease	2 (4)	1
Unknown	5 (10)	
Total	50 (100)	

* Noncardiac operation.

Since aortic stenosis has long been reputed to be a cause of "sudden" death, it is profitable to define what is meant by the term. As we use it here we mean a patient who, when in a status that allows him to be up and around and in no significant distress, suddenly drops dead. The term "unexpected" death seems almost more appropriate. We should differentiate between the patient who drops dead due to sudden cerebral or myocardial insufficiency without previous symptoms and the one who does this after symptoms have been present. This matter is of importance in determining the indications for and the urgency of surgical correction once the diagnosis has been made. We saw no patients who died suddenly in the absence of previous symptoms. The three sudden deaths in our series had had a history of heart failure extending back for three, three, and seven years, respectively. Summaries of them follow.

CASE 1.—The patient was 53 years old at time of death. Twenty years previously he was told he had a "leaky valve." Four years previously dyspnea on exertion proceeded within one year to paroxysmal nocturnal dyspnea for which he was treated in the hospital. Two and a half years previously recurrence took place and did so repeatedly every four months until he suddenly died three years after the first symptom of heart failure.

CASE 2.—This man was 44 years old at time of death. Thirty-five years previously he had rheumatic fever, nine years previously a heart murmur, seven years previously fainting spells, three years previously dyspnea on exertion, and three years previously a left heart catheterization which showed a gradient of 90 mm Hg across the aortic valve and a left ventricular end-diastolic pressure of 14 mm Hg. For the next three years his symptoms were mild on light work until he died suddenly at work at noontime, three years after the diagnosis of heart failure was made at cardiac catheterization.

CASE 3.—This patient was 66 years old at time of death. He had a history of rheumatic fever in childhood; 33 years previously a heart murmur was heard; seven years previously he developed shortness of breath which progressed rapidly to orthopnea and peripheral edema. Over the next seven years he developed angina which was alleviated by medical thyroidectomy with radioactive iodine, but orthopnea and peripheral edema returned intermittently until sudden death occurred seven years after the first diagnosis of cardiac decompensation.

It is thus seen that in those patients who died suddenly, congestive failure had been first recognized prior to death for a longer period than the mean prognosis for life after the onset of heart failure (2.8 years). It is true that five of the 17 patients dying with heart failure did so in their first attack and were therefore eliminated from the possibility of sudden death at a later date. It is of interest that only one of these patients was among the 16 in this series who had had previous attacks of syncope. Five of the patients who died of myocardial infarction or of cerebral vascular accident had had cardiac failure for an average of two years prior to death. Another point of some interest to examine was the duration of the final episodes leading to death. In the patients with cardiac failure the duration of the terminal episode from the onset of failure until death averaged three months (range four days to two years). In those dying from a cerebral vascular accident it was ten days (range 1 to 30 days) and in those dying of myocardial infarction one day.

B. *The Influence of Coronary Disease* (Table 7).—Comparison of 16 patients who had associated coronary disease and 44 patients without coronary disease showed there to be no difference between these two groups except that the mortality in the group without coronary disease was slightly lower (79%) than in the group with it (93%). Predictably, the incidence and duration of angina in the coronary disease group were

TABLE 7.—*Aortic Stenosis: Comparison of the Group With Coronary Disease With That Without Coronary Disease*

	Without Coronary Disease	With Coronary Disease
Total No. of patients	44	16
No. of living patients	9 (21) *	1 (7)
No. of deaths	35 (79)	15 (93)
Mean interval, onset of any symptom to death (yr)	4.3	6.0
Angina		
Incidence	26 (59)	11 (68.8)
Mean duration to death (yr)	3.3	5.2
Mean age at onset (yr)	53.4	57.5

* Parentheses indicate %.

greater (68.8%, 5.25 years) than in the non-coronary disease group (59%, 3.3 years), but the differences were extraordinarily slight.

C. The Influence of Age.—Comparison of the younger group (age at onset of symptoms under 45 years) with the older group (onset at age 45 or over) showed no difference between the two except in two respects: (1) Survival rate was higher (45.5%, or five of the 11 patients) in the younger group than in the older group (10%, or five of 49 patients). (2) The prevalence of these three symptoms was higher but their duration was shorter in the younger group. These differences were not due to a disparity in the mean follow-up periods which were almost the same for both groups (younger group 4.4 years; older group 4.0 years).

Comment

In considering the mean duration of life following the onset of symptoms we have focused principally on those 50 patients who have died. This figure is 4.7 years, quite similar to that culled from the literature (4.3 years). Similarly, the prognosis from onset of individual symptoms until death was not unlike the experience of others. For angina it was slightly over four years both in our group and in those collected from the literature. For syncope it was slightly over three years in the literature, slightly under it in our group. For dyspnea on exertion it was slightly under three years in the literature, slightly over in our group. For cardiac failure, the prognosis was under two years in the experience of others, somewhat longer in our series. Death usually occurred in the seventh decade in the experience of others as well as in our own (mean age 62.5 years). In our series the occurrence of sudden or unexpected death was very low—only three out of 50 deaths, and those three patients had had a history of cardiac failure for at least three years prior to death. This excludes six deaths due to myocardial infarction, all in patients with known coronary disease who died on an average of 24 hours after onset of the attack. Thus the fear of sudden death in the patient who has not had heart failure or coronary disease is small.

The question arises as to whether we have derived from these results useful criteria concerning the timing of operation. Of the 42 patients presenting themselves with heart failure only 17 died of it, but five of these did so in the first attack. On the other hand four are still living at least three years after the first evidence of failure. These living cases were not calculated into the mean figure for prognosis following onset of failure of 2.8 years, which was derived from the dead cases only. The true figure for prognosis should therefore be larger. In the present state of development of operations for aortic stenosis it seems reasonable to state that in the asymptomatic patient it is permissible to postpone operation until symptoms appear, that after they appear one has in the majority of cases about two to four years before failure develops, and after failure develops, the majority of patients will be dead in another three years. Some will live longer, but about 15% will not survive the first attack of failure.

Obviously we must not oversimplify the problem by setting up the onset of heart failure as the earliest sign suggesting the need for operation. The operative mortality under such a policy will be higher than if surgery is undertaken on the appearance of any symptoms. Over-all operative mortalities for pure aortic stenosis in which plastic procedures are employed are now near 10%, and in some hands even those where partial or total valve replacements are done are approaching this low level. It is certain that indications suggested now will be modified soon as techniques continue to improve. Furthermore, little has been said about what the influence on indications might be of the degree of valve narrowing as measured at catheterization, or of the presence of left ventricular strain as assayed by ECG and x-ray. The operative indications for each patient must be individualized against the setting of the surgeon's experience. The information presented merely re-emphasizes the fact that, given no symptoms or mild ones only, there is time to wait for a period until the surgical techniques now available have become even better. Further emphasis is given to the point that when cardiac failure once develops, operation should then be undertaken at the earliest opportunity after a maximal response to medical treatment.

Summary

Sixty-five patients with pure aortic stenosis were admitted to Boston Veterans Administration Hospital and West Roxbury Veterans Administration Hospital between 1948 and 1959.

Sixty of these were followed for at least three years or until death. The mortality was 83%.

The mean prognosis for life following the onset of angina in those that died was 4.4 years, of syncope 3.8 years, of dyspnea on exertion 3.7 years, and of heart failure 2.8 years.

Only three patients died suddenly or unexpectedly; all three had been in heart failure previously.

Inference as to the current indications for surgical relief are drawn.

Richard Warren, MD, Veterans Administration Hospital, Veterans of Foreign Wars Pkwy, West Roxbury 32, Mass.

REFERENCES

1. Anderson, M. W.: The Clinical Course of Patients With Calcific Aortic Stenosis, Proc Mayo Clin 36:439-444, 1961.

2. Baker, C., and Somerville, J.: Clinical Features and Surgical Treatment of 50 Patients With Severe Aortic Stenosis, Guy Hosp Rep 108:101-125, 1959.

3. Bland, E. F., and Jones, T. D.: Rheumatic Fever and Rheumatic Heart Disease: A 20-Year Report on 1,000 Patients Followed Since Childhood, Circulation 4:836-843, 1951.

4. Clawson, B. J.; Bell, E. T.; and Hartzell, T. B.: Valvular Disease of the Heart With Special Reference to the Pathogenesis of Old Valvular Defects, Amer J Path 2:193, 1926.

5. Clawson, B. J.; Noble, J. F.; and Lufkin, N. H.: The Calcified Nodular Deformity of the Aortic Valve, Amer Heart J 15:58-76, 1938.

6. Contratto, A. W., and Levine, S. A.: Aortic Stenosis With Special Reference to Angina Pectoris and Syncope, Ann Intern Med 10:1636-1653, 1937.

7. Cosby, R. S.; Hedge, B.; Amsden, N.; and Mayo, M.: A Critical Review of Aortic Stenosis, Amer J Cardiol 9:203-208, 1962.

8. Edwards, J. E.: Calcific Aortic Stenosis: Pathologic Features, Proc Mayo Clin 36:444-451, 1961.

9. Gardner, F. E., and White, P. D.: Coronary Occlusion and Myocardial Infarction Associated With Chronic Rheumatic Heart Disease, Ann Intern Med 31:1003-1009, 1949.

10. Green, H. D.: The Coronary Blood Flow in Aortic Stenosis, in Aortic Insufficiency and in Arterio-Venous Fistula, Amer J Physiol 115:94-103, 1936.

11. Hufnagel, C. A., and Conrad, P. W.: Calcific Aortic Stenosis, New Eng J Med 266:72-76, 1962.

12. Kennedy, J. H.: Aortic Stenosis: Results of So-Called Conservative Management, Geriatrics 17: 98-102, 1962.

13. Mitchell, A. M.; Sackett, C. H.; Hunzicker, W. J.; and Levine, S. A.: The Clinical Features of Aortic Stenosis, Amer Heart J 48:684-720, 1954.

14. Pfister, C. W.; Plice, S. G.; and Dodsworth, J.: The Co-Existence of Rheumatic Heart Disease and Myocardial Infarction, Dis Chest 37:240-242, 1960.

15. Uricchio, J. F.; Litwak, R.; Denton, C.; Goldberg, H.; and Likoff, W.: A Medical Appraisal of Transaortic Commissurotomy, Ann Intern Med 44:844-860, 1956.

16. Uricchio, J. F.; Sinha, K. P.; Bentivoglio, L.; and Goldberg, H.: A Study of Combined Mitral and Aortic Stenosis, Ann Intern Med 51: 668-678, 1959.

17. Wood, P.: Aortic Stenosis, Amer J Cardiol 1:553-571, 1958.

Major Thermal Burns

A Mortality Appraisal and Review

THOMAS M. JACKSON, MD
AND
WILLIAM H. LEE, JR., MD
MEMPHIS

In the year ending in June, 1959, there were 929,000 individuals who sustained burns serious enough to require medical attention. Of these, 70,000 required hospitalization, and an estimated 11,300 died.[15] An estimated 6,000 hospital beds are constantly occupied by burned patients.

Despite the apparent importance of this problem, progress in the treatment of major thermal burns has failed to keep pace with advances in other areas of medical science. Chemotherapeutic agents have not effectively reduced deaths from sepsis, and improved therapy of acute burn shock has merely prolonged the interval until death in many cases. A slight improvement in the mortality rate of major burns has been reported by some,[2] yet other reports have been less encouraging. Clark and Hanson [6] reported an increase in the mortality rate of major thermal burns at San Francisco City and County Hospital from 40% during 1943-1947 to 69% during 1952-1956. During 1943-1947, a total of 69% of the deaths occurred within 48 hours of admission; during 1952-1956, only 19% of the deaths occurred during the first 48 hours.

The purpose of this study is to review the major burns admitted to John Gaston Hospital in order to classify the causes of morbidity and mortality and to identify problems which are prominently associated with therapeutic failure in major burns.

Materials

During the interval between 1955 to 1960, 629 patients with thermal burns were admitted to John Gaston Hospital, the major City of Memphis Hospital for the treatment of indigent patients, and an affiliated hospital of the University of Tennessee. Two hundred and forty-two of these cases involved burns of 20% or more of the body surface, and 90% of these were flame burns. Because lesser burns do not usually result in prolonged morbidity,

---

Submitted for publication June 15, 1963.

Resident in Surgery (Dr. Jackson) and Assistant Professor of Surgery (Dr. Lee).

Supported in part by the John and Mary R. Markle Foundation (Dr. Lee).

From the Department of Surgery, University of Tennessee School of Medicine.

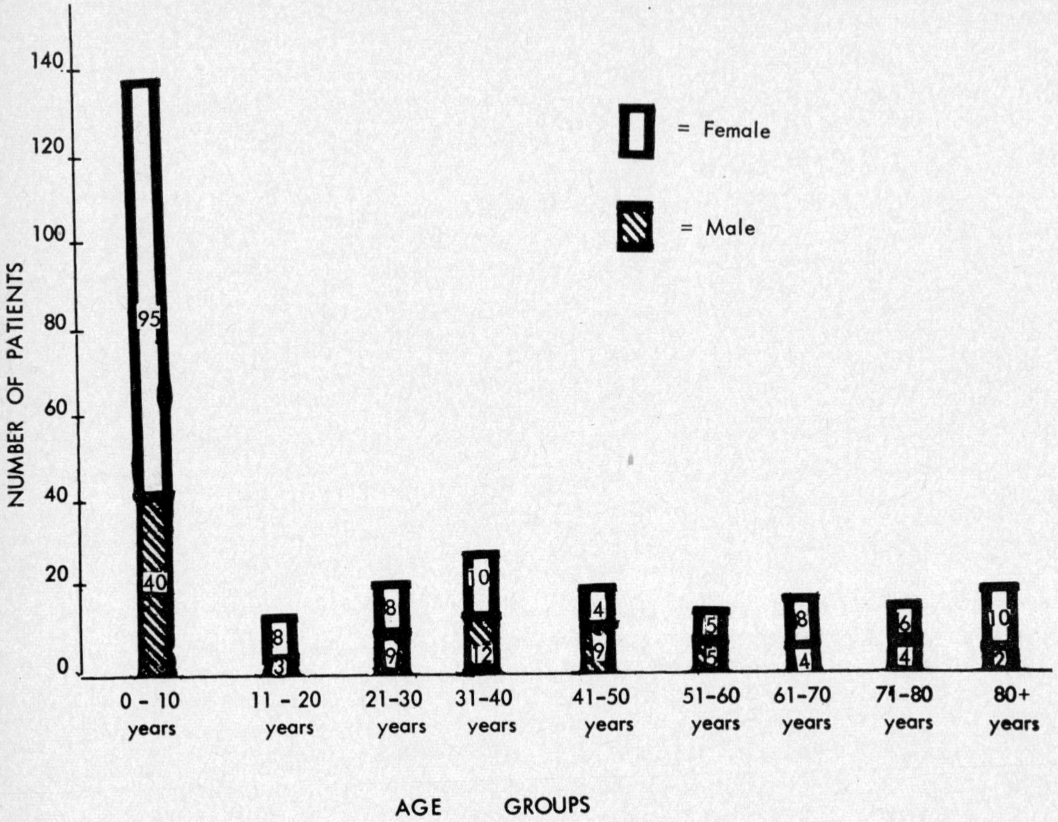

Fig 1.—Age and sex incidence.

or significant mortality, this study is confined to major burns, comprising an analysis of such factors as age, race, sex, etiology, incidence, extent of burn, clinical course, and causes of morbidity and mortality.

Incidence and Distribution

Sixty per cent of these burns occurred in females, most of whom were in the pediatric or geriatric age groups. Fifty-five per cent were children less than ten years of age (Fig 1), with the incidence otherwise distributed almost equally through the other decades. Almost half of the major burns involved only 20% to 30% of the body surface. There was a pronounced seasonal incidence, with 108 of the 242 major burns occurring during the three winter months of December, January, and February. The annual distribution was fairly constant, with a high of 57 admissions in 1957 and a low of 28 in 1956. Negroes, representing the majority of the indigent population in the Mid-South, were involved in 90% of the burns.

Etiology

The typical patient in this series was a small girl whose clothes ignited while standing too close to an open flame heater or "chill-chaser." Almost 40% of the major burns occurred in this manner (Table 1). Another 15% occurred in burning buildings, and about 10% resulted from kerosene explosions. Evaluation of the etiological factors suggests that accident prevention and safety programs have failed to reach those who need it most, eg, the illiterate groups of the lower socioeconomic strata. There is a need to stress a more intensive program of safety and burn prevention, directed to and geared for the attention of these groups, particularly during the winter season when the incidence of "chill-chaser" burn zooms alarmingly.

Table 1.—*Etiology of 242 Major Burns*

	No.
Clothes ignited from open heater or stove	94
Burning house or building	33
Burns from hot liquids	31
Kerosene explosion	19
Miscellaneous or unknown causes	18
Industrial accidents	13
Trash or grass fire	8
Smoking in bed	7
Epileptic or syncope, fell into fire	6
Auto or airplane accidents	5
Attempted murder or suicide	4
Children playing with matches	3
Clothes ignited playing with sparklers	1

Methods of Treatment

The management of burns at John Gaston Hospital, in both adults and children, has been the responsibility of the resident staff under the supervision of the faculty of the Department of Surgery. The general management of the burn cases in this series did not differ greatly from that reported in the recent surgical literature. During most of the study period the Evans formula[8] was used as a guide for fluid and electrolyte therapy during the acute phase of the burn, although other formulas[7,19] were occasionally utilized, depending on the preference of the individual doctors caring for the patient. Since the primary aim in early fluid therapy was the provision of an adequate fluid replacement to combat hypovolemic shock, and to establish stable circulatory and renal hemodynamics, no particular formula was stressed; furthermore, no significant advantage of one burn formula over any other was demonstrated in these cases. However, there has been a definite trend to use much less whole blood during the initial phase of burn treatment, substituting plasma or dextran to provide colloid replacement.

Systemic antibiotics were used during the initial treatment period and altered according to sensitivity studies of bacterial cultures from the wound surface, sputum, and blood stream. All patients received tetanus prophylaxis. Soluble nitrofurazone (Furacin *) fine mesh gauze was used next to the burn surface when dressings were applied; however, the exposure method was preferred when applicable. Tub baths were initiated from the eighth to tenth postburn day and general debridement of the burn eschar initiated. Definitive surgical debridement and skin grafts were usually undertaken by the third or fourth postburn weeks. Homografts were utilized in treating many of the extensive burns, with the usual varying success.

* Produced by Eaton Laboratories.

Classification of Burns

Comparison of data from this study with reports from other hospitals is of limited value because of the chaotic lack of uniformity in format of mortality analysis in the surgical literature.[2,5,10,23] Furthermore, comparison of burn data on the basis of extent of burn alone has little merit since other factors such as distribution and depth of the burn, age, nutrition, and pre-existing disease may be more important, and these vary in each case. A burn classification based on all possible prognostic factors would be valuable in comparison of mortality statistics; however, it would be too complex for practical use. The following classification is simple, and utilizes several important factors related to burn mortality, such as extent *and* depth of burn, presence of significant metabolic problems, and some age factors. Although retrospective, the classification aids *evaluation* of success of burn management.

A. *Type I Burns.*—These (1) are first and second degree burns involving less than 50% of the body surface, (2) have no significant third degree component, (3) cause no challenging metabolic problems and usually do not require parenteral fluid therapy, (4) will not require skin grafts for wound closure, (5) heal with little or no residual scarring, and (6) should have 100% prognosis for recovery.

B. *Type II Burns.*—These (1) are full thickness burns involving less than 20% of the body surface, (2) usually cause no serious metabolic problems, and rarely require parenteral fluid therapy, (3) require skin grafts for closure of wound, (4) can be treated in many cases by immediate excision

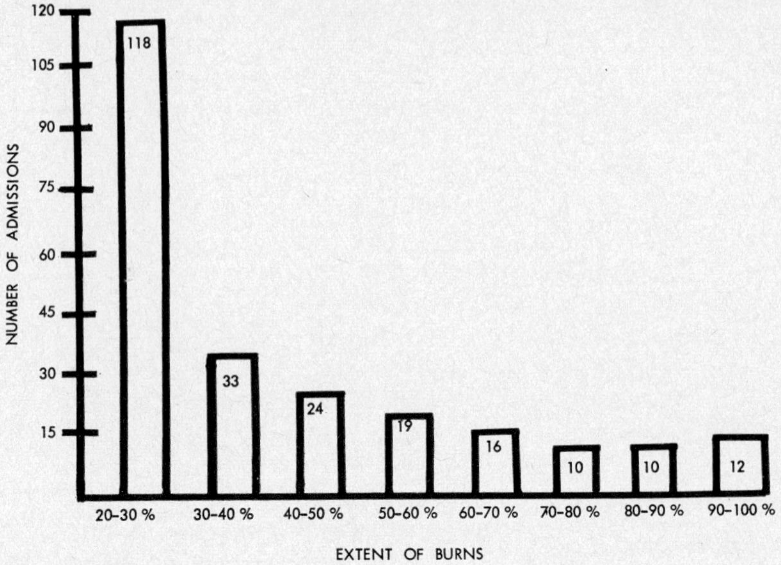

Fig 2.—Extent of burns.

and skin grafting, and (5) have an excellent prognosis, except for significant mortality in neonates, the very elderly, and those with debilitating chronic diseases.

C. *Type III Burns.*—These (1) have full thickness components involving 20% to 40% of the body surface, (2) are characterized by burn shock in acute phase, (3) present significant metabolic alterations, (4) differ from type IV burns in that the majority of the skin surface is available as donor area for skin grafts, (5) are usually too extensive to be treated by early excision and grafting,[13] and (6) have an excellent prognosis for survival in the younger age groups, with relatively higher mortality in the middle-aged patients.

D. *Type IV Burns.*—These (1) have full thickness skin loss involving 40% to 80% of the body surface, (2) are characterized by severe burn shock in the acute phase, (3) are subject to a serious mortality risk from sepsis and bronchopneumonia, (4) are associated with major nutritional and metabolic problems, (5) are frequently candidates for temporary skin coverage with homografts while multiple "crops" of autografts are obtained from the same donor areas, (6) have a mortality rate of 20% to 80% depending on the age, extent of burn, and numerous other factors, with an average mortality of 50%, and (7) represent the group of burns for which advances in treatment can offer the most improvement.

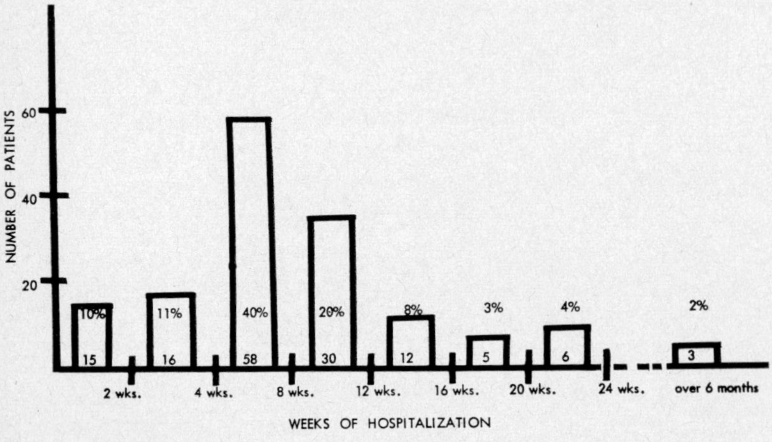

Fig 3. — Duration of hospitalization—survivors—first admission.

E. *Type V Burns.*—These (1) involve over 80% of the body surface, or over 40% of the body surface in patients over the age of 70 years, and (2) have almost 100% mortality rate (thus categorically unsalvagable at the present).

Mortality Studies

The over-all burn mortality will vary considerably in any series, depending on the category of the burns. A large portion of type V burns will elevate the mortality rate—47% of all deaths in this series involve burns of this nature. So far, attempts to save the victims of type V burns have only succeeded in prolonging the interval until death. Thirty per cent of the type V burns in this series survived the immediate postburn period, only to succumb from septic starvation and bronchopneumonia. This group of 30% would theoretically be salvagable if more advanced methods of wound closure, and more effective methods in resisting septic starvation, were available.

Any major burn in the elderly patient carries a grave prognosis because of frequently associated debility from renal, cardiovascular, and other chronic diseases and resultant poor tolerance for sepsis and pneumonia. Only one patient over the age of 70 survived a major burn in this study. Blocker[4] reported that he had not seen a single patient over the age of 60 who survived a burn of 30% or more. The data from this study show a 37% survival rate in patients with major burns between the ages of 60 to 70 years, including a 69-year-old Negro female with a 50% total body burn.

Nevertheless, 97 deaths in this series of 242 major burns—a mortality rate of 40%—seemed excessive. However, comparison with reports from other general hospitals reveals similar results (Tables 2-4), and this is to be expected since the same principles in

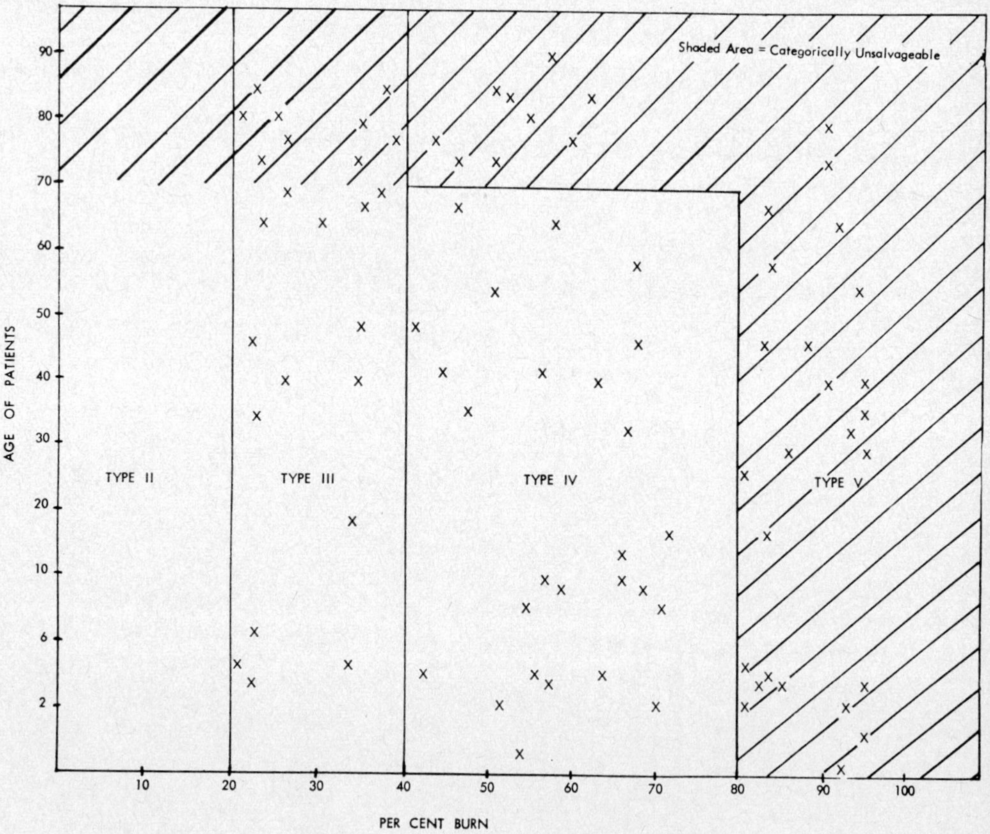

Fig 4.—Burn deaths (97)—John Gaston Hospital.

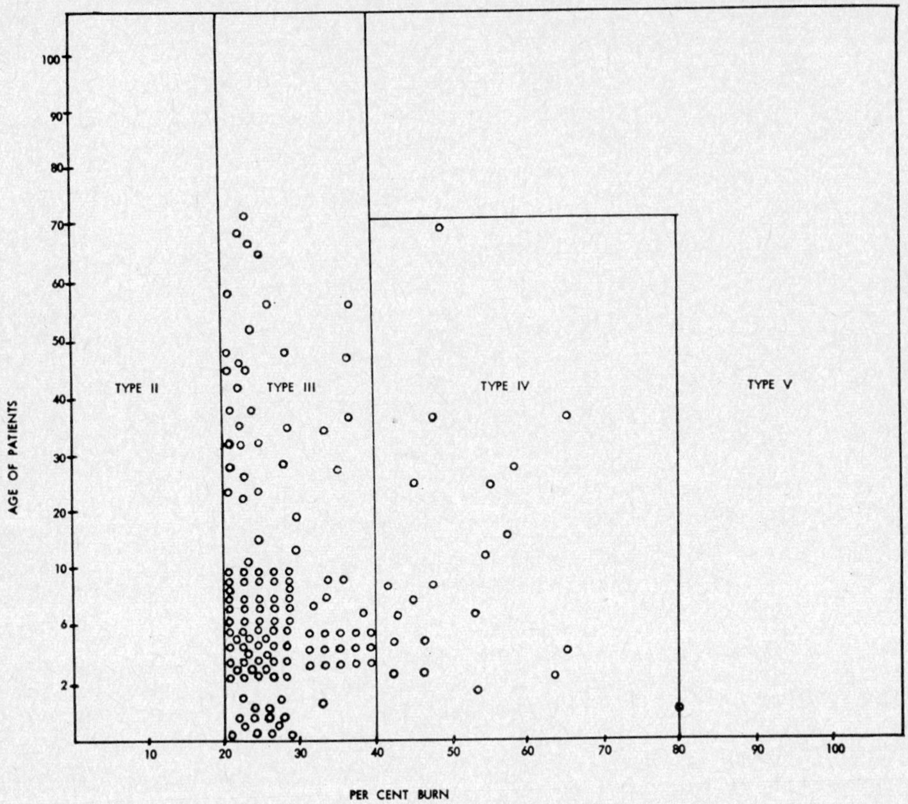

Fig 5.—Burn survivors (145)—John Gaston Hospital.

burn therapy are almost universally employed.

Deaths During the First 48 Hours

There were 17 deaths during the first 48 hours of hospitalization. Fourteen of these patients had almost complete body burns and died in a state of respiratory distress, shock, and anuria. Autopsies obtained on five of these patients revealed pulmonary congestion, edema, focal atelectasis, and intra-alveolar hemorrhage in all, and frank bronchopneumonia in two. Changes in the renal tubular epithelium were invariable. Adrenal cortical hemorrhages were evident in 40%. Other changes include passive congestion of the gastrointestinal tract, liver, and spleen in all patients. Areas of liquefaction necrosis of the brain were seen in two of the five autopsied. Necrosis of the gastrointestinal mucosa was present in one.

There were three deaths in which an almost total body burn was not involved. One was a four-year-old Negro male with a 60% flame burn resulting from ignition of clothes by an open gas heater, who died in a state of shock five hours post burn, with a poor urinary output and hemoglobinuria. Another was a 77-year-old white male with a 50% burn obtained in a burning house, who died 18 hours after being burned, in a state of shock and anuria. He was thought to have received adequate fluid replacement. The other death occurred in a 60-year-old Negro male who received only a 20% burn while re-

TABLE 2.—*Burn Mortality Rates*

Body Surface Burn	Adults, %		Children, %	
	A	B	A	B
<25%	23.5 (34)	32 (59)	2.6 (75)	13 (55)
26%-50%	74 (27)	67 (48)	12 (32)	58 (36)
51%-100%	84 (39)	97 (30)	80 (35)	94 (16)

A indicates John Gaston Hospital mortality rate; B, Medical College of Virginia (Haynes, B. W., reference 10) mortality rate; number in parentheses is total cases treated.

TABLE 3.—*Burn Mortality Rates*

Body Surface Burned, %	% Mortality 0-14 Yr A	B	C	15-44 Yr A	B	C	45-64 Yr A	B	C	65+ Yr A	B	C
20-24	4.8	5	5.5	0	6	16	0	19	15	70	80	46.5
25-34	2.4	14	11.8	0	0	25.2	57	80	27	70	100	61
35-44	18	32	20.5	57	11	36	100	75	41	100	100	73
45-54	42	44	32	60	62	46.5	—	75	56	75	100	85
55-64	72.7	86	45.5	25	100	55	100	—	74	100	100	95
65-74	100	75	61	100	74	67	—	100	91	100	100	100
75-84	88	75	81	100	100	78	100	100	100	—	100	100
85-94	100	100	100	100	89	100	100	100	100	100	100	100

A indicates mortality rate John Gaston Hospital; B, mortality rate Bull and Fisher, Birmingham, England (reference 5); C, mortality rate King County Hospital, Winterscheid and Merendino (reference 23).

trieving clothes and two other people from a burning house. He died seven hours post burn in respiratory distress despite a tracheostomy. The latter two deaths were thought to be due to respiratory burns and inhalation of toxic fumes and smoke, with possible carbon monoxide intoxication.

Deaths in Type III Burns

Since these burns should have an excellent prognosis for recovery, investigation of the contributing factors in the deaths of these patients seemed of unique import. As Phillips and Cope[18] have recently emphasized, respiratory complications were the major contributing cause of death (Table 6). While bronchopneumonia was a suspected cause of death in 50% of cases on clinical impression, it was found to be a major contributing factor in 92% of the cases autopsied (Table 5). Sepsis, alone or associated with bronchopneumonia, was thought to be the major cause of death in 62% of the cases on clinical impression, but evidence of septicemia with multiple metastatic abscesses and infected organs was found in only 16% of cases autopsied.

Gastrointestinal ulcerations ("Curling's ulcers") were evident in three cases (10% of all deaths in this group). Massive hemorrhage was the direct cause of death in a four-year-old Negro male with a 30% burn. Significant bleeding occurred in two other patients but was not considered the chief cause of death.

Fifty-one per cent of the deaths in this group were found to be in people over the age of 60. Autopsy data revealed that preexisting cardiovascular and renal disease was a contributing factor in 55% of these deaths.

The over-all death rate for type III burns for patients under the age of 70 was 10%, but was 7% for patients under the age of 60 and only 4.8% under the age of 30. Our

TABLE 4.—*Burn Mortality Rates*

Body Surface Burned, %	% Mortality 0-15 Yr A	B	C	16-35 Yr A	B	C	36-55 Yr A	B	C	56-100 Yr A	B	C
20-24	4.8 *	0	0	0	0	9	0	25	4.5	71.5	71.5	30.5
25-34	2.4	25	12.5	0	0	18.2	15	33.3	9.1	80	100	75
35-44	16.6	37.5	50	25	0	14.3	33	66.7	50	100	100	100
45-64	47	50	100	20	—	66.6	75	100	85.7	88	100	100
>65	95	50	100	100	100	40	100	100	100	100	100	100

A indicates John Gaston Hospital 1955-1960; B, San Francisco City and County Hospital 1943-1956 (reference 6); C, Massachusetts General Hospital 1939-1954 (reference 2).

* Two deaths—one operative cardiac arrest, the other from viral pneumonitis.

Table 5.—*Cause of Death in Type III Burns*

	Autopsy (13)	Clinical (16)	Total (29)
Acute bronchopneumonia	12	3	15
Septicemia with multiple abscesses	2	3	5
Sepsis plus bronchopneumonia	—	5	5
Septic shock	—	2	2
Severe cardiovascular disease	6	1	7
Severe renal disease	7	2	9
Gastrointestinal ulcerations			
Direct cause: hemorrhage	2	1	3
Associated cause: hemorrhage	—	1	1
Incidental finding	2	—	2
Pulmonary infarcts	3	—	3
Suppurative pericarditis with thrombosis of pulmonary artery	1	—	1
Congestive heart failure, pulmonary edema	—	1	1
Respiratory burn, hypoxic shock	—	1	1
Postoperative cardiac arrest	—	1	1

best results were obtained in the very young. Of 14 type III burns under two years of age, there were no deaths. At the other end of the age scale, of ten patients over the age of 70, only one survived.

All Major Burns

Autopsies were obtained on 40 of the 97 burn deaths in this study (Table 6). The findings incriminate pathology of the respiratory system as major contributing factor in the death of these patients. Acute bronchopneumonia was found in 77%, other major pulmonary pathology in 30%, and pulmonary infarcts in 12%. Most patients with bronchopneumonia ran a septic clinical course. Evidence of septicemia with widespread infections, or multiple metastatic microabscesses, was found in only 12.5%. Diffuse liver necrosis was noted in 5% of the deaths. Severe cardiovascular and renal disease was found in 45% of the autopsies.

One revelation was a very high incidence of gastrointestinal ulcerations, which were found in 37.5% of autopsies (15 cases). Others have reported incidences varying from 0% to 36%, with an average reported incidence of 3.8%.[10,12] Obviously many factors are responsible for the wide variation. Many cases recover after having only minor symptoms and thus are overlooked. In 10 of 15 cases, Curling's ulcers apparently did not contribute to the death of the victim and were

Table 6.—*Cause of Death in Major Burns: 40 Autopsies*

	No.	%
Acute bronchopneumonia	31	77
Pulmonary infarcts	5	12.5
Other pulmonary pathology (atelectasis, pulmonary edema, etc)	12	30
Septicemia with multiple abscesses or multiple organ involvement	5	12.5
Diffuse liver necrosis	2	5
Severe cardiovascular disease	16	40
Severe renal disease	19	47.5
Gastrointestinal ulcerations	15	37.5
Direct cause of death: hemorrhage, perforation	2	5
Associated cause of death: hemorrhage	3	10
Incidental finding at autopsy	10	25

incidental findings at autopsy. In 10 to 15 cases, ulcers were found in only one part of the gastrointestinal tract: five involved the stomach; three involved the esophagus only; two involved the duodenum only; five cases involved multiple organs. Ulcers were found in the stomach in 10 of 15 cases.

Ulcers were more commonly found in the extensively burned patients (all ages) with 12 of 15 cases occurring in type IV and V burns. In those patients with symptoms, the presence of ulcers usually became evident between the 4th and 14th day, with an average of nine days post burn. However, they were present at autopsy in two patients within 24 hours post burn.

Previously, the diagnosis of Curling's ulcers was only made when pain, or evidence of complications such as bleeding or perforation, was apparent. However, the fact that 66% of the cases were not diagnosed clinically provided the incentive to review closely these charts for symptoms or findings which might be clues to the diagnosis of uncomplicated Curling's ulcers. Only one of these patients complained of epigastric pain. Two patients, who subsequently were found to have multiple ulcers of the esophagus, complained of sore throat or difficulty in swallowing. The most consistent finding was the presence of anorexia, frequently with a sudden onset after the patient had been eating well. Almost as frequent was the presence of abdominal distention or gastric dilatation. Subsequent clinical observation has proved that anorexia, especially if associated with abdominal distention, is a useful warning of the presence of Curling's ulcers.

Because of the difficulty in making accurate diagnosis of uncomplicated ulcers, early prophylactic neutralization of gastric acid with antacids in all major burns has been advocated. Review of the records shows that this has not been routine in this group of patients, and none of the patients who subsequently developed ulcers received prophylactic antacids. However, two patients exsanguinated from acute ulcers several days after being placed on strict ulcer regimens, including Sippy diet, antacids, and antispasmodics. The etiology is not understood and may not be dependent upon increased acid-peptic activity.[11,12] Friesen believes these ulcers result in association with hemoconcentration and mucosal congestion.[9] Despite this evidence, very high incidence of gastrointestinal ulcers in this group which did not receive antacid prophylaxis, when compared to much lower incidence in other groups in which antacid prophylaxis is routine, suggests a need for prophylactic neutralization of gastric acid in all major burns.

Comment

Autopsy data indicate that respiratory complications are the most frequent factors in burn deaths. Factors which might contribute to the development of respiratory complications should be emphasized: excessive sedation, delayed treatment of burn shock, mismanagement of the tracheostomy, and excessive parenteral fluid therapy.

One of the most frequent errors noted was usually committed by the first physician to attend the victim of an extensive burn, that is, the administration of large doses of morphine before resuscitative measures were implemented to combat burn shock. Victims of extensive burns are usually lethargic and subdued and experience only moderate pain during the first few hours following the burn. Restlessness and motor excitement are usually the results of cerebral hypoxia due to shock and respiratory insufficiency due to inhalation of hot gases, smoke, and toxic fumes. When this restlessness is misinterpreted as being due to pain, the compassionate doctor administers a large dose of morphine, which further depresses respirations and cardiovascular reflexes. This is certainly equally as dangerous as the administration of large doses of narcotics before resuscitation in other forms of traumatic, hemorrhage, hypovolemic, or hypoxic shock.

Another, but less frequent, error contributing to morbidity and mortality from respiratory complications was the failure to perform early tracheostomy when indicated. Physical examination of the lungs soon after the burn frequently belies the serious nature of the respiratory injury, and in most cases there are no significant findings, such as rales, rhonchi, or wheezes, until several hours later at which time the patient has developed severe hypoxic acidosis. Immediate tracheostomy should be considered in the following instances: (1) any significant burns of the head or neck, (2) burns incurred in a flaming building or inclosed space where hot gases or smoke and toxic fumes were inhaled, (3) other evidence of a respiratory burn such as singed nasal cilia, or burns of the nose, mouth, tongue, or pharynx, (4) physical signs of respiratory burns such as rales, rhonchi, and wheezes, (5) hoarseness, or the expectoration of blood-tinged, purulent, or smoke-stained sputum, (6) the presence of associated injuries of the thoracic cage such as rib fractures, and (7) tracheostomy in conjunction with bilateral relaxing incisions when circumferential deep burns of the chest and upper abdomen markedly restrict ventilatory exchange and pulmonary function.[16,22]

Performance of a tracheostomy does not terminate the necessity for careful attention to the respiratory tract, since there are many complications which attend the tracheostomy in burn patients.[16] Edema and swelling of the neck may cause a short tracheostomy tube to slip out of the trachea, resulting in asphyxiation. Standard tracheostomy care is mandatory to avoid obstruction from excessive secretions which are inevitable after inhalation of flame or irritating fumes. The cannula may erode the irritated trachea causing hemorrhage. The wound itself may serve as a focus of infection, contributing to the development of suppurative tracheobronchitis and bronchopneumonia, and represents a source of generalized sepsis. The frequency of these complications should stimulate the doctor to remove the tracheostomy tube and to allow the wound to close and heal as soon as the respiratory crisis is over, usually after three or four days. At this time patients can cough more effectively and clear the terminal bronchi and bronchioles, whereas suctioning through the tracheostomy can only clear the secretions from the trachea and larger bronchi. While many have emphasized the need for tracheostomies in acute burns, the need to discontinue it at the earliest possible opportunity in order to decrease suppurative tracheobronchitis and bronchopneumonia has not been clearly emphasized.

Excessive parenteral fluids result in plethora and hypotonicity; associated pulmonary vascular congestion contributes to the development of pulmonary edema, atelectasis, and pneumonitis. Complications and morbidity from excessive parenteral fluid therapy have prompted several investigators to recommend only oral fluid therapy, if at all possible.[20-22] Several factors contribute to excessive parenteral fluid therapy: (1) Overestimation of the extent of the burn and strict adherence to a mathematical formula for parenteral fluid therapy are probably the most common causes of error. (2) Overly vigorous attempts to lower the hematocrit to a preselected level may be harmful, since signs and symptoms of shock and reduced renal blood flow are usually relieved before the hematocrit returns to normal. (3) The mistaken concept that urinary output is directly related to the efficacy of parenteral replacement, and efforts to maintain a high urine output in the face of stress-induced antidiuresis, may result in vascular overloading. (4) Young children and the elderly patients, especially those with pre-existing cardiovascular and renal disease, poorly tolerate overinfusion with water and electrolyte solution. Parenteral fluid therapy in the treatment of burn shock cannot be reduced to a simple mathematical formula, and the efficacy of such treatment cannot be assesed by laboratory measurements alone. Frequent bedside observations are mandatory to provide proper therapy for burn shock.

The prevalence of pulmonary complications, especially in patients without related burns of the respiratory tract and in patients who give no history of inhalation of toxic fumes or hot gases, suggests that other factors should be considered. Recent investigations suggest that intrinsic circulatory abnormalities induced by the burn injury may influence the development of pulmonary complications. Steph, as quoted by Wilson and Stirman,[22] noted a marked derangement in respiratory dynamics immediately after experimental scald burns in dogs, as reflected by changes in total lung volume and pulmonary compliance. Baxter and De Cosse [3] demonstrated in burned men that respiratory insufficiency begins early after burning and persists, often causing death several days later. Blood gas studies showed a decreased arterial oxygen saturation with variable carbon dioxide pressure.

Generalized sepsis is a major complication of burns, although necropsy findings fail to substantiate the clinical suggestion of its leading prevalence as a cause of death. Antibiotics have not been the answer to this problem. Sources of infection and sepsis such as septic thrombophlebitis from an infected "cutdown" site, an infected tracheostomy wound, urinary tract infections from neglect of urethral catheters, and exposure to other patients infected with virulent organisms must be avoided. Adherence to sound surgical principles, early debridement, and grafting of the burn wound provide the best defense, until greater understanding of the diffuse biochemical and metabolic derangements of burn trauma is achieved.

Liver pathology varied from parenchymatous swelling of the epithelium and cytoplasmic vacuolization (seen in practically every death secondary to major burns) to diffuse total necrosis of the liver which was the direct cause in 5% of deaths in this series. Hypoxia due to oligemia and blood sludging has been incriminated as a major contributing cause of liver damage, but other factors such as sepsis, serum hepatitis, hepatotoxic drugs, metabolic effects of starvation, etc, must be considered. Arturson [1] found that maximum liver cell damage occurred on the second and third post burn days but that microscopic and biochemical abnormalities were detectable until the convalescent stage of the burn (eg, after the wound was healed).

The profound influence of hepatic damage on the total burn syndrome can be better appreciated when the essential challenges of the burn are considered—shock, sepsis, starvation, and skin loss. Liver damage results in (1) impairment of metabolism of foodstuffs absorbed from the gastrointestinal tract including vitamins, minerals, carbohydrates, lipids, and proteins, (2) loss of sources of energy from lipid and carbohydrate metabolism, depletion of liver glycogen, and impairment of gluconeogenesis, (3) fluid and electrolyte derangements secondary to negative energy balance, and to impaired hormone metabolism and detoxification, (4) impairment of detoxification of bacterial and chemical toxins, (5) impairment of reticuloendothelial function with reduced resistance to infection and decreased antibody and γ-globulin production, (6) impaired metabolism of amino acids and proteins in face of diminished intake and excessive losses in burn exudate, and (7) impaired wound healing secondary to these and other changes.

Liver damage secondary to circulatory abnormalities and other factors adversely influences the clinical course of the burn victim. While massive liver necrosis is relatively uncommon (5% of deaths), detectable microscopic and biochemical abnormalities are present in all major burns.

Adherence to sound surgical principles, vigilance for possible sources of sepsis, and early debridement and grafting of the burn wound provide the best defense against sepsis.

Summary

The charts of 242 patients admitted to John Gaston Hospital between 1955 to 1960 with thermal burns involving more than 20% of the body surface were reviewed. Females and children were most commonly injured, with burns most commonly resulting from ignition of clothing while standing next to open flame heaters. This implies a greater need for a more forceful accident prevention program during the winter months when the accidents most often occur. Ultimate prevention of these accidents may eventually require precise legislation regarding minimum standards of heating systems and pretreatment of clothing fabrics to reduce flammability.

Comparison of our mortality statistics with reports from other hospitals was difficult because of the lack of uniformity in the format of these reports. Therefore a classification based on pathology, treatment, and prognosis of the burn is submitted so that a comparison of similar injuries may be possible in the future. A relatively high incidence of Curling's ulcers was evident in this study. Review of the records shows that the most suggestive symptom indicating the presence of uncomplicated ulcers is the onset of anorexia, especially if associated with gastric dilatation or abdominal distention.

The importance of respiratory complications as the most common factor contributing to death was brought out by the autopsy statistics, and confirms other reports.[18] Some of the more common errors which increase morbidity and mortality from respiratory complications were discussed: (1) injudicious use of large doses of morphine during uncompensated shock phase of the burn, (2) failure to perform early tracheostomy when indicated, (3) failure to discontinue the tracheostomy at the earliest possible time, (4) failure to recognize the importance of the tracheostomy wound as an important factor in the development of purulent tracheobronchitis and bronchopneumonia, (5) overinfusion of parenteral fluids. Specific mechanisms of metabolic, physiologic, and biochemical derangement in each organ system following thermal burn would seem to provide fertile ground for future investigation.

William H. Lee, Jr., MD, Department of Surgery, Medical College of South Carolina, Charleston, S.C.

REFERENCES

1. Arturson, G.: Pathophysiological Aspects of the Burn Syndrome, Acta Chir Scand suppl 274, 1961.

2. Barnes, B. A.: Mortality of Burns at the Massachusetts General Hospital (1939-1954), Ann Surg 145:210, 1957.

3. Baxter, C. R., and De Cosse, J. J.: Pulmonary Function Following Thermal Trauma—Hypoxia, Annual Research Progress Report, US Army Surgical Research Unit, Brooks Army Medical Center, Fort Sam Houston, Texas, 1958.

4. Blocker, T. G., Jr.: Treatment of Burns in Elderly Patients, Geriatrics 12:457, 1957.

5. Bull, J. P., and Fisher, A. J.: A Study of Mortality in a Burns Unit: A Revised Estimate, Ann Surg 139:269, 1954.

6. Clark, A. G., and Hanson, J. H.: Mortality Rates in Patients With Burns, Calif Med 89:210, 1958.

7. Cope, O., and Moore, F. D.: The Redistribution of Body Water and the Fluid Therapy of the Burned Patient, Ann Surg 126:1010, 1947.

8. Evans, E. I.; Purnell, O. J.; Robinett, P. W.; Batchelor, A.; and Martin, M.: Fluid and Electrolyte Requirements in Severe Burns, Ann Surg 135:804, 1952.

9. Friesen, S. R.: The Genesis of Gastroduodenal Ulcer Following Burns, Surgery 28:123, 1950.

10. Haynes, B. W.: Dextran Therapy in Severe Burns, Amer J Surg 99:684, 1960.

11. Howard, J. M.: Gastric and Salivary Secretion Following Injury, Ann Surg 141:342, 1955.

12. Hummel, R. P.; Balikov, B.; and Artz, C. P.: Studies in Curling's Ulcers, Surg Forum 6:306, 1955.

13. Jackson, D.; Topley, E.; Cason, J. S.; and Lowbury, E. J. L.: Primary Excision and Grafting of Large Burns, Ann Surg 152:167, 1960.

14. Mears, F. B.: Autopsy Survey of Peptic Ulcer Associated With Other Diseases: A Review of Related Etiological Factors Concerned, Thesis, University of Minnesota, 1947.

15. Metropolitan Life Insurance Company Bulletin, Oct, 1960.

16. Moncrief, J. A.: Tracheotomy in Burns, AMA Arch Surg 79:45, 1959.

17. Moyer, C. A.: The Sociologic Aspect of Trauma With Particular Reference to Thermal Injury, Amer J Surg 87:421, 1954.

18. Phillips, A. W., and Cope, O.: Burn Therapy: The Revelation of Respiratory Tract Damage as a Principal Killer of the Burned Patient, Ann Surg 155:1, 1962.

19. Reiss, E.; Stirman, J. A.; Artz, C. P.; Davis, J. H.; and Amspacher, W. H.: Fluid and Electrolyte Balance in Burns, JAMA 152:1309, 1953.

20. Rosenthal, S. M., and Millican, R. C.: The Role of Fluids, Electrolytes and Plasma Proteins in Experimental Traumatic Shock and Hemorrhage, Pharmacol Rev 6:489, 1954.

21. Wilkinson, A. W.: The Early Treatment of Burns, Brit J Plast Surg 10:275, 1958.

22. Wilson, B. J., and Stirman, J. A.: Initial Treatment of Burns, JAMA 173:115, 1960.

23. Winterscheid, L. C., and Merendino, K. A.: Etiology and Mortality From Burns at a General Hospital, Amer J Surg 100:375, 1960.

Primary Inguinal Hernioplasty

Our Experience with 3,572 Operations

LOUIS T. PALUMBO, MD
WENDELL S. SHARPE, MD
H. L. GERNDT, JR., MD
E. D. MAGLIETTA, MD
AND
W. B. EIDBO, MD
DES MOINES, IOWA

Introduction

In 1952 and 1954 we reported our results in 1,375 cases of primary inguinal hernioplasty in adult patients.[1,2] This current report is based upon our total experience of 3,572 operations performed during a 16-year period beginning Aug 1, 1946.

A current evaluation of the results of primary repair of inguinal hernia in the adult continues to be one of the most important socioeconomic problems in modern medicine. Even though there are currently a number of anatomically and technically sound surgical procedures for the repair of this congenital and/or acquired disabling defect, the recurrence rate countrywide continues to remain too high. A recent survey of the literature revealed considerable variations in this respect; from a low of 0.85% to 21% with an average of about 7% for indirect and 8.5% for direct type hernias.[3-13] These, however, are reports from groups and centers which have had a broad experience with this condition and therefore does not represent a true index of the actual recurrence rate by all physicians performing this type surgery. It is impossible to estimate accurately the average recurrence rate countrywide, since these figures are not available. It is the opinion of the senior author (L. T. P.) that this rate is closer to 15%-25%. A more accurate estimation can be made, particularly in the younger age group, since the military services have found a recurrence rate of 8.3% in 5,834 young men examined at the time of induction. In 3 million selective service examinations the incidence of inguinal hernia was 5.9%. It is estimated that the incidence of inguinal hernia in the male population of the United States is 5% and is about 1% in the female population.

Generally speaking, there are very few contraindications to the surgical treatment of

Submitted for publication June 17, 1963.

From the Department of Surgery, Veterans Administration Hospital.

Other members of full-time and resident staff participated in this study.

TABLE 1.—*Age Incidence at Time of Surgery*

Age	No.	%
<20	10	0.3
20-29	381	12.1
30-39	511	16.2
40-49	545	17.3
50-59	866	27.4
60-69	735	23.3
70+	107	3.4
Totals	3,155	100.0

inguinal hernia at any age. The morbidity and mortality rates are extremely low and certainly are less than those arising from the group of patients not treated surgically.

If a physician is experiencing a recurrence rate of over 3% in elective cases of primary inguinal hernia repair in the adult, it is important that he re-evaluate his technical capabilities and the type of repair he is using. There are several surgical techniques which, when properly performed, will result in a low recurrence rate. If the physician became proficient in one acceptable method, he could expect a definite and consistent reduction in his recurrence rate.

Purpose of Report

We are presenting the results of our experience covering a 16-year period from Aug 1, 1946, to Aug 1, 1962. In this group we performed the same basic operative procedure on all patients.[1,2] It is the same repair we have used since 1938. This is a series of 3,155 patients, consecutive and unselected, representing 3,572 operations for primary inguinal hernias (all adults).

In all cases nonabsorbable suture cotton or silk (94% were silk) sutures were used. These operations were performed by 70 members of our full-time and house staff, principally the latter. Only in recent years were bilateral hernias repaired at the same time (39 cases).

TABLE 3.—*Location of Hernia*

Side	No.	%
Right	1,960	54.9
Left	1,612	45.1
Totals	3,572	100.0

11.8% bilateral (417 cases).

TABLE 2.—*Type of Hernia*

Type	No.	%
Indirect	2,304	64.5
Direct	686	19.2
Combined	582	16.3
Totals	3,572	100.0

52 (1.4%) cases also had femoral hernia.

Age Incidence

The patients' ages ranged from 18 to 85 years, with the largest numbers occurring in the 50-69 age groups, representing 50.7%. Over 26% were 60 years of age or older (Table 1).

Location and Types of Hernia

All types of inguinal hernia are included in this study. This report represents consecutive and unselected patients both in elective and emergency groups. Also included are patients who had femoral hernia (52 cases), sliding, incarcerated, and strangulated hernias. The incidence of sliding hernia was 3.1%. Seventy-nine patients were operated upon for incarceration and only seven for strangulation. Emergency surgery was performed on 86 (2.7%) patients.

In 64.5% the hernia was indirect, and in 19.2% it was direct in type (Table 2).

TABLE 4.—*Operations Performed at Time of Hernioplasty*

Type	No.
Appendectomy	43
Epigastric hernioplasty	21
Femoral hernioplasty	52
Hydrocelectomy	61
Lipoma, cord (excision)	126
Orchiectomy	27
Spermatocelectomy	7
Spigelian hernioplasty	3
Umbilical hernioplasty	40
Varicocelectomy	31
Total	411

Bilateral hernias were present in 11.8% of the patients. In unilateral cases, the hernia occurred most frequently on the right (54.9%) (Table 3).

Additional Surgical Procedures

In 285 patients (7.9%), 411 additional surgical procedures were performed at time of the hernioplasty (Table 4).

Operative Technique

The same basic technique has been employed in all cases in this survey and in all hernias repaired since 1938. The operation has been only slightly modified and improved since 1942. The technique has resulted from combining and utilizing some of the basic principles as described in the original operations by Bassini,* Halsted,[4] and Andrews.[2] However, in this repair, which also includes several important and special features of our own, muscle is not used at all. Transversalis fascia is utilized as the first line of defense by imbrication (to be described later). An aponeurosis to inguinal ligament and a fascia-to-fascia repair is employed. The sutures are placed without tension and tied so as not to cause constriction or strangulation of the tissue.

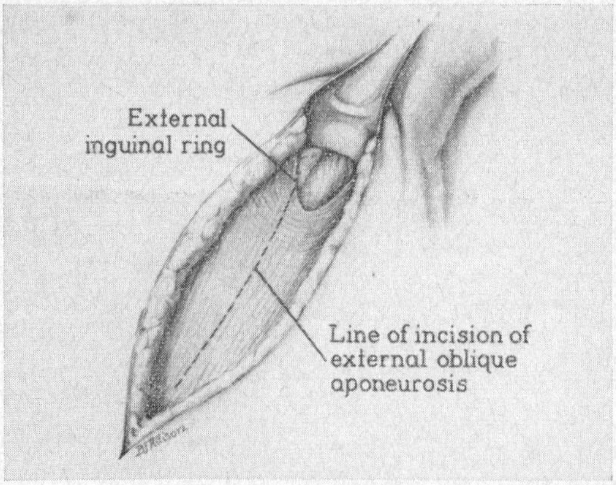

Fig 1.—Dotted line represents the line of incision made in the direction of the fibers of the external oblique aponeurosis along the medial side of the cord. (This and the following illustrations were used through the courtesy of W. B. Saunders Company, *Surgical Clinics of North America* 34:3, 1954.)

* Cited by Summers, J. E.[15]

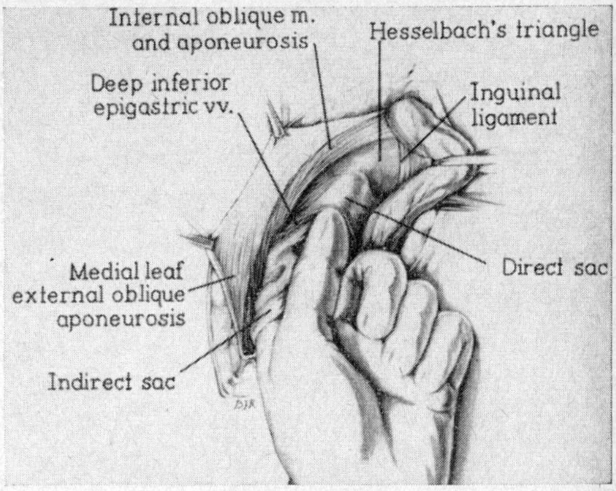

Fig 2.—The external oblique aponeurosis has been divided and the cord displaced from its bed. The indirect sac has been dissected completely from the cord structures. The tip of the index finger is within the direct sac revealing the direct weakness in Hesselbach's triangle.

In 3,361 (94.1%) hernioplasties were performed with the patient under spinal anesthesia; the remaining 211 (5.9%) were accomplished with the use of a general anesthetic agent. In 94% silk was the suture material; in 6% cotton was used.

An oblique skin incision extends from the pubic spine upward to and about 5 cm medial to the anterosuperior iliac spine. The external oblique aponeurosis is divided in the direction of its fibers along the medial side of the external inguinal ring (Fig 1). This

Fig 3.—The first layer of the basic repair is shown with the imbrication of the transversalis fascia with 000 silk. The figure-of-eight or pulley stitch of 00 silk is in place over the pubic spine area to obliterate the weak area at this point. The lower border of the internal inguinal ring is formed by a horizontal mattress of 00 silk approximating internal oblique aponeurosis to the shelving edge of the inguinal ligament.

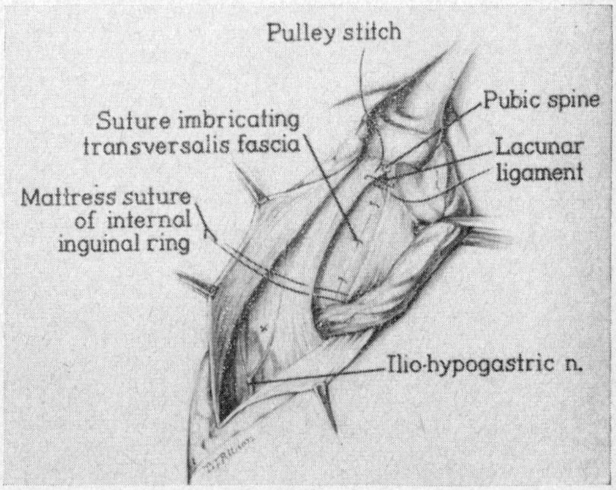

division provides an adequate medial and lateral leaf of the external oblique aponeurosis which is important in the final stages of the repair.

The cord and associated structures are displaced laterally from their bed. The indirect sac, if present, is dissected free from the cord structures high up to the internal ring. If an associated direct weakness or sac is present, it is dissected from the surrounding structures and from the urinary bladder. This maneuver converts the two hernial sacs into one common sac and opening. If an indirect sac is not present, the direct sac is approached at the upper part of Hesselbach's triangle. It is our opinion that a careful and complete dissection of the sac is extremely important. As shown in this series a direct or combined (direct and indirect) hernia occurred in 35% of the patients (Fig 2). The excess portion of the sac is excised, the neck of the sac is closed with a purse-string suture of 00 or 000 silk. In some cases the sac is transplanted and anchored to the abdominal wall.

In all cases, whether or not there is a direct hernia or direct weakness in Hesselbach's triangle, interrupted imbricating sutures of 000 silk are taken in the transversalis fascia. It is our opinion that this is the first line of defense, and taking the relaxation out of this structure helps to form a solid foundation for the hernia repair. Usually three sutures in this area suffice (Fig 3). The superior suture is taken close to the internal inguinal ring and aids considerably in fortifying this weak area. This fascia when properly utilized provides a strong floor and wall in the Hesselbach's triangle, which is the weak area of the abdominal wall.

In order to prevent recurrence immediately superior to the pubic spine area, which represents a normal weak point and a frequent point for direct recurrences, steps are taken to fortify this area. A 00 silk suture is used as a pulley or figure-of-eight stitch approximating Gimbernat's and inguinal ligaments with the anterior rectus sheath. The suturing is begun by passing the needle through the medial aspect of the anterior rectus sheath or the internal oblique aponeurosis above the pubic spine. The next step is to pass the needle through the inguinal ligament at the point where it attaches to the pubic spine. It is important not to place the suture through the periosteum. This same suture is then continued as a parallel stitch, being brought up and through the internal oblique aponeurosis close to the first one taken. The final step of this four-way stitch is to sweep upward behind the area of the pubic spine, the suture being placed through Gimbernat's ligament and coming out at the free margin of the inguinal ligament close to the suture taken above the pubic spine (Fig 3). As this suture is tied, it approximates these structures superior to and over the pubic spine area, closing off this weak angle (Fig 4).

The lower border of the internal inguinal ring is formed with a horizontal mattress suture of 00 silk approximating the free rolled edge of the internal oblique aponeurosis to the shelving edge of the inguinal ligament (Fig 3 and 4). The upper border of this ring is then formed by suturing the same two structures with the same size suture. *The size of the ring* is made according to the size of the cord and its structures and *not by the size of the index finger of the surgeon.* The ring must be small and snug. In none of our cases was the size of the ring

Fig 4.—The second layer of the basic repair is completed. The internal oblique aponeurosis is sutured to the inguinal ligament using 00 silk. The new internal inguinal ring is small, admitting the back end of a small thumb forceps.

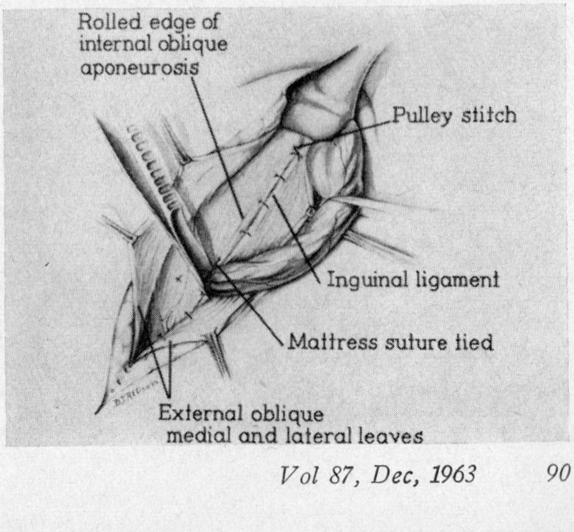

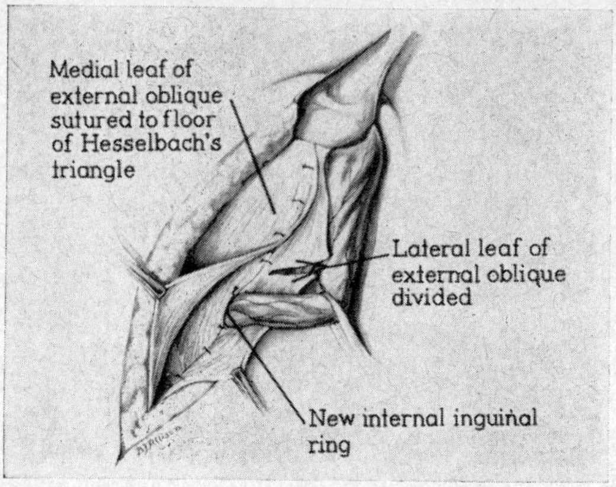

Fig 5.—The medial leaf of the external oblique aponeurosis is sutured with 000 silk to the newly formed floor inferior to the cord. The lateral leaf of the external oblique has been cut toward the inguinal ligament ½ to ¾ in (1.25-1.9 cm) inferior to the internal inguinal ring.

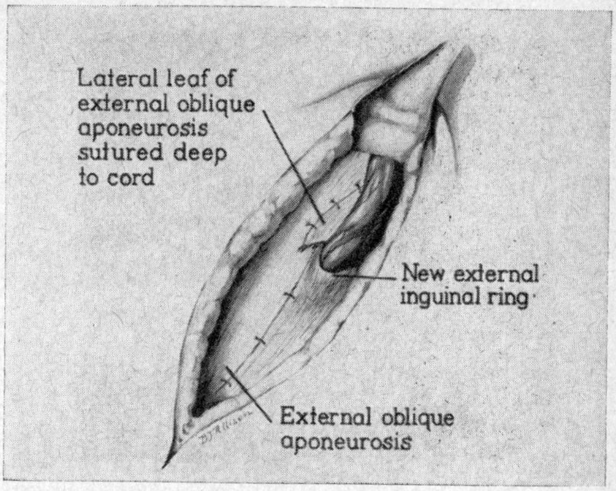

Fig 6.—The lateral leaf of the external oblique is sutured beneath the cord with interrupted 000 silk. The new external inguinal ring is formed ½ to ¾ in (1.25-1.9 cm) inferior to the internal ring. The external oblique is reapproximated superior to the cord.

large enough to admit the tip of the little finger. We feel that it is adequate in size if it will admit the blunt end of an ordinary-sized thumb forceps (Fig 4).

The second layer of the basic repair is then completed by approximating the rolled edge of the internal oblique aponeurosis to the shelving edge of the inguinal ligament superior and inferior to the internal ring, using interrupted 00 silk sutures (Fig 4 and 5).

The lateral leaf of the external oblique aponeurosis is divided at right angles to its fibers down to the inguinal ligament about ¾ in (1.9 cm) below the lower border of the newly formed internal ring (Fig 5). The divided medial and lateral leaves of the external oblique aponeurosis inferior to the internal ring are now imbricated and sutured to the newly formed floor in Hesselbach's triangle, using interrupted 000 silk (Fig 5 and 6). This step completes a four-layer fascial and aponeurotic repair in Hesselbach's triangle.

The new external inguinal ring is then formed ½ to ¾ in (1.25-1.9 cm) inferior to the internal ring by suturing the divided leaves of the external oblique aponeurosis above the cord. The operation is completed by reapproximating the cut leaves superior to the cord, using 000 silk (Fig 6). The superficial fascia is closed with 0000 silk and the skin with mattress and interrupted 000 silk.

Deaths

There were two postoperative deaths, a mortality of 0.05%. The first death occurred on the tenth day in a 42-year-old white male as a result of peritonitis secondary to perforation of the ascending colon. The second death occurred in a 71-year-old white male on the eighth day as a result of bilateral femoral emboli and acute coronary occlusion.

Results

A 1- to 16-year follow-up was obtained in 91.2% of the patients. The data assembled were from a combined survey consisting of questionnaire, recall examination at this hospital, examination by local physician, or result of examination at place of employment. In the event of any doubt concerning the patient, he was recalled for further examination. For those who had recurrences repaired elsewhere, the information was requested from the surgeon including a report of the operative procedure and findings at time of repair.

Recurrences

There were 37 recurrences, or a recurrence rate of 1.04%, in the group in which a

Table 5.—*Recurrence Rate—Age Incidence*

Age	Operations	No.	%
<20	12	0	0
20-29	448	3	0.69
30-39	596	8	1.5
40-49	613	7	1.1
50-59	965	15	1.5
60-69	828	4	0.49
70+	110	0	0
Totals	3,572	37	1.04

follow-up was obtained. The recurrences developed in 4 cases within one year, in 9 within two years, and in 24 three years or after; 75% of the recurrences occurred after the third year. Patients in the 30-39 and 50-59 year age groups had the highest recurrence rate, 15 (1.5%) cases.

A number of these recurrences were due to associated diseases or to the uncooperation of the patient. Those causes or conditions listed below are frequently beyond the control of the surgeon. Several patients had disabling rheumatoid arthritis and silicosis; others had advanced pulmonary changes with a chronic cough. Another of this group had epilepsy and developed a grand mal seizure in the fifth postoperative day; several returned to heavy work—as a truck driver on the tenth day, laborer on the seventh day, machine operator on the seventh day, and painter on the eighth day. In 13 (35%) patients described above of the 37 who developed recurrences, the hernia repair most likely could have remained intact under more favorable circumstances.

Of the 70 surgeons performing this operation, 24 (34%) experienced one to two recurrences in their series.

The recurrence rate occurred fairly equally throughout all decades (Table 5). To date in 110 patients 70 years or older, no recurrences have developed.

Of the 37 recurrences, 21 were indirect, 3 direct, and in 13 the type of recurrence was not classified.

Effects of Early and Late Ambulation

A carefully controlled program was instituted at the inception of this study to determine the effects of early and late ambulation upon the postoperative complication and recurrence rates. In all groups (Table 6) the patients were consecutive and unselected. In group A were 208 patients, 239 hernioplasties, ambulatory after the tenth postoperative day. There were 24 (10.2%) complications and a recurrence rate of 1.7% with a follow-up period of 6 months to 14 years and a 91.8% follow-up. In group B were 508 patients, 590 hernioplasties, ambulatory third to ninth postoperative day. There were 57 (9.8%) complications and a recurrence rate of 1.7% with a follow-up period of 6 months to 14 years and a 93.3% follow-up. In group C were 2,439 patients, 2,743 hernioplasties, ambulatory day of operation or the first postoperative day. There were 151 (5.5%) complications and a recurrence rate of 0.8% with a follow-up of 6 months to 16 years and an 88.6% follow-up (Table 7).

The recurrence rate was low in all three groups. Early ambulation effected a marked reduction (50%) in the postoperative complication rate.

Early ambulation, however, did not increase the recurrence rate. The over-all re-

Table 6.—*Early and Late Ambulation, Results*

	No. Patients	No. Operations	% Follow-Up	Period of Follow-Up	% Complications	% Recurrences
Group A	208	239	91.8	6 mo-14 yr	10.2	1.7
Group B	508	590	93.3	6 mo-14 yr	9.8	1.7
Group C	2,439	2,743	88.6	6 mo-16 yr	5.5	0.8
Totals	3,155	3,572	91.2		6.5	1.04

Group A: ambulatory after tenth postoperative day; group B: ambulatory third to ninth postoperative day; group C: ambulatory first and second postoperative day.

TABLE 7.—*Early and Late Ambulation: Complications*

Type	Group A, 239 Op	Group B, 590 Op	Group C, 2,743 Op	% Complications
Pulmonary	13 (5.5) *	12 (2.1)	63 (2.3)	88 (2.5)
Wound	6 (2.6)	15 (2.6)	47 (1.7)	68 (1.9)
Miscellaneous	5 (2.1)	30 (5.1)	41 (1.5)	76 (2.1)
Totals	24 (10.2)	57 (9.8)	151 (5.5)	232 (6.5)

* Parentheses indicate %.
Group A: ambulatory after tenth postoperative day; group B: ambulatory third to ninth postoperative day; group C: ambulatory first and second postoperative day.

currence rate for patients ambulated late was 1.7% compared to a rate of 0.8% for those ambulated early (Table 6).

Our patients were instructed to refrain from heavy lifting, straining, or athletics for a period of four to six weeks postoperatively. They were permitted to return to sedentary work at the end of 10 to 14 days, moderately heavy work in about 30 days, and heavy work in about 45 days.

Primary Direct Inguinal Hernias

There were 658 patients with direct inguinal hernia. Of this number 28 (4.3%) patients had a bilateral hernia. The age ranged from 19 to 85 years at time of surgery. There were 58 (8.5%) postoperative complications in this group. There were two (0.29%) postoperative deaths which occurred in 42- and 71-year-old males. There were only 11 (1.6%) recurrences. Seven were indirect in type, and these were possibly due to the fact that a small indirect sac was overlooked at the time of the original hernioplasty. In only four (0.6%) instances a direct recurrence occurred.

Inguinal Hernias in the Geriatric Patients

The age ranged from 60 to 85 years. There were 842 patients in this group; in 96 (11.4%) the primary inguinal hernias were bilateral. Therefore, 938 operations were performed with only one (0.11%) postoperative death occurring in a male 71 years old. In 554 (59.1%) the hernia was indirect; in the remaining it was either of the direct or combined type.

There were 79 (8.4%) complications. In the early ambulatory group, the complication rate was 5.7% compared to 16.8% in the late ambulatory group.

There were only four (0.43%) recurrences.

Recurrences in Bilateral Hernioplasty

Bilateral hernias were present in 417 (11.8%) patients. In only 39 patients was bilateral hernioplasty performed at the same time. Two (2.5%) recurrences occurred in this group. The remaining 756 operations performed upon 378 patients were accomplished separately at intervals of six to ten days. In this group, there were only four (0.5%) recurrences; this was five times less frequent than in the group in whom both hernias were repaired at the same time.

Summary and Conclusions

A statistical analysis of the results of 3,572 operations of our type hernioplasty performed for primary inguinal hernias upon 3,155 unselected consecutive male adults with a follow-up of 1 to 16 years in 91.2% of this series is presented.

Recurrence rate of only 1.04%, a total of 37 recurrences, occurred. In 686 direct inguinal hernioplasties, 11 (1.6%) recurrences developed. In only four (0.6%) cases did a direct recurrence occur. In 938 hernioplasties in patients 60 years and older, the recurrence rate was 0.43% (four cases).

Recurrence rate (2.5%) was five times greater in the group upon whom a bilateral hernia repair was accomplished at the same time.

Early ambulation resulted in a 50% reduction in the complication rates in all age groups without increasing the recurrence rate and also aided in a more rapid rehabilitation of the patient and resulted in a great economic savings.

Our same basic technique, a combined modification of Bassini, Halsted II, and Andrews operations, coupled with many of our own refinements has been employed in all types of primary inguinal hernias in the adult male for the past 25 years with a recurrence rate consistently under 2%.

Louis T. Palumbo, MD, Chief, Surgical Service, Veterans Administration Center, Des Moines 8, Iowa.

REFERENCES

1. Andreasen, A. T.: Twenty Years' Experience With Midline Extra-Peritoneal Approach to Hernias of the Inguinofemoral Region, J Int Coll Surg 35:713, 1961.

2. Andrews, E.: A Method of Herniotomy Utilizing Only White Fascia, Ann Surg 80:225, 1924.

3. Estes, W. L., Jr.: Five Year End Results in Treatment of Inguinal Hernia, Western J Surg 68: 269, 1960.

4. Halsted, W. S.: The Radical Care of Inguinal Hernia in the Male, Bull Hopkins Hosp 4:17, 1893.

5. Koontz, A. R.: Personal Technique and Results in Inguinal Hernia Repair, JAMA 164:29, 1957.

6. Lamphier, T. A., et al: Inguinal Hernia-Survey of 977 Cases, J Int Coll Surg 35:451, 1961.

7. Levy, A. H.; Wren, R. S.; and Friedman, M. N.: Complications and Recurrences Following Inguinal Hernia Repair, Ann Surg 133:533, 1951.

8. McVay, C. B., and Anson, B. J.: Inguinal and Femoral Hernioplasty, Surg Gynec Obstet 88:473, 1949.

9. McVay, C. B., and Chapp, J. D.: Inguinal and Femoral Hernioplasty: The Evaluation of a Basic Concept, Ann Surg 148:499, 1958.

10. Marsden, A. J.: Inguinal Hernia: Three Year Review of 1,000 Cases, Brit J Surg 46:234, 1958.

11. Nyhus, L. M.; Condon, R. E.; and Harkins, H. N.: Clinical Experiences With Preperitoneal Hernial Repair for All Types of Hernia of Groin, Amer J Surg 100:234, 1960.

12. Palumbo, L. T.; Paul, R. E.; and Emery, F. B.: Results of Primary Inguinal Hernioplasty, AMA Arch Surg 64:384, 1952.

13. Palumbo, L. T.; Paul, R. E.; and Mighell, S. J.: Primary Inguinal Hernioplasty: A Study of 1,375 Cases, Surg Clin N Amer 34:3, 1954.

14. Telle, L. D.: Inguinal and Femoral Hernia: A Review of 1,694 Cases, Amer J Surg 93:433, 1957.

15. Summers, J. E.: Classical Herniorrhaphies of Bassini, Halsted and Ferguson, Amer J Surg 73:87, 1947.

Systemic Effects of Massive Hepatic Necrosis

I. Acute Effects of Hepatic Infarction on the Kidneys

GUNTHER E. KRAUS, DVS
AND
GIOVANI COSTA, MD
BUFFALO

A relationship between liver disease or damage and kidney function has been observed and was termed the hepatorenal syndrome.[1-3] The exact nature of this relationship has never been delineated and theoretically could involve insufficient liver function; circulatory insufficiency, such as dehydration and hypovolemia; massive outpouring of protoplasmic catabolites from disintegrating liver; or bacterial infection. Shock, alone or combined with any of the above, may be the precipitating factor.[4,5]

It is the purpose of the present study to examine whether severe hepatic damage, in the form of massive liver necrosis, is capable of suppressing renal performance completely or partially, in the absence of dehydration or shock. In another publication [6] it was demonstrated that, in the same experimental model [7] used for the present work, infection of the devitalized liver and hepatic insufficiency [8] play no significant role.

Submitted for publication June 15, 1963.

From the Departments of Experimental Surgery and Medicine A, Roswell Park Memorial Institute, New York State Department of Health.

Supported, in part, by the Public Health Service grant GR 9211.

Materials and Methods

Twelve apparently healthy mongrel dogs of either sex, ranging in age between one and five years, were selected, whose values for blood urea nitrogen (BUN), non-protein nitrogen (NPN), and sulfobromophthalein (Bromsulphalein) retention had been established as within normal limits. A base line urinalysis for each animal was also recorded.

The dogs were randomly assigned to two groups. In the first group (eight animals), approximately 70% of the liver was infarcted by ligation of branches of the hepatic artery and portal vein (major infarction). Pre- and postsurgical antibiotics were employed.[7] Because partial obstruction of the portal vein has been reported to cause transient decrease of urine formation, portal venous pressures were measured in four dogs by means of a polyethylene tube introduced through the splenic vein. These measurements were begun just prior to actual liver surgery and continued for 30 to 90 minutes thereafter. In the second group of four animals infarction of 30% of the liver was produced in the same way (minor infarction).

In the animals of group I, anesthesia was induced and maintained with sodium thiopental until death. A femoral artery was cannulated and connected to a mercury manometer for continuous blood pressure determinations. Vital signs, such as pulse and respiration, were checked every 15 minutes from surgery until death. An EKG was obtained every 30 minutes. Urine was collected every three hours from a suprapubic bladder catheter and analyzed for microscopic changes and for total volume, specific gravity, presence of albumin, hemoglobin, and bile. Blood samples were drawn at intervals of two to four hours, for the determination of BUN, NPN, and blood sugar. Sulfobromophthalein retention was measured at intervals of three to six hours.

In the surviving animals of group II, similar laboratory examinations were carried out twice a week for two weeks. Autopsies were performed on all animals of group I.

Results

Of the eight dogs of group I, six died within 48 hours after surgery. Dogs 7 and 8 were killed as soon as their mean arterial blood pressure was 70 mm of Hg, in order to obtain a histological picture of the kidney unaffected by premortal hypotension. Table 1 gives the data concerning the survival of the dogs and their postoperative management.

TABLE 1.—*Survival and Postoperative Management*

Dog No.	Survival Time, Hr	Postoperative Intravenous Fluids
1	41	no
2	23	no
3	29	10% glucose in water
4	18	10% glucose in water
5	37	10% glucose in water
6	48	10% glucose in water
7	27 *	10% glucose in water
8	27 *	10% glucose in water

* Killed when their mean arterial blood pressure reached 70 mm of Hg.

Portal pressures after laparotomy and prior to liver surgery ranged from 9 to 14 cm of water. Ligation of the left main branch of the portal vein immediately caused an increase of from 22 to 39 cm, followed within 15 minutes by a return to 8 to 17 cm of water. During this short period of portal hypertension the mesenteric tributaries of the portal vein were only moderately filled, and there was no mesenteric cyanosis.

After the major operation three circulatory stages were observed (Fig 1). The first stage lasted from 6 to 21 hours (median 17 hours) and was characterized by arterial blood pressures increased from the normal range between 120 and 130 mm of Hg to

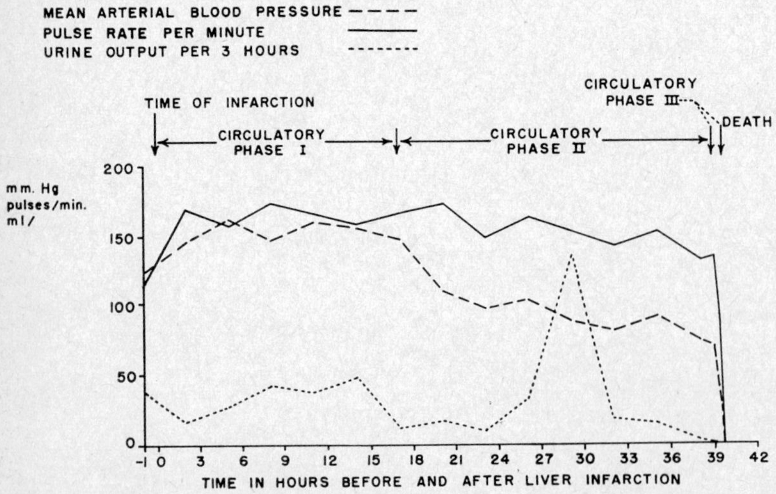

Fig 1.—Median slopes of dogs No. 1 to 6.

values of from 140 to 180 mm of Hg. The elevated blood pressures were associated with increased pulse rates of up to 210 pulses per minute.

During the second phase the high pulse rates were maintained while the blood pressures slowly and irregularly declined. This phase lasted from 9 to 36 hours (median 22 hours). At the end of this phase the arterial blood pressures had fallen to values between 45 and 128 mm of Hg (median 70 mm of Hg). Then, suddenly (third phase), pulse rates and blood pressures declined rapidly and death occurred in 30 to 50 minutes.

A 10% solution of glucose in water was given to dogs 1 and 2 in small amounts to

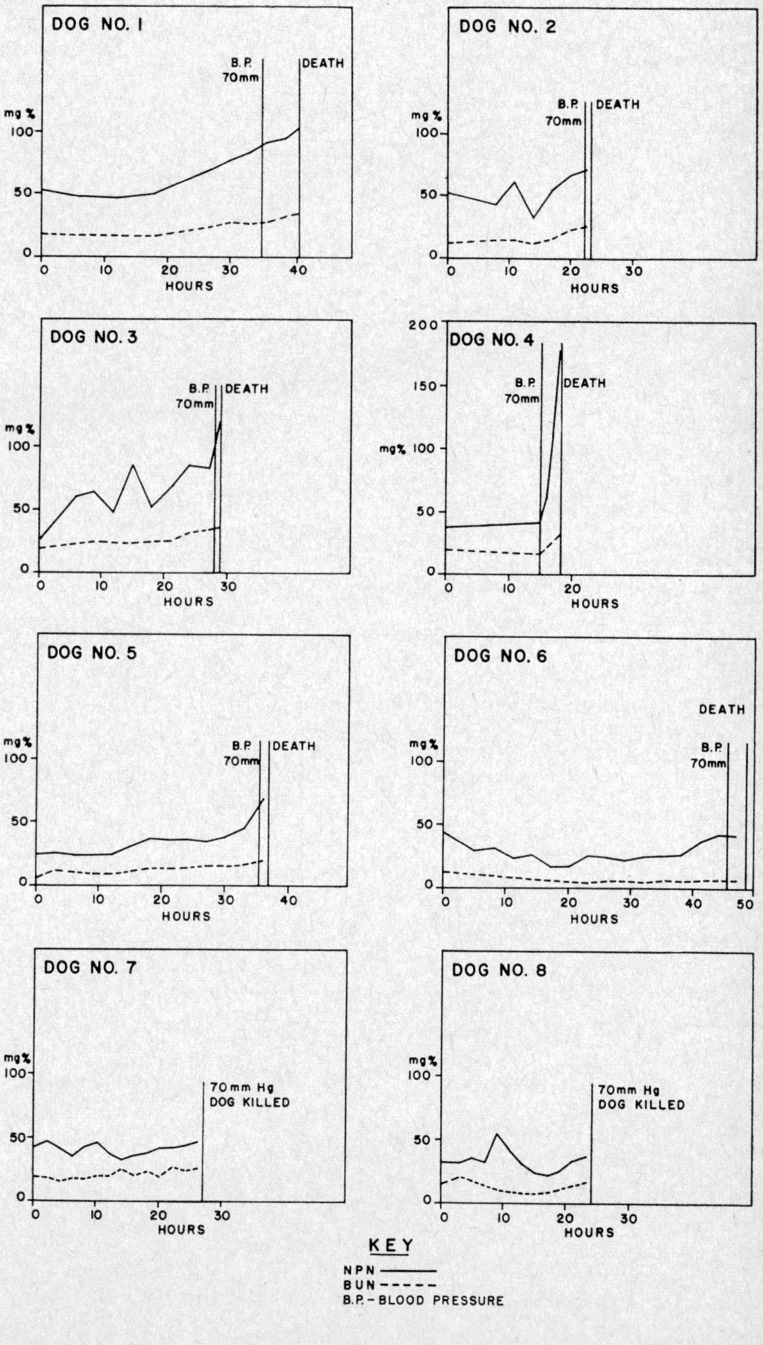

Fig 2. — Changes in levels of BUN and NPN in all eight dogs of group I.

prevent hypoglycemia; dogs 3 to 8 received a continuous drip, at a rate of 6 to 8 ml/kg per hour.

The total urinary output was less than half of the total fluid input. An increase in body weight was noticed in these dogs. There was a tendency toward oliguria in the first and second postoperative circulatory phases. Late in the second phase, a short period of increased urine formation occurred (Fig 1) followed by oliguria and terminal anuria.

Albumin, hemoglobin, and bilirubin appeared in the urine a few hours after surgery. Epithelial cells, erythrocytes, and granular casts followed in the second phase. These findings persisted until death.

The blood of all dogs became hemolysed. The serum hemoglobins were never below 40 mg/100 ml and sometimes as high as 400 mg/100 ml.

Sulfobromophthalein retention increased steadily and became 100% at the end of phase II.

At autopsy, no gangrenous changes were found in the infarcted liver, and clostridia were never detected upon culturing. The rectal temperatures of all dogs were elevated (1 C to 3 C).

Fig 2 shows the changes in the levels of BUN and NPN in all eight dogs of group I. Fig 3 and 4 show the fitted slopes and the confidence limits for NPN and BUN. The presurgical levels of BUN and NPN are within normal ranges. While the BUN levels usually were only minimally increased

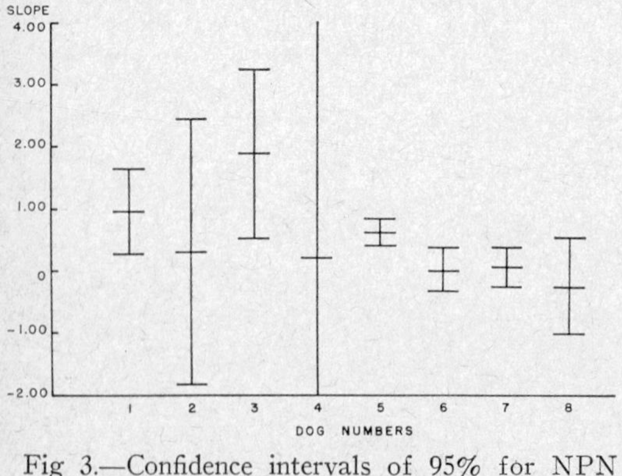

Fig 3.—Confidence intervals of 95% for NPN slopes.

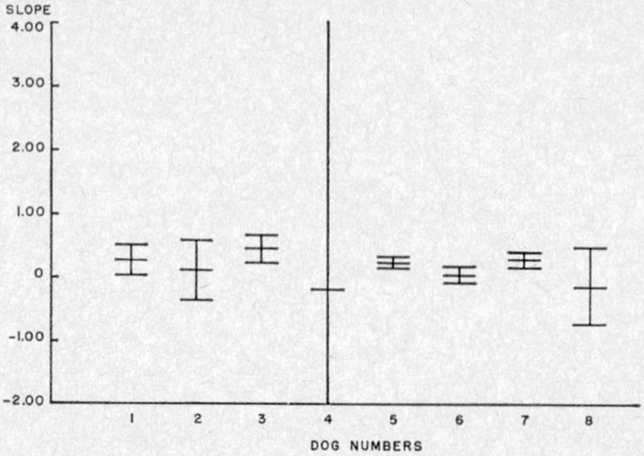

Fig 4.—Confidence intervals of 95% for BUN slopes.

prior to the advent of hypotension, more marked NPN elevations were seen in the dogs 1, 3, and 5.

Three dogs from group II recovered from anesthesia and ate and drank normally within one day. The fourth animal was weak, refused food, and vomited repeatedly after drinking water; after four days it had completely recovered. All four dogs had fever of the intermittent type, lasting from six to nine days (+0.5 C to 1.5 C). The levels of BUN remained unaltered. In the early postoperative period there was a tendency toward moderate hypoglycemia which was treated with dextrose infusions. The mild and transitory urinary deviations are listed on Table 2. All urines were normal eight to ten days after the infarctions.

The kidneys of the dogs of group I appeared macroscopically normal. Histological examination revealed pink-staining material in some glomerular spaces of three dogs (numbers 1, 2, and 5). Similar material was present in a few collecting tubules of most animals of this group. There were no other morphological alterations.

Comments

In the absence of sepsis and before the onset of hypotension, some form of kidney damage occurred. This was evidenced by inconstant increases of BUN and NPN, proteinuria, cylinduria, and a tendency toward oliguria in all dogs. The latter finding is in agreement with the delayed diuretic response toward intravenous fluid loading,

TABLE 2.—*Results of Urinary Analysis During the First Ten Days After Surgery, Group II*

Dog No.	Amt Urine *	Sp G †	Albuminuria	Bilirubinuria	Hemoglobinuria	Casts
1	218-463 cc	0.017-24	+	trace	+	−
2	188-328 cc	0.014-41	++	trace	+	−
3	324-615 cc	0.016-30	+	+	+	−
4	116-398 cc	0.012-28	++	+	++	+ (granular)

* Per 24 hr.
† Upper and lower limits.

found in dogs with ligated hepatic arteries.[11] The elevation of BUN was modest; one might speculate whether its magnitude could have been masked by a probable decrease in BUN synthesis, for which impaired liver function would be responsible. The increase of NPN was more marked. At the moment we have no data concerning the nonureic fractions of NPN, which might account for the difference between BUN and NPN. This was associated with only minor histological changes of the kidneys. Complete renal failure was not evident prior to the advent of hypotension. As hypotension developed, anuria and a rapid increase in BUN and NPN occurred.

At the present status of our investigation, it is still impossible to say whether the moderate impairment of the kidneys, which was present in our dogs prior to hypotension, was due to the progressive disappearance of liver function, or to a toxic effect of autolysing liver. As shown in another publication,[6] hepatic failure did not occur in the same experimental preparation before the end of circulatory phase II; renal impairment, however, was present before this time. For this reason we believe that the cause of renal damage was associated with some products from autolysing liver; an auxiliary factor might have been the presence of free hemoglobin in the serum. Infusions of hemoglobin alone have been shown to have no effect on the kidneys, but renal damage could be produced by the simultaneous actions of hemoglobin and bacterial toxins.[12]

Alterations of hepatic blood flow were reported to reduce renal circulation and to abolish urine formation. Partial obstruction of the portal vein caused reversible anuria only when the portal pressure became elevated.[9] A similar effect on the kidneys could be produced by ligation of the hepatic arteries.[10] Complete ligation of the portal vein caused a decrease of renal blood flow by as much as 90% and was followed by severe general hypotension.[11] In our dogs hypotension appeared during, rarely shortly before, circulatory phase III. The short period of moderate portal hypertension, seen in our dogs, was not accompanied by anuria. The final evaluation of this point would require measurements of renal, portal, and hepatic blood flows and pressures, immediately after ligation of the left portal venous branch.

That complete renal failure can be caused by liver necroses without shock cannot be denied entirely. Possibly more time might be required for the development of completely disturbed renal integrity. Our experimental design pertains only to a relatively rapid sequence of events. Renal, functional, and pathological studies in human fulminant hepatitis,[13] which is characterized by progressive hepatic necrosis, make it doubtful whether a more chronic form of hepatic damage could produce renal failure.

Summary

Large, and acutely fatal, liver infarcts induced renal alterations of the type of toxic glomerulitis, accompanied by light to moderate elevations of BUN and moderate to pronounced increases of NPN levels. These changes were not caused by general hypotension, dehydration, or bacterial infection. It is believed that they were not mediated by a decline of hepatic function. A possible etiologic factor might be the liberation of toxic catabolites from autolysing liver. Smaller liver infarcts were survived and induced mild transitory disturbance of renal function, followed by restoration within eight to ten days.

Miss Xenia Gawrylowski, Miss Janet Kellam, Miss Marsha Wolf, and Mr. Ludwig Ulrich gave technical assistance.

Gunther E. Kraus, DVS, Department of Experimental Surgery, Roswell Park Memorial Institute, 666 Elm St, Buffalo 3, NY.

REFERENCES

1. Helwig, F. C., and Orr, T. G.: Traumatic Necrosis of the Liver With Extensive Retention of Creatinine and High Grade Nephrosis, Arch Surg 24:136, 1932.

2. Pytel, A.: Zur Frage des hepato-renalen Syndroms, Arch Klin Chir 187:27, 1936.

3. Wilensky, A. D.: Occurrence, Distribution and Pathogenesis of So-Called Liver Death and/or the Hepato-Renal Syndrome, Arch Surg 38:625, 1939.

4. Darmady, E. M.: Renal Anoxia and the Traumatic Uremia Syndrome, Brit J Surg 34:262, 1947.

5. Fajers, C. M.: Experimental Studies on the So-Called Hepato-Renal Syndrome: III. On the Effect of Hepatic Necrosis by Itself and Combined With Ten Minutes Unilateral Renal Ischemia on the Kidneys of Hydrated Rabbits; As Judged by Some Renal Function Tests, Acta Path Microbiol Scand 44:5, 1958.

6. Kraus, G. E.: The Toxicity of Autolysing Liver: I. Evidence for a Fatal Termination in the Absence of Infection and/or Liver Insufficiency, in preparation.

7. Kraus, G. E.; Myiares, J.; and Ross, C. A.: Observations on Induced Liver Infarctions in Dogs, Surgery 49:751, 1961.

8. Popper, H., and Schaffer, F.: Liver Structure and Function, New York: McGraw-Hill Book Co., Inc., p 667.

9. Hermann, H.; Lemarchands, H.; and Tanche, M.: Influence d'une obstruction partielle de la veine porte sur le débit urinaire, J Physiol (Paris) 50:316, 1958.

10. Onnis, M.; Shumacker, H. B., Jr.; and Bounous, G.: Response to Occlusion of the Portal Vein: Blood Pressure and Renal Blood Flow, Arch Surg 85:897, 1962.

11. Donovan, A. J., and Child, C. G., III: The Influence of Eck Fistula Upon Diuresis and Antidiuresis in the Dog, Surg Forum 9:546, 1959.

12. Regelson, W.: Personal communication.

13. Lucke, B., and Mallory, T.: The Fulminant Form of Epidemic Hepatitis, Amer J Path 22:867, 1946.

Nonunion of the Clavicle

EINER W. JOHNSON, JR., MD
AND
H. ROYER COLLINS, MD
ROCHESTER, MINN

The clavicle is the bone in the body most frequently fractured, accounting for 5% to 10% of all fractures.[1] Because of the difficulty of completely immobilizing fractures in this region, more than 200 different methods of treatment have been suggested. However, despite the apparent dissatisfaction with methods of fixation, nonunion is rare. Annersten in 1948[2] reviewed 350 cases and found the incidence of pseudarthrosis to be 1.3%. A review of the English-language literature reveals only three studies of 18 or 20 cases each and one of nine cases.[3-6] It has been stated that nonunion is becoming more frequent,[7] but it is not certain whether this is due to an increased severity of injuries (secondary to the increased trauma in accidents associated with higher speeds of vehicles), a complacent attitude about the initial treatment, or more frequent open reduction of fractures.

Of the reports mentioned, one, by Ghormley and co-workers,[4] was of 20 cases examined at the Mayo Clinic in the period January, 1913, to October, 1939. We wish to report 69 additional cases seen here since then.

Clinical Data

Sixty-eight patients with 69 ununited fractures of the clavicle * were examined at the Mayo Clinic in the period October, 1939, to December, 1962. Nonunion was considered to be present if the patient had roentgenographic or clinical evidence, or both, of nonunion four months after injury. Nonunion had existed from 4 months to 45 years except in two cases, in which operation was performed two months after injury, at which time typical pseudarthrosis was found. Thirty-six of the patients were male and 32 female, with ages ranging from 3 to 69 years and averaging 43 years. Thirty-five of the fractures were in the left clavicle and 34 in the right; 36 fractures were in the middle third, 20 in the outer third, 7 involved the junction of the middle and outer thirds, and the location was unknown in 6.

Fourteen of these fractures were treated initially by open reduction, 23 by closed reduction, 4 by later internal fixation (one to three months after injury), 4 had no treatment, and, in 24, the initial treatment was unknown.

Methods and duration of external fixation varied widely: 6 patients were immobilized for three to six weeks, 7 for less than three weeks, 3 had no immobilization, and, in 52, the method and duration of fixation were unknown.

An attempt was made to classify the injuries involved according to degree of severity. Thirty of the fractures were caused by severe injury, such as automobile accidents, and 17 by moderate trauma, such as falls or wrestling. In 20 cases the initial injury was not known, and in two cases there

Read before the 112th Annual Meeting of the American Medical Association, Section on Orthopedic Surgery, Atlantic City, NJ, June 18, 1963.

Section of Orthopedic Surgery (Dr. Johnson); Fellow in Orthopedic Surgery (Dr. Collins).

Mayo Clinic and Mayo Foundation.

* One patient had fracture of both clavicles.

was known to have been no trauma (one of these patients was four months old and congenital pseudarthrosis was possible).

The most common clinical findings were motion, deformity, tenderness, depression, limitation of motion, and, in four cases, neurologic signs such as weakness and paresthesia in the adjacent arm and hand. In 22 cases, no findings were reported on physical examination, but nonunion was found on roentgenograms of the chest. Significant symptoms were pain in 33 cases, weakness in 7, numbness and paresthesia in 10, limitation of motion in 3, a mass at the site of fracture in 2, and, in 28 cases, there were no symptoms and the nonunion was found on thoracic roentgenograms during examination for other reasons.

Treatment

In 47 cases treatment was conservative and, in 22, by operation. Of those cases treated conservatively (physiotherapy such as heat, massage, range-of-motion exercises, shoulder-strengthening exercises, or any other treatment but operation) results were excellent in 23 with no symptoms or complaints, pain continued in one 5 years later, pain occurred with excess activity in one, slight pain was noted after seven years in one, and the end result was unknown in 21 cases. It should be emphasized that those patients treated conservatively had minimal or no symptoms or findings when seen at this clinic; in only five cases were these considered serious enough to warrant surgical treatment (two were advised to have a bone graft, and three were advised to have excision of the outer third of the clavicle).

Of the 22 cases with surgical treatment, two had excision of the nonunion only, with an excellent result in one and a poor result (nonunion) in the other. Six cases of fracture of the outer third of the clavicle were treated by distal fragment excision (Fig 1). In these, three patients had excellent results, one had 20% limitation of motion, one had residual pain, and for one the result was unknown. Five patients were treated by open reduction, onlay bone graft, and intramedullary fixation with a Kirschner wire or Rush nail (Fig 2); solid unions resulted in four and the result was unknown in one. One patient had excision of pseudarthrosis with wire fixation; however, pseudarthrosis recurred despite external fixation with a figure-of-eight bandage for four months. Four patients were treated by onlay bone graft alone with solid union in one, good motion and less pain with questionable union in one, and unknown results in two. The results, in one patient, of treatment by Kirschner-wire fixation alone and, in one, of

Fig 1.—Fracture of distal third of left clavicle in 22-year-old man which occurred when he was playing football. *A*, preoperative view showing nonunion; *B*, appearance five weeks after resection of distal fragment.

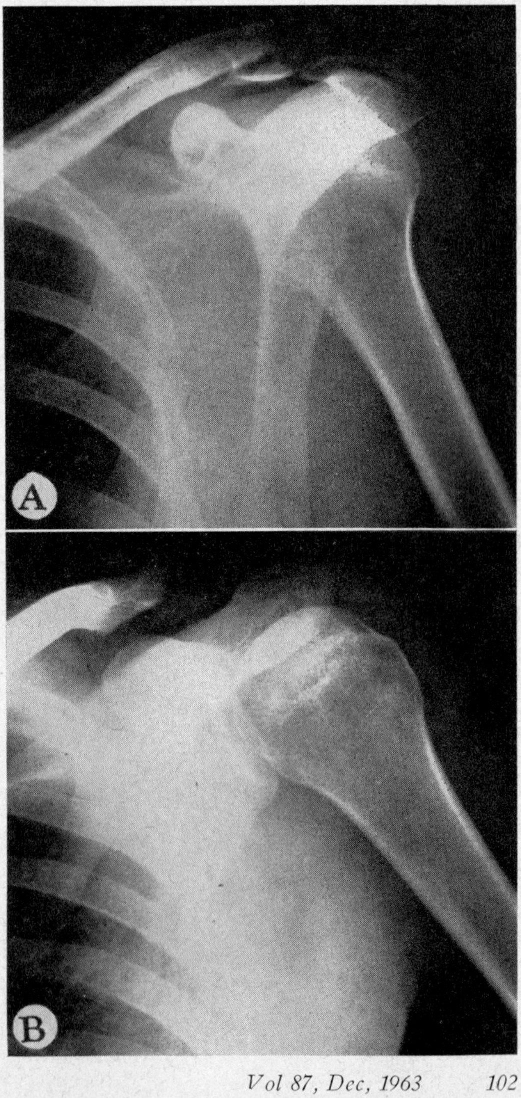

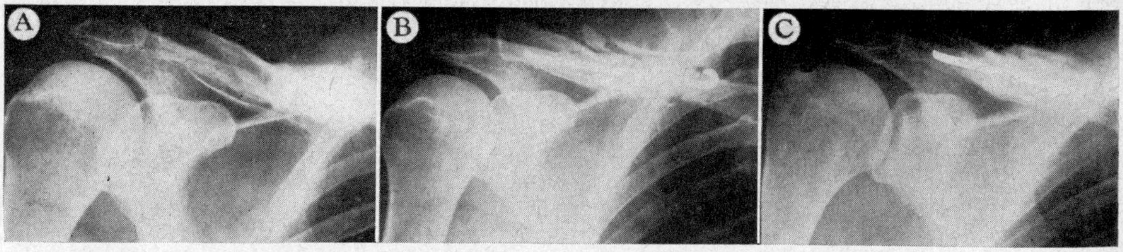

Fig 2.—Fracture of middle third of right clavicle in 45-year-old man. *A,* preoperative view showing nonunion; *B,* postoperative view after resection of pseudarthrosis, intramedullary fixation with Rush nail, and onlay graft with iliac bone; *C,* solid union seen six months postoperatively.

treatment by resection of the proximal third of the bone were not known. In one patient there was good union after treatment by dual onlay bone graft with intramedullary nail fixation and two Parham bands, followed by bed rest for four weeks, and then figure-of-eight bandage and, later, fixation in a cast for a total of three months. One patient was treated by removal of a prior metal fixation but complained of ulnar paresthesia of the right arm postoperatively.

Our patients were immobilized postoperatively for at least five weeks, as advocated by Ghormley and co-workers,[4] with a Velpeau dressing, a figure-of-eight bandage, a plaster splint, or bed rest followed by immobilization with a figure-of-eight bandage and a cast; in two cases, external fixation was maintained for four months.

Comment

It becomes apparent from reviewing these cases that no one factor can be blamed for nonunion. One can say only that nonunion was more common in fractures of the middle third of the clavicle which occurred after severe trauma with considerable distraction and which were treated with open reduction initially. Admittedly, closed reduction with adequate external fixation for a period long enough to allow union is the best method in the majority of cases. Neer [5] has stated that of 2,235 patients with fractures of the middle third of the clavicle treated by closed methods, only three (0.1%) had failure of union, whereas, of 45 treated by immediate open reduction, two (4.6%) had failure of union. It is thought that local tissue damage, stripping of soft parts, removal of valuable bone, inadequate internal fixation, and infection all may increase the chances of nonunion.

Cave [8] has stated that there have been no instances of nonunion in patients treated by open reduction with intramedullary fixation at the Massachusetts General Hospital, provided the pin was left in place for eight to ten weeks. If the pin was taken out too soon, delayed union was noted. Ghormley and co-workers [4] also have stated that open reduction should be considered in cases of fracture caused by severe injury with disruption of the coracoclavicular ligaments or with displacement or gapping which cannot be reduced, or in cases with other injuries which prevent proper splinting. Despite the trend to treat more fractures by open methods,[9] we would like to make a plea for conservative treatment. Under rare and unusual circumstances, open reduction occasionally may be indicated; but, in our experience, almost all fractures of the clavicle can be treated conservatively. If this conservative treatment is managed properly, a favorable result can be expected in an extremely high percentage of cases regardless of the severity of the initial injury.

It is difficult to arrive at any definite conclusions regarding duration of immobilization and type of immobilization used in our series, but it is interesting to note that many of the fractures were not immobilized for very long and several received no treatment at all.

Once nonunion is diagnosed, choice of treatment depends on the findings and symptoms. As mentioned, most of our patients were treated conservatively, and, of those who were operated on, several were given a trial of physiotherapy and other conservative treatment before surgical treatment was undertaken. It is interesting to note that one patient, who was treated elsewhere eight months after accident with intramedullary Kirschner-wire fixation with an iliac bone graft and a cast for six weeks, was seen with resultant nonunion and pain; he was better after several days of physiotherapy and no further surgical treatment was necessary. Also, one patient, treated with external fixation by plaster cast for six weeks, who was seen at this clinic five months later with pain and numbness of the shoulder and adjacent arm, had an excellent result four years later after conservative treatment.

Operation was undertaken only if symptoms such as pain, limitation of motion, weakness, numbness and paresthesia, or deformity were sufficiently severe or disabling to warrant it. Frequently, nonunion is present without the patient's knowing it and without the patient's having any serious disability; and, of course, in these cases, no treatment is necessary. It is our conclusion that the best surgical procedure for nonunion of the middle third of the clavicle is open reduction with intramedullary Kirschner-wire fixation and onlay bone graft followed by fixation with a Velpeau dressing, figure-of-eight bandage, plaster splint, or bed rest for at least five weeks. Fractures of the outer third with nonunion are treated best by excision of the outer third. Excision of the pseudarthrosis alone or inadequate internal fixation at the time of operation seems to predispose to nonunion.

Summary

Sixty-nine cases of nonunion of fracture of the clavicle are summarized. Thirty-six fractures were in the middle third, 20 in the outer third, and 7 at the junction of the middle and outer thirds of the clavicle. Closed reduction with adequate external fixation for a sufficient period is the treatment of choice regardless of the initial injury or damage except under rare and unusual circumstances. Open reduction should be undertaken only with good indications and always accompanied by adequate internal fixation. Severe initial injury and improper immobilization certainly contribute to nonunion.

In 16 of the 22 cases treated surgically, a variety of surgical procedures were used, with union in eight cases and nonunion in two. The result was not known in six cases. In the other six, treatment was excision of the outer third of the clavicle, with excellent results in three, 20% limitation of motion in one, slight residual pain in one, and result unknown in one.

Conservative treatment is advocated if symptoms are not severe. If operation is indicated, onlay bone graft with intramedullary metal fixation followed by external fixation for five weeks is the treatment of choice. With increasing incidence of more severe injuries, it is conceivable that nonunion will become more prevalent than it has been.

Mayo Clinic, Rochester, Minn.

REFERENCES

1. Moore, T. O.: Internal Pin Fixation for Fracture of the Clavicle, Amer Surg 17:580-583 (July) 1951.

2. Annersten, S., quoted by Powell, H. D. W.: Ununited Fractures of the Clavicle, Brit Med J 2:651-652 (Sept 20) 1952.

3. Berkheiser, E. J.: Old Ununited Clavicular Fractures in the Adult, Surg Gynec Obstet 64:1064-1072 (June) 1937.

4. Ghormley, R. K.; Black, J. R.; and Cherry, J. H.: Ununited Fractures of the Clavicle, Amer J Surg 51:343-349 (Feb) 1941.

5. Neer, C. S., II.: Nonunion of the Clavicle, JAMA 172:1006-1011 (March 5) 1960.

6. Sakellarides, H.: Pseudarthrosis of the Clavicle, J Bone Joint Surg 43A:130-138 (Jan) 1961.

7. Bateman, J. E.: "Fractures and Dislocations of the Shoulder Region," in Shoulder and Environs, St. Louis: C. V. Mosby Company, 1955, pp 457-521.

8. Cave, E. F.: Fractures and Other Injuries, Chicago: The Year Book Medical Publishers, Inc., 1958, pp 254-263.

9. O'Donoghue, D. H.: "Injuries to the Shoulder Girdle," in Reynolds, F. C.: The American Academy of Orthopaedic Surgeons: Instructional Course Lectures, St. Louis: C V. Mosby Company, 1960, vol 17, pp 392-406.

Acute Thoracic Compression With Traumatic Asphyxia

Report of Six Cases

JAMES R. SHAMBLIN, MD
AND
DWIGHT C. McGOON, MD
ROCHESTER, MINN

Acute thoracic compression may produce a striking and characteristic syndrome referred to variously as traumatic asphyxia, ecchymotic mask, pressure stasis, traumatic cyanosis, cervicofacial cutaneous asphyxia, and Perthes' symptom complex.[1] It is caused by a crushing injury to the chest or upper abdomen, or both, with a period of apnea. It is characterized by reddish, purplish, or black discoloration of the skin of the face, neck, and shoulders, accompanied by bilateral subconjunctival hemorrhages.

"Traumatic asphyxia," the most common designation of this syndrome, is actually a misnomer. The patients have not been asphyxiated in the usual definition of the term, but instead have suffered from excessive oxygen removal in the cutaneous capillaries due to stasis of blood flow. "Cervicofacial static cyanosis" accurately describes the pathophysiology; but because the term is somewhat cumbersome, "traumatic asphyxia" probably will continue to be used.

Since most recent cases of this entity have been due to accidents involving motor vehicles or heavy machinery, one may expect its frequency to increase in the future. No review of this condition has been published in the past decade. For these reasons, six cases are presented with emphasis on the recognition and treatment of the symptom complex and the associated injuries.

Submitted for publication June 13, 1963.

Fellow in Surgery, Mayo Foundation (Dr. Shamblin); Section of Surgery (Dr. McGoon), Mayo Clinic and Mayo Foundation.

Report of Cases

CASE 1.—In 1943 a 54-year-old man had been pinned beneath an overturned tractor for 20 minutes.[2] The steering wheel had rested on the right side of his chest and abdomen. He had been unconscious when found.

Marked purplish discoloration appeared over the face, head, and neck, extending to the deltoid region of the shoulders. Multiple petechiae were found in this region and in the buccal mucosa. Subconjunctival hemorrhages were present bilaterally, and funduscopic examination revealed a small hemorrhage in the superior nasal portion of the right retina. The eyelids were edematous. The vital signs were normal except for some expiratory slowing. The neck veins were distended, and there was subcutaneous emphysema in the region of the right upper anterior axillary line. Several ribs on the right were fractured posteriorly. The chest roentgenogram showed minimal fluid in the right pleural space. A lumbar puncture three hours after admission evidenced no abnormality. The patient was unconscious, and the position of the head and extremities suggested decerebrate rigidity.

With no specific treatment other than administration of oxygen and mild sedation, he gradually regained consciousness after 18 hours. By the eighth day he was up. On the 12th day he first noticed diplopia, but neurologic examination revealed only weakness of the right external rectus muscle. At dismissal from the hospital on the 16th day, the purplish color was fading and the subconjunctival hemorrhages were resolving. Three months after the accident the diplopia was no longer present and the skin and sclera were of normal color.

CASE 2.—In 1957 a 52-year-old woman had been thrown from her car and her chest had been pinned beneath the edge of the car. For 10 to 15 minutes it had been impossible to free her, and whether she had been unconscious or apneic was not known.

She complained of pain in the anterior part of the chest, lumbar region, and right elbow. Examination revealed bilateral periorbital ecchymoses and subconjunctival hemorrhages. Motion of the neck was painful, and there was tenderness about the manubrium sterni. Roentgenograms revealed a compression fracture of the first lumbar vertebra and elevation of the right side of the diaphragm with adjacent pleural reaction.

Complete rest in bed was prescribed for three weeks, after which only slight discoloration of the sclera remained. Back pain persisted for several months, although the patient wore an orthopedic support.

CASE 3.—A 16-year-old girl had been pinned beneath a car in an automobile accident in 1959. She had not been unconscious or apneic at any time, but had remained under the car 15 to 20 minutes.

When admitted to the hospital she was alert and had normal vital signs. Petechiae were scattered over the face and neck, most prominently on the eyelids; and subconjunctival hemorrhages were noted. There was dried blood in the right nostril. Superficial abrasions were present over both legs, and abrasion and avulsion of the skin was noted in the left lumbar area. Fractures were found in the medial and posterior right malleolus and the midshaft of the right fibula.

The leukocyte count was 16,900 per cubic millimeter, but returned to normal the next day. Roentgenograms of the chest showed nothing abnormal.

Treatment was given for the fractures, and the petechiae had disappeared when the patient was dismissed from the hospital one week after admission. Two and a half months after the accident she was enjoying full activity and the sclerae were normal.

CASE 4.—In 1962 a 37-year-old man had been found unconscious with his chest beneath an overturned tractor at approximately 10 AM, having been there an undetermined length of time. He had been taken to his local hospital, where tracheostomy had been done and intravenous administration of fluids started, after which he had been sent by ambulance to a hospital affiliated with this clinic.

On arrival at 1 PM he was comatose and unresponsive, but occasionally moved all four extremities. His appearance was striking—the head, face, and neck were a deep purple which changed to mottled red over the shoulders and upper arms (Fig 1). The skin color was normal below the nipples and on the forearms. The discolored skin blanched somewhat with pressure, but close inspection also revealed hundreds of petechiae in it. Both eyelids were swollen, obscuring vision, and there was moderate exophthalmos. Massive subconjunctival hemorrhages were present. The pupils were equal and reactive, and the fundi were normal. Blood was present in both external auditory canals, and mucosal ecchymoses were noted. Subcutaneous emphysema was noted in the right side of the neck. No evidence of venous distention was found. Respiration was predominantly normal, with occasional periods of dyspnea; and the breath sounds were normal. Abdominal examination revealed no abnormality. All peripheral reflexes were diminished and Babinski reflexes were positive bilaterally. The blood pressure varied from 150 to 110 mm Hg systolic over 120 to 70 diastolic with a pulse rate of about 110.

The hemoglobin concentration was 17.4 gm per 100 ml of blood, and the leukocytes numbered 38,200 per cubic millimeter with a differential count of 83% segmental forms, 10 lymphocytes, 5 monocytes, and 2 eosinophils. The chest roentgenogram showed no abnormality except an old fracture of the right seventh rib and subcutaneous emphysema. The skull and cervical vertebrae appeared normal roentgenographically. The electroencephalographic pattern was normal.

The patient was given 90 mg of urea intravenously shortly after arrival here. On the evening of admission he moved all extremities and responded to painful stimuli. His fluid intake was restricted to 1,500 ml of glucose solution daily. The day after admission he was responsive, but irrational. On the third hospital day he had sudden, pleuritic chest pain lasting one hour, and a thoracic roentgenogram revealed collapse of the upper lobe of the right lung. The sensorium cleared on the third day, and the findings from neurologic examination at that time were normal. The tracheostomy tube was removed, and ambulation and general diet were prescribed. Skin biopsy from the upper part of the neck revealed extravasation of erythrocytes in the mid and deep layers of the dermis (Fig 2). By the time of dismissal from the hospital, 11 days after admission, the purplish discoloration of the face and neck was much lighter and the chest was normal roentgenographically. One month after the accident the patient had recovered completely except for a slight xanthochromic appearance of the sclerae.

CASE 5.—A 52-year-old farmer had been attempting to repair an approximately 300 lb tractor implement from below when the prop holding it had slipped and the implement had fallen, coming to rest across his body from the left lower part of the chest to the right shoulder. As the machine had fallen slowly, he had had time to cry for help before losing consciousness. His wife had found him within one to two minutes. He had been cyanotic and apneic, with both eyes bulging. It had taken three to four minutes to remove him from under the implement. He then had been given mouth-to-mouth resuscitation; and within a few seconds he had resumed breathing himself and

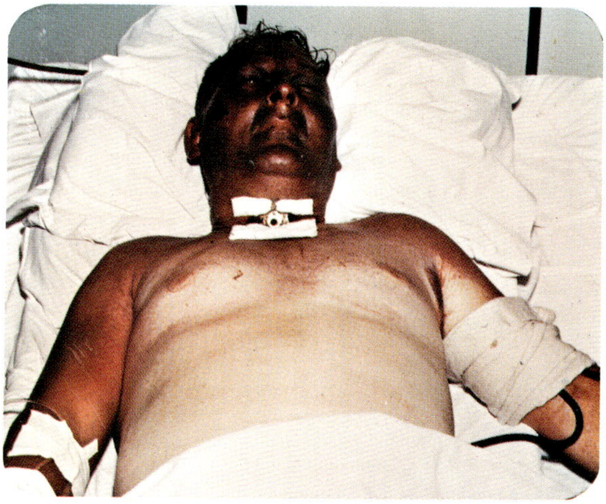

Fig 1 (case 4). — Discoloration of face, shoulder, and upper arms 24 hours after injury. Note also dried blood around nares.

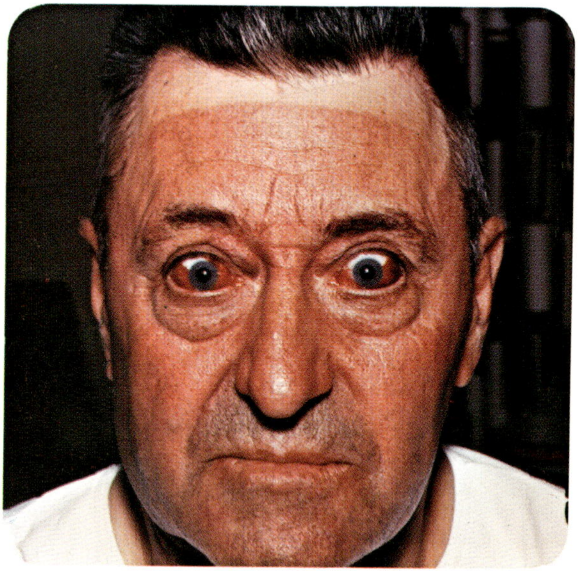

Fig 3 (case 5). — Massive subconjunctival hemorrhage; abrupt limit of redness where hatband crossed forehead.

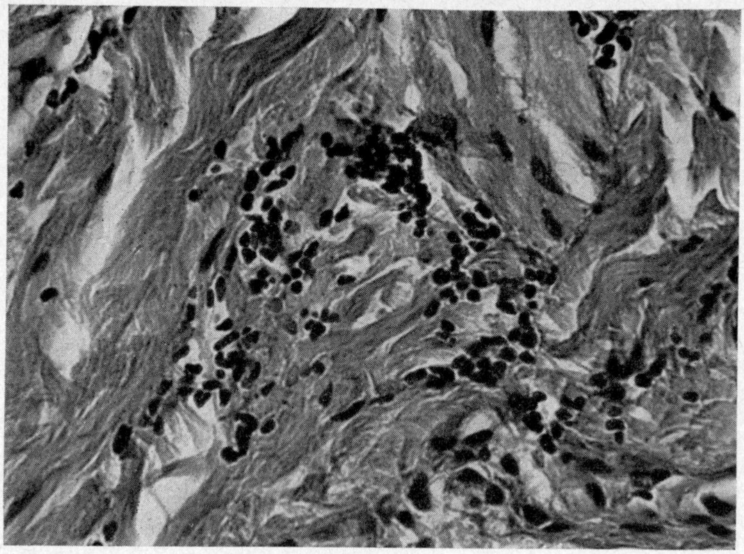

Fig 2 (case 4).—Subcutaneous tissue from neck, showing extravasated erythrocytes. Hematoxylin and eosin; × 400.

had become conscious. He had been brought to the hospital in a private car.

On arrival he was alert and cheerful, and his only complaints were pain in the left lower anterior part of the chest and the right temperomandibular joint. The face and upper part of the chest had the appearance of a fresh, severe sunburn with the redness ending abruptly on his forehead at the level where his hat had been. Close inspection revealed that the redness was caused by petechiae. Both eyes had massive subconjunctival hemorrhages extending even under the palpebrae (Fig 3). The fundi were normal. Prominent ecchymoses were present under the tongue and there was dried blood in both nostrils. An ecchymotic area over the right shoulder and tenderness over the lower left ribs anteriorly were noted. Thorough examination revealed no other abnormalities. The vital signs were stable on admission and remained so during hospitalization.

The hemogram, urinalysis, roentgenograms of chest and mandible, and electrocardiogram indicated normality.

The patient was observed in the hospital for two days and then dismissed. One month after the accident, he had no residua except slight tenderness in the left anterior part of the chest.

Case 6.—A 34-year-old farmer had been crushed under a loaded cornpicker in 1962. The wheels had passed over his chest and then he had been dragged 200 ft before stopping. He had got up unassisted and walked several feet before collapsing. On admission to a local hospital he had been unconscious and the skin from the nipple-line to the head, including the upper extremities in their entirety, had been black. Bilateral subconjunctival hemorrhages and buccal ecchymoses had been present. A chest roentgenogram had revealed multiple rib fractures on the left.

He had a history of asthma and chronic cough.

Supportive care had been given and he had regained consciousnes quickly. On the day after admission, left thoracentesis had removed 150 ml of blood. On the third day, atelectasis of the left lung had been suspected and he had been transferred to a clinic-affiliated hospital.

On admission here, the patient was alert and the vital signs were normal except for a temperature of 102 F (38.9 C) and labored respiration. A bluish discoloration was present over the upper part of the chest and the neck, face, and upper arms. This was rather homogeneous except for linear streaks of normal color in the anterior axillary skin folds (Fig 4). The nail beds were pale and dusky, and slight generalized cyanosis was noted. Slight venous distention was present in the cervical region. Massive subconjunctival hemorrhage and edema involved both eyes. Paradoxical motion was observed in the left side of the chest. Rhonchi and rales were present bilaterally, more prominently on the left. Deep palpation over the abdomen caused some guarding, and the bowel sounds were hypoactive. No neurologic deficit was found.

A chest roentgenogram revealed several rib fractures on the left, contusion of the left lung and a left hemothorax estimated at 1,500 to 2,000 ml. In an arterial blood sample, pH was 7.51 and estimated oxygenation 85%. The pattern of an electrocardiogram was normal.

At tracheostomy performed shortly after admission a No. 6 cuffed tracheostomy tube was inserted, and breathing then was assisted by the Bird respirator. Shortly after assisted ventilation was begun, the paradoxical movement of the left side of the chest ceased. Penicillin and streptomycin were given intramuscularly twice daily.

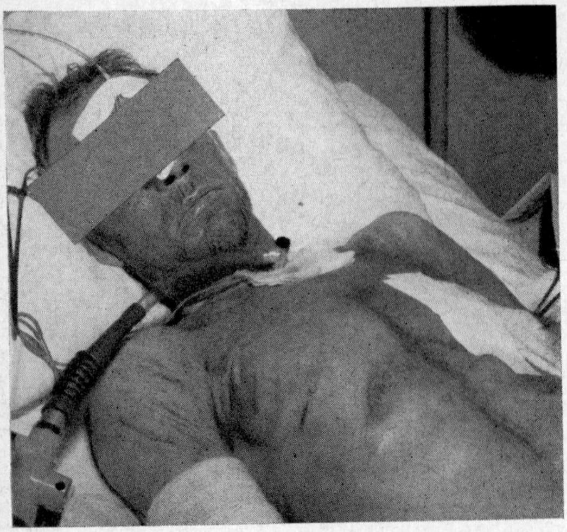

Fig 4 (case 6).—Linear discoloration in axillary folds, 72 hours after injury.

Hemoglobin measured 8.8 gm and leukocytes numbered 15,400. A sputum culture grew *Staphylococcus aureus* and *Pseudomonas*.

The patient's course was stable throughout the next three days except for a spiking fever. On the fourth day inspiratory and expiratory wheezes developed in the chest and the rectal temperature reached 104 F (40 C). Increasingly long periods were required for receiving pure oxygen in the respirator. That evening the pulse rate rose to 160 per minute and he was pale and lethargic. After two units of whole blood were given slowly the pulse rate decreased and the color and respiration improved.

The next morning, however, the patient was less responsive and showed restlessness and air hunger. The pulmonary rales increased and the breathing became irregular. Digitalization was started, but he died shortly after the first dose. Necropsy was not performed.

Comment

Previous Reports.—After necropsy on several people trampled to death in a French riot in 1837, Ollivier [3] described the condition of "masque ecchymotique" but attempted no explanation of it as a process. Perthes [4] in 1900 gave a complete description of the syndrome as we know it today and advanced a hypothesis as to its cause. Heuer [5] collected published reports of 126 cases in 1923 and added one of his own. Dwek,[6] reviewing published accounts in 1946, found 170 cases. The latest review, that of Fred and Chandler [1] in 1960, totaled 179 cases. Subsequent to that, we have been able to find only two additional cases, reported by Quigley [7] in 1961. To these 181, we add five more. (Our case 1 was reported in 1944 by Stickney and Hagedorn.[2])

Etiology.—The cause of traumatic asphyxia is usually a severe, sustained, crushing injury that affects directly the chest or upper part of the abdomen or both. But also it may result from indirect injuries that make the body jackknife with the knees exerting pressure on the abdomen and chest.[6] These injuries occur in industrial, agricultural, or automobile accidents, and in panics where people are trampled.[3,8] Any injury that raises the intrathoracic pressure to high levels may cause this syndrome, and mild cases have been reported after epileptic attacks,[9] difficult delivery,[10] whooping cough,[11] and vomiting.[12]

In our series from a predominantly agricultural region four of the cases were caused by tractors or tractor attachments and two by automobiles.

Perthes,[4] in his description of the syndrome, postulated two mechanisms by which the syndrome is produced: first, a mechanical reflux of blood to the head and neck through the innominate and jugular system of veins where valves are incompetent or absent; and second, contusion of the abdominal sympathetic system which produces vasodilatation of the vessels in the head and neck. Attempts to reproduce the clinical effect in animals by causing crushing injuries of the chest or division of the splanchnic nerves were unsuccessful.[6] However, Reichert and Martin [13] in 1951, working with white dogs, produced all the typical clinical signs by surgically occluding the superior vena cava proximal to the azygos vein for ten minutes.

Perthes' conception of mechanical cephalad reflux through the venous system is now thought by most to be the primary factor in the production of this syndrome. The veins of the innominate and jugular system have either incompetent valves or none. When a severe crushing injury to the chest is sustained, the blood is squeezed out of the right atrium, superior cava, and azygos system and forced in a retrograde manner through the veins and capillaries of the chest, neck, and face. This produces distention followed by atony of the capillary walls, with stasis of blood in these vessels accounting for the bluish discoloration. Where the vessels are not supported by the surrounding tissue, as in the conjunctiva and buccal mucosa, or when the retrograde pressure is excessive, there is actual extravasation of erythrocytes from the vessels with production of petechiae and ecchymoses (Fig 2). Where counterpressure is applied externally by such agents as hat bands, suspenders, or tight collars, the vessels are protected from overdistention and these areas are not discolored (case 5). The infolding of skin in case 6 produced an unusual striped pattern with normal skin alternating with ecchymoses (Fig 4).

At the time of injury, the victim may have momentary or prolonged apnea. This causes temporary hypoxia which may produce a generalized cyanosis that rapidly clears as breathing is resumed but is thought by some to contribute to the atony of the capillaries.[1] The patient in our case 5 was apneic with generalized cyanosis when found; but on examination some 30 minutes later, after a period of spontaneous respiration, no cyanosis was present in the trunk or extremities. In case 6, slight generalized cyanosis was noticeable three days after the accident; but mechanical factors prohibited adequate respiratory function in this patient.

Clinical Characteristics.—The clinical manifestations depend on the severity and duration of the thoracic compression and on other concomitant injuries.

The skin is reddish-purple to black with the discoloration extending over the face, neck, and sometimes the upper part of the chest to the level of the nipples anteriorly, the lower level of the trapezius posteriorly, and usually not farther than the elbows laterally. Close examination reveals many petechiae. If extravasation of erythrocytes is minimal or absent, pressure causes blanching. The color may increase in intensity for a few hours or days and then gradually fade over a period of days or weeks. Xanthochromic changes do not occur unless there has been hemorrhage into the tissues. Administration of oxygen has no appreciable effect on the discoloration unless there is generalized cyanosis. In three of our cases (No. 1, 4, and 6) the color was markedly bluish (or purplish) about the face and gradually faded over the shoulders and upper part of the chest. One patient (case 5) had reddish discoloration limited to the face, neck, and upper shoulders; one (case 3) had it only on the face and neck; and one (case 2) had normal skin color except for bilateral periorbital ecchymoses.

Mild to massive subconjunctival hemorrhages nearly always are present, usually in the exposed portion of the conjunctiva; and we consider them an essential feature of the syndrome. Frequently they are accompanied by periorbital edema and ecchymosis. The color fades gradually, passing through a xanthochromic stage. In most cases there is no damage to the retina or optic nerve, but Heuer[5] found 16 instances of visual disturbance among 127 reported cases. Seven of the 16 patients had immediate and permanent impairment or loss of vision in one or both eyes; six had immediate but transient loss of vision; and three had late visual difficulties. He concluded that immediate loss of vision may occur as a result of retinal edema, with prompt return of vision within hours or days. In those cases with permanent damage, retinal hemorrhage usually was apparent. Hemorrhage into the retrobulbar region, causing exophthalmos and damage to the optic nerve, is possible also. All of our patients had subconjunctival hemorrhages, which were limited to the interpalpebral region in three instances but involved the entire bulbar conjunctivae in the other three. Four patients had edema of the lids, severe enough in one to obscure vision. In the only case with retinal hemorrhage, transient diplopia developed 12 days after the injury.

Bleeding from the nose or ears or into the buccal mucosa usually has subsided by the time of medical examination. Four of our patients had evidence of mucosal hemorrhage, and dried blood was found in the nares of two patients and in the external auditory canals of another. Miliary ecchymosis of the tympanic membrane has been demonstrated in reported cases and transient hearing loss has occurred.

Associated injuries are encountered frequently. Those present in this series are listed in the Table. Rib fractures are the most common, and severe intrathoracic injury must always be suspected. Chest roentgenograms, which showed no damage in half of our cases, may demonstrate contusion of the lung, pneumothorax, hemothorax, subcutaneous emphysema, or fractures of the ribs or vertebrae. Our case 6 showed several of these findings, which resulted in a "flail chest" and later fatal respiratory complications. Injury to the heart and great vessels is rare, but should be suspected in every case and checked by serial roentgenograms, electrocardiograms, and hemoglobin determinations.

Three of our patients were comatose for more than a few hours. Necropsy in cases of traumatic asphyxia has revealed edema of the brain substance but a striking absence of intracerebral or intracranial hemorrhage. It is believed that such hemorrhage is prevented by the rigid cranium, which limits expansion of the vessel walls, and by the large sinuses at the base of the brain, which act as a baffle against the sudden retrograde flow of blood.[6] Cerebral edema plus the temporary hypoxia occurring at the time of injury may cause coma and other signs of cortical irritation such as restlessness, irrationality, or convulsions.[1,2,5] It seems that the extent and duration of the brain injury should be proportional to the magnitude and duration of the venous hypertension plus the duration of the apneic period. Among the collected cases, the time of unconsciousness was brief, and few, if any, neurologic sequelae followed.[1]

Hypotension is not prominent among the usual clinical features and was not significant in any of our cases. If it is present, blood loss from such sources as rupture of the heart or great vessels or laceration of the spleen or liver should be suspected. Abdominal and genitourinary injuries were not encountered in our cases, but do occur rarely. Obviously injury to any part of the body may be encountered after trauma of this severity, and Laird and Borman[8] warned of unsuspected fractures, especially of the vertebrae. The systems affected in our series were summarized in the Table.

Sites of Injury in Presently Reported Series

Site	Cases 1	2	3	4	5	6	Total
Skin	+	0	+	+	+	+	5
Eyes	+	+	+	+	+	+	6
CNS	+	0	0	+	+	0	3
Mouth	+	0	0	+	+	+	4
Skeleton	+	+	0*	0	0	+	3
Nose	0	0	+	0	+	0	2
Respiratory tract	0	0	0	+	0	+	2
Ears	0	0	0	+	0	0	1
Heart	0	0	0	0	0	0	0
Gastrointestinal tract	0	0	0	0	0	?	0?
Genitourinary tract	0	0	0	0	0	0	0
Total	5	2	3	6	5	5?	

* Lower extremity only.

Differential Diagnosis.—Once this condition has been seen, diagnosis in subsequent cases is seldom difficult. However, a similar combination of subconjunctival hemorrhage, periorbital edema, epistaxis, and bleeding from the ears may result from basilar skull fracture. Mediastinal tumors with superior vena caval obstruction may cause edema and cyanosis of the face and neck; but there will be evidence of increased venous pressure in these regions, a condition not present in traumatic asphyxia after the thoracic compression is relieved.

Treatment.—The prominent characteristics of this syndrome—skin discoloration and subconjunctival hemorrhages—require no treatment at all. The administration of oxygen has been shown to have little effect on the facial discoloration. Instead, the clinician's attention should be directed toward diagnosis of associated injuries, especially those involving the brain, thorax, and abdomen.

If the degree of cerebral damage seems severe, intravenous administration of urea with or without hypothermia may be useful. When injury to the chest wall or lung is evident, administration of oxygen usually is indicated, and sometimes tracheostomy may be necessary, with or without assisted ventilation (cases 4 and 6). Specific measures directed toward the associated conditions should be applied as required.

Prognosis.—Among the 143 cases collected by Laird and Borman,[8] 27 patients were dead on arrival at the hospital or died before definitive treatment could be started. An additional 12 died later in the course of their illness; but 104 recovered, though in some cases with residual defects. Thus 73% survived the injury. Stickney and Hagedorn [2] believed that two factors are responsible for the deaths: prolonged compression of the thorax, and associated injuries and their complications. In our series of six hospitalized patients, one died from the associated pulmonary complications and one had a transient residual neurologic defect.

Summary

Traumatic asphyxia is a syndrome consisting of petechiae and purplish discoloration of the skin of the face, neck, and upper part of the chest along with subconjunctival hemorrhages. Usually it is seen in people who have undergone sustained, severe compression of the chest or upper part of the abdomen. Four cases are presented that showed this syndrome in its typical form. The fifth case presented showed only mild cutaneous and conjunctival manifestations and the sixth only periorbital and subconjunctival hemorrhages. Treatment is directed toward the associated conditions, the most serious being rib fractures and pulmonary injury. If the patient survives the initial insult, the prognosis is good. As our rate of automobile and other mechanical accidents rises, it is anticipated that the syndrome will be encountered more frequently.

Mayo Clinic, Rochester, Minn.

REFERENCES

1. Fred, H. L., and Chandler, F. W.: Traumatic Asphyxia, Amer J Med 29:508-517 (Sept) 1960.

2. Stickney, J. M., and Hagedorn, A. B.: Chest Injuries and Traumatic Asphyxia, Proc Mayo Clin 19:207-213 (April 19) 1944.

3. Ollivier: Quoted by Dwek, J.[6]

4. Perthes, G.: Über "Druckstauung," Deutsch Z Chir 55:384-392 (April) 1900.

5. Heuer, G. J.: Traumatic Asphyxia: With Special Reference to Its Ocular and Visual Disturbances, Surg Gynec Obstet 36:686-696 (May) 1923.

6. Dwek, J.: Ecchymotic Mask, J Int Coll Surg 9:257-265 (March-April) 1946.

7. Quigley, W. F.: Acute Superior Vena Caval Compression, Hawaii Med J 20:337-338 (March-April) 1961.

8. Laird, W. R., and Borman, M. C.: Traumatic Asphyxia: With Report of Five Additional Cases, Surg Gynec Obstet 50:578-585 (March) 1930.

9. Alexander, E. G.: A Case of Stasis Cyanosis Following an Epileptic Seizure, Simulating Traumatic Asphyxia, Ann Surg 49:762-766, 1909.

10. Ryerson, E. S.: A Case of Traumatic Asphyxia With Recovery, Canad Pract Rev 32:195-201, 1907.

11. Robertson, L. B.: Traumatic Asphyxia With a Report of Six Cases, Canad Med Ass J 4:501-507 (June) 1914.

12. Bolt, R. A.: Traumatic Asphyxia, With Report of a Case, Cleveland Med J 7:647-659 (Dec) 1908.

13. Reichert, F. L., and Martin, J. W.: Traumatic Asphyxia: Experimental and Clinical Observations With a Report of a Case With Concomitant Paraplegia, Ann Surg 134:361-368 (Sept) 1951.

Histopathological Spectrum of Regional Enteritis

THEODORE R. MEADOWS, MD, AND JOHN G. BATSAKIS, MD, ANN ARBOR, MICH

Since Crohn's original description,[1] the histopathologic criteria for the diagnosis of regional enteritis have not been conspicuously altered. Despite technical refinements and search for specificity of various histologic parameters [2-9] in the disease, it may be said that there are no pathognomonic features in regional enteritis. This is predicated upon the following: (1) the small intestine has, in the majority of instances, a restricted mode of reactivity to various and diverse agents; (2) regional enteritis is a progressive disease with a fluidity of transition between various histopathologic changes; and (3) the appearance of the intestine, at any given time during the clinical course of the disease, is a composite of "primary" and "secondary" reactions with obscuration of the primary lesion by the latter in the progression of biologic time.[5]

The sequence of morphologic changes occurring in regional enteritis may then be considered to represent a spectrum with considerable merging and overlapping, prohibiting a rigid delineation or clinicopathological classification that is intended to correlate with the clinical course of the disease or with duration of symptoms.

In this study of 35 surgical specimens from 29 patients with regional enteritis, we have attempted to (1) demonstrate the histopathologic evolution of regional enteritis from its *earliest recognizable* lesion to the lesion or aberrant lesions at the end of a biologic time spectrum; and (2) evaluate various histopathologic findings, with respect to their primary or secondary nature and specificity.

Read before the 112th Annual Meeting of the American Medical Association, Section on Gastroenterology and Proctology, Atlantic City, NJ, June 19, 1963.

From the Department of Pathology, The University of Michigan.

Methods and Materials

Thirty-five surgical specimens from 29 patients with regional enteritis treated at The University of Michigan Medical Center were selected for microscopic examination. The histologic lesions were divided into three morphologic phases: early, intermediate, and late. Anatomic distribution of the lesions is shown in Table 1. This is more than an arbitrary separation since the early phase represents the *first recognizable* alteration in any portion of resected bowel wall, that coincidentally or in later resected specimens exhibited the more commonly accepted lesions ascribed to regional enteritis. The late phase represents the biologic end point or irreversible stage of pathologic alteration; and the intermediate phase, a transition phase representing progression from the early, but lacking in the severe destructive and productive alterations associated with the late phases. The relative incidence of pyloric metaplasia of epithelium, ulcers, granulomata, and neurovascular changes in each of these phases was ascertained and their histogenetic relation to the primary lesion studied.

Results

Three merging morphologic phases occur in the evolution of regional enteritis: early, intermediate, and late. Three patients (8.8%) showed morphologic changes of the early phase, unaccompanied by other reactions (Fig 1). The major finding of an early phase, that may occur at any time in the chronologic development of the disease,

TABLE 1.—*Anatomic Distribution of Lesions*

	Location			
Phase	Jejunum (%)	Ileum (%)	Ileocolonic (%)	Total (%)
Early	0	3 (100)	0	3 (100)
Intermediate	1 (12)	3 (33)	5 (55)	9 (100)
Late	2 (8.7)	16 (70.6)	5 (21.7)	23 (100)

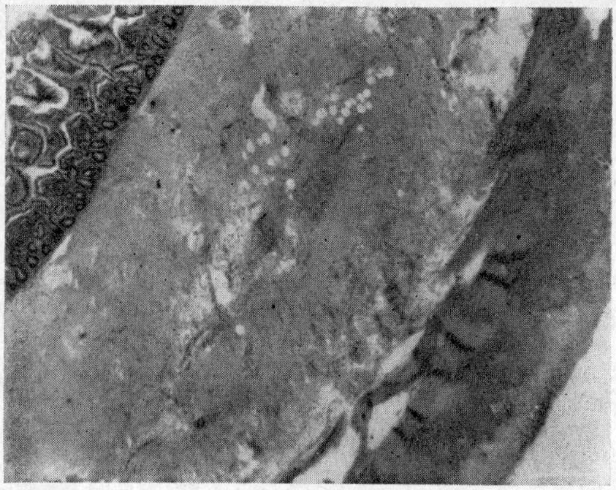

Fig 1.—Earliest recognizable lesion in the evolutionary spectrum of regional enteritis. Note marked submucosal edema with associated hyperemia and telangiectasis. Hematoxylin and eosin; reduced 41% from mag × 40.

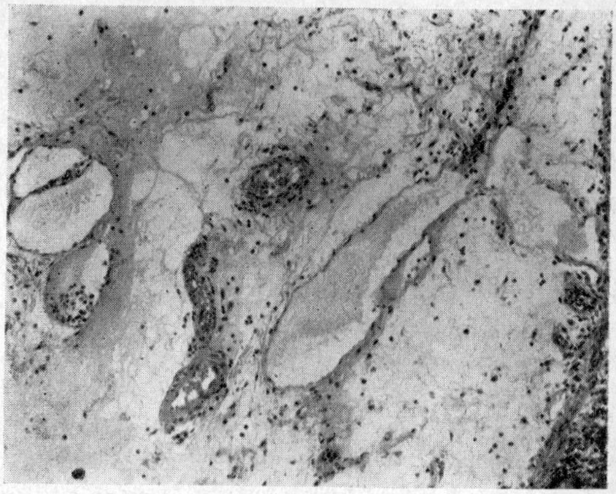

Fig 2.—See legend for Fig 1. Hematoxylin and eosin; reduced 41% from mag × 200.

is a pronounced edema of the entire bowel wall, but especially marked in the submucosa (Fig 2). The edema is accompanied by a hyperemia and lymphangiectasis. Goblet cell population is slightly increased, and a fibrinopurulent exudate is invariably present on the serosal surface. Evidence of biologic chronicity, ie, fibrosis, chronic inflammation, and lymphoreticular hyperplasia and hypertrophy, is notably absent. That this early change may occur without respect to clinical course is emphasized by the finding of an intermediate-phase morphology in an earlier resection in one patient, a preceding late-stage morphology in another, and admixture of all three phases in a third patient.

Nine patients (25%) showed morphologic stigmata of an intermediate phase (Fig 3). The bowel wall is thickened, and although there is persistence of edema and lymphangiectasis, the thickening is more attributable to the fibrosis of the submucosa and subserosa. Villous blunting is more apparent, and there is a definite increase in lamina propria cellularity, with lymphocytes, plasma cells, and eosinophils predominating. There is a notable increase in goblet cell population. Ulcers were found in eight of the nine specimens. These are usually small and focal, and they rarely penetrate beneath the muscularis mucosae. An occasional "slit-ulcer" extended into the submucosa. The mucosa adjacent to these ulcers is generally thinned and shows a heavy infiltrate of plasma cells, lymphocytes, and focal aggregates of eosinophils. No deep ulcers, intramural abscesses, or fistulae are found in this phase. In several examples, a nodular hypertrophy of the muscularis mucosae lay at the base of an ulcer, seemingly preventing submucosal extension. In the submucosa, three distinct alterations occur (Fig 4): fibrosis, initially fine and fibrillar in character; diffuse infiltration of mononuclear cells; and, most prominently, hypertrophy and hyperplasia of lymphoid follicles and aggregates. The neural changes show a direct relationship to the biologic progression of the disease (Table 2). They are subtle in the early phase. The intermediate phase shows a definite, diffuse or nodular hypertrophy of neurilemmal cells as well as an increased number and prominence of ganglion cells, limited to the myenteric plexuses. The submucosal plexus was involved in only one of the nine cases. The muscularis propria is hypertrophic, and the character of the fibrosis and infiltrate in the subserosa and mesentery is like that, and varies with that, found in the submucosa. Three of the nine specimens showed an accompanying morphology of the early phase, two located at the proximal and distal ends of the ileal resection and one throughout the resected specimen.

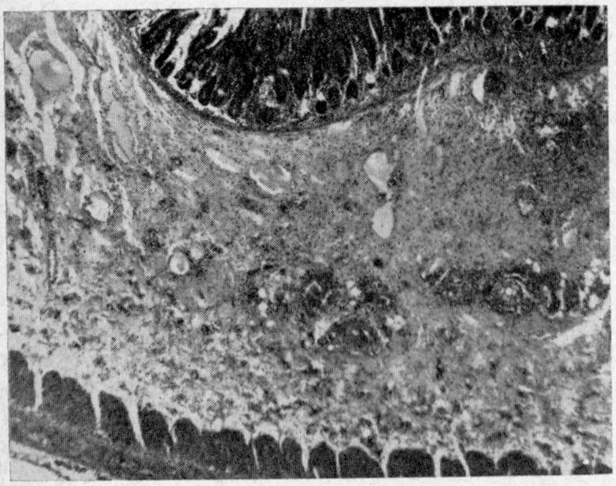

Fig 3.—Intermediate phase. Persistence of edema and telangiectasis, but in addition, fibrillar fibrosis and lymporeticular hyperplasia. Hematoxylin and eosin; reduced 41% from mag × 40.

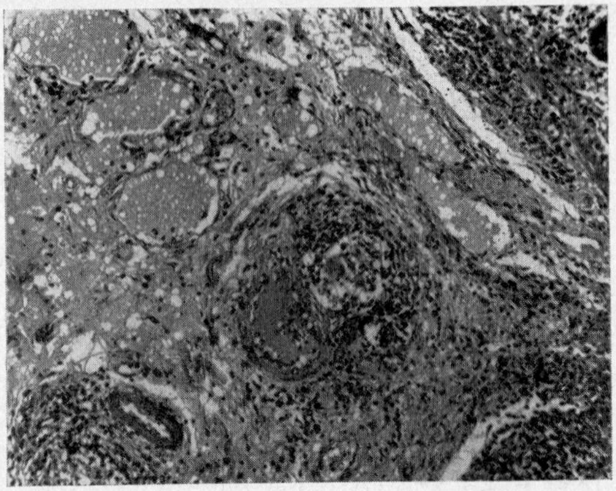

Fig 4.—Fine fibrillary fibrosis, dilatation of lymphatics, and lymphoid aggregates. Note formative granuloma adjacent to small lymphatic. Hematoxylin and eosin; reduced 41% from mag × 200.

Late-stage morphology was found in 23 specimens (66.6%), ten coexisting with early- or intermediate-stage morphology, five of which were found in the proximal end of the specimen.

That the impact of the lesion throughout the biologic course of the disease resides in the submucosa is exemplified by the progressive cicatrization in that zone (Fig 5). Coexistent and perhaps concomitant with this change, ulcers are more severe and expansive. Large areas of epithelial denudation are present, covered by granulation tissue of heavy subacute inflammatory cell infiltration and angiofibroblastic proliferation. Where epithelium persists, it is like that of the intermediate phase. In 12 specimens, pyloric gland metaplasia in the mucosa was identified (Fig 6). This metaplastic lesion is most prominent in areas adjacent to the ulcers, and origin from crypt epithelium can be demonstrated in the majority of instances. Pyloric gland metaplasia, like the neuromatous hypertrophy, becomes progressively more prominent with progression of the disease. The early phase of regional enteritis is devoid of this metaplasia. Only two of nine specimens in the intermediate phase showed pyloric type glands, whereas 12 of 23 late-phase specimens contained metaplastic foci. A generalized hypertrophy of the muscularis mucosae replaces the focal nodular hypertrophy of earlier phases, and in addition broad smooth muscle bands, apparently originating from "splintering" of this muscle layer, course through the thickened submucosa intimately admixed with the hyalinized and collagenized connective tissue. Nodular hypertrophy of the myenteric plexuses is marked and is accompanied by broad bands of neurilemmal sheath cells and increased numbers of swollen ganglion cells in the myenteric plexuses and submucosa (Fig 7). Hypertrophy of the muscularis propria is variable and probably related to compression effects from subserosal and submucosal cicatrization. Lymph nodes were examined in 16 of the total series. All were characterized by a medullary lymphangiectasis and edema. In addition, sarcoidal granulomas were present in four of the late-phase specimens.

Table 2.—*Progression of Neuromatous Hypertrophy* *

Phase	1+	2+	3+	4+
Early	2	0	0	0
Intermediate	4	3	1	0
Late	2	7	7	7

* 1+ indicates slight diffuse hypertrophy of myenteric plexus; 2+, marked nodular hypertrophy of myenteric plexus; 3+, marked nodular hypertrophy of myenteric plexus and slight diffuse hypertrophy of submucosal plexus; 4+, marked nodular hypertrophy of myenteric and submucosal plexuses.

Since the sarcoid-like granulomata have had such an important diagnostic role in regional enteritis, they are best considered

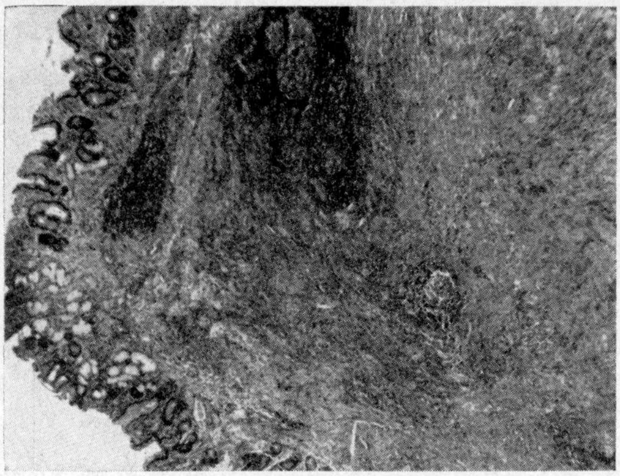

Fig 5.—Maturation of fibrosis in submucosa and increase in the dominance of the lymphoid aggregates. Note pyloric gland metaplasia. Hematoxylin and eosin; reduced 41% from mag × 40.

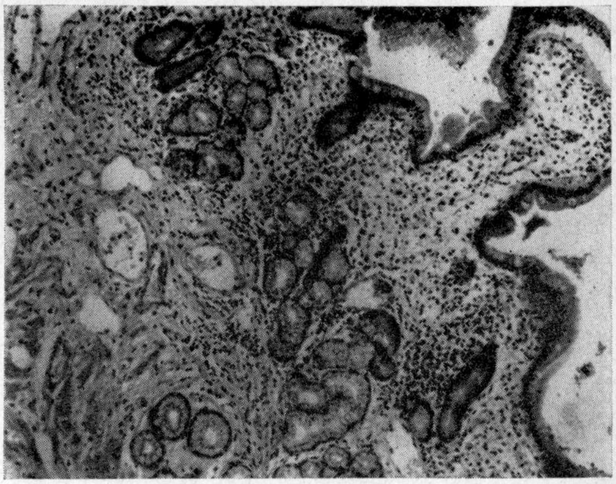

Fig 6.—Pyloric gland metaplasia, a secondary lesion that becomes more prominent with progression in biologic time. Hematoxylin and eosin; reduced 41% from mag × 180.

separately. Our findings are that the granulomata are a secondary reactive process and not essential to the diagnosis. The incidence of granulomata increases with biologic chronicity, and they are not invariably present. The early phase is devoid of granulomata, and unlike other features of the disease they may be found in all stages of development in a given intermediate- or late-phase regional enteritis. In this series granulomata were found in the submucosa, subserosa, mesentery, adjacent lymph nodes, and occasionally in the muscularis propria. No granulomata were present in the mucosa, this latter feature serving as a differential point from ileal tuberculosis, in which mucosal tubercle involvement is the rule.

Two cases exhibited an atypical or aberrant late-stage morphology. Tumor-like masses of mononuclear cells diffusely infiltrated the submucosa and extended into the lamina propria (Fig 8 and 9). These "pseudolymphomatous" lesions were characterized by an admixture of lymphocytes, reticular cells, plasma cells, and eosinophils with variable dominance of cell type in different areas of the lesion. Adjacent sections of small intestine showed variable degrees and stages of the three phases of the regional enteritis spectrum. Adjacent lymph nodes were hyperplastic and reactive in their appearance.

Comment

An appraisal of the histopathologic appearance of regional enteritis must perforce

Fig 7.—Secondary hypertrophy of neurilemmal sheaths in myenteric plexuses. Hematoxylin and eosin; reduced 41% from mag × 180.

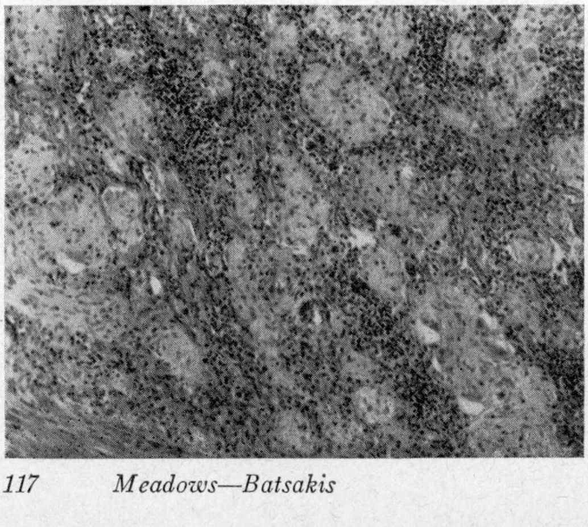

Fig 8.—Aberrant "end stage" leading to formation of pseudolymphoma. Although cells may show atypism, the polymorphous character of the infiltrate is in contrast to the monomorphism of true lymphoma. Hematoxylin and eosin; reduced 41% from mag × 180.

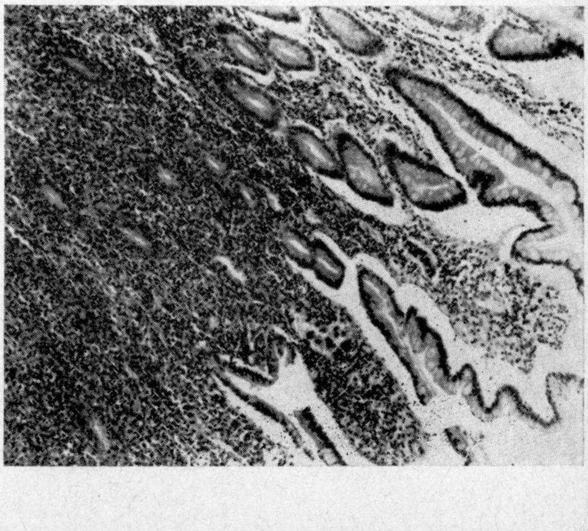

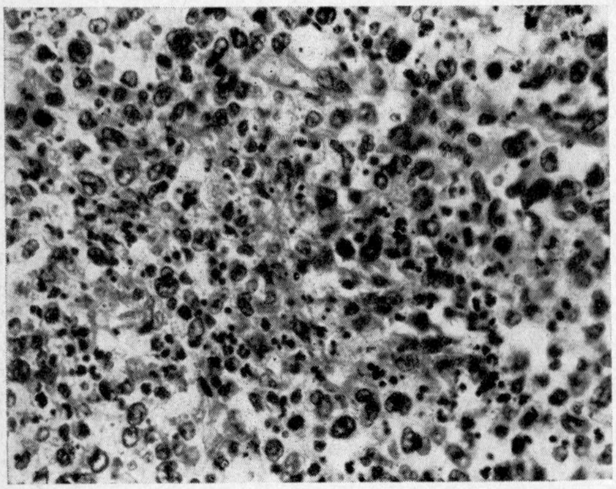

Fig 9.—See legend for Fig 8. Hematoxylin and eosin; reduced 41% from mag × 420.

be consideration of primary and secondary lesions.[5,10] Any histologic classification of the disease is inadequate unless the interplay of these two reactive processes is weighed in a given surgical specimen.[5] Although there exists a considerable difference of opinion as to the amount of stress to be accorded various lesions as being primary or secondary in nature, and although it is true that few cases of the early phase of regional enteritis have been described, this study shows that edema and telangiectasia are the earliest microscopic lesions, occurring in patients, that subsequently evolve into the more classic lesion. Rappaport and his associates commented that the transition from "acute" to "chronic" regional enteritis has never been firmly established on pathological grounds, although such has been postulated on a clinical basis.[4] However, as shown in this study, all stages of the primary disorder and/or its biologic sequelae may be recognized in any suitable state. The transition is never abrupt but more of a fluid nature, which incidentally does not correlate with the chronologic time of clinical symptoms. The present study further illustrates that the primary impact of the microscopic disturbance falls upon the submucosal layer of the small intestine, and that the histopathologic course of the disease is always reflected in that layer. Alterations in the other coats of the intestinal wall are preceded by these changes. Edema and telangiectasia exist for a short period of biologic time and are superseded by direct consequences of their presence, ie, lymphoreticular hyperplasia, granuloma formation, and an increasingly maturing and productive fibrosis of the submucosa. Submucous thickening precedes ulceration, and ulcers may well be a direct consequence of the submucosal lesion since the severity, depth of penetration, and size are in direct correlation with the maturation of the submucosal lesions. Pyloric metaplasia, by the very nature of its genesis and occurrence only in the later phases of the spectrum, can only be considered as a secondary lesion. The same is true for the neuromatous hypertrophy and hyperplasia, and obliterative vascular changes, histogenetically related in part to the preceding submucosal alteration.

Finally, a small yet significant number of patients with regional enteritis do not conform to the usual biologic progression of the disease and by virtue of an aberrant lymphoreticular response present as "pseudolymphomas" of the small intestine.

Throughout the course of this study, it becomes increasingly apparent that regional enteritis, after the initial or early phase, is fundamentally a panhyperplasia of the reticular tissue of the small intestine, occasionally of the colon and the lymph nodes draining these areas. The reticular tissue is composed of fixed primitive reticular cells supported on a fibrillar framework and includes all cells derived from that tissue. The morphologic end result of reactivity by this tissue is in essence the ascendancy or dominance of one or more of the derivatives of the reticular tissue. Fibrosis and cicatrization are the most common end result. Uncommonly the reaction is complex, and in addition to the fibrosis and reticuloendothelial cells, there is a proliferation of reticular stem cells and a profusion of lymphocytes and plasma cells, producing a lesion designated as "pseudolymphoma" in deference to its gross and histologic appearance and to align this small intestinal lesion with similar peculiar reactive processes elsewhere in the alimentary tract.

Differentiation of the pseudolymphoma from true neoplasm is not easy, since gross configuration, rather sharp localization, and regional lymphadenopathy are common to both lesions. Microscopically, too, true lymphomas are separated with difficulty from these atypical reactive lymphoreticular responses. Azzopardi and Menzies [11] point out that these granulomatous tumor-like conditions closely mimic a genuine neoplasm; Jackson and Parker [12] and Ewing [13] are of the same opinion.

Primary lymphomas, with the exception of Hodgkin's disease, are essentially monomorphic neoplasms, ie, one cell type. Pseudolymphomatous lesions have a polymorphous cellular infiltrate, with admixture of macrophages, lymphocytes, eosinophils, and reticuloendothelial cells. Reaction centers and lymphoid follicles may be present in the better defined lesions. Increased vascularity with prominent endothelial cells and an accompanying fibroblastic reaction form the background in which the cells proliferate or infiltrate. Regional adjacent lymph nodes show only hyperplasia.

Summary

Regional enteritis is a progressive disease that evolves through three merging and overlapping morphologic phases, which are composed of both "primary and secondary" lesions.

The earliest lesions are edema and telangiectasia, with the primary impact of the disease in the submucosa of the small intestine. With progression in biologic time, there is obscuration of the primary lesions and ascendancy of the secondary lesions: fibrosis, lymphoreticular hyperplasia, granuloma formation, neuromatous hypertrophy and ulcers, pyloric metaplasia, and fistulae. The usual morphologic end result or so-called late phase of the disease is then the result of interplay between primary and secondary lesions.

A small group of patients deviate from the usual progressive maturation of morphologic changes and by virtue of an aberrant lymphoreticular response present as pseudolymphomas of the small intestine. Differentiation of this lesion from true lymphoma may be difficult, but the polymorphous character of the infiltrate serves to distinguish it from the usually monomorphic lymphomas.

John G. Batsakis, MD, Department of Pathology, The University of Michigan, 1335 E Catherine, Ann Arbor, Mich.

REFERENCES

1. Crohn, B. B.; Ginzburg, L.; and Oppenheimer, G. D.: Regional Ileitis: A Pathologic and Clinical Entity, JAMA 99:1323, 1932.

2. Hadfield, G.: The Primary Histological Lesion of Regional Ileitis, Lancet 2:773, 1939.

3. Warren, S., and Sommers, S. C.: Cicatrizing Enteritis (Regional Ileitis) as a Pathologic Entity: Analysis of 120 Cases, Amer J Path 24:475, 1948.

4. Rappaport, H.; Burgoyne, F. H.; and Smetana, H. F.: The Pathology of Regional Enteritis, Milit Surg 109:463, 1951.

5. Van Patter, W. N.; Bargen, J. A.; Dockerty, M. B.; Feldman, W. H.; Mayo, C. W.; and Waugh, J. M.: Regional Enteritis, Gastroenterology 26:347, 1954.

6. Kawel, C. A., and Tesluk, H.: Brunner-Type Glands in Regional Enteritis, Gastroenterology 28:810, 1955.

7. Davis, D. R.; Dockerty, M. B.; and Mayo, C. W.: The Myenteric Plexus in Regional Enteritis: A Study of the Number of Ganglion Cells in the Ileum in 24 Cases, Surg Gynec Obstet 101:208, 1955.

8. Antonius, J. I.; Gump, F. E.; Lattes, R.; and Lepore, M.: A Study of Certain Microscopic Features of Regional Enteritis, and Their Possible Prognostic Significance, Gastroenterology 38:889, 1960.

9. Ammann, R. W., and Bockus, H. L.: Pathogenesis of Regional Enteritis: Based Upon Histologic Study of 40 Cases, Arch Intern Med 107:504, 1961.

10. Schepers, G. W. H.: The Pathology of Regional Ileitis, Amer J Dig Dis 12:97, 1945.

11. Azzopardi, J. G., and Menzies, T.: Primary Malignant Lymphoma of the Alimentary Tract, Brit J Surg 47:358, 1960.

12. Jackson, H., Jr., and Parker, F., Jr.: Hodgkin's Disease: IV. Involvement of Certain Organs, New Eng J Med 232:547, 1945.

13. Ewing, J.: Neoplastic Diseases, ed 4, Philadelphia: W. B. Saunders Company, 1940.

Left-Sided Gallbladder and Liver Without Situs Inversus

ALFRED M. LARGE, MD
DETROIT

Although situs inversus, partial or complete, occurs perhaps once in every 10,000 individuals, left-sided gallbladder without situs inversus is extremely rare. Indeed, we could find only 16 cases reported in the world literature up to 1956,[1] and all of these occurred in patients whose gallbladders were found under the left lobe of the liver.

The present case report appears to be unique in that both the liver and gallbladder were placed on the left side of the abdomen while the other viscera were in normal position, although incomplete rotation of the large intestine had occurred.

Case Report.—A 68-year-old white woman was first admitted to Grace Hospital in February, 1955, for massive coronary thrombosis with arteriosclerotic heart disease and hypertension. Her progress was satisfactory, and she remained well on limited activity until January, 1962, when she was admitted again to the hospital suffering from diverticulitis of the sigmoid colon with localized perforation and abscess formation; she was also found at this time to be suffering from diabetes mellitus. Operation was performed on Jan 9, 1962. The left colon from the midtransverse area down to the lower sigmoid was resected and an end-to-end anastomosis performed. It was noted that the liver and gallbladder were on the left side of the abdomen, and the gallbladder contained a single good-sized stone. As well as this, the cecum was located in the right upper quadrant, thus indicating that complete rotation of the large bowel had not occurred. Because of the patient's previous heart attack and the magnitude of the colonic resection, it was felt wisest not to disturb the gallbladder at this operation.

The postoperative course was very satisfactory, but within a few months she began to complain of indigestion and left upper abdominal pain. This pain came in attacks radiating arount to the left side and back and also at times radiated downwards to the

Submitted for publication June 25, 1963.

From the Department of Surgery of the Wayne State University College of Medicine and the Grace Hospital.

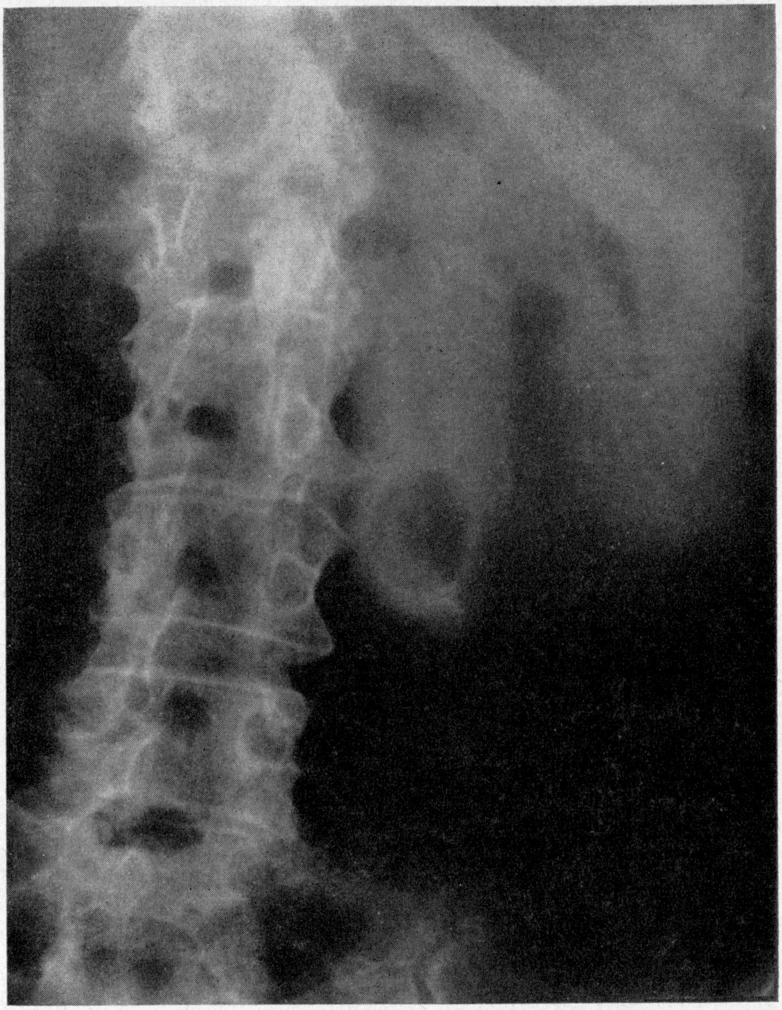

Fig 1.—Cholecystogram showing low lying left-sided gallbladder containing a large solitary stone.

left lower abdomen. Because of increasing discomfort, she returned to the hospital on Feb 10, 1963, at which time cholecystogram (Fig 1) confirmed the impression of a low lying left-sided gallbladder containing a single stone. Upper gastrointestinal x-rays showed the stomach to be in normal position, but the duodenal loop was missing and the duodenum passed straight over into the jejunum on the right side. Chest film confirmed the previously known normal position of the thoracic viscera. At operation on Feb 14, 1963, it appeared that the liver was simply shifted over to the left side of the abdomen. The gallbladder lay in its normal relationship to the right lobe of the liver, but the entire liver and biliary system were located to the left of the midline (Fig 2). A cystic duct cholangiogram showed the common duct passing downward and to the right to enter the duodenum in its midportion (Fig 3). The gallbladder contained a single stone and showed a moderate amount of inflammation of its wall. Cholecystectomy was performed; the appendix also was removed. Postoperative course was uneventful and the patient has been relieved of her attacks of left-sided abdominal pain, although some vague indigestion persists.

Comment

Most of the reported patients with left-sided gallbladder and gallstones have complained of pain on the right side of the abdomen or else in the midepigastric region. It is interesting that in the case reported here,

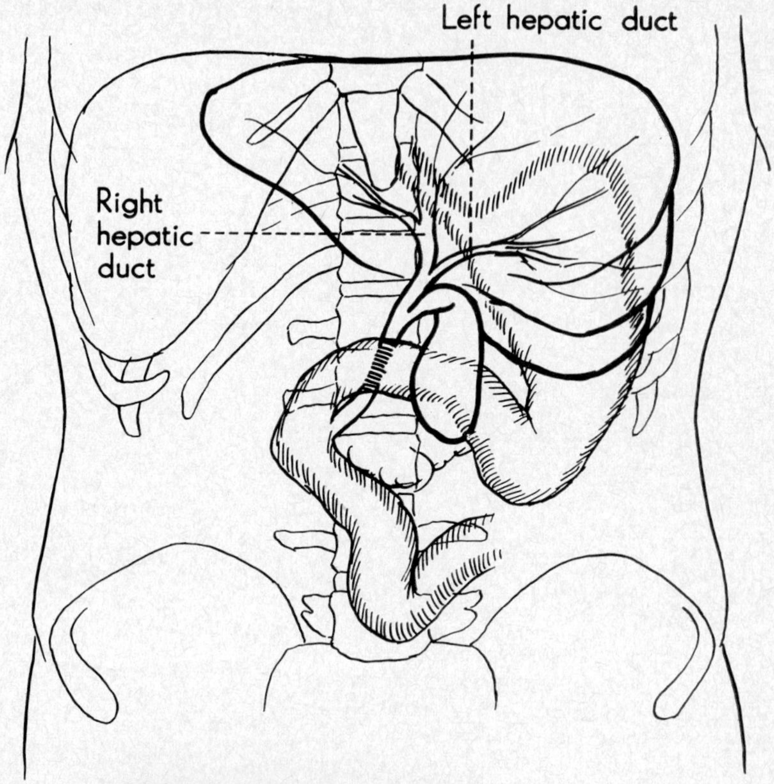

Fig 2.— Drawing of the operative findings. The entire liver is shifted over to the left so that the major portion of the right lobe is located to the left of the midline.

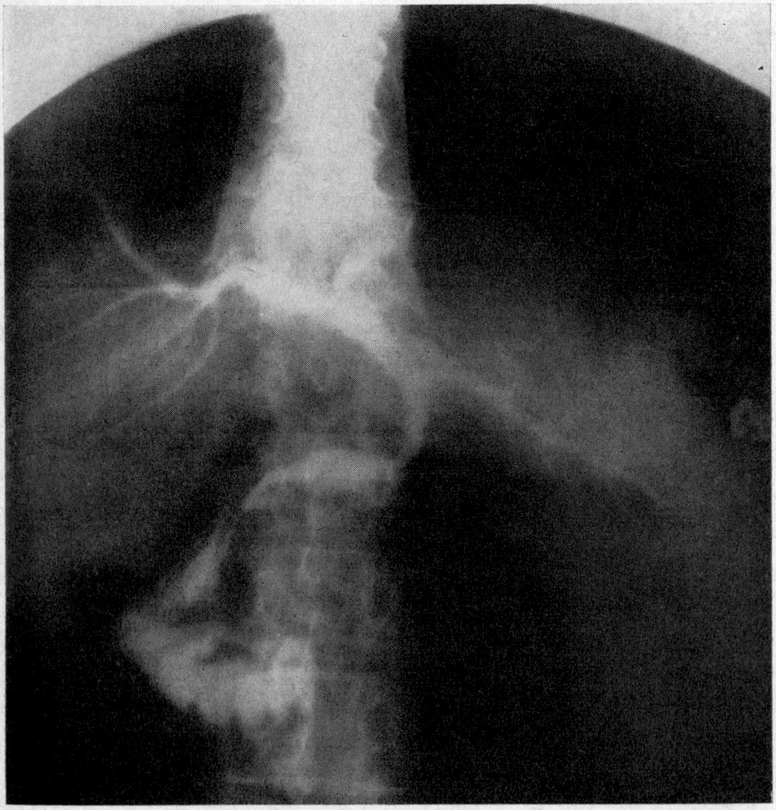

Fig 3. — Cystic duct cholangiogram.

the attacks of pain were always on the left side and sometimes radiated, as well as around to the back, down to the suprapubic area. It was at first thought that this pain might be related to the diverticulitis, which was moderately severe, but when the attacks of pain continued after resection of the diseased colon, it became evident that the gallbladder disease must have been responsible, at least in part, for these symptoms. The rather low lying level of the gallbladder in this case may possibly explain the radiation of the pain to the suprapubic area.

The curious location of the liver and the bile ducts in this patient indicate the importance of operative cholangiography whenever any anomalous condition of the biliary tract is encountered. The common duct in this case was very small; it passed from left to right toward a straightened out duodenum, and it might easily have been damaged had a cystic duct cholangiogram not been performed prior to extirpation of the gallbladder.

No attempt is made to explain the peculiar position of the liver and biliary tract in this patient, with the stomach, spleen, and pancreas in their normal positions directly behind the liver. Despite this unusual position, the liver was of average size and apparently functioned normally, and the biliary tract appeared to be quite normal as well, except for the presence of cholelithiasis and its associated cholecystitis.

Attention is again called to the observation that failure of the gallbladder to visualize in the right upper quadrant need not necessarily indicate gallbladder disease, but in the occasional case, may be related to an anomalous position of the gallbladder even in the absence of situs inversus.

Summary and Conclusions

An unusual case of left-sided liver and gallbladder in the absence of situs inversus, but associated with incomplete rotation of the intestine, is reported. The gallbladder contained a single stone which evidently caused attacks of pain on the left side of the abdomen. These symptoms were relieved by cholecystectomy.

Alfred M. Large, MD, 701 David Whitney Bldg, Detroit 26, Mich.

REFERENCE

1. Flannery, M. G., and Caster, M. P.: Congenital Abnormalities of the Gallbladder: 101 Cases, Int Abstr Surg 103:439-457 (Nov) 1956.

New "One Hand" Double-Loop Method of Tying Knots

H. WRIGHT SEIGER, MD
SANTA MONICA, CALIF

Synthetic sutures such as nylon and Orlon are coming to the fore because they are stronger than silk and, thus, can be used in smaller diameters. Also, claims have been made that these synthetic materials are less irritating.

However, their coefficient of friction is less that that of silk, and if they are tied, even with three or more "squared" single loops, the suture will not hold. Slippage can be prevented by using double-loop ties. But many surgeons are accustomed to tie knots with the so-called one-hand methods to speed up the procedure. Another advantage of "one-hand" tying is that each tie is customarily "squared" in relation to the preceding tie. To tie a knot with a double loop, it has been necessary to use "two-hands" which is much slower. Also, a tight "first" tie can be maintained more easily with a double loop.

Submitted for publication June 30, 1963.

The accompanying photographs describe a "one-hand" method of tying knots with double loops. It is a modification of previous "one-hand" methods, and, similarly, it is much faster than "two-hand" methods.

Double loops can be placed in the first tie only, or alternately in the first and third ties, etc, of a square knot. A single loop, here, is used in the second tie. Using double loops during the first and third ties will even hold slippery materials such as monofilament nylon or Orlon. Even silk will hold better if the first tie uses a double loop. With a little practice, this method can be used almost as fast as the commonly used single-loop "one-hand" methods.

The accompanying photographs (Fig 1-12) depict the different steps of a "one-hand" method of tying a double loop tie followed by a single-loop tie. Finally a double-loop tie repeated as in Fig 1 to 7 may be desirable for a very slippery suture for a third tie.

Note: After making each double-loop tie, turning both hands about 180 degrees clockwise before tightening the tie will straighten the knot and make a neater tie, as is done in Fig 7. This is also true of single-loop "one-hand" ties to make a neat knot.

H. Wright Seiger, MD, 520 Arizona Ave, Santa Monica, Calif.

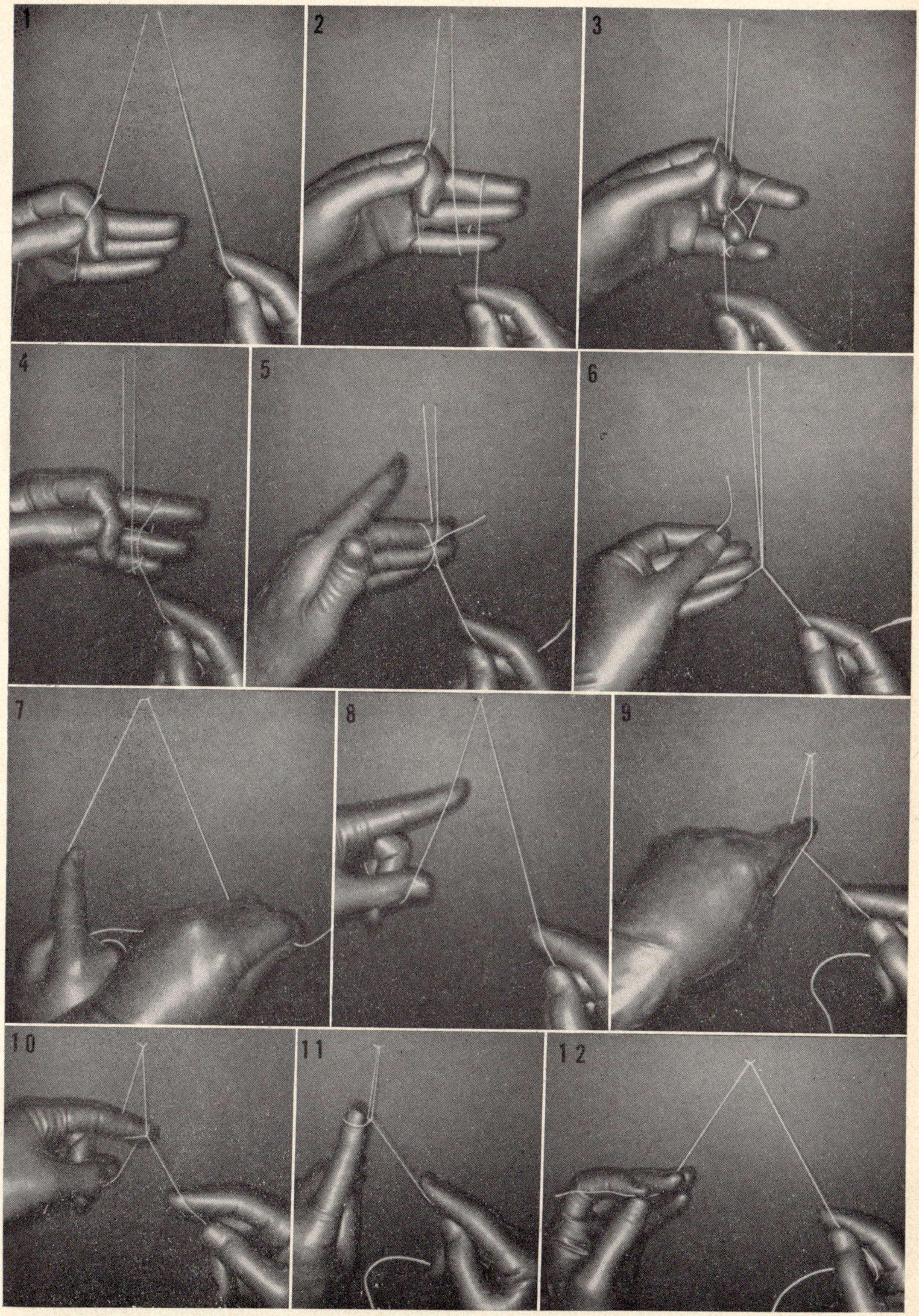
1
2
3
4
5
6
7
8
9
10
11
12

Experimental Pancreatitis

Synchronous Production in Normal and in Ectopic Pancreas

THOMAS R. KELLY, MD
EVERETT P. BRATCHER, MD
WILLIAM H. FALOR, MD
LLOYD CATRON, MD
AND
LEOVIGILDO B. REYES, MD
AKRON, OHIO

The exact genesis of acute hemorrhagic pancreatitis is unknown, although it has been the subject of repeated clinical and experimental study. In 1855 Claude Bernard [1] first attempted to produce hemorrhagic pancreatitis in dogs by injecting bile mixed with sweet oil into the pancreatic duct. Ever since this early study many methods for producing the disease have been employed, none of which completely demonstrate the pathogenesis.

Rich and Duff [2] concluded that obstruction and subsequent distention and rupture of pancreatic ductules with a resultant escape of pancreatic juice into the interstitial tissue is the cause of edematous pancreatitis. They further stated that necrosis of the walls of neighboring arteries and veins transforms edematous pancreatitis into hemorrhagic pancreatitis. Archibald,[3] Cameron,[4] and Opie [5] consider that obstruction at the papilla of Vater by stone or spasm with reflux of bile through a common channel into the pancreatic duct is the usual mechanism of acute pancreatitis. Thal and co-workers [6] convincingly demonstrated the effectiveness of ischemia in producing fulminant lethal hemorrhagic pancreatitis; when the capillaries and venules of the pancreas were made to undergo thrombosis by the local Shwartzman or Arthus phenomenon or were severely constricted by introduction of staphylococcic toxin through the duct, typical diffuse hemorrhagic necrosis ensued. However, in clinical pancreatitis ductal obstruction is rarely demonstrable. In 1949 Hasche-Klünder [7] reported a case of acute pancreatitis in which the acute process was confined to heterotopic pancreatic tissue; the pancreas per se was normal. In 1956 Longmire [8] presented two cases of acute pancreatitis occurring simultaneously in the pancreas and in aberrant pancreatic tissue located in the small intestine. In these cases the reflux of bile could not be responsible for the pancreatitis which developed in the

Submitted for publication June 28, 1963.

From the Surgical Research Department of the Akron City Hospital.

Supported in part by research grants from the National Institutes of Health, H-7253, and from the J. A. Hartford Foundation, Inc.

heterotopic tissue. The findings would indicate that the etiologic factors were extra-pancreatic, possibly involving humoral or, more likely, local neurovascular mechanisms. This particular departure from the common channel concept of etiology stimulated the following investigation into the production of hemorrhagic pancreatitis synchronously in the normal and in the ectopic pancreas.

Methods and Materials

In the dog the pancreas is composed of a rather loosely joined ventral and dorsal lobe. The dorsal component acquires its blood supply from the celiac axis by way of the superior pancreaticoduodenal artery; the ventral component receives blood from the superior mesenteric artery by way of the inferior pancreaticoduodenal artery, finally through the right pancreatic artery. The distal two or three inches of the ventral lobe together with the right pancreatic artery and vein may be separated as a viable anatomic pedunculated organ simply by teasing a cleavage through the fine anastomoses between the two pancreaticoduodenal arteries. After further division of the mesentery up to the right pancreatic neurovascular pedicle (Fig 1), the pancreas thus mobilized may readily be implanted in the subcutaneous tissue of the anterior abdominal wall. To maintain continuity of the autonomic nerves, the areolar envelope of the pedicle is preserved. It should also be noted that a complete separation of the ducts of the two lobes is effected during mobilization of the ventral lobe. The duct of the ventral lobe is not ligated and allowed to drain through the abdominal wall as a cutaneous fistula.

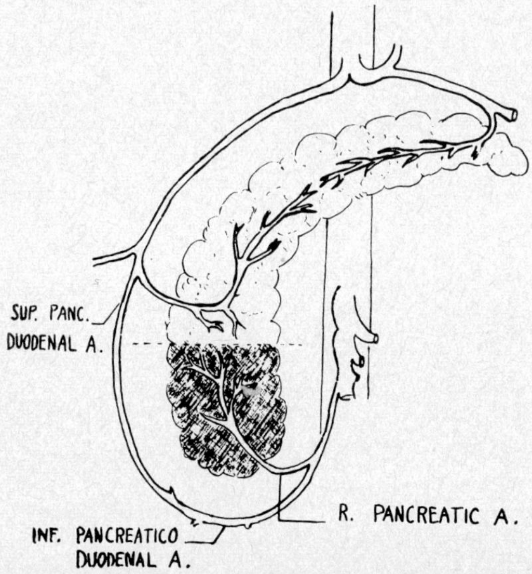

Fig 1.—Drawing of the dog pancreas showing the blood supply of the dorsal and ventral lobes. The shaded ventral lobe is transected at the dotted line and transplanted into the abdominal wall with an intact right pancreatic artery pedicle.

In healthy mongrel dogs heterotopic pancreas was prepared as described. Pancreatitis was produced by the injection of 10 cc of autogenous bile into the pancreatic duct of the dorsal lobe; by a transduodenal approach a polyethylene catheter was passed into the duct by way of the papilla; the bile was injected with pressure sufficient to rupture the pancreatic ductules and under direct vision allow the extravasation of bile into the gland.

Thirty animals were studied in groups of ten, as follows:

Group I: Bile injected into the dorsal lobe without ventral lobe mobilization.

Group II: Ventral lobe mobilization and transplantation to the anterior abdominal wall—ie, creation of a heterotopic pancreas—without injection of bile into the dorsal lobe.

Group III: Ventral lobe mobilization and transplantation accompanied by injection of bile into the dorsal lobe. The dorsal lobe duct is injected at the same time the ventral lobe is transplanted.

At autopsy, performed as soon after death as possible, in the animals with acute hemorrhagic pancreatitis the findings were characteristic and included: (1) a large volume of thin, serosanguinous peritoneal fluid, (2) an edematous, tense, hemorrhagic pancreas, and (3) areas of fat necrosis spread throughout the lesser peritoneal sac and mesentery. The surviving animals, having apparently completely recovered, were sacrificed two or three weeks after operation: there was no residual evidence of fat necrosis; however, the pancreas was indurated and shrunken in size. Histologic examination of pertinent tissues was performed in all animals.

Results

Group I.—All dogs in which the dorsal lobe was injected with bile, but in which no ventral lobe mobilization or transplantation was performed, died 6 to 24 hours postoperatively of acute fulminating hemorrhagic pancreatitis.

Group II.—All dogs subjected to ventral lobe mobilization and transplantation, but without dorsal lobe injection of bile, showed no pancreatitis in either lobe (Fig 2). These animals all had an uneventful postoperative course.

Group III.—All dogs subjected to ventral lobe mobilization and transplantation with dorsal lobe injection of bile died 24 to 48

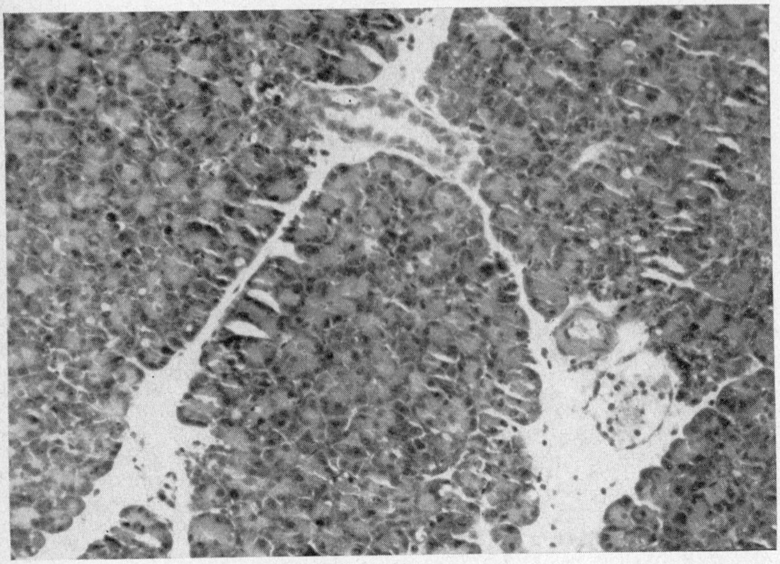

Fig 2.—Photomicrograph from the transplanted ventral lobe of a dog in which no bile was injected into the dorsal lobe duct. Note that the normal lobular architecture is preserved and no evidence of acute pancreatitis is present.

hours after surgery: In all ten dogs acute hemorrhagic pancreatitis involved the in situ dorsal pancreas. In five dogs, 50% of this group, acute hemorrhagic pancreatitis was also found in the ventral isolated pancreatic lobe. Fig 3 shows the gross appearance of the dorsal and ventral lobes of the pancreas in one of the animals of this group. Note the tremendous hemorrhage and edema of both lobes. In the microscopic sections of both lobes (Fig 4 and 5) one notes edema and parenchymal hemorrhage and necrosis, typical of acute hemorrhagic pancreatitis. The remaining five dogs of group III developed hemorrhagic pancreatitis in only the dorsal pancreatic lobes; the ventral transplanted lobes were normal.

Comment

A neurovascular or hormonal etiologic agent would appear to be most likely explanation for the acute hemorrhagic pancreatitis developing in the heterotopic organs in group III. Because the concept of a neurovascular agent only needs as a basis the existence of pancreatitis in some other portion of the organ—the dorsal lobe in group III—it is most readily accepted. Indeed, the opinion that hemorrhagic pancreatitis may result from neurovascular disturbances is not new. Mallet-Guy [9] and Longo [10] produced experimental pancreatitis by transitory disturbance of the blood supply of the pancreas following stimulation of the left splanchnic nerve. Menguy [11] showed in dogs that ligation of the pancreatic ducts in combination with stimulation of the left splanchnic nerve or ligation of major pancreatic arteries or veins caused a severe acute hemorrhagic pancreatitis. Vascular disturbances alone, brought about by ligation of the pancreatic arteries or veins or by stimulation of the left splanchnic nerve, did not suffice to induce acute pancreatitis.

Fig 3.—Dorsal (*A*) and transplanted ventral (*B*) pancreatic lobes from a dog in which bile was injected into the dorsal lobe duct. Note the presence of edema and hemorrhage in both lobes. The neurovascular pedicle (*C*) of the ventral lobe is demonstrated.

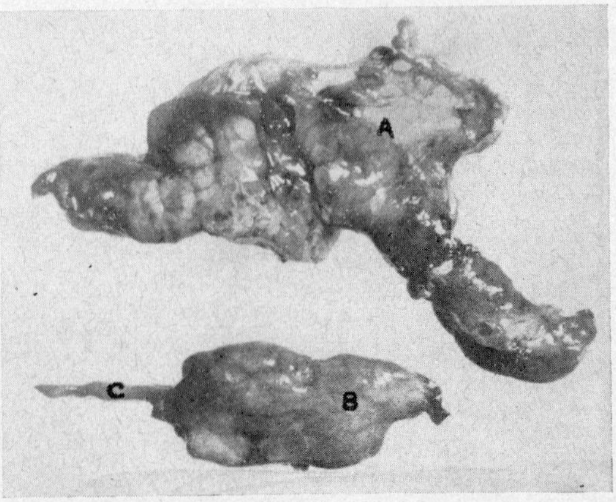

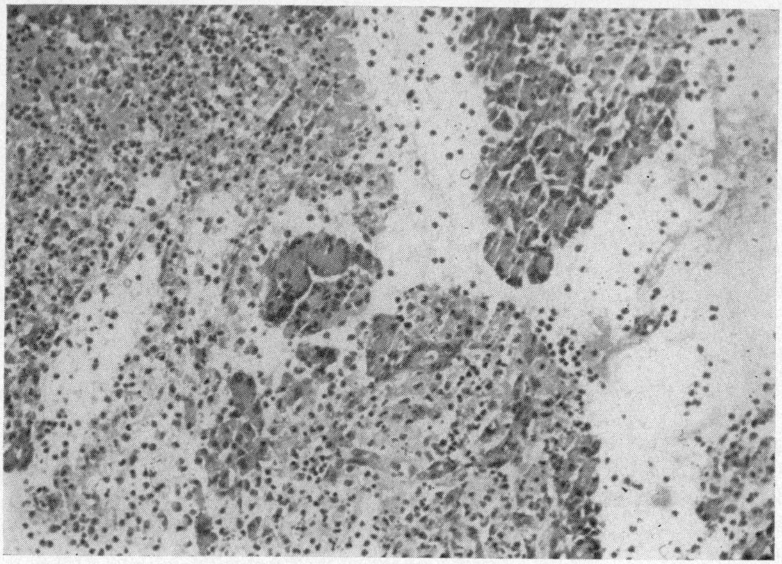

Fig 4.—Photomicrograph from the dorsal lobe (*A*) in Fig 3. Note the parenchymal necrosis, edema, and hemorrhage of acute hemorrhagic pancreatitis.

Thal[12] also presented evidence that suppression of blood flow to the pancreas was an important factor in precipitating hemorrhagic pancreatitis. By using a binocular dissecting microscope and a special transillumination apparatus, observations on the blood flow in the rabbit's pancreas were made after the forcible injection of bile intraductally or into the pancreatic parenchyma. Within a few minutes after the injection of the bile, the capillary circulation became sluggish and the cells closely packed. The veins and arteries supplying the lobule showed areas of segmental spasm alternating with areas of extreme venous distention. After 10 to 15 minutes lobular circulation had virtually ceased; after 20 minutes punctate ruptures of capillary walls with subsequent extravasation of red blood cells occurred, giving the pancreas a hemorrhagic appearance. It was felt that the extreme circulatory stasis was due to the direct action of bile salts on the blood vessel wall.

Nemir and Drabkin[13] state that in the transition from edematous pancreatitis to hemorrhagic pancreatitis the vascular com-

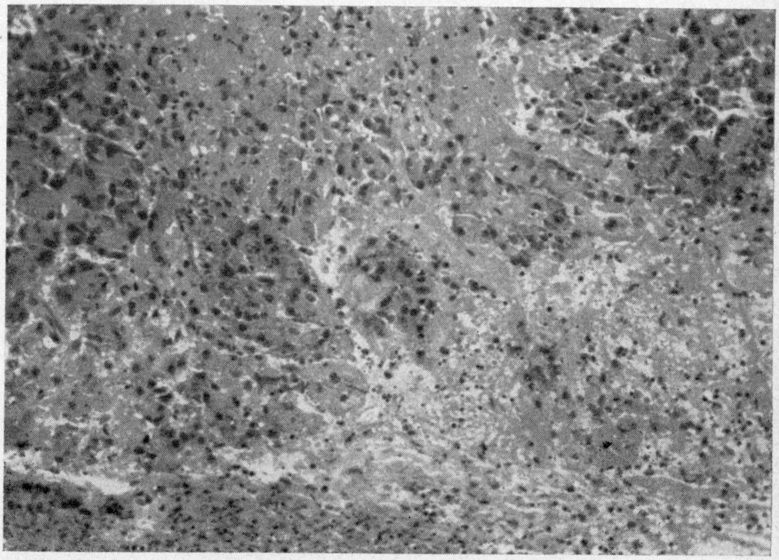

Fig 5.—Photomicrograph from the transplanted ventral lobe (*B*) in Fig 3 showing, as in the dorsal lobe, the parenchymal necrosis, edema, and hemorrhage typical of acute hemorrhagic pancreatitis.

ponent is the principal factor. They relegated to secondary importance the controversy as to whether the ischemia produced in the pancreatic gland is based on obstruction of the capillaries as a result of edema, or on vascular spasm, or on the stasis of blood within the capillaries incident to the action of bile salts. Any of these circumstances, however, would increase capillary wall permeability sufficiently to allow the admixture of blood with pancreatic juice and thus produce a highly toxic menstrum.

It should be noted, however, that Helms and Meredith[14] in experiments similar to those reported herewith could not produce hemorrhagic pancreatitis in the isolated ventral pancreatic lobe. No plausible explanation can be given for this discrepancy.

Mention should be made of the possibility of release from the hemorrhagic pancreas of toxic products which during ultimate circulation into the heterotopic pancreas led to similar disease of that organ. This theory seems far less attractive than does the neurovascular concept. Finally, in the presence of the fat necrosis of pancreatitis, the possibility of fat embolization must at least be mentioned.

Summary

After the introduction of homologous bile into the ductal system of the normal pancreas experimental acute hemorrhagic pancreatitis has been produced synchronously in the normal and in a simulated heterotopic pancreas.

A neurovascular mechanism is proposed as the etiologic agent, acting in the following chain of events: bile injected into the normal pancreas leads to pancreatitis and to violent reflex stimulation of the nerve supply of both the normal and of the heterotopic gland, thus precipitating spasm of the vessels of both glands with a resultant increase in the pancreatitis of the normal gland and the inception of the same disease in the heterotopic gland. Further pancreatitis leads to further reflex vasospasm; the cycle leading to ultimate destruction of the pancreas is thus started.

Thomas R. Kelly, MD, 503 Ohio Bldg, Akron 8, Ohio.

REFERENCES

1. Bernard, C.: Memoire sur le pancréas, Paris: J. B. Bailliere, 1856.

2. Rich, A. R., and Duff, G. L.: Experimental and Pathological Studies on Pathogenesis of Acute Hemorrhagic Pancreatitis, Bull Hopkins Hosp 58: 212, 1936.

3. Archibald, E.: The Experimental Production of Pancreatitis in Animals as the Result of the Resistance of the Common Duct Sphincter, Surg Gynec Obstet 28:529, 1919.

4. Cameron, A. L., and Noble, J. F.: Reflux of Bile up the Duct of Wirsung Caused by an Impacted Biliary Calculus, JAMA 82:1410, 1924.

5. Opie, E. L.: The Relation of Cholelithiasis to Disease of the Pancreas and to Fat Necrosis, Amer J Med Sci 121:27, 1901.

6. Thal, A.: Studies on Pancreatitis: II. Acute Pancreatic Necrosis Produced Experimentally by the Arthus Sensitization Reaction, Surgery 37:911, 1955.

7. Hasche-Klünder, R.: Fettgewebsnekrose im Nebenpankreas eines Meckelschen Divertikels, Chirurg 20:82, 1949.

8. Longmire, W. P.: Pancreatitis Occurring in Heterotopic Pancreatic Tissue, Surgery 40:412, 1956.

9. Mallet-Guy, P.; Feroldi, J.; and Rebaul, E.: Recherches expérimentales sur la pathogénie des pancréatitis auguës: Leur provacation par l'excitation du nerf splanchnique gauche, Lyon Chir 44: 281, 1949.

10. Longo, O. F.; Sosa Gallardo, C. A.; and Ferraris, A.: Contribution â la pathogénie des pancreatites aiguës, Lyon Chir 45:297, 1950.

11. Menguy, R. B.; Hallenbeck, G. A.; Bollman, J. L.; and Grindlay, J. H.: Ductal and Vascular Factors in Etiology of Experimentally Induced Acute Pancreatitis, AMA Arch Surg 74:881, 1957.

12. Thal, A.: Studies on Pancreatitis: IV. Pathogenesis of Bile Peritonitis, Surg Forum 5: 391, 1955.

13. Nemir, P., Jr., and Drabkin, D. L.: The Pathogenesis of Acute Necrotizing Hemorrhagic Pancreatitis: An Experimental Study, Surgery 40: 171, 1956.

14. Helms, C. H., and Meredith, J. H.: Concerning Neurovascular Factors in Pancreatitis, Amer Surg 27:665, 1961.

Progressive Changes in the Depth of Burns

J. RAYMOND HINSHAW, MD
D. Phil (Oxon)
ROCHESTER, NY

Introduction

Can the initial treatment of a burn prevent further tissue destruction during the early postburn period? A definite answer to that question cannot yet be given. However, if tissue destruction is progressive during the first several hours after burning, or if some of the damaged tissue can recover during that period, the initial therapy, eg, immersion in cold water, might well influence the severity.

This study shows that in untreated burns some tissues are progressively destroyed while others recover during the first 48 hours after injury.

Methods

Young Chester White pigs were used as the experimental animals because their skin closely resembles human skin histologically. They were anesthetized with intraperitoneal or intravenous barbiturates.

Shortly before the burns were to be placed the hair was closely clipped from each side, and the skin was gently washed with water and a liquid detergent. The animals were then transferred to an air-conditioned room where the ambient temperature was controlled within narrow limits to prevent wide variations in skin temperature.

The heat source was a modified 24 inch Army carbon arc searchlight[1] which can deliver a predetermined radiant exposure with great accuracy. Half of the burns were produced with a rectangular pulse, ie, one in which the irradiance rises very rapidly to the desired height and then falls very rapidly to the base line at the end of the exposure. The other half were produced with a thermal pulse which simulates that of nuclear weapons,[8] ie, one which rises rapidly to the peak irradiance and then falls increasingly slowly to the base line.

To obtain moderately severe second-degree burns, all injuries were produced with a radiant exposure of 10 calories per square centimeter. The burns were circular and were 1.7 cm in diameter. Burns with the rectangular thermal pulse were produced in one of three exposure times: 0.3, 3.0, or 10.0 seconds. The shortest exposure time results in a true flash burn, but the two longer times have characteristics similar to flame burns. The three exposure times chosen for the simulated nuclear weapon pulse were 1.8, 4.0, and 12.7 seconds; these were selected because they correspond, respectively, with the pulses of 20, 100, and 1,000 kiloton nuclear weapons.

Submitted for publication July 1, 1963.

From the Department of Surgery, University of Rochester School of Medicine and Dentistry.

Biopsies were taken at 4, 24, and 48 hours, and at 4 or 5, 9 or 10, and 14 days after burning. The six exposure times and six biopsy times made up 36 possible combinations of exposure time and biopsy time. These 36 treatments were randomly assigned exposure sites on one side of an animal. The treatment block of 36 exposure and exposure time combinations was replicated 16 times to produce a total of 576 burns. For the study reported here only half of the burns are considered—those biopsied at 4, 24, and 48 hours after injury. Two biopsies were unsuitable for histologic study and were eliminated, leaving 286 burns to be considered. The other 288 burns formed one part of a study on the histology of healing second-degree burns and will be described in a subsequent paper.

The biopsies consisted of blocks of skin and subcutaneous tissue which included not only the entire diameter of the burn but also normal tissue on each side of the burn. They were fixed in formalin and were stained by Hinshaw's modification of Verhoeff's stain[3] which provides differential staining of burned and normal tissues. In addition to a careful study of the individual cellular changes, the characteristics of the different components of skin—epidermis, dermal collagen, hair follicles, dermal and subdermal glands—were examined to detect similarities or differences at the three time intervals after injury. For microscopic evaluation, the central part of each burn, where maximal damage occurs, was the site of the measurements used to estimate burn severity.

The criteria for damage to the epithelial cells (in the epidermis, the hair follicles, and the glands in and beneath the dermis) were differences in staining characteristics as evidenced by a color difference between the damaged and undamaged cells and, more importantly, cellular and nuclear structural alterations. One criterion of damage to dermal collagen was its differential staining. Another was the depth of the zone of increased interfiber spacing, interpreted as edema, beneath the differentially stained collagen. Vascular and neural elements were not evaluated in this study.

In order to be able to compare the histology of the different types of burn and to detect any histologic changes which occur in the burn itself during the first 48 hours after injury, burn damage was also tabulated in these terms:

Epidermis: Not separated, partially separated, or completely separated from the dermis.

Dermal Collagen: Depth of differentially stained collagen (measured in microns with a ruled ocular and also tabulated as being in the upper, the middle, or the lower third of the dermis); characteristics of the differential staining; degree of sharpness of the boundary between damaged and undamaged tissue; physical properties of the collagen fibers; and depth of edema.

Hair Follicles: Relationship of depth of hair follicle damage to depth of dermal collagen injury.

Epithelial Glandular Elements or Adnexae: Disrupted, or apparently not damaged.

Results

As the time between burn and biopsy increases, the measured depth of differentially stained dermal collagen decreases. Table 1

TABLE 1.—*Depth of Differentially Stained Dermal Collagen Measured as Fraction of Total Dermal Thickness*

Exposure Time, Sec	Pulse Type	Biopsy Time, Hr Post Burn	No. of Burns in: Outer Third *	Mid Third †	Deepest Third ‡
0.3	Square	4	10	3	3
		24	16	0	0
		48	12	3	1
3.0	Square	4	1	10	5
		24	8	7	0
		48	11	4	1
10.0	Square	4	8	7	1
		24	14	2	0
		48	15	1	0
1.8	Nuclear weapon	4	6	7	2
		24	12	2	2
		48	12	2	2
4.0	Nuclear weapon	4	6	7	3
		24	10	6	0
		48	12	5	1
12.7	Nuclear weapon	4	8	6	2
		24	14	2	0
		48	16	0	0

* Damaged collagen confined to the outermost third of the dermis.

† Damaged collagen found in the middle third of the dermis but no deeper.

‡ Damaged collagen present in the deepest third of the dermis.

shows that four hours after burning 39 of the 95 burns have evidence of damaged collagen no deeper than the outer third of the dermis, while 16 have injured tissue in the deepest third, and the remaining 40 burns are intermediate in severity. Twenty-four hours after burning, however, 74 burns show damage confined to the outer third of the dermis and in only two is damaged collagen found in the deepest third. At 48 hours the picture is quite similar to that at 24 hours: 78 burns show damage no deeper than the outer third, and in only five is there damage to the deepest third.

Table 2 illustrates the same finding in a different way. The measurements reported here are, no doubt, influenced by the fact that edema occurs, increases for a time, and then decreases during the 48 hours under study. However, since pig skin does not become nearly so edematous after thermal burns as does human skin, the figures are reasonably accurate reflections of the true depths of injury. Damaged dermal collagen is found at greater depths four hours after injury than at either 24 or 48 hours; there is little difference in the location of injured collagen in the 24- and 48-hour biopsies, however.

Variations in the accumulation of edema fluid are shown in Table 3. In general, burn edema is greater at four hours than at 24 and is somewhat less at 48 hours than at 24. Since pig skin does not become very edematous after a burn, the microscopic evaluation of the location and extent of edema is often quite difficult.

TABLE 2.—*Deepest Location of Damaged Collagen*

Exposure Time, Sec	Pulse Type	Biopsy Time, Hr Post Burn	Depth of Collagen Damage, Mm *
0.3	Square	4	0.75
		24	0.49
		48	0.52
3.0	Square	4	1.02
		24	0.75
		48	0.71
10.0	Square	4	0.66
		24	0.45
		48	0.32
1.8	Nuclear weapon	4	0.85
		24	0.71
		48	0.63
4.0	Nuclear weapon	4	0.89
		24	0.63
		48	0.59
12.7	Nuclear weapon	4	0.71
		24	0.48
		48	0.42

* These figures represent the median depth of damage of the 15 or 16 burns in each category.

TABLE 3.—*Depth of Edema*

Exposure Time, Sec	Pulse Type	Biopsy Time, Hr Post Burn	No. of Burns With: Edema Confined to Dermis	Edema in Subcutaneous Tissue
0.3	Square	4	5	11
		24	12	5
		48	14	2
3.0	Square	4	1	15
		24	6	9
		48	12	4
10.0	Square	4	1	15
		24	4	12
		48	10	6
1.8	Nuclear weapon	4	2	13
		24	6	10
		48	12	4
4.0	Nuclear weapon	4	1	15
		24	6	10
		48	11	7
12.7	Nuclear weapon	4	2	14
		24	3	13
		48	7	9

For various technical reasons exact measurements of hair follicle injury have little meaning. Therefore, to determine whether this tissue destruction is progressive or reversible it is necessary to compare the levels of hair follicle and dermal damage. Even with this limitation, however, the results indicate that destruction of hair follicle epithelium progresses at the same time that some of the reversibly damaged collagen is restored to a normal appearance (Table 4).

Table 5 indicates that there is progressive destruction of the epithelial cells in the deep dermal glands during the first 24 hours. Since these observations are independent of the changes in dermal collagen, they are not subject to the same difficulties in interpretation as are the measurements of injured hair follicle epithelium.

Comment

This study shows that some types of burned tissue can recover during the first 48 hours after injury and, perhaps more

TABLE 4.—*Depth of Damage to Hair Follicle Epithelium*

Exposure Time, Sec	Pulse Type	Biopsy Time, Hr Post Burn	Depth to Damaged Dermis <0.3 Mm *	Depth to Damaged Dermis >0.3 Mm †
0.3	Square	4	12	4
		24	7	9
		48	6	9
3.0	Square	4	3	13
		24	1	14
		48	0	16
10.0	Square	4	2	14
		24	2	14
		48	2	13
1.8	Nuclear weapon	4	7	8
		24	3	12
		48	1	14
4.0	Nuclear weapon	4	7	8
		24	0	16
		48	2	15
12.7	Nuclear weapon	4	4	11
		24	1	15
		48	2	14

* Number of burns in which the deepest area of damaged hair ollicle epithelium is less than 0.3 mm deeper than the area of deepest dermal collagen damage.

† Number of burns in which the deepest area of damaged hair follicle epithelium is greater than 0.3 mm deep to the area of deepest dermal collagen damage.

TABLE 5.—*Presence or Absence of Injured Dermal Glands*

Exposure Time, Sec	Pulse Type	Biopsy Time, Hr Post Burn	No. of Burns: With Damaged Glands	No. of Burns: Without Damaged Glands
0.3	Square	4	1	15
		24	2	15
		48	2	12
3.0	Square	4	6	10
		24	8	7
		48	8	8
10.0	Square	4	6	10
		24	5	11
		48	11	5
1.8	Nuclear weapon	4	1	14
		24	4	12
		48	7	9
4.0	Nuclear weapon	4	4	12
		24	8	8
		48	13	5
12.7	Nuclear weapon	4	6	10
		24	11	5
		48	11	5

importantly, other tissues are progressively destroyed during that time. Since the earliest biopsies were not taken until four hours after burning, it is possible that the changes with time are even more striking than have been reported here. Other experiments in our laboratory and elsewhere have also indicated, directly or indirectly, that certain mildly burned tissues are probably rapidly restored to a normal state [4] and that other tissues are destroyed many hours following the thermal insult.[5,9]

These findings suggest the initial treatment of a burn might well be capable of altering the severity of injury either by preventing later tissue destruction or by assisting the body in repairing reversibly damaged tissues. Price and his co-workers,[6,7] Ófeigsson,[10] Schulman,[11] and Ferrer et al [2] have stimulated interest in cold water as an initial treatment for thermal burns. Nobody who has tried the treatment can doubt its effectiveness in relieving pain, and the evidence seems clear that it also decreases edema formation.[2] Can immersion in cold water also decrease tissue destruction? While the study reported here does not attempt to answer the question directly, it does provide evidence that could support this supposition. If a burned area is immersed in cold water within seconds after injury it is quite probable that damage will be decreased simply by the effect of lowering tissue temperatures below those capable of causing irreversible changes. However, it is unlikely that immersion in cold water even several minutes after burning can alter the outcome in this way. On the other hand, cooling the burn, perhaps by temporarily reducing the metabolism of the burned area, may well be able to prevent or mitigate the progressive tissue destruction which occurs even hours after injury, and it might also be of assistance in the repair of reversibly damaged tissue. Further work will, of course, be necessary to learn whether lowering the metabolic requirements of the injured area by cooling does, indeed, affect the outcome in one or both of these ways.

The results reported here indicate that the initial treatment of a burned area can, theoretically, alter the depth or even the degree of the burn. Perhaps more attention should be directed toward discovering what early local or systemic treatments result in the least tissue destruction, or which ones aid the body in restoring reversibly damaged tissues.

One additional, minor suggestion comes from this work. Because the histology of the burned area changes with time, if histologic comparisons are to be made between one burn and another, comparable biopsy times should be selected.

Summary and Conclusions

Comparable radiant energy burns on Chester White pigs were biopsied at 4, 24, or 48 hours after injury.

Between 4 and 24 hours after burning there is histologic evidence that damage to the hair follicles and the dermal glands is progressive.

Between 4 and 24 hours after burning some of the damaged collagen apparently recovers.

Between 24 and 48 hours after injury there is little change in the depth of damage.

Burns do not produce nearly so much edema in pig skin as they do in human skin. In these experimental burns edema is more prominent four hours after injury than at the later biopsy times.

This study shows that destruction of some tissue is progressive while other changes are reversible during the early postburn period. Therefore, it seems likely that the early treatment of a burned area might be capable of altering the ultimate depth, or even the degree, of the burn for better or worse.

Possible effects of initially cooling the burned area are discussed.

The necessity of selecting similar biopsy times for histologic comparison of burns is pointed out.

J. Raymond Hinshaw, MD, University of Rochester School of Medicine and Dentistry, 260 Crittenden Blvd, Rochester 20, NY.

REFERENCES

1. Davis, T. P., and Pearse, H. E.: Use of the Carbon Arc and Burning Magnesium Thermal Sources for Experimental Burns, Ann Surg 149:68, 1959.

2. Ferrer, J. M., Jr.; Crikelair, G. F.; and Armstrong, D.: Some Effects of Cooling on Scald Burns in the Rat, Surg Forum 13:486, 1962.

3. Hinshaw, J. R., and Pearse, H. E.: Histologic Techniques for the Differential Staining of Burned and Normal Tissues, Surg Gynec Obstet 103:726, 1956.

4. Hinshaw, J. R.: Some Effects of Superimposing Two Radiant Energy Thermal Burns on Bare Porcine Skin, Rochester, NY: University of Rochester Atomic Energy Project Report, UR-433, 1956.

5. Hinshaw, J. R.: An Experimental Study of the Degeneration and Regeneration of Nerve Fibers Following a Burn, Surg Gynec Obstet 103:31, 1956.

6. King, T. C.; Reynolds, L. E.; and Price, P. B.: Local Edema and Capillary Permeability Associated With Burn Wounds, Surg Forum 6:80, 1955.

7. King, T. C.; Zimmerman, J. M.; and Price, P. B.: Effect of Immediate Short-Term Cooling on Extensive Burns, Surg Forum 13:487, 1962.

8. Mixter, G., Jr., and Davis, T. P.: A Method of Shaping Thermal Energy Pulses From a Carbon Arc Source, Rochester, NY: University of Rochester Atomic Energy Project Report, UR-387, 1955.

9. Moritz, A. R.: Studies of Thermal Injury: III. The Pathology and Pathogenesis of Cutaneous Burns; An Experimental Study, Amer J Path 23:915, 1947.

10. Ófeigsson, Ó. J.: First-Aid Treatment of Scalds and Burns by Water Cooling, Postgrad Med 30:330, 1961.

11. Schulman, A. G.: Ice Water as Primary Treatment of Burns, JAMA 173:1916, 1960.

Replacement of Segments of the Venous System

RONALD S. TODD, MB, FRCS; EUGENE B. SIVE, MD; LOUIS R. DeJODE, MB, FRCS; CALLISTO DANESE, MD; AND JOHN M. HOWARD, MD, PHILADELPHIA

This paper is a review of the continued experiences, over the past four years in this laboratory, of segmental replacement of both the superior and the inferior venae cavae in the dog. When uniform success in venous substitution is achieved experimentally, there will be adequate opportunity for clinical application in the bridging of major venous defects caused by thrombosis, radical operations for cancer, or as a sequel to injuries of the venous system.

East and Muller,[1] in a review of the literature of the superior vena caval obstruction syndrome, pointed out that its treatment has been discouraging and that although the ideal replacement of the superior vena cava would be a large autogenous vein graft, these grafts are difficult to obtain. In their experimental work they found knitted Teflon grafts to be less liable to occlusion than nylon grafts. More recent reports indicate increasing success both in the experimental animal [2] and in man.[3,4]

There is a growing indication that reliance will have to be placed on synthetic grafts as venous substitutes. Large autografts are usually unobtainable, and homografts have not proved very satisfactory in the venous system. In addition there is mounting evidence to suggest that success in replacement of segments of the venous system depends to some extent on the ability of the graft to maintain a lumen without obstruction due to collapse of its walls. Many venous substitutes have been investigated, but the best results have been reported with autogenous venous grafts in the inferior vena cava of the dog, in which 90% of the grafts remained open.[5] Schauble [6] reported 69% of autografts to remain patent. Deterling and Bhonslay [7] reported poorly functioning autografts when a large-caliber autograft was "constructed" by suturing together several venous segments.

Plastic prostheses have been investigated without uniform success. Moore, Teramoto, and Heimburger [8] replaced the superior vena cava in dogs with grafts of crimped Teflon and achieved encouraging results. They concluded that the relatively rigid nature of the graft served to maintain the lumen in the low-pressure venous channel. Except for particular instances in which the venous pressure might be elevated, as with vena caval obstruction or portal hypertension, grafts will have to be inserted without the advantage of a high venous pressure, for there is no clinical means of safely altering venous pressure in man. The following experiments were thus undertaken in an effort to find a venous replacement that would be an effective substitute in circumstances involving essentially normal venous pressure.

Methods

This study has been an evaluation of superior and inferior venae caval replacements using a variety of materials in a large series of dogs.

Serial postoperative venographic studies were done routinely. Dogs were sacrificed and autopsies performed when venograms demonstrated that the grafts were narrowed or closed. Results were summarized as to the type of graft and length of time the grafts remained patent.

Submitted for publication July 1, 1963.

From the Department of Surgery Hahnemann Medical College.

Supported by grants HE 04182 and HTS 5553 from the National Heart Institute, United States Public Health Service.

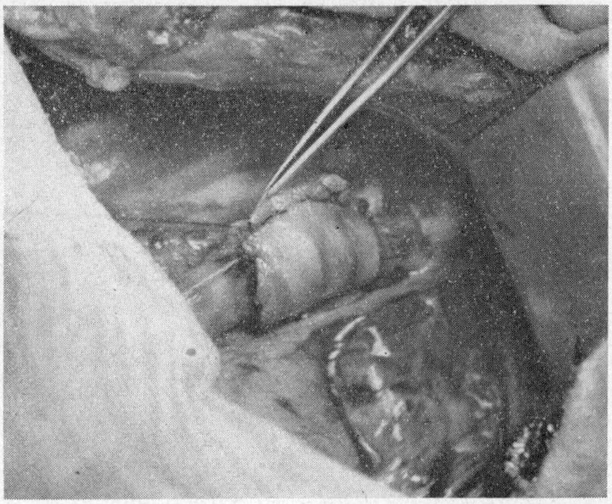

Fig 1.—Tracheal homograft immediately after its insertion into the superior vena cava.

Superior Vena Cava.—Arterial, venous, and tracheal homografts and plastic prostheses in 51 dogs were evaluated. Healthy adult dogs, weighing 25 to 55 lb, were used. In each animal, a right thoracotomy was performed through the fourth intercostal space. The vena cava was dissected free from the right and left innominate veins to the right atrium. The azygos vein was mobilized and ligated. The segment of vena cava immediately proximal (central) to the innominates and distal (craniad) to the azygos was the site used for the replacement procedures.

A dose of 10 mg of heparin was injected into the vena cava at the site of the anticipated anastomosis after first occluding the vena cava craniad to the azygos. The occluded segment of the vena cava was then either transected and allowed to retract or had a 2.5 cm segment removed.

Inferior Vena Cava.—Tracheal and venous homografts, peritoneal autografts, and Dacron grafts (crimped, noncrimped, reinforced, carbonized, or siliconized) were evaluated in 58 dogs.

The abdomen was opened by a midline incision and the small bowel was mobilized by division of the ligament of Treitz. The vena cava, from below the renal veins to the iliac bifurcation, was dissected free and its tributaries ligated. After isolating a segment between vascular clamps a segment, 2-3 cm long, was excised, or in a few instances the vein was simply transected and allowed to retract. Heparin was injected into both proximal and distal segments of the occluded vein.

In both superior and inferior venae cavae, grafts of 2.5-5 cm in length were inserted. Anastomoses were made with continuous sutures of 5-0 Mersilene or silk. Sutures were placed sufficiently close so that anastomotic hemostasis was almost perfect when the clamp was removed.

Materials and Results

Venous Homografts.—Venous homografts were utilized when fresh or after storage under refrigeration (4 C) for one to ten days in saline containing penicillin and streptomycin. In the thoracic study four dogs were still alive with patent grafts (5-14 months) out of an original 17 grafts, a long-term patency record of 24%. In the abdomen one graft of 11 remained patent for four months.

Aortic Homografts.—Aortic homografts, refrigerated similarly to the venous homografts, were used only in the superior vena cava. Of an initial 11 grafts, only one remained patent for an appreciable period of time. This animal was sacrificed after 12 months, at which time marked narrowing of the grafts due to fibrosis was confirmed at autopsy.

Peritoneal Autografts.—These were used only in the inferior vena cava. The posterior sheath of the rectus abdominis was made into a peritoneal lined tube and was used

Fig 2.—Venogram showing patency of a tracheal homograft in the superior vena cava 13 months after its insertion.

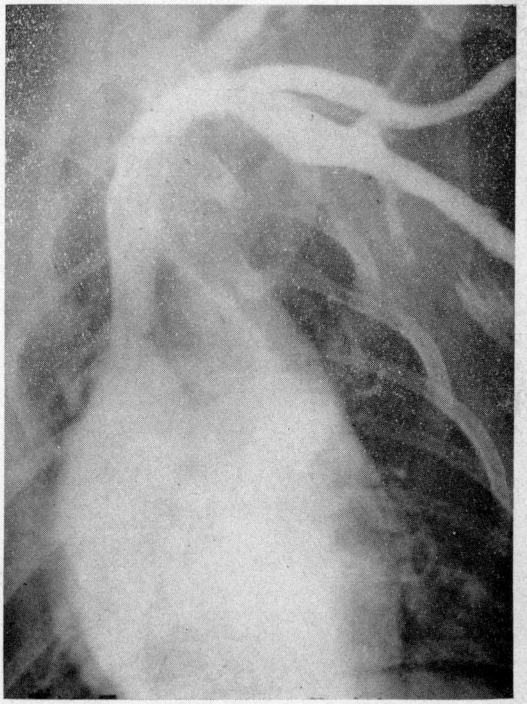

either immediately or after storage for a week as described above. All 14 grafts were occluded within two weeks.

Tracheal Homografts.—Because of their ringed, flexible structure, tracheal homografts were evaluated. The grafts were refrigerated as described above. The posterior membranous portion of the trachea was used as the anterior wall of the graft. This was an essential technique, for by so doing, the pliable membranous wall could be tailored to fit the diameter of the recipient vein, the circumference of the trachea being reduced by externally plicating the membranous portion (Fig 1). In several instances, small sections of the cartilaginous rings were resected in order to make the ends of the graft conform to vena caval size.

In the thorax the best results were obtained with this group. Seven of the 11 grafts remained patent (64%). Four dogs were still alive with completely patent grafts as revealed by venographic studies 8, 9, 11, and 13 months after the superior vena caval replacement (Fig 2). A postmortem specimen of a patent eight-month-old graft is shown in Fig 3.

In the abdomen only one graft of seven remained patent. Autopsy in the majority of instances disclosed that occlusion of the graft was due to thrombosis at the suture line. In one instance, unusually severe degeneration of the tracheal mucosa appeared to have caused occlusion. This was interpreted as a severe tissue response to a homograft.

Plastic Prostheses.—Pilot studies were performed utilizing various prosthetics. These prosthetics were prepared for this study by Edwards * and Pyenson.† Models were designed to vary the rigidity, smoothness, porosity, electrical conductivity (carbonization), and wettability (siliconization) of the grafts.

In the thorax four rigid Teflon tubes were inserted; each was closed within 25 days. All four dogs died from superior

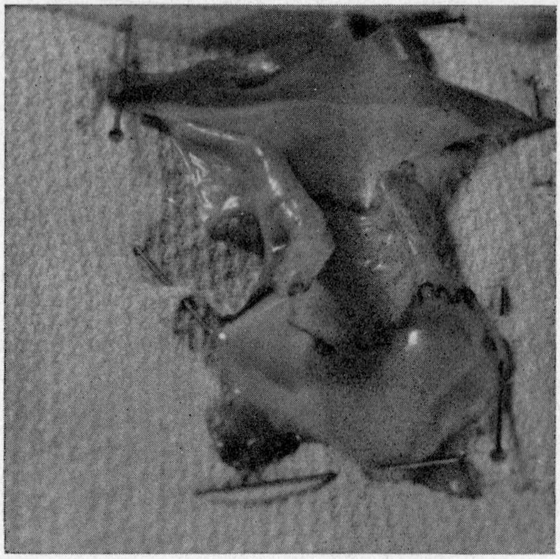

Fig 3.—A patent tracheal homograft as seen at autopsy almost eight months after its insertion.

vena caval occlusion. One Tygon tube was patent at the end of six days, when the dog died from pulmonary atelectasis. Two woven Dacron grafts were occluded at the end of 20 days, when both dags died from acute superior vena caval occlusion. Five crimped Teflon grafts patterned after the trachea with rigid rings incorporated were inserted.‡ Four remained patent 6-12 months later, although narrowed. This graft incorporated the essential principle of the trachea: semirigidity to keep the graft from collapsing, as well as porosity, inherent in the knitted character of the graft, to allow tissue ingrowth so that the graft may be permanently incorporated as part of the vascular system. This architectural pattern may permit a solution to the problem of venous replacement.

In the abdomen a wide variety of plastic and reinforced plastic grafts were tried. These included crimped Dacron (seven dogs), noncrimped Dacron (two dogs), woven carbonized Dacron with an acrylic spiral or ring (seven dogs), Dacron reinforced with Teflon threads (four dogs), siliconized Dacron with rubber rings (three dogs) and polyprophylene grafts (three dogs). Of a total of 26 dogs only three grafts remained patent longer than

* Philadelphia College of Textiles.

† Division of Biophysics, Hahnemann Medical College.

‡ Ethicon, Inc., New Jersey.

TABLE 1.—*Long-Term Patency Rate of Segmental Replacements of The Vena Cava (Open Four Months or Longer)*

Graft Type	No. of Dogs	No. Open	Durat. of Patency, Mo	% Open
Superior Vena Cava				
Tracheal homografts	11	7	4-13	64
Venous homografts	17	4	5-14	24
Aortic homografts	11	1	12	9
Plastic prostheses	7	0	—	0
Plastic prostheses of tracheal design	5	4	6-12	80
Inferior Vena Cava				
Tracheal homografts	7	1	5	14
Venous homografts	11	1	4	9
Peritoneal autografts	14	0	—	0
Plastic prostheses	26	3	7	11

four months. The patent prostheses consisted of a Dacron graft reinforced by Teflon threads in two instances and an acrylic splint on carbonized Dacron in the other.

Low-Molecular-Weight Dextran.—It was thought that low-molecular-weight dextran might prevent red cell aggregation[9] and thereby be of value in preventing early thrombosis in the grafts. Accordingly, an additional 13 dogs were given 1,000 ml of "Rheomacrodex" § (average molecular weight 40,000) on the day of operation. This series had grafts of Dacron reinforced with Teflon threads, polypropylene, or venous homografts inserted into the inferior vena cava. Alternate animals did not receive dextran. An amount of 500 ml of dextran was given during operation, followed by 500 ml six hours later. This had no appreciable effect on the rapidity of occlusion. All but two occluded within three weeks; both of these consisted of Dacron reinforced with Teflon. Two controls remained open for comparable periods of time.

Anticoagulant.—Similarly, an anticoagulant, Warfarin, was given to six dogs for one week after operation. Warfarin, a coumarin derivative, was given to depress the prothrombin level to 20% of normal. Grafts of Dacron with Teflon support were inserted into the inferior vena cava. The results are shown in Table 2. Two of the six dogs bled to death as the result of the anticoagulant.

§ Supplied by Pharmacia Ltd., New York.

Comment

In an attempt to achieve a satisfactory method of venous replacements, various substitutes have been studied in the laboratory during the last four years in a total of 145 dogs.

Early occlusion of the grafts occurred as a result of thrombosis originating at the suture line. Fibrosis with attendant narrowing was a common occurrence in most types of long-term grafts. Narrowing of the graft was less of a problem with the semirigid tracheal grafts. It is believed that a satisfactory venous replacement should retain its tubular configuration without collapsing yet exhibit sufficient pliability and resilience to carry out the function of the vena cava. It should not promote development of thrombosis. The trachea apparently meets several fundamental requirements for such satisfac-

TABLE 2.—*Effects of Low-Molecular-Weight Dextran and Anticoagulant on Thrombosis of Grafts (Inferior Vena Cava)*

Series	No. of Grafts	No. Patent 3 Wk
Control	13	2
Low-molecular-weight Dextran	13	3
Control	4	2
Anticoagulant (warfarin)	6	0

tory graft, but its mucosal separation encourages occlusion. Since the two main factors responsible for occlusion in venous grafts are early intraluminal thrombosis and later stenosis at the suture lines, techniques and grafts have been designed to minimize these factors. An effort has been made to obviate the stenosis by the use of reinforced grafts, and in the thorax this has met with modest success. Results in the inferior vena cava, however, remain disappointing. After the failure of low-molecular-weight dextran to delay thrombosis, six dogs were given intramuscular warfarin sodium as an anticoagulant. Again this was unsatisfactory, and it was noticed that clotting of the graft appeared to take place even when the prothrombin level of the blood was reduced to such a level as to cause death from hemorrhage. In this respect it has been suggested that the dog is a particularly unsuitable animal to use in work of this nature in view of the increased tendency of the blood to clot when compared with blood of man. However, in a large series of canine renal homotransplants carried out in this laboratory, direct venous anastomoses have been routinely performed between the venous homografts (renal vein of graft) and the iliac veins of the recipient animals. In these grafts, early venous thrombosis has seldom occurred.

At the present time a new prosthesis is being evaluated. This consists of bovine collagen reinforced with semi-rigid Dacron rings.|| It has been designed so that the interstices will allow liberal fibroblastic permeation of the graft, and after a period of 6 to 12 weeks the Dacron rings will remain as a permanent support for the intimal lining. Three such grafts, not included in the tabulations of this report, have remained patent for a period of three months.

Conclusions

In a series of 145 vena caval grafts in dogs, tracheal homografts proved superior to other homografts and to most prostheses for replacement of segments of the superior vena cava. Adaptation of the architectural pattern of the trachea to the design of the prostheses offers the most promising lead to continued study. In a series of 36 experiments, neither low-molecular-weight dextran nor anticoagulation was of value in maintaining patency of the graft. Patency of a graft in the superior vena cava was more frequently attained than was patency in the inferior (abdominal) vena cava.

Neither siliconization of the prosthesis nor alteration of its electrical conductivity (carbonization) appeared to alter its tendency to occlude.

Grafts in the venous system occlude by early thrombosis or by late stenosis at the suture line.

Although the incidence of occlusion has been quite high, long-term successful grafts demonstrate the biological feasibility of replacing segments of the venous system. A reasonable basis exists for the conclusion that continued study of techniques and materials will permit the development of a practical clinical method of segmental venous replacement.

|| Ethicon, Inc., New Jersey.

John M. Howard, MD, Professor of Surgery, Hahnemann Medical College and Hospital, 230 N Broad St, Philadelphia 2, Pa.

REFERENCES

1. East, W. M., and Muller, W. H., Jr.: An Experimental Study of Resection and Replacement of the Superior Vena Cava, Amer J Surg 99:6-12, 1960.

2. Hambraeus, G., and Andersen, M. H.: Experimental Vena Cava Replacement With Teflon Prostheses, Arch Surg 85:220, 1962.

3. Allansmith, R.: Surgical Treatment of Superior Vena Cava Obstruction Due to Malignant Tumor, J Thorac Cardiov Surg 44:258-263, 1962.

4. Hardin, C. A.: Bypass Saphenous Grafts for the Relief of Venous Obstruction of the Extremity, Surg Gynec Obstet 115:709, 1962.

5. Bower, R.; Federicci, V.; and Howard, J. M.: Continuing Studies of Replacement of Segments of the Venous System, Surgery 47:132, 1960.

6. Schauble, J. F.; Anlyan, W. G.; and Postlethwait, R. W.: A Study of Grafts in the Venous System, AMA Arch Surg 78:288, 1959.

7. Deterling, R. A., Jr., and Bhonslay, S. B.: Use of Vessel Grafts and Plastic Prostheses for Relief of Superior Vena Caval Obstruction, Surgery 38:1008, 1955.

8. Moore, T. C.; Teramoto, S.; and Heimburger, I. L.: Successful Use of Teflon Grafts for Superior Vena Caval Replacement, Surg Gynec Obstet 111:475-483, 1960.

9. Gelin, L. E.: Studies in Anemia of Injury, Acta Chir Scand suppl 210:1-130, 1956.

Concentrated Preoperative Irradiation Therapy

KOMEI NAKAYAMA, MD
FUMINORI YANAGISAWA, MD
KINICHI NABEYA, MD
TATSUO TAMIYA, MD
SEIICHIRO KOBAYASHI, MD
AND
KOHJI MAKINO, MD
CHIBA, JAPAN

Introduction

Operative mortality in patients with cancer has been greatly reduced, but the incidence of recurrence has not been significantly altered (Fig 1 and 2). Surgical removal and irradiation [18,21] offer the only means of control. Theoretically it would seem that a combination [3-5] of these therapies should offer the best opportunity for a permanent cure. It is surprising how little work [5,7,10-12,17,19] has been done in this regard when the world literature is reviewed. Postoperative irradiation [1,2,3] has had significant trials in cases of uterine, breast, and oral cancer. The value of postoperative radiation in patients with gastrointestinal lesions has been shown to be rather limited.

Submitted for publication July 2, 1963.

Professor of Surgery and Head, Department of Surgery (Dr. Nakayama), Instructor (Dr. Yanagisawa), Assistants (Dr. Nabeya, Dr. Tamiya), Department of Surgery, School of Medicine, Chiba University.

Curiosity was stimulated, however, by noting that in our series of patients with esophageal cancer there were three cases of five-year survival in patients who had received preoperative irradiation. We found this true also in one survivor of a lung cancer who lived for nine years postoperatively. We have therefore embarked on a systematic investigation of the effects of preoperative irradiation in both animals and humans. Our purpose, of course, is to improve the end results in the treatment of the disease. We feared at first that preoperative irradiation would make the surgery more difficult and increase operative morbidity and mortality; therefore, a protracted fractionated dose was employed initially. Subjects and results were carefully evaluated by surgeons, pathologists (Prof Enjiro Takizawa et al), and radiologists (Prof Hirotake Kakei et al) at the Chiba University Hospitals. Concentrated preoperative irradiation has replaced pro-

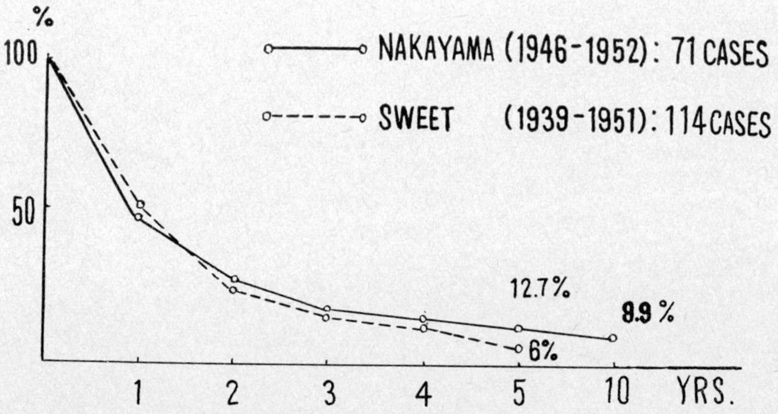

Fig 1.—Follow-up results of cancer of the upper and midthoracic esophagus resected.

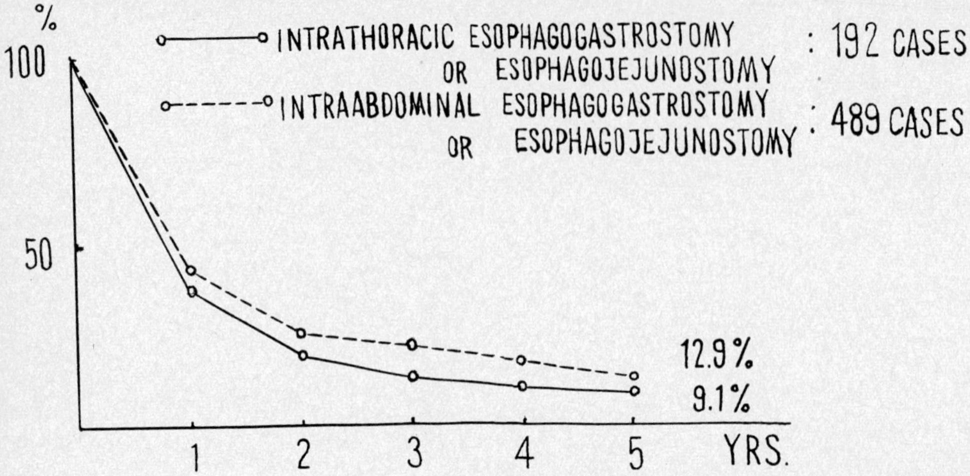

Fig 2.—Follow-up results of cancer of the lower esophagus and the cardiac end of the stomach resected (a survey of those resected from January, 1946, to December, 1952).

tracted fractionated irradiation, and our results have supported the value of this change. Our series of cases includes 490 patients who have received preoperative irradiation up to December of 1962 (Table 1). The accumulated results demonstrate definite advantages and improvement in patients receiving preoperative radiation, particularly when that irradiation is given in concentrated dosage.

Animal Studies [15,16]

The animal's response is not identical with that of man. However, with animals we can rapidly provide a large series of cases and statistical results which are of some significance. Human studies require years. Irradiation factors used in animal studies were: 200 kilovolt peak; filter: 0.3 mm Cu plus 0.5 mm Al; half-value layer: 0.85 mm Cu; focus to skin distance: 40 cm; and air dose at skin: 116 r/min. A shield box was used for irradiation to the optimum area of each animal. Radiation

TABLE 1.—*A Survey of Cases Undergoing Preoperative Irradiation Therapy at Nakayama's Surgery Department up to December, 1962*

Carcinoma Location	No. Cases
Upper & midthoracic esophagus	161
Lower esophagus & cardiac end of the stomach	120
Stomach	140
Rectum	21
Breast	41
Others	7
Total	490

dose in the box was less than 0.18% of the air dose and was negligible.

A. *Experiment 1.*—Ascites hepatoma, M. H. 134, was grafted to the tail of male mice (F 1) offsprings of C3H (male) and D. D. (female). The influences of the various form of therapy on lymph node metastasis were then observed. The mice were divided into the following four groups:

I: Control—M. H. 134 grafted mice.

II: Grafted mice followed by amputation of the tail.

III: Grafted and irradiated.

IV: Grafted, irradiated, and then amputated.

The results are as follows (Table 2):

1. Group II demonstrated that surgical removal of the lesion in the early stage of the disease tended to inhibit nodal metatasis, but that surgical removal in a late stage promoted lymph node metastasis.

2. Group III demonstrated an inhibitory effect on both the primary lesion and the metastatic lesions after heavy irradiation (2,000 r) and that the lapse of time prior to therapy diminished irradiation effect.

3. Group IV showed a marked inhibitory effect to metastasis even when the lesion was irradiated in late stage, and the reduction of metastatic lesions was more notable than in group III.

B. *Experiment 2.*—The factors and animal apparatus in the second experiment were identical with those of the first experiment; however, here the animals were followed for a period of some 60 days in order to observe the prolongation of survival due to preoperative irradiation. The results in this experiment are shown in Table 3. Group II demonstrated that amputation of the lesion without irradiation therapy did prolong survival time if this amputation was done early in the course of the disease. Late in the course of the disease amputa-

TABLE 2.—*Experiment 1: Influence of Irradiation to Lymph Node Metastasis*

Exp. Groups	No. Mice Used	No. Mice With Meta.	Meta. Rate, %
Groups Amputated in an Early Stage (Graft $\xrightarrow{2\ Wk}$ Sacrifice)			
1. Graft only	14	12	85.7
2. Graft $\xrightarrow{4\ days}$ amputation	10	3	30.0
3. Graft $\xrightarrow{4\ days}$ 500 r × 1	10	7	70.0
$\quad\quad$ → 2,000 r × 1	10	4	40.0
4. Graft $\xrightarrow{4\ days}$ 500 r × 1 $\xrightarrow{2\ days}$ amput.	12	6	50.0
$\quad\quad$ → 2,000 r × 1 $\xrightarrow{2\ days}$ amput.	12	3	25.0
Groups Amputated in a Late Stage (Graft $\xrightarrow{2\ Wk}$ Sacrifice)			
1. Graft only	14	12	85.7
2. Graft $\xrightarrow{10\ days}$ amputation	10	10	100.0
3. Graft $\xrightarrow{10\ days}$ 500 r × 1	10	8	80.0
$\quad\quad$ → 2,000 r × 1	9	5	55.5
4. Graft $\xrightarrow{10\ days}$ 500 r × 1 $\xrightarrow{2\ days}$ amput.	12	8	66.6
$\quad\quad$ → 2,000 r × 1 $\xrightarrow{2\ days}$ amput.	12	6	50.0

tion altered survival very slightly. The third group showed that irradiation alone also prolonged survival time to some degree. In group IV, amputation of the primary lesion, in addition to radiation therapy, when performed in the early stages of the disease provided the most satisfactory results with the longest survival times. But here also, when irradiation was given and the lesion amputated in the relatively late stage of the disease, survival time was prolonged considerably, when compared with group II and III.

C. *Experiment 3.*—In this group Ehrlich ascites carcinoma was grafted in mice of the D. D. strain. The influences of irradiation on the carcinoma were observed. The results in this experiment are shown in Table 4. Preoperative irradiation here reduced the per cent of successful grafting and prolonged the retention of ascites. The inhibitory effect was most marked when 3,000 r were given.

TABLE 3.—*Experiment 2: Survival Rate of the Mice With Ascites Hepatoma (M.H. 134) Grafted on Their Tails (Observation for 60 Days)*

Exp. Groups	No. Used	No. Surviving	Survival Rate, %
Groups Amputated in an Early Stage			
1. Graft only	21	0	0
2. Graft $\xrightarrow{4\ days}$ amputation	20	13	65.0
3. Graft $\xrightarrow{4\ days}$ 2,000 r × 1	17	2	11.8
4. Graft $\xrightarrow{4\ days}$ 2,000 r × 1 $\xrightarrow{2\ days}$ amput.	19	12	63.2
Groups Amputated in a Late Stage			
1. Graft only	21	0	0
2. Graft $\xrightarrow{10\ days}$ amputation	19	3	15.8
3. Graft $\xrightarrow{10\ days}$ 2,000 r × 1	18	3	16.7
4. Graft $\xrightarrow{10\ days}$ 2,000 r × 1 $\xrightarrow{2\ days}$ amput.	18	5	27.8

TABLE 4.—*Experiment 3: Influence of Irradiation to Ehrlich Ascites Carcinoma*

Exp. Groups	No. Used	No. Deaths	Succeeding Grafts, %	Ascites Retention Period, Days
Graft without irradiation (control)	10	10	100	7
1,500 r × 1 —1 day→ graft	10	7	70	7-14
3,000 r × 1 —1 day→ graft	10	3	30	14-21

Clinical Experience

Esophageal carcinoma has been the main subject of our studies since we see many patients with this disease. We feel that esophageal carcinoma lends itself well to irradiation therapy. Squamous cell carcinoma is usually susceptible to irradiation, and the esophagus is a fixed organ, relatively free from other radiosensitive structures. In this study we will also review preoperative irradiation therapy in the treatment of carcinoma of the cardiac end of the stomach, the stomach proper, the rectum, and the breast.

A. *Methods of Investigation and Criteria of Effect.*—1. Histological Studies[15,16]: Therapeutic effect was evaluated on the basis of the histology of the surgical specimens. The changes in histology varied with dose-time relationships, as well as the interval between irradiation therapy and surgery. The findings were analyzed in accordance with Takizawa's classification as described in Tables 5, 6, 7, and 8.

Preoperative irradiation therapy caused catabolic changes such as swelling and pyknosis of the nuclei and a reduction in, or

TABLE 5.—*Histological Changes in Carcinomatous Parenchyma After Irradiation (Takizawa's Classification)*

Grade, Morphological Changes	Nuclei	Protoplasm	Changes in Cancer Nests
X_1	Mitosis visible yet partially	Degeneration visible partially	Proliferation visible yet partially
X_2	Mitosis not recognized	Degeneration visible diffusely	Degenerated
X_3	Caryorrhexis	Marked degeneration	Destroyed or disappeared

TABLE 6.—*Histological Classification of Carcinoma According to the Infiltration Grade*

	Carcinoma		
Grade	Esophageal	Gastric	Breast
L_1	Submucous	Submucous	Within mammary gland
L_2	Intramural	Intramural	Fat tissues surrounding mammary gland
L_3	Extramural	Subserosal or serosal	Skin or muscles

TABLE 7.—*Classification of Carcinoma According to the Maturity of Carcinomatous Parenchyma*

	Carcinoma		
Grade	Esophageal	Gastric	Breast
D_1	Differentiated squamous cell Ca	Adenocarcinoma	Adenocarcinoma
D_2	Low differentiated squamous cell Ca	Cuboidal cell Ca	Cuboidal cell Ca
D_3	Carcinoma simplex	Carcinoma simplex	Carcinoma simplex

TABLE 8.—*Histological Changes in Stroma After Irradiation (Takizawa's Classification)*

Grade	Connective Tissues	Regenerative Signs
S_1	Proliferative	Present
S_2	Degenerative	Recognized yet
S_3	Destructive	Not recognized

complete absence of, mitosis. These changes have been arbitrarily classified as X_1, X_2, and X_3, according to the grade of the morphologic change. This is shown in Table 6 and Fig 3. These denote the mildest irradiation change found in a given surgical specimen. Such classification has given the basic criteria of irradiation effects throughout our studies.

2. Other Supplementary Studies. We are presently doing extensive radioisotope studies in our department. The fact that cancer tissues take up a greater quantity of P^{32} has been clearly demonstrated. We find that this is especially true in carcinoma of the esophagus. Radiation therapy can alter the degree of uptake of P^{32}, and sometimes sufficient therapy will reduce this uptake to entirely normal levels. Macro-autographs of surgical specimens have supported this also. Our chemical analysis of the phosphorus fractions of cells has revealed a significant decrease of the DNA and RNA contained in malignant tissues after preoperative irradiation (Table 9). We feel that this indicates a weakening and destructive effect on malignant cells. Those patients undergoing irradiation therapy have been followed closely with periodic re-evaluations by x-ray (Fig 4), endoscopy, hematological studies, and electrolytic evaluation. We have followed the latter two closely in an attempt to evaluate the untoward effects of irradiation therapy. All factors influencing surgical risk and the postoperative course have been carefully analyzed.

B. *Irradiation Factors.*[16]—1. Apparatus: Initially a pendulum irradiation system with high-voltage x-ray was employed for esophageal carcinoma, and a stationary sieve irradiation system or a Tele Co^{60} (air shooter) system for gastric carcinoma. These systems have been replaced by a 2,000 curie

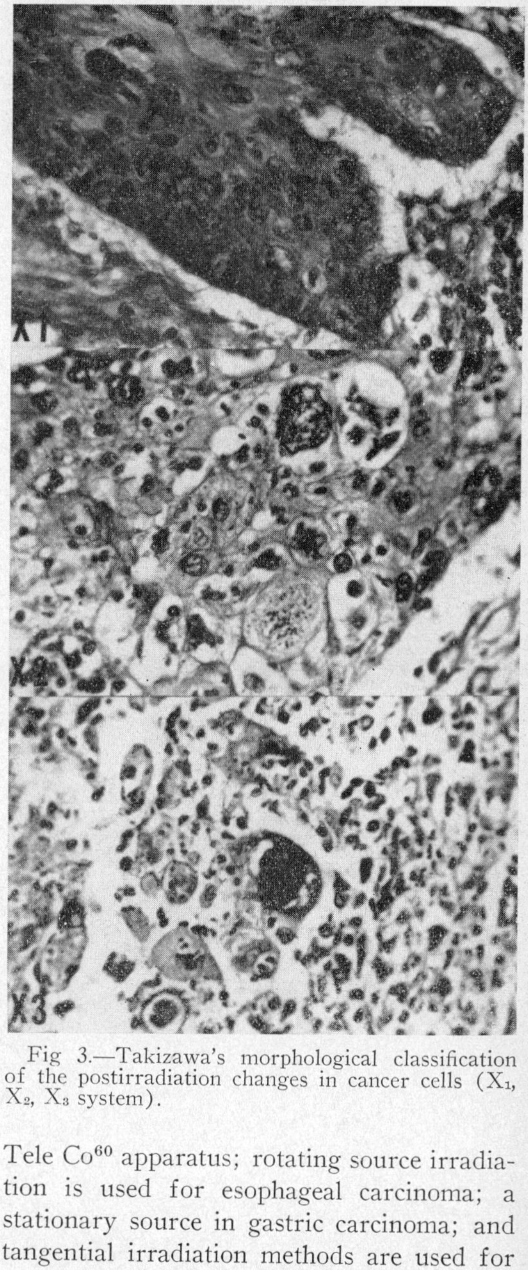

Fig 3.—Takizawa's morphological classification of the postirradiation changes in cancer cells (X_1, X_2, X_3 system).

Tele Co^{60} apparatus; rotating source irradiation is used for esophageal carcinoma; a stationary source in gastric carcinoma; and tangential irradiation methods are used for carcinoma of the breast (including the axilla) and rectum.

2. Irradiation Field: It is obviously desirable that the irradiation cover the total lesion in an attempt to prevent dissemination of malignant cells during surgical manipulation; however, the size of the lesion or the response of the patient to radiation therapy may not permit this. The selection of the field of therapy must be evaluated and chosen

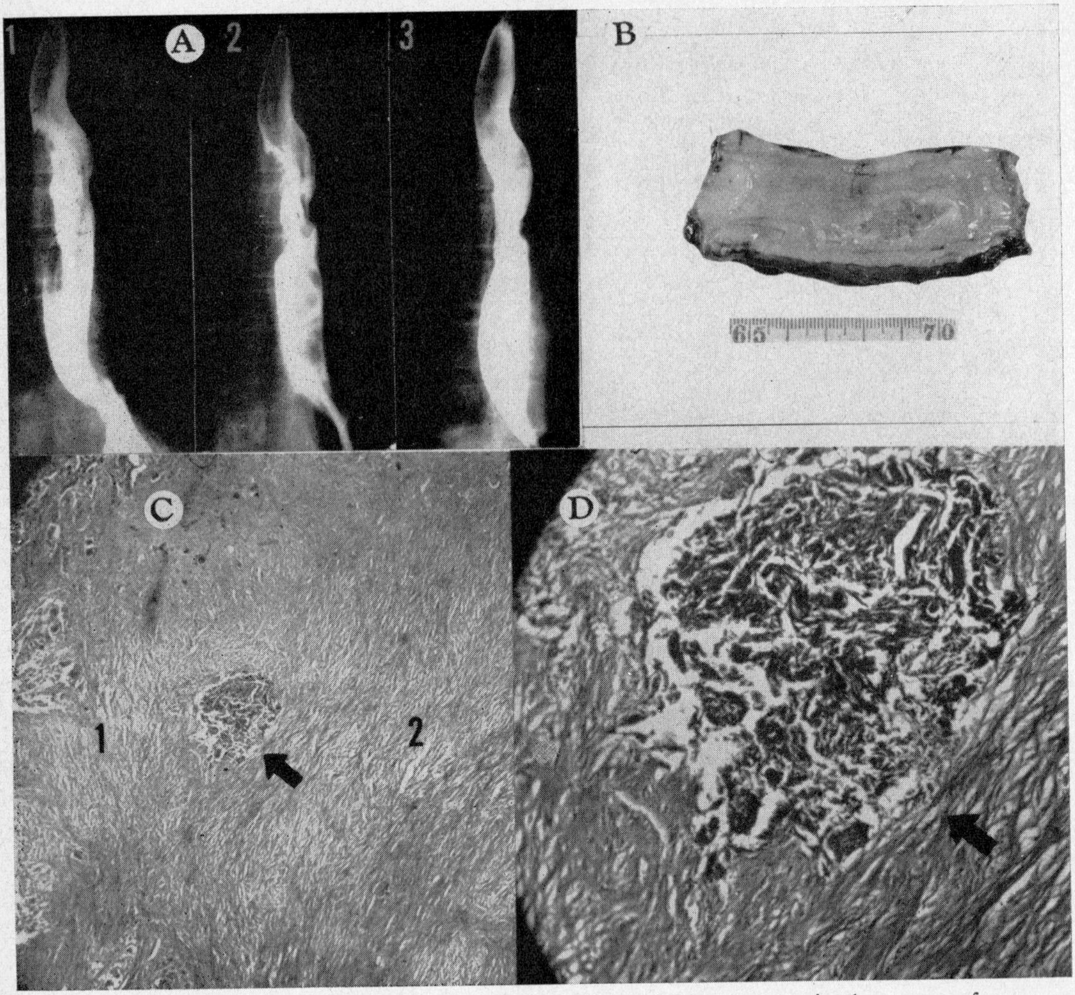

Fig 4.—An example of the progressive improvement shown in x-ray in the course of our preoperative irradiation therapy. protracted irradiation: *1,* before; *2,* 1,200 r given (at six days); *3,* 2,400 r (given at 20 days). *B,* surgical specimen. *C,* microscopic view showing X_3 serosa side. *D,* microscopic view showing X_3 changes; contracted cancer nest shows disappearing process of cancer cells (high power).

in each case. Where the lesion is very large, the area which should prove to be the most difficult to remove should receive the bulk of the therapy. If there is an area which frequently shows postoperative recurrence of tumor, this area must be irradiated. We presently employ a field which measures 5 to 6 cm by 10 to 12 cm for esophageal carcinomas. With lesions of the cardia or body of the stomach, the field measures 7 cm by 10 cm and always includes the celiac axis (Fig 5). The field of similar size is used in carcinoma of the breast, and the axilla is routinely irradiated in these cases.

TABLE 9.—*A Comparative Study for Specific Activity of the Phosphorus Fractions Contained in Cancer Tissues*

P Fractions	Group Not Irradiated	Group Irradiated
acid-soluble P	3.03	0.51
phospholipid	2.80	1.14
DNA	3.32	0.66
RNA	2.51	0.69
phosphoprotein	1.44	1.55

3. Dosage: During this study the total dosage has varied from 300 to 6,000 r. These doses have been fractionated in many ways in an attempt to establish the optimum dosage. At first daily dosage varied from 200 to 300 r; at the suggestion of our con-

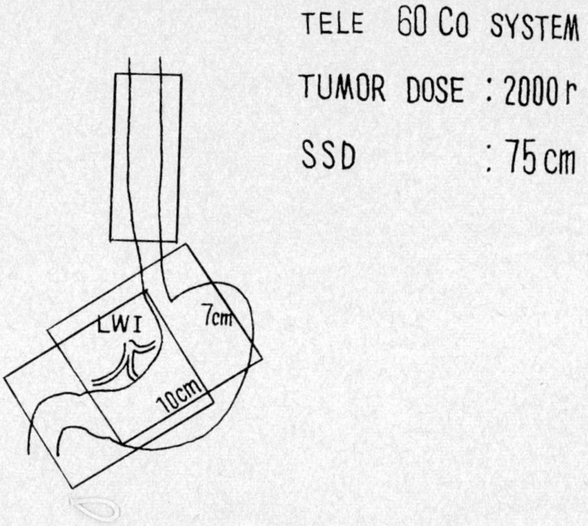

CA. OF UPPER & MID-THORACIC ESOPHAGUS		4~6 cm x 10~12 cm	ROTATION
CA. OF LOWER ESOPHAGUS & CARDIA		7 x 10	STATIONARY
CA. OF STOMACH		7 x 10	"
CA. OF RECTUM		7 x 10	"
CA. OF BREAST	BREAST	6 x 8	" (TANGENTIAL)
	AXILLA	7 x 10	STATIONARY

Fig 5.—Irradiation field.

sultant radiologists, consideration and correlation of the multiple factors and results have shown that from 2,000 to 3,000 r fractionated over a period of from 10 to 14 days is most successful in protracted therapy. (The dosage in our concentrated irradiation will be described later.)

4. Interval From the End of Irradiation to Surgery (Fig 6): We have shown histologically that if this interval is greater than two weeks, there is some retrogression of the therapeutic effect. It is true that this loss is minimal from two weeks to one month, but beyond one month it is marked. We, at present, feel that a four- to seven-day waiting period is ideal. This will allow for preoperative laboratory and physical evaluation prior to surgery.

C. *Results.*—Our follow-up of 490 cases which have received preoperative irradiation therapy covers a period of three years in the majority of our cases. We do feel that the results thus far are significant. Important is the fact that preoperative irradiation has not made the surgery more difficult or increased the operative mortality or morbidity, in those patients where the total dose of radiation has not exceeded 3,000 r (Table 10 and 11). Instead we have been surprised to find that frequently the tumor-bearing organs were removed more easily than we had anticipated. The degree of resectability and the frequency

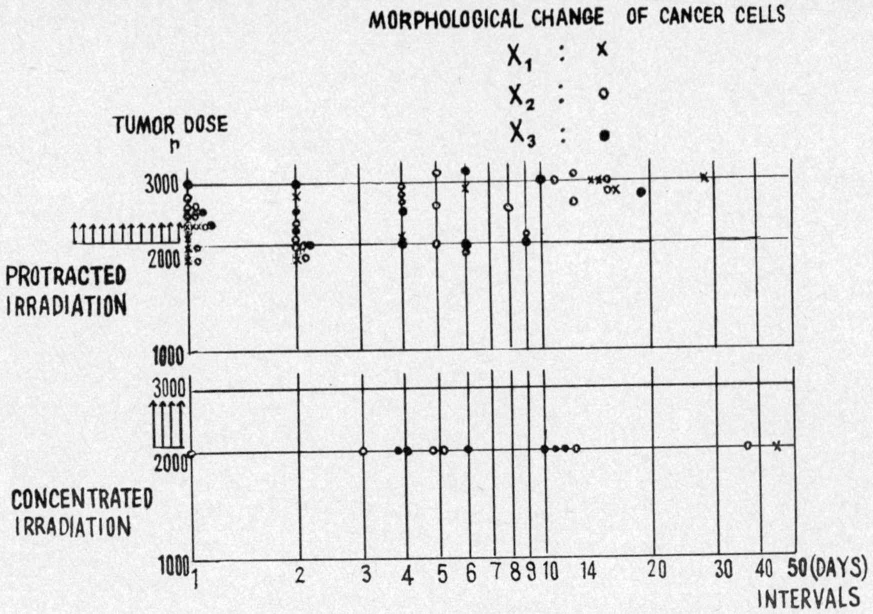

Fig 6.—Intervals between irradiation end and operation.

TABLE 10.—*Operative Results of Carcinoma Undergoing the Preoperative Irradiation Therapy at Nakayama's Surgery Department (1958-1962)*

Carcinoma	Irradiated or Not	No. Cases	Operative Deaths	Operative Mortality, %
Upper & midthoracic esophagus	Yes	161	7	4.4
	No	55	3	5.4
Lower esophagus & cardiac end of stomach	Yes	120	4	3.3
	No	311	12	3.8
Stomach	Yes	140	2	1.4
	No	457	5	1.1

of resectability in lesions of the upper and midthoracic esophagus have definitely increased. It is also our impression that the presence of extraserosal invasion has diminished markedly. At the same time, wound healing and postoperative recuperation have been altered only slightly.

TABLE 11.—*Operative Results of Carcinoma of the Upper and Midthoracic Esophagus Undergoing the Preoperative Irradiation Therapy at Nakayama's Surgery Department*

Total Tumor Dose	No. Cases	Operative Deaths	Operative Mortality %
Less than 2,000 r *	49	1	2.0
2,000-3,000 r	70	1	1.4
More than 3,000 r †	35	4	11.4
Others ‡	7	1	14.5
Total	161	7	4.4

A comparative study for the total tumor dose given.

* Smaller doses for poor risk.

† Larger doses as attempts.

‡ Irradiated at other hospitals; therefore, irradiation factors were unknown or not uniform.

The survival rate in those patients having carcinoma of the esophagus treated by irradiation only was 6.8%. The rate in those patients having only surgery was 21.7%; whereas in those patients having combined therapy irradiation followed by surgery, the survival rate has been 44.4% (Fig 7). It is of interest that in the series of patients having esophageal carcinoma without lymph node metastasis, the three-year survival rate was 35.7% prior to the institution of preoperative irradiation therapy. In the same group of patients (esophageal carcinoma without lymph node metastasis) after the

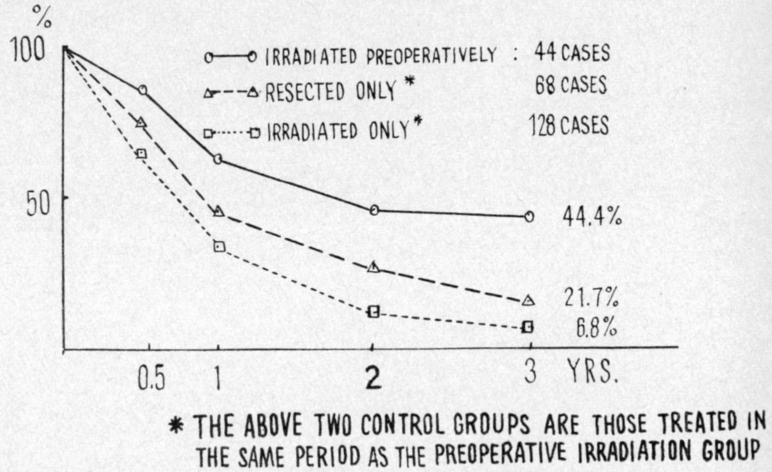

Fig 7.—Follow-up results of cancer of the upper and midthorácic esophagus undergoing our preoperative irradiation therapy (a survey made in 1963).

institution of irradiation therapy, the survival rate to date has been 100% (Fig 8). All seven in this final group are alive. They had received 2,000 to 3,000 r prior to surgery. The two-year follow-up study of patients with carcinoma of the lower esophagus or cardiac end of the stomach and the body or pyloric portion of the stomach (approximately 30 cases in each group) has shown an increase in survival rate from 10% to 20% (Fig 9). Our 30 patients with breast cancer who received preoperative irradiation are all living after two years. This has been true also in ten cases of rectal cancer. Four of the

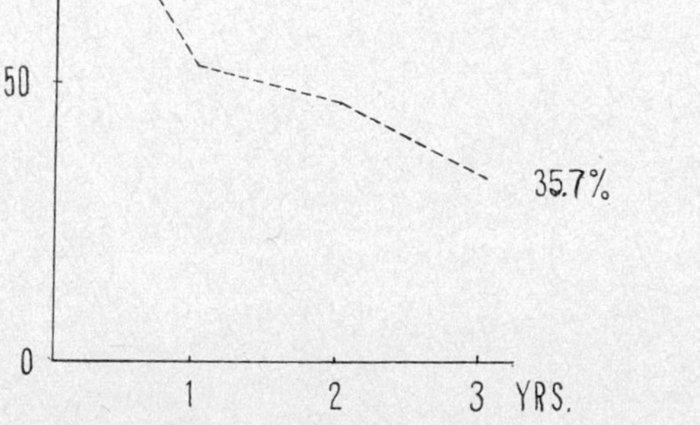

Fig 8.—Follow-up results of cancer of the upper and midthoracic esophagus not accompanying lymph node metastasis.

cases of rectal cancer fell into Duke's grade three.

D. *Concentrated Irradiation.*—When we initiated preoperative irradiation, the therapy was fractionated over a period of from 10 to 14 days in order to decrease the likelihood of damage to normal tissue and to avoid untoward postoperative effects. This pattern has been modified recently, and none of the anticipated serious ill effects has developed (Table 12). The modifications have included a reduction of the time of preoperative therapy with an increase in the daily dosage. The therapeutic effect of irradiation is closely related to the dosage and period over which that dosage is given (Fig 10). Our histological data (X_1, X_2, and X_3) on carcinoma of the upper and midthoracic esophagus have been plotted, and an empirical formula has been obtained from this chart in order to determine a dose-time relationship (Fig 11). The formula is D equals 1,300 r $\times$ $T^{0.32}$, as presented in Table 13. In accordance with this formula, a total single dose of 1,300 r should yield X_3 changes in 100% of the cases.

In May of 1962 we established 2,000 r as a total tumor dose to be given in a period of three days (700 r, 700 r, and 600 r) for carcinoma of the esophagus, cardiac end, and body of the stomach. This three-day plan has reduced the period of waiting prior to surgery which we feel is desirable when dealing with cancers. A single dose of 2,000 r

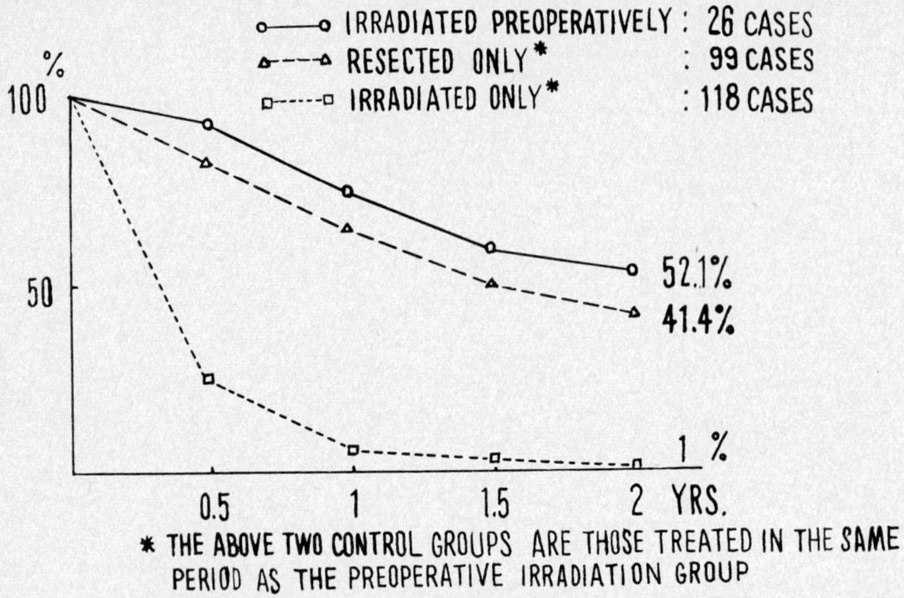

Fig 9.—Follow-up results of cancer of the stomach undergoing our preoperative irradiation therapy (a survey made in 1963).

has been given for carcinoma of the breast and rectum without untoward effect. We feel that a single dose is safe in cancer of these areas because there is no need for an anastomosis to be performed after surgery and the surrounding structures are not of as great significance as in the chest or upper abdomen. Up to February of 1963, 99 patients had undergone concentrated irradiation therapy (Table 14). Histologically we have found 50% of the specimens show X_2 changes, and in the remaining 50%, X_3 changes have been achieved (Fig 12 and 13). The morphologic changes are definitely more significant than when fractionated irradiation is given. It is of particular interest that mature, well differentiated adenocarcinomas responded histologically to concentrated irradiation. This was true although almost no effect had been noted when protracted irradiation therapy was employed. We also feel that there has been a very definite selective damage to cancer cells when compared with normal stromal tissues, and these

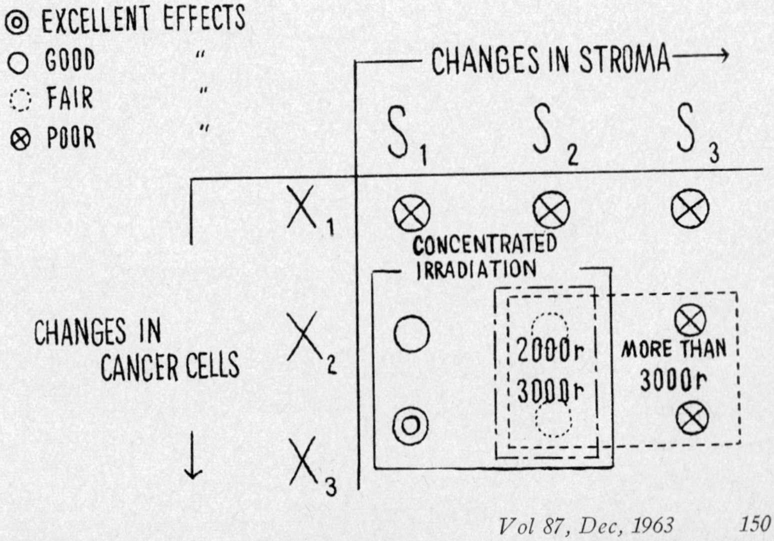

Fig 10.—Determination of optimal radiation factors on the basis of histology.

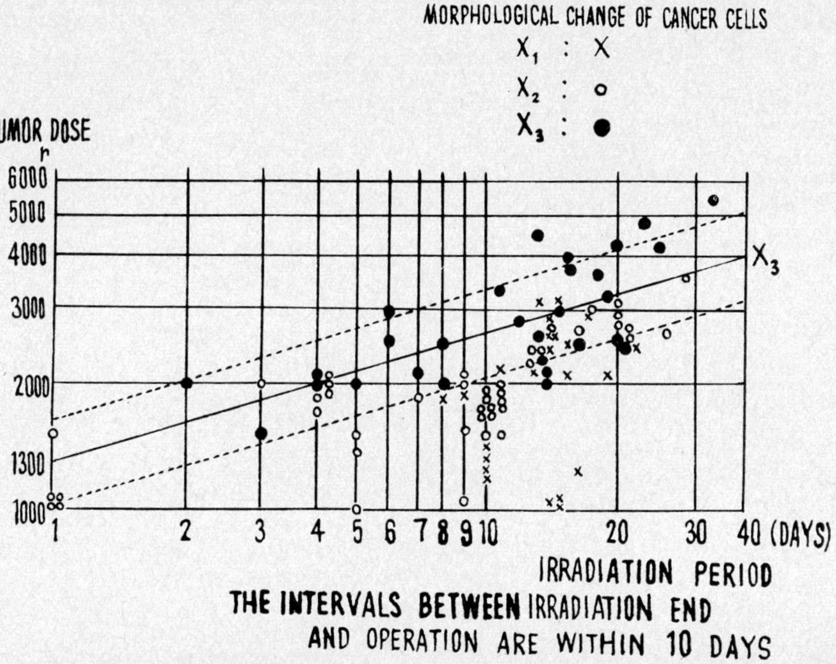

Fig 11.—Dose-time relationship in squamous cell carcinoma of the esophagus treated with preoperative irradiation.

changes are also more significant in the group receiving concentrated irradiation as compared with the group receiving fractionated irradiation. None of the factors has increased surgical risk in our experience to this time.

Comment

The primary aim of preoperative irradiation therapy is the same as all other treatment techniques in the management of carcinoma, that is, an improvement in the end results.

The basic thoughts behind the advantages of preoperative irradiation therapy are summarized as follows: First, fibrosis and cicatrix formation develop postoperatively. They alter the environment of residual cancer cells and diminish the blood supply to the cells. This has been generally accepted to be the main reason for the lowering of susceptibility to carcinoma where postoperative irradiation is used. Secondly, preoperative irradiation reduces the incidence of dissemination by manipulation at the time of

TABLE 12.—*Preoperative Irradiation and Radiation Sickness*

	Concentrated Method				Protracted Method			
Volume Dose, Megagram r	No. Cases	0 (%)	I (%)	II (%)	No. Cases	0 (%)	I (%)	II (%)
Less than 1	15	6 (40)	4 (23)	5 (33)	2		1 (50)	1 (50)
1-2	28	13 (49)	7 (25)	8 (29)	5	3 (60)	1 (20)	1 (20)
2-3	6	1 (17)	3 (50)	2 (33)	16	4 (25)	7 (44)	5 (31)
3-4	2			2 (100)	8	1 (13)	7 (87)	
4-5					6	3 (50)	3 (50)	

0 indicates no ill effects; I, general malaise & anorexia; II, nausea, vomiting, & dizziness.

TABLE 13.—*Our Formula on Dose-Time Relationship for Squamous Cell Carcinoma of the Esophagus*

$D = E \times T^n$

D indicates total tumor dose (to cause changes of grade X_3); E, a single dose (to cause changes of grade X_3); T, irradiation period (days); *n*, recovery index.

Empirically:
$D = 1{,}300\ r \times T^{0.32}$

surgery. This is probably accomplished by the direct effect on cancer cells of irradiation, reducing the tumor cell's ability to reproduce and grow. Also by surrounding tumor cells or nests of tumor cells with connective tissue and fibrosis of the capillary area and the lymphatics systems, the manipulative dissemination is diminished during surgery (Oelssner [17] and Leb [11]). We have studied the degree of manipulative dissemination during operation by placing gauze packs within the abdomen and then examining these packs for malignant cells. Tumor cells were found in 54% of the cases (Table 15). Degenerative cancer cells grade X_3 could not be implanted and grown. These cells have

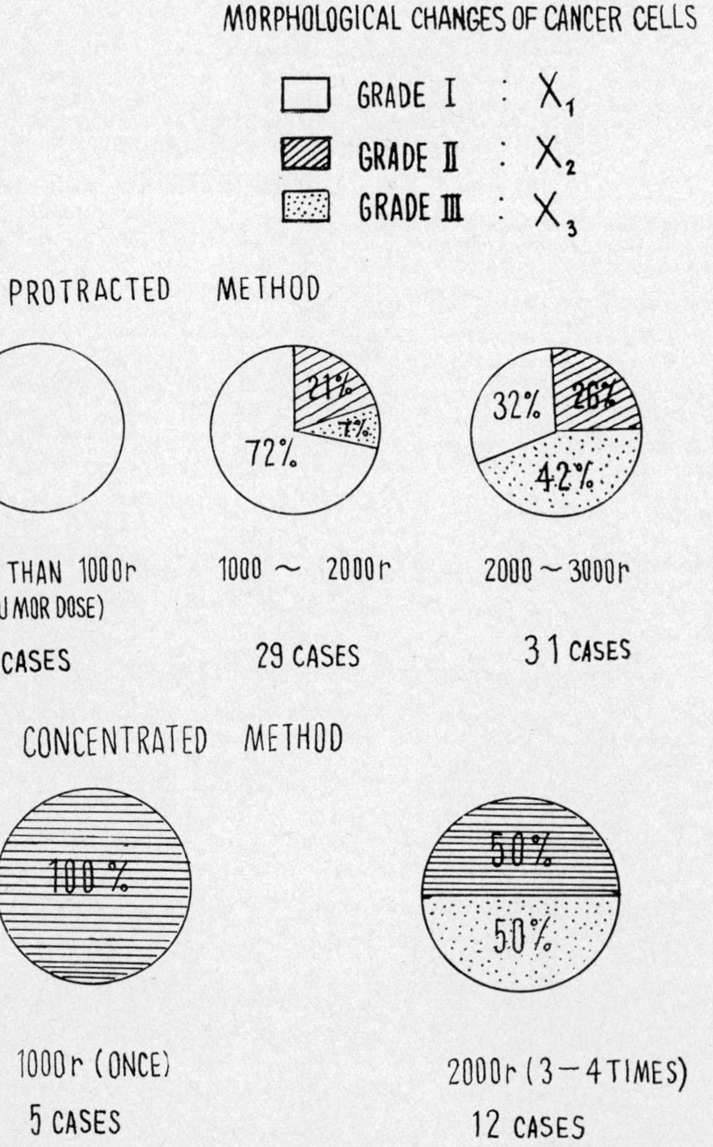

Fig 12.—Tumor dose and irradiation effects to histology (squamous cell carcinoma of the esophagus), operated within two weeks after irradiation end.

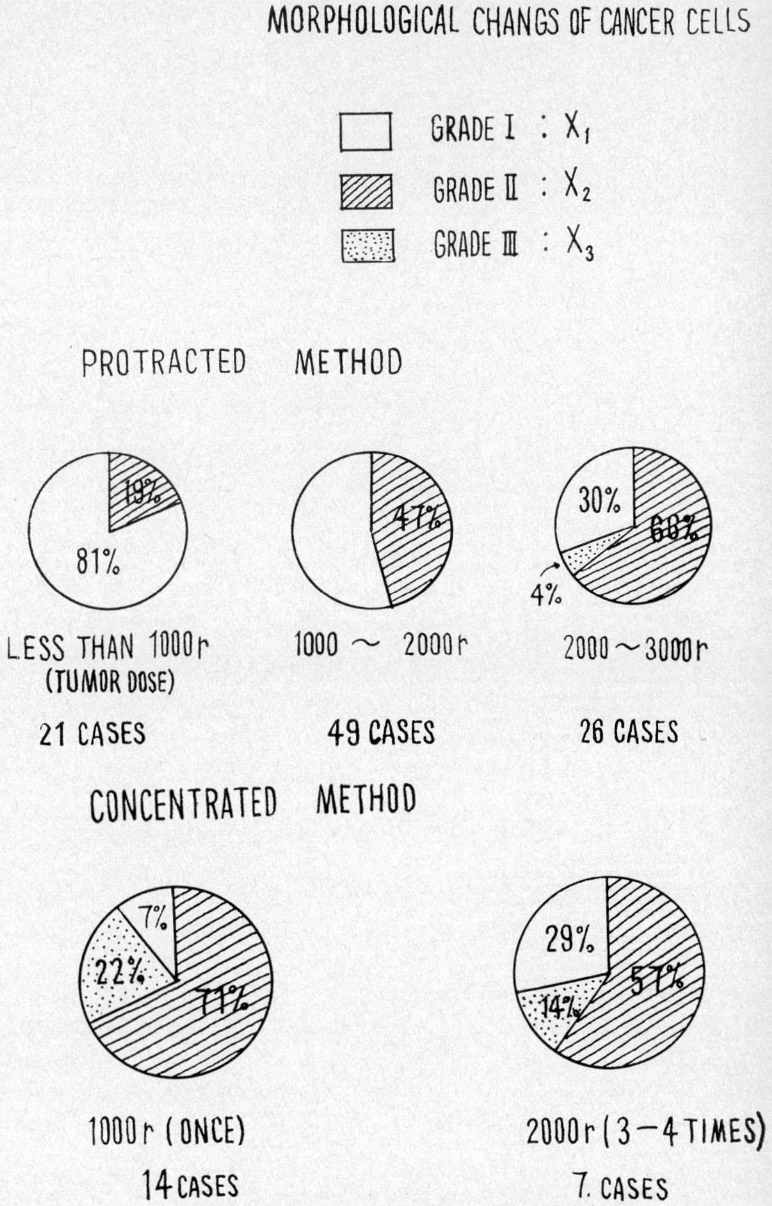

Fig 13.—Tumor dose and irradiation effects to histology (carcinoma of the stomach), operated within two weeks after irradiation end.

TABLE 14.—*Operative Results of the Concentrated Preoperative Irradiation Method at Nakayama's Surgery Department (a Survey in February, 1963)*

Carcinoma	No. Cases	Operative Deaths
Upper & midthoracic esophagus	22	0
Lower esophagus & cardiac end of stomach	31	0
Stomach	14	0
Rectum	7	0
Others	25	0
Total	99	0

been "sterilized." Thirdly, irradiation often reduces the size of malignant lesions and the extent of direct invasion. We feel that this frequently creates a resectable tumor from what would have been previously a nonresectable lesion. At the same time, this reduces the degree and amount of trauma necessary to accomplish the surgical procedure.

There is no doubt that irradiation therapy does produce some untoward effects.

TABLE 15.—*Discovery Rate of Cancer Cells Liberated in the Operative Field*

Cancer * Advance Grade	Total Resection of Thoracic Esophagus (%)	Resection of Lower Esophagus & Cardia (%)	Gastrectomy (%)	Gastrostomy, Jejunostomy, or Gastro-enterostomy (%)	Total (%)
I †	—	—	0/5	—	0
II	3/18	4/9	3/12	—	10/39 (25.6)
III	8/10	4/5	8/12	—	20/27 (74.1)
IV	2/2	5/5	2/2	4/4	13/13 (100)
Total	13/30 (43.3)	13/19 (68.4)	13/31 (41.8)	4/4 (100)	43/79 (54.4)

* According to the classification standardized in Japan.
† Classification criteria are:

	Serosal Infilt.	Periton. or Pleur. Invasion	Node Meta.	Liver Meta.
I	(—)	(—)	(—)	(—)
II	Localized	(—)	Limited to 2nd group, removable	(—)
III	Diffuse	Involving adjacent portion	Limited to 3rd group, removable	(—)
IV	Involving adjacent organ(s)	Involving remote portion also	Not removed or not removable	(+)

Nahmmacher,[13] Jüngling,[8] and others have stressed the importance of radical irradiation in order to render complete destruction of cancer cells prior to surgery. We feel this is not practical. Kohler,[10] Leb,[11] Kaneda,[9] and others feel that a moderate dosage would be preferable since the primary purpose is to prevent liberated cancer cells from implanting during a surgical procedure. Wakabayashi [20] and others have implied that preoperative irradiation therapy may stimulate a protective vital response which thwarts the recurrence of the tumor. Some animal studies [20] have suggested indirect effects of irradiation therapy. However, our clinical experience has not supported this significantly.

We, of course, have attempted to establish a practical and effective technique of preoperative irradiation therapy. This, of course, must be the specific requirement of improvement in the end results. Without affecting operative results, our early findings were encouraging. The use of the total dose between 2,000 and 3,000 r over a period of from 10 to 14 days (200 r to 300 r daily) did yield encouraging results. Modification of this technique and condensing the period of time over which therapy was given have yielded even more encouraging results and have demonstrated a destructive effect on the tumor without compromising surgical risk. In this way our method of concentrated preoperative irradiation therapy was born. The introduction of the Tele Co^{60} unit has significantly reduced skin burns, and concentrated irradiation to the tumor has become technically possible. Radiation sickness has not been a great problem. After a three-day plan, the total dosage of 2,000 r is given in divided doses of 700 r, 700 r, and 600 r consecutively. Complications have been few. In those patients receiving this therapy, supplementary use of glucose solutions, amino acid mixtures, vitamins, and liver protecting agents have controlled any untoward effects.

Our fear expressed by radiologists when using high-dosage irradiation therapy has been the possibility of fistula formation due to rapid necrotic changes. This complication is not encountered in these patients since the area which is being irradiated is surgically removed before such changes can take place. We have established a period of from four to seven days as routine between the end of irradiation and the surgical assault on the tumor.

What we have expected in preoperative irradiation therapy is an improvement of end results of malignancy rather than a cure of the disease. Our data, accumulated particularly on esophageal carcinoma, have suggested that it cures the disease in such an early stage that node invasion is not recognized yet. It was not found generally when surgery alone was employed in our experience. Now, cancer is curable by means of preoperative irradiation, if it is still fairly localized!

We feel that the fact that changes can be demonstrated in well-differentiated adenocarcinomas after concentrated irridiation therapy, and that these changes could not be demonstrated with the fractionated and protracted technique of preoperative therapy is most significant. We have even thought of a single preoperative therapy dose of 1,300 r. The problems inherent in such a technique require careful evaluation, and further studies will be required before any conclusion can be drawn with regard to this type of therapy. We do feel, however, that if we can show that such a technique will not be attended by severe complications, it would seem the ideal future mode of preoperative irradiation therapy.

Summary and Conclusion

Since 1960, a systemic evaluation of preoperative irradiation therapy has been carried on in our department. The purpose of this study was to determine whether or not the end results in treatment of carcinoma could be improved by altering tumor cells with preoperative radiation therapy. Up to December, 1962, a total of 490 cases were treated. Initially a protracted fractionated form of preoperative therapy was given. For a period of from 10 to 14 days 200 to 300 r was administered. The results of this irradiation therapy have been evaluated and recorded regarding the histological status of the irradiated tissue. The classification of these changes has been recorded as X_1, X_2, and X_3. X_3 represents the most desirable form of change accomplished by preoperative therapy. We have established that the ideal tumor dose is from 2,000 r to 3,000 r. The follow-up period with regard to these patients is still quite short. However, we have already noted a prolongation of the survival time, particularly in patients suffering from carcinoma of the upper and midthoracic esophagus, carcinoma of the breast, and cancer of the rectum. All the cases of esophageal carcinoma resected in the absence of node metastasis showed a 100% survival rate in the preoperative irradiation group (at our latest or three-year follow-up). It was not found in the group treated only surgically. Thus, this combined therapy permits us to expect a cure of the localized disease. The possible mechanisms of such improvement are considered here. The preoperative irradiation seems to contribute also by increasing the incidence of resectable lesions. The side effects have not been of great consequence and have been controlled with ease. A formula of the dose-time relationship has been made on histological analysis. We believe that this system, as presented here for the first time, offers a definite advantage and that the new technique of concentrated irradiation offers more than any previously described modes of preoperative treatment. We feel that the Tele Co^{60} system is preferable for this treatment. The concentrated technique of therapy was employed in 99 patients up until February of 1963. No significant untoward effects have been encountered. In fact, such concentrated therapy increases the degree of destruction of tumor cells. The patient is ready for surgery earlier, and we feel that chances for cures are better. At present we are considering the possibility of single-dose preoperative irradiation, and we propose that this possibly will be the final and most desirable method of preoperative irradiation therapy.

Dr. E. Takizawa, Professor of Pathology; Dr. H. Kakei, Professor of Radiology; their colleagues at the Chiba University Hospitals; and Dr. E. Tazaki, Chief of Medical Affairs Section at the National Institute of Radiological Sciences, and his staff aided in this study. Dr. Paul Weiss supervised English usage.

Komei Nakayama, MD, Professor of Surgery, School of Medicine, Chiba University, Chiba, Japan.

Addendum

Recently, 1,800 r has been given for 3 days in gastric cancer only in the following manner: 500, 600, and 700 r, or 700, 600, and 500 r, because the radiation sickness has been found to be considerably strong in some patients receiving 700, 700, and 700 r consecutively.

REFERENCES

1. Adams, H. D.; Hare, H. F.; Davis, W. L.; Trump, J. G.; and Granke, R. C.: Treatment of Carcinoma of Esophagus and Cardia by Resection and Postoperative Supervoltage Roentgen Rays, Ann Surg 138:631, 1953.

2. Buschke, F., and Cantril, S. T.: Results of Supervoltage Roentgen Therapy of Esophageal Carcinoma, J Thorac Surg 26:105, 1953.

3. Buschke, F.: Surgical and Radiological Results in Treatment of Esophageal Carcinoma, Amer J Roentgen 71:9, 1954.

4. Cliffton, E. E., and Blansfield, H. N.: Treatment of Carcinoma of Esophagus by Radiation Therapy and Surgery: Case Report, Surgery 33: 748, 1953.

5. Cliffton, E. E.; Goodner, T. T.; and Bronstein, E.: Preoperative Irradiation for Cancer of the Esophagus, Cancer 13:37, 1960.

6. Dalley, V. M.: Malignant Disease of the Antrum, Brit J Radiol 32:378, 1959.

7. Gadjanski, B., and Jankovic, I.: Vorbestrahlung und Metastasierung bei Mammakarzinom, Strahlentherapie 112:515, 1960.

8. Jüngling, O.: Grundsätzliches zur Frage des präoperativen Bestrahlung, Strahlentherapie 51: 393, 1934.

9. Kaneda, H.: Preoperative Irradiation Therapy for Carcinoma, Jap J Clin (Kyoto) 14:1482, 1952.

10. Kohler, A.: 10 Jahre Praoperative Bestrahlung des Mammacarcinom, Strahlentherapie 88:150, 1952.

11. Leb, A.: Die Indikationen, Technik und Die Resultate der Röntgenvorbestrahlung der malignen Tumoren, Wien Med Wschr 104:835, 1954.

12. Muntean, E.: Die Präoperative Röntgenbestrahlung des Mammakarzinoms, Stuttgart: George Thieme Verlag, 1961.

13. Nahmmacher, F.: Die Erweiterte Behandlung des Mammacarcinoms, Strahlentherapie 30:490, 1928.

14. Nakayama, K.: Erfahrungen bei etwa 3,000 Fällen von Oesophagus und Kardiacarcinom, Langenbeck Arch Klin Chir 295:81, 1960.

15. Nakayama, K.: Die Präoperative Strahlenbehandlung des Oesophaguskrebses und ihre theoretische Grundlage, Chirurg 33:14, 1962.

16. Nakayama, K.: Irradiation Therapy and Operation, Clin Radiol (Tokyo) 7:11, 1962.

17. Oelssner, W.: Frühergebnisse der präoperativen Bestrahlung des Brustkrebses, Strahlentherapie 87:49, 1952.

18. Smithers, D. W.; Clarkson, J. R.; and Strong, J. A.: Roentgen Treatment of Cancer of Esophagus, Amer J Roentgen 49:606, 1943.

19. Streams, M. W.; Deddish, M. R.; and Quan, S. H. Q.: Preoperative Roentgen Therapy for Cancer of the Rectum, Surg Gynec Obstet 109: 225, 1959.

20. Wakabayashi, M.: Studies on Indirect Effects of Radiation, Jap Med J 7-13:1579, 1954.

21. Watson, T. A., and Brown, E. M.: X-Ray Therapy in Carcinoma of Esophagus, J Thorac Cardiov Surg 22:216, 1952.

Neonatal Hirschsprung's Disease

Treatment of Complete Aganglionosis of the Colon by the Duhamel Operation

JEAN G. DESJARDINS, MD, FRCS (C), AND JAMES S. SIMPSON, MD, FRCS (C) FACS, TORONTO

Although Hirschsprung's disease in the neonatal period is being recognized more frequently, complete aganglionosis of the colon is rare [7] and presents a difficult diagnostic problem.[10,16] Treatment of this condition can be successful if the diagnosis is established early.[1,3,4,5,7,8]

The following patient illustrates the problems encountered in such cases and describes a method of definitive treatment in the neonate.

Report of Case

A 13-day-old girl was admitted to the Hospital for Sick Children, Toronto, on April 18, 1963. Her chief signs were vomiting and abdominal distention, which had been noted a few days after birth.

The baby had been born of a gravida IV mother who had had persistent nausea during her pregnancy. Labor and delivery were uneventful.

Birth weight was 7 lb 10 oz (3,459 gm). She was started on breast feedings but did not nurse well. It was difficult to get the infant to take sufficient feedings. There was no spontaneous bowel movement except with enemas. A change of formula was tried, but this failed to improve the infant's condition, and the oral feedings had to be supplemented with interstitial fluids. A blood culture at that time showed a moderate growth of *Staphylococcus pyogenes* and the baby was treated with intravenous tetracycline.

The infant did not appear acutely ill at that time, but her abdomen was distended and she was not thriving. On April 16, 1963, a barium enema was performed which was interpreted as normal. On April 18, 1963, an upper gastrointestinal series was done which showed good emptying of the stomach. However, within hours of the x-ray the infant started to vomit what was described as fecal material and she was transferred to the Hospital for Sick Children, Toronto, the same day.

Physical examination at the time of admission revealed a well-developed infant who was moderately dehydrated. The abdomen was distended but soft. Distended loops of bowel could be palpated, and the abdomen was tympanitic to percussion. Rectal examination revealed a tight anus and an empty rectum. A roentgen study of the abdomen, shortly after admission, revealed a great deal of contrast material within the colon. The rectum and sigmoid colon appeared narrowed, and the proximal portion of the colon was also interpreted as being narrowed. The small bowel contained barium and was distended. This appearance suggested the presence of Hirschsprung's disease involving the entire colon.

Vomiting of feculent material occurred once again, shortly after admission. Rehydration of the infant was started. Gas and stools were obtained with an enema, and the baby had one bowel movement as well. During the night she had no vomiting while on intravenous fluids.

On April 19, 1963, x-ray of the abdomen (Fig 1) showed no change in the amount of barium in the large bowel. These findings were also compatible with a diagnosis of extensive Hirschsprung's disease.

A rectal biopsy was performed by the technique described by Shandling,[15] using no anesthesia, and frozen sections showed an aganglionic rectum.

Laparotomy was performed on April 20, 1963, and at operation the entire small bowel was distended except for the distal 12 cm of ileum which looked narrowed. The entire colon was small. Proximal to the distal portion of the ileum the muscular wall of the small bowel was hypertrophic. Biopsy specimens (Fig 2) were then taken from the narrowed portion of the ileum and from the proximal hypertrophied wall of the ileum. Frozen sections showed the presence of ganglion cells in the proximal hypertrophied ileum only. The distal part of ileum was completely aganglionic.

A resection of about 6 cm of the distal ileum and 6 cm of the proximal normal looking ileum was carried out.

Submitted for publication July 8, 1963.

Former Resident-in-Chief (Dr. Desjardins), Department of Surgery, Hospital for Sick Children, and Assistant Surgeon, Ste. Justine Hospital, Montreal, Canada; Associate (Dr. Simpson), Department of Surgery, University of Toronto, and Assistant Surgeon, Hospital for Sick Children.

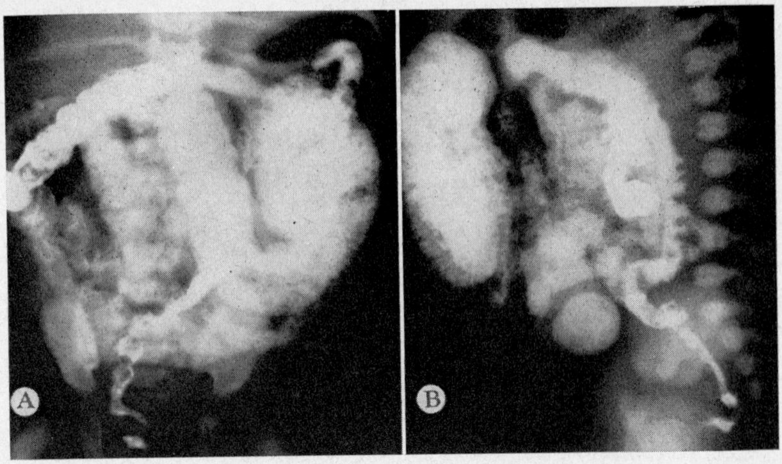

Fig 1 (*A* and *B*).—Postevacuation film, 48 hours postbarium enema and upper gastrointestinal series, showing the distended small bowel full of barium. The colon presents smaller than normal caliber (microcolon).

At that time, because of the age (two weeks) and weight, 7 lb, 10 oz (3,459 gm) of the child, it seemed inadvisable to proceed with a total colectomy. An exclusion of the colon with an ileoanal anastomosis as described by Duhamel[2] and Roviralta[13] was carried out. The distal ileum was brought out in the right lower quadrant of the abdomen (Fig 2) as a cutaneous fistula. The proximal normal ileum was then brought down behind the rectum (Fig 3) and anastomosed to the anus by three posterior interrupted 4-0 silk sutures (Fig 4). Finally the posterior wall of the rectum and the anterior wall of the ileum were approximated by two crushing clamps forming a $\wedge$ (Fig 5).

The infant made an uneventful recovery. The postoperative course was remarkably smooth, and the baby seemed comfortable even with the forceps aprotruding from the anus. There was no urinary retention (the catheter was removed after 24 hours), and she started to pass spontaneous stools the day after the operation. The enterotomy forceps fell out on the third day, and the infant had eight to ten liquid stools a day for the first week, and four to six by the second week. She was discharged two weeks after her operation.

Comment

In infant's Hirschsprung's disease is very often unrecognized[4] and is usually lethal.[5] In this case the colon and about 12 cm of the terminal ileum were aganglionic. The outstanding symptoms on admission were those of intestinal obstruction, but the occasional passage of flatus and feces demonstrated that the obstruction was not complete.[5] The appearance of the colon after a barium enema

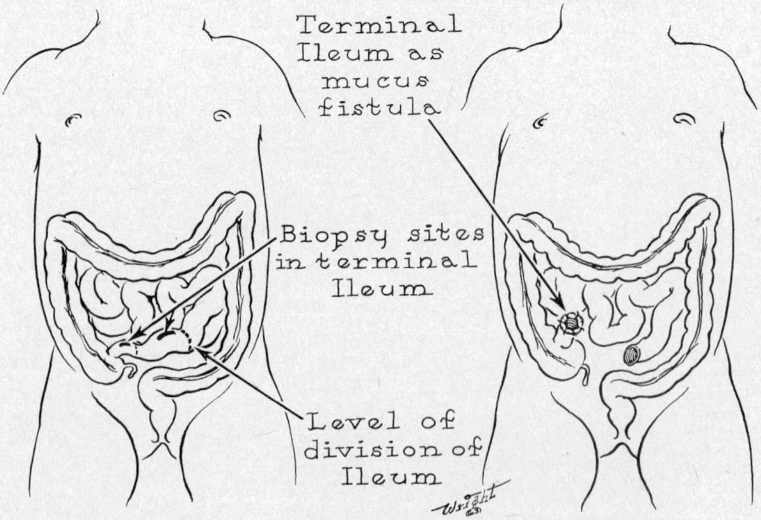

Fig 2

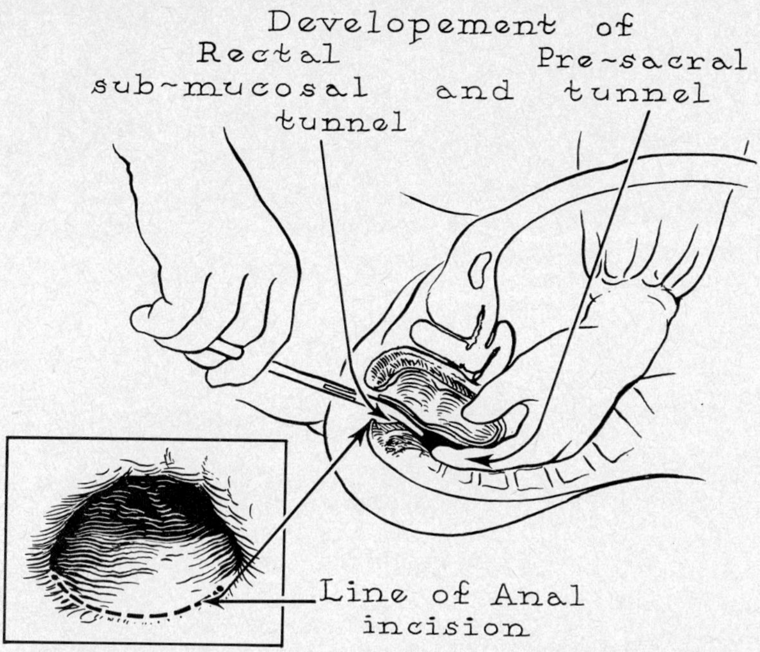

Fig 3

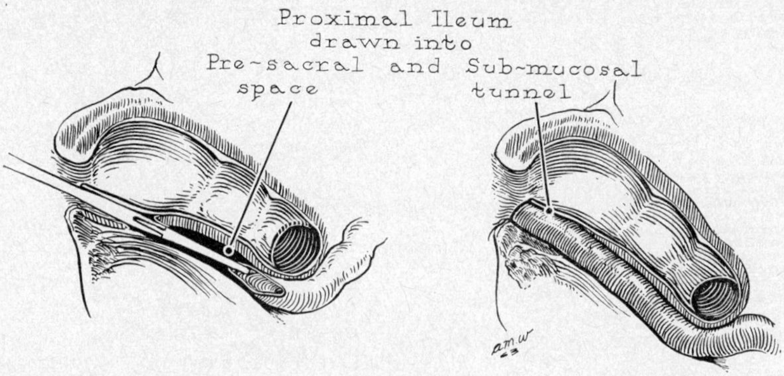

Fig 4

can be very misleading. Because of its small size and the absence of proximal dilatation, it may be interpreted as normal, as happened

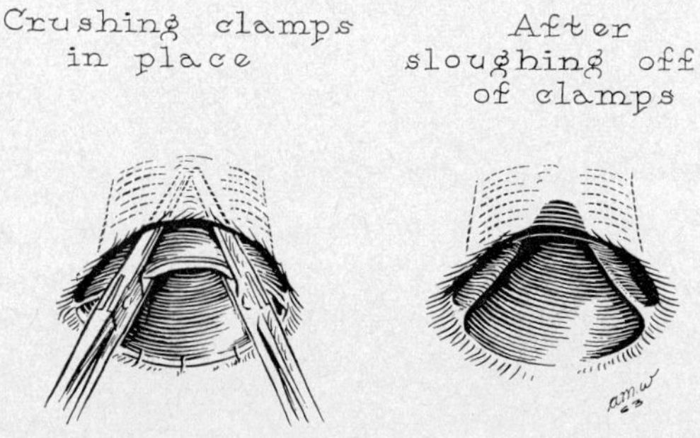

Fig 5

initially in this case. X-rays taken 24 and 48 hours later usually show retention of contrast material in the colon.[11] This should suggest the diagnosis of Hirschsprung's disease, which can be confirmed by a rectal biopsy.

Sandegard [14] in 1953 recorded the first successful treatment of long segment Hirschsprung's disease. In 1955 Swenson [16] reported two cases of complete aganglionosis of the colon and recommended total colectomy and ileoproctostomy. These cases were the first three survivors recorded in the literature, and thereafter this form of treatment was advocated by most authors.[1,3,5,6,7,8,10,12,16,17]

Edelman, et al, in April, 1960,[3] reviewing the literature, found 26 cases. These cases were treated by the method described by Swenson, and the mortality rate was 73%. Since then, eight other cases [5,6,11,12] are reported in the literature treated by the same method, with two survivals. The difficulty of diagnosis is mainly responsible for this high mortality rate.

Duhamel in 1960 [2] described an operation which eliminated the need for ileostomy (or colostomy) and was safe in the first few months of life. Since then, four cases of complete aganglionosis of the colon have been treated successfully by this technique and are reported in the literature.[9,13]

The outstanding features common to all these cases are the simplicity of the operation even in small infants, minimal blood loss, and a remarkably smooth postoperative convalescence.[2,9,13]

Similar findings were observed in the case presented.

Total colectomy may not be necessary in this disease. Roviralta,[13] commenting on two cases treated by Duhamel and one of his own, doubts the necessity of proceeding with a total colectomy at a later date.

Conclusion

A case of complete aganglionosis of the colon treated by a by-pass procedure as described by Duhamel is presented. This operation is recommended as a simple, conservative, and highly satisfactory procedure in cases of extensive Hirschsprung's disease.

Summary

A case of complete aganglionosis of the colon treated by a by-pass procedure as described by Duhamel is presented. This operation is recommended as a simple, conservative, and highly satisfactory procedure in cases of extensive Hirschsprung's disease.

James S. Simpson, MD, The Hospital for Sick Children, 555 University Ave, Toronto 2, Canada.

REFERENCES

1. Adams, B. E., and Adams, R. M.: Hirschsprung's Disease With Extensive Aganglionic Segments, Amer J Surg 98:248-256 (Aug) 1959.

2. Duhamel, B.: A New Operation for the Treatment of Hirschsprung Disease, Arch Dis Child 35:38-39 (Feb) 1960.

3. Edelman, S.; Strauss, L.; Becker, J. M.; and Arnheim, E.: Universal Aganglionosis of the Colon, Surgery 47:667-677 (April) 1960.

4. Gibbons, D.: A Case of Hirschsprung's Disease in the Newborn, Clin Proc Child Hosp (Wash) 18:167-174 (June) 1962.

5. Hallenbeck, G. A.; Brown, P. M.; Waugh, G. M.; and Stickler, G. B.: Surgical Treatment of Hirschsprung's Disease: A Review of 40 Cases, Arch Surg 83:928-933 (Dec) 1961.

6. Herman, R. E.; Izant, R. J.; and Bolande, R. P.: Surgery 53:664 (May) 1963.

7. Howard, H., and McBurney, R. P.: Hirschsprung's Disease: Report of a Case With Complete Aganglia of the Colon, Ann Surg 148:142-144 (July) 1958.

8. Kostia, J.: Results of Surgical Treatment in Hirschsprung's Disease, Arch Dis Child 37:167-168 (April) 1962.

9. Louw, J. H.: The Duhamel Operation for Hirschsprung's Disease, South Afr J Med Sci 35:1033 (Dec) 1961.

10. Bowden, D. H.; Goodfellow, A. M.; and Munn, J. D.: Hirschsprung's Disease in the Neonatal Period, J Pediat 50:321, 1957.

11. Pouyanne, L.; Lasserre, J.; Honton; and Bach: Maladie de Hirschsprung generalisee: Cause de l'echec de traitement d'une atresie congenitale de l'intestin Grele, Arch Franc Pediat 17:1361-1363, (Dec) 1960.

12. Richardson, W. R., and Brown, I. H.: Hirschsprung's Disease in Infants and Children, Amer Surg 28:149 (March) 1962.

13. Roviralta, E.: Nouvelles Orientations chirurgicales dans le traitement du megacolon congenital, Ann Chir Infant 3:155-158 (Sept) 1962.

14. Sandegard, E.: Hirschsprung's Disease With Ganglion Cell Aplasia of the Colon and Terminal Ileum: Report of a Case Treated With Total Colectomy and Ileocecostomy, Acta Chir Scand 106:369, 1953.

15. Shandling, B.: A New Technique in the Diagnosis of Hirschsprung's Disease, Canad J Surg 4:298, 1961.

16. Swenson, O., and Fisher, J. H.: Treatment of Hirschsprung's Disease With Entire Colon Involved in Aganglionic Defect, AMA Arch Surg 70:535 (April) 1955.

17. Wyllie, G. G.: Treatment of Hirschsprung's Disease by Swenson's Operation, Lancet 1:850 (April) 1957.

Management of Spontaneous Pneumothorax

A Comparison of Treatment Methods

HERBERT T. RANSDELL, JR., MD
AND
RICHARD C. McPHERSON, MD
LOUISVILLE

Itard [1] first recognized pneumothorax as a pathological entity and gave it a name in 1803; however, it was Laennec,[2] in 1819, who gave an accurate clinical and autopsy description of spontaneous pneumothorax and first appreciated its possible relationship to emphysema and bleb formation.

Tuberculosis was considered to be the predominant cause of spontaneous pneumothorax by most in the later 19th century and the early 20th century. However, Laennec, in 1819; McDowell,* in 1856; Chauffard,[4] in 1896; and Fussell and Riesman,[5] in 1902, seriously questioned this concept by case reports in which they were unable to demonstrate tuberculosis. It remained for Kjaergaard,[6] in 1933, to establish finally that the large majority of spontaneous pneumothoraces are of a nontuberculous origin and to stimulate further clinical and pathological studies to establish its etiology. Tuberculosis was seldom incriminated as the cause of spontaneous pneumothorax in our patients. Over 80% were due to rupture of small apical blebs in otherwise normal appearing lungs. Of the 46 open thoracotomies performed for pneumothorax, blebs (many of which were leaking air) were demonstrated in 43.

Since 1933, rupture of a vesicle and interstitial air dissection in an area of localized emphysema with resulting escape of air into the pleural space has become firmly established as the usual etiology of spontaneous pneumothorax.

The vesicles or blebs are usually small, localized, and directly beneath the parietal pleura in the extreme apices of the upper lobes. The rupture of these blebs results from a rise of air pressure within the bleb distal to valve-like obstructions in the extreme peripheral bronchial branches, which might occur with postinflammatory changes, bronchospasm, mucus, or exudates. The air

Submitted for publication July 13, 1963.

From the Department of Surgery, University of Louisville School of Medicine, the Louisville General Hospital, and the Louisville Veterans Administration Hospital.

* Cited by Galliard.[3]

from the ruptured bleb may escape directly into the pleural space or occasionally dissect along hilar lung structures into the mediastinum. This then accumulates as a pneumomediastinum which then may rupture through the pleura into the pleural space to produce a pneumothorax.

Some other causes of spontaneous pneumothorax are necrotizing bronchiolitis in infancy, particularly of the staphylococcal type, and rupture of emphysematous blebs arising secondary to reduced lung volume in agenesis, fibrosis, atelectasis, or surgical removal of lung tissue.

Disagreement persists as to the preferred management of patients with spontaneous pneumothorax. The more conservative-minded place the patient on markedly restricted activity or bed rest, sedation, antitussives, and antibiotics for control of infection. Active removal of air is done only when necessary to relieve severe respiratory distress. A "rule of thumb" is that 1% of that air in the filled pleural space will be absorbed daily; eg, a 50% pneumothorax would require 50 days to be absorbed; a 20% pneumothorax, 20 days, etc.

The less conservative-minded believe that more rapid expansion may be obtained by aspiration of sufficient air to establish a slight negative pressure in the pneumothorax space. They occasionally cautiously repeat these aspirations to maintain this negative pressure. Their more conservative colleagues, however, believe that each aspiration threatens empyema, air embolism, "pleural shock," etc, and they are therefore willing to subject the patient to several weeks' hospitalization or markedly restricted activity to avoid these complications.

The so-called radicals advocate complete and rapid expansion of the lung by removal of the air by thoracentesis if possible, but more often by closed tube drainage of the pleural space. They believe infection is much less likely to occur if there is no space and that the patient's period of disability is markedly decreased.

At present our surgical department favors aggressive (or radical) treatment and the medical department has practically abandoned their former conservative treatment. A review of our experience with spontaneous pneumothorax at the Louisville General Hospital and the Louisville Veterans Hospital will help to explain our reasons for this attitude.

Review of Series

From January, 1950, through December, 1961, a total of 213 roentgenographically proven spontaneous pneumothoraces in 170 patients were treated in the Louisville General and Louisville Veterans Hospitals. Fifty-six patients were admitted to the Louisville General Hospital 66 times for 69 bouts of spontaneous pneumothorax. At the Louisville Veterans Hospital, 114 patients were admitted 143 times for 144 bouts of spontaneous pneumothorax. Of these patients, 144 were treated for one bout, 14 for two, 8 for three, 3 for four, and 1 for five episodes.

Fifty (29.4%) of the 170 patients had a good history for a previous spontaneous pneumothorax ipsilaterally prior to admission to the hospital or were treated in our hospitals for two or more bouts of pneumothorax on the same side during the period of this study. Five (3%) of the 170 patients had recurrent pneumothoraces on both sides. Four other patients had been treated elsewhere for spontaneous pneumothorax of the contralateral chest prior to their admission to our hospital.

The usual preponderance of males (4.5 males to 1 female) was prevalent in the Louisville General Hospital series. A larger proportion of older people was noted than in the usual reported series, with 41 (60%) of 69 pneumothoraces at Louisville General Hospital and 90 (62.5%) of 144 pneumothoraces at the Louisville Veterans Hospital occurring in patients over 40 years of age.

Determination of the etiology in this series showed that the majority were the result of small ruptured blebs in the apices of otherwise normal lungs. Several others had pulmonary emphysema, and a few had bronchial asthma. There were a few cases

Summary of Treatment Method

Treatment	Pneumothorax *	Patients *	Successful Re-Expansion, %	Av Collapse, %	Av Days Treatment	Directly Related to Treatment	
						Complications	Deaths
Conservative	92	87	55	25-30	27	0	0
Thoracentesis	103	98	38	60	15	0	0
Closed tube	95	88	74	65-70	11	6	1
Major thoracotomy	46	40	98	—	15	2	1

* Several patients required more than one method of treatment.

of tuberculosis; but even in these cases, blebs distal to active foci, or scarring, were usually seen. Carcinoma of the lung was rarely first brought to our attention by the occurrence of pneumothorax. It is of particular interest that of 46 cases in which thoracotomy was done for spontaneous pneumothorax, 43 had definite blebs. In many of these patients a definite air leak from rupture of the bleb was evident.

We were able to determine activity status at the time of onset of symptoms of pneumothorax in 122 patients. Violent activities such as coughing, heavy labor, or lifting accompanied the onset in 25 (20%). Mild activities such as walking, driving a car, or arising from a bed or chair were associated with the onset of symptoms in 43 (35%). Sedentary activity, as sleeping or sitting quietly, was associated with the onset in 54 (45%).

Conservative Management

Conservative management consisting of restricted activity or bed rest only was chosen as initial therapy in 92 pneumothoraces in 87 patients. It was carried to complete re-expansion in 46 (50%) pneumothoraces in an average of 27 days for an average of 25% to 30% pneumothorax. Five patients were discharged with small apical pneumothoraces present after an average hospitalization of 21 days. Four patients left the hospital after 9.5 days against medical advice and with their pneumothoraces little changed. Two patients were transferred to other facilities a few hours after admission and diagnosis. Conservatism was abandoned for other methods of treatment in 33 pneumothoraces after an average of 15 days. Two patients died; one 25 days after admission for pneumothorax from carcinomatosis; in the other a contralateral pneumothorax was noted in a chest x-ray obtained just prior to the death of the patient being treated by tube drainage for spontaneous pneumothorax.

Thoracentesis

Thoracentesis was used in 103 pneumothoraces in 98 patients. It was used as initial treatment in 89 and after failure of conservative therapy in 14 after an average of ten days' conservative care. In 39 pneumothoraces (38%), with an average of 60% collapse, thoracentesis was successful. Full expansion of the lung was obtained in 26 instances with an average of 15 days' hospitalization, and 13 patients were discharged with small apical pneumothoraces remaining after an average of 12 days' hospitalization. Two patients left the hospital against advice after ten days with little change in their pneumothoraces. In 59 pneumothoraces with an average 70% collapse, thoracentesis was abandoned for other treatment—56 for tube drainage and three for pleural scarification. Thirty-nine had tubes inserted immediately after or within a few hours of the thoracentesis and 17 an average of five days after treatment with thoracentesis. Three had pleural scarification done after an average of six days' treatment with thoracentesis. Three deaths occurred: one comatose, 75-year-old, bedridden invalid died of respiratory acidosis three days after thoracentesis; one 63-year-old patient with pneumothorax and terminal bronchogenic carcinoma died six days after thoracentesis; one 41-year-old patient admitted in terminal state from septicemia and Friedlander's pneumonia died 48 hours after admission and thoracentesis.

Closed Tube Drainage

Tube drainage was used in 95 pneumothoraces in 88 patients—in 34 as initial treatment, and in 61 after conservative care and/or thoracentesis. Complete re-expansion of the lung was obtained in 70 (73.6%) with an average of 65% to 70% collapse with average hospitalization of 11 days following the tube insertion. Failure to obtain expansion was experienced in 14 instances after an average of eight days. In these failures, subsequent open thoracotomy for scarification revealed persistent air leak from a ruptured bleb, many of which were kept open by pleural adhesions. One patient left against advice with pneumothorax still present two days after insertion of a tube. Ten pneumothoraces are listed as treatment failures due to the death of nine patients, even though lung expansion had been obtained in four. One 43-year-old Negro female bedridden invalid suddenly died with a pulmonary embolus 24 hours after bilateral tube drainage for bilateral pneumothorax, with her lungs well expanded. One 83-year-old male died with pulmonary embolus seven days after re-expansion of his lung. One 64-year-old male died from pulmonary and congestive failure six days after lung expansion. One 74-year-old, comatose, uremic, Negro male suddenly died a few hours after tube drainage with a contralateral pneumothorax. Another 74-year-old Negro male died with total empyema eight days after tube drainage for his fourth recurrence of pneumothorax. One 61-year-old male died of progressive pulmonary fibrosis and severe emphysema. One 64-year-old male died from pulmonary embolus. One 60-year-old male died of leukemia. One 22-year-old male died with empyema and carcinomatosis from a primary bronchogenic carcinoma unrecognized until autopsy. Twenty-three of the 95 pneumothoraces required two or more tube insertions. One patient developed severe paralytic ileus; three, severe subcutaneous emphysema; and one, acute gastric dilatation.

Pleural Scarification

Open thoracotomy in seven to ten days with removal of blebs and ablation of the pleural space by pleural scarification is advocated if expansion of the lung has not been obtained by the previously mentioned modalities. Elective scarification is recommended in those patients having had two or more collapses on the same side.

Pleural scarification with resection of blebs was performed 43 times in 37 patients, six of whom had bilateral surgery. Seventeen were scarified because of failure to obtain lung expansion with other measures. Twenty-three had scarification electively due to two or more previous occurrences of pneumothorax on the same side, and three had scarification and removal of large blebs which were compressing the adjacent lung. In the early years of this series, two other patients had parietal pleurectomies; one as an elective procedure for recurrent pneumothorax and one to obtain expansion of an unexpanded lung. Another patient had an upper lobe lobectomy seven days after thoracentesis with incomplete lung expansion. Scarification was successful in 42 instances with an average of 15 days' postoperative hospitalization.

Major complications included one patient with a postoperative lower lobe atelectasis and another patient with a temporary brachial plexus palsy on the side opposite surgery. One patient died of empyema and pneumonia 3½ months after an elective scarification for recurrent pneumothoraces.

Summary of Series

With conservative care in 92 pneumothoraces, re-expansion was obtained in 51 (54.4%) averaging 25% to 30% collapse, with an average of 26 days' hospitalization. Conservative care was unsuccessful or was abandoned for other treatment in 41 (45.6%). Two patients died with their pneumothoraces unchanged.

Thoracentesis in 103 pneumothoraces was successful in 39 (38%) averaging 65% collapse, in an average of 13 days' hospitalization. In 64 pneumothoraces averaging 68% collapse, thoracentesis was unsuccessful or was abandoned for other method of treatment. Three patients died.

Tube drainage in 95 pneumothoraces resulted in complete expansion in 70 (73.6%) in an average of 11 days' hospitalization for an average of 65% to 70% collapse of the lung. Tube drainage was unsuccessful in 25 pneumothoraces. Ten pneumothoraces in nine patients with tube drainage are considered failures due to deaths of the patients, although four of the pneumothoraces were expanded.

Open thoracotomy was utilized in 46 pneumothoraces in 40 patients. Forty-three of these had pleural scarification with excision of blebs. Two patients had parietal pleurectomies and one an upper lobe lobectomy. Average hospitalization was 15 days. Only two major postoperative complications were experienced. One death occurred due to massive empyema 3½ months following surgery.

Comment

Onset of the symptoms of spontaneous pneumothorax in this series commonly occurred during periods of sleep or physical inactivity, 45% of the time, as compared to 20% during strenuous physical activities. We would agree with Klassen [8] that decreased ventilation of physical inactivity results in retention of secretion in the terminal bronchioles. There follows a local atelectasis with overdistention of an adjacent area which can lead to bleb formation and subsequent rupture with resulting pneumothorax.

A comparison in this series of the commonly used treatment modalities for spontaneous pneumothorax tends to favor tube drainage as the treatment of choice for patients with spontaneous pneumothorax.

Conservative care was successful in 54% of those in which it was used but required an average of 26 days' hospitalization for an average 25% to 30% collapse of the lung. Applying the old dictum of 1% re-expansion a day, conservative care could often result in three to four months' disability to the patient who has complete collapse of the lung.

Thoracentesis, although successful in only 36% of those in which it was used, shortened the hospitalization period to 13 days even though the average collapse in which it was successful was 60%.

Complete lung expansion was obtained in 74% of those in which tube drainage was used. An average of 11 days was required for an average 65% to 70% pneumothorax.

If expansion of the lung has not been obtained in seven to ten days, open thoracotomy, usually with removal of ruptured blebs and ablation of the pleural space by dry gauze scarification, should be considered. This study, as well as others, has shown that after two bouts of pneumothorax, 40% of individuals will have recurrent collapses of their lungs. We therefore believe open thoracotomy should be considered in all recurrent pneumothoraces.

Of the several methods advocated for obtaining permanent obliteration of the pleural space, including the various poudrages, chemical irritants, pleurectomies, cross-hatching of the pleural surfaces, etc, we have chosen pleural scarification produced by rubbing with dry gauze as the method of choice. Poudrages, chemical irritants, and cross-hatching procedures give unpredictable results in the number and uniformity of adhesions. Pleurectomy, besides being rather shocking in itself, may present the hazard of hemorrhage. Rather firm massive adhesions which may possibly impair chest motion may be produced, although some experimental dog work and some pulmonary function studies in humans point against this. During the opportunities we have had of reopening a pleural space in which a pleural scarification has been previously done, we have been impressed by the complete uniform obliteration of the pleural space by soft pliable adhesions which paradoxically seem to permit good movement of the underlying lung and overlying chest cage.

Open thoracotomy with bleb excision and pleural scarification was uniformly successful in obtaining re-expansion of the lung in patients in which we had been unable to obtain expansion by other methods.

A patient admitted to the surgical service of the Louisville General Hospital or Louisville Veterans Hospital with spontaneous pneumothorax will be managed as follows: If chest x-ray reveals only 5% to 10% collapse, he will be managed conservatively with no active treatment other than modified bed rest and careful observation. A patient with more than 10% collapse will have a thoracentesis immediately with aspiration of air. If expansion is maintained as observed by physical and x-ray examination, conservative management is continued. If recollapse occurs within a few hours, or air is continuously aspirated by thoracentesis, a moderate-sized catheter is inserted into the pleural space by trocar using local anesthesia. This catheter is connected to a water trap bottle or set of chest suction bottles. Tube drainage is continued for 24 to 48 hours after expansion of the lung has been obtained, and the tube is then removed. If lung expansion has not been obtained after seven to ten days, thoracotomy with excision of the offending blebs and scarification of the pleura is done.

We are strong advocates of thoracotomy with excision of blebs and pleural scarification in recurrent pneumothorax. We believe the likelihood of recurrence increases with each episode of pneumothorax, and few if any recurrences follow operative pleural space obliteration.

Summary

Two hundred and thirteen roentgenographically proven spontaneous pneumothoraces in 170 patients treated in years 1950 through 1961 are reviewed. The commonly recognized modalities of treatment are compared as to success of re-expansion, average hospitalization, and complications of treatment. Closed tube drainage resulted in the best expansion rate and the shortest hospitalization. Pleural space obliteration by scarification was uniformly successful in obtaining lung expansion in those failing to respond to other methods of treatment. Scarification was equally successful as prophylaxis against a recurrence of penumothorax.

Herbert T. Ransdell, Jr., MD, Department of Surgery, University of Louisville School of Medicine, 511 S Floyd St, Louisville 2, Ky.

REFERENCES

1. Itard, J. E.: Dissertation sur le pneumothorax ou les congestions gazeuses qui se forment dans la poitrine, thesis, Paris, 1803.

2. Laennec, R. T.: De l'auscultation médiate, Paris: J. A. Brosson and J. S. Chaudé, 1819.

3. Galliard, L.: Du pneumothorax simple, sans liquide, et de sa curabilité, Arch Gen Med (Paris) 1:75, 1888.

4. Chauffard, A.: Du pneumothorax simple et de son diagnostic par la tuberculine, Sem Med 16:501, 1896.

5. Fussell, M., and Riesman, D.: Spontaneous Nontuberculous Pneumothorax, Amer J Med Sci 124:218, 1902.

6. Kjaergaard, H.: Spontaneous Pneumothorax in the Apparently Healthy, Acta Med Scand suppl 43:1-159, 1932.

7. Kjaergaard, H.: Pneumothorax Simplex, Acta Med Scand 80:93, 1933.

8. Klassen, K. P., and Meckstrath, C. V.: Treatment of Spontaneous Pneumothorax, JAMA 182:1, 1962.

Acid-Base Balance Changes in Citrated Bank Blood

SHLOMO L. SAMUELOFF, MD
EDMUND M. LUTTWAK, MD
AND
BATHSHEVA M. WIGDERHOUSE, MD
JERUSALEM, ISRAEL

Since massive transfusions of citrated bank blood have become a widely accepted practice in surgery, the interest in the changes occurring in the recipient's blood has increased.[3] In connection with this problem some reports on acid-base balance changes resulting from transfusions have been published.[4] Litwin, Smith, and Moore [5] have shown the occurrence of metabolic alkalosis after massive blood transfusions, even though the citrated blood shows a pH of 7.0 (Gibson et al [2]). This post-transfusion metabolic alkalosis has recently been confirmed by Schweizer and Howland.[7] A number of clinical cases under our observation have shown a similar trend after massive transfusions (8-20 units), though, upon infusion of moderate amounts (1-3 blood units), the changes remained in the range of normal variations in acid-base balance.

While data relating to the recipient's blood changes are accumulating, it appears that information pertinent to the acid-base balance characteristics of the citrated blood is limited. The purpose of this study was, therefore, to investigate the effect of the anticoagulant acid citrate dextrose (ACD) solution used for blood storage on the acid-base balance of the donor's blood and its changes during storage.

Methods

Donor's blood was examined at the time of collection and during storage in ACD solution kept under the standard conditions prevailing in the blood bank. Prior to collection, two samples were withdrawn from the donor. One was used for determination of the acid-base status of the donor, the second was diluted with isotonic saline in the proportion used for blood storage with ACD addition. The acid-base characteristic of the diluted blood was determined. After collection, an additional sample was withdrawn from the bottle immediately after mixing with the ACD solution. During the

Submitted for publication July 13, 1963.

Lecturer in Physiology, The Rogoff Laboratory of Physiology, The Hebrew University, Hadassah Medical School (Dr. Samueloff); Lecturer in Surgery, Department of Surgery (Dr. Luttwak); Blood Bank, Hadassah University Hospital (Dr. Wigderhouse).

following 14 days samples were withdrawn from the bottle under sterile conditions.

All blood samples were collected in siliconized 30 ml sterile syringes containing a drop of heparin solution of 5,000 units/ml to which a solution of 10% sodium fluoride, in a final concentration of 0.1%, was added so as to prevent glycolysis and changes in the acid-base balance resulting thereof. Hematocrit values were determined prior to introducing the fluoride solution. Acid-base balance was estimated according to Brewin et al[1]: 5 ml portions of each blood sample were equilibrated in 230 ml tonometers with pCO_2 ranging from 20 to 80 mm Hg in air, during 15 minutes, in a water bath at 37 C. The blood was then withdrawn in an air-free syringe, and its CO_2 content was determined using the manometric Van Slyke apparatus. The pH of the blood was measured by a Cambridge pH meter with a Stadie electrode system at 37 C and buffer at pH 7.37. The pCO_2 of the gas phase in the tonometer was determined in the Haldane gas analysis apparatus. With the results obtained, log pCO_2 was plotted against log vol% CO_2 and against pH. Concomitant shifts in both plots indicated metabolic changes in acid-base balance. For comparative purposes the values of CO_2 combining power and pH at pCO_2 40 mm Hg are shown.

Oxygen capacity was determined in the portion of blood equilibrated at approximately 40 mm Hg pCO_2 in air. Lactic acid concentration in the blood samples was estimated according to the enzymatic method of Wieland.[8]

The acid-base balance characteristic of the ACD solution used by the blood bank was also studied. It consists of the standard solution B* (citric acid 4.4 g; sodium citrate 13.2; dextrose 17.2 to 1,000 ml distilled water). Of solution B, 100 ml were used for the preservation of 300 to 350 cc of whole blood.

Results

The ACD solutions used in this investigation had a pH in the range of 5.04 to 5.07, which remained stable while the change of the pCO_2 was from 20 to 80 mm Hg. The CO_2 combining power at pCO_2 40 mm Hg was found to be 3 to 3½ vol%.

The addition of ACD solution to donor's blood had a severe acidifying effect. The normal blood samples of the donors had a CO_2 combining power ranging from 45.5 vol% to 48.5 vol% and a pH range of 7.37 to 7.41. After mixing with the ACD solution, the CO_2 combining power decreased to less than half of the normal—namely, in the range of 21 to 22 vol%, while the pH fell to 6.91-6.99 at 40 mm Hg pCO_2. A further gradual reduction of the pH occurred during the 14 days of storage, the values reached being as low as pH 6.77 to 6.79 and CO_2 combining power 16 to 17 vol%, respectively.

The acidifying properties of the ACD solution exceeded by far the effect of dilution as seen when the results were compared with those obtained after dilution of the blood with isotonic saline. The low pH of the ACD solution increased the intracellular water content of the erythrocytes. After mixing the donors' blood separately with the ACD solution and with isotonic saline, a similar decrease in O_2 capacity was observed in both mixtures, while the hematocrit values of the citrated blood were higher.

Accumulation of lactic acid occurred during storage. From the initial concentration of 9.8 and 11.6 mg% in the two cases examined, it rose within 14 days to 45.5 and 66.0 mg%, respectively.

The results of all determinations are tabulated in the Table; the Figure represents the plots obtained on one of the examined samples.

Comment

The present study shows that ACD solution has a severe acidifying effect on donors' blood. During storage, further reduction in the pH occurs with the accumulation of lactic acid.

It has repeatedly been shown that the constituents of the anticoagulant ACD solution have a beneficial effect on the viability of red blood cells during storage. Dextrose provides the substrate for cellular metabolism, and its consumption is raised by the alkalinity of sodium citrate. The citric acid and cold storage decrease the rate of glycolysis, thus causing an inhibition in the metabolism. The breakdown of dextrose during storage results in a progressive accumulation of lactate and pyruvate.

Considering the acid-base characteristic of citrated blood it is questionable whether the ACD solution has a strictly detrimental effect on the normal acid-base balance of the

* As accepted by National Institutes of Health.

Results of Determinations

Donor	Date	Conditions	CO_2 Content at 40 Mm Hg pCO_2	pH at 40 Mm Hg pCO_2	O_2 Capacity	Hematocrit	Lactic Acid, Mg %
	23/8/62	Donor's blood	48.0	7.39	21.8	52.0	—
1	23/8/62	Diluted with 0.9% NaCl (3:1)	41.0	7.33	15.7	39.3	—
	23/8/62	ACD blood	22.0	6.98	15.8	44.8	—
	5/9/62	Donor's blood	47.5	7.37	21.3	47.0	13.0
	5/9/62	Diluted with 0.9% NaCl (3:1)	40.5	7.28	15.8	33.8	—
	5/9/62	ACD blood	21.0	6.91	15.6	41.5	9.8
2	7/9/62	" "	20.0	6.85	15.5	41.4	—
	12/9/62	" "	18.5	6.82	15.7	41.0	32.2
	16/9/62	" "	17.2	6.80	15.6	40.5	45.0
	19/9/62	" "	17.0	6.79	15.6	40.4	45.5
	13/9/62	Donor's blood	45.5	7.41	22.5	50.1	17.0
	13/9/62	Diluted with 0.9% NaCl (3:1)	40.0	7.21	17.7	36.4	20.4
	13/9/62	ACD blood	21.0	6.99	16.4	44.0	11.6
3	16/9/62	" "	19.2	6.84	16.7	44.0	36.0
	20/9/62	" "	18.0	6.80	16.5	43.8	41.0
	26/9/62	" "	16.7	6.765	16.7	44.0	62.0
	28/9/62	" "	16.0	6.765	16.7	42.7	66.0

donor's blood. It must be borne in mind that the accumulation of acid products, accompanied by minor changes in pH values, depends on the quantity of available buffer base and the effectiveness of the buffers present. As is well known, buffer systems are more effective at pH values in their pK range. Within this range the concentrations of free acids and the alkali salt of the buffer are equal. The normal pH of blood ranges from 7.37 to 7.42, at which level the buffers present in the blood are far from exerting their maximal capacity.

The maximal power of the main buffers, carbonic acid, bicarbonate, and hemoglobin, is at pH below 7. Phosphate buffer is the only one close to its effective range, but due to its limited quantity, the buffer effect is negligible. It follows that the ACD solution, while taxing the available buffer base, reduces the pH to the level of maximal efficiency of the blood buffers. In addition, the buffer characteristics of the ACD solution per se may balance the effect of the accumulating lactic acid.

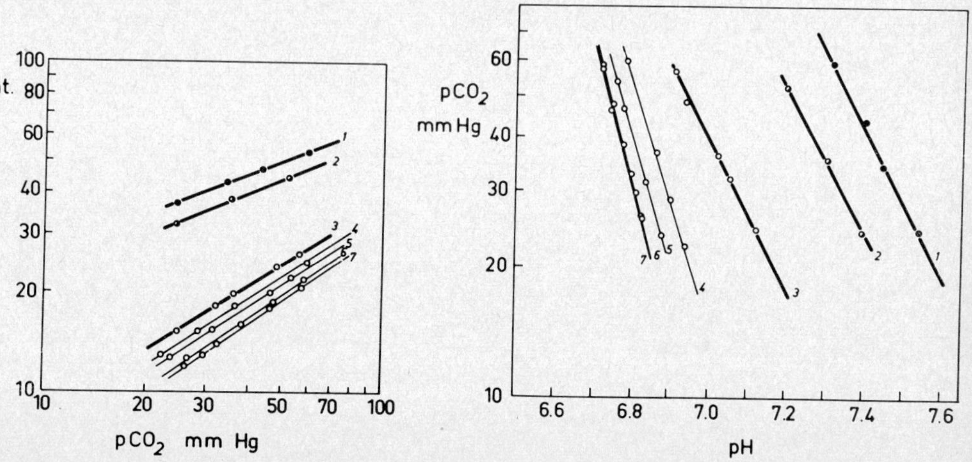

Logarithmic CO_2 dissociation lines and log pCO_2/pH graphs obtained from blood samples of donor No. 3. Solid circle (*1*) indicates donor's blood at the time of collection (Sept 13, 1962). Half-filled circle (*2*) indicates diluted donor's blood (Sept 13, 1962). Open circle (*3-7*) indicates ACD blood samples: examined at time of blood collection (*3*) and 14 day's storage (*4*: Sept 16, 1962; *5*: Sept 20, 1962; *6*: Sept 26, 1962; and *7*: Sept 28, 1962).

One more point which arises is the relation of the lactic acid accumulated during storage to the simultaneous fall in CO_2 combining power expressed in milliequivalents.

$$1 \text{ mEq lactic acid} = \frac{1 \text{ mg lactic acid}}{9}; \text{ and}$$

$$1 \text{ mEq } CO_2 = \frac{\text{vol\% } CO_2}{2.22}$$

It is apparent from the tabled results that no straight correlation exists between lactic acid accumulation during storage and the fall in the CO_2 combining power, thus indicating that acidification during storage cannot be related solely to lactic acid accumulation. Perhaps it could be ascribed to some, as yet unknown, changes occurring in the ACD component under the influence of biological systems.

Summary

The acid-base balance properties of donors' blood were examined at the time of collection and during storage in acid citrate dextrose (ACD) solution.

It resulted that the acidifying properties of the ACD solution exceeded by far the effect of dilution.

During storage, further acidification occurred, which, however, cannot be considered as solely due to lactic acid accumulation.

The influence of the pH on the effectiveness of blood buffers is discussed.

Miss G. Reinharz and Mr. G. Golshani rendered technical assistance, and Mr. S. Ben-Yonah prepared the Figure and the Table.

S. L. Samueloff, M.D., Department of Physiology, Hebrew University, Hadassah Medical, School, POB 1172, Jerusalem, Israel.

REFERENCES

1. Brewin, E. G.; Gould, R. P.; Nashat, F. S.; and Neil, E.: An Investigation of Problems of Acid-Base Equilibrium in Hypothermia, Guy Hosp Rep 104:177, 1955.

2. Gibson, J. G.; Murphy, W. P.; Sheitlin, W. A.; and Rees, S. B.: The Influence of Extracellular Factors Involved in the Collection of Blood in ACD on Maintenance of Red Cell Viability During Refrigerated Storage, Amer J Clin Pathol 26:855, 1956.

3. Howland, W. S.: Cardiovascular and Clotting Disturbances During Massive Blood Replacement, Anesthesiology 19:140, 1958.

4. Howland, W. S.; Bozan, C. P.; and Schweizer, O.: Physiological Observations With Massive Blood Replacement, Surg Gynec Obstet 101:478, 1955.

5. Litwin, M. S.; Smith, L. L.; and Moore, F. D.: Metabolic Alkalosis Following Massive Transfusion, Surgery 45:805, 1959.

6. Peters, J. P., and Van Slyke, D. D.: Quantitative Clinical Chemistry, Baltimore: The Williams and Wilkins Company, 1931, vol 1, p 888.

7. Schweizer, O., and Howland, W. S.: The Effect of Citrated Bank Blood on Acid-Base Balance, Surg Gynec Obstet 114:90, 1962.

8. Wieland, O.: Eine optisch-enzymatische Bestimmung der L-(+)-Milchsäure mit DPN-unabhängiger Milchsäure-Dehydrogenase aus Hefe, Biochem Z 329:568, 1958.

Sigmoid Volvulus

BEREL L. ABRAMS, MD

LOUISVILLE

Dissatisfaction with the accepted treatment and mortality rate of volvulus of the sigmoid colon has prompted us to review this condition and present our experience over the past ten years in an effort to evolve the best approach to this problem.

In the United States, sigmoid volvulus is a relatively infrequent but serious cause of intestinal obstruction comprising about 1% to 3% of all intestinal obstructions.[1,2,3] Still, at the present time it is the second leading cause of colon obstruction in the United States and the number one cause of strangulation obstruction of the large bowel with a reported mortality of from 14% to 50%.[2,4-8] With the known propensity of this entity for the older age group [4,9,10] and the increasing number of aged it would seem that sigmoid volvulus will be encountered with increasing frequency. In Eastern Europe and Russia sigmoid volvulus is a major problem and accounts for about 30% to 50% of all intestinal obstructions.

It is interesting to note that this is a frequent cause of intestinal obstruction in mental hospitals and institutions. In Dean and Murry's series,[6] it constitutes 25% of all cases of intestinal obstruction at the Arkansas State Mental Institution. In Campbell's series [5] half the patients are psychotic.

Classification

Shackelford,[10] Griffin,[11] Hinshaw and Carter,[2] Drapanas and Stewart,[7] all point out that there are two distinct clinical types of sigmoid volvulus.

1. *Acute, Fulminating Type.*—This is characterized by an explosive onset with nausea, vomiting, abdominal pain, and distention. This occurs mostly in younger patients and progresses rapidly to gangrene.

Submitted for publication July 15, 1963.

Formerly Chief Surgical Resident, University of Louisville Hospitals; now Instructor in Surgery, University of Louisville School of Medicine.

From the Department of Surgery, University of Louisville School of Medicine, Louisville General Hospital, and Louisville Veterans Administration Hospital.

2. *Subacute, Chronic Type.*—This characteristically occurs in older patients with a history of previous episodes, associated with abdominal distention and pain, and runs a more insidious course, but if unrelieved, progresses to gangrene.

Pathology and Physiology

The basic pathology is that of a large redundant sigmoid loop with a narrow base of attachment of the mesosigmoid. Axial torsion is produced by rotation of this loop around its mesenteric axis in either a clockwise or counterclockwise manner, resulting in a twist of 180 degrees or more.

The volvulus, if unrelieved, results in venous strangulation with a rise in the intravascular pressure in the segment. This is accompanied by distention and a pooling of fluid in the segment. Because of this continuing influx of arterial blood, some route for escape is necessary. This is accomplished by engorgement of vessels and frank hemorrhage in the bowel lumen and wall. At the same time there is a degeneration of the wall as a result of anoxia and proteolytic activity of the bacteria and their toxins. There is transudation of this material from the strangulated segment, resulting in death due to shock from hypovolemia and by transperitoneal absorption of the bacterial "toxins."[12-14]

Two basic physiological aberrations exist: a closed loop, strangulating obstruction of the sigmoid, and a simple obstruction of the large bowel proximal to the volvulus. In the high percentage of cases where the ileocecal valve remains competent, a double closed loop obstruction results.

Diagnosis

In the acute, fulminating type of sigmoid volvulus the patient presents an intra-abdominal catastrophe simulating a perforated viscus or strangulated bowel, and prompt exploration is indicated.

The chronic type occurs usually in the older patient with a story of previous episodes and long-standing constipation. The most common findings are abdominal distention, pain, and occasionally nausea and vomiting.

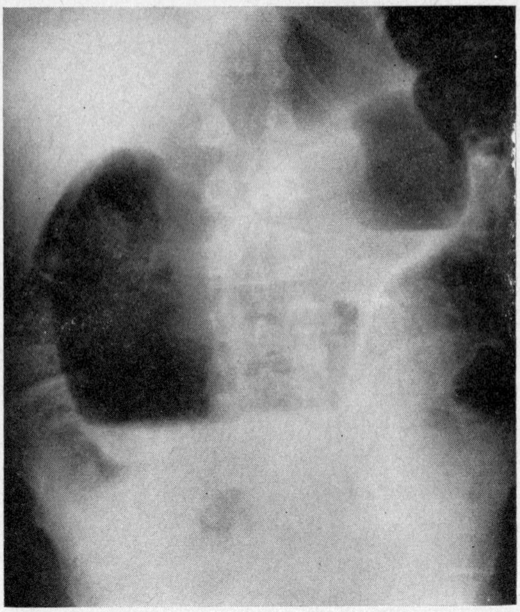

Fig 1.—Picture of classic sigmoid volvulus demonstrating characteristic large loop rising out of the pelvis with the "bent inner tube" effect.

X-ray is a great aid in making the diagnosis.

In addition to the characteristic large loop arising out of the pelvis with the "bent inner tube" effect one may see that the walls of the loop are often relatively thick without haustration. Fluid levels may be seen, one in each limb of the loop, and generally are small and short compared to the overlying accumulation of gas (Fig 1). These x-ray findings are classically described in Frimann-Dahl's monograph.[15] If there is any question about the diagnosis then a barium enema will reveal obstruction to the barium at the twist called a "bird's beak" or "ace of spades" deformity (Fig 2).

Case Analysis

This series is comprised of 23 patients with 27 admissions to the Louisville General Hospital and Louisville Veterans Administration Hospital in the ten-year period from 1950 to 1960. Almost all fall into the subacute, chronic category. There are 18 males and five females in the series with an average age of 65. The overwhelming predominance of males is due to the eight males from the Veterans Hospital, as the ratio of males to females at Louisville General Hospital is two to one in this

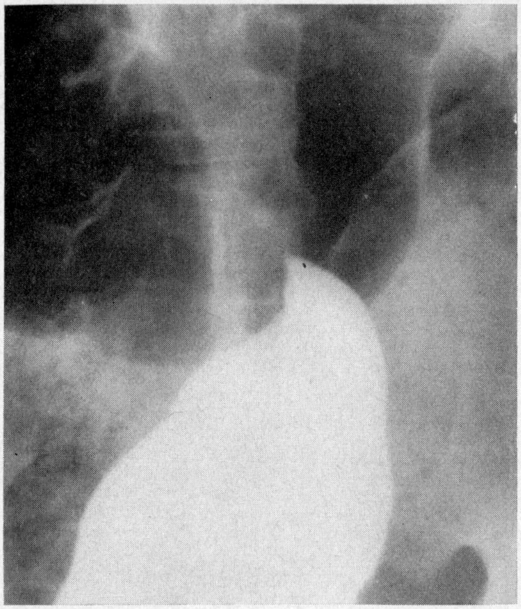

Fig 2.—Barium enema showing obstruction to the flow of barium at the site of the twist with the "bird's beak" deformity.

series. The most common findings are abdominal distention (75%), pain (50%), and nausea and vomiting (25%). These patients usually have a normal white blood cell count, low-grade fever, and relatively normal electrolyte patterns.

There were six deaths among the 23 patients, a mortality of 26%. There was one death among three patients with a gangrenous bowel, a 33% mortality rate. This number is too small to show the true seriousness of this complication which in other series[2,5,6,16,17] led to a mortality of from 65% to 85%.

Among the 27 admissions for primary emergency treatment there were six deaths, a mortality of 22.2% (Table 1). In the seven cases treated with sigmoidoscopic reduction and tube decompression there was one death, a 14% mortality. This death was due to pneumonia and cerebral vascular accident following successful reduction of volvulus. Three patients of this group had definitive surgery during the same hospitalization, one patient refused surgery, and two other patients had no definitive surgery.

There were two deaths among the nine operative detorsions, a 22% mortality. One of these died in the immediate postoperative period in acute pulmonary edema secondary to syphilitic heart disease with aortic insufficiency. The second death was due to cecal perforation and peritonitis. The patient died one day postoperatively.

There were eight obstructive resections with two deaths for a mortality of 25%. One of these deaths was in a patient who suffered cardiac arrest on the table during an exteriorization procedure for gangrenous bowel. Seven of the eight obstructive resections were on viable bowel. These were done earlier in the series, and the practice of doing obstructive resections in the absence of gangrene has been abandoned.

The condition of the patients in the operative group was no different from those in the nonoperative series, with the exception of the three patients with gangrenous bowel who presented "acute abdomens." Excluding these patients the operative mortality was 20% and must be related to the major operative procedure rather than condition of the patient per se.

The definitive surgical procedures are listed in Table 2. There are 16 patients with three deaths for an 18.7% mortality. It is noteworthy that five elective resections were done with no mortality, and one successful Hartmann's procedure * was done on gangrenous bowel extending too far down to exteriorize.

Five cases had recurring volvulus one or more times in the hospital, a 31% recurrence rate. Three required emergency operation, one signed out, and one had no definite surgery. Three of these recurrences followed operative detorsion and two followed nonoperative decompression.

* Division of the sigmoid distal to the gangrenous portion, closure of the distal stump, exteriorization and excision of the proximal gangrenous portion, and creation of a single-barrelled proximal colostomy.

TABLE 1.—*Primary Emergency Treatment (27 Admissions)*

Treatment	Admissions, No.	Viable Bowel	Nonviable	Deaths	% Mortality
Sigmoidoscopic reduction & insertion of rectal tube	7	7	0	1	14
Operative detorsion	9	9	0	2	22
Primary resection	2	1	1	1	50
Obstructive resection	8	7	1	2	25
Hartmann procedure	1	0	1	0	0
Totals	27	24	3	6	22.2

TABLE 2.—*Definitive Treatment (16 Patients)*

Treatment	Patients, No.	Viable Bowel	Nonviable	Deaths	% Mortality
Primary resection	2	1	1	1	50
Obstructive resection	8	7	1	2	25
Hartmann procedure	1	0	1	0	0
Elective resection	5	5	0	0	0
Totals	16	13	3	3	18.7

The following cases illustrate certain features of the disease:

CASE 1.—A 72-year-old white male, a mental defective, was admitted with a one-day history of abdominal swelling and a two-day history of anorexia and obstipation. Blood pressure was 120/70; pulse, 130 irregular; respiration, 30; temperature, 102.2.

The patient was fibrillating with a markedly distended abdomen, tympanitic, with high-pitched bowel sounds. A film of the abdomen revealed a large dilated loop of bowel arising out of the pelvis consistent with volvulus. Exploratory laparotomy revealed a sigmoid volvulus with markedly distended colon above it with perforation of the cecum and a moderate amount of fecal soilage. The volvulus was reduced and a cecostomy done, but the patient died after one day with peritonitis and sepsis.

Comment.—The patient was a mental defective. (In several series [5,11,15] a significant number of cases came from mental institutions.) This case also illustrates the second closed loop obstruction above the volvulus of the colon which, with a competent ileocecal valve, resulted in perforation of the cecum with a fatal outcome.

CASE 2.—A 63-year-old white male was admitted with a one-day history of cramping abdominal pain, abdominal swelling, and vomiting. The patient was afebrile, pulse, 120; blood pressure, 98/82, with a distended, tender abdomen, tympanitic, with no bowel sounds, and a visibly outlined left colon. The white blood cell count was 16,850 with 84 neutrophils. The nonprotein nitrogen was 85. X-ray was consistent with a sigmoid volvulus. Exploratory laparotomy revealed about 18 inches of gangrenous sigmoid. There was not enough length to bring out the distal sigmoid below the gangrene, so a Hartmann procedure was done with creation of a single-barrelled proximal colostomy. The patient had a stormy course but survived. Five months later his colonic continuity was re-established.

Comment.—This case illustrates the seldom-quoted fact that the gangrenous bowel often extends too far distally to exteriorize. Bruusgaard [4] warns against an obstructive resection where the site of the torsion is so distal that it produces too much pull on the efferent loop of the sigmoid which may cause gangrene and peritonitis.

CASE 3.—A 51-year-old white male was admitted with a one-day history of cramping abdominal pain, nausea, and vomiting. Abdomen was soft and slightly distended with generalized tenderness and occasional high pitched bowel sounds. Temperature was 99.2 F (37.3 C); pulse, 92; respiration, 20; blood pressure, 108/70; white blood cell count, 12,900, with 89 neutrophils. X-rays revealed a sigmoid volvulus. Patient had exploratory laparotomy after sigmoidoscopy was abandoned due to the color and friability of mucosa. The patient had sigmoid volvulus with 18 inches of gangrenous bowel. A primary closed resection was done. The patient's postoperative course was uneventful.

Comment.—This patient was considered a good candidate for primary resection. He was relatively young and was well hydrated with normal electrolytes and a pulse below 100. At the operating table he did not show a lot of distention and edema of the bowel proximal to the volvulus. This case is the exception to the general rule but does point out that in selected cases a primary resection can be accomplished. In Dean and Murry's series [6] this was the method of choice. Baronofsky [17] also mentions its feasibility.

CASE 4.—The patient was a 73-year-old Negro female with a 1½-week history of abdominal distention without pain, nausea, or vomiting. Patient gave a long history of constipation. Blood pressure was 200/96; pulse, 56; respirations, 20. Abdomen was distended, mildly tender throughout, and tympanitic. White blood cell count was 7,860 with normal differential. X-rays revealed a sigmoid volvulus. Patient was sigmoidoscoped, decompressed, and a colon tube was passed through the scope and taped in place. The tube was removed the following day. Three days later, on Feb 23, the patient redistended and was sigmoidoscoped and decompressed again; the episode was repeated on March 2, 1960. The patient refused definitive surgery.

Comment.—This case points out the recurring nature of this disorder. The rectal tube should remain in place for 24 hours to obviate against recurring volvulus. While nonoperative decompression is excellent acute treatment, it is not a definitive procedure and should in most cases be complemented by a later elective resection, depending on age and other disease entities.

Comment

In the acute, fulminating type of sigmoid volvulus there is no controversy among surgeons concerning treatment. These patients present an "acute abdomen" characterized by abdominal pain, distention, nausea and vomiting, fever, and leukocytosis. They deserve exploration as soon as they can be adequately prepared for surgery. A few hours delay to prepare the patients properly for anesthesia and surgery reaps dividends in more living patients.

About the emergency treatment for the subacute, chronic type of volvulus there is no such agreement. It would seem that the surgeon should embrace the easiest and safest way to handle the acute problem. In our opinion, this is nonoperative reduction by means of the proctoscope and a tube threaded past the twist and sutured or taped to the perianal skin. This should be left in place for 24 hours to prevent early recurrence. This method has long been championed by Bruusgaard [4] who reported 136 successful treatments with four deaths, a 2.9% mortality rate; perforation was due to instrumentation in one instance, but no gangrenous bowel was overlooked and in only nine attempts was intubation unsuccessful. Immediate laparotomy in his nine cases reveals no untoward effect from the try at intubation. The over-all mortality rate for Bruusgaard's series is 14.2%. The reports of Shapiro and Mason,[19] Isaacson and Greer,[20] Hamlin,[21] and Isaacson [22] further substantiate the efficiency of this method of treatment. Drapanas and Stewart [7] in their excellent article show 98 episodes with 82 successful tube decompressions: an 84% success rate with 1.2% mortality.

On the other side of the ledger, Farringer and Wilson [16] champion operative detorsion. Their mortality rate was 17.6%. Pool and Dunavant [3] believe that surgery is the treatment of choice and should be undertaken as soon as the diagnosis of volvulus is made and the patient is properly prepared. Hinshaw and Carter [2] likewise favor surgery and reserve nonoperative decompression for the occasional patient of the moderately progressive type with no obvious signs of nonviability and whose general condition prohibits laparotomy. The over-all mortality rate in their series is 42%.

The hazard associated with nonoperative reduction must be borne in mind. When proctoscopy and tube decompression are used, the proctoscopist must carefully observe the mucosa and it it appears friable, bloody, or discolored, or it one cannot easily guide the well-lubricated rectal tube past the twist, then proctoscopy should be abandoned and the patient prepared for operative decompression. In our series and others [4,19-22] there was no overlooked gangrenous bowel and there was only one instance of perforation due to instrumentation.

If operative decompression is undertaken a rectal tube may be placed in the rectum preoperatively, and if the bowel is viable, detorsion and guiding of the rectal tube past the twist is all that should be done. We have abandoned operative resection of viable bowel in view of the seemingly high mortality in our early experience. Now only detorsion is done, followed by elective resection in the same hospitalization. Our feeling is supported by the 33% mortality rate reported by Drapanas and Stewart [7] and the 25% mortality rate reported by Hinshaw and Carter [2] for obstructive resection in viable bowel.

There is a 31% hospital recurrence rate in our series. Three follow operative detorsion and two follow nonoperative decompression. Dean and Murry [6] and Drapanas and Stewart [7] both report a 60% recurrence rate. Boggs and Ratcliffe [1] report a 46% recurrence, and the experience of others is similar. In view of this high rate of recurrence and the 14% mortality associated with nonoperative decompression and the 22% mortality with operative detorsion, unless age or other medical conditions make the risk prohibitive, a strong argument can be made for elective resection with its zero mortality rate in our hands to date and the low mortality presented by others.[5,6,21,23] This is particularly true in those cases in which it was necessary to perform operative decompression, because of inability to pass the proctoscope, or because dead bowel was suspected. Survival from one episode in no way protects the patient from potentially lethal second or third episodes.

If the patient is decompressed easily by the proctoscope then one is naturally more hesitant to perform major elective surgery. Again, one must equate the possibility of recurrence with a lethal outcome against the low risk of elective resection and the life expectancy of the patient. One is certainly justified in doing an elective resection in a mentally defective or disturbed patient because of the inability of these patients to take care of themselves properly. Elective resection can be accomplished between seven to ten days following the initial episode without any great technical difficulty or increased morbidity or mortality.

In the face of gangrenous bowel the problem is much more serious. Resection or exteriorization of this segment is mandatory. This can best be accomplished by an obstructive resection with exteriorization of the proximal and distal loop as a double-barreled colostomy. Care must be taken to avoid unnecessary tension on the bowel in attempting to exteriorize a long enough segment. As pointed out by Shackelford,[10] Bruusgaard,[4] and others, the site of the gangrenous twist may be too distal to exteriorize. It is then necessary to divide the sigmoid distal to the gangrenous portion, close the distal stump, bring out and excise the proximal gangrenous portion, and create a proximal colostomy. This was done once in our series and the patient survived.

On occasion, in certain select cases it will be possible to resect the gangrenous bowel and do a primary end-to-end anastomosis. The condition of the patient and the amount of distention and edema of the bowel all have to be taken into consideration. This was done successfully once in our series.

On the basis of our experience a plan for the management of sigmoid volvulus has exolved:

I. Acute, fulminating type requires immediate surgery.

II. Subacute, chronic type:
   - A. Nonoperative decompression with the proctoscope and rectal tube followed in most instances by elective resection in about seven to ten days.
   - B. If unsuccessful or if the mucosa appears friable, discolored, or bloody then immediate laparotomy is indicated.
     - (1) If bowel is viable then detorsion is done with a rectal tube passed above the twist and sutured or taped to the anus. No resections are done in the presence of viable bowel. An elective resection is accomplished after seven to ten days in most instances.
     - (2) If the bowel is nonviable:
       - (*a*) Obstructive resection where anatomically possible.
       - (*b*) Hartmann's procedure for those cases where gangrenous segment is too distal to exteriorize.
       - (*c*) Primary resection in the rare case where the general condition of the patient and the bowel permits.
   - C. For those patients in whom definitive surgery is not indicated, a low-fiber diet and wetting agents may be of benefit.

Summary

A brief review of sigmoid volvulus and our experience with 23 patients with 27 admissions to the Louisville General Hospital and the Veterans Hospital has been presented. The over-all mortality rate was 26%.

On the basis of this review and our experience a plan for the treatment of sigmoid volvulus was established. This plan consists of immediate operation for the acute, fulminating type; and for the subacute, chronic type, nonoperative decompression of the volvulus with the proctoscope and rectal tube, followed in most instances by elective resection in seven to ten days.

Where gangrenous bowel was suspected, where proctoscopic decompression was unsuccessful, or where, at proctoscopy, the mucosa appears friable, discolored, or bloody, laparotomy was indicated. If the bowel was viable, operative detorsion was accomplished, and a rectal tube was passed up past the twist and sutured in place at the anus. If the bowel was gangrenous an obstructive resection was done. If the gangrenous segment was too distal to exteriorize then a Hartmann's procedure was done. In the occasional case where the condition of the patient and bowel permitted a primary resection, an end-to-end anastomosis was accomplished.

In those cases successfully reduced where age or other medical conditions contraindicate surgery, a low-fiber diet and wetting agents were of benefit.

Berel L. Abrams, MD, Department of Surgery, University of Louisville, 511 S Floyd St, Louisville 2, Ky.

REFERENCES

1. Boggs, H. W., Jr., and Ratcliffe, H. H., Jr.: Volvulus of the Sigmoid Colon, Southern Med J 53:1039, 1960.

2. Hinshaw, D. B., and Carter, R.: Surgical Management of Acute Volvulus of the Sigmoid Colon: A Study of 55 Cases, Ann Surg 146:52, 1957.

3. Pool, R. M., and Dunavant, W. D.: Volvulus of Sigmoid Colon, Ann Surg 133:719, 1951.

4. Bruusgaard, C.: Volvulus of the Sigmoid Colon and Its Treatment, Surgery 22:466, 1947.

5. Campbell, L. J., and Musselman, M. M.: Volvulus of Sigmoid Colon, Gastroenterology 24:378, 1953.

6. Dean, G. O., and Murry, J. W.: Volvulus of Sigmoid Colon, Ann Surg 135:830, 1952.

7. Drapanas, T., and Stewart, J. D.: Acute Sigmoid Volvulus: Concepts in Surgical Treatment, Amer J Surg 101:70, 1961.

8. Levin, I. A.: Volvulus of Sigmoid Colon, J Louisiana Med Soc 111:116, 1959.

9. Maingot, R.: Abdominal Operations, ed 4, New York: Appleton-Century-Crofts, Inc., 1961.

10. Shackelford, R. T.: Surgery of the Alimentary Tract, Philadelphia: W. B. Saunders Company, 1955, vol 2, pp 1489-1497.

11. Griffin, W. D.; Barton, G. R.; and Meyer, K. A.: Volvulus of Sigmoid Colon: Report of 25 Cases, Surg Gynec Obstet 81:287, 1945.

12. Cohen, I., Jr.: Strangulation Obstruction, Springfield, Ill: Charles C Thomas, Publisher, 1961.

13. Nemir, P., Jr.; Hawthorne, H. R.; Cohen, I., Jr.; and Drabkin, D. L.: The Cause of Death in Strangulation Obstruction: An Experimental Study, Ann Surg 130:874, 1949.

14. Nemir, P., Jr.; Hawthorne, H. R.; and Drabkin, D. L.: The Pathogenesis of Strangulation Intestinal Obstruction: An Experimental and Clinical Study, Gastroenterology 32:249, 1957.

15. Frimann-Dahl, J.: Roentgen Examinations in Acute Abdominal Diseases, Springfield, Ill: Charles C Thomas, Publisher, 1960.

16. Farringer, J. L., Jr., and Wilson, H.: Volvulus of Sigmoid Colon, Amer J Surg 90:588, 1955.

17. Hilton, H. D., and Waugh, J. M.: Volvulus of Sigmoid Colon, AMA Arch Surg 62:437, 1951.

18. Baronofsky, I. D.: Primary Resection and Asceptic End-to-End Anastomosis for Acute and Subacute Large Bowel Obstruction, Surgery 27: 664, 1950.

19. Shapiro, S. W., and Mason, E. E.: Ileus As a Cause of Volvulus of the Sigmoid: Review of Results of Management, Surgery 41:512, 1957.

20. Isaacson, N. H., and Greer, D.: Conservative Treatment of Acute Form of Sigmoid Volvulus, Surgery 31:544, 1952.

21. Hamlin, F. J., Jr.: Nonoperative Reduction of Acute Volvulus of Sigmoid, New Eng J Med 247:835, 1952.

22. Isaacson, N. H.: Sigmoid Volvulus: Treatment by Proctoscopic Reduction and Elective Resection, Amer J Proctol 9:309, 1958.

23. Halligan, E. J.; Hamdan, F.; and Baer, J. J.: Volvulus of the Sigmoid Colon, Amer J Proctol 9:453, 1958.

Distal Antrectomy With Vagectomy for Duodenal Ulcer

Review of 450 Cases

LOUIS T. PALUMBO, MD
AND
WENDELL S. SHARPE, MD
DES MOINES, IOWA

Introduction

The surgical pendulum is swinging toward universal adoption of the recent more conservative type surgical procedures which have been developed in a number of surgical centers during the past 20 years. As a result of the findings of several investigators, particularly the monumental work of Dragstedt and associates, the basic altered gastric physiology in the pathogenesis of duodenal ulcer is now known and understood. By the clinical application of these basic physiologic principles, several surgeons have patterned conservative surgical procedures to control duodenal ulcer without affecting, to any serious degree, the normal gastric functions or nutritional status of the patients. In addition, several of these procedures have reduced the incidence and severity of many of the undesirable postoperative sequelae associated with many of the older and time-tested surgical procedures for this chronic disease.

Submitted for publication July 15, 1963.

From the Department of Surgery, Veterans Administration Hospital.

These patients will be included in a cooperative peptic ulcer study which the Veterans Administration Research in Surgery is conducting.

It has been definitely established by careful research studies that there are two major physiologic phases which control and influence gastric secretory function, particularly in the production of pepsin, free hydrochloric acid, and total gastric secretory volume. These two phases are controlled and influenced by a cephalic phase, entirely neurogenic via the vagus nerves to the stomach, and by a humoral or hormonal phase, through the liberation of gastrin from the gastric antrum. Each in itself is almost wholly independent though they affect each other to some degree.

Very few surgeons doubt that the pathogenesis of a duodenal ulcer is primarily overactivity of the gastric glands secreting digestive juices through the hyperactivity of vagal stimulation to the stomach. This results in hypersecretion of the gastric juices, particularly of free hydrochloric acid in both total volume output as well as the concentration of free acids measured in milliequivalents. In conjunction with this, there is hypermotility and pylorospasm, both of which contribute to a vicious cycle of increased acid production. As the ulcer diathesis develops, the vagal stimulation continues unabated at night during the normal gastric secretory resting phase. Under normal circumstances, the total gastric secretory volume during a 12-hour night resting phase is under 350 cc and with less than 20 mEq of free hydrochloric acid; in patients with a chronic duodenal ulcer, this secretion will average about 1,000 cc. Some patients secrete over 3,000 cc.

The other important gastric secretory control is mediated by the gastric antrum which occupies about 25%-35% of the distal portion of the stomach. The hormone (gastrin) secreted by this portion of the stomach is capable by local action of stimulating the acid glands in the body and fundus of the stomach. Antral stimulation is affected by the presence of an alkaline gastric content, by mechanical or chemical irritation, by distention, by hypermotility, by puddling of food, and by *delayed gastric emptying.* Any one of these factors can augment the antral stimulatory phase and thereby enhance the total gastric secretory volume as well as the amount of free hydrochloric acid.

In order adequately to control duodenal ulcer diathesis and to prevent recurrent ulceration and/or stomal ulcer formation, these two major functions should be eliminated.

Purpose

In 1949, it was our opinion that a minimal gastric resection, distal antrectomy—25% or less—with a bilateral vagectomy might prove to be the ideal surgical procedure for duodenal ulcer; and that it may, because of conservation of all of the normal reservoir capacity of the stomach, eliminate most of the undesirable postoperative sequelae associated with other older and currently advocated surgical procedures. However, at that time we were not prepared to start such a study and evaluation program, for all the evidence concerning antral functions was not known or fully understood.

By 1953, we were convinced by the reports of Dragstedt and associates of the important role of the antrum in the pathogenesis of duodenal ulcer. From 1953 through 1957 we performed this procedure upon 20 patients as a pilot study. During this four-year period a careful follow-up program was carried out. The results in this early group were so outstanding that on July 1, 1957, we discontinued the performance of all other surgical procedures for duodenal ulcer and began to perform a distal antrectomy (resecting 25% or less of the distal end of the stomach) with a bilateral vagectomy in all patients coming to surgery for a duodenal ulcer. The first 350 operations were performed on consecutive and unselected adult males.

Up to May 1, 1963, a total of 450 antrectomies were performed. Since January, 1961, an additional 28 other gastric procedures were performed for this condition. These will be discussed later.

The selection of patients for surgical intervention was based upon the generally accepted criteria: hemorrhage, obstruction, pain, intractability, perforation, and recurrent ulceration. Throughout this entire period, the program has been carefully and closely supervised by one Chief of Surgery (L.T.P.). We have applied the same basic indications for surgical treatment and all other factors concerning pre- and postoperative management, operative technique, and every ancillary factor to all patients. The methods of follow-up studies and evaluation have been likewise standardized.

Follow-Up Program

The patients are recalled at the end of the first six months after surgery. If the patient has no complaints or problems, he is recalled at the end of the first year for admission to the hospital for a complete evaluation which includes gastric analyses, 12-hour night rest-

TABLE 1.—*Age Distribution*

Age	No.	%
20-29	14	3.1
30-39	92	20.5
40-49	131	29.1
50-59	93	20.7
60-69	100	22.2
70 and over	20	4.4
Totals	450	100

TABLE 2.—*Indications for Operation* *

Cause	No.	%
Hemorrhage	240 †	53.3
Intractability	115	25.5
Obstruction	45	10.0
Prior perforation	48	10.7
Acute perforation	2 †	0.5
Totals	450	100

* A number of patients had more than one of these complications or indications for operation.

† In this group 64 (14.2%) emergency for massive hemorrhage; and 66 (14.7%) operated upon for emergency.

ing secretory volume determinations, upper gastrointestinal roentgenographic studies including motor meal, routine blood and urine examinations, and complete entries in the protocol. This latter covers every phase and represents a multipaged review, so that a thorough evaluation of the patient's status can be readily made.

The patients are recalled every two years thereafter, and the same studies conducted. A five-year follow-up has been obtained in 126 patients and a three-year follow-up in 208 patients. Of the patients, 96% have been followed to date.

Age Incidence.—The average age was 50.7 years; the youngest was 24, and the oldest was 76. The greatest number, 131 (29.1%), were in the 40- to 49-year-old age group; however, 120 (26.6%) were over 60 years of age, and 213 (47.3%) were over 50 years old.

Indications for Surgery.—A great number of patients had more than one indication for surgery. The most common indications are intractability and bleeding. In both these categories there is considerable overlap. Hemorrhage, in our series, is greater than in many series reported by others. In this group are all patients with a history of bleeding or who were hemorrhaging at the time of admission, at which time definitive surgery was performed (Table 2). Sixty-four (14.2%) patients were operated upon as an emergency for massive hemorrhage.

Duration of Symptoms and Preoperative Gastrointestinal Bleeding.—The average duration of symptoms prior to definitive surgery was 14.2 years.

Bleeding or hemorrhage occurred in 240 (53.3%) cases. Of the group with a history of bleeding or hemorrhage at the time of hospital admission during the period of hospitalization, 122 (50.8%) cases were classified as massive, 82 (34.2%) as moderate, and 36 (15%) as minimal (Table 3). Of the patients who bled, 177 (73.8%) had hemorrhaged more than once. In 102 (42.5%), hemorrhage had occurred three or more times before the patient had been referred for surgical treatment (Table 4).

Preoperative Gastric Analysis.—In the first 350 patients, excluding those hemor-

TABLE 3.—*Age Incidence and Degree of Hemorrhage*

Age	Total No. Patients (%)	Minimal (%)	Moderate (%)	Massive (%)
20-29	13 (5.5)	2 (15.4)	4 (30.8)	7 (53.8)
30-39	63 (26.2)	12 (19.0)	28 (44.4)	23 (36.6)
40-49	58 (24.2)	8 (13.8)	14 (24.1)	36 (62.1)
50-59	56 (23.3)	7 (12.5)	20 (35.7)	29 (51.8)
60-69	29 (12.1)	4 (13.8)	8 (27.6)	17 (58.6)
70 and over	21 (8.8)	3 (14.3)	8 (38.1)	10 (47.6)
Totals	240 (53.3)	36 (15.0)	82 (34.2)	122 (50.8)

TABLE 4.—*Age Incidence and Occurrence of Hemorrhage*

Age	Total No. Patients (%)	Initial Episode (%)	Second Episode (%)	Third or More (%)
20-29	13 (5.4)	3 (23.1)	3 (23.1)	7 (53.8)
30-39	63 (26.8)	15 (23.8)	17 (27.0)	31 (49.2)
40-49	58 (24.2)	15 (25.9)	23 (39.7)	20 (34.4)
50-59	56 (23.3)	17 (30.4)	17 (30.4)	22 (39.2)
60-69	29 (12.1)	7 (24.1)	8 (27.6)	14 (48.3)
70 and over	21 (8.8)	6 (28.6)	7 (33.3)	8 (38.1)
Totals	240 (53.3)	63 (26.2)	75 (31.3)	102 (42.5)

rhaging at the time of hospitalization or who had pyloric obstruction, total night gastric secretory volume studies were carried out in addition to free hydrochloric acid determination on the resting gastric specimen, after betazole (Histalog) injection and after the Hollander's insulin test. Most patients had 30 or more milliequivalents of free hydrochloric acid. The average night secretory volume was 890 cc with a maximum of 3,400 cc.

Type of Operation Performed.—The procedure was accomplished through a supraumbilical, elliptical, transverse or right subcostal, oblique transrectus abdominal incision. The bilateral vagectomy was performed after mobilization of the lower esophagus through the esophageal hiatus. The vagus nerves and their branches are completely dissected free for a distance of 3-4 inches along the esophagus down to the stomach. This portion of the vagal pathways was resected. The vagal resection, *including all branches, must be complete.* Variations in the branches and pattern of distribution in this area occur and should be known by the surgeon.

A distal antrectomy was performed, removing 25% or less of the stomach. The resection is carried distal to the pyloric ring so as to avoid leaving any antrum in the duodenal stump.

The duodenal ulcer was left in situ in 30% of the cases. The ulcer was removed in those patients who were hemorrhaging at the time of surgery or in whom a safe duodenal closure could not be obtained.

An antecolic gastrojejunal anastomosis, Billroth II, Polya, or Hofmeister type, was accomplished, the type depending upon the width of the antral canal. However, no attempt was made to form a small stoma. The afferent jejunal loop was short—4 to 5 inches in length.

TABLE 5.—*Postoperative Complications 440 Living Patients*

	Patients (%)		No.	% of Total	Incidence, %
	4 (0.9)	Cardiopulmonary			
		Atelectasis	2		
		Infarction (pulmonary)	1		
		Pneumonia	1		
			4	7.7	0.9
	9 (2.0)	Wound			
		Abscess	6		
		Dehiscence	4		
		Infection	2		
			12	23.1	2.7
	18 (4.0)	Intra-abdominal			
		Gastric atony	5		
		Abscess, subhepatic	4		
		Hepatitis	4		
		Leak, duodenal stump	4		
		Pancreatitis, acute	3		
		Peritonitis	1		
		Intestinal obstruction	1		
			22	42.3	4.9
	14 (3.1)	Miscellaneous			
		Diarrhea, specific	4		
		Hypoprothrombinemia	1		
		Jaundice, homologous serum	3		
		Jaundice, transient	4		
		Psychosis	1		
		Thrombophlebitis	1		
			14	26.9	3.1
Totals	45 (10.0)		52	100.0	11.6

* Several patients had more than one complication.

TABLE 6.—*Mortality—Complications*

	Patients (%)		No. (%)
Cardiopulmonary (ages: 61-65-67-69-70)	5 (1.1)	Atelectasis	2
		Infarction (pulmonary)	2
		Infarction (cardiac)	3
2 elective		Pneumonia	3
3 emergency		Esophageal perforation	1
			11 (2.4)
Intra-abdominal (ages: 51-65-76)	3 (0.7)	Hepatitis	1
		Leak, duodenal stump	1
2 elective		Necrotizing pancreatitis	1
1 emergency		Traumatic pancreatitis	1
			4 (0.9)
Miscellaneous (ages: 33-70)	2 (0.5)	Oliguric uremia	1
		Toxemia, *C Welchii*	1
1 elective			
1 emergency			2 (0.5)
Total	10 (2.2)		17 (3.8)

* Several patients had more than one complication.

The abdominal wounds were closed by approximating the anterior and posterior rectus sheaths with interrupted fine silk sutures. The majority of patients was ambulatory on the first day.

Results

Postoperative Complications.—Fifty-two (11.6%) complications developed in 45 (10%) of the 440 patients who survived. The most frequent types of complications occurred within the abdominal cavity (Table 5).

Postoperative Deaths.—The *over-all mortality* was ten (2.2%) deaths. This includes all deaths (related or unrelated to surgery) occurring within 30 days after surgery (Table 6). There were 384 elective cases with five (*1.3%*) deaths and 66 emergency cases with five (*7.6%*) deaths.

Excluding three deaths unrelated to surgery, the over-all mortality was 1.5%, and in the emergency group it was 3%.

Three of the five deaths in the elective series of 384 cases were in connection with technique. In two patients, death occurred from pancreatitis. In both instances the ulcer was resected, the resection requiring considerable dissection about the head of the pancreas. Our current policy is to leave these ulcers in situ to avoid this type of complication.

Three are deaths due to complications which are common to most all types of major general surgery. These are not necessarily attributed to the specific type of procedure performed. These are acute coronary occlusion, pulmonary embolism, pneumonia, and atelectasis. In this series of 450 operations, there were four deaths caused by the factors mentioned above.

One rare and unusual complication occurred in a 70-year-old male, elective procedure, on the third postoperative day and resulted in rapid downhill course and death in a matter of hours—a *Clostridium welchii* (gas bacillus) infection of the abdominal wall.

Postoperative Gastric Analysis.—Of the 440 patients who survived and in whom follow-up was obtained, 431 were tested postoperatively for free hydrochloric acid and total night resting secretory volume determinations. The average total volume was 260 cc. *No free acids* were present in 416 (96.4%) cases. This has persisted on repeated follow-up determinations. Only 15 (3.6%) cases showed free acids. In ten of these, the free acids were within normal range, being less than 20 mEq. In the other five, the free hydrochloric acid exceeded 20 mEq.

Of 126 patients followed five years or longer, 116 were without any free acids, 6 had free acids less than 20 mEq, and 4 had free acids in excess of 20 mEq (30, 25, 34, and 34 mEq) with total night secretion volume of 600, 1,350, 1,200 and 900 cc. One patient in this group developed a marginal ulcer; on reoperation, vagus resection was completed; this patient had a third medium-sized trunk intact. The patient made a complete recovery and, upon repeated follow-up studies, has only 130 cc 12-hour night volume secretions and a persistent absence of free hydrochloric acid.

Of 208 patients followed three years or longer, 204 have no free acids upon repeated examinations. Four have less than 20 mEq (14, 10, 10, and 12) with total night volume of 775, 900, 200, and 210 cc. Only one patient in this group has more than 20 mEq (38) with a night volume of only 280 cc.

In the entire group, only two (0.45%) patients developed a marginal ulcer.

The second patient with marginal ulcer had 1,175 cc 12-hour night resting phase secretory volume with 52.9 mEq of free hydrochloric acid. Patient was reoperated upon, vagal area not exposed because of adhesions. A resection of distal two thirds of the stomach with an antecolic Hofmeister gastrojejunostomy was accomplished. Gastric analysis and secretory volume measurements were performed on the second postoperative day with the following results: 950 cc volume and 4.9 mEq free hydrochloric acid.

In both cases of marginal ulcer formation, the patients developed symptoms and findings of a marginal ulcer within six months after the original procedure, and both were reoperated within nine months. In both cases, it is our opinion that an incomplete vagus resection was the cause.

Postoperative Gastrointestinal Roentgenographic Studies.—Repeated postoperative follow-up gastrointestinal roentgenographic examinations revealed a satisfactory functioning stoma in 285 patients examined. The average emptying time of the gastric remnant six months after operation was 75 minutes. After one year, the emptying time was normal, with complete emptying in 30 to 40 minutes.

Repeated motor meal roentgenographic studies of the small bowel in 100 cases revealed clumping, segmentation, puddling, and motility disturbances in 40% of the patients. However, even though these changes were seen on roentgenograms, the patients had no signs or symptoms related to a disturbed motor function. By the end of the first year, a repeat examination in 90% of the 100 patients revealed the motor meal studies to be within normal range without any further evidence of disturbed motility or pattern.

Evaluation of Follow-Up Studies.—The ability to gain weight is no problem after this procedure. In 94% of the patients, the average gain in weight was 12 lb (5.4 kg) by the end of the first year. In the remaining 6%, the patients voluntarily lost weight or their weight remained unchanged. In addition to this favorable response, after one year all patients maintained themselves on three meals a day without any major dietary restrictions. Diarrhea does not occur. In fact, after a period of adjustment, there were no cases of persistent or recurrent episodes of diarrhea except in three (0.7%) cases of mild diarrhea.

The dumping syndrome has been practically eliminated. In only six patients (1.3%) it occurred early after surgery and was mild (Table 7). Of the 440 patients, only two (0.46%) developed a marginal ulcer.

TABLE 7.—*Results of Follow-up Studies*

Type	%
Weight:	
Gain	93.9
Stationary or loss	6.1
Dumping syndrome: mild, transient	1.3
Diet: regular, 3 meals	100.0
Diarrhea: mild	0.7
Marginal ulcer	0.46

The over-all evaluation of the results in 422 patients with follow-up studies was considered excellent to good in 97% of cases.

Comment

This procedure continues to be superior to and has proved more effective in producing the desired results in the surgical management of patients with chronic duodenal ulcer than any other operation we have employed in the past. It can be accomplished with a lower morbidity and mortality than most other procedures currently being used. It can be performed in practically all patients requiring surgery for duodenal ulcer.

In over 90% of these patients the operation was performed by the senior house officers under the direct supervision of the full-time surgical staff. The operating time is shorter than that of previous procedures, and the patient's hospital stay is shortened by 25%, with a more rapid convalescence and rehabilitation period than before.

It has eliminated practically all of the undesirable postoperative sequelae usually seen with other surgical procedures. The major significant favorable factors are weight gain (no patient has lost weight because of the type of operation), no bowel disturbances, no dietary restrictions (all patients on three meals a day), freedom from any symptoms or signs usually seen after other surgical procedures, no dumping syndrome, and practically all patients completely satisfied with this operation.

It is readily apparent from these studies that a resection of the stomach greater than 25% is unnecessary provided that the bilateral vagectomy is complete. Persistent absence of free hydrochloric acid in over 96% and a total night resting secretory volume of less than 300 cc (normal level) will occur, and because of this fact, recurrent or stomal ulcers will not occur. This is sufficient evidence to substantiate the fact that both major physiologic acid-producing functions are controlled and eliminated; thereby, the pathogenesis of duodenal ulcer in these patients is controlled. There is no need or physiologic indication for a higher or greater type gastric resection than 25%. A higher type resection adds nothing to an already controlled gastric hormonal phase but will in turn lead to the occurrence of many undesirable postoperative sequelae which have plagued a variety of surgical procedures currently and formerly used in the treatment of duodenal ulcer. The smaller the gastric remnant is, the greater are the number and intensity of the sequelae. By a conservative resection of the distal portion of the stomach, removing most of the antrum as we have practiced during the past ten years, we have demonstrated in this group of patients that the larger this gastric remnant is, the less chance there is of producing disturbed gastric functions resulting in undesirable sequelae. There appears to be no sound justification for resecting any greater amounts of stomach than 25% if combined with a complete bilateral vagectomy. With the type of anastomosis we have used, delayed emptying of the gastric remnant has not occurred, so that any small amount of antrum which may remain along the lesser curvature side of the gastric remnant has not presented any problem and has not shown any evidence of gastric secretory stimulating activity.

The presence of free hydrochloric acid in the fasting stomach postoperatively, in only 3.6% of the cases, most likely is due to an incomplete vagus resection rather than from the antrum remaining in the gastric remnant. Only in 1.2% of the entire series are the free acid determinations above the normal level of 20 mEq.

Nasogastric suction is discontinued as soon as bowel sounds are heard; this usually occurs about the second or third day. Prolonged suction is no longer used even in the presence of delayed gastric emptying. Even though in some patients gastric content is 1,000 cc or more, suction is discontinued. If the patient has distress as a result of overdistention from delayed gastric emptying, intermittent gastric aspiration is performed. With this procedure, prolonged delayed emptying of the gastric remnant has not been a problem. With a more rapid progression and greater liberalization in food intake and with the need of nasogastric suction for only a short period of time, we have not found it advisable or desirable to use gastrostomy. We believe the risks involved are much greater than the program outlined above. The need for prolonged gastric decompression as required by others using different types of operative procedures is not a necessity with our type procedure.

The mortality rate is considered low, in view of the fact that this series does not represent selectivity and has included all deaths occurring within 30 days after surgery; this includes deaths related and unrelated to surgery. Since January, 1961, an additional 28 other operations were performed on very poor risk patients with massive hemorrhage and/or obstruction. These were: 13 pyloroplasty with vagectomy—one death; 2 pyloroplasty without vagectomy—one death; 10 gastroenterostomy with vagectomy—one death; 1 hemigastrectomy with vagectomy and 2 partial gastrectomies without vagectomy—no deaths.

Summary and Conclusions

Distal antrectomy (25% or less) with bilateral vagectomy, Billroth II, antecolic gastrojejunostomy with short afferent jejunal limb continues to be our operation of choice for chronic duodenal ulcer. This is based upon a ten-year experience with 450 operations with a follow-up of over five years in 126 patients and of three years in 208 patients.

The procedure eliminates the two major gastric acid stimulatory phases: neurogenic (cephalic phase) via the vagal pathways and the humoral or hormonal (gastrin) phase via antral stimulation. The pathogenesis of duodenal ulcer is controlled with a minimal disturbance in gastric physiology, function, and gastric reservoir capacity and without practically any undesirable postoperative sequelae. The salutory results are evidenced by lower morbidity and mortality, more rapid rehabilitation, fewer side effects, no dietary restrictions, no diarrhea or dumping syndrome, ease in gaining weight, shorter operating time and hospital stay, least chance for recurrent or marginal ulcer formation, and over-all results superior to those of practically all other operative procedures.

Louis T. Palumbo, MD, Chief Surgical Service, Veterans Administration Center, Des Moines 8, Iowa.

REFERENCES

1. Palumbo, L. T.; Sharpe, W. S.; Lulu, D. J.; Vespa, R.; and Colon-Bonet, J.: Antrectomy With Vagectomy for Chronic Duodenal Ulcer, Surgery 46:1005 (Dec) 1959.

2. Palumbo, L. T.; Sharpe, W. S.; Lulu, D. J.; Vespa, R.; and Colon-Bonet, J.: Antrectomy With Vagectomy or Partial Gastrectomy for Chronic Duodenal Ulcer: A Comparative Analysis, Surg Clin N Amer 39:1697 (Dec) 1959.

3. Palumbo, L. T.; Sharpe, W. S.; Lulu, D. J.; and Vespa, R.: Antrectomy With Bilateral Vagectomy for Chronic Duodenal Ulcer, Scientific Exhibit, Postgrad Med 30:591 (Dec) 1961.

4. Palumbo, L. T.; Sharpe, W. S.; Lulu, D. J.; Bloom, M. H.; and Porter, H. R.: Results in 300 Cases of Antrectomy With Bilateral Vagectomy for Chronic Duodenal Ulcer, Surgery 51:289 (March) 1962.

5. Palumbo, L. T., and Sharpe, W. S.: Antrectomy With Vagectomy for Chronic Duodenal Ulcer, Clin Med 69:1131 (May) 1962.

6. Dragstedt, L. R.: The Etiology of Gastric and Duodenal Ulcers, Postgrad Med 15:99, 1954.

7. Dragstedt, L. R.: Physiology of Gastric Antrum, AMA Arch Surg 75:552, 1957.

8. Dragstedt, L. R.; Oberhelman, H. A., Jr.; Zubiran, J. M.; and Woodward, E. R.: Antrum Motility as a Stimulus for Gastric Secretion, Gastroenterology 24:71, 1953.

Blind Intestinal Loops in Dogs

Effect on Heidenhain Pouch Secretion

JOHN H. LANDOR, MD
W. KERMIT BAKER, MD
AND
DENNIS F. HITE, BA
COLUMBIA, MO

Recent reviews [1,2] have called attention to the blind loop syndrome as a cause for vitamin B_{12} (cyanocobalamin) deficiency and, less commonly, steatorrhea. This syndrome may arise whenever stasis is produced in the small intestine, either by surgical creation of a segment of bowel which does not empty properly or by disease processes such as inflammatory stricture or multiple diverticulae. The clinical manifestations of this entity can usually be controlled, at least temporarily, by the administration of broad-spectrum antibiotics such as chloramphenicol and those of the tetracycline group, and it is felt that an overgrowth of bacteria in the poorly emptying intestinal segment is responsible for the deranged physiology.

Few reports of such cases have included data on gastric secretion, although it has been noted that some patients with the blind loop syndrome who present with a pernicious anemia-like picture have free acid in the stomach aspirate. The following experiment was undertaken in order to determine if the construction of blind intestinal loops in dogs would result in a significant change in gastric pouch secretion and to attempt to elucidate the mechanisms involved in the observed gastric secretory changes.

Submitted for publication July 22, 1963.

From the Department of Surgery, University of Missouri School of Medicine.

This work was supported by grant No. AM-03836-04 from the United States Public Health Service.

Method

A total of 16 mongrel dogs weighing between 12.0 kg and 21.4 kg was utilized. In 12 of these dogs the chronic effect of a blind intestinal loop on the secretion from Heidenhain pouches was measured, and in four dogs a series of acute experiments was performed to test the effect of distention of the small bowel on Heidenhain pouch secretion.

Chronic Experiment.—A Heidenhain pouch was constructed in each of 12 dogs. After recovery from operation the animals were placed on a standard diet of pelleted meal and horsemeat with the daily addition of 5 to 10 gm of sodium chloride. Secretions from the Heidenhain pouches were collected daily. The volume of each specimen was measured carefully, and the free acidity was ascertained by titration with 0.1 N sodium hydroxide to the Toepfer's reagent end point. The daily output of free acid in milliequivalents was then calculated by multiplying the volume in liters by the free acidity in clinical units. After a minimum of 30 such collections the dogs were divided into three groups and subjected to a second surgical procedure.

Group A: In this group of four dogs a "self-filling" blind loop of jejunum was formed. The jejunum was divided approximately 1½ ft distal to the ligament of Treitz, and the proximal end was closed by infolding. The distal end was anastamosed end-to-side to the jejunum at a point 1 ft proximal to the blind end of jejunum, thus creating a "self-filling" blind jejunal loop 1 ft in length. When the animals had recovered from this procedure and were eating normally, the daily output of free acid from the Heidenhain pouches was again determined for a minimum of 30 days. The dogs were then started on oxytetracycline, 250 mg per os three times daily for periods of time ranging between 18 and 33 days. Twenty-four-hour collections of pouch secretions were continued throughout this period and for 14 to 40 days after the antibiotics had been discontinued.

Group B: The four dogs of this group had a similar operation performed except that a 1 ft segment of terminal ileum just proximal to the ileocecal valve was utilized for construction of the "self-filling" blind intestinal loop. After a minimum of 30 daily Heidenhain pouch collections the animals were started on oxytetracycline 250 mg per os three times daily for 21 to 28 days. The postantibiotic observation period varied from 41 to 44 days in this group.

Group C: Two of the four animals in this group were provided with a "self-emptying" blind jejunal loop by dividing the jejunum just distal to the ligament of Treitz, infolding the distal end, and anastomosing the proximal end to the side of the jejunum approximately 1 ft distal to the point of division. In the remaining two dogs a similar "self-emptying" intestinal loop was fashioned from the terminal ileum just proximal to the ileocecal valve. Daily collections of Heidenhain pouch secretions were resumed after recovery from the operations and were continued for 27 to 45 days.

Acute Experiments.—Four dogs were provided with Heidenhain pouches, and, in addition, a segment of small intestine approximately 18 inches in length was completely isolated with intact blood supply. Intestinal continuity was restored by end-to-end anastomosis. The distal end of the isolated segment was closed by an inverting suture, and the proximal end was exteriorized through a stab wound in the abdominal wall so that it formed a cutaneous mucous fistula. In two of the dogs the proximal jejunum was utilized for the isolated segment, and in the remaining two, the distal ileum was isolated. After the animals had recovered from this procedure, they were subjected to a series of experiments in which the effect of saline distention of the isolated segment on pouch secretion was measured. After an 18-hour fast the animals were placed in a stand and rubber balloons were attached to the Heidenhain pouch cannulae for collection of gastric juice. The balloons were emptied at half-hour intervals, and the volume and free acidity of each specimen were determined. After the first one-half hour a Foley catheter was inserted into the cutaneous fistula and the balloon was inflated with 3 to 5 cc of water. The catheter was then connected by means of rubber tubing to a reservoir of isotonic saline which was held at a measured distance above the level of the cutaneous fistula. These distances ranged between 20 and 35 cm. Collections were continued for

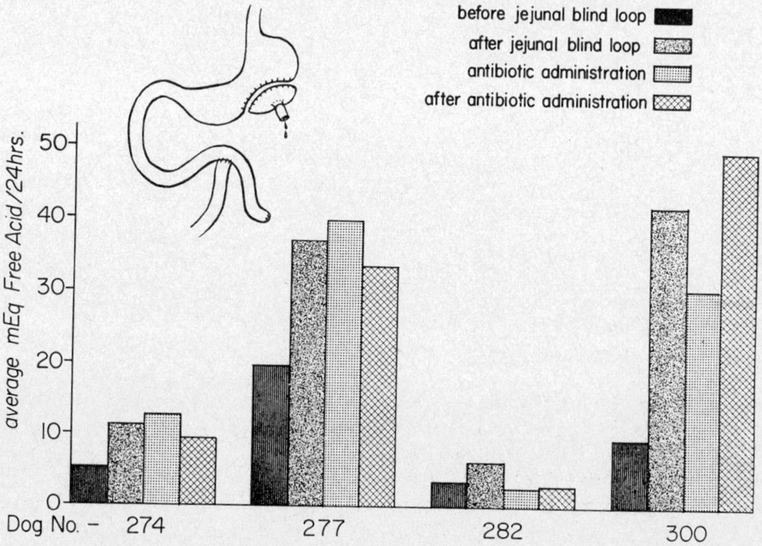

Fig 1.—Average daily secretion in milliequivalents of free acid from Heidenhain pouches in dogs with "self-filling" blind jejunal segments. Secretion during and after antibiotic administration is also depicted.

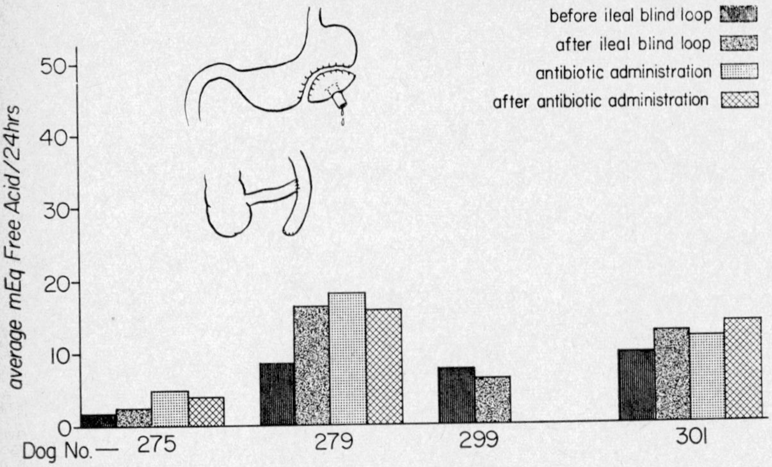

Fig 2.—Average daily secretion in milliequivalents of free acid from Heidenhain pouches in dogs with "self-filling" blind ileal segments. Secretion during and after antibiotic administration (oxytetracycline) is also depicted.

two to four hours, and, in those instances where gastric secretory responses were obtained, the secretion was usually followed after discontinuing the saline distention. In all, 20 such experiments were performed.

Results

Chronic Experiment.—As seen in Fig 1, all four animals who underwent construction of a "self-filling" blind jejunal loop had a significant increase in Heidenhain pouch secretion after this procedure. The average daily secretion for the four dogs was 10.5 mEq of free acid prior to creation of the blind loop and 24.1 mEq of free acid after. Two dogs exhibited a decrease in gastric secretion while receiving oxytetracycline but in only one of these was there a return of secretion to previous levels after cessation of antibiotic therapy. Fig 2 gives the results in the group with "self-filling" ileal blind loops. Here the "preloop" secretion averaged 6.6 mEq of free acid and the "postloop" secretion averaged 9.2 mEq of free acid. Dog No. 299 died before oxytetracycline therapy was instituted, and the remaining animals showed no consistent change in Heidenhain pouch secretion during oxytetracycline therapy. Fig 3 illustrates the secretory results in the animals with "self-emptying" jejunal and ileal loops. There was no significant change in secretion in any of the dogs in this group.

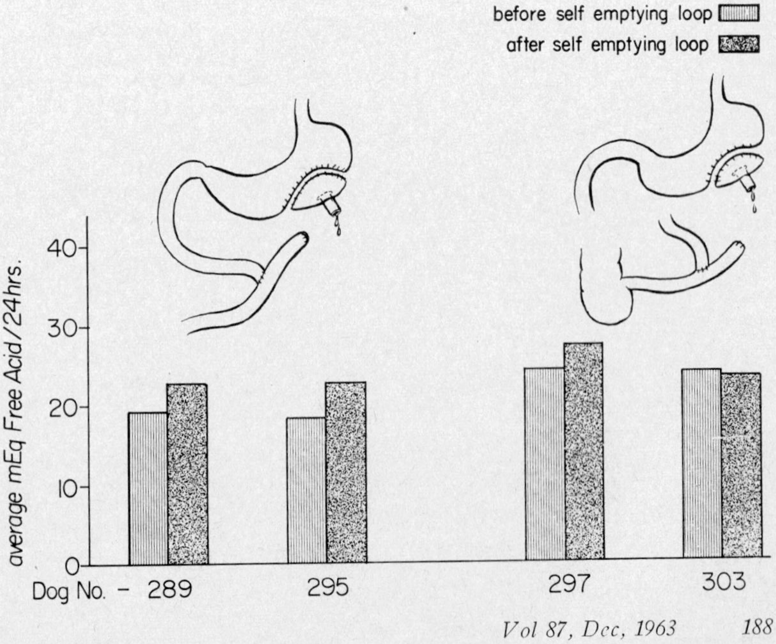

Fig 3.—Average daily secretion in milliequivalents of free acid from Heidenhain pouches in dogs with "self-emptying" jejunal (No. 289 and 295) and ileal (No. 297 and 303) blind segments.

Acute Experiment.—Isolated jejunal loops were distended a total of 11 times, and ileal loops were distended nine times. A positive secretory response was obtained from the Heidenhain pouches in five of the experiments with jejunal distention and in five of the experiments with ileal distention. In those experiments where a gastric secretory response was not obtained there was usually evidence of nausea (increased salivation and restlessness), and in some experiments there was frank retching. In general, nausea and a negative secretory response were more likely to occur when the level of saline in the reservoir was placed higher than 25 cm above the cutaneous fistula, although there were rather marked individual differences among the dogs in their ability to tolerate distention in the higher pressure ranges. A representative experiment in which a positive secretory response was obtained is depicted in Fig 4.

Comment

Although there was little or no increase in Heidenhain pouch secretion after construction of a "self-filling" blind loop of ileum, striking increase in pouch secretion occurred in all dogs after creation of a similar blind loop of jejunum. This increase in acid secretion can be assumed to be humoral rather than nervous in origin because of the lack of vagal innervation in the stomach

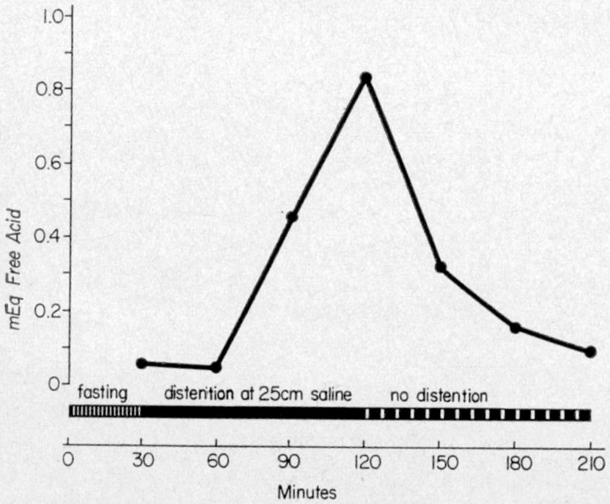

Fig 4.—Representative secretory response of a Heidenhain pouch to distention of an isolated segment of jejunum with saline. The output of free acid in milliequivalents is plotted for successive 30-minute periods.

pouches utilized. In seeking an explanation for the gastric hypersecretion seen in association with blind jejunal loops, factors which deserve consideration as possible inciting causes are: (1) overgrowth of intestinal bacteria in the blind jejunal segments; (2) removal of a short segment of jejunum from its normal location in the intestinal stream; and (3) chronic distention of the blind portion of small intestine.

Administration of a broad-spectrum antibiotic usually suppresses bacterial overgrowth in blind loops, thereby alleviating the vitamin B_{12} deficiency and/or steatorrhea seen clinically in the blind loop syndrome. Since the giving of oxytetracycline failed to abolish consistently the gastric hypersecretion seen in the dogs with jejunal blind loops, it would seem unlikely that the increase in gastric secretion was dependent upon the altered bacterial flora generally found in such blind intestinal segments. That the observed gastric hypersecretion did not result from removal of a segment of small bowel from normal continuity is apparent from the fact that creation of "self-emptying" loops of jejunum and ileum failed to bring about significant augmentation of Heidenhain pouch secretion in any of the four animals in which this procedure was carried out.

On the other hand, acute distention of small bowel is known to exert a stimulatory influence on gastric secretion,[3,4] and it may well be that chronic distention of a "self-filling" blind loop would have a similar gastric secretory effect. That distention did indeed occur is attested to by the finding of marked elongation and dilatation in the majority of such loops at autopsy. The acute experiments reported herein confirm the fact that small bowel distention is an adequate stimulus to gastric secretion. Of particular relevance is the fact that these acute studies were carried out by fluid distention of isolated loops which resembled the "self-filling" blind loops utilized in the chronic secretory experiments, ie, the distal end of the segment was closed and proximal end was open for ingress of fluid.

Attractive as is the hypothesis that chronic distention of the blind jejunal loops provided the stimulus for gastric hypersecretion, it must be admitted that this explanation has by no means been proved conclusively by the above observations. Somewhat in conflict with the stated hypothesis is the observation that acute distention of both jejunum and ileum led to an increase in gastric pouch secretion whereas chronic increases in secretion were seen only in dogs with jejunal blind loops and not in those with ileal blind loops. Another finding which, at first glance, appears to be inconsistent with the theory of small bowel distention as a cause for gastric hypersecretion is the failure to obtain positive gastric secretory responses in all experiments with saline distention of isolated bowel segments. However, nausea was noted in the majority of the negative experiments, and, as shown by Grossman et al,[5] nausea acts as a potent inhibitor of gastric secretion, apparently via a hormonal or vascular mechanism. It is possible that, in those few instances where saline distention yielded negative gastric secretory responses in the absence of overt nausea, subclinical nausea without outward manifestation was present to a degree sufficient enough to suppress gastric secretion. Sircus [3] has previously shown that balloon distention of a Thiry-Vella loop of duodenum or jejunum at 15-30 mm of mercury pressure caused a gastric secretory response, whereas distention at pressures above 30 mm of mercury produced restlessness or nausea and no gastric response.

Despite these inconsistencies it is our feeling that chronic jejunal distention most likely accounted for the gastric hypersecretion associated with "self-filling" blind jejunal loops. We have no satisfactory explanation for the fact that gastric hypersecretion was not observed after formation of similar blind loops of ileum, although it is possible that changes in the consistency of intestinal chyme between the proximal jejunum and distal ileum may account for this difference. Whether chronic distention of blind loops of small bowel in patients could result in increases in gastric secretion of a magnitude sufficient to produce peptic ulceration or contribute to the peptic ulcer diathesis remains a matter for speculation. Careful gastric secretory studies on patients before and after surgical correction of intestinal abnormalities responsible for the blind loop syndrome would be of great interest.

Summary

Surgical creation of "self-filling" blind jejunal loops in dogs with Heidenhain pouches brought about a marked increase in gastric pouch secretion. Such an increase in secretion was not observed when similar blind loops of ileum were formed, nor was it seen in animals with "self-emptying" segments of jejunum or ileum. The administration of a broad-spectrum antibiotic (oxytetracycline) did not consistently abolish the gastric hypersecretion seen in the animals with "self-filling" blind jejunal segments. Since distention of isolated segments of small bowel with saline brought about an increase in Heidenhain pouch secretion, it is postulated that chronic distention of the jejunal segments provided the stimulus for the increased Heidenhain pouch secretion observed in the animals with "self-filling" blind loops of jejunum.

Mr. Robert Ziervogel of Charles Pfizer and Co., Inc., supplied the oxytetracycline (Terramycin) used in this experiment.

John H. Landor, MD, Department of Surgery, University of Missouri Medical Center, Columbia, Mo.

REFERENCES

1. Reilly, R. W., and Kirsner, J. B.: Blind Loop Syndrome, Gastroenterology 37:491, 1959.

2. Starzl, T. E.; Butz, G. W., Jr.; and Hartman, C. F.: The Blind-Loop Syndrome After Gastric Operations, Surgery 50:849, 1961.

3. Sircus, W.: The Intestinal Phase of Gastric Secretion, Quart J Exp Physiol 38:91, 1953.

4. Nagano, K.; Johnson, A. N., Jr.; Cobo, A.; Oberhelman, H. A., Jr.; and Dragstedt, L. R.: The Effect of Distention of the Duodenum on Gastric Secretion, Surg Forum 10:152, 1959.

5. Grossman, M. I.; Woolley, J. R.; Dutton, D. F.; and Ivy, A. C.: The Effect of Nausea on Gastric Secretion and a Study of the Mechanism Concerned, Gastroenterology 4:347, 1945.

Pancreatitis as a Complication of Operation

CHARLES F. FREY, MD
AND
JOHN M. BEAL, MD
NEW YORK

Pancreatitis is a serious complication in the postoperative period which has been associated with a high mortality rate. The incidence of postoperative pancreatitis is uncertain, although it has been considered to be infrequent. The recent appearance of a number of reports raises some questions as to its rarity.[3-5,9,15,16]

The experience of the pavilion service of The New York Hospital has been reviewed to study the clinical features of postoperative pancreatitis and to assess factors that seem to contribute to a fatal outcome.

Clinical Material

Pancreatitis occurred in 52 patients who had been subjected to a variety of surgical procedures from 1939-1960. Thirty-one patients were women, and 21 were men. Their average age was 52 years.

The operations that preceded the onset of pancreatitis have been listed in Table 1. The development of this complication was encountered in 40 patients after intra-abdominal procedures and in seven patients after procedures upon the urinary tract. In five patients the operation did not involve entry into the peritoneal cavity.

Postoperative pancreatitis was encountered most frequently when the pancreas was the site of the initial operation. There was little numerical difference in the incidence of this complication after operations upon the stomach, kidney, and biliary tract. However, when the frequency of these operations is considered, the actual frequency of pancreatitis after operations upon the biliary tract was low.

Submitted for publication Aug 1, 1963.

The Department of Surgery, The New York Hospital-Cornell Medical Center.

Evidence of pancreatitis was present from the first postoperative day to 60 days later. The average interval of the onset of symptoms which were attributed to pancreatitis was five days after operation, though unrecognized symptoms may have been present sooner. Relationship could not be established between the onset of symptoms and the subsequent course of the patient, with the exception of

TABLE 1.—*Pancreatitis as a Complication of Operation*

Site of Operation and Procedure		No. Patients
Biliary tract		9
Cholecystectomy	6	
Cholecystectomy & choledochotomy	3	
Stomach		7
Partial gastrectomy with gastrojejunostomy	7	
Pancreas		15
Radical pancreatoduodenectomy	7	
Biopsy	5	
Enucleation of islet cell tumor	2	
Splenectomy and biopsy of pancreas	1	
Miscellaneous intra-abdominal		9
Splenectomy	1	
Adrenalectomy	1	
Resection of hepatic flexure of colon	1	
Appendectomy with drainage	1	
Endarterectomy, superior mesenteric artery and small bowel resection	1	
Colostomy	2	
Ileostomy	1	
Portocaval shunt	1	
Urinary tract		7
Pyeloureteroplasty	3	
Transurethral resection of prostate	2	
Segmental resection of bladder	2	
Miscellaneous		5
Therapeutic abortion	1	
Craniotomy	1	
Cocaine reaction	1	
Thyroidectomy	1	
Biopsy	1	
Total		52

pseudocyst formation where symptomatology was often delayed in onset.

Pain is often difficult to assess after abdominal operations, particularly with an upper abdominal incision. However, pain which seems to be out of proportion to the operative procedure, together with unexplained fever and significant distention of ileus is a symptom complex in which postoperative pancreatitis must be included in the differential diagnosis. Tachycardia or the presence of an abdominal mass were often noted in association with these findings.

Associated systemic diseases were present in 31 patients. These problems included marked obesity in five, hypertensive cardiovascular disease in five, and Laennec's cirrhosis in two. Diabetes mellitus was present in two patients, and tuberculous peritonitis in one. Chronic cholecystitis and cholelithiasis was found in four of the patients who had postmortem examinations and in one patient at the time of a subsequent laparotomy.

Intra-abdominal neoplasms were present in 11 patients. These consisted of carcinoma of the ampulla of Vater in three, benign islet cell tumors of the pancreas in two, and carcinoma of the duodenum, stomach, liver, and parathyroid in one instance each. Intra-abdominal carcinomatosis was found in one patient, and lymphosarcoma of the stomach in another.

Diagnosis

Establishment of the diagnosis of pancreatitis in the postoperative period is difficult. This complication was detected prior to autopsy or laparotomy in less than half of the 52 patients in this series. Often the clinical impression was that some other acute abdominal problem was present, such as peritonitis, perforated viscus, or acute cholecystitis. The similarity between the manifestations of pancreatitis and other acute intra-abdominal diseases is a factor in the difficulty of differential diagnosis. The clinical course and determination of serum amylase levels can be correlated with and may establish the presence of pancreatitis in most of these patients. Appearance of a pancreatic fistula or abdominal mass representing a pseudocyst of the pancreas made diagnosis obvious in a few patients. The patients with pseudocysts usually had symptoms of nausea, vomiting, abdominal pain, and tachycardia early in their course. These symptoms usually preceded the development of a mass or fistula.

Laboratory Data

White blood cell counts were elevated above 10,000 cu mm in 41 of 44 patients. Eight patients did not have white blood cell counts during the immediate postoperative period. Serum amylase levels were elevated in 27 of 29 patients. Twenty-three patients did not have amylase determinations. Albuminuria was present in 31 of 35 patients whose urine was examined during the postoperative period.

Blood urea nitrogen levels were normal in 18 of 23 survivors of postoperative pancreatitis. Determinations of blood urea nitrogen were not obtained in three patients, while elevated levels were found in two survivors. Sixteen of 25 patients who died of postoperative pancreatitis demonstrated blood urea nitrogen retention after the onset of postoperative pancreatitis. Normal values had been established preoperatively in ten of these patients. Five patients who died had normal blood urea nitrogen levels before and after operation. There were four patients in whom blood urea nitrogen values were not obtained.

Course and Treatment

Survivors.—Twenty-seven of 52 patients with postoperative pancreatitis survived hospitalization. Four of these patients later died after leaving the hospital. When the four patients that died after leaving the hospital are excluded, 16 of the remaining 23 survivors were subjected to additional laparotomy prior to discharge because of the symptomatology which resulted from postoperative pancreatitis (Table 2).

Six of those who required another operation had pseudocysts of the pancreas. Pseudocysts developed subsequent to biopsy of the pancreas in three patients, after an enucleation of an islet cell tumor and after transection of the pancreas for carcinoma. One patient who suffered damage to the tail of the pancreas at the time of left adrenalectomy was found to have black silk sutures at the base of a pseudocyst. External drainage or marsupialization was carried out in four of these patients, and primary excision was

TABLE 2.—*Secondary Operations in Patients With Postoperative Pancreatitis*

Organ or Anatomical Area Initially Operated Upon	Operative Procedure Performed at Re-Exploration	No. Patients	Pancreatic Pathology
	Group Surviving Hospitalization		
Cholecystectomy	Exploratory laparotomy	2	Acute (2)
	Gastrojejunostomy for pyloric obstruction	1	Acute (1)
Partial gastrectomy	Exploratory laparotomy	4	Chronic (1) Acute (3)
	Cholecystojejunostomy for common duct injury	1	Acute (1)
Pancreas	Exploratory laparotomy		
	Incision and drainage	3	Pseudocyst (3)
	Excision	2	Pseudocyst (2)
	Radical pancreatoduodenectomy for Ca. ampulla of Vater	1	Acute (1)
Other Abdominal Organs	Exploratory laparotomy; incision and drainage	1	Pseudocyst (1)
Urinary Tract	Cholecystectomy	1	Acute (1)
	Group That Died		
Postmortem			
Partial gastrectomy	Exploratory laparotomy	1	Acute (1)
Pancreas	Exploratory laparotomy	1	Hemorrhagic (1)
Death, but no postmortem			
Pancreas	Exploratory laparotomy; incision and drainage	1	Pseudocyst (1)
	Exploratory laparotomy; excision sinus tract	1	Pancreatic fistula (1)
	Death After Hospital Discharge		
Pancreas	Exploratory laparotomy	1	Acute (1)
	Incision and drainage	1	Pseudocyst (1)
	Excision sinus tract	1	Pancreatic fistula (1)

undertaken in two. Pancreatic drainage persisted for from two to six months in the patients with external drainage or marsupialization of the pseudocyst. Primary excision was successful in one patient. The other developed a pancreatic fistula which closed after four months.

Four patients underwent procedures designed to improve the nutrition of the patient or removal of the causes of pancreatic or common duct obstruction or biliary disease. These procedures were gastrojejunostomy for pyloric canal obstruction, cholecystojejunostomy for common duct obstruction, cholecystectomy for cholelithiasis, and radical pancreatoduodenectomy for carcinoma of the ampulla of Vater. Six patients were subjected to exploratory laparotomy, at which time the diagnosis of pancreatitis was made but specific therapy did not seem indicated. Eight patients with postoperative pancreatitis were treated by conservative measures only, which consisted of nasogastric tube decompression, intravenous fluids, and antispasmodics.

Death After Hospital Discharge.—Four patients after surviving hospitalization died three days to two years after hospital discharge. Two of these patients had carcinoma of the ampulla of Vater, one carcinoma of the pancreas, and one a pseudocyst of the pancreas.

Three of these patients had been subjected to secondary laparotomy before leaving the hospital. A pancreatic fistula was excised in one patient, and a pseudocyst marsupialized in another. Exploratory laparotomy alone was performed in the third patient.

Hospital Deaths.—Twenty-five patients did not leave the hospital but died from postoperative pancreatitis. Postmortem examination was performed on all but two patients. Only four of these patients were subjected to secondary laparotomy. Incision and drainage of a pseudocyst was performed in one patient and excision of a pancreatic fistula in another. Laparotomy alone was performed in two patients.

In order to determine if additional surgery might have salvaged some of the 23 patients who died, the postmortem findings were reviewed for evidence of untreated biliary abscesses, fistulae, or cholelithiasis. Of the 23 patients examined at autopsy five had cholelithiasis and chronic cholecystitis, one a pancreatic and biliary fistula, and another a perforation of the duodenum. A pancreatic fistula was present in one patient, and another had pancreatic hemorrhage. It was considered that operative correction could have been beneficial to six of these patients. However, the majority of patients who died did not have pancreatic biliary obstruction, biliary disease (unrecognized) or fistulae, or other surgical conditions that appeared suitable for correction by further operation.

Pathologic Studies

The pancreas of 23 patients examined at autopsy showed hemorrhagic changes in ten, acute necrotic changes in three, acute edematous changes in four, and predominantly chronic changes in six patients. The average survival of these groups of patients was 17, 18, 5, and 44 days after the onset of pancreatitis. Pancreatitis was the chief cause of death in all patients but five, in whom other conditions contributed significantly. These conditions were superior mesenteric artery thrombosis, *Escherichia coli* septicemia, secondary pyelonephritis, metastatic carcinoma of the parathyroid, generalized peritonitis secondary to colon perforation, and abdominal carcinomatosis.

Of the 23 patients examined at autopsy, 11 showed gross and microscopic evidence of liver dysfunction. Fatty metamorphosis of the liver was noted in six patients, cirrhosis of the liver in two, and central necrosis of the liver in two. One patient with abdominal carcinomatosis had extensive liver metastases.

Nine patients showed gross and microscopic evidence of renal disease. Five additional patients had oliguria and elevated blood urea nitrogen levels during life, though gross and microscopic findings in the kidneys were considered normal. The kidneys at autopsy demonstrated tubular necrosis in three patients, arterionephrosclerosis in two, and, in one patient each, pyelonephritis and thromboembolism with renal infarcts, and nephrolithiasis, pyelonephritis, and renal cysts.

Eight of the ten patients with hemorrhagic pancreatitis demonstrated elevation of the blood urea nitrogen levels (seven patients) and/or anatomical evidence of renal disease (six patients). Of these eight patients, four had liver disease manifested by cirrhosis in two, necrosis in one, and fatty metamorphosis in the other. One patient who had liver necrosis without anatomical renal disease did not have a blood urea nitrogen determination. One patient with a normal blood urea nitrogen test demonstrated no anatomical liver or renal disease.

All three patients with acute necrotic pancreatitis demonstrated elevation of the blood urea nitrogen (two) or anatomical evidence of renal disease (two). Two of these three patients also had fatty metamorphosis of the liver.

One of the four patients with acute edematous pancreatitis demonstrated both elevation of the blood urea nitrogen levels and anatomical renal disease. Of three patients who did not have anatomical renal disease, two had normal blood urea nitrogen levels, while the third was not tested. Two of the three patients without renal disease showed fatty metamorphosis of the liver.

Five of the six patients in whom changes of chronic pancreatitis predominated demonstrated either elevation of the blood urea nitrogen (four) or anatomical renal disease (three). One of these patients also demonstrated fatty metamorphosis of the liver. The one patient without renal dysfunction showed fatty metamorphosis of the liver.

Comment

The mortality rates associated with postoperative pancreatitis have been related to three general factors: difficulty in diagnosis, frequency of hemorrhagic necrosis in established cases, and the lack of specific therapy.

The mortality rate of 48% in the present series is comparable to other reports,[6,8,13] but the validity of this figure may be questioned when it is noted that the diagnosis was made at autopsy in approximately half of the cases. Presumably many cases of postoperative pancreatitis not serious enough to cause death also went undiagnosed clinically. The original operation appeared to influence survival. Only seven (22%) of the 31 patients died when they developed pancreatitis after operations upon the biliary tract, pancreas, or stomach. In contrast, pancreatitis was least suspected after operations on organs outside the peritoneal cavity or not contiguous to the pancreas and was associated with a fatal outcome in 16 (80%) of 21 patients.

The serious nature of established severe pancreatitis was emphasized by the autopsy findings. Thirteen of the 23 patients who were examined had marked pathological changes in the pancreas, hemorrhagic changes in ten and acute necrosis in three. The frequency of hepatic and renal disease was striking in the patients that died. It is difficult to correlate precisely the changes in the liver and kidneys with the degree of pancreatitis, but the incidence of pathological hepatic and renal changes was greater in patients with hemorrhagic pancreatitis. An increase in blood urea nitrogen levels accompanied the onset of pancreatitis in 83% of the fatal cases. Thus, pancreatitis in patients with liver and kidney disease was associated with an increased mortality rate.

Often the signs and symptoms of postoperative pancreatitis are nonspecific or atypical. Consequently, an awareness of conditions which may predispose to the development of pancreatitis is important. Direct surgical trauma to the pancreas during procedures on this organ or organs in close proximity may lead to postoperative pancreatitis. Injury, inflammation, edema, obstructing the common or pancreatic duct by stone, and obstruction of the afferent limb of a gastrojejunostomy have also been noted as events which may be followed by pancreatitis.

Pancreatitis after procedures on organs not contiguous to the pancreas may be of vascular origin in some patients. Thrombi were often noted in veins or capillaries in fatal pancreatitis by Thal.[14] Development of pancreatic thrombi in patients whose operations are spatially distant from the pancreas have been noted in patients with red cell hemolysis after transurethral resection [8] or transfusion reactions.[1]

The effects of aging on the pancreatic ductal system and the increasing viscosity of pancreatic secretions during periods of dehydration associated with the operative period may predispose to pancreatitis. Berman, with the use of vinyl acetate casts, has demonstrated that the pancreatic ductal system becomes tortuous, kinked, and partially obstructed with increasing age.[2] Viscous plugs of secretion may develop in the pancreatic ducts when patients are not receiving oral intake. When oral feeding is begun, the combination of a secreting gland and an obstructed ductal system may lead to pancreatitis.

Reduction in mortality rate should follow the prompt institution of therapy when the diagnosis of pancreatitis is made soon after the signs and symptoms appear. The initial therapy is directed toward the control of secretion by the administration of anticholinergic drugs. This is supplemented by vasogastric decompression, adequate fluid, albumin and/or plasma, and whole blood replacement.[7,11,12] The frequent occurrence of renal and liver dysfunction in fatal pancreatitis suggests the importance of maintenance of adequate nutrition and of an effective circulating blood volume. Prevention of shock may help protect liver and kidney function, particularly in the more severe forms of pancreatitis.

Complications associated with postoperative pancreatitis which could have been corrected surgically were present in at least six of the 23 patients examined at autopsy. The group that was treated by laparotomy had a much lower mortality rate than those who were not. This indicates the advisability of surgical intervention if conservative measures are not followed by clinical and laboratory improvement. The analysis of our experience has indicated that the mortality rate of postoperative pancreatitis could have been reduced by earlier diagnosis and a more aggressive surgical approach.

Summary

The clinical, laboratory, and postmortem findings in 52 patients with postoperative pancreatitis have been discussed. It is suggested that the incidence of postoperative pancreatitis is higher and the mortality rate lower than is commonly reported in the literature.

Mortality is increased with the hemorrhagic form of pancreatitis and with hepatic and renal dysfunction, present in 83% of the patients who died.

Treatment may be improved if a clinical diagnosis of pancreatitis is established, attention directed to fluid and nutritional requirements, and complications amenable to surgery recognized and treated.

John M. Beal, MD, Department of Surgery, Northwestern University Medical School, 303 E Chicago Ave, Chicago 11, Ill.

REFERENCES

1. Ackerman, L. V.: Acute Pancreatitis Following Blood Transfusions, Arch Path 34:1065-1069, 1942.

2. Berman, L. G.; Prior, J. T.; Abramow, S. M.; and Ziegler, D. D.: A Study of the Pancreatic Duct System in Man by Use of Vinyl Acetate Casts of Postmortem Preparations, Surg Gynec Obstet 110:391-403, 1960.

3. Boles, T.: Postoperative Pancreatitis, Bull Mason Clin 8:15-26, 1954.

4. Burnett, W. E.; Rosemond, G. P.; Caswell, H. T.; Beauchamp, E. W., Jr.; Tyson, R. R.; and Wright, W. C.: Studies on So-Called Postgastrectomy Pancreatitis, Trans Southern Surg Ass 70:145-154, 1958.

5. Burton, C. C.; Eckman, W. G., Jr.; and Haxo, J.: Acute Postgastrectomy Pancreatitis, Amer J Surg 94:70-79, 1957.

6. Diffenbaugh, W. G., and Strohl, L. L.: Acute Hemorrhagic Pancreatitis Following Biliary Tract Procedures, AMA Arch Surg 72:931-941, 1956.

7. Elliot, D. W.: The Mechanism of Benefit Derived From Concentrated Human Serum Albumin in Experimental Acute Pancreatitis, Surg Forum 5:384-390, 1954.

8. Ferris, D. O.; Lynn, T. E.; Cain, J. C.; and Baggenstoss, A. H.: Fatal Postoperative Pancreatitis, Ann Surg 146:263-273, 1957.

9. Frieden, J. H.: Postoperative Acute Pancreatitis, Surg Gynec Obstet 102:139-144, 1956.

10. Hardaway, R. M., and McKay, D. G.: Production of Acute Hemorrhagic Pancreatitis in Dogs by Means of an Episode of Intravascular Clotting in the Pancreas, Surgery 45:557-561, 1959.

11. Keith, L. M., and Watman, R. N.: Blood Volume Deficits in Pancreatitis, Surg Forum 5:381-384, 1954.

12. Kenwell, H. N., and Wels, P. B.: Acute Hemorrhagic Pancreatitis: Report of 11 Consecutive Cases Treated With Human Serum Albumin, Surg Gynec Obstet 96:169-170, 1953.

13. Ponka, J. L.; Landrum, S. E.; and Chaikof, L.: Acute Pancreatitis in the Postoperative Patient, Arch Surg 83:475-486, 1961.

14. Thal, A. P.; Perry, J. F.; and Egner, W.: A Clinical and Morphologic Study of 42 Cases of Fatal Acute Pancreatitis, Quart Rev Obstet Gynec 15:10-12, 1958.

15. Thompson, J. A.; Howard, J. M.; and Vowles, D. J.: Acute Pancreatitis Following Choledochostomy, Surg Gynec Obstet 105:706-710, 1957.

16. Warren, K. W., and Cattell, R. B.: Pancreatic Surgery, New Eng J Med 261:280-288 and 333-340, 1959.

Influence of Direction of Aortic Perfusion on Regional Blood Flow

WORTHINGTON G. SCHENK, JR., MD
LAWRENCE A. POLLOCK, MD
KJARTAN B. KJARTANSSON, MD
AND
N. ANDERS DELIN, MD
BUFFALO

Whole body perfusion has been carried out by using several arteries for the inflow site, most often a femoral or subclavian artery. Use of a femoral artery for inflow results in retrograde flow through the aorta, while subclavian cannulation permits flow in the conventional direction except to the more proximal aortic arch outflow. The varying angle formed by aortic branches in leaving the aorta suggests the possibility that this angle is of importance in determining distribution of aortic outflow, and hence such distribution might be altered by changing direction of aortic flow. This study was designed to determine whether alteration in distribution to aortic outflow branches occurred on changing from antegrade to retrograde perfusion.

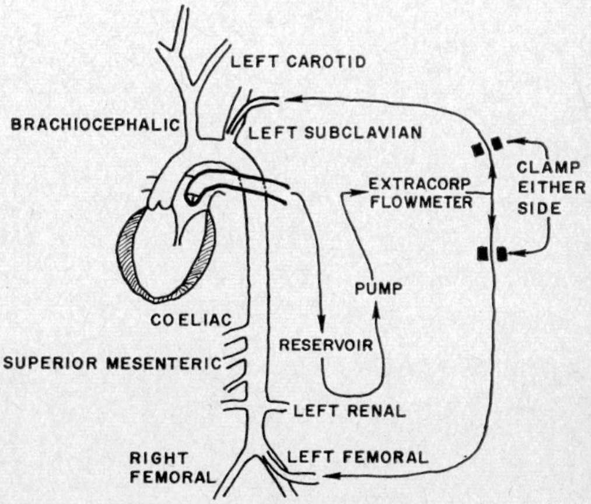

Schema of experimental setup.

Submitted for publication Aug 19, 1963.

From the Department of Surgery, State University of New York at Buffalo, and the Edward J. Meyer Memorial Hospital.

Supported in part by United States Public Health Service grant No. HE 03181 of the National Heart Institute.

Results of Experiments

Exp. No.	Wt/Kg	Carotid: SC Fem.	Carotid: % Change	Femoral: SC Fem.	Femoral: % Change	L. Renal: SC Fem.	L. Renal: % Change	Sup. Mes.: SC Fem.	Sup. Mes.: % Change
1	19	224→224	0	66.5→ 38	42 ↓	155→155	0		
		212←198	7 ↑			155←155	0		
2 *	20	241←241	0	133←133	0			666→640	4 ↑
		245→245	0	133→114	14 ↓			699←699	0
3 *	18	111←124	10 ↓	49→ 34	30 ↓	118→112	5 ↓		
		155→136	12 ↓	34→ 49	30 ↑	124←124	0		
4	25			76← 70	9 ↑	149←149	0		
				76→ 61	20 ↓	161→161	0		
5 †	18	157→185	9 ↑	49.5← 46.5	6 ↑				
		164←170	3 ↓						
6 †	24								
7	25	250←250	0	70← 70	0	120→120	0		
		100→100	0	40← 40	0	60→ 60	0		
8 *	27	495←495	0	210→248	18 ↑	245→224	4 ↓		
9 †	17	207→244	18 ↑	63→ 61	3 ↓				
		178←216	18 ↓						
Mean change			6		14		1		2

(Regional Vessel Being Studied: Carotid, Femoral, L. Renal, Sup. Mes.; SC / Fem. = Vessel Used For Inflow)

* Ascending aorta clamped.
† Heart fibrillating.
→ indicates direction inflow switched.

Methods

Under light intravenous sodium pentobarbital anesthesia, left thoracotomy was performed in nine mongrel dogs. Gravity drainage of the left atrium was carried out by inserting a large stainless steel cannula through the left atrial appendage. The left subclavian and left femoral arteries were cannulated with thin-wall stainless steel cannulas of identical internal diameter. After heparinization, left ventricular bypass was performed as shown schematically in the Figure. With this system it was possible to make a virtually instantaneous shift from femoral to subclavian inflow, thus reversing the flow through the aorta. Flow was measured through each of the labeled vessels by using the squarewave electromagnetic flowmeter * of Denison and Spencer,[2] and miniature noncannulating probes.† Total perfusion was measured from the extracorporeal probe. Rapid switching from one probe to another was possible by use of a special probe switch-box.‡ In most instances, flow through specific vessels of distribution was made during switch of inflow from subclavian to femoral and back to subclavian again, or the reverse, in random fashion. The renal and splanchnic arteries were exposed through a retroperitoneal approach in the left flank. Different groups of vessels were studied in different experiments for technical reasons of vessel exposure. Most animals were perfused in excess of 100 cc/kg/min and none less than 80 cc/kg/min.

* Carolina Medical Electronics, Winston-Salem, NC.

† Electromagnetic Probe Co., Winston-Salem, NC.

‡ Carolina Medical Electronics, Winston-Salem, NC.

Results

In only rare instances did total perfusion flow alter on switch from one input site to the other. Regional flow data are included only if total perfusion was unchanged after switching of inflow site. All the regional flow data are shown in the Table. In no instance was there a significant or reproducible redistribution of flow on reversal of aortic flow through the perfusion circuit.

In three animals the ascending aorta was clamped during the experiment to be sure the left ventricle was not contributing to aortic flow. In three animals the experiment was performed with the heart fibrillating throughout the study. No alteration in distribution occurred in either instance. Reduction of pump flow as in experiment 7 reduced branch flow but not distribution according to the site of inflow.

Celiac Axis		Brachiocephalic		
S C Fem.	% Change	S C Fem.	% Change	Pump Flow, Cc/Min
				3,200
325←325	0			2,200
112←128	12↓			
134←168	14↓			2,400
180←180	0	335→335	0	2,600
180→180	0	335←335	0	
				1,600
		465→416	10	1,900
				3,200
				2,400
				2,800
				1,400
	6		3	

Comment

We are only aware of one other study aimed at investigating this specific point, that performed by Camishion, Ota, and Gibbon,[1] in which flow through the superior mesenteric artery was measured with antegrade and retrograde aortic perfusion. The findings here reported support their evidence—that direction of inflow produced no alteration in superior mesenteric artery flow. From this evidence it would appear that direction of inflow is of no consequence during perfusion, at least for short periods of time.

Summary

Blood flow in the carotid, femoral, renal, superior mesenteric, celiac, and brachiocephalic arteries was studied during sudden switching from subclavian to femoral artery inflow in a left ventricular bypass perfusion circuit.

No significant or consistent alteration in flow occurred in any of the vessels studied on switching from antegrade to retrograde aortic flow or vice versa.

Worthington G. Schenk, Jr., MD, 462 Grider St, Buffalo 15, NY.

REFERENCES

1. Camishion, R. C.; Ota, Y.; and Gibbon, J. H., Jr.: Blood Flow Thru the Superior Mesenteric Artery With Antegrade and Retrograde Perfusion of the Aorta, Circulation 24:900, 1961.

2. Denison, A. B., Jr., and Spencer, M. P.: Squarewave Electromagnetic Flowmeter Design, Rev Sci Instruments 27:707, 1956.

Bacteriological Studies in Pulmonary Atelectasis

W. G. JAMIESON, MD
AND
A. M. LANSING, MD., PhD,
FRCS (C)
LONDON, ONT, CANADA

Previous experiments in dogs demonstrated that the fever in experimental atelectasis was caused by sympathetic vasoconstriction stimulated by bacterial infection in the collapsed segment.[1] The tachycardia was also of sympathetic origin, while the tachypnea was caused partly by bacterial infection and partly by the associated decreased arterial oxygen saturation and decreased lung volume. Certain questions remained to be answered, however. These included the importance of species variation; the role of inadvertant bronchial contamination at the time of plug insertion; and the effect of prolonged antibiotic administration on the bacterial flora in the atelectatic segment. The earlier bacteriological studies in dogs have been extended and observations in cats and humans added in an attempt to answer these problems.

Submitted for publication Aug 12, 1963.

MRC Fellow in Physiology, Resident in Surgery (Dr. Jamieson); Markle Scholar in Medical Science, presently Associate Professor of Surgery, University of Louisville School of Medicine, Louisville, Ky (Dr. Lansing).

From the Departments of Physiology and Surgery, University of Western Ontario, London, Canada.

The investigation was supported by an Ontario Heart Foundation Research Grant.

Methods

The experimental animals were devocalized mongrel dogs of both sexes weighing 20 to 40 lb and cats of both sexes weighing 5 to 12 lb. Anesthesia was induced with hexobarbital, 15 mg/lb, administered intravenously in the dogs and intraperitoneally in the cats. Complete recovery from anesthesia occurred in 30 to 60 minutes at most, although the animals responded to bronchoscopic stimulation within five minutes.

Atelectasis was produced by insertion of an absorbent cotton plug into the left main bronchus. Biopsy forceps were used for its insertion through a No. 8 Nygus bronchoscope in the dogs and a No. 5 bronchoscope in the cats. Care was taken to occlude the bronchus completely, one to four cotton plugs being inserted in each animal. Although in the first few animals the instruments and cotton plugs were merely clean, in most of the experiments a sterile technique was employed.

Criteria for production of the syndrome consisted of a significant rise in temperature, pulse rate, and respiratory rate within 12 hours, a decrease in arterial oxygen saturation, and at times radiological and histological evidence of atelectasis. The cotton plugs were removed 24 to 48 hours after insertion except when the effect of prolonged occlusion was investigated.

Cultures were taken from the cotton plug and from the bronchus and trachea prior to its insertion. When the plug was removed, both it and the seromucinous exudate in the distal bronchial tree were cultured. The media used for the cultures included blood plates, blood agar plates, McKonkies' plate, and Brewers' media, the subcultures being taken from the latter. Both aerobic and anaerobic conditions were used for the cultures. Blood cultures were obtained from the foreleg vein of nine dogs at the height of the clinical response to atelectasis, 20 cc of blood being drawn under sterile conditions and immediately inoculated into an agar broth medium.

In five dogs atelectasis was produced by transthoracic ligation of the left main bronchus without the administration of antibiotics. Twenty-four hours later the animal was sacrificed, the lung removed, and the bronchial contents distal to the ligature were cultured using a sterile technique.

Two injections of 1 cc of gas gangrene antitoxin * were administered intramuscularly to five dogs 12 hours and one hour prior to insertion of the plug. Each cubic centimeter contained 2,000 units *Clostridium perfringens (welchii)* antitoxin, 2,000 units *C vibrion septique* antitoxin, and 300 units of *C oedematiens* antitoxin. A control group of five dogs received two injections of 1 cc each to determine the effect of the antitoxin itself.

Intramuscular penicillin and streptomycin were administered to another group of dogs in a dose of 300,000 IU of penicillin G procaine, 100,000 IU of penicillin G potassium, 0.25 gm of dihydrostreptomycin, and 0.25 gm of streptomycin base. In one group of six dogs the antibiotics were administered only at the time of insertion of the bronchial plug, while in a second group of four dogs the plug was left in place and antibiotics were administered both at the time of its insertion and daily until the completion of the experiment.

* Parke, Davis & Co.

Cross transfusion experiments were carried out in five pairs of dogs. A sterile plug was inserted into the bronchus of one of the pair without the administration of antibiotics. After the usual fever had developed, 50 cc of venous blood was withdrawn from the foreleg under sterile conditions, clotting was prevented by a small amount of heparin in the syringe, and the blood was immediately injected into the second animal of the pair.

To compare the experimental results with observations in humans, 115 recorded cases in the categories of postoperative atelectasis and postoperative pneumonia were reviewed in the clinical records of Victoria Hospital in London.

Results

Insertion of a cotton plug into the left main bronchus of dogs resulted in the classical clinical picture of pulmonary atelectasis. Within 12 hours, the rectal temperature rose to 103-105 F, the heart rate increased to 110-160 beats per minute, and the respiratory rate rose to 25-50 per minute. The same course has occurred on each occasion regardless of whether the conditions used for insertion of the plugs were clean or sterile. The animals rarely coughed out the plug and at the height of the response appeared to be very ill. Beyond the plug, the bronchial tree was filled with a thick mucopurulent exudate. Removal of the plug 24 to 48 hours later was always followed by a return to normal conditions within 8 to 12 hours.

Cultures were taken from the trachea and bronchus prior to insertion of the plug and at the time of its removal. Cultures of the bronchus, trachea, and plug in 12 dogs prior to insertion of the plug were all sterile. Cultures were obtained from the plug and the bronchial exudate in 26 dogs after the plug had been in place for 24 hours. Of these, 24 (92%) grew pathogenic organisms and 2 (8%) were sterile. The types of organisms grown were *C welchii* (16), *Streptococcus* (12), *Escherichia coli* (2), *Staphylococcus* (2), and *Aerobacter aerogenes* (2). External ligation of the left main bronchus was carried out at thoracotomy in five dogs. Twenty-four hours later pathogenic organisms were cultured from the distal bronchial tree in all five, these being *C welchii* (5), *Streptococcus* (2), *Neisseria* (1), and a diphtheroid (1).

Blood cultures taken under sterile conditions from foreleg veins at the height of clinical response were positive in five of nine animals (55%). The organisms cultured included *Streptococcus* (2), *C welchii* (2), *Aerobacter* (2), *Bacillus subtilis* (2), and *E coli* (1). Injection into a normal recipient of 50 cc of venous blood withdrawn from an animal at the height of fever was carried out five times. In two of these a marked rise in temperature, heart rate, and respiratory rate occurred in the recipient within five minutes, the reaction completely subsiding within three hours. Twenty-four hours after the bronchial plug had been removed and the experimental animal had returned to normal, injection of its blood into the same recipient caused no reaction.

Gas gangrene antitoxin administered to a series of five control dogs caused no fever. In five dogs with atelectasis, the usual increases in temperature, heart rate, and respiratory rate associated with bronchial occlusion were not altered by prior antitoxin therapy. In these dogs the organisms cultured from the bronchus were *Strep viridans* (3), beta-hemolytic *Streptococcus* (4), *E coli* (3), *C welchii* (2), *A aerogenes* (2), *Staphylococcus* (1), and a Gram-positive bacillus (1).

The modification of the response to atelectasis by the administration of antibiotics at the time of insertion of the plug has been previously reported[1] and was confirmed again in another six dogs. With this treatment, the bronchial cultures were sterile and only very slight rises in temperature and heart rate were observed, although the respiratory rate was still increased. In four other dogs, intramuscular penicillin and streptomycin were given at the time of insertion of the plug and daily while the plug was left in the bronchus. The animals remained afebrile for about two weeks, but were weak and lethargic and coughed constantly. Overnight they became well and stopped coughing. Bronchoscopy revealed that the plugs had been coughed out and the distal bronchial tree, although inflamed, was clear and patent. Cultures at this time were not obtained.

Similar results were found when cats were the experimental animals. Within 12 hours the rectal temperatures rose to 102-104 F, the heart rate increased to 120-160 beats per minute, and the respiratory rate rose to 25-50 per minute. Removal of the plug was followed by a return to normal conditions in 8 to 12 hours. Cultures taken from the bronchi of five cats after the plug had been in place for 24 hours demonstrated pathogenic bacteria in each case. The organisms identified were *Streptococcus* (4), *A aerogenes* (1), an unidentified anaerobic bacillus (1), and a Gram-negative bacillus (1).

A review of postoperative atelectasis and pneumonia in humans substantiated the experimental findings. The onset of fever in human atelectasis occurred in as short a period as three hours after operation. While the fever usually developed within 24 hours, it could be masked for several days by antibiotic therapy, although tachypnea was still present. A dramatic improvement in the clinical picture took place within hours of removal of the offending bronchial plug, and the temperature, heart rate, and respiratory rate returned to normal in 6 to 12 hours. In the few cases in which cultures were obtained, pathogenic bacteria were always found. If a patient developed the clinical syndrome of atelectasis while receiving antibiotics, the organisms were usually resistant to those employed. Two illustrative case histories follow:

CASE 1.—A 72-year-old white male was admitted with arterial insufficiency of both legs. Aortofemoral bypass graft was performed, the operation concluding at 4 PM, and intramuscular chloramphenicol, 1.0 gm every six hours, was administered. At midnight, eight hours postoperatively, his temperature rose to 102.6 F (39.2 C). The fever remained at 102-105.2 F (38.9-40.7 C) for four days, during which time atelectasis was obvious with tachypnea, tachycardia, and copious amounts of thick green sputum. Penicillin therapy was added on the third day. Culture of the bronchial suction on the fourth day revealed *Staph aureus* resistant to penicillin but sensitive to chloramphenicol and *Pseudomonas* resistant to both antibiotics.

CASE 2.—A 1½-year-old female was admitted to hospital because her mother thought she had aspirated something. The child was well until 1 PM, at which time the mother noticed that she became extremely short of breath and hot and had a nonproductive cough. In hospital, three hours later, the child's temperature was 102.4 F (39.1 C), heart rate 136 per minute, and respiratory rate 40 per minute. Penicillin therapy was started, but two days later her temperature was 104 F (40 C), heart rate 150, and respiratory rate 60. At bronchoscopy an inspissated mucous plug in the right main bronchus was removed. Culture of the plug revealed *Diplococcus pneumoniae.* Twelve hours after its removal her temperature was 98.4 F (36.9 C), heart rate 100, and respiratory rate 20.

Comment

The present experiments have confirmed the previous observation that bacterial infection is almost universally present (92%) within 24 hours in the obstructed bronchi of experimental atelectasis in the dog. It has been shown again that antibiotic therapy suppresses the fever and tachycardia and partially reduces the tachypnea, thus providing further evidence of the bacterial stimulus for these changes. The dramatic cure obtained by removal of the plug without antibiotic therapy has also continued without exception.

The experiments have also shown that this phenomenon is not confined to the dog. A comparable physiological situation has been produced in cats, and here cultures of the mucous distal to the plug grew pathogenic bacteria in every case. In those humans with postoperative atelectasis in whom cultures were obtained, pathogens were present, even within four hours of the onset of bronchial obstruction.

The significance of clostridial infection in dogs was investigated. First, it must be stated that this was the predominant organism in the occluded bronchi in only 50% of the cases and was found as a secondary organism in 12%. There was no apparent difference in the physiological disturbance between the cases in which the dominant organism was a *Clostridium* and those in which it was absent. *Clostridium* as a secondary organism was seldom found in cats and never in humans, although other organisms were cultured and the clinical picture was the same. Finally, administration of a polyvalent clostridial antitoxin to five dogs did not alter the course of events after bronchial obstruction, although *C welchii* was cultured in two of them.

Although sterile instruments and cotton plugs were used, the possibility of contamination of the bronchi by oropharyngeal organisms during insertion of the bronchoscope could not be completely ruled out despite negative bronchial cultures at this time. External bronchial ligation, however, resulted in atelectasis, fever, tachycardia and tachypnea, and culture of the distal bronchi 24 hours later revealed pathogenic organisms in each case. It could not be determined whether these organisms were present in the bronchi at the time of bronchial obstruction in numbers too few to culture and proliferated under the favorable conditions of bronchial stasis, or whether they entered later from the blood stream.

Prolonged antibiotic therapy in the presence of bronchial obstruction suppressed the fever and tachycardia for two weeks until the plug was coughed out by the animal, at which time a dramatic clinical recovery occurred within a few hours. It was hoped that the obstruction could be maintained until a septic course occurred so that the antibiotic sensitivity of the pathogenic bacteria could be determined. An analogous situation, however, was found in human cases of clinical atelectasis previously treated with antibiotics: under these conditions, the organisms in the atelectatic segment were usually resistant to the antibiotics being administered. Frequently, the case was classified as a postoperative pneumonia occurring seven to ten days after surgery, when actually it was probably a case of atelectasis in which the early acute manifestations of fever and tachycardia had been suppressed by antibiotic therapy.

The mechanism by which bacterial infection in the bronchi brings about sympathetic stimulation has not been completely elucidated. Afferent nervous stimulation from the lung has been previously excluded,[1] and the response to antibiotic therapy precludes an action of the accumulated bronchial mucus itself. The failure of clostridial antitoxin to prevent the changes does not rule out an effect of exotoxins of other bacteria, but endotoxins are unlikely in view of the protective action of antibiotic therapy. The dramatic effect of transfusion of blood from a dog with clinical atelectasis into a normal dog supports the hypothesis that the stimulus is blood-borne. While the responsible factor may be an endogenous pyrogen produced in the atelectatic lung, the finding of a positive blood culture in five of nine dogs suggests that bacterial invasion of the blood stream must be highly regarded as the causative agent. The septic swinging course of the fever also supports the bacteremic hypothesis, showers of bacteria being superimposed on continuous invasion from the area of infection.

Summary

The tachycardia, tachypnea, and fever of experimental pulmonary atelectasis in dogs and cats are caused by bacterial infection in the distal bronchial tree. A survey of clinical cases of atelectasis and postoperative pneumonia provides supportive evidence for the importance of this mechanism in humans as well.

The infection is not caused by bronchial contamination at the time of experimental obstruction. Pathogens cannot be cultured from the bronchi at the time of insertion of the plug but are present within 24 hours even when external bronchial ligation is employed to produce atelectasis.

Clostridial antitoxin administered to dogs does not prevent the physiological changes associated with atelectasis. Continued antibiotic therapy in the presence of atelectasis suppresses the changes for about two weeks in dogs until the plug is coughed out. Removal of the obstruction without antibiotic therapy restores the temperature, heart rate, and respiratory rate to normal in a few hours.

Prof R. G. E. Murray and Miss Marion Luney of the Department of Bacteriology gave assistance. Dr. R. B. Passi actively participated in the technical aspects of the project.

A. M. Lansing, MD, Department of Surgery, University of Louisville School of Medicine, 511 S Floyd St, Louisville 2, Ky.

REFERENCE

1. Lansing, A. M., and Jamieson, W. G.: Mechanisms of Fever in Pulmonary Atelectasis, Arch Surg 87:168, 1963.

AUTHOR AND TITLE INDEX TO VOLUME 87

In this Index in alphabetical order are the names of the authors of all articles, followed by the title of the article and the page numbers on which their articles begin. Page numbers in the Index refer to bold face (dark) numbers in the text.

For Subject Index see page [*225*-**1079**].

A

Ablaza, S. G. G.; Raber, G. T.; Blanco, G.; Morse, D. P.; Adam, A.; and Nichols, H. T.: Intentional hemodilution: use of rotating disc oxygenator primed with acid citrate dextrose blood and low molecular weight dextrin; preliminary report, 548 (O)

Abrams, B. L.: Sigmoid volvulus, 1033 (D)

Adam, A.: See Ablaza, S. G. G., jt. auth.

Adashek, E. P., and Adashek, W. H.: Blood transfusion hepatitis in open-heart surgery, 792 (N)

Adashek, W. H.: See Adashek, E. P., jt. auth.

Alexander, J. W.: See Altemeier, W. A., jt. auth.

Alexander, M. J.: See Snyder, C. A., jt. auth

Altemeier, W. A., and Alexander, J. W.: Pancreatic abscess: study of 32 cases, 80 (Jl)

Anastasi, G. W.; Wertheimer, H. M.; and Brown, J. R.: Popliteal aneurysm with osteochondroma of femur, 636 (O)

Anderson, R. E.: See Strohl, E. L., jt. auth.

Arena, S.: See Conley, J., jt. auth.

Asada, S.; Itaya, H.; Nakamura, K.; Isohashi, T.; and Masuoka, S.: Radical pancreatoduodenectomy and portal vein resection: report of two successful cases with transplantation of portal vein, 609 (O)

Asch, T.: See Moody, F. G., jt. auth.

Ashbaugh, D. G., and Owens, J. C.: Intestinal complications following irradiation for gynecologic cancer, 100 (Jl)

Austen, W. G.: See Bender, H. W., jt. auth.

Avola, F. A., and Gonnella, J. P.: Intraperitoneal hemorrhage due to uterine fibroid: report of case in late pregnancy, 666 (O)

B

Bagshaw, M. A.: See Nelsen, T. W., jt. auth.

Baker, W. K.: See Landor, J. H., jt. auth.

Barber, K. W., Jr.; ReMine, W. H.; Priestley, J. T.; and Gage, R. P.: Critical evaluation of total gastrectomy, 23 (Jl)

Batsakis, J. G.: See Meadows, T. R., jt. auth.

Beal, J. M.: See Frey, C. F., jt. auth.
See Moody, F. G., jt. auth.

Beck, W. C., and Carlson, W. W.: Aseptic barriers, 288 (Ag)

Becker, J. M.; Schneider, K. M.; and Fischer, A. E.: Pyloric atresia, 413 (S)

Bell, J. W.: See Strandness, D. E., Jr., jt. auth.

Bender, H. W.; Austen, W. G.; Tsunekawa, T.; and Ebert, P. A.: Effects of hypothermia on myocardial contractile force, 464 (S)

Benson, J. W.; Kiehn, C. L.; and Holden, W. D.: Cancer chemotherapy by arterial infusion, 125 (Jl)

Bergan, J. J., and Trippel, O. H.: Management of juxta-renal aortic occlusions, 230 (Ag)

Bernardo, P.: See Hopkins, R. W., jt. auth.

Bernatz, P. E.: See Hopkins, D. M., jt. auth.

Berns, A. W.: See Blumenthal, H. T., jt. auth.

Bernstein, E. F.; McFee, A. S.; Goodale, R. L., Jr.; Madsen, A. J.; and Wangensteen, O. W.: Treatment of postgastrectomy stomal ulcer by gastric freezing, 13 (Jl)

Berry, R. E. L., and Sanislow, C. A.: Clinical manifestations and treatment of congestive atelectasis, 153 (Jl)

Beven, E. B.: See Humphries, A. W., jt. auth.

Blanco, G.: See **Ablaza, S. G. G.**, jt. auth.

Block, M. A., and Whitehouse, F. W.: Below-knee amputation in patients with diabetes mellitus, 682 (O)

Block, M. A.; Horn, R. C., Jr.; and Miller, J. M.: Unilateral thyroid nodules with lymphocytic thyroiditis: surgical problems and management, 280 (Ag)
See **Duhamel, P. A.**, jt. auth.

Blount, S. G., Jr.: See **Swan, H.**, jt. auth.

Blumenthal, H. T.; Probstein, J. G.; and Berns, A. W.: Interrelationship of diabetes mellitus and pancreatitis, 844 (N)

Bounous, G.; Hampson, L. G.; and Gurd, F. N.: Regional blood blow and oxygen consumption in experimental hemorrhagic shock, 340 (Ag)

Bowers, R. F., and Henley, W. H.: Carcinoma of tongue, buccal mucosa, and mandible: results from surgical treatment, 516 (S)

Bozer, A. Y.; Schuster, S. R.; and Kiernan, E. R.: Closure of established Potts anastomosis: experimental method, 722 (N)

Bradley, R. L.: See **Carey, J. P.**, jt. auth.

Bradham, G. B., and Buxton, J. T., Jr.: Successful resection of syphilitic aneurysm of aortic arch, 521 (S)

Bratcher, E.: See **Kelly, R. R.**, jt. auth.

Brown, J. R.: See **Anastasi, G. W.**, jt. auth.

Burnham, P. J.: Acute carpal tunnel syndrome: median artery thrombosis as cause, 645 (O)

Bussmann, D. W.; Reddy, V.; and Hanlon, C. R.: Direct auscultation of heart, 257 (Ag)

Buxton, J. T., Jr.: See **Bradham, G. B.**, jt. auth.

C

Camp, F. A.: See **McDonald, K. E.**, jt. auth.

Carey, J.: See **Zuhdi, N.**, jt. auth.

Carey, J. P., and Bradley, R. L.: Chemodectoma: review with two new cases, 879 (D)

Carlson, W. W.: See **Beck, W. C.**, jt. auth.

Catron, L.: See **Kelly, T. R.**, jt. auth.

Chun, B. K.: See **Doberneck, R. C.**, jt. auth.

Claman, M. A.: Acute intestinal obstruction caused by food: case report, 422 (S)

Clatworthy, H. W., Jr.: See **Schultz, L. R.**, jt. auth.

Clemente, E.: See **Tice, D. A.**, jt. auth.

Cohn, I., Jr.: See **Cotlar, A. M.**, jt. auth.

Collins, H. R.: See **Johnson, E. W., Jr.**, jt. auth.

Collins, N. P.: Intestinal hemorrhage in von Recklinghausen's disease: neurogenic tumors as cause, 374 (S)

Conley, J., and Arena, S.: Parotid gland as focus of metastasis, 757 (N)

Cooley, J. C., and McIntosh, C. L.: Myocardial contractile force in experimental hemorrhagic shock: some observations, 330 (Ag)

Corbus, H. F.: See **Hibner, R. W.**, jt. auth.

Costa, G.: See **Kraus, G. E.**, jt. auth.

Cotlar, A. M., and Cohn, I., Jr.: Iodophor for preoperative skin preparation, 857 (N)

Covell, J.: See **Lancaster, J. R.**, jt. auth.

Cranley, J. J.: See **Krause, R. J.**, jt. auth.

Crutcher, R. R.: See **Gryboski, W. A.**, jt. auth.

Csanaky, G.: See **Mester, Z.**, jt. auth.

Cullen, D.: See **Zuidema, G. D.**, jt. auth.

Cutter, J.: See **Zuhdi, N.**, jt. auth.

D

Danese, C.: See **Todd, R. S.**, jt. auth.

Dearing, W. H.: See **Santschi, D. R.**, jt. auth.

DeJode, L. R.: See **Todd, R. S.**, jt. auth.

Delin, N. A.: See **Schenk, W. G., Jr.**, jt. auth.

Desjardins, J. G., and Simpson, J. S.: Neonatal Hirschsprung's disease: treatment of complete aganglionosis of colon by Duhamel operation, 1019 (D)

deWolfe, V. G.: See **Humphries, A. W.**, jt. auth.

Diffenbaugh, W. G.: See **Strohl, E. L.**, jt. auth.

Doberneck, R. C.; Nunn, D. B.; Johnson, D. G.; and Chun, B. K.: Iron metabolism after portacaval shunt in dogs. 751 (N)

Dragstedt, L. R.: Influence of geography on duodenal ulcers (editorial), 193 (Ag)
See **Woodward, E. R.,** jt. auth.

Drapanas, T.; Shim, W. K. T.; and Stewart, J. D.: Studies of fibrinolytic activity after hepatectomy, 64 (Jl)

Duhamel, P. A.; Block, M. A.; and Haubrich, W. S.: Are benign gastric ulcers really benign? 391 (S)

DuVal, M. K., Jr.: See **Price, W. E.,** jt. auth.

E

Ebert, P. A.: See **Bender, H. W.,** jt. auth.
See **Greenfield, L. J.,** jt. auth.

Eckert, C.: See **Leather, R. P.,** jt. auth.

Effler, D. B.; Westcott, R. N.; Groves, L. K.; and Scully, N. M.: Surgical treatment of ventricular aneurysm: report of ten cases, 249 (Ag)

Eidbo, W. B.: See **Palumbo, L. T.,** jt. auth.

Eigenbrodt, E. H.: See **Nelsen, T. S.,** jt. auth.

Eiseman, B.: See **Gryboski, W. A.,** jt. auth.
See **Moore, T. C.,** jt. auth.

Eisenberg, M. M., and Woodward, E. R.: Gastric cancer: midcentury look, 810 (N)

Enquist, I. F.: See **Golding, M. R.,** jt. auth.

Epstein, O.: See **Mester, Z.,** jt. auth.

Ernst, R. W.: See **Luna, R.,** jt. auth.

F

Falor, W. H.: See **Kelly, T. R.,** jt. auth.
See **Meyer, E. G.,** jt. auth.

Farrell, J. J.: See **Lighterman, I.,** jt. auth.

Feller, I., and Hill, C. C.: Surgical wire welding, 866 (N)

Firestein, A.: See **Morel, A. S.,** jt. auth.

Fischer, A. E.: See **Becker, J. M.,** jt. auth.

Foley, W. T.: See **Qureshi, M. A.,** jt. auth.

Foster, J. H.: See **Killen, D. A.,** jt. auth.

Freckman, H. A.: See **Mendez, F. L.,** jt. auth.

Frey, C. F., and Beal, J. M.: Pancreatitis as complication of operation, 1053 (D)

Friendenberg, M. J.: See **Stokes, J. M.,** jt. auth.

Fulmer, H. F.: See **Hibner, R. W.,** jt. auth.

G

Gage, R. P.: See **Barber, K. W., Jr.,** jt. auth.

Gaisford, W. D.: See **Zuidema, G. D.,** jt. auth.

Gardner, R. J.; Henegar, G. C.; and Preston, F. W.: Staphylococcus enterocolitis, 58 (Jl)

Gazel, G.: See **McKibbin, B.,** jt. auth.

Geraci, C. L.: New iodine compound for degerming skin surface, 560 (O)

Gerber, B. C.: Hereditary pancreatitis: role of surgical intervention, 70 (Jl)

Gerndt, H. L., Jr.: See **Palumbo, L. T.,** jt. auth.

Gerwig, W. H., Jr., and Ghaphery, A.: Experimental attempt to delay alimentary transit after small bowel exclusion, 34 (Jl)

Ghaphery, A.: See **Gerwig, W. H.,** jt. auth.

Gilchrist, R. K.: See **Yang, J.,** jt. auth.

Giordano, R. P.: See **Miscall, L.,** jt. auth.

Gittes, R. F., and Kartchner, M. M.: Posttraumatic temporal artery aneurysm: recurrent surgical curiosity, 398 (S)

Glenn, F.: See **Moody, F. G.,** jt. auth

Goade, W. J., Jr.: See **Malt, R. A.,** jt. auth.

Golding, M. R.; Oberlander, L. K.; and Enquist, I. F.: Cartilage speeds healing in diabetic wounds, 647 (O)

Gonnella, J. P.: See **Avola, F. A.,** jt. auth.

Goodale, R. L., Jr.: See **Bernstein, E. F.,** jt. auth.

Goodman, H. O.: See **Wray, J. B.,** jt. auth.

Grant, G. N.: See **Kelley, H. G.,** jt. auth.

Greenfield, L. J., and Ebert, P. A.: Cardiac denervation effect in hypoxia and hypercapnia: effect of total denervation of cardiovascular response, 717 (N)

Greer, A.: See **Zuhdi, N.,** jt. auth.

Gresham, R. B.; Perry, V. P.; and Thompson, V. K.: Practical methods of short-term storage of homografts, 417 (S)

Griffith, B. H.: See **Sutton, W. T.,** jt. auth.

Groves, L. K.: See **Effler, D. B.,** jt. auth.

Gurd, F. N.: See **Bounous, G.,** jt. auth.

Gryboski, W. A.; Crutcher, R. R.; Holloway, J. B.; Mayo, P.; Segnitz, R. H.; and Eiseman, B.: Surgical aspects of histoplasmosis, 590 (O)

H

Hafner, C. D.: See Krause, R. J., jt. auth. **See Qureshi, M. A.,** jt. auth.

Haimovici, H.; Zinicola, N.; Noorani, M.; and Hoffert, P. W.: Vein grafts in venous system: experimental evaluation of autogenous veins used as bypass implants, 542 (O)

Haines, C. R.: See Hanson, D. J., Jr., jt. auth.

Hallaba, M. A. S.: See Krause, R. J., jt. auth.

Halstead, W. S.: Ligature and suture material, 216 (Ag)

Hampson, L. G.: See Bounous, G., jt. auth.

Hanlon, C. R.: See Bussman, D. W., jt. auth.

Hanson, D. J., Jr.; Soule, A. B.; Peterson, O. S., Jr.; Haines, C. R.; and Janney, C. D.: Liver photoscanning in evaluation of cancer chemotherapy, 442 (S)

Hardin, R. A.; Shumacker, H. B., Jr.; and Su, C. S.: Studies on portal venous oxygen saturation, 831 (N)

Hardy, J. D., and Yelverton, R. L.: "Spontaneous rupture" of spleen: one mechanism: routine splenectomy challenged, 468 (S)

Harkins, H. N.: See Savage, L. E., jt. auth.

Harris, L. E.: See Peck, D. A., jt. auth.

Haubrich, W. S.: See Duhamel, P. A., jt. auth.

Hayasaka, H.; O'Malley, J. F.; and Howard, J. M.: Antitoxic effect of aldosterone on cats in endotoxic shock: further studies, 861 (N)

Henegar, G. C.: See Gardner, R. J., jt. auth.

Henley, W. H.: See Bowers, R. F., jt. auth.

Hertel, R. C.: See Morgan, H. C., jt. auth.

Hibner, R. W.; Corbus, H. F.; and Fulmer, H. F.: Myxoma of left atrium: presenting as embolus to femoral artery, 525 (S)

Hill, C. C.: See Feller, I., jt. auth.

Hinshaw, J. R.: Progressive changes in depth of burns, 993 (D)

Hite, D. F.: See Landor, J. H., jt. auth.

Hoffert, P. W.: See Haimovici, H., jt. auth.

Holden, W. D.: See Benson, J. W., jt. auth.

Holloway, J. B.: See Gryboski, W. A., jt. auth.

Holt, M. H., and Lewis, F. J.: Internal cooling for general hypothermia, 471 (S)

Holzman, D.: See Takeda, J., jt. auth.

Hopkins, D. M., and Bernatz, P. E.: Experimental replacement of cervical esophagus, 265 (Ag)

Hopkins, R. W.; Sabga, G.; Bernardo, P.; Penn, I.; and Simeone, F. A.: Significance of post-traumatic and postoperative oliguria, 320 (Ag)

Hoppe, E.: See McKibbin, B., jt. auth.

Horn, R. C., Jr.: See Block, M. A., jt. auth.

Howard, J. M., and Singh, L. M.: Peritoneal fluid pH after perforation of peptic ulcers: myth of "acid-peritonitis," 483 (S)
See Hayasaka, H., jt. auth.
See Miller, S., jt. auth.
See Todd, R. S., jt. auth.

Huizenga, K. A.: See Santschi, D. R., jt. auth.

Hume, M.: Pulmonary embolism: historical aspects, 709 (O)

Humphrey, L. J.: See Swerdlow, M., jt. auth.

Humphries, A. W.; Young, J. R.; deWolfe, V. G.; LeFevre, F. A.; and Beven, E. B.: Severe ischemia of lower extremity due to arteriosclerosis obliterans, 175 (Jl)

I

Inada, K.: See Sunada, T., jt. auth.

Isohashi, T.: See Asada, S., jt. auth.

Itaya, H.: See Asada, S., jt. auth.

J

Jackson, F. C.: "Directional" flow patterns in portal hypertension: assessment by spleen pressure and percutaneous splenoportography, 307 (Ag)

Jackson, J. M.: Annular pancreas and duodenal obstruction in the neonate: review, 379 (S)

Jackson, T. M., and Lee, W. H., Jr.: Major thermal burns: mortality appraisal and review, 937 (D)

Jamieson, W. G., and Lansing, A. M.: Bacteriological studies in pulmonary atelectasis, 1062 (D)
See Lansing, A. M., jt. auth.

Janney, C. D.: See Hanson, D. J., Jr., jt. auth.

Jennings, E. M.: See Kinman, L. M., jt. auth.

Johnson, D. G.: See Doberneck, R. C., jt. auth.

Johnson, E. W., Jr., and Collins, H.: Nonunion of clavicle, 963 (D)

Juardo, J.: See Phelan, J. T., jt. auth.

Just-Viera, J. O.: See Lewers, D. J., jt. auth.

K

Kaiser, G. C.: See Lempke, R. E., jt. auth.

Kartchner, M. M.: See Gittes, R. F., jt. auth.

Katz, I.: See Luna, R., jt. auth.

Kelley, H. G.; Grant, G. N.; and Elliott, D. W.: Massive gastroduodenal hemorrhage: changing concepts of management, 6 (Jl)

Kelly, T. R., and Troyer, M. L.: Pancreatic ducts and postoperative pancreatitis, 614 (O)
Bratcher, E. P.; Falor, W. H.; Catron, L.; and Reyes, L. B.: Experimental pancreatitis: synchronous production in normal and in ectopic pancreas, 988 (D)

Kiehn, C. L.: See Benson, J. W., jt. auth.

Kiernan, E. R.: See Bozer, A. Y., jt. auth.

Kiesewetter, W. B.: See Sieber, W. K., jt. auth.

Killen, D. A., and Foster, J. H.: Severity of renal injury incident to abdominal aortography: effect of concentration of contrast solution, 650 (O)

King, R. D.: See Lempke, R. E., jt. auth.

Kinman, L. M., and Jennings, E. M.: Control of bleeding in suprapubic prostatectomy: use of bilateral ligation of hypogastric arteries, 887 (D)

Kitzerow, E.: See Wagner, M., jt. auth.

Kjartansson, K. B.: See Schenk, W. G., Jr., jt. auth.

Klein, D. E., and Persky, L.: Renal hypertension, heart failure, and azotemia: report of case treated successfully by nephrectomy, 530 (S)

Kobayashi, S.: See Nakayama, K., jt. auth.

Komoto, Y.: See Sunada, T., jt. auth.

Kowalczyk, R. S.: See Zuidema, G. D., jt. auth.

Kozoll, D. D., and Meyer, K. A.: Laboratory findings in massively bleeding gastroduodenal ulcers: review of 2,008 cases, 916 (D)

Kraus, G. E., and Costa, G.: Systemic effects of massive hepatic necrosis: I. acute effects of hepatic infarction on kidneys, 957 (D)

Krause, R. J.; Cranley, J. J.; Hallaba, M. A. S.; Strasser, E. S.; and Hafner, C. D.: Caval ligation in thromboembolic disease, 184 (Jl)

Kretchmar, L. H., and McDonald, D. F.: Urine sediment in acute appendicitis, 209 (Ag)

L

Laine, J. B.: See Miller, S., jt. auth.

Lancaster, J. R.; Stewart, P. B.; Lennertz, J.; Covell, J.; and Moulder, P. V.: Effect of hypoxia on pulmonary vasculature of dog, 485 (S)

Landor, J. H.; Baker, W. K.; and Hite, D. F.: Blind intestinal loops in dogs: effect on Heidenhain pouch secretion, 1048 (D)

Lansing, A. M., and Jamieson, W. G.: Mechanisms of fever in pulmonary atelectasis, 168 (Jl)
See Jamieson, W. G., jt. auth.

Large, A. M.: Left-sided gallbladder and liver without situs inversus, 982 (D)

Lari, A. A.: See Parsonnet, V., jt. auth.

Lary, B. G.: Effect of endocardial incisions on myocardial blood flow, 424 (S)

Laufman, H.: See Nora, P., jt. auth.

Leather, R. P., and Eckert, C.: Hyperbaric oxygenation and mechlorethamine effectiveness, 144 (Jl)

Lee, W. H., Jr.: See Jackson, T. M., jt. auth.

LeFevre, F. A.: See Humphries, A. W., jt. auth.

Lempke, R. E.; King, R. D.; and Kaiser, G. C.: Lateral pancreaticojejunostomy, 90 (Jl)

Lennertz, J.: See Lancaster, J. R., jt. auth.

Lepley, D., Jr.: See O'Connor, T., jt. auth.

Lett, J. C.: See Mazuji, M. K., jt. auth.

Lewers, D. T.; Just-Viera, J. O.; and Yeager, G. H.: Lethal properties of rapidly polymerizing adhesive: product used in nonsuture surgery, 627 (O)

Lewis, F. J.: See Holt, M. H., jt. auth.

Liechty, R. D., and Raterman, L.: Villous adenoma, a surgical dilemma, 107 (Jl)

Lighterman, I., and Farrell, J. J.: Mandibular fractures treated with plastic polymers, 868 (N)

Luna, R.; Katz, I.; and Ernst, R. W.: Intrathoracic pheochromocytoma: case report, 369 (S)

Luttwak, E. M.: See Samueloff, S. L., jt. auth.

Lynn, H. B.: See Peck, D. A., jt. auth.

Mc

McDonald, D. F.: See Kretchmar, L. H., jt. auth.

McDonald, K. E.; Camp, F. A.; and Schenk, W. G., Jr.: Comparison of three mechanical ventilators: effects on pulmonary blood flow, 796 (N)

McEachern, C. G., and Sullivan, R. E.: Perforation of gallbladder: analysis of twenty-one cases, 489 (S)

McFee, A. S.: See Bernstein, E. F., jt. auth.

McGoon, D. C.: See Shamblin, J. R., jt. auth.

McIntosh, C. L.: See Cooley, J. C., jt. auth.

McKibbin, G.; Gazet, J.; Hoppe, E.; and Schwab, C.: Chemical irrigation of wounds inoculated with cancer cells, 877 (N)

McKittrick, J. B.: See Miscall, L., jt. auth.

McLachlin, A. D.: Surgical training in Canada, 1 (Jl)

McPherson, R. C.: See Ransdell, H. T., jt. auth.

M

Mackay, W. D., and Matheson, N. A.: Nasogastric tube and pulmonary ventilation, 673 (O)

Madsen, A. J.: See Bernstein, E. F., jt. auth.

Maglietta, E. D.: See Palumbo, L. T., jt. auth.

Mahaley, M. S., Jr.; Odom, G. L.; and Woodhall, B.: Histological changes after regional chemotherapy: brain and face tumors, 765 (N)

Makino, K.: See Nakayama, L., jt. auth.

Malt, R. A.; Olken, H. G.; and Goade, W. J., Jr.: Renal tubular necrosis after oral cholecystography, 743 (N)

Martin, H.: Proposed glossary of cancer, 534 (S)

Masuoka, S.: See Asada, S., jt. auth.

Matheson, N. A.: See Mackay, W. D., jt. auth.

Maurer, E. R. P.: See Mendez, F. L., Jr., jt. auth.

Mayo, P.: See Gryboski, W. A., jt. auth.

Mazuji, M. K., and Lett, J. C.: Siliconized Dacron as pericardial patch, 446 (S)

Meadows, T. R., and Batsakis, J. B.: Histopathological spectrum of regional enteritis, 976 (D)

Meagher, S. W.: Post-traumatic vasospasm: role of thermal measurement, 539 (O)

Mendez, F. L., Jr.; Maurer, E. R. P.; and Freckman, H. A.: Effect of chemical agents on bronchogenic cancer, 147 (Jl)

Messina, E. J.: See Tice, D. A., jt. auth.

Mester, Z.; Csanaky, G.; Mocsay, L.; and Epstein, O.: Anatomy of duodenal papilla and genesis of pancreatic reflux, 775 (N)

Meyer, E. G., and Falor, W. H.: Coronary artery pressure in perfused heart, 805 (N)

Meyer, K. A.: See Kozoll, D. D., jt. auth.

Miller, J. M.: See Block, M. A., jt. auth.

Miller, S.; Laine, J. B.; and Howard, J. M.: Lymphatic pressures in extremities of dogs, 881 (N)

Miscall, L.; McKittrick, J. B.; Giordano, R. P.; and Nolan, R. B.: Stenosis of trachea resection and end-to-end anastomosis: report of two cases, 726 (N)

Mocsay, L.: See Mester, Z., jt. auth.

Moody, F. G., and Beal, J. M.: Carcinoma of cecum associated with intussusception, 836 (N)

Asch, T.; and Glenn, F.: Intrahepatic cholangiography, 475 (S)

Moore, T. C.; Normell, L.; and Eiseman, B.: Effect of serotonin loading on histamine release and blood flow of isolated perfused liver and lung, 42 (Jl)

Morel, A. S., and Firestein, A.: Repair of traumatic fistulas of parotid duct, 623 (O)

Morgan, H. C.; Hertel, R. C.; and Stamp, W. G.: Quantitative barrier of synovium to penicillin, 450 (S)

Morse, D. P.: See **Ablaza, S. G. G.,** jt. auth.

Moulder, P. V.: See **Lancaster, J. R.,** jt. auth.

N

Nabeya, K.: See **Nakayama, K.,** jt. auth.

Nadler, S. H.: Gastric ulcers—management, 619 (O)

Nakamura, K.: See **Asada, S.,** jt. auth.

Nakanishi, M.: See **Sunada, T.,** jt. auth.

Nakayama, K.; Yanagisawa, F.; Nabeya, K.; Tamiya, T.; Kobayashi, S.; and Makino, K.: Concentrated preoperative irradiation therapy, 1003 (D)

Nelsen, T. S.; Eigenbrodt, E. H.; and Bagshaw, M. A.: Low-flow fail-safe intraarterial infusion, 640 (O)

Nichols, H. T.: See **Ablaza, S. G. G.,** jt. auth.

Nolan, R. B.: See **Miscall, L.,** jt. auth.

Noorani, M.: See **Haimovici, H.,** jt. auth.

Nora, P., and Laufman, H.: Effects of various drugs on exotoxin (Cl perfringens) toxicity: pretreatment with chlorpromazine, phenoxybenzamine, heparin, and cortisone, 53 (Jl)

Normell, L.: See **Moore, T. C.,** jt. auth.

Nunn, D. B.: See **Doberneck, R. C.,** jt. auth.

Nyhus, L. M.: See **Savage, L. E.,** jt. auth.

O

Oberlander, L. K.: See **Golding, M. R.,** jt. auth.

O'Connor, T.; Watson, R.; Lepley, D., Jr.; and Weisel, W.: Esophageal prosthesis for palliative intubation: further evaluation of 378 patients, 275 (Ag)

Odom, G. L.: See **Mahaley, M. S., Jr.,** jt. auth.

Ohin, A.: See **Peden, J. C., Jr.,** jt. auth.

Olken, H. G.: See **Malt, R. A.,** jt. auth.

O'Malley, J. F.: See **Hayasaka, H.,** jt. auth.

Orloff, M. J., and Thomas, H. S.: Pathogenesis of esophageal varix rupture: study based on gross and microscopic examination of esophagus at time of bleeding, 301 (Ag)

Owens, J. C.: See **Ashbaugh, D. G.,** jt. auth.
See **Swan, H.,** jt. auth.

P

Palmer, J. M.: Portacaval transposition in experimental hypertension: effect on blood pressure, 500 (S)

Palumbo, L. T., and Sharpe, W. S.: Distal antrectomy with vagectomy for duodenal ulcer: review of 450 cases, 1040 (D)
Sharpe, W. S.; Gerndt, H. L., Jr.; Maglietta, E. D.; and Eidbo, W. B.: Primary inguinal hernioplasty: our experience with 3,572 operations, 949 (D)

Park, C. L., Jr.: See **Woodward, E. R.,** jt. auth.

Parsonnet, V.; Lari, A. A.; and Shah, I. H.: New stent for support of veins in arterial grafts, 696 (O)

Peck, D. A.; Lynn, H. B.; and Harris, L. E.: Congenital atresia and stenosis of colon, 428 (S)

Peden, J. C., Jr.; Ohin, A.; Williams, P. T.; and Weathers, H.: Intravenous protein hydrolysates: favorable influence on postoperative nitrogen balance, 401 (S)

Penn, I.: See **Hopkins, R. W.,** jt. auth.

Persky, L.: See **Klein, D. E.,** jt. auth.

Perry, V. P.: See **Gresham, R. B.,** jt. auth.

Peterson, O. S., Jr.: See **Hanson, D. J., Jr.,** jt. auth.

Phelan, J. T., and Juardo, J.: Moh's chemosurgery for basal cell carcinoma of chin and cheek areas of face, 212 (Ag)

Phillips, R. S.: Prognosis in deep venous thrombosis, 732 (N)

Podolak, E.: See **Simmers, M. H.,** jt. auth.

Pollock, L. A.: See **Schenk, W. G., Jr.,** jt. auth.

Pool, P. E.: See **Swan, H.,** jt. auth.

Porter, R. W.: See **Wild, W. O.,** jt. auth.

Preston, F. W.: See **Gardner, R. J.,** jt. auth.
See **Sutton, W. T.,** jt. auth.

Price, W. E., and DuVal, M. K., Jr.: Regional lymph node dissection and malignant melanoma: effect on survival, 747 (N)

Priestley, J. T.: See Barber, K. W., Jr., jt. auth.

Probstein, J. G.: See Blumenthal, H. T., jt. auth.

Q

Qureshi, M. A.; Foley, W. T.; and Hafner, C. D.: Adenocarcinoma of appendix: report of four cases, 453 (S)

R

Raber, G. T.: See Ablaza, S. G. G., jt. auth.

Rader, L.: See Zuhdi, N., jt. auth.

Ransdell, H. T., Jr., and McPherson, R. C.: Management of spontaneous pneumothorax: comparison of treatment methods, 1023 (D)

Raterman, L.: See Liechty, R. D., jt. auth.

Redy, V.: See Bussmann, D. W., jt. auth.

Redisch, W.: See Tice, D. A., jt. auth.

Reed, G. E.: See Tice, D. A., jt. auth.

Reed, W. H.: See Strohl, E. L., jt. auth.

Reis, L. D.: Visceral lesions in acute pancreatitis: experimental study, 604 (O)

ReMine, W. H.: See Barber, K. W., Jr., jt. auth.

Reyes, L. B.: See Kelly, T. R., jt. auth.

Roe, B. B.: Are postoperative narcotics necessary? 912 (D)

Roper, C. L.: See Spector, G. W., jt. auth.

Rydell, W. B., Jr.: Inguinal and femoral hernias, 493 (S)

S

Sabga, G.: See Hopkins, R. W., jt. auth.

Sabiston, D. C., Jr.: See Sheil, A. G. R., jt. auth.

Samueloff, S. L.; Luttwak, E. M.; and Wigderhouse, B. M.: Acid-base balance changes in citrated bank blood, 1029 (D)

Sanislow, C. A.: See Berry, R. E. L., jt. auth.

Santschi, D. R.; Huizenga, K. A.; Scudmore, H. H.; Dearing, W. H.; and Waugh, J. M.: Bile ascites, 851 (N)

Savage, L. E.; Stavney, L. S.; Stevenson, J. K.; Harkins, H. N.; and Nyhus, L. M.: Secretory studies in frozen Heidenhain pouches, 690 (O)

Schapiro, H.: See Woodward, E. R., jt. auth.

Schenk, W. G., Jr.; Pollock, L. A.; Kjartansson, K. B.; and Delin, N. A.: Influence of direction of aortic perfusion on regional blood flow, 1059 (D)
See McDonald, K. E., jt. auth.

Schneider, A. J.: See Zeidman, H., jt. auth.

Schneider, K. M.: See Becker, J. M., jt. auth.

Schultz, L. R., and Clatworthy, H. W., Jr.: Esophageal strictures after anastomosis in esophageal atresia, 120 (Jl)

Schumer, W.: Sodium oxacillin in surgical infections: clinical evaluation, 507 (S)

Schuster, S. R.: See Bozer, A. Y., jt. auth.

Schwab, C.: See McKibbin, B., jt. auth.

Scudamore, H. H.: See Santschi, D. R., jt. auth.

Scully, N. M.: See Effler, D. B., jt. auth.

Segnitz, R. H.: See Gryboski, W. A., jt. auth.

Seiger, H. W.: New "one hand" double-loop method of tying knots, 986 (D)

Shah, I. H.: See Parsonnet, V., jt. auth.

Shamblin, J. R., and McGoon, D. C.: Acute thoracic compression with traumatic asphyxia: report of six cases, 967 (D)

Sharpe, W. S.: See Palumbo, L. R., jt. auth.

Sheil, A. G. R., and Sabiston, D. C., Jr.: Experimental venous thrombosis and thrombectomy, 408 (S)

Shenkin, H. A., and Somach, F. M.: Scalenotomy in patients with and without cervical ribs; analysis of surgical results, 892 (D)

Shim, W. K. T.: See Drapanas, T., jt. auth.

Shoemaker, W. C.: Studies on viscosity alterations in shock: I. effect of high and low viscosity dextrans upon plasma and red cell volume, 355 (Ag)

Shumacker, H. B., Jr.: See Hardin, R. A., jt. auth.

Sieber, W. K., and Kiesewetter, W. B.: Duhamel's operation for Hirschsprung's disease, 111 (Jl)

Sigel, B.: Partial hepatectomy in dog: revised technique based on anatomic considerations, 788 (N)

Simeone, F. A.: See **Hopkins, R. W.,** jt. auth.

Simmers, M. H., and Podolak, E.: Effect of simulated gallstones on guinea pig gallbladders, 583 (O)

Simpson, J. S.: See **Desjardins, J. G.,** jt. auth.

Singer, A.: Segmental distribution of peripheral atherosclerosis, 384 (S)

Singh, L. M.: See **Howard, J. M.,** jt. auth.

Sive, E. B.: See **Todd, R. S.,** jt. auth.

Smith, L.: Ceramic-plastic material as bone substitute, 653 (O)

Snyder, C. A., and Alexander, M. J.: Peptic ulcer in Africa, 206 (Ag)

Somach, F. M.: See **Shenkin, H. A.,** jt. auth.

Soule, A. B.: See **Hanson, D. J., Jr.,** jt. auth.

Spector, G. W.; Roper, C. L.; and Spratt, J. S., Jr.: Chemodectoma of mediastinum, 903 (D)

Spinuzza, S. J.: See **Yang, J.,** jt. auth.

Spratt, J. S., Jr.: See **Spector, G. W.,** jt. auth.

Stamp, W. G.: See **Morgan, H. C.,** jt. auth.

Stavney, L. S.: See **Savage, L. E.,** jt. auth.

Stein, L.: Granular cell myoblastoma of breast, 703 (O)

Stevenson, J. K.: See **Savage, L. E.,** jt. auth.

Stewart, J. D.: See **Drapanas, T.,** jt. auth.

Stewart, P. B.: See **Lancaster, J. R.,** jt. auth.

Stokes, J. M.; Friendenberg, M. J.; and Sunshine, H.: Comparison of methods used to diagnose renal hypertension: renal arteriography versus individual ureteral catherization, 238 (Ag)

Strandness, D. E., Jr., and Bell, J. W.: Portal hypertension from postbulbar duodenal ulcer, 440 (S)

Strasser, E. S.: See **Krause, R. J.,** jt. auth.

Strohl, E. L.: Johnannes Scultetus (1595-1645), 395 (S)

Reed, W. H.; Diffenbaugh, W. G.; and Anderson, R. E.: Carcinoma of bile ducts, 567 (O)

Su, C. S.: See **Hardin, R. A.,** jt. auth.

Sullivan, R. E.: See **McEachern, C. G.,** jt. auth.

Sunada, T.; Inada, K.; Nakanishi, M.; and Komoto, Y.: Left superior vena cava with anomalous inferior vena cava: report of case with associated atrial septal defect and pulmonic stenosis, successfully corrected, 632 (O)

Sunshine, H.: See **Stokes, J. M.,** jt. auth.

Sutton, W. T.; van Hagen, F.; Griffith, B. H.; and Preston, F. W.: Drug effects on survival of homografts of skins, 840 (N)

Swan, H.: How cardiac surgery transformed surgery (editorial), 365 (S)

Kamongo and anabolone (editorial), 715 (N)

Owens, J. C.; Pool, P. E.; Vogel J. H. K.; and Blount, S. C., Jr.: Absent left pulmonary artery and right-sided patent ductus arteriosus, 196 (Ag)

Swerdlow, M., and Humphrey, L. J.: Fibrocystic disease and carcinoma of breast, 457 (S)

T

Taitel, A.: See **Wagner, M.,** jt. auth.

Takeda, J.; Warren, R.; and Holzman, D.: Prognosis of aortic stenosis: special reference to indications for operative treatment, 931 (D)

Tamiya, T.: See **Nakayama, K.,** jt. auth.

Thomas, H. S.: See **Orloff, M. J.,** jt. auth.

Thompson, V. K.: See **Gresham, R. B.,** jt. auth.

Thompson, W. R.: Cast syndrome: case report, 662 (O)

Tice, D. A.; Reed, G. E.; Messina, E. J.; Clemente, E.; and Redisch, W.: Lumbar sympathectomy: effects on vascular responses in lower extremity of patients with arteriosclerosis obliterans, 461 (S)

Todd, R. S.; Sive, E. B.; DeJode, L. R.; Danese, C.; and Howard, J. M.: Replacement of segments of venous system, 998 (D)

Trippel, O. H.: See **Bergan, J. J.,** jt. auth.

Troyer, M. L.: See **Kelly, T. R.,** jt. auth.

Tsunekawa, T.: See **Bender, H. W.,** jt. auth.

Tyson, R. R.: See **Wright, G. F.,** jt. auth.

V

van Hagen, F.: See Sutton, W. T., jt. auth.

Vogel, J. H. K.: See Swan, H., jt. auth.

W

Wagner, M.; Kitzerow, E.; and Taitel, A.: Vertebral artery insufficiency, 885 (D)

Wangensteen, O. H.: See Bernstein, E. F., jt. auth.

Warren, R.: In summary (editorial), 194 (Ag)
See Takeda, J., jt. auth.

Watson, M. R.: Primary nonspecific ulceration of small bowel, 600 (O)

Watson, R.: See O'Connor, T., jt. auth.

Waugh, J. W.: See Santschi, D. R., jt. auth.

Weathers, H.: See Peden, J. C., Jr., jt. auth.

Weisel, W.: See O'Connor, T., jt. auth.

Wertheimer, H. M.: See Anastasi, G. W., jt. auth.

Westcott, R. N.: See Effler, D. B., jt. auth.

Whitehouse, F. W.: See Block, M. A., jt. auth.

Wigderhouse, B. M.: See Samueloff, S. L., jt. auth.

Wild, W. O., and Porter, R. W.: Metastatic epidural tumor of spine: study of 45 cases, 825 (N)

Williams, P. T.: See Peden, J. C., Jr., jt. auth.

Wolfman, E. F., Jr.: See Zuidema, G. D., jt. auth.

Woodall, B.: See Mahaley, M. S., Jr., jt. auth.

Woodward, E. R.; Park, C. L., Jr.; Schapiro, H.; and Dragstedt, L. R.: Significance of Meissner's plexus in gastrin mechanism, 512 (S)
See Eisenberg, M. M., jt. auth.

Wray, J. B., and Goodman, H. O.: Postfracture vascular changes and healing process, 801 (N)
See Zeidman, H., jt. auth.

Wright, G. F., and Tyson, R. R.: Oxidized regenerated cellulose for hepatic hemostasis, 669 (O)

Y

Yanagisawa, F.: See Nakayama, K., jt. auth.

Yang, J.: Spinuzza, S. J.; and Gilchrist, R. K.: Aneurysm of splenic artery with calcification, 676 (O)

Yeager, G. H.: See Lewers, D. T., jt. auth.

Yelverton, R. L.: See Hardy, J. D., jt. auth.

Young, J. R.: See Humphries, A. W., jt. auth.

Z

Zeidman, H.; Wray, J. B.; and Schneider, A. J.: Alterations in vascular volume after long bone fracture, 907 (D)

Zinicola, N.: See Haimovici, H., jt. auth.

Zuhdi, N.; Carey, J.; Cutter, J.; Rader, L.; and Greer, A.: Intentional hemodilution, 554 (O)

Zuidema, G. D.; Cullen, D.; Kowalczyk, R. S.; and Wolfman, E. F., Jr.: Blood ammonia reduction by potassium exchange resin: experimentation in Eck-fistula dogs, 296 (Ag)
Gaisford, W. D.; Kowalczyk, R. S.; and Wolfman, E. F., Jr.: Whole-body hypothermia in ammonia intoxication: effect on monkeys with portacaval shunts, 578 (O)

SUBJECT INDEX TO VOLUME 87

The following Index is an alphabetical list of significant subjects presented in this volume. Page numbers in the Index refer to the bold face (dark) numbers in the text.

A

Abnormalities
absent left pulmonary artery and right-sided patent ductus arteriosus [Swan et al], 196 (Ag)
atrial septal defect, auscultation in [Bussmann et al], 260 (Ag)
congenital atresia and stenosis of colon [Peck et al], 428 (S)
esophageal strictures after anastomosis in esophageal atresia [Schultz & Clatworthy], 120 (Jl)
left-sided gallbladder and liver without situs inversus [Large], 982 (D)
pyloric atresia [Becker et al], 413 (S)
ventricular septal defect, auscultation in [Bussmann et al], 261 (Ag)

Abscess
pancreatic: study of 32 cases [Altemeier & Alexander], 80 (Jl)

Adenocarcinoma
of appendix: report of four cases [Qureshi et al], 453 (S)

Africa
peptic ulcer in [Snyder & Alexander], 206 (Ag)

Aldosterone
antitoxic effect of [Hayasaka et al], 861 (N)

Alkylating agents
effects on survival of homografts [Sutton et al], 840 (N)

American Medical Association
call for papers, scientific exhibits, and motion pictures for the 113th Annual Meeting, June 21-25, 1964, 756 (N)

Ammonia
blood, reduction by potassium exchange resin [Zuidema et al], 296 (Ag)
hypothermia for ammonia intoxication [Zuidema et al], 578 (O)

Amputation
below-knee, in patients with diabetes mellitus [Block & Whitehouse], 682 (O)
rehabilitation of patients with below-knee amputations [Block & Whitehouse], 687 (O)
techniques employed in below-knee amputations [Block & Whitehouse], 684 (O)

Anastomosis
closure of established Potts anastomosis: experimental method [Bozer et al], 722 (N)
iron metabolism after portacaval shunt in dogs [Doberneck et al], 751 (N)
stenosis of trachea resection and end-to-end anastomosis [Miscall et al], 726 (N)

Anatomy
of duodenal papilla and genesis of pancreatic reflux [Mester et al], 775 (N)
partial hepatectomy in dog: revised technique based on anatomic considerations [Sigel], 788 (N)

Anesthesia
and portal venous oxygen saturation [Hardin et al], 831 (N)

Aneurysm
of splenic artery [Yang et al], 676 (O)
popliteal [Anastasi et al], 636 (O)
post-traumatic temporal artery [Gittes & Kartchner], 398 (S)
surgical treatment of ventricular aneurysm: report of ten cases [Effler et al], 249 (Ag)
syphilitic, of aortic arch: successful resection of [Bradham & Buxton], 521 (S)
ventricular: clinical features [Effler et al], 251 (Ag)
ventricular: evaluation of patient for surgical treatment [Effler et al], 253 (Ag)
ventricular: pathologic features [Effler et al], 249 (Ag)

Antibiotics
effect on survival of homografts [Sutton et al], 840 (N)
penicillin, quantitative barrier of synovium to [Morgan et al], 450 (S)
sodium, oxacillin, in surgical infections: clinical evaluation [Schumer], 507 (S)

Antimetabolites
effect on survival of homografts [Sutton et al], 840 (N)

Aorta
influence of direction of aortic perfusion on regional blood flow [Schenk et al], 1059 (D)
juxtarenal aortic occlusions, management of [Bergan & Trippel], 230 (Ag)

Aorta—continued
prognosis of aortic stenosis: special reference to indications for operative treatment [Takeda et al], 931 (D)
successful resection of syphilitic aneurysm of aortic arch [Bradham & Buxton], 521 (S)

Aortography
abdominal [Killen & Foster], 650 (O)

Anuria
significance of post-traumatic and postoperative oliguria [Hopkins et al], 320 (Ag)

Apparatus and instruments
nasogastric tube and pulmonary ventilation [Mackay et al], 673 (O)
new stent for support of veins in arterial grafts [Parsonnet et al], 696 (O)
rotating disc oxygenator [Ablaza et al], 548 (O)

Appendicitis
urine sediment in acute appendicitis [Kretchmar & McDonald], 209 (Ag)

Appendix
adenocarcinoma of [Qureshi et al], 453 (S)

Arteries
absent left pulmonary artery and right-sided patent ductus arteriosus [Swan et al], 196 (Ag)
acute carpal tunnel syndrome: median artery thrombosis as cause [Burham], 645 (O)
aneurysm of splenic artery with calcification [Yang et al], 676 (O)
atherosclerosis, peripheral, segmental distribution of [Singer], 384 (S)
cancer chemotherapy by arterial infusion [Benson et al], 125 (Jl)
coronary artery pressure in perfused heart [Meyer & Falor], 805 (N)
hypogastric, bilateral ligation of [Kinman & Jennings], 887 (D)
low-flow fail-safe intra-arterial infusion [Nelsen et al], 640 (O)
management of juxtarenal aortic occlusions [Bergan & Trippel], 230 (Ag)
myxoma of left atrium: presenting as embolus to femoral artery [Hibner et al], 525 (S)
new stent for support of veins in arterial grafts [Parsonnet et al], 696 (O)
popliteal aneurysm with osteochondroma of femur [Anastasi et al], 636 (O)
post-traumatic temporal artery aneurysm [Gittes & Kartchner], 398 (S)
vertebral, insufficiency [Wagner et al], 885 (D)

Arteriography
renal, versus individual ureteral catheterization [Stokes et al], 238 (Ag)

Arteriosclerosis
segmental distribution of peripheral atherosclerosis [Singer], 384 (S)

Arteriotomy
pulmonary, used in closure of established Potts anastomosis [Bozer et al], 722 (N)

Ascites
bile [Santschi et al], 851 (N)

Asphyxia
acute thoracic compression with traumatic asphyxia [Shamblin & McGoon], 967 (D)

Atelectasis
bacteriological studies in pulmonary atelectasis [Jamieson & Lansing], 1062 (D)
congestive [Berry & Sanislow], 153 (Jl)
diagnosis [Berry & Sanislow], 163 (Jl)
mechanisms of fever in pulmonary atelectasis [Lansing & Jamieson], 168 (J1)
pathologic anatomy, physiology [Berry & Sanislow], 159 (Jl)
See Lung diseases

Auscultation
direct, of heart [Bussmann et al], 257 (Ag)
See Heart sounds

B

Bacteriology
bacteriological studies in pulmonary atelectasis [Jamieson & Lansing], 1062 (D)

Bandages
gutta percha used as [Halsted], 226 (Ag)
silver foil used as dressing [Halsted], 225 (Ag)

Barriers
aseptic [Beck & Carlson], 228 (Ag)
operative field, surgical drapes and gowns [Beck & Carlson], 293 (Ag)
specifications and testing [Beck & Carlson], 290 (Ag)

Bile ducts
anatomy of duodenal papilla and genesis of pancreatic reflux [Mester et al], 775 (N)
carcinoma of [Strohl et al], 567 (O)

Blood
acid-base balance changes in citrated bank [Samueloff et al], 1029 (D)
ammonia reduction by potassium exchange resin: experimentation in Eck-fistula dogs [Zuidema et al], 296 (Ag)
control of bleeding in suprapubic prostatectomy [Kinman & Jennings], 887 (D)

Blood—continued
- effect of serotonin loading on histamine release and blood flow of isolated perfused liver and lung [Moore et al], 42 (Jl)
- flow, effect of endocardial incisions on myocardial [Lary], 424 (S)
- influence of direction of aortic perfusion on regional blood flow [Schenk et al], 1059 (D)
- intentional hemodilution: use of rotating disc oxygenator primed with acid citrate dextrose blood and low molecular weight dextran; preliminary report [Ablaza et al], 548 (O)
- laboratory findings in [Kozoll & Meyer], 916 (D)
- oxidized regenerated cellulose for hepatic hemostasis [Wright & Tyson], 669 (O)
- pathogenesis of esophageal varix rupture: study based on gross and microscopic examination of esophagus at time of bleeding [Orloff & Thomas], 301 (Ag)
- portacaval transposition in experimental hypertension: effect on blood pressure [Palmer], 500 (S)
- postfracture vascular changes and healing process [Wray & Goodman], 801 (N)
- regional blood flow and oxygen consumption in experimental hemorrhagic shock [Bounous et al], 340 (Ag)
- results of intentional hemodilution [Zuhdi et al], 554 (O)
- studies on portal venous oxygen saturation [Hardin et al], 831 (N)

Blood cells
- increase or decrease of after long bone fracture [Zeidman et al], 907 (D)

Blood circulation
- comparison of three mechanical ventilators: effects on pulmonary blood flow [McDonald et al], 796 (N)
- vertebral artery insufficiency [Wagner et al], 885 (D)

Blood coagulation
- studies of fibrinolytic activity after hepatectomy [Drapanas et al], 64 (Jl)

Blood pressure
- portacaval transposition in experimental hypertension: effect on blood pressure [Palmer], 500 (S)

Blood system
- chemodectoma of [Carey & Bradley], 897 (D)
- replacement of segments of [Todd et al], 998 (D)

Blood transfusion
- hepatitis in open-heart surgery [Adashek & Adashek], 792 (N)

Blood vessels
- chemodectoma of mediastinum [Spector et al], 903 (D)
- deep venous thrombosis, prognosis in [Phillips], 732 (N)
- injury to, in thoracic compression [Shamblin & McGoon], 967 (D)

Blood volume
- alterations in vascular volume after long bone fracture [Zeidman et al], 907 (D)

Body temperature
- internal cooling for general hypothermia [Holt & Lewis], 471 (S)

Bone
- acute carpal tunnel syndrome: median artery thrombosis as cause [Burnham], 645 (O)
- alterations in vascular volume after long bone fracture [Zeidman et al], 907 (D)
- substitute, ceramic-plastic material as [Smith], 653 (O)

Brain tumors
- histological changes after regional chemotherapy [Mahaley et al], 765 (N)

Breast
- fibrocystic disease and carcinoma of breast [Swerdlow & Humphrey], 457 (S)
- granular cell myoblastoma of [Stein], 703 (O)
- preoperative irradiation therapy of cancer of [Nakayama et al], 1003 (D)

Bronchi
- effect of chemical agents on bronchogenic cancer [Mendez et al], 147 (Jl)

Burns
- classification of [Jackson & Lee], 937 (D)
- major thermal burns: mortality appraisal and review [Jackson & Lee], 937 (D)
- progressive changes in depth of [Hinshaw], 993 (D)

C

Cancer
- bronchogenic, effect of chemical agents on [Mendez et al], 147 (Jl)
- chemical irrigation of wounds inoculated with cancer cells [McKibbin et al], 877 (N)
- chemotherapy by arterial infusion [Benson et al], 125 (Jl)
- chemotherapy, liver photoscanning in evaluation of [Hanson et al], 442 (S)
- effect of simulated gallstones [Simmers & Podolak], 583 (O)
- experimental work with gastric [Eisenberg & Woodward], 812 (N)

Cancer—continued
gastric cancer: midcentury look [Eisenberg & Woodward], 810 (N)
intestinal complications following irradiation for gynecologic cancer [Ashbaugh & Owens], 100 (Jl)
premalignant conditions [Eisenberg & Woodward], 813 (N)
proposed glossary of [Martin], 534 (S)
results of arterial infusion chemotherapy for [Benson et al], 137 (Jl)
squamous cell, metastatic [Conley & Arena], 759 (N)
stomach, diagnostic techniques for [Eisenberg & Woodward], 817 (N)

Carbon dioxide
cardiac denervation effect in hypoxia and hypercapnia [Greenfield & Ebert], 717 (N)

Carcinoma
basal cell, of chin and cheek areas of face: Mohs' chemosurgery technique for [Phelan & Juardo], 212 (Ag)
of bile ducts [Strohl et al], 567 (O)
of breast: fibrocystic disease and [Swerdlow & Humphrey], 457 (S)
of cecum associated with intussusception [Moody & Beal], 836 (N)
of esophagus, effect of preoperative irradiation of [Nakayama et al], 1003 (D)
of stomach, diagnosis of [Eisenberg & Woodward], 817 (N)
of tongue, buccal mucosa, and mandible: results from surgical treatment [Bowers & Henley], 516 (S)
treatment for gastric carcinoma [Eisenberg & Woodward], 817 (N)
treatment of bile duct carcinoma [Strohl et al], 571 (O)

Cardiovascular system
effect of total denervation on cardiovascular responses [Greenfield & Ebert], 717 (N)

Cartilage
speeds healing in diabetic wounds [Golding et al], 647 (O)

Casts
body, mechanical obstruction cause of cast syndrome [Thompson], 662 (O)
cast syndrome: case report [Thompson], 662 (O)

Catheterization
ureteral, individual: renal arteriography versus [Stokes et al], 238 (Ag)

Cellulose
oxidized regenerated [Wright & Tyson], 669 (O)

Central Surgical Association
surgical training in Canada (presidential address) [McLachlin], 1 (Jl)
twentieth annual meeting, Chicago, Feb 21-23, 1963; papers read, 1-192 (Jl); 193-364 (Ag)

Cervical ribs
scalenotomy in patients with and without [Shenkin & Somach], 892 (D)

Chemistry, pharmaceutical
chemical irrigation of wounds inoculated with cancer cells [McKibbin et al], 877 (N)

Chemotherapy
arterial infusion [Benson et al], 125 (Jl)
complications of arterial infusion chemotherapy [Benson et al], 141 (Jl)
effect of chemical agents on bronchogenic cancer [Mendez et al], 147 (Jl)
histological changes after regional chemotherapy [Mahaley et al], 765 (N)
liver photoscanning in evaluation of cancer chemotherapy [Hanson et al], 442 (S)
selection of patients for arterial infusion chemotherapy [Benson et al], 134 (Jl)

Chin
Mohs' chemosurgery technique for based cell carcinoma of [Phelan & Juardo], 212 (Ag)

Chlorpromazine
effect on exotoxin [Nora & Laufman], 54 (Jl)

Cholangiography
clinical study of cholangiograms [Moody et al], 480 (S)
intrahepatic [Moody et al], 475 (S)

Cholecystectomy
bile ascites after [Santschi et al], 851 (N)

Cholecystography
renal tubular necrosis after oral cholecystography [Malt et al], 743 (N)

Choledochostomy
bile ascites after [Santschi et al], 851 (N)

Cholelithiasis
effect of simulated gallstones on guinea pig gallbladders [Simmers & Podolak], 583 (O)

Clavicle
nonunion of [Johnson & Collins], 963 (D)

Clostridium perfringens
effects of various drugs on exotoxin (Cl perfringens) toxicity [Nora & Laufman], 53 (Jl)
See Clostridium welchii

Cold
effect of, on progressive changes in

Cold—continued
depth of burns [Hinshaw], 993 (D)
See also Body temperature

Colitis
staphylococcus enterocolitis [Gardner et al], 58 (Jl)

Colon
congenital atresia and stenosis of [Peck et al], 428 (S)
treatment of aganglionosis of [Desjardins & Simpson], 1019 (D)

Coronary artery
pressure in perfused heart [Meyer & Falor], 805 (N)

CORRESPONDENCE
for whom the bell tolls [Laforet], 538; [Millard], 538 (S)

D

Dacron
siliconized, as pericardial patch [Mazuji & Lett], 446 (S)

Dextran
use of rotating disc oxygenator primed with acid citrate dextrose blood and low molecular weight dextran [Ablaza], 548 (O)

Dextrose
acid citrate, use of rotating disc oxygenator primed with [Ablaza et al], 548 (O)

Diabetes
cartilage speeds healing in diabetic wounds [Golding et al], 647 (O)
conservative attitude in management of foot problems in [Block & Whitehouse], 682 (O)
mellitus, below-knee amputation in patients with [Block & Whitehouse], 682 (O)
mellitus, interrelationship of, and pancreatitis [Blumenthal et al], 844 (N)

Dissection
of regional lymph node [Price & DuVal], 747 (N)

Dressings: See Bandages

Drugs
effects of various drugs on exotoxins (Cl perfringens) toxicity: pretreatment with chlorpromazine, phenoxybenzamine, heparin, and cortisone [Nora & Laufman], 53 (Jl)

Duodenal ulcers: See Peptic ulcers

Duodenum
anatomy of duodenal papilla and genesis of pancreatic reflux [Mester et al], 775 (N)
massive gastroduodenal hemorrhage [Kelley et al], 6 (Jl)
obstruction, duodenal, annular pancreas and [Jackson], 370 (S)

Duodenum—continued
radical pancreatoduodenectomy and portal vein resection [Asada et al], 609 (O)
See Intestines, small

Dura mater
metastatic epidural tumor of spine [Wild & Porter], 825 (N)

E

EDITORIALS
how cardiac surgery transformed surgery [Swan], 365 (S)
kamongo and anabolone (editorial) [Swan], 715 (N)

Embolism
mechanism of death from pulmonary embolism [Hume], 710 (O)
myxoma: presenting as an embolus to femoral artery [Hibner et al], 525 (S)
pulmonary [Hume], 709 (O)
treatment for pulmonary embolism [Hume], 711 (O)

Enteritis, regional
histopathological spectrum of [Meadows & Batsakis], 976 (D)

Enterocolitis: See under Colitis

Esophagus
acid-peptic hypothesis: evidence [Orloff & Thomas], 302 (Ag)
cervical, experimental replacement of [Hopkins & Bernatz], 265 (Ag)
esophageal prosthesis for palliative intubation: further evaluation of 378 patients [O'Connor et al], 275 (Ag)
esophageal strictures after anastomosis [Schultz & Clatworthy], 120 (Jl)
esophageal varix rupture, pathogenesis [Orloff & Thomas], 301 (Ag)

Exercise
effects of, on portal venous oxygen saturation [Hardin et al], 831 (N)

Extremities
lymphatic pressures in extremities of dogs [Miller et al], 881 (N)

F

Face
Mohs' chemosurgery technique for basal cell carcinoma of chin and cheek areas of face [Phelan & Juardo], 212 (Ag)

Facial tumors
histological changes after regional chemotherapy for [Mahaley et al], 765 (N)

Femoral nerve
chemodectoma of [Carey & Bradley], 897 (D)

Femur
popliteal aneurysm with osteochondroma of [Anastasi et al], 636 (O)

Fever
mechanisms of, in pulmonary atelectasis [Lansing & Jamieson], 168 (Jl)
See Body temperature

Fibrinolysis
after hepatectomy [Drapanas et al], 64 (Jl)
See Blood coagulation

Fistulas
repair of traumatic fistulas of parotid duct [Morel & Firestein], 623 (O)

Food
acute intestinal obstruction caused by [Claman], 422 (S)
effect on portal venous oxygen saturation [Hardin et al], 831 (N)
experimental attempt to delay alimentary transit after small bowel exclusion [Gerwig & Ghaphery], 34 (Jl)

Fracture
alterations in vascular volume after long bone [Zeidman et al], 907 (D)
mandibular, treated with plastic polymers [Lighterman & Farrell], 868 (N)
nonunion of clavicle [Johnson & Collins], 963 (D)
postfracture vascular changes and healing process [Wray & Goodman], 801 (N)

G

Gallbladder
bile ascites [Santschi et al], 851 (N)
left-sided, and liver without situs inversus [Large], 982 (D)
perforation of: analysis of twenty-one cases [McEachern & Sullivan], 489 (S)

Gallbladders
effect of simulated gallstones on guinea pig gallbladders [Simmers & Podolak], 583 (O)

Gastrectomy
associated surgery with total gastrectomy [Barber et al], 25 (Jl)
restoration of gastrointestinal continuity after total [Barber et al], 25 (Jl)
total, critical evaluation of [Barber et al], 23 (Jl)

Gastrointestinal hormones
significance of Meissner's plexus in gastrin mechanism [Woodward et al], 512 (S)

Genetics
hereditary pancreatitis: role of surgical intervention [Gerber], 70 (Jl)

Geography
influence of geography on duodenal ulcers (editorial) [Dragstedt], 193 (Ag)

Geriatrics
inguinal hernias in geriatric patients [Palumbo et al], 953 (D)

Gloves
and masks, barrier effects of [Beck & Carlson], 292 (Ag)

Gloves, surgical
use of [Halsted], 223 (Ag)

Glycosuria
of diabetes mellitus and pancreatitis [Blumenthal et al], 844 (N)

Grafts and grafting
drug effects on survival of homografts of skins [Sutton et al], 840 (N)
experimental replacement of cervical esophagus [Hopkins & Bernatz], 265 (Ag)
new stent for support of veins in arterial grafts [Parsonnet et al], 696 (O)
practical methods of short-term storage of homografts [Gresham et al], 417 (S)
replacement of segments of venous system [Todd et al], 998 (D)
vein grafts in venous system: an experimental evaluation of autogenous veins used as bypass implants [Haimovici et al], 542 (O)

H

Heart
aneurysm, ventricular, surgical treatment for [Effler et al], 249 (Ag)
auscultation, direct, of [Bussmann et al], 257 (Ag)
cardiac denervation effect of hypoxia and hypercapnia: effect of total denervation on cardiovascular responses [Greenfield & Ebert], 717 (N)
coronary artery pressure in perfused heart [Meyer & Falor], 805 (N)
effect of endocardial incisions on myocardial blood flow [Lary], 424 (S)
effects of hypothermia on myocardial contractile force [Bender et al], 464 (S)
how cardiac surgery transformed surgery (editorial) [Swan], 365 (S)
left superior vena cava with anomalous inferior vena cava [Sunada et al], 632 (O)
myocardial contractile force in experimental hemorrhagic shock: some observations [Cooley & McIntosh], 330 (Ag)
myxoma of left atrium: presenting as embolus to femoral artery [Hibner et al], 525 (S)

Heart—continued
renal hypertension, heart failure, and azotemia [Klein & Persky], 530 (S)
siliconized Dacron as pericardial patch [Mazuki & Lett], 446 (S)

Heart defects, congenital
absent left pulmonary artery and right-sided patent ductus arteriosus [Swan et al], 196 (Ag)

Heart sounds
in patent ductus arteriosus [Bussmann et al], 258 (Ag)
in pulmonary valvar stenosis [Bussmann et al], 258 (Ag)

Hemoglobin
and massively bleeding gastroduodenal ulcers [Kozoll & Meyer], 916 (D)

Hemorrhage
caused by thoracic compression [Shamblin & McGoon], 967 (D)
control, ligature and suture material [Halsted], 216 (Ag)
experimental hemorrhagic shock: myocardial contractile force in [Cooley & McIntosh], 330 (Ag)
experimental hemorrhagic shock, treatment for [Cooley & McIntosh], 332 (Ag)
in acute pancreatitis [Kelly et al], 988 (D)
in pancreatitis as complication for operation [Frey & Beal], 1053 (D)
intestinal, in von Recklinghausen's disease: neurogenic tumors as cause [Collins], 374 (S)
intraperitoneal, due to uterine fibroid: report of case in late pregnancy [Avola & Gonnella], 666 (O)
laboratory findings in [Kozoll & Meyer], 916 (D)
operative procedures for gastroduodenal [Kelley et al], 6 (Jl)
regional blood flow and oxygen consumption in experimental hemorrhagic shock [Bounous], 340 (Ag)

Hemorrhage, gastrointestinal
massive gastroduodenal hemorrhage: changing concepts of management [Kelley et al], 6 (Jl)

Hemostasis
oxidized regenerated cellulose for hepatic hemostasis [Wright & Tyson], 669 (O)
See also Blood coagulation

Heparin
effect on exotoxin [Nora & Laufman], 54 (Jl)

Hepatectomy
partial, in dog [Sigel], 788 (N)
studies of fibrinolytic activity after [Drapanas et al], 64 (Jl)

Hepatitis
blood transfusion hepatitis in open-

Hepatitis—continued
heart surgery [Adashek & Adashek], 792 (N)

Heredity: See Genetics

Hernia, inguinal
primary inguinal hernioplasty: our experience with 3,572 operations [Palumbo et al], 949 (D)
recurrences of [Palumbo et al], 953 (D)

Hernias
inguinal and femoral [Rydell], 493 (S)
mortality and morbidity [Rydell], 494 (S)

Hernioplasty
early and late ambulation after [Palumbo et al], 953 (D)
primary inguinal [Palumbo et al], 949 (D)

Hirschsprung's disease
Duhamel's operation for [Sieber & Kiesewetter], 111 (Jl)
neonatal: treatment of complete aganglionosis of colon by the Duhamel operation [Desjardins & Simpson], 1019 (D)

Histamine
release, effect of serotonin loading on [Moore et al], 42 (Jl)

Histopathology
of regional enteritis [Meadows & Batsakis], 976 (D)

Histoplasmosis
surgical aspects of [Gryboski et al], 590 (O)

Homografts
storage of [Gresham et al], 417 (S)

Hormones
anabolic, anabolone (editorial) [Swan], 715 (N)

Hydrocortisone
effect on exotoxin [Nora & Laufman], 54 (Jl)

Hyperglycemia
in diabetes mellitus and pancreatitis [Blumenthal et al], 844 (N)

Hypertension
comparison of methods used to diagnose renal hypertension: renal arteriography versus individual ureteral catheterization [Stokes et al], 238 (Ag)
"directional" flow patterns in portal hypertension: assessment by spleen pressure and percutaneous splenoportography [Jackson], 307 (Ag)
nephrogenic, requiring both renal angiography and differential renal clearance tests for proper evaluation [Stokes et al], 245 (Ag)
portal, five classes of collateral flow patterns [Jackson], 310 (Ag)

Hypertension—continued
portal, from postbulbar duodenal ulcer [Strandness & Bell], 440 (S)
renal, correlation of tests for [Stokes et al], 244 (Ag)
renal, heart failure, and azotemia: report of case treated successfully by nephrectomy [Klein & Persky], 530 (S)
renal, surgery for [Bergan & Trippel], 232 (Ag)

Hypothermia
effects of [Bender et al], 464 (S)
general, internal cooling for [Holt & Lewis], 471 (S)
indications for in stomal ulcers [Bernstein et al], 14 (Jl)
secretory studies in frozen Heidenhain pouches [Savage et al], 690 (O)
techniques used in gastric freezing [Bernstein et al], 14 (Jl)
treatment of postgastrectomy stomal ulcer by gastric freezing [Bernstein et al], 13 (Jl)
use in closure of anastomosis [Bozer et al], 722 (N)
whole-body, in ammonia intoxication: effect on monkeys with portacaval shunts [Zuidema et al], 578 (O)

I

Infant, newborn
annular pancreas and duodenal obstruction in neonate: review [Jackson], 379 (S)

Infection
pulmonary, and thermal burns [Jackson & Lee], 937 (D)
surgical, sodium oxacillin in [Schumer], 507 (S)

Infusion
arterial, cancer chemotherapy by [Benson et al], 125 (Jl)
arterial, technical aspects of [Benson et al], 126 (Jl)
low-flow fail-safe intra-arterial [Nelsen et al], 640 (O)

Injury
thoracic compression [Shamblin & McGoon], 967 (D)

Intestinal obstruction
sigmoid volvulus [Abrams], 1033 (D)

Intestines
acute intestinal obstruction caused by food: case report [Claman], 422 (S)
blind intestinal loops in dogs: effect on Heidenhain pouch secretion [Landor et al], 1048 (D)
congenital atresia and stenosis of colon [Peck et al], 428 (S)
hemorrhage, intestinal, in von Recklinghausen's disease [Collins], 374 (S)
histopathological spectrum of regional enteritis [Meadows & Batsakis], 976 (D)

Intestines, large
carcinoma of cecum associated with intussusception [Moody & Beal], 836 (N)

Intestines, small
experimental attempt to delay alimentary transit after small bowel exclusion [Gerwig & Ghaphery], *34 (Jl)
lateral pancreaticojejunostomy [Lempke et al], 90 (Jl)
primary nonspecific ulceration of [Watson], 600 (O)
pyloric atresia [Becker et al], 413 (S)
radical pancreatoduodenectomy and portal vein resection: report of two successful cases with transplantation of portal vein [Asada et al], 609 (O)

Intussusception
carcinoma of cecum associated with [Moody & Beal], 836 (N)

Iodine
comparative actions of iodine compound and hexachlorophene [Geraci], 563 (O)
compound, new, for degerming skin surface [Geraci], 560 (O)

Ion exchange resins
blood ammonia reduction by potassium exchange resin [Zuidema et al], 296 (Ag)

J

Jaws
reactions to plastic polymers used in experimental fractures of [Lighterman & Farrell], 868 (N)

Jejunum
pancreaticojejunostomy [Lempke et al], 90 (Jl)

Johannes Scultetus
[Strohl], 396 (S)

K

Kidneys
acute effects of hepatic infarction on [Kraus & Costa], 957 (D)
management of juxtarenal aortic occlusions [Bergen & Trippel], 230 (Ag)
renal hypertension, heart failure, and azotemia [Klein & Persky], 530 (S)
renal tubular necrosis after oral cholecystography [Malt et al], 743 (N)
severity of renal injury incident to abdominal aortography [Killen & Foster], 650 (O)
visceral lesions in acute pancreatitis: experimental study [Reis], 604 (O)

Knots
new "one hand" double-loop method of tying [Seiger], 986 (D)

L

Laboratory
findings in bleeding ulcers [Kozoll & Meyer], 916 (D)

Liver
blood ammonia reduction by potassium exchange resin [Zuidema et al], 296 (Ag)
effect of serotonin loading on histamine release and blood flow of isolated perfused liver and lung [Moore et al], 42 (Jl)
fibrinolytic activity after hepatectomy [Drapanas et al], 64 (Jl)
intrahepatic anatomy [Moody et al], 475 (S)
intrahepatic cholangiography [Moody et al], 475 (S)
left-sided gallbladder and liver without situs inversus [Large], 982 (D)
necrosis, effect of [Kraus & Costa], 957 (D)
oxidized regenerated cellulose for hepatic hemostasis [Wright & Tyson], 669 (O)
photoscanning in evaluation of cancer chemotherapy [Hanson et al], 442 (S)
visceral lesions in acute pancreatitis [Reis], 604 (O)

Lung
absent left pulmonary artery [Swan et al], 196 (Ag)
associated atrial septal defect and pulmonic stenosis [Sunada et al], 632 (O)
bacteriological studies in pulmonary atelectasis [Jamieson & Lansing], 1062 (D)
comparison of three mechanical ventilators: effects on pulmonary blood flow [McDonald et al], 796 (N)
congestive atelectasis, clinical manifestations and treatment [Berry & Sanislow], 153 (Jl)
effect of hypoxia on pulmonary vasculature of dog [Lancaster et al], 485 (S)
effect of serotonin loading on histamine release and blood flow of isolated perfused liver and lung [Moore et al], 42 (Jl)
hemodilution, intentional, in pulmonary embolectomy [Zuhdi et al], 554 (O)
management of spontaneous pneumothorax: comparison of treatment methods [Ransdell & McPherson], 1023 (D)
mechanisms of fever in pulmonary atelectasis [Lansing & Jamieson], 168 (Jl)
nasogastric tube and pulmonary ventilation [Mackay et al], 673 (O)
pulmonary embolism: historical aspects [Hume], 709 (O)

Lung—continued
surgical aspects of histoplasmosis [Gryboski et al], 590 (O)

Lymph
lymphatic pressures in extremities of dogs [Miller et al], 881 (N)

Lungfish
kamongo and anabolone (editorial) [Swan], 715 (N)

M

Mandible
carcinoma of tongue, buccal mucosa, and [Bowers & Henley], 516 (S)

Mechlorethamine
effectiveness [Leather & Eckert], 144 (Jl)

Mediastinum
chemodectoma of [Spector et al], 903 (D)

Megacolon
Duhamel's operation for Hirschsprung's disease [Sieber & Kiesewetter], 111 (Jl)
See Hirschsprung's disease

Melanoma
metastasis to parotid gland [Conley & Arena], 758 (N)
regional lymph node dissection and malignant melanoma: effect on survival [Price & DuVal], 747 (N)

Membrane
carcinoma of tongue, buccal mucosa, and mandible [Bowers & Henley], 516 (S)
effect of endocardial incisions on myocardial blood flow [Lary], 424 (S)
significance of Meissner's plexus in gastrin mechanism [Woodward et al], 512 (S)

Meninges
metastatic epidural tumor of spine [Wild & Porter], 825 (N)

Metabolism
iron, after portacaval shunt in dogs [Doberneck et al], 751 (N)

Metastasis
to parotid gland from malignant tumors [Conley & Arena], 761 (N)

Mortality
major thermal burns, mortality appraisal of [Jackson & Lee], 937 (D)

Muscles
scalenotomy in patients with and without cervical ribs [Shenkin & Somach], 892 (D)

Myoblastoma
granular cell, of breast [Stein], 703 (O)

Myocardium
effect of endocardial incisions on myo-

Myocardium—continued
cardial blood flow [Lary], 424 (S)
effects of hypothermia on myocardial contractile force [Bender et al], 464 (S)
myocardial contractile force in experimental hemorrhagic shock: some observation [Cooley & McIntosh], 330 (Ag)

N

Narcotics
are postoperative narcotics necessary? [Roe], 912 (D)

Necrosis
renal tubular [Malt et al], 743 (N)
systemic effects of massive hepatic necrosis: I. acute effects of hepatic infarction on kidneys [Kraus & Costa], 957 (D)

Nephrectomy
renal hypertension, heart failure, and azotemia [Klein & Persky], 530 (S)

Nerves
cardiac denervation effect in hypoxia and hypercapnia [Greenfield & Ebert], 717 (N)

Nervous system
lumbar sympathectomy [Tice et al], 461 (S)
significance of Meissner's plexus in gastrin mechanism [Woodward et al], 512 (S)

Neurofibromatosis
intestinal hemorrhage in von Recklinghausen's disease: neurogenic tumors as cause [Collins], 374 (S)

Nitrogen
intravenous protein hydrolysates: favorable influence on postoperative nitrogen balance [Peden et al], 401 (S)

Nitrogen mustards
histological changes after regional use of [Mahaley et al], 765 (N)

Node
regional lymph node dissection and malignant melanoma: effect on survival [Price & DuVal], 747 (N)

Nutrition
experimental attempt to delay alimentary transit after small bowel exclusion [Gerwig & Ghaphery], *34 (Jl)
See also Food

O

Oxygen
cardiac denervation effect in hypoxia [Greenfield & Ebert], 717 (N)
effect of hypoxia on pulmonary vasculature of dog [Lancaster et al], 485 (S)
hyperbaric oxygenation and mechlorethamine effectiveness [Leather & Eckert], 144 (Jl)
in experimental hemorrhagic shock [Bounous et al], 340 (Ag)
studies on portal venous oxygen saturation [Hardin et al], 831 (N)

P

Pain
are postoperative narcotics necessary? [Roe], 912 (D)

Pancreas
abscess, pancreatic [Altemeier & Alexander], 80 (Jl)
anatomy of duodenal papilla and genesis of pancreatic reflux [Mester et al], 775 (N)
annular, and duodenal obstruction in neonate: review [Jackson], 379 (S)
experimental pancreatitis: synchronous production in normal and in ectopic pancreas [Kelly et al], 988 (D)
hereditary pancreatitis: role of surgical intervention [Gerber], 70 (Jl)
interrelationship of diabetes mellitus and pancreatitis [Blumenthal et al], 844 (N)
pancreatic ducts and postoperative pancreatitis [Kelly & Troyer], 614 (O)
pancreaticojejunostomy [Lempke et al], 90 (Jl)
radical pancreatoduodenectomy and portal vein resection: report of two successful cases with transplantation of portal vein [Asada et al], 609 (O)

Pancreatitis
as complication of operation [Frey & Beal], 1053 (D)
experimental [Kelly et al], 988 (D)
hereditary [Gerber], 70 (Jl)
interrelationship of diabetes mellitus and [Blumenthal et al], 844 (N)
pancreatic ducts and postoperative [Kelly & Troyer], 614 (O)
visceral lesions in acute pancreatitis: experimental study [Reis], 604 (O)

Paraganglia
chemodectoma of [Carey & Bradley], 897 (D)

Parotid gland
anatomy [Conley & Arena], 757 (N)
as focus of metastasis [Conley & Arena], 757 (N)
repair of traumatic fistulas of parotid duct [Morel & Firestein], 623 (O)

Pathology
of carcinoma of bile ducts [Strohl et al], 569 (O)
of sigmoid volvulus [Abrams], 1033 (D)

Penicillin
quantitative barrier of synovium to [Morgan et al], 457 (S)

Peptic ulcers
are benign gastric ulcers really benign? [Duhamel et al], 391 (S)
distal antrectomy with vagectomy for [Palumbo & Sharpe], 1040 (D)
in Africa [Snyder & Alexander], 206 (Ag)
influence of geography on duodenal ulcers (editorial) [Dragstedt], 193 (Ag)
laboratory findings in massively bleeding gastroduodenal ulcers: review of 2,008 cases [Kozoll & Meyer], 916 (D)
peritoneal fluid pH after perforation of [Howard & Singh], 483 (S)
radiological and laboratory findings [Nadler], 619 (O)
treatment and pathology of [Nadler], 619 (O)

Perfusions
intentional hemodilution [Zuhdi et al], 554 (O)

Pericardium
pericardial patch, siliconized Dacron as [Mazuji & Lett], 446 (S)

Peritoneum
peritoneal fluid pH after perforation of peptic ulcers: myth of "acid-peritonitis" [Howard & Singh], 483 (S)

Peritonitis
"acid-peritonitis," myth of [Howard & Singh], 483 (S)

Phenoxybenzamine
effect on exotoxin [Nora & Laufman], 54 (Jl)

Pheochromocytoma
intrathoracic [Luna et al], 369 (S)

Phlebograms
use in study of prognosis in venous thrombosis [Phillips], 732 (N)

Plasma
and red cell volume, effect of high and low viscosity dextrans on [Shoemaker], 355 (Ag)
effect of high and low viscosity dextrans upon [Shoemaker], 355 (Ag)

Plastics
ceramic-plastic material as bone substitute [Smith], 653 (O)
new stent for support of veins in arterial grafts [Parsonnet et al], 696 (O)

Pneumothorax
conservative management of spontaneous [Ransdell & McPherson], 1023 (D)
spontaneous, pleural scarification for [Ransdell & McPherson], 1023 (D)

Poisons and poisonings
lethal properties of rapidly polmerizing

Poisons and poisoning—continued
adhesive: product used in nonsuture surgery [Lewers et al], 627 (O)

Polyethylenes
esophageal prosthesis for palliative intubation [O'Connor et al], 275 (Ag)
See Plastics

Polymers
mandibular fractures treated with plastic polymers [Lighterman & Farrell], 868 (N)

Portacaval anastomosis
effect of hypothermia in ammonia intoxication on monkeys with portacaval shunts [Zuidema et al], 578 (O)
iron metabolism after [Doberneck et al], 751 (N)

Pregnancy
late, intraperitoneal hemorrhage due to uterine fibroid in [Avola & Gonnella], 666 (O)

Prognosis
in metastasis to parotid gland [Conley & Arenal], 757 (N)

Prostatectomy
control of bleeding in suprapubic prostatectomy: use of bilateral ligation of hypogastric arteries [Kinman & Jennings], 887 (D)

Prostheses
esophageal, for palliative intubation [O'Connor et al], 275 (A)
experimental replacement of cervical esophagus [Hopkins & Bernatz], 265 (Ag)
replacement of segments of venous system [Todd et al], 998 (D)

Protein
hydrolysates, intravenous: favorable influence on postoperative nitrogen balance [Peden et al], 401 (S)

Pylorus
pyloric atresia [Becker et al], 413 (S)

Pyuria
urine sediment in acute appendicitis [Kretchmar & McDonald], 209 (Ag)

R

Radiation
animal studies of effect of preoperative irradiation therapy [Nakayama et al], 1003 (D)
concentrated preoperative irradiation therapy [Nakayama et al], 1003 (D)
intestinal complications following irradiation for gynecologic cancer [Ashbaugh & Owens], 100 (Jl)

Radiography
intrahepatic cholangiography [Moody et al], 475 (S)

Roentgenograms
findings in deep venous thrombosis [Phillips], 732 (N)

Roentgenography
assessment of spleen pressure and percutaneous splenoportography [Jackson], 307 (Ag)

Respiratory tract infections
and histoplasmosis [Gryboski et al], 591 (O)

S

Scalenotomy
in patients with and without cervical ribs: analysis of surgical results [Shenkin & Somach], 892 (D)

Secretion
blind intestinal loops in dogs: effect on Heidenhain pouch [Landor et al], 1048 (D)
secretory studies in frozen Heidenhain pouches [Savage et al], 690 (O)

Serotonin
loading, effect of [Moore et al], 42 (Jl)

Shock
antitoxic effect of aldosterone on cats in endotoxic shock [Hayasaka et al], 861 (N)
hemorrhagic, experimental [Cooley & McIntoch], 330 (Ag)
hemorrhagic, regional blood flow and oxygen consumption in [Bounous], 340 (Ag)
of major thermal burns [Jackson & Lee], 937 (D)
studies on viscosity alterations in shock: I. effect of high and low viscosity dextrans upon plasma and red cell volumes [Shoemaker], 355 (Ag)

Skin
drug effects on survival of homografts of skin [Sutton et al], 840 (N)
iodine compound for degerming [Geraci], 560 (O)
iodophor for preoperative skin preparation [Cotlar & Cohn], 857 (N)
iodophor (Ioprep) and thimerosal (Merthiolate) in preoperative skin preparation [Cotlar & Cohn], 857 (N)

Solution
effect of concentration of contrast solution [Killen & Foster], 650 (O)

Spasm
vasospasm, post-traumatic: role of thermal measurement [Meagher], 539 (O)

Spine
metastatic epidural tumor of [Wild & Porter], 825 (N)

Spleen
aneurysm of splenic artery with calcification [Yang et al], 676 (O)

Spleen—continued
"spontaneous rupture" of spleen; one mechanism: routine splenectomy challenged [Hardy & Yelverton], 468 (S)

Splenectomy
routine, challenged [Hardy & Yelverton], 468 (S)

Stains and staining
histoplasmosis and [Gryboski et al], 590 (O)

Stenosis
aortic [Takeda et al], 931 (D)

Stomach
distal antrectomy with vagectomy for duodenal ulcer: review of 450 cases [Palumbo & Sharpe], 1040 (D)
hemorrhage, massive gastroduodenal [Kelley et al], 6 (Jl)
nasogastric tube and pulmonary ventilation [Mackay et al], 673 (O)
preoperative irradiation therapy of cancer of [Nakayama et al], 1003 (D)
pyloric atresia [Becker et al], 413 (S)
secretory studies in frozen Heidenhain pouches [Savage et al], 690 (O)

Surgery
for congenital atresia and stenosis of colon [Peck et al], 428 (S)
for fulminating type of sigmoid volvulus [Abrams], 1033 (D)
hereditary pancreatitis: role of surgical intervention in [Gerber], 70 (Jl)
how cardiac surgery transformed surgery (editorial) [Swan], 365 (S)
intentional hemodilution in open-heart surgery [Ablaza et al], 548 (O)
nonsuture: lethal properties of polymerizing adhesive [Lewers et al], 627 (O)
open-heart, blood transfusion hepatitis [Adashek & Adashek], 792 (N)
sodium oxacillin in surgical infections: clinical evaluation [Schumer], 507 (S)
surgical training in Canada [McLachlin], 1 (Jl)
surgical wire welding [Feller & Hill], 866 (N)
villous adenoma, surgical dilemma [Liechty & Raterman], 107 (Jl)

Suture
ligature and suture material [Halsted], 216 (Ag)

Sutures
use of catgut as [Halsted], 216 (Ag)
use of silk as [Halsted], 216 (Ag)

Sympathectomy
lumbar: effects on vascular responses in lower extremity of patients with arteriosclerosis obliterans [Tice et al], 461 (S)

Synovial membrane
quantitative barrier of synovium to penicillin [Morgan et al], 450 (S)

Syphilis, cardiovascular
successful resection of syphilitic aneurysm of aortic arch [Bradham & Buxton], 521 (S)

T

Temperature
post-traumatic vasospasm: role of thermal measurement [Meagher], 539 (O)

Thoracentesis
in management of spontaneous pneumothorax [Ransdell & McPherson], 1023 (D)

Thorax
acute thoracic compression with traumatic asphyxia: report of six cases [Shamblin & McGoon], 967 (D)
intrathoracic pheochromocytoma: case report [Luna et al], 369 (S)

Thrombectomy
experimental venous thrombosis and [Sheil & Sabiston], 408 (S)

Thrombosis
experimental venous, and thrombectomy [Sheil & Sabiston], 408 (S)
management of juxtarenal aortic occlusions [Bergan & Trippel], 230 (A)
median artery [Burham], 645 (O)
prognosis in deep venous thrombosis [Phillips], 732 (N)

Tissue
changes in burns [Hinshaw], 993 (D)
ligature and suture material [Halsted], 216 (Ag)
practical methods of short-term storage of homografts [Gresham et al], 417 (S)

Tissues
lethal properties of rapidly polymerizing adhesive [Lewers et al], 627 (O)

Toxicity
exotoxin, effect of various drugs on [Nora & Laufman], 53 (Jl)
lethal properties of rapidly polymerizing adhesive [Lewers et al], 627 (O)

Toxins and antitoxins
antitoxic effect of aldosterone on cats in endotoxic shock: further studies [Hayasaka et al], 861 (N)

Trachea
stenosis of trachea resection and end-to-end anastomosis: report of two cases [Miscall et al], 726 (N)

Tracheostomy
use in stenosis of trachea [Miscall et al], 726 (N)

Transplantation
portacaval transposition in experimental hypertension: effect on blood pressure [Palmer], 500 (S)

Transplants
experimental replacement of cervical esophagus [Hopkins & Bernatz], 265 (Ag)

Trauma
post-traumatic vasospasm [Meagher], 539 (O)
repair of traumatic fistulas of parotid duct [Morel & Firestein], 623 (O)
See Wounds and injuries

Tuberculosis
and associated histoplasmosis [Gryboski et al], 593 (O)

Tumors
adenoma, villous [Liechty & Raterman], 107 (Jl)
are benign gastric ulcers really benign? [Duhamel et al], 391 (S)
chemodectoma of mediastinum [Spector et al], 903 (D)
chemodectoma: review with two new cases [Carey & Bradley], 897 (D)
fibroid, uterine, intraperitoneal hemorrhage due to [Avola & Gonnella], 666 (O)
inoperable, low-flow fail-safe intra-arterial infusion [Nelsen et al], 640 (O)
metastatic epidural tumor of spine: study of 45 cases [Wild & Porter], 825 (N)
myxoma of left atrium [Hibner et al], 525 (S)
neurogenic [Collins], 374 (S)
pheochromocytoma, intrathoracic [Luna et al], 369 (S)

U

Ulcers
chronic gastric ulcers [Eisenberg & Woodward], 810 (N)
duodenal, portal hypertension from [Strandness & Bell], 440 (S)
gastric ulcers—management [Nadler], 619 (O)
primary nonspecific [Watson], 600 (O)
See Peptic ulcers
stomal, results of gastric freezing [Bernstein et al], 17 (Jl)
stomal, treatment of by gastric freezing [Bernstein et al], 13 (Jl)

Uremia
renal hypertension, heart failure, and azotemia [Klein & Persky], 530 (S)

Urine
sediment in acute appendicitis [Kretchmar & McDonald], 209 (Ag)
See also Pyuria
significance of post-traumatic and post-

Urine—continued
operative oliguria [Hopkins et al], 320 (Ag)

V

Vagus nerve
chemodectoma of [Carey & Bradley], 897 (D)
vagectomy for duodenal ulcer [Palumbo & Sharpe], 1040 (D)

Vascular system
effect of hypoxia on pulmonary vasculature of dog [Lancaster et al], 485 (S)
lumbar sympathectomy: effects on vascular responses in lower extremity of patients with arteriosclerosis obliterans [Tice et al], 461 (S)

Veins
"directional" flow patterns in portal hypertension [Jackson], 307 (Ag)
experimental evaluation of autogenous veins used as bypass implants [Haimovici et al], 542 (O)
experimental venous thrombosis and thrombectomy [Sheil & Sabiston], 408 (S)
intravenous protein hydrolysates: favorable influence on postoperative nitrogen balance [Peden et al], 401 (S)
portacaval transposition in experimental hypertension: effect on blood pressure [Palmer], 500 (S)
thrombosis of, prognosis in [Phillips], 732 (N)
transplantation of portal vein [Asada et al], 609 (O)

Venae cavae
left superior vena cava with anomalous inferior vena cava: report of case with associated atrial sepal defect and pulmonic stenosis, successfully corrected [Sunada et al], 632 (O)

Ventilation
nasogastric tube and pulmonary ventilation [Mackay et al], 796 (N)

Ventilators
comparison of three mechanical ventilators [McDonald et al], 796 (N)

Viscosity
alterations in shock [Shoemaker], 355 (Ag)

Volvulus
sigmoid [Abrams], 1033 (D)

W

Wounds and injuries
chemical irrigation of wounds inoculated with cancer cells [McKibbin et al], 877 (N)
post-traumatic and postoperative oliguria [Hopkins et al], 320 (Ag)
post-traumatic temporal artery aneurysm: recurrent surgical curiosity [Gittes & Kartchner], 398 (S)
severity of renal injury incident to abdominal aortography: effect of concentration of contrast solution [Killen & Foster], 650 (O)

Writing, medical
in summary (editorial) [Warren], 194 (Ag)